Revised & Enlarged

21ST. CENTURY EDITION

MEDICAL DICTIONARY

ENGLISH INTO ENGLISH AND URDU

by

WAHAB AKHTAR AZIZ

M.Sc., L.M.B.

Head of Biology Department

Government College, Civil Lines, Multan.

Dr. MOHAMMAD MUNEER SANDHU

M.B.B.S-M.D (TURKEY)

Ex- Research Medical Officer G. Surgery

BURSA UNIVERSITY TURKEY

Registarar Deptt. of Neurosurgery

Kantons hospital-9000 St. Gallan Switzerland

Dr. MOHAMMAD RAFIQUE SANDHU

DTL (TURKEY)

M.B.B.S - M.D. (Doctor of Medicine) Turkey

M.D.F.M. (Lahore)

R.M.P. (Punjab)

Dr. LUBNA SHAHPER

M.B.B.S.

M. SUQLAIN BHATTI

I.H.H.

EDUCATIONAL PUBLISHING HOUSE, DEHLI-6

Revised & Enlarged

21ST. CENTURY EDITION

MEDICAL DICTIONARY

Vth Edition : 2007
Price : Rs. 200/-
ISBN : 81-86232-38-9
Printed at : Afif Printers, Delhi-6

Published by

EDUCATIONAL PUBLISHING HOUSE

3108, Vakil Street, Kucha Pandit, Lal Kuan, Delhi-6
Ph. : 3214465, 3216162, Fax. : 91-011-3211540
E-Mail : ephdelhi@yahoo.com

PREFACE

This Dictionary aims at providing latest medical terms that are commonly used in various branches of Medical field. The book has been compiled to cater for a need widely felt by the students of Medical Colleges. The total number of terms in this volume is approximately 8,000. The principal bracnches of Medical Science covered by this Dictionary are Anatomy, Physiology, Pathology, Biochemistry, Surgery, Psychology, Alchemy, Bio-engineering, Bacteriology, Actionobiology, Embryology, Genetics, Gynaecology, Immunology, Medicine, Neurology, Obstetrics, Pharmacology, Radiobiology, Serology, Enzymology, Cardiology, Meteria medica, Neuropathology, Ophthalmology, Paediatrics, Radiotherapy and others.

Urdu equivalents of medical terms have been sought wherever available and every effort has been made to present Urdu version in a simple way. A new Urdu word for a term was coined only when I failed to find it anywhere else.

I am highly indebeted to the following for their valuable suggestions:

1. Dr. Feroze Shah Afroz, Layyah
2. Dr. Rafiq Ahmad Azia, Layyah
3. Dr. Masood Ahmad, Eden (Australia)
4. Dr. Farida Naeem, Lahore.
5. Dr. Zahid Kamal, bahawal Pur.
6. Dr. Imtiaz Ahmad Khan, Multan.
7. Miss Dr.Ghazala Yasmeen Akhtar, MBBS.
   K.E. Medical College, Lahore.

WAHAB AKHTAR AZIZ,
M.S.c, L.M.B
HEAD OF BIOLOGY DEPARTMENT
GOVERNMENT COLLEGE, CIVIL LINES,
MULTAN.

ABOUT THE AUTHOR

Son of a Physician and surgen. His family is known as Doctor's family as most of his family members are associated with medicine. Born in 1939. Passed SSc Examination from Board of Secondary Education, Punjab and got training in **First Aid.** He attended many patients with his father. Studied at Multan, Lahore and Jamshoro. He studied **BIOCHEMIC MEDICINE.** Served as Lecturer in Biology for many years. He has been Officer-in-Charge of College **DISPENSARY** for several years and gave **MEDICAL TREATMENT** to thousands of students. Then, he was promoted as Assistant Professor and serves as Principal at several Places. Gave training in Population Census in 1981. He was interested in **MEDICINAL PLANTS.** Author of many books including Dictionary of Botany, Dictionary of Zoology and Dictionary of Science. Chairman ANTI NARCOTIC Association, Chairman Biologists Forum, Head of Biology Department anmd Member of **CANCER** Society, Multan.

Guide to Pronunciation: Consonants

ch (= tsh) as in cheese (chez),
stitch (stich),
picture (pik'-cher).

j (dzh)judge (juj),
rigid (rij' id').

sh dish,
lotion (lo'shun).

zh vision (vizh'-n).

ng sing,
think (thingk)

g Always hard as in good.

r This letter is often left unsounded or is slurred into the preceding vowel. In the combination 'er' (see Vowels) the 'r' is rarely trilled or marked. Where it receives its full consonantal value it is usually placed preceding a vowel; in most other cases its face is determined by individual taste and custom.

th No attempt has been made to distinguish between the breathed sound as in 'think' and the voiced sound as in 'them'.

Accent: The accented syllable is indicated by a slanting stroke at its termination, e.g. fibrositis (fi-brō-si'-tis).

Guide to Pronunciation: Vowels

a	as in fat, back, tap.
ā	lame, brain (brān). vein (vān).
a	far, calf (kaf), heart (hart), coma (kō'ma).
e	flesh, deaf (def), said (sed).
ē	he, tea (tē), knee (nē), anaemia (an-ē'-mi-a).
e	there, air (er), area (er'-i-a).
i	sit , busy (biz'-i)
i	spine, my, eye, tie.
o	hot, cough (kof).
ō	bone, moan (mōn), dough (dō).
u	gum, love (luv), tough (fuf), colour (kul'-er).
ū	mute, due, new, you, rupture (rup'-tūr).
aw	saw, gall (gawl), caul (kawl), water (waw'ter).
oi	loin, boy.
oo	foot, womb (woom) , wound (woond), rude (rood).
ow	cow, sound (sownd), gout (gowt).

When followed by 'r' , 'e' is often sounded as in 'her' or as 'u' in 'fur' (for example, 'ferment'); in '-er' as a final unaccented syllable, the 'e' is some-times more or less elided (drawer, tower). See also consonant 'r'

Abbreviations used in definitions

adj	Adjective
adv.	Adverb
Ar.	Arabic
A.S.	Anglo-Saxon
ef.	[L. *confer*] Compare
dim.	Diminution of
dub.	Dubious
E.	English
e.g.	[L. *exempli gratia*] For example
Etym.	Etymology
F.	French
G.	Greek
i.e.	[L. *id est*] That is
it.	Italian
L.	Latin
L.L.	Late Latin
M.E.	Middle English
n.	Noun
N.L.	New Latin
O.N.	Old Norse
Opp.	Opposite to
per se	As such
Pg.	Portuguese
pl.	Plural
q.v.	[L. *quod vide*] Which see
Sing.	Singular
Syn.	Synonym
v.	Verb
v.i.	Intransitive verb
v.t.	Transitive verb

A

Abacterial *(a-bak-te-ri-al)* [G. *a*, negative; *bacterion*, rod]. Having no bacteria, bacteria-less.

بے جراثیمی، بے بیکٹیریا: بیکٹیریا کے بغیر۔ جراثیم سے پاک۔

Abasia *(aba'-zha)* [G. *a*, negative; *basis*, step]. Inability to walk.

معذور: چلنے کے قابل نہ ہونا۔ یونانی الفاظ 'اے' بمعنی نہیں اور ''بسیز'' بمعنی قدم سے ماخوذ ہے۔

Abdomen *(ab-do'-men)* [L. belly]. The major central part of the body. It is in cavity shape and starts immediately below the thorax, and diaphragm separates it. Muscles and facia are present in wall of it, which make it capable of changing size and shape. Internally serous membrane is present called peritonium. This acts as a covering over most of its internal organs.

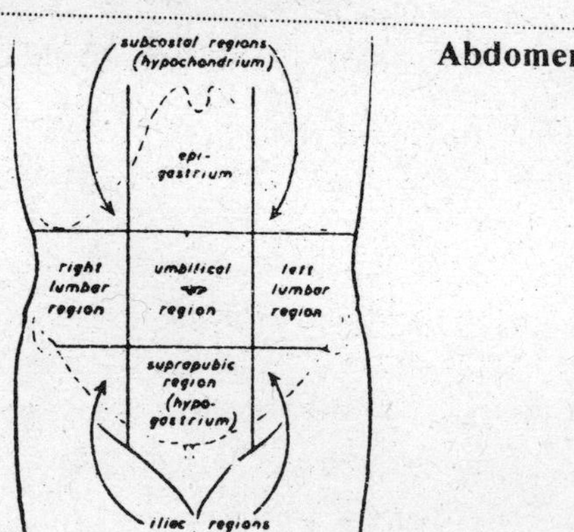

Abdomen

شکم: جوف۔ معدہ۔ بطن۔ لاطینی زبان کا لفظ ہے جس کے معنی پیٹ ہیں۔ جسم کا سب سے بڑا کہفہ جو چھاتی کے نیچے واقع ہوتا ہے اور اسے حجاب حاجز الگ کرتا ہے۔ یہ حصہ سینے کے بعد اور پچھلی ٹانگوں کے درمیان واقع ہوتا ہے۔ اس حصہ کو جوف شکم بھی کہتے ہیں۔ اس کے اندر آنتیں، جگر، گردے وغیرہ پائے جاتے ہیں۔ یہ حصہ دل اور پھیپھڑوں سے جدا ہوتا ہے۔ یعنی یہ اعضاء اس میں نہیں ہوتے۔ بالائی جانب اسے ڈایافرام علیحدہ کرتا ہے۔

Abdominopelvic *(ab-dom'-in-o-pel'vik)* [L. *abdomen*, belly; *pelvis*, basin]. The term shows the relation between abdomen and pelvic cavity.

شکمی عانی: لاطینی زبان کا لفظ ہے جو ''ایبڈومن'' اور ''پیلوس'' کا مرکب ہے، جن کے معانی بالترتیب ''پیٹ'' اور ''حوض'' کے ہیں۔ پیٹ اور کولہے یا ہیکل عانی سے متعلق۔

Abdominoperineal *(ab-dom'-in-o-per-ine'al)* [G. *perineos*, the space between the anus and scrotum]. Term showing the relation of abdomen to perineum.

شکمی عجانی: یہ اصطلاح لاطینی لفظ ''ایبڈومن'' بمعنی ''پیٹ'' اور یونانی لفظ ''پیری نیوس'' بمعنی مقعد اور خصیوں کا درمیانی حصہ'' کا مرکب ہے۔ شکم اور عجان سے متعلق۔ مقعد اور خصیوں کے درمیانی حصہ کے متعلق۔

Abduct *(ab-dakt)* To divert away from the median line of the body. It is opposite to adduct.

تبعید کرنا: جسم کے وسطی حصہ سے الگ کرنا۔

Abductor *(ab-duk'-tor)* [L. *abducere*, to lead away]. A muscle which, on contraction. draws a part away from the median line of the body. Opp. to adducor.

باعد، عضلہ مُبعدہ، دور کنندہ۔ ایسا عضلہ جس کے سکڑنے سے جسم کا وسطی حصہ دوسرے سے جدا ہوتا ہے، یا رگ جو ایسے عضلے یا پٹھے کو جاتی ہے۔

Aberration *(ab-er-ra-shun)* [L. *aberrare*, to wander from]. A deviation from normal. ***Mental a.***, a mild mental abnormality. ***Optical a.***, imperfect focus of light rays by a lens - **aberrant** *adj*.

انحراف، ضلالت، خلل دماغ۔ نارمل سے ہٹا ہوا یا منحرف۔ ذہنی انحراف معمولی دماغ خلل کو کہتے ہیں۔ اسے خبطِ دماغ بھی کہا جاتا ہے۔ بصری یا مناظری ضلالت سے مراد عدسے سے نوری شعاعوں کا نامکمل ارتکاز ہے۔

Ablation *(ab-la-shun)* [L. *ablatio*, take away]. Removal. In surgery, excision or amputation - **ablative** *adj*.

قطع عضو۔ جسم کے کسی عضو کا عمل جراحی سے کاٹ دینا۔ مثلاً ہاتھ، بازو، ٹانگ کاٹ دینا

Abort *(ab-awrt')* [L. *abortus*, premature birth]. To terminate before full development.

ساقط ہونا، حمل گرنا، اسقاط۔ اندامِ نہانی سے خون جاری ہو جاتا ہے۔ اور رحم میں تشنج شروع ہو جاتا ہے۔ آخرکار جنین خارج ہو جاتا ہے۔ اس کے علاوہ یہ صورت بھی ہوتی ہے کہ پہلے غشا امینون پھٹ جانے سے جنین خارج ہو جاتا ہے، بعد میں پردے نکل جاتے ہیں۔ جب اسقاط مکمل ہو جاتا ہے تو خون بند ہو جاتا ہے۔ ابتدائے حمل میں جنین عموماً پورا خارج ہوتا ہے لیکن دوسرے ماہ کے بعد رحم کی گردن کے راستے سے جنین گزر نہیں سکتا چنانچہ جب تک رحم کی گردن پورے طور پر نہیں کھلے گی، جنین رحم میں پڑا رہے گا۔ رحم کے تشنجی دوروں سے اس کی گردن پھیلتی جائے گی اور خون بھی کثرت سے نکلے گا۔ حمل گر جانے کی حالت میں حاملہ کو زیادہ تکلیف ہوتی ہے۔ زیادہ خون بہنے سے عورت کی جان کا خطرہ ہوتا ہے۔ جب اسقاطِ حمل مکمل ہو، خون رک جائے عورت کو بخار نہ ہو اور درد بھی نہ ہو تو عورت چند دن میں چلنا پھرنا شروع کر دیتی ہے۔

Abortifacient *(ab-awr'-ti-fa'-shi-ent)* [L.abortus, premature birth; facere, to make]. Causing abortion. Drug or agent inducing expulsion of a nonviable fetus.

مسقط:- دوا یا کسی عمل سے، حمل کا ساقط ہونا، حمل گرانے والی شے۔

Abortion *(ab-awr-ti-fa-shi-ent)* [L. *abortus*, premature birth] 1. Abrupt termination of a process. 2. Expulsion from uterus of product of conception before it is viable, i-e. before the end of the 28th week. **complete a.,** the entire contents of the uterus are expelled. criminal a., intertional evacuation of uterus on any other than medical grounds. habitual a,. preferable syn. recurrent a., term used when abortion recurs in successive pregnancies incomplete a,. part of the pregnancies. incomplete a., part of the fetus or placenta is retained within the uterus. induced a. (also called 'artificial'), intentional evacuation of uterus. **inevitable a.,** one which has advanced to a stage where termination of pregnancy cannot be prevented. **missed a.,** early signs and symptoms of pregnancy disappear and the fetus dies, but is not expelled for some time. See MOLE under which carneous mole is defined. **septic a.,** one associated with uterine infection and rise in body temperature. **therapeutic a.,** intentional termination of a pregnancy which is a hazard to the mother's life and health. **threatened a.,** slight blood loss per vaginam whilst cervix remains closed. **tubal a.,** a tubal pregnancy that dies and is expelled from the fimbriated end of the Fallopian tube--abortive, adj.

اسقاط۔ لاطینی لفظ ابارٹس سے ماخوذ جس کے معنی ہیں قبل از وقت پیدائش (1) کسی عمل کا اچانک خاتمہ (2) اگر حمل کے دوران بچہ ضائع ہو جائے یعنی ماں کی یوٹرس سے باہر آ جائے تو اسے اسقاط حمل کہتے ہیں۔ اسقاط خون آنا شروع ہو جاتا ہے۔ اس میں دردزہ اسی طرح ہوتا ہے جس طرح بچے کی پیدائش کے وقت ہوتا ہے۔ لیکن اس میں درد کی شدت کم ہوتی ہے۔ ماں کی احتیاط اسی طرح کی جانی چاہیے جس طرح زچہ کی بچہ کی پیدائش کے بعد احتیاط رکھی جاتی ہے۔ جنین کے قبل از وقت اخراج کو اسقاط کہا جاتا ہے۔ اسقاط حمل سے مراد جنین کی ایسے وقت میں ولادت ہے کہ وہ ابھی ماں کے جسم سے باہر زندہ رہنے کیلئے کافی نشو و نما نہ پا چکا ہو یعنی حمل کے ساتویں قمری مہینے سے پہلے۔ بیشتر اسقاط دوسرے اور تیسرے مہینوں میں ہوتے ہیں۔ اس امر کی اولین علامت کہ اسقاط ہونے والا ہے' خون کا بہنا ہے۔ اگر حمل کے دوران اندام نہانی سے خون آتا ہے یا پانی نکلتا ہے تو ڈاکٹر کی ہدایت موصول ہونے تک لیٹ جانا قرین مصلحت ہے۔ حمل گرنے کی مندرجہ ذیل وجوہات دیکھی گئی ہیں: آتشک و سوزاک' رحم کی رسولیاں' رحم کی کمزوری' رحم کا ورم' کثرت جماع' زیادہ اچھل کود' جلاب' ہارمون کی کمی بیشی' آر۔ ایچ فیکٹر اور

ذہنی پریشانی حادثاتی اسقاط کسی حادثہ کی وجہ سے ہوتا ہے۔ اسقاط ارادی سے مراد جان بوجھ کر حمل گرانا ہے۔ پورا بیضہ خارج ہو جائے تو اسے اسقاط مکمل کہتے ہیں۔ بلاضرورت طبی حمل گرانا اسقاط مجرمانہ کہلاتا ہے۔ اسقاط عادی سے مراد بار بار حمل گرنا' اسقاط ناقص سے مراد آنول کا کچھ حصہ رحم میں رہ جانا' اسقاط ارادی جان بوجھ کر حمل گرانا اور اسقاط ناگزیر اسقاط سے مراد طبی مشورہ پر مجبورا اسقاط کرانا ہے۔ نامکمل اسقاط سے مراد یوٹرس میں جنین کے کسی حصے کا رہ جانا ہے۔ بعض دفعہ جنین رحم میں مر جاتا ہے لیکن دیر سے خارج ہوتا ہے' اسے مسڈ اسقاط کہتے ہیں۔

Abortus fever. See BRUCELLOSIS.

اسقاطی تپ۔ اسقاطی بخار۔ دیکھئے مالٹا بخار یعنی بروسیلوسیس۔ بروسیلا کی ایک نوع سے ہونے والی چھوت کی مرض۔ ایک صنعتی مرض۔

Abrasion (ab-ra`-zhun) [*L. abradere, to scrape off*].Superficial injury to skin or mucous membrane from scraping or rubbing; excoriation -- abrade, v.t; to undergo abrasion, v.i.

خراش۔ خراشیدگی۔ جلد کا رگڑ سے چھل جانا۔ عموما چوٹ گہری نہیں ہوتی۔ بروز میں اوپر سے جلد کا چھل جانا۔ یہ کند آلات کی چوٹ سے' گرنے' دانتوں سے کاٹنے یا ناخن لگنے سے ہوتی ہے۔ خراشیں قاتل و مقتول کے درمیان کشمکش کا پتہ دیتی ہیں۔

Abreaction *(ab-re-ak`-shun)* [L. ab, away; re-, again; agere, to do]. An emotional reaction resulting from reccall of past painful experiences relived in speech and action during psychoanalysis or under the influence of light anaesthesia, or drugs. See NARCOANALYSIS, CATHARSIS.

تحلیل نفسی۔ ماہر نفسیات کے سامنے ماضی کی تلخ یادوں کو ذہن سے کھرچ ڈالنا۔ گزشتہ تلخ واقعات کا ردعمل۔ نفسیاتی تجزیہ۔

Abscess *(ab`-ses)* [L. *abscessus,* a going away]. Localized collection of pus produced by pyogenic organisms. May be acute or chronic. **alveolar a.,** at the root of a tooth. **Brodie's a.,** chronic osteomyelitis (q.v.) occurring without previous acute phase. **cold a.,** one occurring in the course of such chronic inflammation as may be due to the tubercle bacillus *(Mycobacterium tuberculosis).* **psoas a.,** a cold abscess in the psoas muscle, resulting from tuberculosis of the lower dorsal or lumbar vertebrae.

پھوڑا۔ ناسور۔ کسی پھوڑے یا غدود کا مخصوص جراثیم کی وجہ سے ابھرنا۔ جسم کے کسی حصے میں مقامی طور پر پیپ کا جمع ہونا۔ اس کی کئی اقسام ہیں۔ مثلاً ہاد پھوڑا یا عام پھوڑا مسوڑھے کا پھوڑا' مقعد کے قریب پھوڑا' دانت کا جڑ کا راسی پھوڑا' پھوڑا جس کا منہ ہو' پستان کا پھوڑا جو دودھ کی نالی پر اثر انداز نہ ہو' رفتہ رفتہ بڑھنے اور مندمل ہونے والا پھوڑا' سوزش کی جگہ ہٹ کر نمودار ہونے والا پھوڑا' برازی پھوڑا' سوراخ بول پھوڑا' چھوٹے پھوڑوں کا مجموعہ' سابقہ سوزش کی جگہ کے نزدیک کا پھوڑا' خناریزی پھوڑا' ثانوی پھوڑا نس کے غلاف میں پھوڑا' ایسا پھوڑا جو ابتدائی مرکز سے دور کسی مقام پر نمودار ہو' کیسی پھوڑا' پستانی پھوڑا۔

Abstem *(ab`-stem).* Citrated calcium carbimide. Analogue of disulfiram (q.v.).

Acapnia *(a-kap`-ni-a)* [G.a-, not; *kapnos,* smoke]. Absence of CO_2 in the blood, sometimes used synonymously with hypocapnia (q.v.); can be produced by hyper-ventilation--acapnial, adj.

بے دخانی۔ خون میں کاربن ڈائی آکسائیڈ کی کمی واقع ہونا۔

Acatalasia *(a-kat-al-az`-i-a)* Absence of the enzyme catalase; predisposes to oral sepsis.

Accommodation *(ak-kom-mo-da`-shun)* [L. *accommodare,* to adapt]. Adjustment ,e.g. the power of the eye to alter the convexity of the lens according to the nearness of distance of objects.

تطابق۔ موزونیت۔ تطبیق:۔ لاطینی زبان کے لفظ اکموڈیر سے ماخوذ جس کے معنی ڈھالنا ہے۔ دور یا نزدیک دیکھنے کے آنکھ کی موزونیت یعنی پتلی کو پھیلایا اور سکڑایا جاتا ہے۔ روشنی کی شعاعیں پردہ شبکیہ پر مرکوز ہوتی ہیں۔ وہ اشیاء جن عکس پردہ شبکیہ پر بنتا ہے' دور و نزدیک ہوتی ہیں۔ لیکن عدسہ اور شبکیہ کا درمیانی فاصلہ تبدیل نہیں ہوسکتا اس لئے عدسہ کا طول ماسکہ تبدیل ہوتا ہے طول ماسکہ کی تبدیلی میں معلقی رباط کی امداد شامل ہوتی ہے۔ عدسہ کے محدب پن میں اس کی بیشی کو تطبیق کہتے ہیں۔

Accuchement *(ak-koosh -mong)* [F.]. Delivery in childbirth. Confinement

زچگی:۔ عمل ولادت۔ حمل۔ بچے کی پیدائش کا عمل۔

Accoucheur *(ak-koo-sher)* [F.]. A man skilled in midwifery; an obstetrician.

جناوڑا۔ قابل مرد:۔ بچے کی پیدائش میں مددگار مرد۔ مرد جو بچے کی ولادت میں مدد دے۔ آبسٹریشن

Accoucheuse *(ak-koo-shez`)* [F.]. A midwife; a female obstetrician.

دایہ۔ذائی۔قابلہ:۔مڈوائف۔دائی

Accretion *(ak-kre`-shun)* [L. accrescere, to grow]. An increase of substance or deposit round a central object; in dentistry, an accumulation of tartar round the teeth--accrete, adj., v.t. and i.; accretive,adj.

ترقی۔اضافہ:۔لاطینی لفظ اکریسیر سے ماخوذ جس کے معنی بڑھنا ہیں۔کسی مرکزی شے کے گرد کسی چیز کی تہہ جمنا۔دانتوں کے گرد میل جمنا۔

Acebutolol *(ac-bu`-to-lol)*. A B-adrenoceptor blocking agent used in cardiac dysrhythmias, angina pectoris and hypertension.

Acephalous *(a-kef`-a-lus)* [G.a-,not; *kephate,* head]. Without a head.

بے سر۔بریدہ:۔دو یونانی الفاظ اے اور کفالے سے ماخوذ جن کے معانی نہیں اور سر ہیں۔سر کے بغیر

Acetabuloplasty *(as-et-ab`-ul-o-plas-ti)* [L. *acetabulum,* vinegar cup; G.*plassein* to form].An operation to improve the depth and shape of the hip socket (acetabulum); necessary in such conditions as congenital dislocation of the hip and osteoarthritis of the hip -acetabuloplastic, adj.

فنجانی پلاسٹی:۔یہ لاطینی لفظ ایسیٹیبولم بمعنی سرکے کا کپ اور یونانی لفظ پلیسین بمعنی تنا سے ماخوذ ہے۔فنجان یعنی ران کی ہڈی کے جوڑ پر کوئی پلاسٹک اپریشن۔

Acetabulum *(as-et-ab`-ul-um)* [L.].Acup-like socket on the external surface of the innominate bone, into which the head of the femur fits to form the hip joint...acetabula pl.

فنجان،حرقفی،کاسہ ران:۔ہرلا اسی کے تقریباً درمیان میں بیرونی جانب ایک پیالہ نما گہرا کھفہ ہوتا ہے جسے فنجان کہتے ہیں۔یہ لاطینی زبان کا لفظ ہے اور اس کے معنی ہیں سرکے کا پیالہ۔کولہے کی ہڈی کی بیچ میں ایک پیالہ نما جوف جس میں ران کی ہڈی کا گول کنارہ رہتا ہے۔

Acetarsol *(a-set-ar`-sol)*. An organic compound of arsenic, used in amoebiasis (q.v.), usually to supplement emetine.

ایسیٹارسول:۔آرسینک کا نامیاتی مرکب جو فرج میں رکھنے والی بتی یا شیاف کے لیے مقامی طور پر استعمال کیا جاتا ہے۔

Acetate *(as`-e-tat)*. A salt of acetic acid.

ایسی ٹیٹ۔نمک سرکہ:۔ایسٹیک ایسڈ کے نمک۔نامیاتی مرکبات مثلاً کرومیم ایسی ٹیٹ، ایتھائل ایسی ٹیٹ، کیلشیم ایسی ٹیٹ۔

Acetazolamide *(a-set-az-ol`-a-mid)*. Diuretic. Inhibits action of carbonic anhydrase, the kidney enzyme controlling excretion of bicarbonate; results in excretion of increased amount of alkaline urine. As the body has limited reserves of bicarbonate, acetazolamide is self-limiting in action. Also used in glaucoma and epilepsy.

ایسیٹازولائیڈ:۔مرکب جو کاربونک ہائیڈریس کے عمل کو روکتا ہے امراض مرگی میں مفید ہے۔الکلائن پیشاب کی زائد مقدار کو خارج کرتا ہے۔

Acetic acid *(as-e-tic-as`-id)*. The acid present in vinegar. Three varieties are used medicinally; (1) glacial acetic acid, sometimes used as a caustic; (2) ordinary acetic acid, used in urine testing; (3) dilute acetic acid, used occasionally in cough mixtures.

ایسیٹک ایسڈ۔سرکے تیزاب:۔ایتھانوئک ایسڈ۔سرکے تیزاب کا ایک جزو۔ایتھائل الکحل کی تکسید سے کاربوکسائیلک ایسڈ CH3COOH حاصل ہوتا ہے۔آتش گیر نقطہ اشتعال 43 ڈگری سنٹی گریڈ، مائع آنکھوں اور جلد کو جلا دیتا ہے۔ایک نامیاتی مرکب' کیمیائی فارمولا ربڑ میں سرکہ ڈال کر ربڑ کی ترتیب کی جاتی ہے۔دوائیوں میں اس کی تین اقسام استعمال کی جاتی ہیں(1) گلیشل سرکے کا تیزاب بعض اوقات کاسٹک کے طور پر استعمال کیا جاتا ہے(2) عام سرکے کا تیزاب پیشاب ٹیسٹ کرنے میں استعمال ہوتا ہے (3) ہلکا سرکے کا تیزاب بعض اوقات کھانسی کے مکسچر میں شامل کیا جاتا ہے یہ پیشاب کے اخراج کو بڑھاتا ہے۔

Acetoacetic acid *(as-e`-to as-e`-tik as`-id)*.
Syn., diacetic acid. A monobasic keto acid. Produced at an interim stage in the oxidation of fats in the human body. In some metabolic upsets, e.g.acidosis and diabetes mellitus, it is present in excess in the blood and escapes in the urine.

ایسیٹو ایسیٹک ایسڈ:۔ڈائی ایسیٹک ایسڈ یک اساسی کیٹو تیزاب انسانی جسم میں چکنائیوں کی تکسید سے پیدا ہوتا ہے۔ذیابیطس میں خون میں زیادہ مقدار میں موجود ہوتا ہے اور پیشاب کے ذریعہ خارج ہوتا ہے۔اگر پیشاب کو ساکن رکھا جائے تو یہ ایسیٹون میں تبدیل ہو جاتا ہے۔خون میں زائد تیزاب کو پیدا کرسکتا ہے۔

Acetohexamide *(as-et-o-heks`-a-mid)*. One of the sulphonylureas. Antidiabetic agent.

ایسیٹو ہیکسا مائیڈ :- دافع ذیابیطس عامل۔

Acetomenaphtone *(a-set-o-men-af-thon)*. A synthetic form of vitamin K (q.v). It is active orally; used in the treatment of obstructive jaundice and in prophylaxis against neonatal haemorrhage.

ایسیٹو مینافتھون :- حیاتین کی قسم کے' جریان خون کو روکنے میں موثر۔ کیپی ان۔ بواسیر یا پائمنر کے علاج کے لئے ایک گولی صبح ایک دوپہر ایک شام۔

Acetonaemia *(as-e-to-ne`-mi-a)* [L. acenam, vinegar; G.haima, blood]. Acetone bodies in the blood--acetonaemic, adj.

ایسیٹو نیمیا :- لاطینی زبان کے لفظ ایسینم بمعنی سرکہ اور یونانی لفظ ہیما بمعنی خون سے مرکب اصطلاح خون میں ایسیٹون اجسام۔ ایسیٹون اجسام میں ایسیٹون' ایسیٹو ایسیٹک ایسڈ اور بیٹاہائیڈروکسی بیوٹاریک ایسڈ شامل ہیں۔

Acetone *(as`-e-ton)*: Inflammable liquid with characteristic odour; valuable as a solvent. a. bodies, a term which includes acetone, acetoacetic acid and B-hydroxybutyric acid. See KETOSIS.

ایسیٹون :- پروپینون ایک بے رنگ کیٹون مائع خلل کے طور پر استعمال کیا جاتا ہے۔ نقطہ سبعوش 56.1 ڈگری سینٹی گریڈ' 94.6 ڈگری سنٹی گریڈ پر ٹھوس ہو جاتا ہے۔ کیمیائی فارمولا CH3COCH3 آتش گیر' مخصوص بو۔ ایسیٹون اجسام میں ایسیٹون' ایسیٹو ایسیٹک ایسڈ اور بیٹاہائیڈروکسی بیوٹا ایٹرک ایسد شامل ہیں۔

Acetonuria *(as-e-to-nu`-ri-a)* [L. *acetum*, vinegar; G.*ouron*, urine]. Excess ecetone bodies in the urine causing a characteristic sweet smell acetonuric, adj.

ایسیٹون بولی :- ایسیٹون اجزاء کا پیشاب میں بکثرت ہونا۔ لاطینی لفظ ایسیٹم بمعنی سرکہ اور یونانی لفظ اورون پیشاب کا مرکب لفظ۔

Acetophenetidin *(a-set-o-fen-et`-id-in)*. Phenacetin (q.v.).

ایسیٹون فنیسڈین :- فناسٹین۔

Acetylochline *(as-et-il-ko`-len)*. Chemical substance released from nerve endings to activate muscle, secretory glands and other nerve cells. The fibres releasing this chemical are termed 'cholinergic.'

ایسی ٹائل کولین :- ایک نامیاتی مرکب جس کے استعمال سے دل کی دھڑکن کی شرح کم ہو جاتی ہے۔ رگوں کے سروں سے خارج ہونے والا مرکب جو عضلات کے عمل کو تیز کرتا ہے۔ شدید عضلاتی کمزوری میں اس کی پیداوار کم ہو جاتی ہے۔

Acetylcysteine *(as-et-il-sis`-ten)*. A mucolytic agent, invaluable in mucoviscidosis (q.v.).

ایسی ٹائل سسٹین :- میوکولائیٹک عامل۔

Acetylsalicylic acid *(a-set-il-sal`-is-il-ik)*. Aspirin; an extensively used mild analgesic. It forms the basis of a large number of proprietary analgesic tablets. Gastric irritant Can cause haematemesis. Aspirin (q.v.) is now the official BP name.

ایسی ٹائل سیسیلک ایسڈ :- اسپرین۔ سر درد' نزلہ' زکام بخار میں عام استعمال ہونے والی دوائی۔ سفید ٹھوس۔ معدے میں جلن پیدا کرتی ہے۔ 5 گرین کو گولی: بیچئے نقطہ پگھلاؤ 133° س۔

Achalasia *(ak-a-la`-zi-a)* [G.a-, not; *chalasis* relaxation]. Failure to relax.cardiac a., food fails to pass normally into stomach, though there is no obvious obstruction. The oesophagus does not demonstrate normal waves of contraction after swallowing; this prevents the normal relaxation of the cardiacsphincter. Associated with loss of ganglion cells within muscle layers of at least some areas of the affected oesophagus.

ناکشادگی :- بیماری جس میں غذا معدہ میں پہنچنے میں ناکام رہتی ہے۔ بظاہر کوئی رکاوٹ نہیں ہوتی۔ نگلنے کے بعد پیرسٹالٹک حرکات نہیں ہوتیں۔

Achilles tendon *(ak-il`-ez ten`-don)* [G.*Achilles;* L. *tendo*, tendon]. The tendinous termination of the soleus and gastrocnemius muscles inserted into the heil bone (os calcis).

گوتر عرقوب۔ ایڑی کی نس۔ اخیلی وتر :- گھٹنے سے ایڑی تک پنڈلی کا بڑا مضبوط اور طاقتور پٹھا۔ یونانی لفظ اکلیز اور لاطینی لفظ ٹنڈو بمعنی پٹھا یا بندھن سے مرکب اصطلاح۔

Achillorrhaphy *(ak-il-or`-af-i)* [G. *Achilles;* rhaphe, a seam]. The operation of stitching the Achilles tendon.

اکلورافی :- وتر عرقوب یا ایڑی کی نس کو جوڑنے کا اپریشن۔

Achillotomy *(ak-il-ot`-om-i)* [G.*Achilles; tome,*

a cutting]. Subcutaneous division of Achilles tendon

اخیل شگافی :- یونانی الفاظ اکلیز اور ٹوم بمعنی کاٹنا سے ماخوذ اصطلاح۔ ایڑی کی نس کی زیر جلدی قسمت یا تقسیم

Achlorhydria *(a-klor-hi`-dri-a)* [G.a-,not; *chloros,* green; *hydrios,* from *hydor,* water]. The absence of free hydrochloric acid in the stomach. Found in pernicious anaemia and gastrio cancer--achlorhydric, adj.

اکلور ہائیڈریا :- یونانی الفاظ اے، کلوروس اور ہائیڈر سے ہائیڈروس سے مرکب اصطلاح جن کے معانی بالترتیب نہیں یا بغیر، سبز اور پانی ہیں۔ معدہ میں آزاد نمک کے تیزاب کی غیر موجودگی۔ الکانیت اور تیزابیت کا توازن درست نہ رہنا۔ گیسٹرک جوس کی پی ایچ کا چھ سے نیچے گرنے میں ناکامی یہ حالت معدہ کے کینسر میں پائی جاتی ہے۔

Acholia *(a-kol`-i-a)* [G. a-, not; chole, bile]. Absence of bile--acholic, adj.

لاصفراویت :- یونانی الفاظ اے اور کول سے مرکب اصطلاح جن کے معانی بالترتیب بغیر اور بائیل ہیں۔ بائیل کی غیر موجودگی۔

Acholouria *(a-kol-u'-ri-a)* [G. a- not: chole, bile; *ouron,* urine] Absence of bile pigment from the urine. See JAUNDICE-acholuric adj.

اَکولُوریا :- یونانی الفاظ اے اورون سے مرکب جن کے معانی بالترتیب بغیر، بائیل اور پیشاب ہیں۔ پیشاب میں بائیل پگمنٹ کی غیر موجودگی۔

Achondroplasia *(a-kon-dro-pla-zi-a)* [G.a-, not; *chondros,* cartilage' plassein, to form]. An inherited condition characterized by arrested growth of the long bcnes resulting in dwarfism. The intellect is not impaired. Syn, fetal rickets- achondroplastic, adj.

صغرُ الجوارح :- ہڈیوں کی نشوونما میں خرابی پیدا ہونا یا رکاوٹ ہونا، بونا پن، ٹھگنا ہونا، یونانی الفاظ اے، کانڈرس اور پلیسین سے مرکب جن کے معانی بالترتیب بغیر، نرم ہڈی اور بنا ہیں۔ بونا پن میں طویل ہڈیوں کی محدود نشونما

Achromatopsia *(a-kro-mat-op-zi-a)* [G.a-, not; *chroma,* colour; *opsis,* vision] complete colour blindness as only monochromatic grey is visible.

رنگ کوری :- یونانی الفاظ اے، کلوروس اور ہائیڈر سے ہائیڈروس سے مرکب اصطلاح جن کے معانی بالترتیب بغیر رنگ اور نظر ہیں۔ رنگوں میں تمیز نہ کرنا۔ رنگ دکھائی نہ دینا۔

Achromycin *(ak-ro-mi-sin).* Tetracycline (q.v.)

ایکرومائی سِن :- ٹیٹراسائیکلین۔ کسی دوسرے جسیے کی نشونما کو روکنے والی دوا۔ آتشک یا سِفلس کے علاج کے لئے اس کے دو کیپسول ہر چھ گھنٹے بعد بیس دنوں تک۔ سپڑ ابواسیر یا پائلز کے علاج کے لئے ایک کیپسول ہر چھ گھنٹے بعد ۔اسی طرح برائے اَنلارجڈ پراسٹیٹ اور نمونیا

Achylia *(a-ki-li-a)* [G. a-, not;' *chylos,* juice] Absence of chyle (q.v.) achylic, adj.

اے کائیلیا یلا کرِس :- یونانی الفاظ اے اور کائیلوس سے مرکب جن کے معانی بغیر اور رس کے ہیں۔ کائیل کی غیر موجودگی۔

Acid (as'-id) [L. *acidus,* sour]. Any substance which in solution gives rise to an excess of hydrogen ions. Identified (1) by turning blue litmus paper red; (2) by being neutralized by an alkali with the formation of a salt. (In popular jargon, any substance with a sour taste.

ایسڈ۔ تیزاب :- لاطینی لفظ ایسڈس بمعنی کھٹا سے ماخوذ۔ ایسی شے جو پانی میں ہائیڈروجن آئن H^+ کی مقدار بڑھا دے، ایسڈ یا تیزاب کہلاتی ہے۔ مثلاً $Hci+ H_2O---- H_3O+ctl$ کلورین آئن ہائیڈرونیم آئن پانی نمک کا تیزاب ۔تیزاب کا ذائقہ ترش ہوتا ہے۔ نیلے لٹمس کو الکلی سے مل کر نمک بناتا ہے۔

Acidaemia *(as-id-e-mi-a)* [L. *acidus,* sour, G. *haima.* blood] giving increased hydrogen ions, and a below normal pH (q.v.) respiratory a,. caused by poor ventilation and increasing carbon dioxide. metabolic a,. caused by increased lactic acid production in muscles. See ACIDOSIS- acidaemic, adj.

خون کا ترشاوَ۔ تیزابی دمویت :- لاطینی لفظ ایسڈ بمعنی تُرش کھٹا اور یونانی لفظ ہیما بمعنی خون سے مرکب اصطلاح۔ خون کی غیر معمولی تیزابیت، ہائیڈروجن آئنز کی زیادتی اور نارمل پی ایچ سے کم۔ تنفسی تیزابی دَمویت تازہ ہوا کی کمی اور کاربن ڈائی آکسائیڈ کی زیادتی کی وجہ سے ہوتی ہے۔ میٹابالک تیزابی دمویت عضلات میں زیادہ لیکٹک ایسڈ پیدا ہونے سے ہوتی ہے۔

Acid-base BALANCE Equilibrium between the acid and base elements of the blood and body fluids.

توازن تیزابیت :- توازن یا تناسب جو خون اور جسمانی رطوبتوں کے درمیان ہوتا ہے۔

Acid-fast In bacteriology, describes an organism which, when stained. does not become decolo(u)rized when subjected to dilute acids, e.g. *Mycobacterium tuberculosis*.

ایسڈ فاسٹ :- علم الجراثیم میں ایک مستعمل اصطلاح جو ایک ایسے جسیمے کو بیان کرنے کے لئے استعمال ہوتی ہے جسے ہلکے تیزاب میں ڈالنے سے بھی رنگ نہ اڑے۔ مثلاً تپ دق کا جرثومہ۔

Acid-alcohol-fast Stained bacteria, resistant to decolo(u)rization by alcohol as well as acid.

Acidity *(as-id-it-i)* [L. *acidus,* acid]. The state of being acid or sour. The degree of acidity can be determined and interpreted on the pH scale. pH 6.9 denoting a very weak acid and pH I a caustic acid.

تیزابیت ۔ تُرشیت ۔ تُرشی :- لاطینی لفظ ایسیڈس سے ماخوذ جس کے معنی ہیں ایسڈ یا تیزاب۔ تیزاب ہونا یا ترش ہونا تیزابیت کا درجہ پی ایچ سکیل پر معلوم کیا جاتا ہے۔ پی ایچ 6،9 بہت کمزور تیزاب کو ظاہر کرتا ہے اور پی ایچ ایک، کاسٹک ایسڈ کو ظاہر کرتا ہے۔ اس کی علامات دل بیٹھنا، کھٹی ڈکار اور سینے کی جلن ہیں۔ کسی عنصر سے ہائیڈروجن کا ٹوٹنا۔

Acidosis (*as-id-o-sis*) [L. *acidus,* sour; G. *-osis* condition]. Depletion of the body's alkali reserve, with resulting disturbance of the acid-base balance. Acidaemia. **renal tubular a.**, metabolic abnormality. See KETOSIS-acidotic, adj.

تیزابی دمویت ۔ خون کا ترشاؤ: لاطینی لفظ ایسیڈس بمعنی ترش اور یونانی لفظ اوسس بمعنی حالت کا مرکب۔ جسمانی الکلی کا ذخیرہ کم ہونا جس سے توازن تیزابیت بگڑ جاتا ہے۔

Acid Phosphatase (*fos-fa-taz*) Enzyme in seminal fluid. Secreted by prostate gland.

ایسڈ فاسفیٹیز : منی میں موجود خامرہ

Aciduria *(as-id-u-ri-a)* [L. *acidus,* sour; G. *-osis,* condition]. Excretion of an acid urine. Current work suggests there might be some association with mental subnormality.

ایسڈوریا ۔ تیزابی حالت : لاطینی لفظ ایسیڈس بمعنی ترش اور یونانی لفظ اوسس بمعنی حالت سے مرکب۔ تیزابی پیشاب کا اخراج۔

Acini (as'-in-i) [L]. Minute saccules or alveoli, lined or filled with secreting cells. Several acini combine to form a lobule-**acinus, sing.; acinous, acinar,** adj.

خوشے : ایک لاطینی لفظ ۔ ننھے خانے جن میں اخراج کرنے والے خلیے

ہوتے ہیں۔

Acme (*ak'-me*) [G. *akme,* prime]. 1. Highest point. 2. Crisis or critical state of a disease.

اوج ۔ بحران : نقطۂ عروج ۔ بیماری کا نازک حد تک بڑھ جانا یونانی زبان کا لفظ۔

Acne, acne vulgarisak'-ne vul-gar'-is). A skin condition common in adolescence, in which blackheads (comedones) are associated with a papular and pustular eruption of the pilosebaceous follicles. Usual sites are the face, neck and upper part of chest and back. **See ROSACEA.**

دانہ ۔ کیل : چہرے کے دانے ایک جلدی بیماری جس میں ناک اور منہ پر کیل اور مہاسے نکل آتے ہیں۔

Acniform (*ak-ne'-i-form*). Resembling acne.

دانہ نما: مہاسوں سے مشابہ۔

Acriflavine (*ak-ri-fla'-ven*). Orange-red, soluble powder. Powerful antiseptic, used as a 1:1000 solution for wounds, and 1:4000 to 1:8000 for irrigation. Acrufavine emulsion is a bland wound dressing containing liquid paraffin. Proflavine and euflavine are similar compounds

ایکریفلیون : زردی مائل سرخ حل پزیر سفوف۔ طاقت ور دافع تعفن۔ زخموں کے لئے ۱۰۰۰: محلول استعمال کیا جاتا ہے اور آبپاشی کے لئے ۴۰۰۰:۱ تا ۸۰۰۰: ا محلول استعمال کیا جاتا ہے۔ ایکریفلیون ایملشن بشمول مائع پیرافین زخموں کی ڈریسنگ کے لئے استعمال کیا جاتا ہے۔ پروفلیون اور یوفلیون ایسے ہی مرکبات ہیں۔ جلی ہوئی جگہ پر گاز پر لگا کر لگایئے۔

Acroarthritis (*ak-ro-arth-ri-tis*) [G. *akron,* extremity; *arthorn,* joint; *-itis,* inflammation]. Inflammation of the joints of hands or feet.

ایکرآرتھریٹس : ہاتھ پاؤں کے جوڑوں پر ورم ہونا یا ان کا سوج جانا۔

Acrocephalia:acrocephaly (*ak-ro-kef-a-li-a*) [G. *akron,* extremity; *kephale* head]. A congenital malformation whereby the top of the head is pointed - acrocephalic, acrocephalous, adj.

نوک سری : یونانی الفاظ ایکرون بمعنی اختتام یا حد اور کفالے بمعنی سر سے مرکب اصطلاح۔ سنکھ ایسے سر والا۔

Acrocephalosyndactyly(*ak-ro-kef-a-lo-sin-dak'-til-i*) [G. *akron,* extremity; *kephale,* head; *syn.* with; *daktylos,* digit]. A congenital malformation consisting of a pointed top of head, with webbed hands and feet. Acrocephalosyndactylism. See SYNDACTYLY.

نوک سری جڑی انگلیاں: یونانی الفاظ ایکرون بمعنی آخری حد' کفالے بمعنی سر' سن بمعنی ہمراہ یا ساتھ اور ڈیکٹا ڈیکٹا ئیلوس بمعنی انگلی سے مرکب اصطلاح۔ نکھ ایسے سر والا جس کی ہاتھ پاؤں کی انگلیاں جھلی دار ہوں۔

Acrocyanosis (*ak-ro-si-an-o-sis*) [G. *akron*, extremity; *kyanos* blue; *-osis*, condition]. Coldness and blueness of the extremities due to circulatory disorder - acrocyanotic, adj.

سر زراق: یونانی الفاظ ایکرون بمعنی آخری حد' کیانوس بمعنی نیلا اور اوسس بمعنی حالت سے مرکب اصطلاح۔ سردی میں ہاتھوں اور پیروں کا سرد ہونا اور ایڑیوں کا پھٹنا۔ سردی سے ہاتھ پاؤں نیلے پڑ جاتے ہیں۔

Acrodynia (*ak-ro-din-i-a*) [G. *akron*, extremity; *odyne*, pain]. Painful reddening of the extremities such as occurs in pink disease (q.v).

ایکروڈائینا۔ وجع الجوارح عفریتیت یونانی الفاظ ایکرون بمعنی آخری حد اور اڈائین بمعنی درد سے مرکب اصطلاح۔ ہاتھ پاؤں کا درد سے سرخ ہونا۔

Acromegaly (*ak-ro-meg'-a-li*) [G. *akron*, extremity; *megas*, large]. Enlargement of the hands, face and feet, occurring in an adult due to disturbed function of the pituitary gland -- acromegalic, adj.

ایکرومیگالی۔ کبرالجوارح: یونانی الفاظ ایکرون بمعنی آخری حد اور میگاس بمعنی بڑا سے مرکب اصطلاح۔ کسی بالغ میں ہاتھوں اور چہرے کا بڑا ہو جانا۔ امامی بلغمی میں فعلیت کی خرابی کی وجہ سے بچپن میں فعلیت کی تیز رفتاری کا

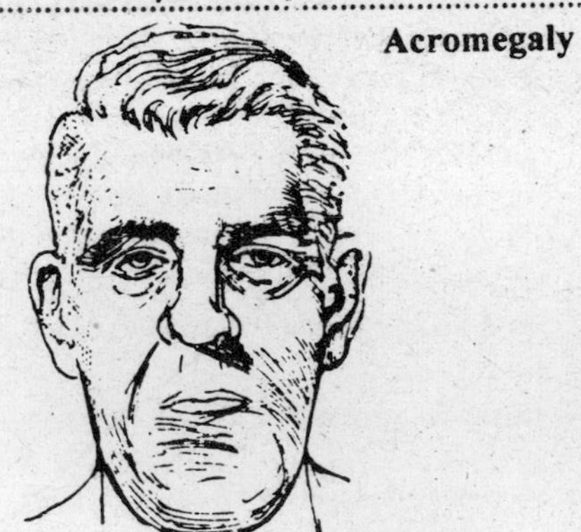

Acromegaly

نقص پیدا ہو جاتا ہے۔ جس سے بچوں میں دیوہیکل پن کی بیماری ہو جاتی ہے۔

رطوبت کے زائد اخراج کی وجہ سے ہڈیاں طویل ہو جاتی ہیں۔ مریض عموماً نو عمری میں فوت ہو جاتا ہے۔ اگر زندہ رہے تو جنسی اشتہا کی کمی ہوتی ہے۔ اگر بڑی ہونے پر غدود میں فعلیت کی تیز رفتاری کا نقص پیدا ہو تو ایکرومیگالی کی خرابی پیدا ہو جاتی ہے جس میں ڈھانچے کے کچھ حصے بہت بڑھ جاتے ہیں۔ مثلاً ہاتھ کافی لمبے ہو جاتے ہیں۔ بازو بھی کافی لمبے ہو جاتے ہیں اور جبڑے باہر نکل آتے ہیں۔ علاج کے لئے ایکسرے' اپریشن اور تھائی رائسین

Acromicria (*ak-ro-mik'-ri-a*) [G. *akron*. extremity; *mikros*, small]. Smallness of the hands, face and feet, probably due to deficiency of growth hormone from the pituitary gland.

ایکرومکریا۔ صغرالجوارح۔ بوناپن: یونانی الفاظ ایکرون بمعنی سرا' نوک یا حد اور مکروس بمعنی چھوٹا سے مرکب اصطلاح۔ بلغمی کی فعلیت میں خرابی کی وجہ سے بچپن میں فعلیت کے بعد اس نقص کے نتیجہ میں فرد بوناپن کا شکار ہو جاتا ہے۔ کارکردگی سست پڑ جاتی ہے۔ خون میں شکر کی کمی' پٹھوں کی کمزوری' خون کی کمی وغیرہ ایسے امراض ہو جاتے ہیں۔

Acromioclavicular I(*ak-ro-mi-o-kla-vi'-ku-lar*) [G *akron*, extremity; *omos*, shoulder; L. *clavicula*, dim. of clavis, key]. Pertaining to the acromion process (of scapula) and the clavicle.

ایکرومیوکلیویکولر: سکیپولا اور کلیویکل کے ایکرومیئن پروسس سے متعلق۔

Acromion (*Ak-ro-mi-on*) [G. *akron*, extremity; *omos*, shoulder]. The point of summit of the shoulder; the triangular process at the extreme outer end of the spine of the scapula - acromial, adj.

نوک شانہ' اخرمہ: یونانی الفاظ ایکرون بمعنی نوک' سرا یا حد اور اموس بمعنی شانہ سے مرکب اصطلاح۔ کندھے کا ابھار۔ شانے کی ہڈی کا اونچا حصہ۔

Acronyx (*ak'-ro'niks*) [G. *akron*, extremity; *onyx*, nail]. Ingrowing of a nail.

چور ناخن: یونانی الفاظ ایکرون بمعنی نوک' حد یا سرا اور اونکس بمعنی ناخن سے مرکب اصطلاح۔ ہاتھوں اور پیروں کے ناخنوں کا اندرونی جانب مڑا ہونا عموماً پاؤں کی انگلیوں میں ایسا ہوتا ہے۔

Acroparaesthesia (*ak-ro-par-es-the'-zi-a*) [G. *akron*, extremity; *paroesthesis*, misperception]. Tingling and numbness of the hands.

انگلیوں کی سنسناہٹ: ہاتھ پاؤں کا سن ہونا۔

Acrophobia (*ak-ro-fo-bi-a*) [G. *akron*, extremity; *phobos*, fear]. Morbid fear of being at a height.

ایکروفوبیا۔ فرازترسی: یونانی الفاظ ایکرون بمعنی نوک' سرا یا حد اور فوبس بمعنی ڈر یا خوف سے مرکب اصطلاح۔ بلندی سے زیریں جانب دیکھ کر خوف کی حالت۔ اونچائی کا خوف۔

Acrylics (*a-kril'-iks).* A group of thermoplastic substances used in making prostheses-- acrylic, adj.

ایکرائیلکس: تھرموپلاسٹک اشیاء کا ایک گروہ۔

ACTH.. Corticotrophin (q.v).

اے۔سی۔ٹی۔ایچ: امامی بلغمی سے بننے والا ایک ہارمون جو ایڈرینل کارٹیکس میں تہیج پیدا کرتا ہے اور اس کی رطوبت کو بڑھاتا ہے۔ ۱۵۰ ملی گرام روزانہ بذریعہ عضلاتی ٹیک برائے ہیم فی گس۔

Acthar gel (*ak-tha jel*). Given in units to suppress disseminated sclerosis.

Actifed (*ak'-ti-fed).* Pseudoephedrine (q.v) and triprolidine (q.v).

Actinic Dermatoses Skin conditions (such as xeroderma pigmentosum, summer prurigo (q.v) and others) in which the integurnent is abnormally sensitive to ultraviolet light.

Actinism (*ak'-tin-izm)* [G. *aktis,* ray]. The chemical action of spectral rays.

کیمیائی شعاعیت: یونانی لفظ ایکٹس سے ماخوذ جس کے معنی شعاع ہیں۔ طیفی شعاعوں کا کیمیائی عمل۔

Actinobiology (*ak'-tin-o-bi-ol-oj-i)* [G. *aktis* ray; *bios,* life; *logos,* discourse]. The study of the effects of radiation on living organisms.

ایکٹینوبیالوجی۔ تنویری حیاتیات: یونانی الفاظ ایکٹس بمعنی شعاع' بایوس بمعنی زندگی اور لوگوس بمعنی مطالعہ' دلیل یا بحث سے مرکب اصطلاح۔ جانداروں پر اشعاع کے اثرات کا مطالعہ۔

Actinomycin C. (*ak-tin-o-mi-sin).* A cytostatic antibiotic useful in Hodgkin's disease and for suppression of the immune reaction in organ transplants.

ایکٹینو مائیسین ''ج'': عام مستعمل دوا۔

Actinomycin D (*ak-tin-o-mi-sin).* An intravenous cytostatic agent especially useful in Wilms' tumour. Also used in Burkitt's lymphoma.

ایکٹینو مائیسین ''د'': عام استعمال ہونے والی دوا۔

Actinomycosis (*ak-tin-o-ko-sis)* [G. **aktis,** ray; ***mykes,*** fungus; *-osis,* condition]. A disease caused by Actinomyces, the sites most affected being the lung, jaw and intestine. Granulomatous tumours form which usually suppurate, discharging a thick, oily pus containing yellowish granules ('sulphur granules') - actinomycotic, adj.

لٹی دار جبڑا۔ کرن فطریت: یونانی الفاظ ایکٹس بمعنی شعاع' مائیکس بمعنی سماروغ یا فنگس اور اوسس بمعنی حالت سے مرکب اصطلاح۔ ایکٹینو مائی سیز کی وجہ سے پیدا ہونے والی بیماری جو سب سے زیادہ پھیپھڑے جبڑے اور آنت کو متاثر کرتی ہے۔ ناسور گندھکی دانوں پر مشتمل گاڑھی' چکنی پیپ خارج کرتے ہیں۔

Actinotherapy (*ak-tin-o-the'-rap-i)* [G. *aktis,* ray; *therapeia,* theraphy]. Treatment radiations, similar to those in natural sunlight, but produced by artificial means.

کیمیا شعاعی علاج: غیر آیونائزنگ اشعاع کے ذریعہ علاج خصوصاً الٹراوائلٹ یا انفراریڈ شعاعوں کے ذریعہ۔

Action (*ak'-shun)* [L. *actio,* from agere, to do or to perform]. The activity or function of any part of the body. **antagonistic a.,** performed by those muscles which limit the movement of an opposing group. **compulsive a.,** performed by an individual at the supposed instigation of another's dominant will, but against his own, **impulsive a.,** resulting from a sudden urge rather than the will. **reflex a.,** a specific, involuntary motor or secretory response to a sensory stimulus. **sexual a.,** coitus, cohabitation, sexual intercourse. **specific a.,** that brought about by certain remedial agents in a particular disease, e.g. salicylates in acute rheumatism. **specific dynamic a.,** the stimulating effect upon the metabolism produced by the ingestion of food, especially proteins, causing the metabolic rate to rise above basal levels, **synergistic a.,** that brought about by the co-operation of two or more muscles, neither of which could bring about the action alone.

عمل۔ فعل: جسم کے کسی حصے کا فعل۔ اعضاء کی حرکات۔ ارادی یا غیر ارادی عمل۔ جنسی یا جنسی مباشرت خوراک کا انہضام وغیرہ سب افعال میں۔

Activator [L. *activus*]. A substance which **renders** something else active, e.g. the **hormone** secretin, the enzyme enterokinase. **An enzyme** activator is called 'co-enzyme' or **'kinase'** -- activate, v.

محرک۔ عامل کار: لاطینی لفظ ایکٹیوس سے ماخوذ۔ دوسرے کے عمل کو تیز کرنے والا۔ خامرہ اور ہارمون سے متعلق مستعمل اصطلاح مثلاً سیکریٹین' ایک ہضمی ہارمون جو لبلبہ کو سرگرم کرتا ہے۔ خامرہ کے عمل کو تیز کرنے والا کو ایزائیم کہلاتا ہے۔

Active [L. *activus*, active]. Energetic. Opp. to passive (q.v) **a. hyperaemia,** see HYPERAEMIA **a. immunity,** see IMMUNITY. **a. movements,** those produced by the patient using his neuromuscular mechanism. **a. principle,** an ingredient which gives a complex drug its chief therapeutic value, e.g. atropine is the active principle in belladonna.

مستعد۔ سرگرم۔ عامل۔ سریع التاثیر: لاطینی لفظ ایکٹیوس سے ماخوذ جس کا مطلب ہے۔ عامل۔ طاقتور یا قوی عمل۔ قوت مدافعت یا ایکٹوامیونٹی سے مراد ہے کہ اینٹی ٹاکسن اور اینٹی سیرم جراثیموں کے زہر اور پرورش کردہ جراثیموں کو کسی حیوان مثلاً گھوڑے وغیرہ کی وریدوں میں انجکشن سے داخل کر دیا جاتا ہے اس سے حیوان بیمار معلوم ہوتا ہے۔ پھر مختلف اوقات میں ٹاکسن کی مقدار رفتہ رفتہ زیادہ کر کے بذریعہ جلدی پچکاری جسم میں داخل کرتے رہتے ہیں۔ اس طریقہ سے جانور میں اینٹی ٹاکسن پیدا ہو جاتے ہیں جو انسانی جسم میں داخل کئے جاتے ہیں۔ وہ مقام یا جگہ جہاں خامرہ کا سالمہ یا مالیکیول عمل کرتا ہے' اسے مقام عاملیعہ کہتے ہیں۔ سالمات یعنی مالیکولوں یا آئینوں کا ارتکاز کے خلاف جھلی کے پار جانے کا ایکٹو ٹرانسپورٹ کہا جاتا ہے۔ اس میں توانائی کا اصراف ہوتا ہے۔

Actrapid (*ak-tra-pid*) Neutral insulin injection BP.

اکٹریپڈ: ٹیکہ لگنے کی جگہ پر حل پذیر انسولن کی تیزابی پی' ایچ کی وجہ سے تکلیف میں مفید۔

Acuity (*ak-u-it-i*) [L. *acucre*, to sharpen]. Sharpness, clearness, keenness, distinctness. **auditory a.,** ability to hear clearly and distinctly. Tests include the use of tuning fork, whispered voice and audiometer. In infants, simple sounds, e.g. **bells,** rattles, cup and spoon are utilized, **visual a.,** extent of visual perception dependent on the clarity of retinal focus, integrity of nervous elements and cerebral interpretation of the stimulus. Usually tested by Snellen's test types (q.v) at 6 meters.

شدت۔ تیزی: لاطینی لفظ ''اکوئر'' سے ماخوذ جس کے معنی ہیں تیز کرنا۔ تیزی' صفائی یا نمایاں ہونا۔ سمعی تیزی سے مراد قوت سامعہ کا تیز ہونا ہے۔ صاف اور واضح طور پر سننے کی اہلیت۔ اسے ٹیسٹ کرنے کے لیے ٹیوننگ فورک' آہستہ آواز اور آڈیومیٹر استعمال کئے جاتے ہیں۔ بچوں میں قوت سماعت کو سادہ آوازوں سے ٹیسٹ کیا جاتا ہے۔ مثلاً گھنٹی یا پیالے اور چمچ کی آوازوں سے۔ تیز نظری یا بصری تیزی سے مراد دو قریبی نقاط کو علیحدہ علیحدہ دیکھنے کی آنکھ کی اہلیت ہے۔ بینائی کو ٹیسٹ کرنے کے لئے بیس فٹ کے فاصلہ سے چارٹ پڑھوایا جاتا ہے۔

Acupuncture (*ak-u-punk-tur*) [L. *acus*, needle; *punctura*, a pricking]. 1. The incision or introduction of fine, hollow tubes into oedematous tissue for the purpose of withdrawing fluid. 2. A technique of insertion of special needles into particular parts of the body for the treatment of disease, relief of pain or production of anaesthesia.

سوزن زنی: لاطینی الفاظ ''ایکس'' بمعنی سوئی اور ''پنکوا'' بمعنی چبھونا یا چبھن سے مرکب اصطلاح۔ سیال کھینچنے کے لئے باریک اور کھوکھلی نلیوں کا دخول۔

Acute (*a-kut'*) [L.*acutus*, sharp]. Short and severe; not long drawn out or chronic. **a. defibrination syndrome,** (hypofibrinogenaemia). excessive bleeding due to maternal absorption of thrombolastins from retained blood clot or damaged placenta within the uterus. A missed abortion, placental abruption, amniotic fluid embolus, prolonged retention in utero of a dead fetus and the intravenous administration of dextran can lead to **ADS. a. dilatation of the stomach,** sudden enlargement of this organ due to paralysis of the muscular wall. See PARALYTIC ILEUS. **a.heart failure,** cessation or impairment of heart action, in previously undiagnosed heart disease, or in the course of another disease. **a. yellow atrophy,** acute diffuse necrosis of the liver; icterus gravis; malignant jaundice.

نوکدار۔حادہ: لاطینی لفظ ''اکوٹس'' سے ماخوذ۔مختصر و تیز مرض میں شدت خون کا زیادہ بہنا جو یوٹرس سے بہتا ہے۔اسقاط کی وجہ سے خون کا جاری ہونا۔ رحم مادر میں جنین کے مرنے سے خون کا جاری ہونا۔معدے کا اچانک بڑھاؤ۔ ہارٹ فیل ہونا۔

۲- پتے کے راس کی مخصوص شکل جس میں راس نوکیلا ہوتا ہے۔مثلاً آم۔

۳- ایسازاویہ جو قائمہ زاویہ یا ۹۰ ڈگری سے کم نہ ہو۔

Acyanosis (*a-si-an-o'-sis*) [G. *a-*, not; *kyanos*, blue; -osis, condition]. Without cyanosis.

اسائی انوسس: یونانی الفاظ ''اے'' بمعنی بغیر،بلا،بے کیانس'' بمعنی نیلا یا نیلی اور ''اوسس'' بمعنی حالت سے مرکب اصطلاح جو امراض قلب کے لئے مستعمل ہے۔

Acyanotic (*a-si-an-ot'-ik*) Without cyanosis; term used to differentiate congenital cardiovascular defects.

اسائی انوٹک: پیدائشی امراض قلب کے لئے مستعمل اصطلاح ایسا مریض جو پیدائشی امراض قلب میں مبتلا ہو۔

Acyesis (*a-si-e'-sis*) [G. *a-*, not; *kyesis*, pregnancy]. Absence of pregnancy acyetic, adj.

بانجھ پن۔عدم حمل: یونانی الفاظ ''اے'' بمعنی نہیں، بلایا کے بغیر اور ''کائیسس'' بمعنی حمل سے مرکب اصطلاح حمل نہ ہونا۔حمل کی غیر موجودگی۔

Acystia *(a-sis'-ti-a)* [G. *a-*, not; *kystis*, bladder]. Congential absence of the bladder -- acystic, adj.

بے مثانگی: یونانی الفاظ ''اے'' بمعنی نہیں، بلایا کے بغیر اور کسٹس بمعنی بولیڈر سے مرکب اصطلاح۔بلیڈر کی غیر موجودگی۔

Adam's Apple The laryngeal prominence in front of the neck, especially in the adult male, formed by the junction of the two wings of the thyroid cartilage.

گھنڈی۔کنھطا۔ٹینٹوا: گلے کی گھنٹی کا ابھرنا جس سے آواز میں بھاری پن آجاتا ہے۔نر میں سن بلوغت کی پہچان۔حجرہ یا آلۂ صوت ٹھوڑی سے دوانچ نیچے ہاتھ سے محسوس کیا جاسکتا ہے۔

Adaptability (*ad-apt'-a-bil-it-i*) [L. adaptare, to adjust]. The ability to adjust mentally and physically to circumstances.

توافق: لاطینی لفظ اڈیپٹیر سے ماخوذ جس کا مطلب ڈھالنا ہے۔ذہنی و جسمانی طور پر حالات کے مطابق ڈھالنے کی اہلیت۔حالات سے سمجھوتہ۔

Adcortyl *(ad-kor'-til)*. Triamcinalone (q.v) **a. in orabase,** emollient dental paste for mouth ulcers.

Addict *(ad'-ikt)* [L. addictum, from addicere, to devote]. One who is unable to resist indulgence in some habit, such as the drug (q.v) habit -- addict, v.t., v.i.; addiction, n.

علتی۔معتاد: لاطینی۔جو کسی عادت کو نہ چھوڑ سکے۔نشہ آور ادویات کا عادی۔

Addison's Disease Deficient secretion of aldosterone and cortisol from the adrenal cortex, causing electrolytic upset, diminution of blood volume, lowered blood pressure, marked anaemia, hypoglycaemia, great muscular weakness, gastrointestinal upsets and pigmen- tation of skin. [Thomas Addison, English physician, diagnostician and teacher, 179- 3-1860].

مرض ایڈیسن: ایک انگریز فزیشن تھامس ایڈیسن کے نام پر بیماری کا نام رکھا گیا ہے۔کم خونی دباؤ یعنی لو بلڈ پریشر، خون کی کمی، شدید اعصابی کمزوری۔اس میں مریض عام خوراک کھاسکتا ہے۔اس میں زائد نمک کی ضرورت نہیں۔

Adduct *(ab-dukt')* [L. ad, to; ducere, to lead]. To draw towards the midline of the body. Opp. to abduct.

تقریب۔جموعہ: لاطینی جسم کے درمیانی حصہ کی جانب کھینچنا۔سادہ طریقوں سے ملاپ۔

Adduction *(ad-duk'-shun)* [L. ad, to; ducere, to lead]. The act of adducting, drawing towards the midline. Opp. to adduction.

تقرب: لاطینی۔جسم کے درمیانی حصے کی طرف کھینچنے کا عمل۔

Adductor *(ad-duk'-tor)* [L. ad. to; ducere, to lead]. Any muscle which moves a part toward the median axis of the body. Opp. to adductor.

مقربہ۔قریب کنندہ: لاطینی ایسا عضلہ جس کا کچھ حصہ جسم کے درمیانی حصے کی طرف حرکت کرے۔وہ پٹھے جو بازو یا ٹانگوں کو جسم کی طرف لاتے ہیں، ندر لانے والے پٹھے کہلاتے ہیں۔

Adenectomy *(ad-en-ek'-to-mi)* [G. aden, gland; ektome, excision]. Surgical removal of a gland.

غدہ برادی: یونانی الفاظ ایڈن بمعنی غدا اور ایکٹومی بمعنی قطع سے مرکب

اصطلاح۔ سرجری کے ذریعہ کسی غدکا کاٹنا۔

Adenitis *(ad-en-i-tis)* [G. aden, gland; itis, inflammation]. Inflammation of a gland or lymph node, **hilar a.**, inflammation of bronchial lymph nodes.

ورم غدہ: یونانی الفاظ ایڈن بمعنی غد اور ائس بمعنی سوج یا ورم سے مرکب اصطلاح۔ غدود کا سوجنا۔

Adenocarcinoma *(ad-en-o-kar-sin-o'-ma)* [G. aden, gland; karkinos, crab; omos, raw flesh]. A malignant growth of glandular tissue -- adenocarcinomatous, adj; adenocarcinomata, pl.

غدی سرطانی سلعہ: یونانی الفاظ ایڈن' کرکینوس داموس سے مرکب اصطلاح جن کے معانی بالترتیب غد' کریب یا کچا گوشت ہیں۔ غدود کی بافت کا بڑھ جانا۔ بدن پر زائد غیر ضروری غدود یہ بافت کا نمایا ہونا۔

Adenofibroma *(ad-en-o'-fi-bro-ma)* See FIBROADENOMA.

اڈینوفائبروما: دیکھئے فائبرواڈینو۔

Adenoid *(ad'-en-oid)* [G. aden, gland; eidos, form]. Resembling a gland. See ADENOIDS.

اڈینائڈ۔ غدہ نما: یونانی الفاظ ایڈن وایڈوس سے مرکب اصطلاح جن کے معانی بالترتیب غد اور بننا کے ہیں۔

(۱) نیزوفیرنکس میں لمفی بافت کا حد سے زیادہ بڑھ جانا (۲) غدود سے مشابہہ۔

Adenoidectomy *(ad-e-noid-ek'-to-mi)* [G. aden, gland; eidos, form; ektome, excision]. Surgical removal from nasopharynx of adenoid tissue.

قطع غدودہ۔ غدودہ تراشی: یونانی الفاظ ایڈن' ایڈوس و ایکٹومی سے مرکب اصطلاح جن کے معانی بالترتیب غد' بننا و قطع ہیں۔ اڈینائڈ بافت کلے نیزوفیرنکس سے سرجری کے ذریعہ قطع و برید۔ زائد غدود کو اپریشن سے نکالنا۔

Adenoids *(ad'-en-oidz)* [G. aden, glan; eidos, form]. Enlarged mass of lymphoid tissue in the nasopharynx which can obstruct breathing and interefere with hearing.

Adenoma *(ad-en-o'-ma)* [G. aden, gland; omos, raw flesh]. A non-malignant tumour of glandular tissue adenomatous,adj.;adenomata, pl.

غدوما: یونانی الفاظ ایڈن و اموس سے مرکب اصطلاح جن کے معانی بالترتیب غد' عضلہ اور کچا گوشت ہیں' عضلے اور غدودی اجزاء پر مشتمل ناسور۔

Adenomyoma *(ad-en-o-mi-o'-ma')* [G. aden, gland; mys, muscle; omos, raw flesh]. A non-malignant tumour composed of muscle and glandular elements, e.g. an adenomyoma of the uterosacral ligaments is composed of smooth muscle in which islands of aberrant endometrium are found -- adenomyomatous, adj.; adenomyomata, pl.

Adenomyosis uteri *(ad-en-o-mi-o'-sisu'-te-ri)* [G. aden, gland; mys, muscle; -osis, condition]. A general enlargement of the uterus due to overgrowth of the myometrium, in which there is a benign invasion of endometrium.

اڈینومی اوسس یوٹری: یونانی الفاظ ایڈن' مائس اور اوسس سے مرکب اصطلاح جن کے معانی بالترتیب غد' عضلہ اور حالت ہیں۔ یوٹرس کا حد سے زیادہ بڑھ جانا یہ مایومیٹریم کے زائد بڑھاؤ کی وجہ سے ہوتا ہے۔

Adenopathy *(ad-en-op'-a-thi)*[G. aden, gland; pathos, disease]. Any disease of a gland, especially a lymphatic gland -- adenopathic, adj.

غدی مرض: یونانی الفاظ ایڈن و پیتھوس سے مرکب اصطلاح جن کے معانی بالترتیب غد اور مرض کے ہیں۔ کسی غد لیکن خصوصاً لمفی غد کی کوئی بیماری۔

Adenosclerosis *(ad-en-o-skle-ro-sis)* [G. aden, gland; sklerosis, a hardening]. Hardening of a gland with or without swelling, usually due to replacement by fibrous tissue or calcification -- adenosclerotic, adj.

صلابت غدہ: یونانی الفاظ ایڈن وسکلیروسس سے مرکب اصطلاح جن کے معانی بالترتیب غد اور سخت ہونا ہیں۔ ورم کے ساتھ یا ورم کے بغیر غدود کا سخت ہونا۔

Adenosine Diphosphate *(ad-en-o'-sin di-f-os'-fat)* ADP. A derivative of phosphoric acid; plays a part in cellular energy currency. After release of some of its enery, ADP becomes adenosine monophosphate; with addition of energy, ADP becomes ADENOSINE TRIPHOSPHATE.

اڈینوسین ڈائی فاسفیٹ: خونی پلیٹوں کو اکٹھا کرتا ہے۔ ایک غیر متوازن مرکب جو اے ایم' پی میں فاسفیٹ کے ایک گروپ کی شمولیت سے بنتا ہے۔

AdenosineTriphosphate *(ad-en-o'-sin tri-fos'-fat)* ATP. A derivative of phosphoric acid. The ATP molecule carries the chemical energy released in the body by the breakdown of large molecules from food (catabolism).

Adenotonsillectomy *(ad-en-o-ton-sil-ek'-to-mi)* [G. aden, gland; L. tonsilloe, tonsils; G. ektome, excision]. Surgical removal of the adenoids and tonsils.

اڈینوٹانسلیکٹومی: یونانی لفظ ایڈن' لاطینی لفظ ٹونسلی اور یونانی لفظ ایکٹومی سے مرکب اصطلاح جن کے معانی بالترتیب غد' گلے اور قطع ہیں۔ سرجری کے ذریعہ اڈینائڈز اور گلے کاٹنا۔

Adenovirus *(ad-en-o-vi'-rus)* [G. aden, gland; L. virus, poison]. A group of DNA-containing viruses composed of 47 serologically distinct types: 31 serotypes have been found in man, and many in various animal species. Some cause upper respiratory infection, others pneumonia, others epidemic keratoconjunctivitis.

غدی یا غدہ وائرس: یونانی لفظ ایڈن اور لاطینی لفظ وائرس سے مرکب اصطلاح جن کے معانی بالترتیب غدا اور زہر ہیں وائرس کا ایک گروپ جن میں ڈی این' اے پایا جاتا ہے۔ یہ وائرس آدمی اور جانوروں میں مختلف بیماریاں پیدا کرتے ہیں۔

Adermin *(ad'-er-min)* See PYRIDOXIN

Adexolin *(ad-eks'-o-'lin)*. Proprietary mixture of vitamin A and D.

ایڈکسولین: حیاتین الف اور (د کا مکسچر یا آمیزہ' ہڈیوں کی کمزوری' نزلہ' زکام' کھانسی' ٹی بی وغیرہ کے لئے مفید۔

ADH Antidiuretic hormone (q.v.).

Adhesion *(ad-he'-zhun)* [L. ad, to; haerere, to stick]. Abnormal union of two parts, often after inflammation; a band of fibrous tissue which joins such parts. In the abdomen such a band may cause intestinal obstruction; in joints it restricts movement; between two surfaces of pleura it prevents complete pneumothorax -- **adherent, adj**.; **adherence**, n.; adhere, v.t. v.i.

چسپیدگی۔ چیک یا چپکاؤ کی قوت: لاطینی زبان کا لفظ۔ دو حصوں کا غیر معمولی اتحاد۔ ایسے ریشہ دار نسیج کی پٹی جو اس قسم کے حصوں کو باہمی جوڑتی ہے۔ پیٹ میں اس سے آنت کی رکاوٹ ہو سکتی ہے۔ جوڑوں میں یہ حرکت کو محدود کر دیتا ہے۔

Adiaphoretic ***(a-di-a-for-et'-ik)*** [G. a-, not; diaphoretikos, promoting perspiration]. Preventing or reducing perspiration -- adiaphoresis, n.

قاطع پسینہ: یونانی الفاظ "اے" اور "ڈایافریٹیکوس" کا مجموعہ جن کے معانی بالترتیب نہیں اور تنفس کو ترقی دینا ہیں۔ تنفس کو روکنا یا کم کرنا۔

Adipose *(ad'-ip-oz)* [L.adeps, lard]. Fat; of a fatty nature.

چربیلا۔ شحمی: چکنائی یا چربی۔ چربیلی فطرت کا۔

Adiposity *(ad-i-pos'-it-i)* [L. adeps, lard; G.-osis, condition]. Excessive accumulation of fat in the body.

فربہی: جسم میں چربی کا زیادہ جمع ہو جانا۔

Adiposuria *(ad-i-pos-u'-ri-a')* [L. adeps, lard; G. ouron, urine]. See LIPURIA.

شحماب: پیشاب میں چربی۔

Aditus *(ad'-it-us)* [L]. In anatomy, an entrance or opening.

نالی۔ موری: سوراخ یا اندر جانے کا راستہ۔

Adjustment 1. The mechanism used in focusing a microscope. 2. In psychology, the establishment of a satisfactory relationship between the individual and his environment.

تطابق۔ ترتیب: ا- وہ میکانیت جس سے خوردبین کی ٹیوب کو اوپر اٹھایا ہے یا نیچے کیا جاتا ہے تاکہ دیکھی جانے والی شے واضح طور پر نظر آ سکے۔
۲- نفسیات میں فرد اور اس کے ماحول کے درمیان تعلق کی استواری۔

Adjuvant *(ad'-joo-vant)* [L. adjuvare, to assist]. A substance included in a prescription to aid the action of other drugs, **a. therapy**, supportive measures in addition to main treatment.

مساعد۔ معاون۔ ممد: لاطینی لفظ "ایڈجویئر" سے ماخوذ جس کا مطلب ہے مدد کرنا۔ ایسی شے جو دوسری ادویات کے عمل میں مدد دے۔

Adler's theory *(ad'-ler)*. The idea that neuroses arise from feelings of inferiority either social or physical. [Alfred Adler, Austrian psychiatrist, 1870-1937]

نظریہ آڈلر: سماجی یا جسمانی احساس کمتری۔ ایک آسٹروی ماہر نفسیات الفریڈ ایڈلر کے نام پر اس نظریہ کا نام رکھا گیا ہے جس کا زمانہ ۱۸۷۰ء تا ۱۹۳۷ء ہے۔

Adnexa *(ad-neks'-a')* [L. ad, to; nectere, to bind]. Structures which are in close proximity to a part. **a. oculi**, the lacrimal apparatus, **a.**

uteri, the ovaries and Fallopian tubes -- adnexal, adj.

ملحقات: وہ ساختیں جو کسی حصے کے سرے کے بالکل قریب ہوں۔ ایڈنکسا آ کولائی سے مراد لیکریمل سامان ہے۔ انڈنکسا یوٹرائی سے مراد بیضہ دان اور فلوپی نالیاں ہیں۔

Adolescence *(ad-o-les'-sens)* [L. adolescere, to grow up]. The period between puberty and full maturity; youth- adolescent, adj., n.

عنفوان شباب۔ نوبلوغ: ایک لاطینی لفظ ایڈ ویسئر سے ماخوذ جس کا مطلب بڑھنا یا نشو ونما پانا ہے۔ اس کا مطلب ہے نوجوانی یا مکمل طور پر بالغ ہونا۔

Adoral *(ad-awr'-al)* [L. ad. to; os, mouth]. Near the mouth.

نزدہن: لاطینی الفاظ ایڈ اور اوس سے ماخوذ جن کے معانی بالترتیب کی طرف اور منہ میں۔ منہ کے نزدیک۔

ADP. Adenosine diphosphate (q.v).

اے ڈی پی۔ اڈف: دیکھیئے اڈینوسین ڈائی فاسفیٹ

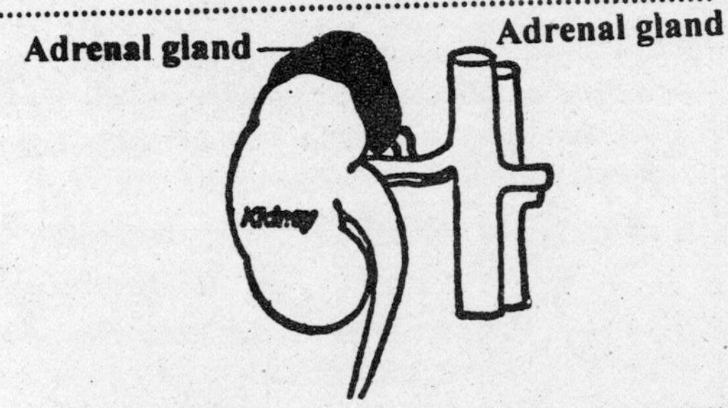

Adrenal *(ad-re'-nal)* [L. ad, to; renes, kidneys]. Near the kidney, by custom referring to the adrenal glands, one lying above each kidney. The **a. cortex** secretes mineral and glucocorticoids which control the chemical constitution of body fluids, metabolism and sexual characteristics. Functionally closely related to the pituitary and other endocrine glands. The **a. medulla** secretes noradrenaline. See ADRENALECTOMY.

"برگردہ: لاطینی الفاظ ایڈ اور یہ رینیز کا مجموعہ جن کے معانی بالترتیب کی طرف اور گردے ہیں۔ گردے کے قریب۔ گردے کے نزدیک چھوٹی اینڈوکرائین غدجو ہر گردے کے اوپر واقع ہوتی ہے۔

Adrenalectomy *(ad-re-nal-ek'-to-mi)* [L. ad. to; renes, kidney; G. ektoıne, excision]. Removal of an adrenal gland, for tumour or for treatment of hypertension, malignant disease of breast, etc. If both adrenal glands are removed, replacement administration of cortical hormones is required.

سرگردہ تراشی: لاطینی الفاظ ایڈ اور رینیز اور یونانی لفظ ایکٹوم سے مرکب جن کے معانی بالترتیب کی طرف، گردہ اور قطع ہیں۔ ایڈرینل گلینڈ کو ختم کرنا جو کسی ناسور یا چھاتی کی بیماری کی وجہ سے کرتے ہیں۔

Adrenaline *(ad-ren'-a-lin)*. A hormone, produced by the adrenal medulla in mammals. It can be prepared synthetically, Solutions may darken in colour and lose activity if stored for long periods. Applied locally as liquor adrenaline (1:1000) in epistaxis; given by subcutaneous injection, it is invaluable in relieving serum sickness, asthmatic attacks, urticaria and other allergic states.

برگردی مادہ: اس سے خونی دباؤ یا بلڈ پریشر زیادہ ہوتا ہے۔ یہ حیوانی غدود سے حاصل کیا جاتا ہے یا مصنوعی طور پر تیار کیا جاتا ہے۔ کئی بیماریوں میں مفید ہے۔ زیادہ عرصہ ذخیرہ کرنے سے ناکارہ ہو جاتا ہے اور رنگت میں گمراہ ہو جاتا ہے۔ اسے ریفریجریٹر میں رکھا جاتا ہے دمہ میں مفید علاج برائے الرجی۔

Adrenergic *(ad-ren-er'-jik)* [L. ad, to; renes, kidney; G. eron, work]. Term applied to sympathetic nerves which liberate adrenaline and noradrenaline from their terminations. Opp. to cholinergic.

ایڈری نرجک: لاطینی الفاظ ایڈ، رینیز اور یونانی لفظ ارگون کا مرکب جن کے معانی بالترتیب کی طرف، گردہ اور کام یا فعل ہیں۔ یہ اصطلاح سمپیتھٹک اعصاب کے لئے مستعمل ہے جو ایڈرینالین اور نارایڈرینالین چھوڑتے ہیں۔

Adrenocorticotrophic *(ad-ren'-o-kor-ti-ko-trot'-ik)* [L. ad, to; renes, kidney; corlex, bark; G. trephein, to nourish]. Having an effect on the adrenal cortex. See CORTICOTROPHIN.

ایڈرینو کارٹیکوٹروفک: لاطینی الفاظ ایڈ، رینیز، کارٹیکس اور یونانی لفظ ٹریفین سے مرکب جن کے معانی بالترتیب کی طرف، گردہ، چھال اور غذا دینا میں ایڈرینل کارٹیکس پر اثر ہونا۔ ایڈرینو کاٹیکوٹروفک ہارمون ایک پولی پیپٹائیڈ ہارمون ہے جسے امامی پیچوایٹری گلینڈ خارج کرتی ہے۔

Adrenogenitalsyndrome *(ad-ren-o-jen'-it-al sin'-drom)* [L. ad, to; renes, kidney; genitalis genital]. 17-Hydroxycorticosteroids in a 24 hour collection of urine is high. Glucocorticoid secretion is deficient and ACTH secretion is stimulated. Steroid intermediates pile up behind the block due to enzyme deficiency and are converted via the remaining unblocked pathways to androgens. Treatment with glucocorticoids inhibits ACTH secretion, thus preventing the abnormal secretion of androgens and other steroids. Hereditary pattern not precise, determined by an autosomal recessive gene. A female child will show enlarged clitoris and possibly labial fusion, perhaps being confused with a male. The male child may show public hair and enlarged penis. In both male and female there is rapid growth, muscularity and advanced bone age.

برگردی تناسلی سنڈروم: خامراتی اقدامات میں نقص جس سے ہائیڈرو کارٹیسون کی کمی ہو جاتی ہے۔ بچی میں بظر بڑھ جاتا ہے اور فرجی لب بھی باہم ملنے کا امکان ہے۔ بچے میں عضو تناسل بڑھ جاتا ہے۔ مادہ اور نر دونوں میں نشوونما تیزی سے ہوتی ہے۔ عضلات اور ہڈیاں بھی تیزی سے بڑھتے ہیں۔ ایسوں کو قازیست کارٹیسون دیا جائے۔

Adrenolytic *(ad-re-no-li'-tic)* [L. ad, to; renes, kidney; G. lysis, dissolution]. That which antagonizes the action or secretion of adrenaline and noradrenaline.

ایڈرینولائی ٹک: ایڈرینالین کے اخراج کوروکنے والا۔

Adriamycin *(ad-ri-a-mi'-sin)*. Antitumour antibiotic of the anthracycline group, particularly effective in childhood maligancies. Similar to daunorubicin, but has less cardiotoxic effect.

ایڈریامائی سین: دافع ناسور اینٹی بیاٹک رسولیوں کے خلاف مستعمل دوا۔

Adsorbents *(Ad-sawrb'-ents)* [L. ad, to; sorbere, to suck]. Solids which attract gases or dissolved substances, to their surfaces, as a film. Charcoal absorbs gases and acts as a deodorant. Kaolin absorbs bacterial and other toxins, hence used in food poisoning.

جاہذ: لاطینی الفاظ ایڈ اور ساربیئر سے ماخوذ جن کے معانی بالترتیب کی طرف اور چوسنا ہیں۔ ایسے ٹھوس جو گیسوں یا حل شدہ اشیاء کو اپنی سطوح کی طرف کشش کر کے فلم بنا دیتے ہیں۔ یہ جراثیم کے زہر کو جذب کرتے ہیں اور اندرونی استعمال سے آنتوں کے لئے مفید ہیں۔ مثلاً کے اولین۔

Adsorption *(ad-sorp'-shun)* [L. ad, to; sorbere, to suck]. The preprty of a substance to attract and to hold to its surface a gas or a liquid -- adsorptive, adj.; adsorb, v.t., v.i.

جذب: لاطینی الفاظ ایڈ اور ساربیئر سے ماخوذ جن کے معانی بالترتیب کی طرف اور چوسنا ہیں سطحی ٹینشن کے نتیجہ میں کسی گیس یا مائع کا کسی سطح پر ارتکاز کسی سیال میں حل شدہ نامیاتی مادے سطحی ٹینشن کو کم کرتے ہیں۔

Advancement An operation to remedy squint. The muscle tendon opposite to the direction of the squint is detached and sutured to the sclera anteriorly.

فروغ: سکنٹ دور کرنے کے لئے اپریشن یا عمل جراحی۔

Adventitia *(ad-ven-tish'-i-a)* [L. adventicius, foreign]. The external coat, especially of an artery or vein -- adventitious. adj.

(بیرونی) غلاف رگ: لاطینی لفظ ایڈونٹیشیس سے ماخوذ جس کا مطلب ہے بیرونی۔ بیرونی پرت خصوصاً کسی شریان یا ورید کی۔

Aedes *(a-e'-dez)* [G. a-, not; edos, pleasure]. A genus of mosquitoes that includes Aedes aegypti, the principal vector of yellow fever and dengue.

ایڈیز: یونانی الفاظ اے بمعنی نہ یا نہیں اور اوڈس بمعنی خوشی یا مسرت کا مجموعہ۔ مچھر کی ایک جنس۔ ایڈیز اچپٹی سے پیلا یا زرد بخار ہوتا ہے۔

AEG. Air encephalography. See PNEUMOENCEPHALOGRAPHY.

Aerive *(a'-er-ob)* [G. *aer*, air; *bios*, life]. A micro-organism which requires O_2 to maintain life -- aerobic, adj.

اروب۔ ہوا جرثومہ۔ ہوا باش: یونانی الفاظ بمعنی ہوا اور بیوس بمعنی زندگی کا مجموعہ۔ ایسا خورد جسیمہ جسے زندہ رہنے کیلئے آکسیجن درکار ہوتی ہے۔ وہ جاندار جو ہوا کی موجودگی میں زندہ رہ سکتے ہوں اور ان میں نشوونما بھی ہوتی ہو ایروب یا ہوا باش کہلاتے ہیں۔

Aerogenous *(a'-er-oj'-en-us)* [G. aer, air; genesis, production]. Gas producing.

ہوا آفریں: یونانی الفاظ ایئر اور جینیسس کا مجموعہ جن کے معانی بالترتیب ہوا اور پیداوار ہیں۔ گیس پیدا کرنے والا۔ جیسے جو کاشت کرنے پر گیس پیدا کرتے ہیں۔

Aerogram *(a-er-o-gram)* [G. aer, air; gramma, letter]. X-ray of tube or hollow viscus after introduction of air or gas. Especially useful after barium meal or enema, when aerogram shows the mucosa coated with a thin layer of barium.

ہوا لاشعاعی تصویر۔ ہوائی تصویر: یونانی الفاظ ایئر بمعنی ہوا اور گریما بمعنی مکتوب کا مجموعہ۔ ہوا یا گیس کے دخول کے بعد نکلی کا ایکسرے۔

Aerophagia-Aerophagy *(a-er-o-faj'-i-a: a-er-of'-a-ji)* [G. aer, air; phagein, to eat]. Excessive air swallowing (as in hysteria).

ادراک باد: یونانی الفاظ ایئر بمعنی ہوا اور فیجین بمعنی کھانا کا مجموعہ۔ ہوا نگلنا۔

Aerosol *(a'-er-o-sol)*. Atomized particles; can be packaged under pressure and from such a source can be used: (1) as inhalation therapy: (2) to sterilize the air: (3) in insect control: (4) as a deodorant or other skin application.

ہوا سم۔ ایروسول: ہوا میں معلق ایٹم زدہ ذرات۔ یہ ہوا کو صاف کرنے' مچھروں یا حشرات کو کنٹرول کرنے یا جلد پر لگانے میں استعمال کیے جاتے ہیں۔ کسی گیس میں ٹھوس کے چھوٹے ذرات یا مائع کے ننھے قطروں کا انتشار۔

Aerosporin *(a-er-o-spor-in)*. Polymyxin B sulphate (q.v).

ایروسپورین: دیکھیے پولیمکسین ب سلفیٹ۔ کان بہنے یا ایس او ایم میں اس کے قطرے دن میں ۳ یا ۴ بار کان میں ڈالیے۔

Aetiology *(e-ti-ol'-o-ji)* [G. aitia, cause; logos, discourse]. A science dealing with the causation of disease. Also spelt etiology -- aetiological, adj.; actiologically, adv.

علم اسباب اللمرض: سائنس جو مرض کی وجہ کے ساتھ بحث کرتی ہے۔

Afebrile *(a-feb'-ril)* [G. a-, not; L. febris, fever]. Without fever.

بے تپ: یونانی لفظ اے اور لاطینی لفظ فیبرس کا مرکب جن کے معانی بالترتیب بلا اور بخار کے ہیں۔ بخار کے بغیر۔

Affect *(af'-ekt)* [L. afficere, to affect]. Feeling; refers to the general emotional state of a person and includes mood.

ماثر: لاطینی لفظ ایفیسیئر بمعنی اثر کرنا سے ماخوذ کسی شے کی طرف احساس۔ ذہن کی وہ سمت جس کا تعلق جذبات یا موڈ کے ساتھ ہے۔

Afferent *(af'-er-ent)* [L. afferre, to bring]. Conducting inward to a part or organ; used to describe nerves, blood and lymphatic vessels. Opp. to efferent.

Afferent

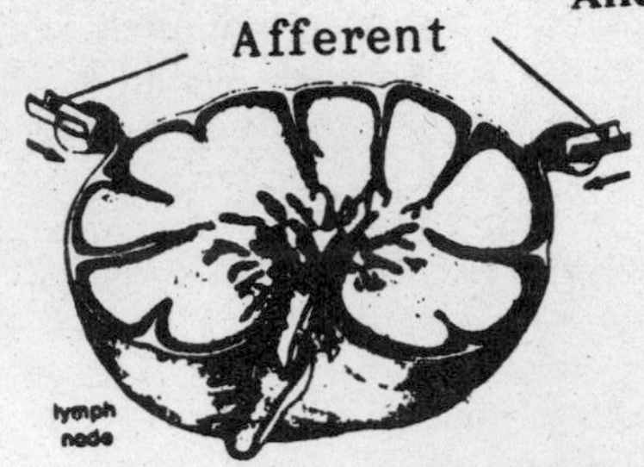

درآور۔ حسی: لاطینی لفظ افیئر سے ماخوذ جس کا مطلب ہے لانا۔ اعصاب اور خونی لمفی رگوں کے لئے مستعمل اصطلاح۔ کسی عضو یا جسم کے بیرونی حصوں سے مرکز کی طرف ظاہر کرتی ہے۔ جو اعصاب پیغامات باہر سے دماغ کو لاتے ہیں انہیں سینسری یا افرنٹ نزدیا اعصاب کہتے ہیں۔

Affiliation *(af-fil-i-a'-shun)*. Settling of the paternity of an illegitimate child on the putative father.

ولدیت: کسی حرامی بچے کی ولدیت قائم کرنا۔

Affinity *(af-in'-i-ti)* [L. affinis, adjoining]. A chemical attraction between two substances, e.g. oxygen and haemoglobin.

رالف: دو مادوں کے درمیان کیمیائی الف یا کشش مثلاً ہیموگلوبن اور آکسیجن میں کیمیائی الف موجود ہے۔ کیمیائی مسافت یوں ہوگی۔ ہیموگلوبن + آکسیجن = آکسی ہیموگلوبن

Afibrinogenaemia *(a-fi-brin'-o-jen-e'-mi-a)* [G. a-, not; L. fibra, fibre; G. genein, from gignesthai, to be born; haima, blood]. More specifically fibrinogenfibrin conversion syndrome; a serious disorder of coagulation in which it is thought that placental thromboplastin causes this conversion -- afibrinogenaemic, adj.

اے فائبر وجینما: گردشی کون میں فائبرینوجن کی کمی۔ اس کی عام وجہ مستور حادثاتی خون بہاؤ ہے۔

Aflatoxin *(af-la-toks'-in)*. Carcinogenic metabolite of certain strains of Aspergillus flavus that infect peanuts.

افلاٹاکسن: اے سماروغ اسپرجلس کے ایک سٹرین کا میٹابولائٹ۔ یہ سماروغ گیلی یا نمدار مقامات پر اگتا ہے۔

Afterbirth [A.S. aefter; M.E. burth]. The placenta, cord and membranes which are expelled from the uterus after childbirth.

آنول ۔ نال: زچہ کی یوٹرس سے بچے کی پیدائش کے بعد خارج ہونے والا مواد جس میں پلیسنٹا' کارڈ اور جھلیاں شامل ہیں۔ بچے کی پیدائش کے بعد زچہ کو درد ہوتے ہیں اور آنول باہر آتی ہے۔

Aftercare A term used in the NHS Act. It denotes the care given during convalescence and rehabilitation. It need not be medical or nursing.

احتیاط مابعد: ہوش میں لانے کے لئے کی جانے والی احتیاط۔

Afterimage [A.S. aefter; L. imago, image]. A visual impression of an object which persists after the object has been removed. This is called 'positive' when the image is seen in its natural bright colours; 'negative' when the bright parts become dark, while the dark parts become light.

پس دید: اینگلو سیکسن لفظ ایفٹر اور لاطینی لفظ امیگو بمعنی عکس کا مجموعہ۔ کسی شے کو ہٹا لینے کے بعد بھی اس کا مرئی تاثر۔

Afterpains [A.S. aefter; M.E. pain, from O.F. peine]. The pains felt after childbirth, due to contraction and retraction of the uterine muscle fibres.

پس درد ۔ زچگی: بچے کی پیدائش کے بعد ہونے والے درد جو کہ یوٹرس کے عضلاتی ریشوں کے سکڑنے اور پھیلنے سے ہوتے ہیں۔ علاج کے لئے کوڈین کمپاؤنڈ کی گولیاں ایک صبح ایک دوپہر ایک شام یا سیلی سیلامائیڈ گولیاں درد میں ایک یا میتھائل ارگومیٹرین گولیاں ایک صبح ایک دوپہر ایک شام۔

Agalactia (*a-gal-ak'-ti-a'*) [G. a-, not; gala, milk]. Non-secretion or imperfect secretion of milk after childbirth - agalactic, adj.

بے شیری: یونانی الفاظ اے بمعنی بغیر اور گیلا بمعنی دودھ کا مجموعہ۔ بچے کی پیدائش کے بعد دودھ کا خارج نہ ہونا یا دودھ کا نامکمل اخراج۔

Agammagiobulinaemia (*a-gam-a-glob'-ul-in-em'-i-a*). Absence of gammaglobulin in the blood, with consequent inability to produce immunity to infection. **Bruton's a.**, a congenital condition in boys, in which B-lymphocytes are absent but cellular immunity remains intact. See DYSGAMMAGLOBULINAEMIA --agammaglobulinaemic, adj.

اے گیموگلوبولی نیمیا: خون میں گیما گلوبولن کی غیر موجودگی۔ اس سے امراض کے خلاف قوت مدافعت ختم ہو جاتی ہے۔

Aganglionosis (*a-gang-li-on-o'-sis*) [G. a-, not; ganglion, swelling; -osis, condition]. Absence of ganglia, as those of the distant bowel, See MEGACOLON.

ایگینگلیونوسس: یونانی الفاظ اے بمعنی بغیر' گینگلیاں بمعنی ابھار اور اوسس بمعنی حالت کا مجموعہ۔ گینگلیا یا ابھاروں کی غیر موجودگی۔

Agar (*a'-gar*). A gelatinous substance obtained from certain seaweeds. It is used as a bulk-increasing laxative, and as a solidfying agent in bacterial culture media.

اگر: جراثیم اگر پر بستیاں بناتے ہیں۔ ایک جلاٹینی مادہ۔

Age: chronological a person's actual age in years. **mental a.,** the age of a person with regard to his mental development; this can be determined by a series of tests. If a woman of 30 can only pass the test for a child of 12, she is said to have a mental age of 12. **physiological a.,** the term applied to age as assessed from appearance and behaviour, thus some people are old at 40, while others are young at 60.

عمر زمانی: کسی شخص کی سالوں میں عمر۔ ذہنی عمر سے مراد کسی شخص کی وہ عمر ہے جو اس کی ذہنی تکمیل سے متعلق ہے۔ اس کا تعین ٹیسٹوں کے ذریعے کیا جا سکتا ہے۔ فعلیاتی عمر سے مراد وہ عمر ہے جو اس کی ظاہری شکل وشباہت اور رویہ سے متعین کی جائے۔

Agenesis (*a-jen-es'-is*) [G. a-, not; genesis, productional]. Incomplete and imperfect development -- agenetic, adj.

بانجھ پن ۔ نامردی: یونانی الفاظ اے بمعنی بغیر اور جینیسس بمعنی پیداوار کا مجموعہ۔ نامکمل تکمیل۔

Agglutination (*a-gloo'-tin-a'-shun*) [L. agglutinare, to glue]. The clumping of bacteria or, red blood cells as effected by the specific immune antibodies called 'agglutinins,' developed in the blood serum of a previously infected or sensitized person -- agglutinable, agglutinative, adj.; agglutinate, v.t. and i.

الزاقین ۔ اگلوٹینن: خون میں موجود مخصوص عوامل جو جسیموں یا پروٹینی مادہ

کو اکٹھا کرتے ہیں۔ لاطینی لفظ اگلوٹینیئر بمعنی چپکنا سے ماخوذ۔

Agglutinins *(a-gloo'-tin-inz)* [agglutinare, to glue]. Specific factors present in sera which agglutinate or clump organisms or particulate protein matter. See ANTIBODIES.

الزاقین زا: لاطینی لفظ اگلوٹینیئر بمعنی چپکنا سے ماخوذ۔ ایک عامل جو اگلوٹینین کی پیداوار تیز کرتا ہے۔ جو قوت مدافعت پیدا کرنے میں استعمال کیا جاتا ہے۔

Agglutinogen *(a-gloo'-tin-o-jen)* [agglutinare, to glue; G. genesthai, to be produced]. A factor which stimulates production of a specific agglutinin, used in the production of immunity, e.g. dead bacteria as in vaccine, particulate protein as in toxoid.

مادہ جارحیت: بعض جراثیم سے پیدا ہونے والا مادہ جو میزبان کے خلاف حملہ میں استعمال ہوتا ہے۔

Aggressin *(a-gress'-in)* [L. agressus, attacked]. A metabolic substance, produced by certain bacteria to enhance their agressive action against their host.

جارحیت: لاطینی لفظ اگریسس بمعنی 'حملہ کیا' سے ماخوذ، کسی کا دھمکی آمیز رویہ یا دوسرے پر حملہ کرنا عموماً احساس کمتری کی وجہ سے ایسا مظاہرہ کیا جاتا ہے۔

Agression *(a-gre'-shun)* [L. agression, from aggredi, to attack]. An attitude of animosity or hostility, usually resulting from frustration or a feeling of inferiority -- agressive, adj.

Agitated Depression *(aj'-i-ta-ted de-pre'-shun)*. Marked restlessness, continual activity, despondency and apprehension. Often associated with menopause.

ارتجاقی پریشانی: نمایاں بے آرامی۔ لگاتار سرگرمی کا مظاہرہ اور سوجھ بوجھ۔

Aglossia *(a-glos'-i-a')* [G. a-, not; glossa, tongue]. Absence of the tongue -- aglossic, adj.

بےلسانی: یونانی الفاظ اے بمعنی بغیر اور گلاسا بمعنی زبان کی غیر موجودگی۔

Aglutition *(a-gloo-ti'-shun)* [G. a-, not; L. glutire, to swallow]. See DYSPHAGIA.

نگل نہ سکنا: یونانی لفظ اے بمعنی بغیر اور لاطینی لفظ گلوٹائر بمعنی نگلنا کا مرکب۔ نگلنے کی نااہلیت یا نگلنے میں دقت۔ مشکل سے نگلنا۔

Agnosia *(ag-no'-ze-a')* [G. a-, not; gnosis, recognizing]. Inability to understand sensory impressions -- agnosic, adj.

لاادراکیت۔ عدم شناخت: مسنری تاثرات کو سمجھنے کی نااہلیت۔ یونانی الفاظ اے بمعنی بغیر اور گنوسس بمعنی پہچاننا کا مجموعہ۔

Agonist *(ag'-on-ist)* [G. agonisters, combatant]. Muscle that shortens to perform a movement. See ANTAGONIST.

متنازع: عضلہ جو حرکت کرنے کے لئے چھوٹا ہوا جاتا ہے۔ یعنی سکڑتا ہے۔

Agoraphobia *(ag-or-a-fo'-bi-a')* [G. agora, market place; phobos, fear]. Morbid fear of being alone in large open places -- agoraphobic, adj.

فضاترسی: یونانی الفاظ اگورا بمعنی منڈی کی جگہ اور فوبوس بمعنی ڈر یا خوف کا مجموعہ۔ بڑی وسیع و عریض جگہوں پر اکیلا ہونے کا خوف۔

Agranulocytosis *(a-gran-u-lo-si-to'-sis)* [G. a-, not; L. granulum, a small grain; G. kytos, cell;-osis, condition]. Marked reduction in or complete absence of granulocytes or polymorphonuclear leucocytes. Usually results from bone marrow depression caused by (1) hypersensitivity to drugs, (2) cytotoxic drugs or (3) irradiation -- agranulocytic adj.

قلت خلیات خون: یونانی لفظ اے بمعنی بغیر، لاطینی لفظ گرینولم بمعنی چھوٹا دانہ، یونانی لفظ کائیٹوس بمعنی خلیہ اور اوسس بمعنی حالت کی مرکب اصطلاح گرینولوسائیٹس یا پولی مارفونکلیائی لیوکوسائیٹس کی مکمل غیر موجودگی یا نمایاں تخفیف

Agraphia *(a-graf'-i-a)* [G. a-, not; graphein, to write]. Inability to express the thoughts in writing -- agraphic, adj.

ناکاتبی۔ لاتحریریت: یونانی الفاظ اے بمعنی بغیر یا نہیں اور گریفین بمعنی لکھنا کا مجموعہ اپنے خیالات کو ضابطۂ تحریر میں لانے کی نااہلیت۔

Ague *(a'-gu)* [F. aigu, sharp, from L. acutus]. See MALARIA.

نوبیہ۔ تپ لرزہ: ملیریا۔ ایک مرض جسے پھیلانے کے ذمہ دار مچھر ہیں۔ اسے باری کا بخار بھی کہتے ہیں۔ کیونکہ یہ لگاتار وقفوں کے ساتھ اترتا اور چڑھتا ہے۔

AHG. Antihaemophilic globulin (q.v).

اے۔ ایچ۔ جی/ اہ گ: دیکھیئے اینٹی ہیموفلک گلوبولن۔ پلازما کے خون جمنے میں ملوث ایک عامل۔

AID. Artificial insemination (q.v) of a female with donor semen.

اے آئی ڈی۔ مصنوعی افزائش نسل: مادہ کو مصنوعی طور پر زرخیز کرنا۔ یعنی حمل ٹھہرانا کسی معطی کی منی مادہ کے جسم میں داخل کرنا جو ٹیوب کے ذریعے کیا جاتا ہے۔ اس طرح پیدا ہونے والا بچہ "ٹیسٹ ٹیوب بے بی" کہلاتا ہے۔

AIH. Artificial insemination (q.v) of a female with her husband's semen.

اے آئی ایچ: مادہ کے جسم میں اس کے شوہر کا مادۂ تولید مصنوعی طور پر داخل کرنا۔

Air [G. aer, air]. The gaseous mixture which makes up the atmosphere surrounding the earth. It consists of approximately 78 per cent nitrogen, 20 per cent oxygen, 0.04 per cent carbon dioxide, 1 per cent argon, and traces of ozone, neon, helium, etc. and a variable amount of water vapour. **a. bed,** a rubber mattress inflated with air. **Complemental a.,** the extra air that can be drawn into the lungs by deep inspiration. **a. hunger,** inspiratory and expiratory distress characterized by sighing and gasping; due to anoxia (q.v) **residual a.,** that which still remains in the alveoli of the lung after forced expiration, **stationary a.,** that which remains after normal expiration. **Supplemental a.,** the extra air that can be expired with effort. **a. swallowing,** see AEROPHAGIA. **tidal a.,** that which passes in and out of the lungs in normal breathing.

ہوا: یونانی لفظ ایئر بمعنی ہوا سے ماخوذ۔ ہوا نائیٹروجن اور آکسیجن کا آمیزہ ہے۔ ان کے علاوہ قلیل مقدار میں دوسری گیسیں بھی شامل ہیں۔ ہوائی بستر سے مراد ہوا سے بھرے جانے والے گدے ہیں۔ کمپلیمنٹل ہوا سے مراد ہے گہرے سانس لینے سے زائد ہوا جو پھیپھڑوں میں جاتی ہے۔ بچی کھچی ہوا سے مراد پھیپھڑوں میں باقی رہ جانے والی ہوا ہے۔ ساکن ہوا سے مراد سانس باہر لینے کے بعد بقایا ہوا ہے۔ ٹائیڈل ہوا سے مراد عام ہوا ہے جو سانس کے ذریعے اندر اور باہر جاتی ہے۔

Airbron *(er'-bron)* Acetylcysteine (q.v).

ایئر بران: میوکو لائٹک نیولائیزر

Akathisia *(ak'-ath-i-zi-a)* [G. a-, not; kathisis, a sitting down]. Inability to sit still. A state in which the patient feels a distressing inner restlessness.

تعودترسی: یونانی الفاظ اے بمعنی بغیر اور کتھیسس بمعنی بیٹھنا کا مجموعہ۔ خاموشی سے بیٹھنے کی نااہلیت۔ ایسی حالت جس میں مریض اندرونی بے آرامی محسوس کرتا ہے۔

Akinetic *(a-kin-et'-ik)* [G. a-, without: kinesis, motion]. Without movement. **a. epilepsy,** epileptic fits where instead of a tonic and clonic phase the patient is limp, the whole body remains flaccid until consciousness returns. **a. catatonia** occurs in schizophrenia. **a. mutism,** sustained periods of unconscitousness in which the patient appears to be rela- xed and asleep, but he can only be roused for a few moments; occurs in tumours of third ventricle, midbrain and thalamus -- akinesia, n.

حرکی: یونانی الفاظ اے بمعنی بغیر اور کائی نیسس بمعنی حرکت کا مجموعہ۔ حرکت کے بغیر۔

Alastrim *(al-as'-trim)* [Pg. from alastrar, to spread, cover]. A less virulent form of smallpox known as variola minor, which may be confused with chickenpox.

جدری کاذب: پرتگالی لفظ السٹرار بمعنی پھیلانا یا ڈھکنا سے ماخوذ۔ چیچک کی ایک معمولی قسم۔

Albamycin *(al-ba-mi'-sin).* Novobiocin, (q.v).

ایلبامائی سین: دیکھیئے نو دو بائیوسین۔ اس کے ۲ کیپسول صبح ۲ شام برائے سینڈفلائی بخار، پیئین آفتھیل مائی ٹس، آسٹیومائی لائی ٹس یعنی گھمبیر۔

Albee's Operation *(al'-bez).* For producing ankylosis of the hip. Upper surface of head of femur is removed, and corresponding edge of acetabulum. **A.'s bone graft,** operation for spinal fixation. Spinous processes of diseased area are exposed and split. Graft from tibia is placed in raw area. [Fred Houdlett Albee, New York surgeon, 1876-1945.]

البی کا اپریشن: ایک عمل جراحی جس میں فیمر کے ہیڈ کی بالائی سطح ہٹائی جاتی ہے۔ اس کے ساتھ ہی ایسٹیبولم کا کنارہ بھی ہٹایا جاتا ہے۔ البی کے استخوانی پیوند میں سپائن کو فکس کرنے کے لئے آپریشن کیا جاتا ہے۔ بیمار جگہ کے زائدے کھلے اور علیحدہ رکھے جاتے ہیں۔ ٹبیا سے پیوند کو اس خام جگہ رکھا جاتا ہے۔ اس کا نام نیویارک کے سرجن فریڈ ہوڈلٹ البی کے نام پر رکھا گیا ہے۔ اس کا عرصۂ حیات ۱۸۷۶ء تا ۱۹۴۵ء ہے۔

Albers-schonberg Disease A spotty calcifying of the bones, which fracture spontaneously. 'Marble bones.' Syn., osteopetrosis. [Heinrich Ernst Albers-Schonberg, German surgeon, [1865-1921.]

البرزشون برگ مرض: ہڈیوں ایک بیماری جس میں اچانک ٹوٹ جاتی ہیں۔اس کا نام ایک جرمن سرجن ہنرخ ارنسٹ البرزشونبرگ کے نام پر ہے۔ جس کا عرصۂ حیات ۱۸۶۵ء تا۱۹۲۱ء ہے۔

Albinism *(al-bin-ism)* [L. albus, white]. Failure of the tyrosine system to oxidize tyrosine through dopa to melanin, so that the skin is fair, the hair white and the eyes pink.

برصیت: پگمنٹ کی غیر موجودگی۔لاطینی لفظ البس بمعنی سفید سے ماخوذ۔اس میں ٹائیروسین نظام ناکام ہو جاتا ہے۔ٹائیروسین کی تکسید ہو کر ملینن نہیں بنتا۔ اس وجہ سے جلد دودھ ایسی سفید ہو جاتی ہے۔بال بھی سفید ہو جاتے ہیں۔ آنکھوں کی پتلیاں گلابی دکھائی دیتی ہیں۔یہ اس صورت میں ہوتا ہے جب برصیت مکمل طور پر پائی جاتی ہے۔

Albino *(al-be' no)*[L. albus, white]. A male affected with albinism -- albinotic, adj.; albiness, female.

بھورا۔ابیض۔زال (آدمی): لاطینی لفظ البس بمعنی سفید سے ماخوذ برصیت کا شکار نر۔

Albucid *(al-bu'-sid)*. Sulphacetamide (q.v).

البوسڈ: دیکھئے سلفاسیٹامائڈ۔علاج چشم کے لئے ایک مرکب۔اس کا ایک قطرہ دن میں ۴ مرتبہ برائے ٹرے کو مایا گکرے۔

Albumen *(al-bu'-men)* [L. albumen, albuminis, white of an egg]. Also spelt albumin. A variety of protein found in animal and vegetable matter. It is soluble in water and coagulates on heating. **serum a.,** the chief protein of blood plasma and other serous fluids. Lactalbumen is the albumen found in milk -- albuminous, albuminoid, adj.

بیضین۔البومن: لاطینی لفظ جس کے معنی میں انڈے کی سفیدی پروٹین کی ایک قسم جو حیوانی و نباتی مادہ میں پائی جاتی ہے۔یہ پانی میں حل پذیر ہے۔اور گرم ہونے پر جم جاتی ہے۔سیرم البومن سے مراد خون پلازما اور دوسرے سیالوں کی بڑی پروٹین ہے۔لیکٹ البومن سے مراد دودھ میں پائی جانے والی البومن ہے۔

Albuminometer *(al-bu-min-om'-et-er)* A graduated test-tube in special stand for estimating quantity of albumen in a fluid. Esbach's (q.v) is the most familiar pattern.

بیضین پیما: کسی سیال میں بیضین ماپنے کا آلہ۔

Albuminuria *(al-bu-min-u'-ri-a')* [L. albus, white; G. ouron, urine]. The presence of albumen in the urine. The condition may be temporary and clear up completely, as in many febrile states. **Chronic a.** leads to hypoproteinaemia (q.v) **orthostatic or postural a.** is an abnormality of little importance in which albumen depends on the upright posture, and is absent in the urine secreted during sleep (the morning specimen) albuminuric, adj.

بول زلالی: لاطینی لفظ البس اور یونانی لفظ اور دن سے مرکب اصطلاح جن کے معانی بالترتیب سفید اور پیشاب ہیں۔پیشاب میں بیضین یا البومن کی موجودگی۔یہ صورت عارضی بھی ہو سکتی ہے۔

Albumose *(al'-bu-moz)*. An early product of proteolysis. It resembles albumen, but is not coagulated by heat.

البوموز: پروٹیولائیسس کا اولین پروڈکٹ یا حاصل بیضین کے ساتھ مشابہہ لیکن گرمی یا حرارت سے نہیں جمتا۔

Albumosuria *(al-bu-moz-u'-ri-a')*. The presence of albumose in the urine -- albumosuric, adj.

البوموس بولی: پیشاب میں البوموز کی موجودگی۔

Alcohol *(al'-ko-hol)* The principal constituent of wines and spirits. **Absolute alcohol is occasionally used by injection for the relief of trigeminal neuralgia and other intractable pain; rectified spirit (90 per cent alcohol) is widely used in the preparation of tinctures: methylated spirit contains 95 per cent alcohol with wood naphtha and is for external application only. Enhances the action of barbiturates and tranquillizers. Intravenous alcohol therapy has been tried in premature labour to delay birth. It is thought to prevent release of substances which stimulate uterine contraction. Alcohol inhabits the milk ejection reflex is humans. a. psychosis,** see KORSAKOFFS SYNDROME.

الکحل: الکینز کے ایک یا زیادہ ہائیڈروجن ایٹموں کو ہائیڈروکسل گروہوں

سے بدلنے پر جو مرکبات بنتے ہیں' الکوحلو کہلاتے ہیں۔ الکحل کاربن' ہائیڈروجن اور اکسیجن کا مرکب ہے۔ یہ نشاستہ یا شکر میں خمیر پیدا ہونے سے بنتا ہے۔ مثلاً میتھے نول' ایتھے ذل' پروپے نول' بیوٹے نول۔

Alcohol-fast A bacteriological term used when alcohol fails to decolo(u)rize a stained organism

الکحل فاسٹ: جب الکحل کسی رنگدار جسیمے کو بے رنگ کرنے میں ناکام ہو جائے تو یہ جراثیمی اصطلاح استعمال کی جاتی ہے۔

Alcoholics Anonymous. A fellowship of people previously addicted to alcohol. Their main aim is curing others of alcoholism.

الکحل گمنام: الکحل کے پہلے سے عادی لوگوں کی فیلوشپ۔ ان کا بنیادی مقصد دوسروں کو الکحل سے نجات دلانا ہے۔

Alcoholism *(al'-ko-hol-izm).* Alcoholic poisoning. In its chronic form it causes severe disturbances of the nervous and digestive systems.

الکوحلیت ۔ شراب خوری۔ اثرالکوحل: الکحل کی وجہ سے زہر آلودگی۔ پرانی قسم میں عصبی اور ہضمی نظاموں کو شدید طور پر ابتر کر دیتی ہے۔

Alcoholuria *(al-ko-hol-u'-ri-a')* Alcohol in the urine. Basis of one test for fitness to drive after drinking alcohol.

الکحلو ریا: پیشاب میں الکحل کی موجودگی۔ الکحل پینے کے بعد گاڑی چلانے کی اہلیت کے لئے ایک ٹیسٹ کی بنیاد۔

Alcopar *(al'-ko-par).* Bephenium hydroxynaphthoate (q.v).

ایلکو پار: دیکھیے بفینیم ہائیڈروکسی نفتھوایٹ۔

Aldactone A *(al-dak'-ton).* Spironolactone (q.v).

الڈیکٹون: دیکھیے سپائیرونولکٹون۔

Aldomet Methyldopa (q.v).

ایلڈومیٹ: دیکھیے میتھائل ڈوپا۔ ہائی بلڈ پریشر کے لئے ۱ تا ۳ گولیاں روزانہ حسب ضرورت۔

Aldosterone *(al-dos-ter'-on).* An adrenocortical steroid which, by renal control, regulates electrolyte metabolism; hence described as a 'mineralocorticoid'. Secretion is regulated by the reninangiotensin system. It increases excretion of potassium and conserves sodium and chloride. Primary aldosteronism is a condition resulting from tumours of the adrenal cortex in which this electrolyte imbalance is marked and alkalosis and tetany may ensue.

الڈوسٹیرون: ایک ہارمون جو ایڈرینل غدود کی کارٹیکس خارج کرتی ہے۔ یہ سٹیرائڈ ہے۔ سوڈیم اور پوٹاشیم آئینز کے ارتکاز کو کنٹرول کرتا ہے۔ پوٹاشیم کے اخراج کو زیادہ کرتا ہے۔ پانی کے اخراج کو کنٹرول کرتا ہے۔

Aleppoboil. See LEISHMANIASIS.

ALEUDRIN *(al'-u-drin)* Isoprenaline (q.v).

الیوڈرین: دیکھیے آئیسوپرینالین۔

Aleukaemic *(a-lu-ke'-mik)* [G. a-, not; leukos, white; haima, blood]. See LEUKAEMIA.

Alevalire *(al'-e-ver)* A solution of glycerine, sodium bicarbonate and a detergent which helps to liquefy tenacious sputum. The patient inhales it as a fine mist produced by passing O_2 through a nebulizer containing Alevaire.

الیور: ایک محلول جس میں گلسرین' سوڈیم بائی کاربونیٹ اور ایک ڈیٹرجنٹ شامل ہے۔

Alexia *(al-leks'-i-a)* [G.a-, not; lexis, word]. Word blindness; loss of the ability to interpret the significance of the printed or written word, but without loss of visual power. Due to a brain lesion -- alexic, adj.

ناخواندنی۔ لفظ کوری: یونانی الفاظ اے بمعنی بغیر اور لیکسس بمعنی لفظ کا مجموعہ۔ لفظ کا اندھاپن۔ کسی طبع شدہ یا تحریر کردہ لفظ کی اہمیت کو واضح کرنے کی اہلیت کا کھویا جانا لیکن بصری قوت ضائع کئے بغیر۔

Algesia *(al-je'-zi-a)* [G. algesis, sense of pain]. Excessive sensitiveness to pain; hyperaesthesia -- algesic, adj. Opp. to analgesia.

درد حسی: یونانی لفظ الجیسز بمعنی احساس درد سے ماخوذ۔ درد کے لئے زیادہ حساس۔ تکلیف یا درد کا شدید احساس۔

Algesimeter *(al-jez-im'-et-er)* An instrument which registers the degree of sensitiveity to pain.

درد حسی پیما: ایک آلہ جو درد کا احساس کے درجے کو رجسٹر کرتا ہے۔

Algid *(al'-jid)* [L. algidus, cold]. Cold. Description of severe attack of fever, especially malaria, with collapse, extreme coldness of the body, suggesting a fatal termination. During this stage the rectal temperature may be high.

لرزہ زدہ : لاطینی لفظ الجیڈس بمعنی سردیس سے ماخوذ۔ سردی۔ ملیریا بخار کے دوران سردی سے جسم کا کانپنا جبکہ جسم کا درجہ حرارت زیادہ ہوتا ہے خصوصاً ریگٹم کا۔

Alginates *(al'-jin-atz)*. Seaweed derivatives which, when applied locally, encourage the clotting of blood. They are available in solution and in specially impregnated gauze.

الجی نیٹز : بحری پودوں کے حاصلات جو کسی جگہ لگانے سے خون کو جما دیتا ہے۔ محلول میں دستیاب ہیں۔

Alidine (a'-li-din). Anileridine (q.v.).

الیڈین : دیکھئے انیلیر یڈین۔ محلول میں دستیاب ہیں۔

Alienation *(a'-li-en-a'-shun)* [L. alienatio, alienation]. In psychiatry, mental illness.

الینیشن ۔ دماغی : ذہنی بیماری۔

Alienist *(a'-li-en-ist)* [L. alienus, of another]. One skilled in treatment of mental disorders, Psychiatrist (q.v)

ماہر امراض دماغی : ماہر نفسیات۔ ذہنی بیماروں کا علاج کرنے میں ماہر۔

Alimentary *(al-i-ment'-a-ri)* [L. alimenta, nourishment, food]. Pertaining to food.

غذائی : لاطینی الیمنٹا بمعنی خوراک سے ماخوذ۔

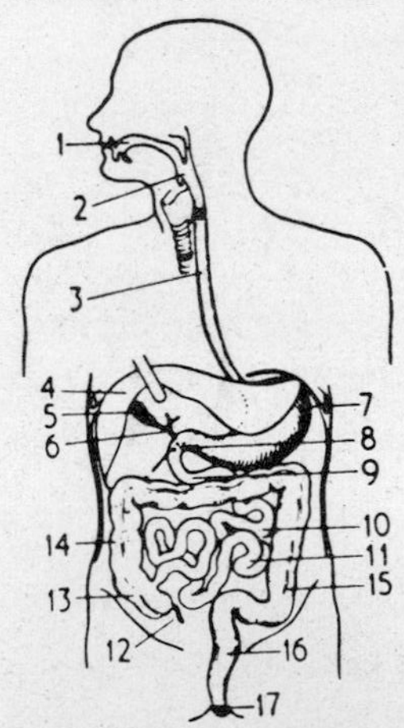

Alimentary canal alve olus

1. Oral cavity. 2. Pharynx. 3. Oesophagus. 4. Liver (turned back). 5. Gall bladder. 6. Bile duct. 7. Stomach. 8. Pylorus. 9, 10, 11. Small intestine (9. duodenum: 10. jejunum: 11. ileum). 12. Vermiform appendix. 13, 14, 15. Large intestine (13, caecum; 14, ascending colon; 15, descending colon). 16. Rectum. 17. Anus

خوراک سے متعلق۔

Alimentation *(al-i-men-ta'-shun)* [L. alere, to nourish]. Act of nourishing with food; feeding.

تغذیہ : لاطینی لفظ الیئر بمعنی خوراک دینا سے ماخوذ خوراک دینے کا عمل۔ کھلانا۔

Aliquot *(al'-i'kwat)* [L. some, so many]. Part contained by the whole an integral number of times. The sample withdrawn from a 24-hour specimen.

عاد : لاطینی لفظ بمعنی کچھ یا بہت زیادہ۔ کئی دفعہ میں سے ایک حصہ ۲۴ گھنٹوں میں سے ایک نمونہ لیا جاتا ہے۔

Alkalaemia *(al-kal-e'-mi-a)* [Ar. alqili, ashes of saltwort; G. haima, blood]. Alkalosis (q.v.)-- alkalaemic, adj.

قلوی دمویت : دیکھئے الکوسس یا بیش قلویت (Alkalosis) جسم میں الکلی کی زیادتی یا ترشوں میں کمی۔ الکلی کی زیادہ خوراک لینے سے زیادہ قے یا زیادہ اسہال کی وجہ سے یہ مرض لاحق ہو جاتا ہے۔

Alkali *(al'-kal-i)* Ar. al-qili, ashes of saltwort]. A series of soluble corrosive bases analogous to and including soda, potash and ammonia which neutralize acids forming salts. Alkaline solutions turn red litmus blue -- alkalis, pl. **a.reserve,** a biochemical term denoting the amount of buffered alkali (normally bicarbonate) available in the blood for the neutralization of acids (normally CO_2) formed in or introduced into the body.

الکلی : اساس یا الکلی وہ اشیاء ہیں جو محلول کی حالت میں OH آئن دیتی ہیں اور یہ آئین تیزابوں کے ہائیڈروجن آئن سے مل کر پانی بنا دیتے ہیں۔ پانی میں حل ہو کر آسانی سے آئن بنانے والے اساس طاقتور اساس کہلاتے ہیں۔ طاقتور اساسوں کو الکلی بھی کہا جاتا ہے۔ الکلی چند دھاتوں کے ساتھ مل کر ہائیڈروجن خارج کر دیتی ہیں۔ یہ خاصیت اساسوں میں نہیں پائی جاتی۔

Alkaline *(al'-kal-in)* [Ar. al-qili, ashes of saltwort]. 1. Possessing the properties of or pertaining to an alkali. 2. containing an excess of hydroxyl over hydrogen ions.

الکلوی: جس میں الکلوی موجود ہو۔ اکلائن گولیوں میں میگنیشیم آکسائیڈ ۲۰ گرین اور کیلشیم کاربونیٹ ۲۰ گرین ہوتا ہے۔ بدہضمی اور معدہ میں تیزاب کے لئے مفید۔

Alkalinuria *(al-kal-in-ur'-i-a)* [Ar. al-qili, ashes of saltwort; G. ouron, urine]. Alkalinity of urine -- alkalinuric, adj.

قلوی بولیت: پیشاب میں الکلی ہونا۔

Alkaloid *(al'-kal-oid)*. Resembling an alkali. A name often applied to a large group of organic bases found in plants and which possess important physiological actions. Morphine, quinine, caffeine, atropine and strychnine are well-known examples of alkaloids -- alkaloidal, adj.

قلیا۔ قلی نما: زہریلے، ناحل پذیر، قلمی، نامیاتی مرکبات جو پودوں میں پائے جاتے ہیں۔ مثلاً افیم، کونین، مارفین وغیرہ۔ الکلی سے مشابہہ، موثر نائیٹروجنی مرکبات۔ عموماً امونیا کے مرکبات جن میں امونیا کے ایک یا دونوں ہائیڈروجن جوہروں کی جگہ کوئی اور ریڈیکل شامل ہوتا ہے۔ یہ تیزابوں کے ساتھ مل کر نمکیات بناتے ہیں جو قلموں کی صورت میں ہوتے ہیں اور اس کیمیائی تعامل کے دوران پانی نہیں بنتا۔ الکلائڈ کھاری صفات کے حامل ہیں اور سرخ لٹمس کے کاغذ کو نیلا کرتے ہیں۔ چند الکلائڈز مائع شکل میں ہیں مثلاً نکوٹین، سپارٹین وغیرہ جن میں صرف کاربن، نائیٹروجن اور ہائیڈروجن ہوتے ہیں۔ ٹھوس الکلائڈرز میں آکسیجن بھی شامل ہوتی ہے اور وہ سفید اور قلمی ہوتے ہیں۔ الکلائڈز پانی کم اور الکحل میں جلدی حل ہو جاتے ہیں۔ اکثر الکلائڈز کے محلول ذائقے میں کڑوے ہوتے ہیں۔

Alkalosis *(al-kal-o'-sis)* [Ar. al, qili, ashes or saltwort; G. -osis, condition]. Alkalaemia. Excess of alkali or reductions of acid in the body. Develps from a variety of causes such as overdosage with alkali, excessive vomiting or diarrhoea, and hyperventilation. See HYPERPNOEA. Results in neuromuscular excitability expressed clinically as tetany (q.v).

بیش قلویت۔ الکلوسز: جسم میں الکلی کی زیادتی یا ترشوں میں تخفیف۔ الکلی کی زیادہ خوراک لینے سے، زیادہ قے آنے سے یا زیادہ اسہال کی وجہ سے یہ بیماری ہوتی ہے نمکین لسی وغیرہ کے ذریعے نمکیات پلائیے۔ نارمل سیلائن ڈرپ لگائیے۔ کیلشیم سینڈوز کا ۱۰ سی سی کا وریدی ٹیکہ صبح وشام۔ امونیم کلورائیڈ یا نوشادر ۱۵ گرین ایک پڑیا دن میں ۳ مرتبہ۔

Alkaptonuria *(al-kap-ton-ur'-i-a)*.The presence of alkaptone (homogentisic acid) in the urine, resulting from only partial oxidation of phenylalanine and tyrosine. Condition usually noticed because urine goes black in the nappies, or when left to stand. Apart from this, and a tendency to arthritis in later life, there are no ill-effects from **a.**

الکپٹو نیوریا: پیشاب میں الکپٹون کی موجودگی۔ اگر پیشاب ایک جگہ کھڑا رہے تو سیاہ ہو جاتا ہے۔ اس کے زیادہ برے اثرات نہیں ہیں۔

Alkeran *(al'-ker-an)*. Melphalan (q.v).

الکیرین: دیکھئے میلفالان۔

Alkylating Agents Disrupt the process of cell division by affecting DNA in nucleus, by addition of alkyl groups. Alternatively called nitrogen mustard compounds. Used as cytotoxic drugs in neoplastic disorders.

الکائی لیٹنگ عوامل: یہ عوامل مرکزے میں ڈی این اے پر اثر کر کے تقسیم خلیہ کے عمل کو ختم کر دیتے ہیں۔

Allegron. Nortriptyline. Similar to amitriptyline (q.v). See ANTIDEPRESSANT.

الگرون: دیکھئے ضد مسکن۔ نار ٹرپٹائی لین۔ ایمی ٹرپٹائی لین سے مشابہ۔

Allelomorphs *(a-le'-lo-morfz)* [G. allelon, of one another; morphe, form]. Inherited characteristics which are alternative and contrasting (typical of artifical selection), such as tallness or shortness. The basis of Mendel's law of dominants and recessives -- allelomorphic, adj.; allelomorphism, n.

متبادل شکلے۔ متبادل الشکل: یونانی الیلون بمعنی ایک دوسرے کا اور مارف بمعنی قسم کا مجموعہ۔ جین جو متضاد خصوصیات والے جوڑے کو ظاہر کرے، اسے الیلز یا، متبادل شکلے کہتے ہیں۔ ہر جوڑے کی ایک خاصیت غالب اور دوسری مغلوب ہوتی ہے۔ مینڈل نے متضاد خواص کے ہر جوڑے کے دو افراد کو الیلو مارف کا نام دیا اور ان پر الگ الگ تجربات کئے۔

Allergen *(al'-er-jen)* [G. allos, other; ergon, activity; genesis, production]. Any agent capable of producing state or manifestation of allergy -- allergenic, adj.; allergenicity, n.

حساسیہ: یونانی الفاظ ایلوس بمعنی دوسرا، ارگون بمعنی عاملیت اور جینیسس بمعنی پیداوار کا مجموعہ الرجی پیدا کرنے کا اہل کوئی ایجنٹ۔

Allergy *(al'-er-ji)* [G. allos, other; ergon, work]. An altered or exaggerated susceptibility to various foreign substances or physical agents which are harmless to the great majority of individuals. It is due to an antigen-antibody reaction, though the antibody formed is not always demonstrable. Hay fever, asthma, urticaria and infantile eczema are allergic conditions and are familial in origin -- allergic, adj. See ANAPHYIAXIS and SENSITIZATION

الرجی ۔ تیز حسست: یونانی الفاظ ایلوس بمعنی دوسرا اور ارگون بمعنی کام کا مجموعہ۔ بیرونی مادوں کے خلاف ہونا۔ خواہ وہ بے ضرر ہوں کہ خاص دوائی' خوشبو' گرد' دھواں وغیرہ کے لئے غیر معمولی حساسیت

Allocheiria *(a-lo-chir'-i-a)* [G. allos, other; cheir, hand]. An abnormality of tactile sensibility under test, wherein patient refers a given stimulus to the other side of the body.

دگردستی: یونانی الفاظ ایلوس بمعنی دوسرا اور چیئر بمعنی ہاتھ کا مجموعہ۔ چھونے کے حس کی ایک غیر معمولی قسم۔

Allograft *(al'-lo-graft)* [G. allos, other; graphein, to write]. Transplantation of part of one person to another. The term **non-viable a.** is used when skin (which cannot regenerate) is taken from a cadaver. See LYOPHILOZED SKIN.

Allonal *(al'-on-al)*. Amidopyrine (q.v).

Allopurinol *(al-lo-pu'-rin-ol)*. A substance which prevents the formation of deposits of crystals from insoluble uric acid. Diminishes tophi in gout and substantially reduces the frequency and severity of further attacks. Can cause skin rash.

الوپوری نیل: ایسا مادہ جو ناحل پذیر یورک ایسڈ سے جمع شدہ قلموں کی باوٹ کو روکتا ہے۔

Aloes *(al'-oz)*. The dried juice from the cut leaves of a tropical plant. Powerful purgative with an intensely bitter taste.

ست صبر: کسی استوائی پودے کے کٹے ہوئے پتوں کا خشک رس۔ اس کا ذائقہ کڑوا ہوتا ہے۔ اور دست آور ہے۔

Alopecia *(al-o-pe'-si-a)* [L. from G. alopekia, fox-mange]. Baldness which can be congenital, premature or senile, **a. areata,** a patchy baldness, usually of a temporary nature. Cause unknown, but shock and anxiety are common precipitating factors. Exclamation mark hairs are diagnostic. **a. cicatrisata,** syn. pseudopelade, progressive alopecia of the scalp in which tufts of normal hair occur between many bald patches. Folliculitis decalvans is an alopecia of the scalp characterized by pustulation and scats.

طاسی ۔ بال کورہ ۔ گنج : گنجاپن ۔ بالوں کا نہ اگنا ۔ پیدائشی یا وقت سے پہلے گنجاپن ۔ سلفر کا گندھک مقامی طور مفید ہے۔

Alophen *(al'-o-fen)*. Compound containing phenolphthalein (q.v).

ایلوفین : فینالفتھلین پر مشتمل مرکب۔

Aloxiprin *(al-oks'-i-prin)*. Aluminium aspirin. Causes less gastric irritation than aspirin; broken down in small intestine to release aspirin. See ACETYLSALICYLIC ACID.

Alphachymotrypsin *(al-fa-ki-mo-trip'-sin)*. A pancreatic enzyme which disolves the capsular ligament and allows the lens to be extracted through the pupil and out of the wound without undue physical manipulation. Anti-inflammatory agent when taken orally.

alphafetoprotein *(al-fa-fe'-to-pro'-tin)*. Present in maternal serum and amniotic fluid in cases of fetal abnormality.

Alphosyl *(al'-fo-sil)*. Colourless preparation of coal tar.

کولتاری کی بے رنگ تیاری۔

Alprenolol *(al-pren'-o-lol)*. An adrenergic blocker. Acts in angina pectoris by decreasing cardiac work; decreases heart rate, cardiac output and arterial pressure.

Al.S Antilymphocyle serum. Immunosuppressive, which appears to act mainly on lymphocytes in the blood stream. It appears to diminish the number of circulating lymphocytes, thereby, giving a transplanted organ a better chance of survival in the reccipient. It does not interfere with the body's general defence mechanism.

اے ایل ایس : خون میں لمفوسائیٹس پر عمل کرتا ہے اور ان کی تعداد کم

کرتا ہے۔ جسم کی عام مدافعتی میکانیت میں مدافعت نہیں کرتا۔

Althesin *(al'-the-sin)*. Induces anaesthesia.

Alum Potassium or ammonium aluminium sulphate. Used for its astringent properties as a mouthwash (1 per cent) and as a douche (1/2 per cent) aslo for precipitating toxoid. See APT.

پھٹکری : پھٹکری پوٹاشیم سلفیٹ اور ایلومینیم سلفیٹ کا دوہرا نمک ہے۔ پھٹکری کی سفید اور ٹھوس قلمیں پانی میں حل پذیر ہیں۔ جب اسے گرم کیا جائے تو آب قلماؤ نکل جاتا ہے اور مسام دار مادہ رہ جاتا ہے۔ پانی یا ہلکے اساسی محلول سے ایلومینیم آئن "Al^{+3}" کی آب پاشیدگی ہو جاتی ہے اور سفید چپکنے والی رسوب بن جاتی ہے جو کیمیائی رنگوں کی جاذب ہے۔ اس لئے پھٹکری بطور رنگ چسپ یا مارڈینٹ استعمال ہوتی ہے۔ رنگ چسپ کیمیائی رنگ کو غیر حل پذیر بنا دیتی ہے۔

ایلومینیم آئن "Al^{+3}" کی وابستگی کی طاقت بہت زیادہ ہوتی ہے۔ اس لئے یہ گدلے پانی کو مصفا کرنے، دباغت (چمڑا کمانے) اور کاغذ کو کلف لگانے (سائیزنگ) کے لئے استعمال ہوتی ہے۔

پوٹاشیم یا امونیم کا ایلومینیم سلفیٹ۔ اس کا ایک فیصد محلول منہ کو صاف کرنے کے لئے استعمال کیا جاتا ہے۔ ٹوکسائیڈ کو رسوب بنانے کے لئے بھی استعمال کیا جاتا ہے۔

Aluminium hydroxide. An antacid with a prolonged action used in the treatment of peptic ulcer. It is usually given as a thin cream or gel. There is no risk of alkalosis with long treatment, as drug is not absorbed.

ایلومینیم ہائیڈروکسائیڈ : ایک سفید سفوف جو آگ بجھانے میں کام آتا ہے اور رنگ سازی میں مارڈینٹ یا رنگ چسپ کے طور پر استعمال کیا جاتا ہے۔ ناسور کے علاج میں استعمال کیا جاتا ہے۔ یہ جسم میں جذب نہیں ہوتا اس لئے بے ضرر ہے۔

Aluminium Paste. A mixture of aluminium powder, zinc oxide and liquid paraffim, used as a skin protective in ileostomy. This paste is sometimes known as 'Baltimore paste'.

ایلومینیم پیسٹ : ایلومینیم سفوف، زنک آکسائیڈ اور مائع پیرافین کا آمیزہ۔ جلد کی حفاظت کے لئے استعمال کیا جاتا ہے۔ اسے بالٹی مور پیسٹ بھی کہا جاتا ہے۔

Alupent *(al'-u-pent)*. Orciprenaline sulphate (q.v).

ایلوپینٹ : دیکھئے آرسیپرینالین سلفیٹ۔

Alveolar-Capillary block syndrome. A rare syndrome of unknown aetiology characterized by breathlessness, cyanosis and right heart failure, due to thickening of the alveolar walls of the lungs, thus impairing diffusion of oxygen.

جوفیزی شعری بلاک سنڈروم : سنڈروم کی ایک قسم۔

Alveolitis *(al-ve-ol-i-tis)* [L. alveolus, air sac; G. itis, inflammation]. of alveoli, by custom usually referring to those in the lung; when caused by inhalation of an allergen such as pollen, it is termed **extrinsic allergic a.**

Alveolus *(al-ve'-o-lus)* [L.]. 1. An air vesicle of the lung. 2. A tooth socket. 3. A gland follicle or acinus -- alveoli, pl.; alveolar, adj.

جوفیزہ۔ جوف دندان : انہیں ہوائی تھیلیاں بھی کہتے ہیں۔ یہ بہت باریک ہوتے ہیں۔ ان میں عروق شعریہ کا جال بچھا ہوتا ہے جن کے ذریعہ

Alveolus

Artery
Bronchiole
Vein
Alveolar duct
Alveoli

پھیپھڑوں میں ناقص خون پہنچتا ہے۔ ایک لاطینی لفظ دانت میں خالی جگہ کو بھی کہا جاتا ہے۔ ایک غدودی فولیکل۔

Alzheimer's Disease A form of presenile [dementia caused by atrophy of the prefrontal areas of the brain. [Alois Alzheimer, German physician, [1864-1915].

مرض الزیمر : ایک جرمن فزیشن الائس الزیمر کے نام پر اس کا نام رکھا گیا ہے جس کا عرصہ حیات ۱۸۶۴ء تا ۱۹۱۵ء تھا۔ ایک بیماری۔

Amlagam *(a-mal'-gam)* [G. malagma, emollient]. An alloy of mercury. **dental a.,** used for filling teeth, contains mercury, silver and tin.

ملغم۔ املگم : پارے کا بھرت جو کہ کسی دوسری دھات یا دھاتوں کے ساتھ مل کر بنتا ہے۔ دانتوں کا املگم دانت بھرنے کے کام آتا ہے۔ اس میں

پارہ، چاندی اور قلعی شامل ہیں۔

Amantadine *(am-an'-ta-din)* An antiviral agent (influenza A_2) which is now used mainly in the management of some patients with Parkinson's disease.

ایمینٹڈن ہائیڈروکلورائیڈ : ہانگ کانگ فلو کی بیماری کی طوالت میں تخفیف کرتا ہے۔

Amastia *(a-mas-'ti-a)* G. a-, not; mastos, breast]. Congenital absence of the breasts.

امیسٹیا : یونانی الفاظ بمعنی بغیر اور مسٹوس بمعنی چھاتی کا مجموعہ۔ چھاتیوں کا موجود نہ ہونا سینے کے ابھار کی غیر موجودگی، ایک پیدائشی نقص۔

Amaurosis *(am-aw-ro'-sis)* [G.amauros, dim]. Partial or total blindness.

ترمراکمنت : یونانی الفاظ اماروس بمعنی مدھم سے ماخوذ جزوی یا مکمل اندھاپن۔

Amaurotic Familial idiocy A form of familial mental subnormality with spastic paralysis of the legs which commences in infancy or childhood. Later, the upper limbs are similarly affected and vision is lost. Tay-Sach's disease.

گنگی ابلہی : ذہنی کیفیت کی ایک قسم۔ بچپن میں ٹانگوں پر اثر ہوتا ہے۔ بعد میں بازو بھی متاثر ہوتے ہیں۔

Ambidextrous *(am-bi-deks'-trus)* [L. ambo, both; dexter, right]. Able to use both hands equally well -- ambidexter, adj.; ambidexterity, n.

ذوالیمینین : لاطینی الفاظ ایمبو بمعنی دونوں اور ڈیکسٹر بمعنی ٹھیک کا مجموعہ۔ دونوں ہاتھ مساوی طور پر استعمال کرنے کے قابل۔

Ambilhar, Niridazole (q.v).

Ambivalence *(am-biv'-al-ens)* [L. ambo, both; valere, to be powerful]. Coexistence in one person of contradictory and opposing emotions at the same time, e.g. love and hate -- ambivalent, adj.

ایمبل ہار : دیکھئے نریڈازول۔

Ambivalent *(am-biv'-al-ent)* [L. ambo, both; valere, to be powerful]. A normal type of personality varying between introversion and extroversion (q.v).

دوجذباتی : متضاد جذبات کا حامل شخص۔

Amblyopia *(am-bli-o'-pi-a)* [G. amblys, dulled; ops, eye]. Defective vision approaching blindness. **tobacco a.**, smoker's blindness, due to absorption of cyanide in the nicotine of the smoke. The sight gets worse, colour vision goes, the victim can go blind. Recently it was discovered that the cyanide prevents absorption of vitamin A. When this vitamin was injected the blindness was halted and cured -- amblyopic, adj.

کم نظری : ضعف بصارت کا اتنا ہونا کہ نابینا پن کے قریب ہو۔ تمباکو نوشی کی وجہ سے ضعف بصارت تمباکو کے نکوٹین میں میانائڈ کی وجہ سے حیاتین الف کا انجذاب نہیں ہوتا۔

Amboceptor *(am-bo-sep'-tor)* [L. ambo, both; capere, to take]. The antibody developed in immune serum which, in association with complement, cause lysis of the specific bacteria or other antigen to which the host has been sensitized. See ANTIBODIES.

ذوالطین : لاطینی الفاظ ایمبو بمعنی دونوں اور کیپئر بمعنی لینا کا مجموعہ۔ امیون سیرم میں اینٹی باڈی بن جاتی ہے۔

Ambulant *(am'-bu-lant)* [L. ambulare, to go about, walk]. Able to walk.

انتقالی : لاطینی لفظ ایمبولیئر سے ماخوذ جس کا مطلب ہے چلنا۔ چلنے کے قابل۔

Ambulatory *(am'-bu-la-tor-i)* [L. ambulare]. Mobile. Walking about. **a. treatment,** method of treatment which insists on keeping the patient on his feet as much as possible, as in Charcot's joint (q.v).

سیار : لاطینی لفظ ایمبولیئر سے ماخوذ چلنا متحرک اس قسم کے علاج میں مریض کو اپنے پاؤں پر کھڑا کرنے کی کوشش کی جاتی ہے۔

Amelia *(a-me'-li-a)* [G. a-, not; melos, a limb]. Congenital absence of a limb or limbs. **complete a.,** absence of both arms and legs.

امیلیا۔ بے جوارحی : یونانی الفاظ اے بمعنی بغیر اور میلس بمعنی جارح۔ جوارح کی غیر موجودگی۔ مکمل امیلیا سے مراد دونوں بازوؤں اور ٹانگوں کی غیر موجودگی۔

Amelioration *(a-me-li-or-a'-shun)* [L. melius, better]. Reduction of the severity of symptoms. Improvement in the general condition.

طاصلاح بہبودی : لاطینی لفظ میلس بمعنی بہتر سے ماخوذ اصطلاح۔ علامات کی شدت میں تخفیف عام حالت کی بہتری۔

Amenorrhoea *(a-men-o-re'-a)* [G. a-, not; men, month; rheein, to flow]. Absence of the menses. **primary a.,** when menstruation has not been established at the time when it should first appear. **secondary a.,** absence of the menses after they have once commenced -- amenorrhoeal, adj.

جبس الطمث : یونانی الفاظ اے بمعنی نہ، مین بمعنی ماہ یا مہینہ اور رین بمعنی بہنا کا مجموعہ۔ حیض کی غیر موجودگی۔ اگر پہلی دفعہ حیض نہ آئی تو اول اور اگر بعد میں بند ہو جائے تو ثانوی قسم ہوگی۔

Amentia *(a-men'-shi-a)* [L. madness]. Mental subnormality; to be distinguished from 'dementia'.

بھولا پن : لاطینی لفظ پاگل پن۔

Amethocaine hydrochloride *(a-meth'-o-kan).* A synthetic substance with some of the properties of cocaine. Used for surface infiltration and spinal anaesthesia; more potent and more toxic than procaine,Lozenges for use before gastroscopy contain 65 mg, and this should be regarded as a maximum dose.

امیتھوکین ہائیڈروکلورائیڈ : ایک تالیفی مرکب جس میں بعض خواص کوکین کے ہیں۔ سطحی دخول اور سپائن کو سن کرنے کے لئے مستعمل ہے۔ پروکین سے زیادہ زہریلا چوسنے والی گولیوں کی شکل میں دستیاب۔

Amethopterin *(am-eth-op'-ter-in)* Antifolic acid drug. Inhibits the enzyme which converts folic acid to its biologically active form, and is thus predominantly active against cells in division, having little effect in the resting stage. Used in treatment of choriocarcinoma, **Burkitt's lymphoma and acute leukaemia of childhood.**

امیتھواپٹیرن : اینٹی فولک ایسڈ دوا۔ اس خامرے کی عاملیت کو روکتا ہے جو فولک ایسڈ کو عامل میں تبدیل کرتا ہے۔ اس طرح تقسیم میں ملوث خلیوں کے خلاف سرگرم رہتا ہے۔

Ametria *(a-met-ri'-a)* [G. a-, not; metra, womb]. Congenital absence of the uterus.

بے رحمی : بچہ دانی یا یوٹرس کی غیر موجودگی۔

Ametropia *(a-met-ro'-pi-a)* [G. a-, not; metron, a measure; ops, eye]. Defective sight due to imperfect refractive power of the eye--ametropic, adj.; ametrope, n.

تیرہ نگاہی : ناقص بصارت جو آنکھ کی انعطافی طاقت کے نامکمل ہونے کی وجہ سے ہے۔

Amicar *(am-i'-kar).* Epsilon aminocaproic acid (q.v).

امی کیر : دیکھئے اپسیلون امینوکیپرونک ایسڈ تیزاب کی ایک قسم۔

Amidone *(ami-e-don).* Methadone (q.v)

ایمیڈون : دیکھئے میتھاڈون۔

Amikacin *(am-ik'-a-sin).* Antibiotic for especial use in serious Gram-negative gentamicin-resistant infections; a semi-synthetic derivative of **Ranamycin,** it has been altered structurally to resist degradation by bacterial enzymes.

Amikin *(am;-i-kin)* Amikacin (q.v).

Amiloride *(am-il-or'-id).* Less powerful diuretic, but has unusual potassiu-tmconserving properties, and when it is used, potassium supplements are rarely required.

ایمیلورائیڈ : پیشاب آور۔ پوٹاشیم ذخیرہ کرنے کی خصوصیات کا حامل۔ جب یہ دوائی استعمال کی جارہی ہو تو مزید پوٹاشیم کی ضرورت نہیں ہوتی۔

Aminoacidopathy *(am-en'-o-as-id-op'-ath-i).* Disease caused by imbalance of amino acids.

Amino Acids *(am-en'-o as-idz).* Organic acids in which one or more of the hydrogen atoms are replaced by the amino group, NH_2. They are the end product of protein hydrolysis and from them the body resynthesizes its protein. Ten cannot be elaborated in the body and are therefore essential in the diet-arginine, histidine, isoleucine; leucine, lysine, methionine, phenylalanine, threonine, treptophane, and valine. The remainder are designated non-essential amino acids.

امینوایسڈز : اس نامیاتی مرکب میں ایک امینوگروہ اور ایک کاربوکسل گروہ دونوں ایک کاربن ایٹم کے ساتھ کیمیائی طور پر متحد ہوتے ہیں۔ جگر امینو ایسڈز کی وافر مقدار یوریا میں تبدیل کرتا ہے جو گردوں کی ذریعے جسم سے باہر نکال دیا جاتا ہے۔

Aminoaciduria *(am-en'-o-as-id-u'-ri-a).*

Increase in urinary excretion of amino acids in Fanconi syndrome, in which there is a congenital defect in the metabolism of protein, and the reabsorptive functions of the kidney are abnormal amino aciduric, adj.

امینوایسی ڈیوریا : فنکونی سنڈروم میں پیشاب کے ذریعے امینوایسڈز کے اخراج میں اضافہ۔ اس میں گردے صحیح طور پر کام نہیں کرتے۔

Aminocrine *(am-en'-o-crin)*. Non-staining acridine antiseptic similar to acriflavine, and used for similar purposes in similar strength.

امینوکرن : رنگ نہ دینے والی دافع جراثیم ایکریدین۔ ایکریفلیوین سے مشابہ اور اسی طاقت کی انہی مقاصد کے لئے مستعمل ہے۔

Aminophenazole *(am-en'-o-fen'-a-zol)*. An analeptic with a marked stimulant action on the respiratory centre.

امینوفینازول : یہ دوائی تنفسی مرکز پر اثر کرتی ہے۔

Aminophylline *(am-in-of'-i-lin)*. The ophylline with ethylene-diamine. A soluble derivative of theophylline, widely used in the treatment of asthma, congestive heart failure, and cardiac oedema. Available as tablets 0.1 g, ampoules (intramuscular) 0.5 g, ampoules (intravenous) 0.25 g, suppositories 0.36 g.

امینوفلین : تھیوفائی لین کا ایک حل پذیر حاصل۔ یہ دوائی دل کے دورہ اور دمہ میں استعمال کی جاتی ہے۔ ایتھائیلین ڈائی امین کے ساتھ تھیوفائی لیں۔ پلمونری ایمبولزم میں مفید۔ اس کی گولیاں دستیاب ہیں۔ دل کے دورہ کے لئے ایک گولی صبح ایک دوپہر ایک شام ایک رات کو سوتے وقت۔ اگر سانس کا دورہ شدید ہو تو اس کا ۱۰ سی سی کا ٹیکہ ۲۵ فیصد گلوکوس ۲۵ سی سی میں ملا کر لگایئے۔ دمہ قلبی اور کن جیسٹو ہارٹ فیلیور میں اس کی ایک گولی صبح ایک دوپہر ایک شام۔

Aminoplex 14 *(am-en'-o-pleks)*. Synthetic preparation of those amino acids normally ingested as protein in egg. meat and fish.

Aminosalicylic acids. *(am-in-o-sal-is-il'-ik)*. Has a bacteriostatic action when given in tuberculous disease. High blood levels essential; owing to rapid elimination, frequency of dose is essential. Given with other antitubercular drugs to reduce drug resistance. Has nauseating taste, therefore best given as cachets or tablets.

امینوسیلی سائیلک ایسڈ : یہ دوائی تپ دق میں دی جاتی ہے۔ جراثیم کی پیدائش کو روکتی ہے چونکہ اس کا ذائقہ متلی والا ہے اس لئے گولیوں کی شکل میں دی جاتی ہے۔

Aminosol *(am-in'-o-sol)*. A solution of amino acids that can be given orally or intravenously. Preparations containing glucose, fructose, and ethyl alcohol are available.

ایمائنوسول : امینوایسڈز کا محلول۔

Amiphenazole See AMINOPHENAZOLE.

Amithiozone *(am-i-thi'-o-zon)*. Antileprotic.

ایمی تھیوزون : جذام یا کوڑھ کے خلاف استعمال ہونے والی دوائی۔

Amitosis *(a-mi-to'-sis)* [G. a-, not; mitos, thread; osis, condition]. Multiplication of a cell by direct fission amitotic, adj.

براہ راست تقسیم۔ بلاواسطہ تقسیم : یونانی الفاظ اے بمعنی بغیر، مائیٹوسس بمعنی دھاگہ اور اوسس بمعنی حالت کا مجموعہ۔ خلوی تقسیم کا ایک طریقہ جس میں ایک خلیہ دو خلیوں میں تقریباً برابر تقسیم ہو جاتا ہے۔

Amtriptyline *(am-i-trip-ti-len)*. A trieyclic antidepressant similar to imipramine but possessing a pronounced sedative effect which is of particular value in the agitated depressive.

امی ٹرپٹائی لین : یہ دوائی امیپرامین سے مشابہ لیکن کچھ فینا تھیازین کی طرح عمل کرتی ہے۔ دافع مسکن۔

Ammonia See A. SOLUTION.

امونیا : دیکھئے امونیا محلول۔ (۱) امونیا بے رنگ گیس ہے اس میں خاصی چبھتی ہوئی بو پائی جاتی ہے۔ امونیا کا مالیکیول چار پہلوؤں والے منشور کی شکل کا ہے جس کے چوٹی پر نائیٹروجن کا ایٹم ہے۔ ہوا سے ہلکی ہے اس کی کثافت 0.7708 گرام فی لیٹر ہے۔ (۲) نائیٹروجن کے تمام مرکبات کی تیاری میں امونیا بنیادی حیثیت رکھتی ہے۔ (۳) امونیا نائیٹروجن اور ہائیڈروجن کا مرکب ہے جو انسانی پیشاب میں موجود ہوتا ہے۔ (۴) پروٹینز یا لحمیات کے ٹوٹنے سے امونیا پیدا ہوتی ہے۔ یہ مرکب زہریلا ہونے کی وجہ سے جانور کے جسم میں نہیں رہنا چاہئے۔ تازہ پانی میں رہنے والی مچھلیوں میں پانی اوسموسس کے ذریعے اندر جاتا رہتا ہے جس میں امونیا حل ہو کر جسم سے باہر نکل جاتی ہے دوسرے جانوروں میں امونیا اور نائیٹروجنی مرکبات یوریا اور یورک ایسڈ میں تبدیل ہو کر جسم سے خارج ہو جاتے ہیں۔ (۵) موجودہ دور کے ماہرین کا خیال ہے کہ زمین کی اولی فضا میں امونیا گیس موجود تھی۔ اس کے علاوہ میتھین، ہائیڈروجن اور آبی بخارات بھی تھے۔ بجلی کے شرارے اور الٹراوائلٹ شعاعوں

کے زیراں کے باہمی ملاپ سے کوئی ایسا مادہ پیدا ہو گیا جس میں زندگی کی خصوصیات تھیں۔

Ammoniumbicarbonate. Widely used in cough mixtures as a mild expectorant, and occasionally as a carminative in flatulent dyspepsia.

نوشادر۔ امونیم کلورائڈ : پیشاب کی تیزابیت میں اضافہ کرنے کے لئے یہ دوائی استعمال کی جاتی ہے۔ بعض دفعہ بلغم خارج کرنے کے لئے بھی استعمال کی جاتی ہے۔ نوشادر کا کیمیائی نام ایک سفید قلمی ٹھوس مرکب۔ الکلوسز میں ۱۵ گرین ایک پڑیا دن میں ۳ مرتبہ کھانسی کے لئے امونیم کلورائڈ کف سیرپ (پلمونیکس) کا ایک چمچہ ہر ۴ گھنٹے بعد۔

Ammonia Solution Liq. ammon. Colourless liquid with a characteristic pungent odour. Used in urine testing ammoniated, ammoniacal, adj.

امونیا کا محلول : ناگوار بو والا بے رنگ مائع۔ پیشاب ٹیسٹ کرنے میں استعمال کیا جاتا ہے۔

Amnesia *(am-ne'-si-a)* [G. a-, not; mnesis, memory]. Partial or complete loss of memory. Occurs following concussion, in dementia, hysteria and following electrotherapy (q.v) amnesic, adj. **anterograde a.,** loss of memory for recent events since an accident, etc. **retrograde a.,** loss of memory for past events before an accident, etc.

نسیان : یادداشت کا جزوی یا کلی ضیاع۔ یونانی الفاظ اے بمعنی بغیر اور مینسس بمعنی یادداشت کا مجموعہ ہسٹیر یا وغیرہ میں یادداشت چلی جاتی ہے۔

Amniocentesis *(am-ni-o-sen-te'sis)* [G. amnio, fetal membrane; kentesis, a prickling]. Aspiration of liquor amnii from its sac. The liquor contains increased haemoglobin break-down products in rhesus incompatibility, es, pl.

امینو سنٹیسس : بچے کی تھیلی سے پانی یا مائع کا امتصاص۔

Amniography *(am-ni-og'-ra'fi)*. [G. amnio, fetal membrane; graphein, to write]. X-ray of the amniotic sac after injection of opaque medium into same: out-lines the umbilical cord and placenta--amniogram, n; amniographical, adj.; amniographically, adv.

امینوگرامی : یونانی الفاظ امینو بمعنی غلاف جنین اور گریفین بمعنی لکھنا کا مجموعہ۔ جنینی تھیلی کا ایکسرے۔

Amnion *(am'-ni-on)* [G.]. The innermost membrane enclosing the fetus and containing the amniotic fluid (liquoramnii). It ensheaths the umbilical cord and is connected with the fetus at the umbilicus--amnionic, amniotic, adj.

غلاف جنین۔ آمینوس۔ انفس : سب سے اندرونی جنینی جھلی۔ یونانی لفظ۔

Amnioscopy *(am-ni-so'-ko-pi)* [G. amnio, fetal membrane; skopein; to examine]. Amnioscope allows inspection of the forewaters through the intact membranes. Clear, colourless fluid is normal; yellow or green staining is due to meconium and occurs in cases of fetal hypoxia--amnioscopic; adj.; amnioscopically, adv.

انفس سکوپی : یونانی الفاظ امینو بمعنی جنین جھلی اور سکوپین بمعنی جانچنا کا مجموعہ۔ امینوسکوپ سے جھلیوں میں پانی کا معائنہ کیا جاتا ہے۔ صاف اور بے رنگ سیال صحیح ہوتا ہے۔

Amniotic Fluid Embolism Formation of an embolus in the amniotic sac and its transference in the blood circulation of mother to lung or brain. A rare complication of pregnancy. May occur at any time after rupture of the membranes.

سیال انفسی ایمبولزم : جنینی تھیلی میں ہوائی بلبلہ یا ٹھوس مادہ کا بننا جو ماں کے گردشی خون میں جاتا ہے اور وہاں سے پھیپھڑوں یا دماغ میں جا سکتا ہے۔ حمل کے دوران ایسا کم ہی ہوتا ہے۔ جھلیوں کے پھٹنے کے بعد کسی بھی وقت ہو سکتا ہے۔

Amniotic Fluid Infusion *(am-ni-ot'-ik)*. Escape of amniotic fluid into the maternal circulation.

گانتقال سیال انفسی : ماں کے خون میں انفسی سیال کا پہنچنا۔

Amniotome *(am'-ni-ot-om)* [G. amnio, fetal membrane; tomos, cutting]. An instrument for rupturing the fetal membranes.

انفس شگاف : یونانی الفاظ امینو بمعنی جنینی جھلی اور ٹموس بمعنی کاٹنا کا مجموعہ۔ ایک آلہ جس سے جنین جھلیاں پھاڑی جاتی ہیں۔

Amniotomy *(am-ni-ot'-o-mi)* [G. amnio, fetal membrane; tome, a cutting]. Artificial rupture of the fetal membranes to in.luce or expedite labour.

انفس شگافی : یونانی الفاظ امینو بمعنی جنینی جھلی اور ٹموس بمعنی کاٹنا کا مجموعہ۔ دردزہ زیادہ کرنے یا شروع کرنے کے لئے جنینی جھلیوں کا مصنوعی طور پر پھٹنا۔

Amodiaquine *(a-mo-di'-a-kwin)*. Potent antimalarial compound similar in action tc chlorcquine.

ایموڈیاکوئن : ملیریا کے خلاف استعمال ہونے والی دوائی۔ یہ اثر میں کلوروکوئین کی طرح ہے۔

Amoeba *(am-e'-ba)* [G. amoibe, change]. A protozoon. One of the elementary, unicellular forms of life. The one cell is capable of ingestion and absorption, respiration, excretion, movement and reproduction by simple fission. One form, Entamoeba histolytica, is a parasitic pathogen producing amoebic dysentery (q.v) in man--amoebae, pl.; amoebic, adj.

امیبا : یونانی لفظ امابۓ بمعنی تبدیلی سے ماخوذ۔ ایک پروٹوزون۔ بڑے سائز کا امیبا صرف ایک ذرہ نظر آتا ہے۔ اس کے عین درمیان میں مرکوزہ ہوتا ہے جو کہ شفاف ہوتا ہے۔ سائیٹو پلازم دو حصوں میں ممیز ہوتا ہے۔ بیرونی حصہ شفاف ہوتا ہے اور ایکٹو پلازم کہلاتا ہے۔ اندرونی حصہ انڈو پلازم کہلاتا ہے۔ انڈو پلازم میں مرکزے کے قریب آبی سیال ہوتا ہے جسے انقباضی خالیہ کہتے ہیں انڈو پلازم میں اس کے علاوہ غذائی خالیے بھی ہوتے ہیں۔ اس کی ایک قسم اینٹ امیبا یک خلوی جانور ہے جو صرف انسانی آنت کے اندر پرورش پاسکتا ہے اور اس کی پیچش میں مبتلا کر دیتا ہے جسے امیبائی پیچش کہتے ہیں۔

Amoebiasis *(am-e-bi'-a-sis)* [G. amoibe, change; N.L. -iasis, condition]. Infestation of large intestine by the protozoon Entamoeba histolytica, where it causes ulceration by invasion of the mucosa. This results in passage per rectum of necrotic mucous membrane and blood, hence the term 'amoebic dysentery'. If the amoebae enter the portal circulation they may cause liver necrocrosis (hepatic abscess). Diagnosis is by isolating the amoeba in the stools.

امیباسس : یونانی لفظ امابۓ بمعنی تبدیلی اور نیولاطینی لفظ ایاسس بمعنی حالت کا مرکب۔ بڑی آنت میں اینٹ امیبا ہسٹو لائیٹکا کے حملہ سے امیبائی پیچش ہو جاتی ہے۔ یہ پروٹوزون خون میں بھی داخل ہو سکتا ہے۔

Amoebicide *(am-e'-bi-sid)* An agent that kills amoebae--amoebicidal, adj.

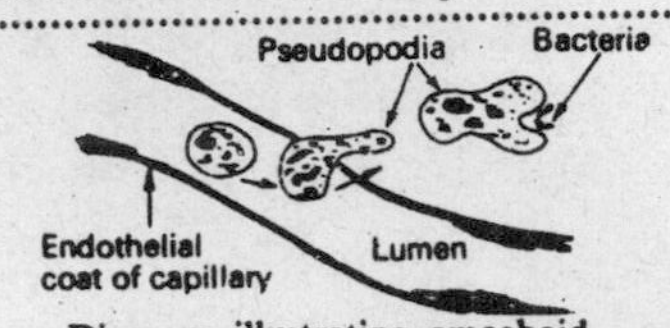

Diagram illustrating amoeboid movement of white blood cells

amoeboid

امیبی سائیڈ : ایک ایجنٹ جو امیبا کو مارتا ہے۔

Amoeboid *(am-e'-boid)* [G. amoibe, change; eidos, form]. Resembling an amoeba in shape or in mode of movement, e.g. white blood cells.

امیبی۔ امیبانما : جو امیبا سے مشابہت رکھتا ہو۔ خواہ شکل میں یا حرکت میں مثلاً سفید خونی خلیے۔

Amorphous *(a-mor'-fus)* [G. a-, not; morphe, form]. Having no regular shape.

نقلما: یونانی الفاظ اے بمعنی بغیر اور مارف بمعنی شکل کا مجموعہ جس کی باقاعدہ شکل نہ ہو۔ کسی نمایاں شکل کے بغیر، ٹھوس جس کی قلمی ساخت نہیں ہوتی۔ غیر قلمی۔ بے قاعدہ شکل والا۔

Amoxycillin *(am-oks-i-sil'-lin)*. Antibiotic; penetrates bronchial secretion more readily than ampicillin independent of the level of purulence, therefore preferable in chronic lower respiratory tract infections. In acute infections the sole advantage is its greater absorption and high blood levels for an equivalent dose.

Amphetamine *(am-fet'-a-mer)*. A sympathomimetic agent (strucutrally related to adrenaline) which is a potent CNS stimulant. It was formerly used as an appetite suppressant and in the treatment of depression but, because of its addictive potential and frequent abuse, is now restricted to use in narcolepsy and certain psychiatric states under specialist supervision.

ایم فیٹامین: ایک طیران پذیر مائع۔ اگر ناک بند ہو تو اسے سونگھ کر یعنی اندر کی طرف سانس لے کر کھولتے ہیں۔ مفید برائے شدید عضلاتی کمزوری، نلار جذیر اسٹیٹ۔

AmphotericinB *(am-fo-ter'-i-sen)*. Antifungal agent given by i.v. infusion to treat serious systemic infections, e.g. histoplasmosis, candidiasis. It is used to eradicate Candida from mouth (lozenges), vagina (cream or pessaries) and gut (tablets).

ایمفوٹیری سین: سماروغ کش۔

Ampicillin *(am-pi-sil'-lin)*. Active against many, but certainly not all, strains of E.coli, Proteus, Salmonella and Shigella; these are bacteria against which benzylpenicillin is far less active. Ampicillin is also effective against benzylpenicillin sensitive (but no resistant) staphylococci, streptococci and other Gram-positive bacteria. It has a wide range of activity and is a broad spectrum antibiotic. Given orally and by injection.

ایمپی سلن: جراثیم کش دوا۔ کئی جراثیم کے خلاف یہ دوائی عمل کرتی ہے۔ یہ اینٹی بیاٹک ہے۔ یہ دوائی منہ سے بھی کھلاتی ہے اور ٹیکے کے ذریعہ بھی جسم کے اندر پہنچائی ہے۔ پلمونری ایمبولزم میں ایک کیپسول ہر چھ گھنٹے یا ٹیکہ صبح و شام۔

Ampiclox *(am'-pi-kloks)*. Mixture of ampicillin (q.v) and cloxacillin (q.v).

ایمپی کلاکس: ایمپی سلین اور کلاکسا سلیں کا مکسچر۔

Ampoule *(am'-pool)* [L. ampulla, bottle]. A small, hermetically sealed glass phial containing a single sterile dose of a drug.

امپول۔ بندنلی: لاطینی لفظ ایمپولا بمعنی بوتل سے ماخوذ دوائی کی ایک خوراک کے لئے چھوٹی شیشی جو بند ہوتی ہے۔ شیشے کی نلکیاں۔

Ampulla *(am-pool'-a)* [L. bottle]. Any flask-like dilatation. **a. of Vater,** the enlargement formed by the union of the common bile duct with the pancreatic duct where they enter the duodenum--ampullae, pl.; ampullar, ampullary, ampullate, adj. [Abraham Vater, German anatomist, 1684-1751.]

امپول۔ بندنلی۔ فراخہ: لاطینی لفظ۔ بوتل۔ کوئی صراحی دار یا صراحی نما۔ اندرونی کان میں نصف دائرہ نما نالیاں ہوتی ہیں جو ایک دوسرے کے ساتھ واقع ہوتی ہیں۔ ہر نالی کا ابھرا ہوا سرا۔

Amputation *(am-pu-ta'-shun)* [L. amputare, to cut away]. Removal of an appending part, e.g. breast, limb. **a. bandage,** applied to produce a coneshaped stump.

قطع عضو: لاطینی لفظ ایمپوٹیئر بمعنی کاٹنا سے ماخوذ کسی عضو کا کاٹنا مثلاً چھاتی یا جوارح کا کاٹنا عمل جراحی کے ذریعہ جسم کے کسی حصے کا کاٹا جانا۔

Amputee *(am'-pu-te)* [L. amputare, to cut away]. A person who has had amputation of one or more limbs.

ایمپیوٹی: لاطینی لفظ ایمپوٹیئر بمعنی کاٹنا سے ماخوذ۔ ایک یا زیادہ جوارح کٹا ہوا شخص۔

Amylase *(am'-i-laz)*. [G. amylon, starch]. Any enzyme which converts starches into sugars. **pancreatic a.,** amylopsin (q.v). **salivary a.,** ptyalin (q.v).

امائلیس۔ امائلز: یونانی لفظ ایمائی لان بمعنی نشاستہ سے ماخوذ۔ ایک خامرہ جو نشاستہ کو شکر میں تبدیل کرتا ہے۔ لبلبی امائلیز ایمی لاپسن ہے جبکہ سلوری امائلیز ٹایالن ہے۔ لعابی غدود لعاب افراز کرتے ہیں جس میں موجود خامرہ امائلیس نشاستہ کو شکر میں تبدیل کرتا ہے۔

Amyl nitrite *(am'-il-nit'-rit* Volatile rapid-acting vasodilator, useo by inhalation from crushed ampoules. Its action is brief, and its main use is in the treatment of angina.

امائیل نائیٹرائیٹ: طیران پزیر تیزی سے عمل کرنے والا باسط شرائین اس کا عمل مختصر ہوتا ہے۔ عموماً درد گلو یا درد سینہ کے علاج کے لئے اس دوائی کو استعمال کیا جاتا ہے۔

Amylobarbitone *(am-il-o-bar'-bit-on)* Barbiturate of medium intensity and duration of action. The sodium salt has a more rapid but less prolonged action.

امائیلو باربی ٹون: عمل اور شدت میں درمیانہ باربیٹوریٹ۔

Amyloid *(am'-i-loid)* [G. amylon, starch; eidos, form]. A starch which is wax-like in appearance. **a. disease or degeneration,** formation and deposit of amyloid in any organ, notably the liver and kidney. It can occur in the terminal phase of any prolonged toxic condition Amyloidosis.

مومی مادہ: یونانی الفاظ ایمائیلون بمعنی نشاستہ اور ایڈوس بمعنی شکل کا مجموعہ۔ ایسا نشاستہ جو شکل میں موم کی طرح دکھائی دے۔

Amyloysis, *(am-il-ol'-is-is)* [G. amylon, starch; lysis, a loosening]. The digestion of starch--amylolytic, adj.

نشاستہ پاشی: یونانی الفاظ ایمائیلون بمعنی نشاستہ اور لائسس بمعنی ڈھیلا کا مجموعہ۔نشاستہ کا ہضم ہونا۔

Amylopsin *(am'-i-lop-sin)*. A pancreatic enzyme, which in an alkaline medium, converts insolube starch into soluble maltose.

نشاستہ ہاضمین: ایک لبلبی خامرہ جو الکلائن واسطہ میں ناحل پذیر نشاستہ کو حل پذیر مالٹوز میں تبدیل کرتا ہے۔

Amylum *(am'-il-um)* [G.]. Starch.

نشاستہ: یونانی لفظ نشاستہ یا سٹارچ۔

Amytal *(am'-i-tal)*. Amylobarbitone (q.v).

امائی ٹیل: دیکھئے امائیلو باربیٹون۔

Anabol *(an'-a-bol)*. Steroid preparation that increases anabolism and is a protein sparer.

سٹیرائڈ جو تجمع کو بڑھاتا ہے اور پروٹین کو الگ کرتا ہے۔

Anabolic compound *(an-ab-ol'-ik)*. Chemical substance which causes a synthesis of body protein. Useful in convalescence. Many of the androgens come into this category.

تجمعی مرکب: کیمیائی مادہ جو جسمانی پروٹین کی تالیف کرتا ہے۔

Anabolism *(an-ab'-ol-izm)* [G. anabole, throwing up]. The series of chemical reactions in the living body requiring energy to change simple substances into complex ones. See ADENOSINE DIPHOSPHATE and TRIPHOSPHATE. METABOLISM.

تجمع: دیکھئے میٹابولزم۔سادہ اشیاء سے پیچیدہ یا مخلوط اشیاء کا بننا جن میں توانائی جذب ہوتی ہے اور توانائی کا ذخیرہ کیا جاتا ہے یہ میٹابولزم کا ایک حصہ ہے۔اینابولزم یا تجمع ایک تعمیری عمل ہے۔مثلاً ضیائی تالیف جس میں سادہ، غیر نامیاتی مرکبات (کاربن ڈائی آکسائیڈ اور پانی) سے پیچیدہ، نامیاتی مرکبات (گلوکوس) بنتے ہیں یہ عمل ضیائی تالیف سبز پودوں میں سورج کی روشنی میں ہوتی ہے۔کیمیائی تعامل کو مساوات کے ذریعہ ظاہر کیا جاتا ہے۔کاربن ڈائی آکسائیڈ + پانی کلوروفل + دھوپ گلوکوس + پانی + آکسیجن مادۂ حیات یا پروٹوپلازم کا بننا بھی ایک تعمیری عمل ہے۔

Anacidity *(an-as-id'-it-i)* [G. a-, not; acere, to be sour]. Lack of normal acidity, especially in the gastric juice. See ACHLORHYDRIA.

بے تیزابی: یونانی الفاظ اے بمعنی نہیں اور ایسیئر بمعنی کھٹا ہونا کا مجموعہ۔تیزابیت کی کمی خصوصاً گیسٹرک جوس میں۔

Anacrotism *(an-ak'-rot-izm)* [G. ana, up; krotos, rattling noise]. An oscillation in the ascending curve of a sphygmographic pulse tracing, occurring in aortic stenos- is an-acrotic, adj.

شہوفیت: ایورٹک سٹینوسس میں واقع سفائیگموگرافک نبض کے خم میں اہتزاز۔

Anaemia *(an-e'-mi-a)* [G. a-,not; haima, blood]. A deficiency of haemoglobin concentration in the blood due to lack of red blood cells and/or their haemoglobin content. Produces clinical manifestations arising from hypoxaemia. **Addisonian pernicious a.** results from failure to absorb food vitamin B_{12} so that erythropoiesis becomes megaloblastic. Treated with vitamin B_{12}. **haemolytic a.,** associated with excessive destruction of red blood cells and haemolytic jaundice. See ACHOLURICJAUNDICE.**iron deficiency a.,** the commonest **type;** due to blood loss, lack of dietary iron or poor iron absorption. Very common in pregnancy when iron requirement increased. **megaloblastic a.,** associated with diminished and abnormal production of red blood cells due to deficiency of vitamin B_{12} or folic acid. Peripheral blood shows **macrocytic a.,** i.e. large red cell picture--anaemic, adj.

قلب خون۔قلت الدم۔بھس: یونانی الفاظ اے بمعنی بغیر اور ہیما بمعنی کون کا مجموعہ۔اس اصطلاح کا مطلب خون کی کمی ہے۔دراصل خون میں سرخ خلیوں کی کمی واقع ہو جاتی ہے۔جگر میں حیاتین ب۱۲ جو سرخ خونی خلیے بناتے ہیں' کی کمی سے یہ بیماری ہو جاتی ہے یا غذا میں لوہے کی کمی کی وجہ سے ہوتی ہے۔علاج کے لئے فیرس فیومریٹ ۱ تا ۲ گولیاں دن میں ۳ دفعہ اور وٹامن بی کمپلیکس و وٹامن ب۱۲ ۱۰۰۰ ملی گرام ایک سی سی عضلاتی ٹیکہ روزانہ لگائیے۔

Anaerobe *(an'-er-ob)* [G. a-, not; aer, air; bios, life]. A micro-organism which will not grow in the presence of molecular oxygen. When this is strictly so, it is termed an 'obligatory anaerobe'. The majority of pathogens are indifferent to atmospheric conditions and will flourish in the presence or absence of oxygen and are therefore termed 'facultative anaerobes'--anaerobic. adj.

ناہواباش۔ناہوائی نامیہ: یونانی الفاظ اے بمعنی بغیر ایئر بمعنی ہوا اور بایوس بمعنی زندگی کا مجموعہ۔وہ جاندار جو آزاد آکسیجن کی غیر موجودگی میں رہتے ہیں۔

Anaesthesia *(an-es-thez'-i-a)* [G. anaisthesia, lack of sensation]. Loss of sensation. **general a.**, loss of sensation with loss of consciousness. In **local a.** the nerve conduction is blocked and painful impulses fail to reach the brain. **spinal a.** may be caused by (1) injection of an anaesthetic into the spinal subarachnoid space; (2) a lesion of the spinal cord.

بے حسی: جس کا ضیاع۔ایسی حالت جس میں احساس نہ ہو۔خصوصاً چھونے کی حس ختم ہو جاتی ہے۔درد کا احساس ختم کرنے کے لئے بے ہوش یا مقامی طور پر کوئی حصہ سن کر دیا جاتا ہے جو کوکین سے کیا جاتا ہے۔آجکل صرف آنکھ کی سرجری میں مستعمل ہے۔چھوٹے اپریشنوں میں باربیٹوریٹس کے محلول ٹیکے کے ذریعہ ورید میں داخل کئے جاتے ہیں۔ٹیکے کے دوران مریض سو جاتا ہے اور دوسری ادویات دی جاتی ہیں۔فقدان حس۔

Anaesthesiology *(an-es-thez-i-ol'-o-ji)* [G. anaisthesia, lack of sensation; logos, discourse]. The science dealing with anaesthetics, their administration and effect.

اینس تھیز یالوجی: سائنس کی وہ شاخ جس میں بے حسی آور کا مطالعہ کیا جاتا ہے۔

Anaesthetic *(an-es-thet'-ik)* [G. anaisthesia, lack of sensation]. 1. A drug which produces anaesthesia. 2. Causing anaesthesia. 3. Insensible to stimuli. **general a.**, a drug which produces general anaesthesia by inhalation or injection. **local a.**, a drug which injected into the tissues or applied topically causes local insensibility to pain. See SPIN- AL--anaesthetize. v.t.

مخدر۔بے حسی آور: وہ دوائی جو بے حسی پیدا کرے۔ادویات بے ہوشی مثلاً کلوروفارم ایتھر۔ذہنی یا بذریعہ ٹیکہ۔سنگھانیسے بھی بے ہوشی طاری کرتی ہیں۔اپریشنوں میں مستعمل۔

Anaesthetist *(an-es'-the-tist)* [G. anaisthesia, lack of sensation]. One who administers anaesthetics.

تخدیر کار: وہ شخص جو بے حسی پیدا کرے۔

Anafranil *(an-af'-ran-il)*. Clomipramine (q.v.).

اینف رینل: دیکھئے کلوی پرامین۔

Analeptic *(an-al-ep'-tik)* [G. analepsis, restoration]. Restorative. Most analeptics stimulate the central nervous system. 'Household' analeptics include smelling salts, sal volatile, whisky and brandy.

مسکن۔مقوی: مرکزی عصبی نظام کو بیدار کرتا ہے۔بگڑی حالت کو بہتر بناتا ہے۔تنفس کی کمزوری کو ٹھیک کرتا ہے۔بلڈ پریشر کی کمی میں بھی فائدہ دیتا ہے۔

Analgesia *(an-al-je'-zi-a)* [G. a-, not; algos, pain]. Loss of painful impressions without loss of tactile sense--analgesic, adj.

بے حسی درد: یونانی الفاظ اے بمعنی بغیر اور الگوس بمعنی درد کا مجموعہ۔چھونے کی حس کے ضیاع کے بغیر درد کے احساس کا فقدان۔

Analgesic *(an-al-je'-zik)* Insensible to pain; alleviating pain; a drug which relieves pain. Syn anodyne.

دافع درد۔مسکن (دوا) : درد محسوس نہ کرنا۔درد کو آرام پہنچانے والی دوا۔مثلاً اسپرین۔

Analogous *(an-al'-o-gus)* [G. analogia, conformity]. Similar in function, but not in origin.

ہم فعل مشابہ۔مماثل : فعل میں یکساں مگر ان کے ماخذ مختلف ہوں سطحی مشابہت والی ساختیں۔

Analysis *(an-al'-i-sis)* [G. a loosening]. A term used in chemistry to denote the determination of the composition of a compound substance--analyses, pl.; analytic, adj.; analytically, adv. See PSYCHOANALYSIS.

تجزیہ۔تحلیل۔تشریح : یونانی لفظ جس کے معنی ڈھیلے ہونا ہیں۔کیمیا میں استعمال ہونے والی اصطلاح جس سے کسی کیمیائی مرکب کی کیمیائی ترکیب معلوم کی جاتی ہے۔اجزاء میں تقسیم کرنا۔پانی کے تجزیہ کو آب پاشیدگی کہا جاتا ہے۔

Analyst *(an'-a-list)* [G. analyein, to unloose]. A person experienced in performing analyses.

تجزیہ کار : تجزیہ کرنے کا ماہر شخص۔

Anaphrodisiac *(an-af-ro-diz'-i-ak)* [G. a-, not; aphrodisiakos, sexual]. See ANTAPHRODISAIC.

Anaphylactoid *(an-a-fil-ak'-toid)* [G. ana, up; phylaxis, protection]. Pertaining to or resembling anaphylaxis.

استبدادی غِ : یونانی الفاظ اینا بمعنی اوپر اور فائیلیکسس بمعنی حفاظت کا مجموعہ۔ اینافائیلیکسس سے مشابہہ یا اس سے متعلق۔

Anaphylaxis *(an-a-fil-aks'-is)* [G. ana, up; phylaxis, protection]. A hypersensitive state of the body to a foreign protein (e.g. horse serum) so that the injection of a second dose after ten days brings about an acute reaction which may be fatal; in lesser degree it produces breathlessness, pallor and collapse--ana-phylactic, adj. See ALLERGY and SENSITIZATION.

اینافائیلیکسس زود حسی : یونانی الفاظ اینا بمعنی اوپر اور فائیلیکسس بمعنی حفاظت کا مجموعہ۔ جسم کی ایک حالت جو بیرونی پروٹین کے داخل ہونے پر ہوتی ہے۔ دس روز کے بعد دوسری خوراک کا ٹیکہ انتہائی ردعمل پیدا کرتا ہے اس لئے مہلک ہو سکتا ہے۔

Anaplasia *(an-a-plaz'-i-a)* [G. anaplassein, to remould]. Loss of the distinctive characteristices of a cell, associated with proliferative activity as in cancer--anaplastic, adj.

قہقری تکوین : کسی خلیے کی نمایاں خصوصیات کا ضیاع۔

Anasarca *(an-a-sark'-a)* [G. ana, up; sarx, flesh]. Serous infiltration of the cellular tissues and serous cavities; generalized oedema; dropsy--anasarcous, adj.

استسقاء لحمی : یونانی الفاظ اینا بمعنی اوپر اور سارکس بمعنی گوشت کا مجموعہ۔ خلوی بافتوں کا دخول۔

Anastomosis *(an-as-to-mo'-sis)* [G. anastomoein, to furnish with a mouth]. 1. The intercommunication of the branches of two or more arteries or veins. 2. In surgery, the establishment of an intercommunication between two hollow organs, vessels or nerves--anas-tomoses, pl.; anastomotic, adj.; anastomose, v.i., v.t.

Ansstomosis

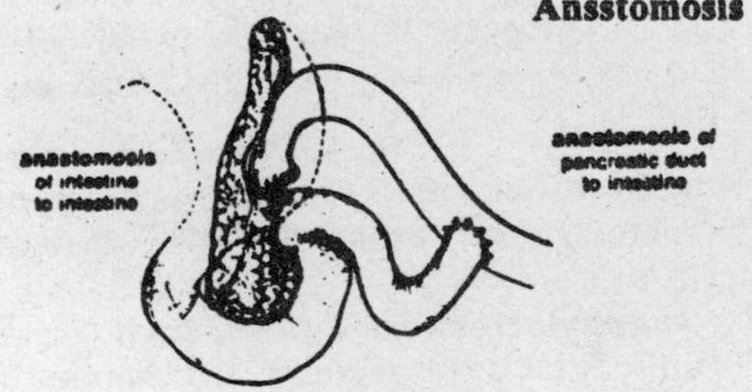

منہ بننا : یونانی لفظ اناسٹومین جس کا مطلب منہ مہیا کرنا ہے۔ (۱) دو یا زیادہ شریانوں یا وریدوں کی شاخوں کے درمیان باہمی تبادلہ۔ (۲) سرجری میں دو کھوکھلے اعضاء، رگوں یا اعصاب کے درمیان باہمی رابطہ کا قیام۔

Anatomy *(a-nat'-o-mi)* [G. anatome, dissection]. The science which deals with the structure of the body by means of dissection--anatomical, adj.; anatomically, adv.

علم تشریح : یونانی لفظ اینا ٹوم بمعنی چیر پھاڑ سے ماخوذ سائنس کی وہ شاخ جس میں جسم کی اندرونی ساخت کا مطالعہ کیا جاتا ہے۔ جسم کو چیر کر اندر سے دیکھا جاتا ہے۔

Ancolan. Antihistamine useful in hyperemesis gravidarum.

اینکولان : اینٹی ہسٹامین۔

Ancrod *(an'-krod)* Anticoagulant obtained from the venom of the Malayan pit viper. It destroys fibrinogen, so depleting the blood of its essential factor for fibrin formation. Being a foreign protein it induces antibody formation so that after a few weeks, patients develop resistance to its action. Ancrod can therefore be used only for short term effects.

این کراڈ : ملایا کے سانپ کے زہر سے حاصل ہونے والا جس سے خون نہیں جمتا۔ اس کی وجہ سے خون فائبرن نہیں بنا سکتا۔

Ancylostoma *(ang-ki-lo-sto'-ma).* Human hookworm. Ancylostoma duodenale is predominantly found in southern Europe and the Middle and Far East. Necator americanus is found in the New World and tropical Africa. Mixed infections are not uncommon. Only clinically significant when infestation is moderate or heavy. As hookworms suck blood, it may be necessary to treat encuing anaemia. Worm inhabits duodenum and upper jejunum, eggs are passed in stools, hatch in moist soil and produce larvae which can penetrate bare feet and reinfect people. Prevention is by wearing shoes and using latrines. See ANKYLOSTOMIASIS.

اینکائیلوسٹوما : انسانی ہک ورم۔ یہ ورم ڈیوڈینم میں ہوتا ہے۔ اس کے انڈے فضلے کے ساتھ باہر آتے اور گیلی زمین پر بچے نکلتے ہیں۔ اس کے لاروے ننگے پاؤں میں سے جسم میں داخل ہوتے ہیں۔ اس کی احتیاطی تدابیر

ہیں کہ ننگے پاؤں نہ پھرا جائے بلکہ جوتے پہنے جائیں اور لیٹرین استعمال کرنا ضروری ہے۔

Andria *(an'-dri-a)* [G. aner, pseudo-male hermaphrodite (q.v), i.e. one in whom the male characteristics predominate.

مکمل مرد : یونانی لفظ ایز بمعنی آدمی سے ماخوذ جس میں نر کی خصوصیات غالب ہوں۔ مردانہ خواص کا حامل۔

Androgens *(an'-dro-jens)* [G. aner, man; genesis, production]. Hormones secreted by the tests and adrenal cortex or synthetic substances which control the building up of protein and the male secondary sex characteristics, e.g. distribution of hair and deepening of voice. When given to females they have a masculinizing effect--androgenic, androgenous, adj. See TESTOSTERONE.

نرزا : یونانی الفاظ اینڈر بمعنی مرد اور جینیسس بمعنی پیداوار کا مجموعہ۔ خصیوں اور ایڈرینل کارٹیکس سے خارج ہونے والے ہارمون جو ثانوی مردانہ خصوصیات کو کنٹرول کرتے ہیں۔

Androgyna *(an-dro-gi'-na)* [G. aner, man; gyne, woman]. A pseudofemale hermaphrodite (q.v), i.e. one in whom the female characteristics are predominant--androgynous, adj.

عورت ہیجڑا: یونانی الفاظ اینڈر بمعنی مرد اور گائن بمعنی عورت کا مجموعہ۔ جس میں زنانہ خصوصیات غالب ہوں۔

Androphobia *(an-dro-fo'-bi-a)* [G. aner, man; phobos, fear]. A morbid dislike or fear of men--androphobic, adj.

نرگریزی۔ نرترسی : یونانی الفاظ ایز بمعنی مرد اور فوبوس بمعنی ڈر یا خوف کا مجموعہ۔ مردوں سے نفرت یا مردوں کا ڈر یا خوف۔

Andursil *(and'-ur-sil)*. Aluminium hydroxide with magnesium hydroxide and carbonate. Antacid and antiflatulent.

Anencephaly *(an-en-kef'-a-li)* [G. a-, not; egkephatos, brain]. Absence of the brain. A term used in connection with fetal monsters. The condition is incompatible with life--anencephalous, anencephalic, adj.

عدم دماغی : یونانی الفاظ اے بمعنی بغیر اور اِنگکفالوس بمعنی دماغ کا مجموعہ۔ دماغ کی غیر موجودگی۔

Anethaine *(an-e-than')* Amethocaine. *(q.v.)*.

اینی تھین : دیکھئے امیتھوکین۔

Aneurine *(an'-u-rin)* . Thiamine or vitamin B_1. Concerned in carbohydrate metabolism; indicated therapeutically in aneurine deficiency disorders such as beri-beri, and some forms of neuritis; also as adjunct to oral antibiotic therapy.

انورین : تھیامین یا حیاتین ب ا۔ اس کا تعلق کاربوہائیڈریٹ میٹابولزم سے ہے۔

Aneurysm *(an'-ur-izm)* [G. aneurysma, dilation]. Local dilatation of a blood vessel, usually artery, due to local fault in the wall through defect, disease or injury, producing a pulsating swelling over which a murmur may be heard. True aneurysms may be saccular, fusiform, or dissecting where the blood flows between the layers of the arterial **wall, false a.** follows rupture of the wall and consists of a cavity lined by blood clot surrounded by the adjacent tissues. **Arteriovenous a.,** an abnormal direct connection between an artery and a vein, usually following injury and sometimes producing delated pulsating veins, **cirsoid a.** (q.v)--aneurysmal, adj.

شریانی پھیلاؤ : خونی رگ کا پھیلنا عموماً شریان پھیلتی ہے جو کسی نقص، بیماری یا زخم کی وجہ سے ہوتی ہے۔

Angiectasis *(an-ji-ek'-ta-sis)* [G. aggeion, vessel; ektasis, extension]. Abnormal dilatation of blood vessels, Telangiectasis (q.v)--angiectatic, adj.

رگوں کا تناؤ: خونی رگوں کا غیر معمولی پھیلاؤ۔

Angiitis *(an-ji-i'-tis)* [G. aggeion, vessel;-itis, inflammation]. Inflammation of a blood or lymph vessel--angitic, adj.

ورم عرق: یونانی الفاظ اجیون بمعنی رگ اور آئیٹس تورم کا مجموعہ۔ خونی یا لمفی رگ کا تورم۔

Angina *(an-ji'-na)* [L. angere, to strangle]. Sense of suffocation or constriction. **Ludwig's a.,** see CELLULITIS. **a. pectoris,** severe but temporary attack of cardiac pain which may radiate to the arms. Results from myocardial ischaemia. Often the attack is induced by exercise (angina of effort). **Vincent's a.** is infection of mouth or throat by a spirochaete and a bacillus in synergis-m--anginal, adj.

دردسینہ۔ دردگلو: گلا گھٹنے یا بند ہونے کا احساس۔ انجائنہ پیکوٹورس یا دل کا درد سیر شدہ چکنائیاں زیادہ مقدار میں کھانے سے ہوتا ہے۔

Angiocardiogram *(an-ji-o-kar'-di-o-gram)* [G. aggeion, vessel; kardia; heart; gramma, letter]. Film demonstrating the heart and great vessels after injection of opaque medium.

انجیو کارڈیوگرام: دل اور بڑی رگوں کو دکھانے والی فلم۔

Angiocardiography *(an-ji-o-kar-di-og'-raf-i)* [G. aggeion, vessel; kardia, heart; graphein, to write]. Demonstration of heart and great vessels by means of injection of opaque medium into cardiac circulation--ang- iocardiographic, adj.; angiocardiographically, adv.

انجیو کارڈیوگرافی: یونانی الفاظ اجیون بمعنی رگ کارڈیا بمعنی دل اور گریفین بمعنی لکھنا کا مجموعہ۔ کارڈیائی گردش میں غیر شفاف واسطہ کے ٹیکے کے ذریعہ بڑی رگوں اور دل کا مظاہرہ۔ عمل تقلیح سے افعال قلب کا مظاہرہ۔

Angiogram *(an'-ji-o-gram)* [G. aggeion, vessel; gramma, letter]. Film demonstrating the arterial system after injection of opaque medium.

دعا نگارش: غیر شفاف واسطہ کے ٹیکے کے ذریعہ شریانی نظام کا مظاہرہ کرنے کے لئے فلم۔

Angiography *(an-ji-og'-raf-i)* [G. aggeion, vessel; graphein, to write]. Demonstration of the arterial system by means of injection of opaque medium--angiographic, adj.; angiographically, adv.

دعا نگاری: یونانی الفاظ اجیون بمعنی رگ اور گریفین بمعنی لکھنا کا مجموعہ۔ غیر شفاف واسطہ کے ٹیکے کے ذریعہ شریانی نظام کا مظاہرہ۔

Angiology *(an-ji-ol'-o-ji)* [G. aggeion, vessel; logos, discourse]. The science dealing with blood and lymphatic vessels--angiological, adj.; angiologically, adv.

دعائیات۔ عروقیات: سائنس کی وہ شاخ جس میں خونی اور لمفی رگوں کا مطالعہ کیا جاتا ہے۔

Angioma *(an-ji-o'-ma)* [G. aggeion, vessel; -oma, tumour]. A non-malignant tumour formed of blood vessels, usually capillaries, **cavernous a.**, when larger spaces are occupied by blood--angiomatous, adj.; angiomata, pl.

دعائی سلعہ: یونانی الفاظ اجیون بمعنی رگ اور اوما بمعنی رسولی کا مجموعہ۔ خونی رگوں کی بننے والی رسولی۔

Angioneurotic oedema *(an-ji-o-nu-rot'-ik-e-d-e'-ma)* [G. aggeion, vessel; neuron, nerve; -osis, condition; oidema, swelling] A severe from of urticaria which may involve the skin of the face, hands or genitals and the mucous membrane of the mouth and throat: oedema of the glottis may be fatal. Occasionally forms part of the clinical picture in anaphylaxis and penicillin sensitization. Immediate cause is an abrupt local increase in vascular permeability, as a result of which fluid escapes from blood vessels into surrounding tissues. Swelling may be due to an allergic hypersensitivity reaction to drugs, pollens or other known allergens, but in many cases no cause can be found. Runs a benign course with spontaneous remission.

دعائی عصبی ابھار: یونانی الفاظ اجیون بمعنی رگ' نیورون بمعنی عصب' اوسس بمعنی حالت اور ایڈما بمعنی ابھار کا مجموعہ۔ پتی کی بیماری۔ اس میں چہرے' ہاتھوں اور تولیدی اعضاء کی جلد متاثر ہوتی ہے اور خارش ہوتی ہے۔ پنسلین سے ردعمل۔

Anioplasty *(an-ji-o'-plast-i)* [G. aggeion, vessel; plassein, to form]. Plastic surgery of blood vessels--anioplastic, adj.

دعائی پیوندکاری: خونی رگوں کی پلاسٹک سرجری۔

Angiosarcoma *(an-ji-o'-sar-ko'-ma)* [G. aggeion, vessel; sarkoma, fleshy excrescence]. A malignant tumour arising from blood vessels--angiosarcomatous, adj,; angiosarcomata, pl

دعائی لحمی سلعہ: خونی رگوں سے ابھرنے والی دانہ دار رسولی۔

Angiospasm *(an-ji-o'-spazm)* [G. ageion, vessel; spasmos, spasm]. Constricting spasm of blood vessels--angiospastic, adj.

دعائی تشنج : یونانی الفاظ اجیون بمعنی رگ اور سپازموس بمعنی تشنج یا اینٹھن سے ماخوذ اصطلاح۔خونی رگوں کی اینٹھن۔

Angiotensin *(an-ji-o-ten'-sin)* [G. aggeion, vessel; teno, to stretch]. A polypeptide formed by the action on a plasma substrate of the enzyme renin (q.v.) found in the kidney. It is the most potent pressor substance known and has been synthesized; available commercially.

انجیوٹنسن : ایک پولی پیپٹائڈ۔مارکیٹ میں دستیاب ہے۔

Angstrom Unit *(ang'-strom).* Measure of wavelength of any radiatio [A.J.Angstrom, Swedish physicist, 1814-74.]

انگسٹر وم اکائی : لمبائی کی ایک اکائی۔اشعاع کی طول موج ناپنے کی اکائی۔یہ 10 میٹر کے برابر ہے۔

Anhidrosis *(an-hi-dro'-sis)* [G. a-, not; hidros, sweat; -osis, condition]. Deficient sweat secretion--anhidrotic, adj.

قلت پسینہ۔کم عرقیت : یونانی الفاظ اے بمعنی بغیر، ہڈروس بمعنی پسینہ اور اوسس بمعنی حالت سے ماخوذ اصطلاح۔پسینے کے اخراج میں کمی۔

Anhidrotics *(an-hid-rot'-iks).* Agents which reduce perspiration.

مانع عرق : وہ ایجنٹس جو پسینے میں تخفیف کرتے ہیں۔

Anhydraemia *(an-hid-rem'-i-a)* [G. a-, not; hydor, water; haima, blood]. Deficient fluid content of blood--anhydraemic, adj.

نابیدگی : یونانی الفاظ اے بمعنی بغیر، ہائیڈر بمعنی پانی اور ہیما بمعنی خون سے ماخوذ اصطلاح خون کے سیال حصے کی کمی۔

Anhydrous *(an-hid'-rus)* [G. a-, not; hydor, water]. Entirely without water, dry.

نابیدہ۔بے آب : یونانی الفاظ اے بمعنی بغیر اور ہائیڈر بمعنی پانی سے ماخوذ۔بالکل خشک۔پانی کے بغیر۔

Anileridine *(an-il'-er-i-din).* Analgesic that is useful pre- and post-operatively.

اینی لیری ڈین : اپریشن سے پہلے اور بعد میں مفید۔

Anicteric *(an-ik'-ter-ik)* [G. a-, not; icteros, jaundice]. Without jaundice.

اینک ٹیرک : یونانی الفاظ اے بمعنی بغیر اور اکٹیر س بمعنی یرقان سے ماخوذ یرقان کے بغیر۔

Aniline *(an'-il-en)* An oily compound obtained from the dry distillation of coal and much used in the preparation of dyes.

انیلین : ایک تیلیا مرکب جو کوئلہ کی خشک کشید سے حاصل ہوتا ہے۔رنگوں، پلاسٹک اور ادویات کی تیاری میں استعمال کیا جاتا ہے۔فینائل امین۔امینو بنزین۔ایک بے رنگ مائع۔نقطۂ جوش ۱۸۴٫۴س، یہ نائیٹرو بنزین کی تخفیف کر کے بنایا جاتا ہے۔

Aniridia *(an-i-rid'-e-a)* [G. a-, not; tris, rainbow]. Lack or defect of the iris; usually congenital.

لاقزحیت : یونانی الفاظ بمعنی بغیر اور ٹرس بمعنی قوس قزح سے ماخوذ اصطلاح، قزحیہ یا آئرس کا نقص۔

Anisocoria *(an-e-so-kor'-e-a)* p[G. anisos, unequal; kore, pupil]. Inequality in diameter of the pupils.

نابرابر مردمیت : یونانی الفاظ اینیسوس بمعنی غیر مساوی اور کور بمعنی پتلی سے ماخوذ اصطلاح۔پتلیوں کے قطر میں نابرابری۔

Anisocytosis *(an-e-so-si-to'-sis)* [G. anisos, unequal; kytos, cell; -osis, condition]. Inequality in size of red blood cells.

این آئیسوسائی ٹوسس : یونانی الفاظ اینیسوس بمعنی غیر مساوی، کائیٹوس بمعنی خلیہ اور اوسس بمعنی حالت سے ماخوذ اصطلاح خلیوں کے سائز میں نابرابری خصوصاً سرخ خونی خلیے۔

Anisomelia *(an-e-so-me'-li-a)* [G. anisos, unequal; melos, limb]. Unequal length of limbs--anisomelous, adj.

اختلاف الجوارح : یونانی الفاظ اینیسوس بمعنی غیر مساوی اور میلس بمعنی جارح سے ماخوذ اصطلاح جوارح کی غیر مساوی طوالت۔

Anisometropia *(an-e-so-me-tro'-pi-a)* [G. anisos, unequal; metron, a measure; ops, eye]. A difference in the refraction of the two eyes--anisometropic, adj.

بھینگا پن : دونوں آنکھوں کے انعطاف میں فرق۔

Ankle Clonus A series of rapid muscular contractions of the calf muscle when the foot is dorsiflexed by pressure upon the sole.

ٹخنے کا جھٹکا، کعبی رعشہ : جب پاؤں ایڑی پر دباؤ سے بطنی طور پر جھکے تو کاف عضلے کی تیز عضلاتی سکڑنے والی حرکت کا سلسلہ۔

Ankyloblepharon *(ang-ki-lo-blef'-a-ron)* [G. agkylos, crooked; blepharon, eyelid]. Adhesion of the ciliary edges of the eyelids.

التصاق الاجفان۔ پلکیں چپکنا: آنکھ کے پپوٹوں کے ہدبی کناروں کا چپکاؤ۔

Ankylosis *(ang-ki-lo'-sis)* [G. agkyle, a thong]. Stiffness or fixation of a joint--ankylose, v.t., vi.; ankylosed, adj.

جساۃ: کسی جوڑ کا سخت ہونا۔

Ankylostoma *(ang-ki-lo-sto'-ma)* [G. agkylos, crooked; stoma, mouth]. Ancylostoma (q.v.).

انکیلوسٹوما۔ کج دہنہ : دیکھئے این کائیلوسٹوما۔

Ankylostomiasis *(ang-ki-los-tom-i'-a-sis)* [G. agkylos, crooked; stoma, mouth; N.L. -iasis, condition]. Infestation of the human intestine with Ankylostoma, giving rise to malnutrition and severe anaemia. Hookworm disease.

کج دہنی۔ مرض ہک ورم : انسانی آنت میں انکیلوسٹوما ہونا جس سے غذائی کمی اور قلت خون کی بیماریاں ہوتی ہیں۔ ہک ورم والی بیماری۔

Annular *(an'-u-lar)* [L. annulus, ring]. Ring-shaped. **a. ligaments,** found surrounding the ankle and proximal and distal ends of radius.

چھلےدار۔ حلقہ دار : چھلے یا حلقے کی شکل کے۔ لاطینی اینولس بمعنی چھلا سے اصطلاح۔ اندرونی و بیرونی چھلے دار جگہ کہا جاتا ہے۔

Anodyne *(an'-o-din)* [G. a-, not; odyne, pain]. A remedy which relieves pain. Analgesic.

درد ربا۔ مسکن دوا : یونانی الفاظ اے بمعنی بغیر اور اوڈائن بمعنی درد سے ماخوذ اصطلاح جس سے درد کو آرام آئے۔

Anogenital *(a-no-jen'-it-al)* [L. anus; G. genesis, descent]. Pertaining to the anus and the genital region.

مبرزی (مقعدی) تولیدی : مقعد اور تولیدی حصے سے متعلق۔

Anomaly *(an-on'-a-li)* [G. anomalia, irregularity]. That which is unusual or differs from --anomalous, adj.

خلاف قاعدگی : یونانی لفظ اینومیلیا بمعنی بے قاعدگی سے ماخوذ اصطلاح۔ وہ جو غیر معمولی ہو یعنی معمول سے ہٹ کر ہو۔

Anomia *an-o'-mi-a)* [G. a-, not; onoma, name]. Inability to name objects or persons. Same as nominal aphasia.

نام فراموشی : یونانی الفاظ اے بمعنی بغیر اور انوما بمعنی نام سے ماخوذ اصطلاح۔ اشیاء یا اشخاص کے نام لینے کی ناقابلیت۔

Anomie *(an'-om-e)* Sociological term applied or a person who is lonely because he cannot relate with others, consequently he no longer identifies with them.

Anonychia *(an-o-nik'-i-a)* [G. a-,not; onyx, nail]. Absence of nails.

بے ناخنی : یونانی الفاظ اے بمعنی بغیر اور اونکس بمعنی ناخن سے ماخوذ اصطلاح۔ ناخنوں کی غیر موجودگی۔

Anoperineal *(a'-no-per-in-e'-al)* [L. anus; G. perineos, space between anus and scrot- um]. Pertaining to the anus and perineum.

مبرزی عجانی: لاطینی لفظ انیس بمعنی مقعد اور یونانی لفظ پرینوس بمعنی مقعد وسکروٹم کی درمیانی جگہ، سے مرکب اصطلاح۔ مقعد اور پیرینیم سے متعلق۔

Anopheles *(an-of'-i-lez)* [G. anopheles, harmful]. A genus of mosquito. The females are the host of the malarial parasite, and their bite is the means of transmitting the disease to man. See MALARIA.

انافلیز۔ ملیریا مچھر: مچھر کی ایک نوع جس کے کاٹنے سے انسان ملیریا بخار میں مبتلا ہو جاتا ہے۔ یہ مچھر انسان کا طفیلی ہے اور اس کا خون چوستا ہے۔ اس مچھر کے کاٹنے سے پلازموڈیم یا ملیریائی طفیلی اس سے انسانی خون میں منتقل ہو جاتا ہے۔ مادہ مچھر جنسی اختلاط کے بعد انڈے دیتی ہے۔ وہ ساکن پانی میں انڈے دیتی ہے۔ انڈوں سے لاروے نکلتے ہیں۔ بعد میں لاروا پیوپا بن جاتا ہے۔ پھر پیوپا سے بالغ ہو جاتا ہے۔ لاروا اور پیوپا پانی میں رہتے ہیں جبکہ بالغ مچھر پانی سے اڑ کر انسانی خون چوستا ہے۔ ملیریا پھیلانے کے ذمہ دار یہی مچھر ہیں۔ یونانی لفظ انافلیز کے معنی ہیں نقصان دہ ہے۔ مچھر کا ایک جنس مادہ مچھر ملیریائی طفیلی کے لئے میزبان ہے جس کے کاٹنے سے انسان کو ملیریا ہو جاتا ہے۔

Anorchus *(an-awr'-kus)* [G. a-, not; orchis, testis]. Without testicles. A male with congenital absence of testes in the scrotum.

این آرکس : یونانی الفاظ اے بمعنی بغیر اور آرکس بمعنی خصیہ سے ماخوذ اصطلاح۔ خصیوں کے بغیر۔ ایسا نر جس کے سکروٹم میں خصیے موجود نہ ہوں۔

Anorectal *(a-no-rek'-tal)* [L. anus, anus; rectus, straight]. Pertaining to the anus and rectum, as a fissure (q.v.).

مبرزی مقعدی : لاطینی الفاظ انیس بمعنی مقعد اور ریکٹس بمعنی سیدھا سے ماخوذ اصطلاح۔ مقعد یا مبرز اور ریکٹم سے متعلق۔

Anorectic *(an-o-rek'-tik)* [G. a-, not; orexis, appetite]. Appetite depressant.

اینور یکلٹک : یونانی الفاظ اے بمعنی بغیر اور اور یکسس بمعنی بھوک سے ماخوذ اصطلاح۔ بھوک کم کرنے والی دوا۔

Anorexia *(an-o-reks'-i-a)* [G. a-, not; orexis, appetite]. Loss or deficiency of appetite for food. **a. nervosa,** hysterical aversion of food leading to atrophy of stomach--anorexic, anorectic, adj.

عدم اشتہا : یونانی الفاظ اے بمعنی بغیر اور اور یکسس بمعنی بھوک سے ماخوذ اصطلاح۔ خوراک کھانے کے لئے بھوک کی کمی یا بھوک نہ ہونے۔ کثرت تمباکو نوشی یا چائے نوشی اس کی وجہ ہے۔

Anosmia *(an-oz'-mi-a)* [G. a-, not; osme, smell]. Absence of the sense of smell anosmic, anosmatic, adj.

عدم شامہ : سونگھنے کی حس کی غیر موجودگی۔ سونگھنے کی حس نہ ہونا۔

Anovular *(an-ov'-u-lar)* [G. a-, not; L. ovum, egg]. **a. bleeding** is uterine bleeding which has not been preceded by ovulation. e.g. in metropathia haemorrhagica. An endometrial biopsy following an **a. cycle** shows no progestational changes.

عدیم البویضی : یونانی لفظ اے بمعنی بغیر اور لاطینی لفظ اووم بمعنی انڈا یا بیضہ سے مرکب اصطلاح۔ عورتوں میں خارج ہونے والا خون جو یوٹرس سے خارج ہوتا ہے۔

Anoxaemia *(an-oks-e'-mi-a)* [G. a-, not; oxys, sharp; haima, blood]. Literally no oxygen in the blood. Usually used to indicate hypoxaemia (q.v.)--anoxaemic, adj.

بے آکسیجنی : یونانی الفاظ اے بمعنی بغیر آکسس بمعنی تیز اور ہیما بمعنی خون سے ماخوذ اصطلاح خون میں آکسیجن نہ ہونا یا خون میں آکسیجن کی کمی۔

Anoxia *(an-ok'-si-a)* [G. a-, not; oxys, sharp]. Literally no oxygen in the tissues. Usually used to signify hypoxia (q.v.)--anoxic, adj.

قلت آکسیجن : یونانی الفاظ بمعنی بغیر اور آکسس بمعنی تیز سے اصطلاح۔ نسیج یا بافتوں میں آکسیجن کی غیر موجودگی۔

Ansolysen *(an'-zo-li-sen)*. Pentolinium (q.v.).

اینسو لائی سن : دیکھئے پنٹولنیم۔

Antabuse *(ant'-a-bus)* Disulfiram (q.v.).

اینٹابیوس : دیکھئے ڈائی سلفائیرم

Antacid *(ant-as'-id)* [G. anti, against; L. acidus, sour]. A substance which neutralizes or counteracts acidity. Commonly used in alkaline stomach powders and mixtures.

ترشہ توڑ : یونانی لفظ اینٹی بمعنی خلاف اور لاطینی لفظ ایسیڈس بمعنی کھٹا سے مرکب اصطلاح۔ تیزابیت کو ختم کرنے والا مادہ۔

Antagonism *(an-tag'-on-izm)* [G. antagonizesthai, to struggle against]. Active opposition; a characteristic of some drugs, muscles and organisms--antagonistic, adj.

تضاد العمل : بھرپور مخالفت۔ چند ادویات، عضلات اور جسیموں کی خصوصیت۔ استخوانی عضلات کی ترتیب۔

Antagonist *(an-tag'-on-ist)* [G. antagonistes, adversary]. A muscle that relaxes to allow the agonist (q.v.) to perform a movement. When applied to drug it is one which blocks, nulifies or reverses the effects of another drug.

مخالف عضلہ : ایک عضلہ جو دوسرے کو حرکت دینے کے لئے ڈھیلا ہوتا ہے۔ ایسی دوائی جو دوسری دوائی کے اثرات کو ختم کرے۔

Antaphrodisiac *(ant-af-ro-diz'-i-ak)* [G. anti, against; aphrodisiakos, sexual]. An agent that diminishes sexual desire; absence of sexual impulse. Also ANAPHRODISIAC.

قاطع باہ : یونانی الفاظ اینٹی بمعنی خلاف اور افروڈزیاکوس بمعنی جنسی سے ماخوذ اصطلاح۔ ایسا ایجنٹ جو جنسی خواہش کو کم کر دے۔ جنسی حس کی غیر موجودگی۔

Antazoline *(an-ta'-zo-lin)*. An antihistamine with local anaesthetic properties. Mostly used locally.

اینٹازولین : ایک اینٹی ہسٹامین اے زیادہ تر مقامی طور پر استعمال کیا جاتا ہے۔ دافع حس دوائی۔ الرجی میں استعمال کی جاتی ہے۔

Anteflexion *(an'-te-flek'-shun)* [L. ante, before; flectere, to bend]. The bending forward of an organ. Commonly applied to the position of the uterus. Opp. to retroflexion.

پیش خمیدگی : لاطینی الفاظ اینٹے بمعنی پہلے یا آگے اور فلکٹیئر بمعنی جھکنا سے ماخوذ اصطلاح۔ کسی عضو کا آگے کی طرف جھکنا۔ عموماً اس اصطلاح کا اطلاق یوٹرس کی پوزیشن ظاہر کرنے کے لئے کیا جاتا ہے۔

Antemortem *(an'-te-mawr'-tem)* [L]. Before death. Opp. to postmortem.

قبل از مرگ : لاطینی لفظ موت سے پہلے۔ پوسٹ مارٹم کا متضاد۔ قبل از موت۔

Antenatal *(an-te-na'-tal)* [L. ante, before natus, birth]. The period between conception and delivery of the child. The term prenatal is now preferred. Normally 40 weeks or 280 days.

قبل پیدائش: لاطینی الفاظ اینٹی بمعنی پہلے اور نیٹس بمعنی پیدائش سے ماخوذ اصطلاح۔ حمل ٹھہرنے اور بچے کی پیدائش کا درمیانی عرصہ۔ عموماً یہ عرصہ ۴۰ ہفتے یا ۲۸۰ دن ہوتا ہے۔

Antepar *(an'-te-par)* Elixir and tablets containing piperazine (q.v.).

اینٹی پار: پائپرازین پر مشتمل گولیاں۔ مقوی دوا۔ آنتوں کے کیڑے مارنے والی دوائی۔

Antepartum *(an'-te-par-tum)* [L.]. Before birth. More generally confined to the three months preceding full-term delivery, i.e. the 6th to 9th month. See PLACENTA.

قبل ولادت: لاطینی لفظ پیدائش سے پہلے وضع حمل کے پہلے تین ماہ۔

Anterior *(an-te-ri-er)* [L. foremost, former]. In front of; the front surface of; ventral--anteriorly, adv. **a. chamber of the eye,** the space between the posterior surface of the cornea and the anterior surface of the iris. See AQUEOUS. **a. tibial syndrom,** severe pain and inflammation over anterior tibial muscle group, with inability to dorsiflex the foot.

اگلا مقدم: لاطینی لفظ جس کے معنی میں سب سے پہلا' سب سے آگے والا یا پہلے والا۔ کے آگے۔ سامنے والی سطح۔ بطنی یا پیٹ کی طرف آنکھ کے اگلے خانے سے مراد آئرس کی اگلی سطح اور قرینہ کی خلفی سطح کی درمیانی جگہ ہے۔ اگلا سرا

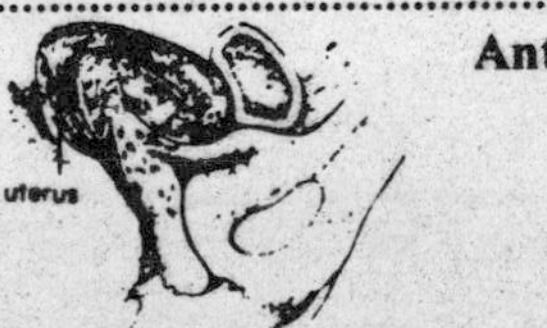

Anteflexon

Anterograde *(an'-ter-o-grad)* [L. anterior, foremost; gradi, to go]. Proceeding forwsard. See AMNESIA.

پیش رواں: لاطینی الفاظ اینٹیر یئر بمعنی اگلا اور گریڈی بمعنی جانا سے ماخوذ اصطلاح آگے بڑھنا۔

Anteversion *(an'-te-ver'-shun)* [L. ante, before, bvertere, to turn]. The forward tilting or displacement forward of an organ or part. Opp. to retroversion--anteverted, adj.; antevert, v.t., v.i.

تقدم رحم: لاطینی الفاظ اینٹی بمعنی پہلے اور ورٹیئر بمعنی مڑنا سے ماخوذ اصطلاح۔ کسی حصے یا عضو کے آگے کی طرف جھکنا۔

Anthelmintic *(an-thel-min)* [G. anti, against; helminus, worm]. Any remedy for the destruction or elimination of intestinal worms.

کرم کش (دوا): یونانی الفاظ اینٹی بمعنی خلاف اور ہیلمنس بمعنی کیڑا۔ آنتو کے کیڑوں کو ختم کرنے والی دوائی۔

Anthiomaline *(an-thi-om'-a-lin)* Antimony lithium thiomalate (q.v.).

اینتھیو مالن : دیکھئے اینٹی لیتھیم تھیومیلیٹ۔

Anthiphen *(an'-thi-fen).* Dichlorophen (q.v.)

اینتھی فین : دیکھئے ڈائی کلوروفین۔

Anthisan *(an'-thiz-an).* Mepyramine (q.v.).

اینتھی زین : دیکھئے میپیرامین۔

Anthracaemia *(an-thra-sem'-i-a)* [G. anthrax. malignant, pustule; haima, blood]. Anthrax septicaemia-anthracaemic, adj.

جمرہ دمویت۔ فحمی اختناق : انتھریکس سپٹسمیا۔

Anthracosis *(an-thra-ko'-sis).* [G. anthrax, coal; -osis, condition]. Black pigmentation of lungs due to inhalation of carbon particles; causes chronic inflammation. A form of pneumoconiosis (q.v.)--anthracotic, adj.

شش فحمیت۔ خبیث قرحہ: یونانی لفظ انتھریکس بمعنی کوئلہ اور اوسس بمعنی حالت سے ماخوذ اصطلاح۔ پھیپھڑوں میں سیاہ پگمنٹ کی موجودگی۔ کیونکہ کاربنی ذرات سانس کے ذریعے اندر چلے جاتے ہیں۔

Anthrax *(an'-thraks)* [G.] A contagious disease of cattle, which may be transmitted to man by inoculation, inhalation and ingestion, causing malignant pustule, woolsorter's disease and gastrointestinal anthrax respectively. Causative organism is Bacillus anthracis (q.v.) Preventive measures include prophylactic immunization of cattle and man.

انتھریکس۔ راج پھوڑا۔ ہزار چشمہ: مویشیوں کی چھوت والی بیماری

جوانسان کو بھی لگ سکتی ہے۔ ایک یونانی لفظ۔ ایک جراثیمی بیماری جو ایک جرثومے بےسلس انتھریس سے ہوتی ہے۔

Anthropology *(an'-thro-pol'-o-ji)* [G. anthropos, a human being; logos, discourse]. The study of mankind. Divided into various branches, such as criminal, cultural and physical anthropology--anthropological, adj.; anthropologically, adv.

انسانیات ۔ بشریات ۔ قدیم انسانیات : یونانی الفاظ انتھروپس بمعنی انسان اور لوگوس بمعنی بحث سے ماخوذ اصطلاح۔ انسان کا مطالعہ۔ انسانی جسم کی ساخت، طریقے، رواج اور جرائم کے بارے میں علم۔

Antiadrenaline *(an-ti-ad-ren'-al-in)* Neutralizing or lessening the effects of adrenaline, e.g. piperoxane.

اینٹی ایڈرینالین : ایڈرینالین کے اثرات کو ختم کرنا یا کم کرنا اور اس کی دوا۔

Antialdosterone *(an-ti-al-dos-ter'-on)*. Any substance that neutralizes or destroys aldosterone, e.g. spironoloact one.

اینٹی ایلڈوسٹیرون : ایسا مادہ جو ایلڈوسٹیرون کو ختم کرتا ہے۔

Antiallergic *(an-ti-al-er'-jik)* [G. anti, against; allos, other; ergon, activity; genesis, production]. Preventing or lessening allergy.

اینٹی الرجک : الرجی کم کرنا یا الرجی کو روکنا۔ اس کے لئے دوائی۔

Antianabolic *(an-ti-an-ab-ol'-ik)* [G. anti, against; anabole, throwing up]. Preventing the synthesis of body protein.

اینٹی انابولک: جسمانی پروٹین کی تالیف روکنا۔

\ntianaemic *(an-ti-an-em-ik)* [G. anti, against; a-, not; haima, blood]. An agent,e.g. vitamin K (q.v.), used to prevent haemorrhage.

اینٹی انیمک : قلت خون کو روکنے والا ایجنٹ۔

Antibacterial *(an'-ti-bak-ter'-i-al)* [G. anti, against; bakterion, little staff]. Any agent which destroys bacteria.

دافع جراثیم ۔ ضد جراثیم : جراثیم کو تباہ کرنے والا ایجنٹ۔

Antiberi-beri *(an-ti-ber'-e-ber'-e)* [G. anti, against; Singhalese, beri, weakness]. Against beri-beri (q.v.). The aneurine portion of vitamin B complex.

اینٹی بیری بیری: بیری بیری کے خلاف۔ حیاتین ب کمپلیکس کا آئینورین حصہ۔

Antibilharzial *(an-ti-bil-har'-ze-al)*. Against bilharziasis. See SCHISTOSOMIASIS.

اینٹی بلہارزیل: بلہارزی ایسس کے خلاف۔

Antibiosis *(an-ti-bi-os'-is)* [G. anti, against; bios, life]. An association between organisms which is harmful to one of them.

ضد زیستی: یونانی الفاظ اینٹی بمعنی خلاف اور بایوس بمعنی زندگی سے ماخوذ اصطلاح۔ جسیموں کے درمیان ایسوسی ایشن جو ان میں سے ایک کے لئے نقصان دہ ہوتی ہے۔

Antibiotics *(an-ti-bi-ot'-iks)* n. Antibacterial substances derived from fungi and bacteria, exemplified by penicillin (q.v.). Later antibiotics such as tetracycline (q.v.) are active against a wider range of organisms, and are also effective orally. Others, such as neomycin and bacitracin, are rarely used internally owing to high toxicity, but are effective when applied topically, and skin sensitization is uncommon.

ضد نامیات جراثیم کش ادویات ۔ اینٹی بائیوٹکس: ایسے مرکبات جو بعض جاندار بناتے ہیں اور جراثیم کے لئے مہلک ہیں۔ یہ کسی پھپھوندی سے حاصل ہوتے ہیں۔ مثلاً پنسلین وغیرہ۔

Antibodies *(an'-ti-bod-iz)* [G. anti, against; A.S. bodig, body]. Specific substances produced in the blood as a reaction to an antigen. They cause agglutination, flocculation, inactivation or lysis of the antigen. See DYSGAMMA-GLOBULINAEMIA.

ضد جسم: یونانی لفظ اینٹی بمعنی خلاف اور اینگلو سیکسن لفظ باڈگ بمعنی جسم سے مرکب اصطلاح۔ یہ پروٹین میں جو خون کے مائع حصے یا سیرم میں پائی جاتی ہیں۔ اینٹی جن کی ردعمل کے طور پر پیدا ہوتی ہیں۔

Anticholinergic *(an-ti-kol-in-erj'-ik)* [G. anti, against; chole, bile; ergon, work]. Inhibitory to the action of a cholinergic nerve (q.v.) by interfering with the action of acetylcholine, a chemical by which such a nerve transmits its impulses at neural or myoneural junctions.

اینٹی کولی نرجک: کولینرجک عصب کے عمل کو روکنے والا۔ پیٹ کے درد کو آرام پہنچاتا ہے۔ مثلاً بیلاڈونا ایٹروپین۔

Anticholinesterase *(an-ti-kol-in-es'-ter-az)* Enzyme that destroys acetylcholine at nerve endings. Used for reversing the effects of muscle relaxant drugs.

اینٹی کولین سیٹر یٹر : خامرہ جو عصبی سروں پر ایسی ٹائل کولین کو تباہ کرتا ہے۔

Anticoagulant *(an-ti-ko-ag'-ul-ant)* [G. anti, against; L. coagulare, to curdle]. An agent which prevents or retards clotting of blood. Small amount made in human body. Uses: (1) to obtain specimens suitable for pathol- ogical investigation and chemical analyses where whole blood or plasma is required instead of serum; the anticoagulant usually is oxalate. (2) To obtain blood suitable for transfusion, the anticoagulant usually being sodium citrate. (3) as a therapeutic agent in the treatment of coronary thrombosis; phlebothrombosis (thrombophlebitis), etc. when aspirin should not be given.

اینٹی کوگولینٹ : ایسا ایجنٹ جو خون کے انجماد کو کم کرتا ہے۔ بار و کتا ہے۔ انسانی جسم میں اس کی خفیف مقدار پائی جاتی ہے۔

Anticonvulsant *(an-ti-kon-vul'-sant)* [G. anti, against; L. convulsus, shaken]. An agent which stops or prevents convulsions--anticonvulsive, adj.

اینٹی کنولسینٹ : ایسا ایجنٹ جو بے ہوشی کے دوروں کو روکتا ہے۔

Anti D. Anti-Rho. A gammaglobulin (q.y.).

اینٹی ڈی اینٹی آر ایچ : ایک گاما گلوبولن۔

Antidepressant *(an-ti-de-pres'-ant)* [G. anti, against; L.depressus, from deprimere, to depress]. Name given to drugs that reduce depression. Divided into two categories; (1) Mainly for endogenous depression: imipramine (Tofranil) and amitriptyline (Tryptizol, Saroten, Laroxyl), desipramine (Pertofran), nortriptyline (Allegron, Aventyl), ancorotriptyline all have a similar action, more rapid than the MAOLs.(2) The monoamine oxidase inhabitors (Niamid, Nardil, Marplan, Actomol, Marsilid, and Parnate) prolong or increase the action of serotonin by interfering with enzyme activity; catecholamines in brain increase. Cheese potentiates these substances and must be avoided during treatment. This group are mainly for exogenous or reactive depression.

ضد مسکن: اضمحلال کم کرنے والی ادویہ۔

Antidiabetic *(an-ti-di'-ab-et-ik)* [G. anti, against; dia, through; bainein, to go]. Literally against diabetes.' Used to describe therapeutic measures in diabetes mellitus; the hormone insulin (q.v.); tolbutamide (q.v.).

دافع ذیابیطس : یونانی الفاظ اینٹی بمعنی خلاف' ڈایا بمعنی میں سے اور بینین بمعنی جانا سے ماخوذ اصطلاح ذیابیطس کے خلاف۔ ہارمون انسولن۔

Antidiphtheritic *(an-ti-dif-ther-it'-ik)* [G. anti, against; diphthera, leather, membrane]. Against diphtheria. Describes preventive measures such as immunization; therapeutic measures; serum used to give passive immunity.

دافع خناق: یونانی الفاظ اینٹی بمعنی خالف اور ڈفتھر ا بمعنی چمڑا یا جھلی سے ماخوذ اصطلاح۔ خناق کے خلاف مزاحمت یا مدافعت پیدا کرنے کے مستعمل سیرم۔

Antidiuretic *(an-ti-di-u-ret'-ik)* [G. anti, against; dia, through; ouron, urine]. Reducing the volume of urine. Against diuresis. **a. hormone,** secreted by the posterior pituitary gland. ADH. See DIABETES.

ضد پیشاب آور: یونانی الفاظ اینٹی بمعنی خلاف' ڈایا بمعنی میں سے اور اوروں بمعنی پیشاب سے ماخوذ اصطلاح پیشاب کی مقدار کم کرنے والے۔

Antidote *(an'-ti-dot)* [G. anti, against; didonai, to give]. A remedy which counteracts or neutralizes the action of poison.

تریاق : یونانی الفاظ اینٹی بمعنی خلاف اور ڈیڈونئی بمعنی دنیا سے ماخوذ اصطلاح۔ زہر کے عمل کو ختم کرنے والا۔

Antiemetic *(an-ti-e-met'-ik)* [G. anti, against; emetikos, provoking sickness]. Against emesis (q.v.). Any agent which prevents nausea and vomiting.

مانع قے۔ دافع قے: متلی قے یا الٹی روکنے والا ایجنٹ۔

Antienzyme *(an'-ti-en'-zim)* [G. anti, against; en, within; zyme, leaven]. A substance which exerts a specific inhibiting action on an enzyme. Antienzymes are found in the digestive tract to prevent digestion of its lining, in blood where they act as antibodies (q.v.).

دفع خامرہ : ایسا مادہ جو خامرہ پر عمل کر کے اسے بے اثر کر دے۔ یہ نظام انہضام میں پائے جاتے ہیں تا کہ اس نظام کا حصہ ہضم نہ ہو۔ خون میں بطور اینٹی باڈیز عمل کرتے ہیں۔

Antiepileptic *(an-ti-ep-i-lep'-tik)* [G. anti, against; epilepsis, seizure]. Name given to drugs that reduce the frequency of epileptic attacks.

دافع صرع : ایسی ادویات جو صرعی یا مرگی کے حملوں کو روکتی ہیں۔

Antifebrile *(an-ti-feb'-ril)* [G. anti, against; L. febris, fever]. Any agent which reduces or allays fever.

دافع تپ۔ دافع بخار : یونانی لفظ اینٹی بمعنی خلاف اور لاطینی لفظ فیبرس بمعنی بخار سے مرکب اصطلاح ایسا ایجنٹ جو بخار کو کم کرتا ہے۔

Antifibrinolytic *(an-ti-fi-brin-o-lit'-ik)* [G. anti, against; L. fibra, fibre; G. lysis,a loosening]. Any agent which prevents fibrinolysis (a pos sible cause of haemorrhage).

Antifols *(an'-ti-fols)* A group of substances used in combination with a sulpha drug or a dapsone as an anti malarial compound.

دافع ملیریا: ایسی اشیاء کا گروہ جو سلفا ادویہ کی ساتھ ملا کر استعمال کی جاتی ہیں اور ملیریا کے خلاف استعمال ہوتی ہیں۔

Antifungal *(an-ti-fung'-al)*. Any agent which destroys fungi.

ضد فطر : ایسا ایجنٹ جو فنجائی یا سماروغ کو تباہ کرتا ہے۔

Antigen *(an'-ti-jen)* [G. anti, against; genos, birth]. Any substance which, under favourable conditions, can stimulate the production of antibodies (q.v.) See D-VACANTIGEN--antigenic, adj.

تریاق زا۔ صد جسم زا : یونانی الفاظ اینٹی بمعنی خلاف اور جینوس بمعنی پیدائش سے ماخوذ الفاظ۔ ایسی شے جو اینٹی باڈیز کی پیداوار شروع کرتی ہے۔ یہ پروٹین میں جو خون کے سرخ جسیموں میں پائی جاتی ہے۔

Antihaemophilic globulin *(an-ti-he-mo-fil'-ik glob'-u-lin)* (AHG). Factor VIII involved in bloodclotting, present in plasma; absent from serum; deficient in haemophilia (q.v.)

اینٹی ہیموفلک گلوبولن : پلازما میں موجود خون جمنے میں ملوث ایک عامل سیرم سے غیر موجود۔

Antihaemorrhagic *(an-ti-hem'-or-aj-ik)* [G. anti, against; haima, blood; rhegnynai, to burst forth]. Any agent which prevents haemorrhage. Pertaining to vitamin K (q.v.).

اینٹی ہیموریجک : ایسا ایجنٹ جو خون کا بہاؤ روکتا ہے۔ حیاتین 'کے' سے متعلق۔

Antihistamines *(an-ti-hist'-a-menz)* [G. anti, against; histos, tissue; ammoniakon, resinous gum]. Drugs which suppress some of the effects of released histamine, and are widely used in the palliative treatment of hay fever, urticaria, angioneurotic oedema and some forms of prutitus. They also have antiemetic properties, and are effective in motion and radiation sickness. Side effects include drowsiness; which is most marked with diphenhydramine, and least with phenindamine and cyclizine.

اینٹی ہسٹامائنز : ایسی ادویات جو خارج ہونے والی ہسٹامین کے کچھ اثرات کو دبا دیتی ہے۔ حرکت اور تابکاری کی بیماری میں موثر ہے۔ الرجی' خارش' پتی اچھلنے اور ٹیکوں کے ردعمل میں مفید ہیں۔

Antihypertensive *(an-ti-hi-per-ten'-siv)* [G. anti, against; hyper, above; tenders, to stretch]. Any agent which reduces high blood pressure.

اینٹی ہائپرٹنسو : ایسا ایجنڈ جو خونی دباؤ یا بلڈ پریشر کو کم کرتا ہے۔ مثلاً سرپاسل' اڈلفین' اسے لین۔

Anti-infective [G. anti, against; L. infectus, to infect]. Any agent which prevents infection. Pertaining to vitamin A (q.v.).

اینٹی انفیکٹو : ایسا ایجنٹ جو بیماری کو روکتا ہے۔ حیاتین الف سے متعلق۔

Anti-inflammatory *(an-ti-flam'-at-o-ri)* [G. anti, against; L. inflammare, to set on fire]. Any agent which prevents inflamation.

آگ روک : یونانی لفظ اینٹی بمعنی خلاف اور لاطینی لفظ انفلیمئر بمعنی آگ لگنا سے مرکب اصطلاح۔ ایسا ایجنٹ جو آگ کو روکتا ہے۔

Antileprotic *(an-ti-lep-rot'-ik)* [G. anti, against; lepros, scaly]. Any agent which prevents or cures leprosy.

دافع کوڑھ : ایسا ایجنٹ جو جذام یا کوڑھ کو روکتا ہے یا آرام دیتا ہے۔

Antiluetic *(an-ti-loo-et'-ik)* [G. anti, against; L. lues, plague]. Any agent which prevents or cures syphilis (lues).

دافع آتشک : یونانی لفظ اینٹی بمعنی خلاف اور لاطینی لفظ لوئس بمعنی طاعون سے مرکب اصطلاح۔ ایسا ایجنٹ جو آتشک کو آرام کرتا ہے یا روکتا ہے۔

Antimalarial *(an-ti-mal-ar'-i-al)* [G. anti, against; It mala aria, bad air]. Any meausre taken to prevent or suppress malaria.

مانع ملیریا : یونانی لفظ اینٹی بمعنی خلاف اور اطالوی لفظ ملا اریا بمعنی گندی ہوا سے مرکب اصطلاح۔ ایسا اقدام جو ملیریا کو ختم کرنے کے لئے کیا جائے۔ مانع ملیریا ادویات ملیریائی طفیلی کو مارنے والی ادویات ہیں۔

Antimetabolite *(an-ti-met-ab'-ol-itz)* [G. anti, against; metabole, change]. A compound which is sufficiently similar to the chemicals needed by a cell to be incorporated into the nucleoproteins of that cell, thereby preventing its development. Examples are methotrexate, a folic acid antagonist, and mecraptopurine, a purine antagonist. They are used in the treatment of leukaemia.

اینٹی میٹابولائٹس : یونانی الفاظ اینٹی بمعنی خلاف اور میٹابول بمعنی تبدیلی سے ماخوذ اصطلاح۔ ایسے مرکبات جو خلیے کو چاہئیں لیکن وہ خلیے کی مزید تکمیل روک دیتے ہیں۔ شدید لقوے میں فولک ایسڈ، امینوپٹرن اور امیتھوپٹرن ذہنی طور پر دیئے جاتے ہیں۔

Antimicrobial *(an-ti-mi-kro'-bi-al)* [G. anti, against; mikros, small; bios, life]. Against microbes.

اینٹی مائیکروبیل : یونانی الفاظ اینٹی بمعنی خلاف، مائیکروس بمعنی چھوٹے اور بائیوس بمعنی زندگی سے ماخوذ اصطلاح۔ خوردجسیموں یا مائیکروبز کے خلاف۔

Antimigraine *(an-ti-me'-gren)*. Against migraine, e.g. Ergodryl, methysergide.

Antimitotic *(an-ti-mi-tot'-ik)* [G. anti, against; mitos, thread; -osis, condition]. Any agent which prevents reproduction of a cell by mitosis.

ضد مائیگرین : مائیگرین کے خلاف۔

Antimony and potassium tartrate *(an-tim'-on-i-pot-as'-si-um tar'-trat)*. Tartar emetic. An old drug, now used mainly in leishmaniasis (q.v.) and other tropical diseases--antimonial. adj.

سرمہ اور پوٹاشیم ٹارٹریٹ : قے آور طرطیر۔ ایک پرانی دوائی۔

Antimony lithium thiomalate *(an-tim'-on-i lith'-i-um-thi-om'-al-at)* Antibilharzial, (q.v.) Administered by intramuscular injection.

اینٹی منی لتھیم تھایومیلیٹ : ایک دوائی جس کا ٹیکہ لگایا جاتا ہے۔

Antimycotic *(an-ti-mi-kot`-ik)* [G. anti, against; *mykes,* a fungus]. Any agent which destroys fungi.

مانع فطیریت : یونانی الفاظ اینٹی بمعنی خلاف اور مائیکس بمعنی ساروغ سے ماخوذ اصطلاح ساروغ کو تباہ کرنے والا ایجنٹ

Antineuritic *(an-ti,-nu-rit`-ik)* [G. anti, against; neuron, tendon; -itis, inflammation]. Any agent which prevents neuritis. Specially applied to vitamin B complex (q.v.)

دافع التہاب عصب : اعصابی درد یا نیوریٹس کو روکنے والا ایجنٹ۔ اس کا اطلاق خصوصاً حیاتین ب کمپلیکس پر ہوتا ہے۔

Antioxidants *(an-ti-oks`-id-ants)* [G. anti, against; *oxys,* sharp]. Any substances which delay the process of oxidation.

تکسید روک : یونانی الفاظ اینٹی بمعنی خلاف اور آکسس بمعنی تیز سے ماخوذ اصطلاح۔ ایسی اشیاء جو تکسید کے عمل کو جلد نہ ہونے دیں۔ یہ نامیاتی اشیاء تکسید کے عمل کو روکتی ہیں۔

Antiparasitic *(an`-ti-par-a-sit`-ik)* [G. *anti,* against; *parasitos,* parasite]. Any agent which prevents or destroys parasites.

طفیلی کش : یونانی الفاظ اینٹی بمعنی خلاف اور پیراسٹیوس بمعنی طفیلی سے ماخوذ اصطلاح۔ ایسا ایجنٹ جو طفیلیوں کو روکتا یا تباہ کرتا ہے۔

Anti-Parkinson (ism) *(an-ti-par`-kin-sonizm)*. Name given to drugs, e.g. benzhexol, orphenadrine, that counteract the side effects of antidepressants.

اینٹی پارکنسن : یہ نام چند ایسی ادویات کو دیا گیا ہے جو اضمحلال کم کرنے والی ادویہ کے سائیڈ اثرات کو زائل کرتی ہیں۔

Antipellagra *(an-ti-pel-a`-gra)* [It. *pelle,* skin; *ogro,* rough]. Against pellagra. Pertaining to the nicotinic acid portion of vitamin B complex.

ضد پیلگرا : اطالوی لفظ پیلے بمعنی جلد یا کھال اور ایگرو بمعنی رف سے ماخوذ اصطلاح۔ پیلگرا کے خلاف۔

Antiperiodic *(an-ti-per-i-od`-ik)* [G. *anti,* against; *periodikos,* periodical]. Any agent which prevents the periodic return of a disease, e.g. the use of quinine in malaria.

ضد نوبیہ : ایسا ایجنٹ جو کسی بیماری کی واپسی کو روکتا ہے مثلاً ملیریا میں کونین کا استعمال۔

Antiperistalsis *(an-ti-pe-ri-stal`-sis)* [G. *anti,* against; *peri,* around; stalsis, constriction]. A reversal of peristaltic action--antiperistaltic, adj.

ضد حرکت انقباضی : کسی عمل کا دوبارہ ہونا۔

Antiphlogistine *(an-ti-flo-jis`-tin)* [G. *anti,* against; *phlogistos,* burnt, roasted]. A proprietary preparation containing kaolin, glycerine, antiseptic and aromatic substances. It is used for poultices, acting as an antiseptic, analgesic and counterirritant in cases of deep seated inflammation.

اینٹی فلوجسٹین : یونانی الفاظ اینٹی بمعنی خلاف اور فلوجسوس بمعنی بھنا سے ماخوذ اصطلاح۔ ایک دوا جس میں کئی اشیاء شامل ہیں۔ مثلاً کولن، گلسرین، جراثیم کش اور معطر اشیاء۔ اسے پلٹس کے لئے استعمال کیا جاتا ہے۔

Antiprothrombin *(an-ti-pro-throm'-bin).* Arrests blood clotting by preventing conversion of prothrombin into thrombin. Anticoagulant.

اینٹی پروتھرومبن : خون کے جمنے کو روکتا ہے۔ کیونکہ پروتھرومبن کو تھرومبن میں تبدیل کر دیتا ہے۔

Antipruritic *(an-ti-proo-rit'-ik)* [G. anti, against; L. pruritus, itching]. Any agent which relieves or prevents itching.

دافع خارش : ایسا ایجنٹ جو خارش یا کھجلی کو روکتا ہے یا آرام پہنچاتا ہے۔

Antipurpura *(an-ti-pur'-pu-ra)* [G. anti, against; L. purple]. Against purpura. Pertaining to vitamin P (hesperidin).

دافع پرپیورا : پرپیورا کے خلاف۔ حیاتین پی سے متعلق۔

Antipyretic *(an-ti-pi-ret'-ik)* [G. anti, against; pyretos, fever]. Any agent which allays or reduces fever.

دافع تپ (دوا) : یونانی الفاظ اینٹی بمعنی خلاف اور پائرٹوس بمعنی بخار سے ماخوذ اصطلاح۔ ایسا ایجنٹ جو بخار کو کم کرتا ہے۔ مثلاً اسپرین وغیرہ۔

Antirabic *(an-ti-ra'-bik)* [G. anti, against; L. rhabies, madness]. Any agent which prevents or cures rabies.

مانع کلب : یونانی لفظ اینٹی بمعنی خلاف اور لاطینی لفظ بمعنی پاگل پن سے ماخوذ اصطلاح۔ ایسا ایجنٹ جو پاگل پن کو آرام کرتا ہے یا اس میں کمی کر دیتا ہے۔

Antirachitic *(an-ti-rak-it'-bik)* [G. anti, against; rachis, spine]. Any agent preventing or curing rickets. Pertaining to vitamin D (q.v.).

نافع کساحت : ملاست عظام یا کساح کو آرام کرنے والا ایجنٹ حیاتین دی سے متعلق۔

Antireflux *(an-ti-re'-fluks)* [G. anti, against; L. re, back; fluxus, to flow]. Against backward flow. Usually refers to re-implantation of ureters into bladder in cases of chronic pyelonephritis (q.v.), See LEADBETTER-POLITANO OPERATION.

خلاف ری فلکس : یونانی لفظ اینٹی بمعنی خلاف، لاطینی لفظ ری بمعنی واپس اور لاطینی لفظ فلکس بمعنی بہنا سے ماخوذ اصطلاح۔ واپس بہنے کے خلاف۔

Antirheumatic *(an-ti-roo-mat'-ik)* [G. anti, against; rheuma, flow, flux]. Any agent which prevents or lessens rheumatism.

دافع گٹھیا : یونانی الفاظ اینٹی بمعنی خلاف اور ریوما بمعنی سے ماخوذ اصطلاح۔ ایجنٹ جو گٹھیا یا جوڑوں کے درد کو کم کرتا ہے یا روکتا ہے۔

Antiscorbutic *(an-ti-skawr-bu'-tik)* [G. anti, against; L. scorbutus, scurvy]. Any agent which prevents or cures scurvy (q.v.). Pertaining to vitamin C (q.v.).

دافع اسکربوط : ایسا ایجنٹ جو اسکربوط کو آرام کرتا ہے یا روکتا ہے۔ وٹامن سی سے متعلق۔

Antisecretory *(an-ti-se-cret'-o-ri)* [G. anti, against; L. secretus, separate]. Any agent which inhibits secretion.

مانع اخراج : یونانی لفظ اینٹی بمعنی خلطاف اور لاطینی لفظ سیکریٹس بمعنی علیحدہ سے ماخوذ اصطلاح۔ وہ ایجنٹ جو اخراج کو روکتا ہے۔ یعنی افراز نہ ہونے دے۔

Antisepsis *(an-ti-sep'-sis)* [G. anti, against; sepsis, decay]. The prevention of sepsis; introduced into surgery in 1880 by Lord Lister, who used carbolic acid.

دافع عفونت : سپسس کی رکاوٹ۔ لارڈ لسٹر نے ۱۸۸۰ء میں اسے سرجری میں متعارف کرایا جس نے کاربالک ایسڈ استعمال کیا۔

Antisera See SERUM.

antiseptics. Substances which destroy or inhibit the growth of micro-organisms. They can be applied to living tissues.

دافع تعفن۔ عفونت ربا۔ مانع عفونت : وہ اشیاء جو خورد جسیموں کی نشو ونما کو روکتی ہیں یا انہیں تباہ کر دیتی ہیں۔ ان کا اطلاق جاندار بافتوں پر کا کیا جاسکتا ہے۔ وہ ادویات جن سے ہم جراثیم کے عمل کو روک کر چیزوں میں بدبو پیدا ہونے سے روک سکتے ہیں۔ مثلاً بورک ایسڈ' فینول وغیرہ۔

Antisialagogue *(an-ti-si'-al-a-gog)* [G. anti, against; sialon, saliva; agogos, leading]. Inhibits salivation.

تھوک کم کرنے والی دوا : یہ لعاب دہن بننے سے روکتا ہے۔

Antiserotonin *(an-ti-se'-ro-ton-in)*. Neutralizes or lessens the effect of serotomin (q.v.), e.g. methysergid given for migraine.

دافع سیروٹونن : سیروٹونن کے اثر کو کم کرتا ہے یا زائل کرتا ہے۔

Antisocial *(an-ti-so'-shal)* [G. anti, against; L. socius, comrade]. Against society. A term used to denote a psychopathic state in which the individual cannot accept the obligations and restraints imposed on a community by its members--antisocialism, n.

سماج دشمن : سوسائٹی یا معاشرہ کے خلاف۔ ایک اصطلاح جو ایسے فرد کے لئے استعمال کی جاتی ہے جو سوسائٹی کے رسم ورواج اور قواعد وضوابط کو قبول نہ کرے۔

Antispasmodic *(an-ti-spaz-mod'-ik)* [G. anti, against; spasmos, spasm]. Any measure used to relieve spasm occuring in muscle.

دافع تشنج : ایسا اقدام جو عضلے میں سپازم کو آرام پہنچائے۔

Antistatic *(an-ti-stat'-ik)* [G. anti, against; statikos, causing to stand]. Any measures taken to prevent or deal with the collection of static electricity.

اینٹی سٹیٹک : یونانی الفاظ اینٹی بمعنی خلاف اور سٹیٹیکوس بمعنی کھڑا کرنا سے ماخوذ اصطلاح۔ ایسے اقدام جو برق سکونی کے جمع کرنے متعلق ہوں یا روکتے ہوں۔

Antisterility *(an-ti-ster-il'-it-i)* [G. anti, against; L. sterilitas, infertile]. Pertaining to vitamin E (q.v.).

دافع بانجھ پن : یونانی لفظ اینٹی بمعنی خلاف اور لاطینی لفظ سٹیریلیٹس بمعنی بانجھ سے مرکب اصطلاح۔ وٹامن ای سے متعلق۔

Antistin *(an-tis'-tin)*.Antazoline, one of the milder antihistamines (q.v.).

اینٹس ٹین : اینٹازولین۔ معمولی محرک برائے حس۔

Antistreptolysin *(an-ti-strep-to-li'sın)* [G. anti, against; streptos, curved; lysis, a lossening]. Against streptolysin, (q.v.). A raised antistreptolysin titre in the blood is indicative of recent streptococcal infection.

دافع سٹرپٹولائی سن : یونانی الفاظ اینٹی بمعنی خلاف' سٹرپٹوس بمعنی خمیدہ اور لائیسس بمعنی ڈھیلا سے ماخوذ اصطلاح۔ سٹرپٹولائیسین کے خلاف۔

Antisyphilitc *(an-ti-sif-il-it'-ik)*. Any measures taken to combat syphilis (q.v.).

دافع آتشک : آتشک کا مقابلہ کرنے کے لئے اقدامات۔

Antithrombin *(an-ti-throm'-bin)* [G. anti, against; thrombos, clot]. Antithrombin or antithrombins are substances occuring naturally in the blood, e.g. heparin. See THROMBIN.

مانع دلمہ مادہ : یہ خون میں قدرتی طور پر پائی جاتی ہے۔

Antithrombotic *(an-ti-throm-bot'-ik)* [G. anti, against; thrombos, clot]. Any measures that prevent or cure thrombosis.

اینٹی تھرومبوٹک : تھرمبوس کو روکنے والے اقدامات۔

Antithyroid *(an-ti-thi'-roid)* [G. anti, against; thureoeides, sheild-shaped]. Any agent used to decrease the activity of the thyroid gland.

اینٹی تھائیرائڈ : تھائیرائڈ گلینڈ کی عاملیت کم کرنے والا ایجنٹ۔

Antitoxic sera *(an-ti-toks'-ik-se'-ra)*. The serum of horses which have been immunized by injections of pathogenic bacterial toxins, such as tetanus and gas gangrene. Such serum contains antib- odies or antitoxins, and after injection confers a temporary immunity against the original toxin. The therapeutic use of antitoxic sera declined after the discovery of the sulph- onamides and antibiotics.

ضد سمیات خون آب : جراثیموں کے زہر کو ختم کرنے کے لئے سیرم جو گھوڑے کا ہوتا ہے۔

Antioxin *(an-ti-toks'-in)* [G. anti, against; toxikon, poison]. An agent which neutralizes a given toxin. It is elaborated in the body, in direct response to the invasion by bacteria, or the injection of a small dose of treated toxin--antitoxic, adj.

ضد سمیات ۔ انٹی ٹاکسن ۔ مانع سمیت : یونانی الفاظ اینٹی بمعنی خلاف اور ٹوکسیکون بمعنی زہر سے ماخوذ اصطلاح ۔ انسانی خون میں کچھ کیمیائی مادے ٹاکسن کے اثر کی تعدیل کرتے ہیں جنھیں اینٹی ٹاکسن کہتے ہیں۔

Antituberculosis *(an'-ti-tu-ber-ku-lo'-sis)*. Any measures used to prevent or cure tuberculosis--antitubercular, adj.

مانع تپ دق : تپ دق کو آرام کرنے یا روکنے والے اقدامات۔

Antitumour *(an-ti-tu'-mor)* [G. anti, against; L.]. Against tumour formation, Inhibits growth of tumour.

مانع رسولی: رسولی بننے کے خلاف ۔ رسولی کی نشو ونما کو روکتا ہے۔

Antitussive *(an-ti-tew-siv)* [G. *anti,* against; L. *tasus,* cough]. Pre-cautions to cough.

دافع کھانسی : یونانی لفظ اینٹی بمعنی خلاف اور لاطینی لفظ ٹسس بمعنی کھانسی سے مرکب اصطلاح ۔ کھانسی کو دبانے والے اقدامات۔

Antivenin *(an-ti-ven'-in)* [G. anti, against; L. venenum, poison]. A serum prepared from animals injected with the venom of snakes; used as an antidote in cases of poisoning by snakebite.

تریاق زہر مار : یونانی لفظ اینٹی بمعنی خلاف اور لاطینی لفظ وینیم بمعنی زہر سے مرکب اصطلاح ۔ جانوروں سے تیار شدہ سیرم جسے سانپوں کے زہر کے ساتھ جسم میں داخل کیا جاتا ہے ۔ سانپ کے کاٹنے سے زہر کا تریاق۔

Antiviral *(an-ti-vi-ral)* [G. anti, against; L. virus, poison]. Acting against viruses.

ضد وائرس : یونانی لفظ اینٹی بمعنی خلاف اور لاطینی لفظ وائرس بمعنی زہر سے مرکب اصطلاح ۔ وائرس کے خلاف عمل۔

Antivitamin *(an-ti-vit'-a-min)* [G. anti, against; L. vita, life; ammoniacum, resinous gum].A substance interfering with the absorption or utilization of a vitamin, e.g. avidin.

ضد وٹامن : ایسی شے جو وٹامن کے استعمال یا انجذاب میں مداخلت کرے۔

Antrectomy *(an-trek'-to-mi)* [G. antron, cave; eklome, exision]. Excision of pyloric antrum of stomach thus removing the source of the hormone gestrin in the treatment of duodenal ulcer.

مغارہ برآری : معدہ کا پائیلورک سرے کا قطع ہونا۔

Antrenyl *(an'-tren-il)* Oxyphenonium. An antispasmodic (q.v.).

اینٹرینل : آکسی فینونیم۔

Antrobuccal *(an-tro-buk'-al)* [G. antron, cave; L. bucca, cheek]. Pertaining to the maxillary antrum and the mouth. **a. fistula** can occur after extraction of an upper molar tooth, the root of which has protruded into the floor of the antrum.

مغاری دہنی : یونانی لفظ انٹرون بمعنی غار اور لاطینی لفظ بکا بمعنی رخسار سے ماخوذ اصطلاح ۔ منہ سے متعلق۔

Antrostomy *(an-tros'-to-mi)* [G. antron, cave; stoma, mouth]. An artificial opening from nasal cavity to antrum of Highmore (maxillary sinus) for the purpose of drainage.

مغاری تفویہ : یونانی الفاظ انٹرون بمعنی غار اور سٹوما بمعنی منہ سے ماخوذ اصطلاح ۔ ناک کے کہفہ میں ایک عارضی سوراخ۔

Antrum *(an'-trum)* [L.]. A cavity especially in a bone, e.g. the **a. of Highmore** in the superior maxillary bone--antral, adj. [Nathaniel Highmore, English physician, 1613-85].

مغارہ : لاطینی لفظ ۔ ایک کہفہ یا جوف ۔ خاص طور پر ہڈی میں۔

Antrypol *(an'-tri-pol)* Suramin (q.v.).

اینٹری پول : دیکھئے سرامن۔

Antuitrin *(an'-tu-it-rin)*. Proprietary extract of the anterior pituitary gland.

پیش نخامین : اگلی پیٹوایٹری گلینڈ کا ست۔

Anturan *(an'-tu-an)*. Sulphinpyrazone (q.v.).

انٹورین : دیکھئے سلفن پائیرازون۔

Anuria *(an-u'-ri-a)* [G. a-, not; ouron, urine]. Absence of secretion of urine by the kidneys. See SUPPRESSION--anuric, adj.

لمبی پیشاب : یونانی الفاظ اے بمعنی بغیر اور ورن بمعنی پیشاب سے ماخوذ اصطلاح ۔ گردوں سے پیشاب کے افراز کی غیر موجودگی ۔ پیشاب کم آنا یا بالکل نہ آنا۔

Anus *(a'-nus)* [L.]. The end of the alimentary canal, at the extreme termination of the rectrum. It is formed of a sphincter muscle which relaxes to allow faecal matter to pass through. **artifical a.,** one produced surgically in some higher part of the bowel in cases of obstruction through any cause. **imperforate a.,** one which has not opening; atresia ani. It is often due to a congenital defect--anal, adj.

سندانی ہڈی :انکس۔درمیانی کان کی تین چھوٹی ہڈیوں میں سے درمیان والی۔

Anxiety *(ang-zi'-et-i)* [L. anxiotas, anxiety]. Feelings of fear, apprehension **a. state,** a neurosis characterized by recurrent acute anxiety attacks (panies). The attacks consist of all the sings and symptoms of fear, leading up to fear of impending collapse and some times death. **'free floating a.** is used to indicate that the apprehension has no source in the external world.

تشویش :لاطینی زبان کالفظ اینگزیٹاس جس کے معنی ہیں پریشانی سے ماخوذ اصطلاح۔خوف یاڈر کا احساس۔تجسس۔

Anxiolytics *(ang-zi-o-lit'-iks)* [L. anxietas, anxiety; G. lysis, a lossening]. Agents that reduce anxiety.

دافع تشویش :بےقراری یاپریشانی کوکم کرنے والے ایجنٹس۔

Aorta *(a-or'-ta)* [G. aorte, the great artery]. The main artery arising out of the left ventricle of the heart.

Aorta

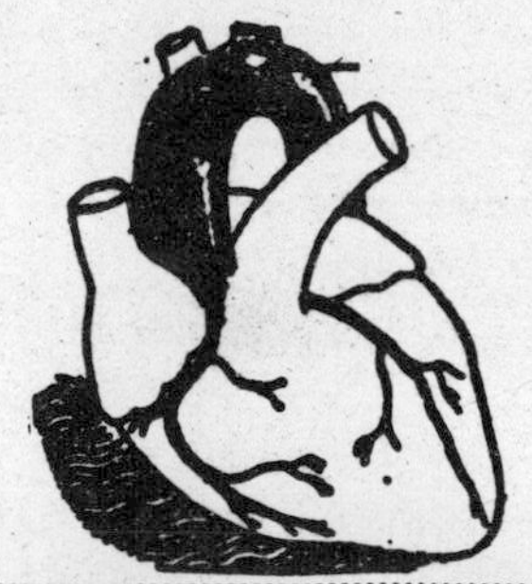

ایورٹا۔اورطہ۔شریان کبیر :یونانی لفظ ایورٹے سے ماخوذ جس کے معنی عظیم شریان ہیں۔دل کے بائیں بطین سے ابھرنے والی بڑی شریان۔

Aortic *(a-or'-tik)* [G. aorte, great artery].. Pertaining to the aorta. **a. aneurysm** see ANEURYSM. **a. incompetence,** regurgitation, resulting from rheumatic or syphilitic disease and allowing reflux of blood from aorta back into the left ventricle. **a. murmur,** abnormal heart sound heard over aortic area; a systolic murmur alone is aortic stenosis, a diastolic, the murmur of aortic incompetence. Advanced syphilitic valvular disease causes abnormality of both the first and second sounds, the so-called 'to and fro' aortic murmur. **a. stenosis,** narrowing of aortic valve found as result of rheumatic heart disease. The aortic valve can also be damaged by the presence of a congenital bicuspid valve which predisposes to the deposit of calcium; by syphilitic aortitis, ankylosing spondylitis, and in Marfan's syndrom where there is deficiency of elastic tissue.

اورطی :ایورٹا سے متعلق۔

Aortitis *(a-or-ti'-tis)* [G. aorte, great artery; -itis, inflammation]. Inflammation of the aorta.

ورم اورطہ : یونانی الفاظ ایورٹے بمعنی عظیم شریان اور ائٹس بمعنی تورم یا سوزش سے ماخوذ اصطلاح ایورٹا کی سوزش یا جلن۔

Aortogram *(a-or'-to-gram)*. See ARTERIOGRAM.

آؤرطوگرام : دیکھئے آرٹیریوگرام۔دل کی حرکات کا جائزہ لینے کے لیے برقی آلہ مثلاً ای سی جی الیکٹروکارڈیوگرام۔

Aortography *(a-or-tog'-raf-i)* See ARTERIOGRAPHY--aortographic, adj.; aortographically, adv.

آؤرطوگرافی :دیکھئے آرٹیریوگرافی۔

Apathy *(a'-pa-thi)* [G. a-, without; pathos, feeling]. In psychiatry abnormal listlessness and lack of activity--apathetic, adj.

بے حسی: یونانی الفاظ اے بمعنی بغیر اور پیتھوس بمعنی احساس سے ماخوذ اصطلاح۔طب دماغی میں سرگرمی کی کمی۔جذبات سے عاری۔

Aperients *(a-per'-i-ents)*. [L. aperire, to open]. Drugs which stimulate evacuation of the bowel. May be further classified as lubricants, laxatives, purgatives and drastic purgative (q.v.).

ملیں (دوائیں) :لاطینی لفظ اپرائر بمعنی کھولنا سے ماخوذ اصطلاح۔ادویات جن سے قبض دور ہوتی ہے۔

Aperistalsis *(a-per-is-tal'-sis)* [G. a-, not; peri, around; stalsis, constriction]. Absence of peristaltic movement in the bowel. Characterizes the condition of paralytic ileus (q.v.)--aperistaltic, adj.

عدم حرکت ویرانی : آنت میں پیرسٹالٹک حرکت کی غیر موجودگی۔

Apert's syndrome *(ap-ertz)*. Congenital craniosyntosis (q.v.) accompanied by deformities of the hands, syndactyly. [Eugene Apert, Paris paediatrician, [1868-1940].

Apex *(a'-peks)* [L. the extreme end]. The summit or top of anything which is cone-shaped. **a. beat,** in a heart of normal size the a. beat (systolic impulse) can be seen or felt in the 5th left intercostal space in the mid-clavicular line. It is the lowest and most lateral point at which an impulse can be detected and provides a rough indication of the size of the heart--apical, adj.; apices, pl.

راس : لاطینی لفظ جس کے معنی آخری سرا ہیں۔ مخروط کا بالائی سرا یا اوپر کا سرا۔ دل کی دھڑکن۔

Apgar score *(ap'-gar)*. Introduced by Dr. Virginia Apgar in 1952. Used for assessing the newborn. Numerical values are given to; Appearance--colour; Pulse--heart rate; Grimac-certain reflexes; Activity--tone; Respiration--breathing.

اپگار سکور : نئے پیدا ہونے والے بچے کا اندازہ لگانے کے لئے مستعمل۔ اس کی شکل، رنگت، دل کی دھڑکن کی شرح، تنفس وغیرہ۔

Aphagia *(a-fa'-ji-a)* [G. a-, not; phakos, lentil]. Absence of the crystalline lensaphakic, adj.

لاعدسیت : قلمی عدسے غیر موجودگی۔

Aphasia *(a-fa'-zi-a)* [G. a-, not phasis, speech]. Disorder of speech due to a brain lesion. There are many recognized varieties. **motor a.,** loss of ability to articulate **sensory a.,** loss of power to recognize the written or spoken word. Aphasia is defined by the College of Speech. Therapy as the absence of recognition and use of verbal expression due to impairment of the dominant cerebral hemisphere subserving the special intellectual functions concerned with the use of language--aphasic, adj.

فتور نطق : یونانی الفاظ اے بمعنی بغیر اور فیسس بمعنی تقریر سے ماخوذ اصطلاح۔ دماغی خلل کی وجہ سے تقریر نہ کر سکنا۔ بے ربط گفتگو۔

Aphonia *(a-fo'-ni-a)* [G. a-, not; phone, voice]. Loss of voice from a cause other than a cerebral lesion--aphonic, adj.

بے صوتی۔ فقدان آواز : یونانی الفاظ بمعنی بغیر اور فون بمعنی آواز سے ماخوذ اصطلاح۔ آواز کا ضیاع۔

Aphrodisiac *(af-ro-diz'-i-ak)*. An agent which stimulates sexual excitement.

شہوت انگیز۔ مبہی (دوا) : ایسا ایجنٹ جو جنسی جوش پیدا کرے۔

Aphthae *(af'-the)* [G. thrush]. Small grey areas surrounded by a ring of erythema; they occur in the mouth; ulceration is inevitable.

برفک۔ قلاع (مرض) : منہ میں واقع خاکی دھبے۔

Apicectomy *(ap-i-sek'-to-me)* [L. apex, top; G. ektome, excision]. Excision of the root of a tooth.

سن راس برآری : لاطینی لفظ ایپکس بمعنی چوٹی یا بالائی سرا اور یونانی لفظ ایکٹوم بمعنی قطع سے مرکب اصطلاح۔ دانت کی جڑ کا اخراج۔

Apicolysis *(ap-ik-ol'-i-sis)* [L. apex, top; G. lysis, a loosening]. The parietal pleura is stripped from the upper chest wall to ensure collapse of the lung apex when it contains a tuberculous cavity.

اس ریہ پاشی : بالائی چھاتی کی دیوار سے بغلی پلیورا کو چھیل دیا جاتا ہے۔

Aplasia *(a-pla'-zi-a)* [G. a-, not plassein, to form]. Incomplete development of tissue; absence of growth.

فطری ذبول : کسی بافت یا نسیج کی نامکمل تکمیل۔ نشوونما کی غیر موجودگی۔

Aplastic *(a-plas'-tik)* [G. a-, not; plassein, to form]. 1. Without structure or form. 2. Incapable of forming new tissue. **a.**

بے صورت۔ غیر تکوینی : یونانی الفاظ اے بمعنی نہیں اور پلیسین بمعنی بنا سے ماخوذ اصطلاح۔ (۱) ساخت کے بغیر۔ (۲) نئی بافت بنانے کے ناقابل۔

Anaemia, the result of complete bone marrow failure.

Apnoea *(ap-ne'-a)* [G. a-, not pnein, to breathe]. A transitory cessation of breathing as seen in Cheyne-Stokes respiration (q.v.). It is due to lack of the necessary CO_2 tension in the blood for stimulation of the respiratory centre--apnoeic, adj.

حبس دم : سانس کی عبوری بندش۔ یہ خون میں کاربن ڈائی آکسائیڈ کی کمی کی وجہ سے ہوتی ہے۔ کیونکہ تنفسی مرکز کو تحریک نہیں ہوتی۔

Apocrine *(ap'-o-krin)* [G. apo, from; krinein, to separate]. Modified sweat glands, especially in axillae, genital and perineal regions. Responsible after puberty for body odour.

بدر غدہ : یونانی الفاظ اپیو بمعنی سے اور کرینین بمعنی الگ کرنا سے ماخوذ اصطلاح۔ ترمیم شدہ پسینے کی غدود۔ جسمانی بو کی ذمہ دار۔

Apodia *(a-po'-di-a)* [G. a-, not pous, foot]. Congenital absence of the feet.

بے پائی : یونانی الفاظ اے بمعنی بغیر اور پاؤس بمعنی پاؤں سے ماخوذ اصطلاح۔ پاؤں کی غیر موجودگی۔

Apomorphine *(a-po-mor'-fen)*. Powerful emetic when injected. Effective when gastric irritant emetics are useless, as in phenol poisoning.

مارفین نما : طاقتور قے آور دوا۔ ایک قلمی الکلائڈ جو مارفین سے اخذ کیا جاتا ہے۔

Aponearosis *(ap-o-nu-ro'-sis)* [G. apo, from; neuron, tendon;-osis, condition]. A broad glistening sheet of tendon-like tissue which serves to invest and attach muscles to each other, and also to the parts which they move--aponeuroses, pl.; aponeurotic, adj.

اپیونیوروسس۔ صفاق : ٹنڈان نما بافت کی ایک چوڑی چمکیلی شیٹ۔

Aponeurositis *(ap-o-nu-ro-si'-tis)* [G. apo, from; neuron, tendon;-osis, condition; -itis, inflammation]. Inflammation of a aponeurosis.

ورم صفاق : اپیونیوروسس کی سوزش۔

Apophysis *(ap-of'-is-is)* [G.]. A projection, protuberance or outgrowth. Usually used in connection with bone.

برون نامیہ : یونانی لفظ ابھار۔ بڑھاؤ۔ عموماً ہڈی سے متعلق استعمال کیا جاتا ہے۔

Apoplexy *(ap-o-pleks'-i)* [G. apoplessein, to cripple by a stroke]. Stroke, Sudden unconsciousness usually caused by cerebral embolism, haemorrhage, or thrombosis. There is stertorous breathing, incontinence of urine and faeces and a varying degree of hemiplegia (q.v.)--apoplectic, apoplectiform. adj.

سکتہ۔ فالج : سٹروک۔ اچانک بے ہوشی۔ مرگی۔ دماغ کی رگ پھٹ جانا۔

Appendicectomy *(ap-pen-di-sek'-to-mi)* [L. appendix, appendage; G. ektome, excision]. Excision of the appendix vermiformis (q.v.).

زائد براری : اپنڈکس یا زائد آنت کا قطع۔

Appendicitis *(ap-pen-di-si'-tis)* [L. appendix, appendage; G. -itis, inflammation]. Inflammation of the appendix vermiformis (q.v.).

ورم زائدہ : لاطینی لفظ اپنڈکس بمعنی زائدہ اور یونانی لفظ ائٹس بمعنی سوزش سے مرکب اصطلاح۔

Appendicostomy *(ap-pen-di-kos'-to-mi)* [L. appendix, appendage; G. stoma, mouth]. An operation in which the appendix is brought to the surface and an opening made into it. This admits a catheter via which the large bowel can be irrigated.

زائدی تفوییہ : لاطینی لفظ اپنڈکس بمعنی زائدہ اور یونانی لفظ سٹوما بمعنی منہ سے مرکب اصطلاح۔ ایک اپریشن جس میں اپنڈکس کو سطح پر لایا جاتا ہے اور اس میں ایک سوراخ کیا جاتا ہے۔ اس میں سے کیتھیٹر کو گزارتے ہیں جس کے ذریعہ بڑی آنت کو دھویا جاتا ہے۔

Appendix *(ap-pen'-diks)* [L.]. An appendage. **a. vermiformis,** a worm-like appendage of the caecum about the thickness of a pencil and usually measuring from 50.8 to 152.4 mm in length. Its position is variable and it is apparently functionless--appendices, pl.; appendicular, adj.

ضمیمہ۔ زائدہ اعور : لاطینی لفظ ایک زائدہ۔ چھوٹی آنت جو کہ آدمی میں تکلیف کا باعث بنتی ہے۔ سیکم کا کیڑا نما زائدہ جس کی موٹائی پنسل جتنی ہوتی ہے اور لمبائی ۵۰٫۸ تا ۱۵۲٫۴ ملی میٹر ہوتی ہے۔ یہ ظاہری طور پر بے فائدہ ہے۔

Apperception *(ap-per-sep'-shun)* [L. ad, to; percipere, to perceive]. Clear perception of a sensory stimulus, in particular where there is identification or recognition--apperceptive, adj.

ادراک۔ نفس شناسی : سنسری تحریک کا صاف دکھائی دینا۔

Applicator *(ap'-li-ka-tor)* [L. applicare, to apply]. An instrument for applying local remedies, e.g. radium.

ملساق : مقامی ادویات لگانے کا آلہ۔

pposition *(ap-o-zish'-un)* [L. ad, to; ponere, to place]. The approximation or bringing together of two surfaces or edges.

اضافہ : دوسطوح یا کناروں کو اکٹھے لانا۔

praxia *(a-praks'-i-a)* [G. a-, not; prassein, to do]. Inability to deal effectively with or manipulate objects as a result of a brain lesion--apraxic, apractic, adj.

فاسد فعلی ۔ بے بصیرتی : یونانی الفاظ اے بمعنی نہیں اور پریسین بمعنی کرنا سے ماخوذ اصطلاح۔ موثر طور پر نبٹنے کے ناقابل۔

prinox *(ap'-rin-oks)* Bendrofluazide (q.v.).

اپیری نوکس : دیکھئے بینڈروفلوازائیڈ۔ ہائپرٹینشن یا بلڈ پریشر اور جگہ کی سختی میں اس کی ایک گولی روزانہ ناشتہ کے بعد۔

protinin *(a-pro'-tin-in)* Concentrated extract of bovine lung tissue. Acts as a strong protease inhibitor. Useful in acute pancreatitis, hyperplasminaemia and as prophylaxis in pancreatic surgery.

اپروٹینین : بووین پھیپھڑوں کے نسیج کا مرتکز ست۔ بیل کے پھیپھڑوں سے حاصل کردہ جوہر پتے کے درد میں مفید۔

PT. Alum precipitated diphtheria toxoid. A diphtheria prophylactic used mainly for children.

اے پی ٹی: پھٹکڑی یا ایلم جو خناق میں بچوں کو دیا جاتا ہے۔ پھٹکڑی سے حاصل ہوا رسوب۔

ptin *(ap'-tin).* Alprenolol (q.v.).

ptitude *(ap'-ti-tud).* Natural ability and facility in performing tasks, either mental or physical.

رغبت ۔ صلاحیت: جسمانی یا ذہنی کام کرنے کی قدرتی اہلیت۔

pyrexia *(a-pi-reks'i-a)* [G. a-, not pyretos, fever]. Absence of fever--anyrexial, adj.

عدم تپ رفع بخار : یونانی الفاظ اے بمعنی بغیر یا نہیں اور پائرٹوس بمعنی بخار سے ماخوذ اصطلاح۔ بخار کی غیر موجودگی۔

pyrogen *(a-pi'-ro-jen)* A brand of sterile distilled water in hermetically sealed ampoules. It is free from pyrogen (q.v.). Used to make up drugs supplied in powder form, when they are to be given by injection.

ایپائیروجن : بند شیشوں میں کشید شدہ پانی۔ اس میں پائیروجن نہیں ہوتی۔ ٹیکہ تیار کرنے کے لئے سفوف کو اس پانی میں حل کیا جاتا ہے۔

Aqua *(ak'-wa)* [L.]. Water. **a. destillata.** distilled water. **a. fortis,** nitric acid. **a. menthae piperitae,** peppermint water.

عرق ۔ آب ۔ پانی : لاطینی لفظ۔ پانی۔ آب مقطر۔ شورے کا تیزاب عرق پودینہ۔

Aquamephyton *(ak-wa-mef'-i-ton).* Vitamin K. Antagonist to anticoagulants (not heparin).

Aquamox *(ak'-wa-mocks)* Quinethazone. See CHOLOROTHIAZIDE.

Aqueduct *(ak'-wi-dukt)* [L. aqua, water; ducere, to lead]. A canal. **a. of sylvius,** the canal connecting the 3rd and 4th ventricles of the brain; aqueductus cerebri. [Francois Sylvius de la Boe, French anatomist, [1614-72].

قنات آبی : ایک قنال۔ دماغ کے تیسرے اور چوتھے کہفے کو جوڑنے والی قنال۔

Aqueous *(a'-kwi-us)* [L. aqua, water]. Watery. **a. humor,** the fluid contained in the anterior and posterior chambers of the eye.

آبی : پانی والا۔ پانی میں تیار کیا ہوا محلول۔ لاطینی ایکوا بمعنی پانی سے ماخوذ اصطلاح۔ آنکھوں کا پانی۔ آنسو۔ آبی ہیومر آنکھ میں عدسہ اور قورینہ کے درمیان پانی۔

Ara-C. See CYTOSINE ARABINOSIDE.

Arachidonic Acid *(ar-ak'-ik-on-ik as'-id).* One of the essential fatty acids. Found in small amounts in human and animal liver and organ fats. A growth factor.

اریکی ڈونک ایسڈ :لازمی فیٹی ایسڈ میں سے ایک۔ انسانی اور حیوانی جگر میں معمولی مقدار میں پایا جاتا ہے۔

Arachis oil *(ar'-ak-is).* Oil expressed from groundnuts. Similar to olive oil.

مونگ پھلی کا تیل : مونگ پھلیوں سے نکالا ہوا تیل۔ مونگ پھلی کا پودا پیپلیونیسی خاندان کا رکن ہے۔

Arachnodactyly *(a-rak-no-dakt'-il-i)* [G. arachne, spider; daktylos, finger]. Congenital abnormality resulting in spider fingers.

عنکب انگشتی :یونانی الفاظ ارکنے بمعنی مکڑی اور ڈیکٹائیلوس بمعنی انگلی سے ماخوذ اصطلاح۔ معمول کے خلاف جو مکڑی انگلیوں میں منتج ہوتا ہے۔

Arachnoid *(ar-ak'-noid)* [G. arachne, spider; eidos, form]. Resembling a spider's web. **a. membrane,** a delicate membrane enveloping the brain and spinal cord, lying between the pia mater internally and the dura mater externally; the middle serous membrane of the meninges--arachnoidal, adj.

غشاء عنکبوتی : مکڑی کے جالے سے مشابہہ۔

Aramine Metaraminol (q.v.).

Arborization *(ar-bor-i-za'-shun)* [L. arbor, tree]. An arrangement resembling the branching of a tree. Characterizes both ends of neurone, i.e. the dendrons and the axon as it supplies each muscle fibre.

تشجر : لاطینی لفظ آربر بمعنی درخت سے ماخوذ۔ درخت کی شاخ داری سے مشابہ ترتیب۔

Arboviruses *(ar-bo-vi'-rus-es)* [L. arbor, tree; L. poison]. An abbreviation for viruses transmitted by arthropods. Members of the mosquito-borne group include yellow fever, dengue and viruses causing infections of the CNS. Sandflies transmit sandfly fever. The tickborne viruses can cause haemorrhagic fevers.

آربووائرس : آرتھروپوڈا کے ذریعہ پھیلنے وائرس۔

Arcus Senilis *(ar'-kus-sen-il'-is)* [L. arcus, an arch; L. senilis, aged]. An opaque ring round the edge of the cornea, seen in old people.

قوس پیری : لاطینی الفاظ آرکس بمعنی قوس اور سنیلس بمعنی معمر الفاظ کا مجموعہ۔ معمر لوگوں میں پایا جانے والا قرینہ کے کنارے کے گرد ایک غیر شفاف چھلا۔

Areola *(ar-e'-o-la)* [L. area, area]. The pigmented area round the nipple of the breast. **secondary a.,** a dark circle of pigmentation which surrounds the primary areola in pregnancy--areolar, adj.

اریولا۔ ہالہ۔ ہالیزہ : لاطینی لفظ اریا بمعنی ایریا یا علاقہ سے ماخوذ لفظ۔ پستان کے نپل کے گرد پگمنٹ والا ایریا۔ ثانوی اریولا سے مراد پگمنٹیشن کا سیاہ دائرہ جو وضع حمل میں اولی اریولا کے گرد ہوتا ہے۔ عورت کی چھاتیوں کے نپل کے گرد نیلا نشان۔

ARF. Acute respiratory failure. See RESPIRATORY FAILURE.

Arfonad *(ar-fo-nad')*. Trimetaphan (q.v.).

رفونیڈ : مختصر العمل بلاک کرنے والا ایجنٹ۔

Arginase *(ar'-jin-az)*. An enzyme found in the liver, kidney and spleen. It splits arginine into ornithine and urea.

رجی نیز: جگر، گردے اور سپلین یا تلی میں پایا جانے والا خامرہ۔ یہ آرجنین لو اور نتھین اور یوریا میں تبدیل کر دیتا ہے۔

Arginine *(ar'-jin-en)*. One of the essential amin acids (q.v.). Used in treatment of acute live failure to tide patient over acute ammoni intoxication.

رجی نینوسکسی نیوریا : پیشاب میں آرجنین اور سکسینک ایسڈ کی وجودگی۔

Argyll Robertsonpupil *(ar-gil' rob'-ert-son)* One which reacts to accommodation, but no to light. Diagnostic sign in neurosyphilis, bu not all examples are syphilitic. Other impor tant causes include disseminated sclerosis an diabetes mellitus. In the non-syphilitic grou the pupil is not small, but often dilated an unequal and is called atypical. {D.M.C.L. Ar gyll Robertson, Scottish physician 1837-1909].

رگائیل رابرٹ سن پتلی : تطبیق کے خلاف ردعمل کرنے والا لیکن وشنی کے خلاف نہیں۔ عصبی آتشک کی نمایاں علامت دماغی امراض میں پتلی لی بے قراری۔

Ariboflavinosis *(a-ri'-bo-flav-in-os'-is)* [G. a- not L. ribes, currant; flavus, yellow; G. -osis condition]. A deficiency state caused by lac of riboflavine and other members of th vitamin B complex. Characterized b cheilosis, seborrhoea, angular stomatitis, glc ssitis and photophobia.

یبوفلیوی نوسس : ریبوفلیون اور وٹامن بی کمپلیکس کے دوسرے ارکان کی می سے ہونے والی کمی کی شکایت۔ ان کی کمی سے کئی امراض ہو جاتے ہیں۔

Arithmomania *(ar-ith-mo-ma'-ni-a)* [G. ar thmos, number; mania, madness]. A form c insanity in which there is an obsession wit numbers.

ارمانیا : یونانی الفاظ ارتھموس بمعنی عدد اور مانیا بمعنی پاگل پن سے ماخوذ طلاح۔ پاگل پن کی ایک قسم جس میں اعداد کے متعلق صحیح پتہ نہیں چلتا۔

Arlef *(ar'-lef)*. Flufenamic acid (q.v.).

Arrectores Pilorum *(ar-ek'-tor-ez-pi-lor-um)* [L. arrectus from; arrigere, to erect]. Internal, plain.

موخیز (عضلات) : لاطینی الفاظ اریکٹس بمعنی سے اریجیر بمعنی سیدھا کرنا سے ماخوذ اصطلاح۔ اندرونی پلین غیر ارادی عضلات جو بالوں کے فولیکلو کے ساتھ ملحق ہوتے ہیں۔ جو سکڑ کر فولیکلو کو سیدھا کرتے ہیں۔ اس طرح رونگٹے کھڑے ہو جاتے ہیں۔

Arrhenoblastoma *(a-ren-o-blas-to'-ma)* [G. arren, male; blastos, germ; -oma, tumour]. A masculinizing tumour of the ovary.

ارینو بلاسٹوما : یونانی الفاظ ارن بمعنی نر بلاسٹوس بمعنی جرثومہ اور اوما بمعنی رسولی سے ماخوذ اصطلاح بیضہ دان کی رسولی کی ایک قسم۔ اس سے عورت میں مردانہ خواص پیدا ہو جاتے ہیں۔

Arteriectomy *(ár-ter-i-ek'-to-mi)* [L. arteria, artery; G. aktome, excision]. Excision of an artery or more usually part of an artery.

Arrhythmia *(a-rith'-mi-a)* [G. a-, not; rhythmos, rhythm]. Any deviation from rhythm, e.g. of the heart. **sinus a.**, increase of the pulse rate on inspiration, dec- rease on expiration. Appears to be normal in some children.

آرتھمیا : معمول کی ردم سے ہٹاؤ۔ مثلاً دل کی دھڑکن۔

Arruga suture *(a-ru'-ga)*. Purse-string suture placed around eye in the treatment of detached retina.

آروگا سیوچر : ریٹنا کے علیحدہ ہونے کی صورت میں آنکھ کے گرد پرس کی ڈوری ایسا سیوچر۔

Arsenic *(ar'-se-nik)*. Occasionally used with iron as a tonic. Usually prescribed as Fowler's solution or liquor arsenicalis. See NEOARSPHENAMINE.

سنکھیا : بعض اوقات لوہے کے ساتھ ملا کر ٹانک کے طور پر استعمال کیا جاتا ہے۔ سنکھیا کا ست جوہری عدد ۳۳۔

Artane *(ar'-tan)*. Benzhexo! (q.v.).

آرٹین : دیکھئے بینز ہکیسول۔ اس کی ایک گولی صبح ایک دوپہر ایک شام برائے علاج پارکن سونزم یعنی رعشہ۔

Artefact *(art'-i-fakt)* [L. ars, art; factus, made]. Any artificial product resulting from a physical or chemical agency; an unnatural change in a structure or tissue.

مصنوعہ : لاطینی الفاظ آرس بمعنی آرٹ اور فیکٹس بمعنی بنا ہوا سے ماخوذ اصطلاح۔ کسی ساخت یا بافت میں غیر قدرتی تبدیلی۔

Arteralgia *(ar-ter-al'-ji-a)* [L. arteria, artery; G. algos, pain]. Pain in an artery.

آرٹیریلجیا : لاطینی لفظ آرٹیریا بمعنی شریان اور یونانی لفظ الجوس بمعنی درد سے مرکب اصطلاح۔ شریان میں درد۔

Arteriogram *(ar-ter'-i-o-gram)* [L. arteria, artery; G. gramma, letter]. Film demonstrating arteries after injection of opaque medium.

شریان نگارش : غیر شفاف واسطے کے انجکشن کے بعد شریانوں کا مظاہرہ کرنے والی فلم۔

Arteriography *(ar-ter-i-og'-raf-i)* [L. arteria, artery; G. graphein, to write]. 1. Graphic recording of the pulse. 2. Demonstration of the arterial system by means of injection of opaque medium arteriographic, adj.; arteriographically, adv.

شریان نگاری : لاطینی لفظ آرٹیریا بمعنی شریان اور یونانی لفظ گریفین بمعنی لکھنا سے مرکب اصطلاح۔ (۱) نبض کی گرافی ریکارڈنگ۔ (۲) غیر شفاف واسطہ کے انجکشن کے ذریعے شریانی نظام کا مظاہرہ۔

Arteriopathy *(ar-ter-i-op'-ath-i)* [G. arteria, artery; pathos, disease]. Disease of any artery--arteriopathic, adj.

مرض شریان : یونانی الفاظ آرٹیریا بمعنی شریان اور پیتھوس بمعنی مرض سے ماخوذ اصطلاح۔ شریان کی ایک بیماری۔

Arterioplasty *(ar-te'-ri-o-plas-ti)* [L. arteria, artery; G. plassein, to form]. Plastic surgery applied to an artery--arterioplastic, adj.

تکوین الشریان: لاطینی لفظ آرٹیریا بمعنی شریان اور یونانی لفظ پلیسین بمعنی بنانا سے مرکب اصطلاح۔ پلاسٹک سرجری جس کا اطلاق شریان پر ہوتا ہے۔

Arteriole *(ar-ter'-i-ol)* [L. arteriola, small artery]. A small artery, joining an artery to a capillary.

شریانک : لاطینی لفظ آرٹیری اولا بمعنی چھوٹی شریان سے ماخوذ اصطلاح۔ ایک چھوٹی شریان جو شریان کو نس کے ساتھ ملاتی ہے۔

Arteriorrhaphy *(ar-te'-ri-or-raf-i)* [L. arteria, artery; G. rhaphe, suture]. A plastic procedure on an artery, such as obliteration of an aneurysm.

شریان دوزی : شریان پر پلاسٹک طریق۔

Arteriorrhaphy *(ar-te-ri-o-skler-o'-sis)* [L. arteria, artery; G. sklerosis, a hardening]. Degenerative arterial change associated with advancing age. Primarily a thickening of the media and usually associated with some degree of atheroma. **cerebral a.,** a syndrome which may include a shuffling gait, tendency to lean backwards, muscle rigidity, loss of memory, mental confusion and incontinence--arteriosclerotic. adj.

تصلب شریان۔شرائین کی سختی : عمر کی زیادتی کے ساتھ انحطاط پذیر شریانی تبدیلی۔شریانوں اور پٹھوں میں سختی۔

Arteriotomy *(ar-te-ri-ot'-o-mi)* [L. arteria, artery; G. tome, a cutting]. Incision of an artery.

فصد : لاطینی لفظ آرٹیریا بمعنی شریان اور یونانی لفظ ٹوم بمعنی تراشہ سے مرکب اصطلاح۔شریان کا قطع۔

Arteriovenous *(ar-te'-ri-o-ven-us)* [L. arteria, artery; vena, vein]. Pertaining to an artery and a vein.

متعلقہ ورید۔شریانی وریدی : لاطینی الفاظ آرٹیریا بمعنی شریان اور وینا بمعنی ورید سے ماخوذ اصطلاح۔شریان اور ورید سے متعلق۔

Arteritis *(ar-te-ri'-tis)* [L. arteria, artery; G. itis, inflammation]. Inflammation of an artery. The cause may be infective, traumatic, chemical or metabolic. Involvement of the ophthalmic arteries, or aortic arch may lead to blindness, **cranial a.,** a collagen (q.v.) disorder Early use of steroids may prevent blindness, **temporal a.,** inflammation with possible occlusion, most often in carotid arteries and branches; alternative name giant cell-a.See ENDARTERITIS. PERIARTERITIS--arteritic. adj.

ورم مفصل : لاطینی لفظ آرٹیریا بمعنی شریان اور یونانی لفظ اٹس بمعنی سوزش سے مرکب اصطلاح۔شریان کی سوزش۔اس کی وجہ کیمیائی رسولی یا کوئی اور وجہ ہو سکتی ہے۔

Artery *(ar'-te-ri)* [L. arteria, artery]. A vessel carrying blood from the heart of the various tissues. The internal endothelial lining provides a smooth surface to prevent clotting of blood. The middle layer of plain musc and elastic fibres allows for distension : blood is pumped from the heart. The oute mainly connective tissue layer preven overdistension. The lumen is largest neare to the heart; it gradually decreases in size. **forceps,** haemostatic (q.v.) forceps--arteria adj.

ریان : لاطینی لفظ آرٹیریا بمعنی شریان سے ماخوذ رگ جو خون دل سے رے حصوں کو لے جاتی ہے۔

Arthralgia *(arth-ral'-ji-a)* [G. arthron, join algos, poin]. Pain in a joint, used especial when there is no inflammation. Syn. articul neuralgia, arthrodynia (q.v.). **Intermittent periodic a.** is the term used when there pain usually accompanied by swelling of th knee at regular intervals arthralgic. adj.

ڑوں کا درد : یونانی الفاظ آرتھرون بمعنی جوڑ اور الجوس بمعنی درد سے وذ اصطلاح۔جوڑ میں درد۔یہ اصطلاح عموماً اس وقت استعمال کی جاتی ہے ب سوزش نہ ہو۔بلاسوزش جوڑوں کا درد۔

Arthrectomy *(arth-rek'-to-mi)* [G. arthro joint; ektome, excision]. Excision of a joint.

صل براری : یونانی الفاظ آرتھرون بمعنی جوڑ اور ایکٹوم بمعنی قطع سے وذ اصطلاح۔جوڑ کا قطع۔

Arthritis *(arth-ri'-tis)* [G. arthron, joint; -iti inflammation]. Inflammation of a joint. **deformans juvenilis,** Still's disease (q.v. See PERTHES DISEASE. **a. deforman neoplastica,** osteitis fibrosa (q.v.) **a. nodos (a. uratica)** gout--arthritic, adj.

م مفصل : یونانی الفاظ آرتھرون بمعنی جوڑ اور اٹس بمعنی سوزش سے ماخوذ طلاح۔جوڑ کی سوزش۔

Arthroclasia *(arth-ro-kla'-zi-a)* [G. arthro joint; klaein, to break]. Breaking down adhesions within the joint cavity to produce wider range of movement. Arthroclasis.

ق جساۃ : یونانی الفاظ آرتھرون بمعنی درد اور کلین بمعنی توڑنا سے ماخوذ طلاح۔حرکت پیدا کرنے کے لئے جوڑ کے کہفہ میں چپکاؤ کا ٹوٹنا۔

Arthrodesis *(arth-ro-de'-sis)* [G. arthro

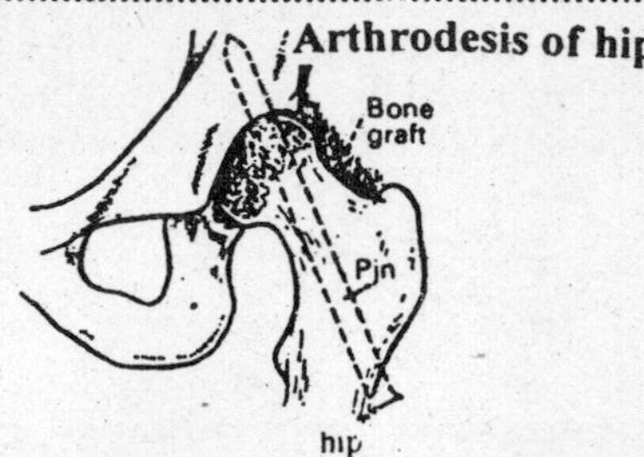

Arthrodesis of hip

joint; desis, a binding together]. The stiffening of a joint by operative means.

تبثیت منفصل : یونانی الفاظ آرتھرون بمعنی جوڑ اور ڈیسس بمعنی اکٹھے باندھنا سے ماخوذ اصطلاح۔ اپریشن کے ذریعہ جوڑ کی سختی۔ بذریعہ جراحی یا پلاسٹک سرجری جوڑ کا علاج۔

Arthrodynia *(arth-ro-din'-i-a)* [G. arthron, joint; odyne, pain]. Pain in a joint. See ARTHRALGIA--arthrodynic, adj.

دردمفاصل : یونانی الفاظ آرتھرون بمعنی جوڑ اور اوڈائن بمعنی درد سے ماخوذ اصطلاح جوڑ میں درد۔

Arthroendoscopy *(arth-ro-end-os'-kop-i)* [G. arthron,joint;endon,within;skopein,to examine].Visualization of the interior of a joint using an endoscope(q.v.)-- arthroendoscopic, adj.; arthroendoscopically, adv.

آرتھراینڈوسکوپی : یونانی الفاظ آرتھرون بمعنی جوڑ، انڈوں بمعنی اندر ہی اور سکوپین بمعنی جانچنا سے ماخوذ اصطلاح۔ انڈوسکوپ استعمال کر کے درد کا اندرونی منظر۔

Arthrogram *(arth'-ro-gram)*. [G. arthron, joint; gramma, letter]. An X-ray film demonstrating a joint.

آرتھروگرام : جوڑ کا درد ظاہر کرنے کے لئے ایکس رے فلم

مفاصل نگاری۔ مفاصلیات: یونانی الفاظ آرتھرون بمعنی جوڑ اور گریفین بمعنی لکھنا سے ماخوذ اصطلاح۔ درد کا ایکس رے۔

Arthrography *(arth-rog'-raf-i)* [G. arthron, joint; graphein, to write]. X-ray of a joint,sometimes after injection of air or radio-opaque material--arthrographic, adj.; arthrographically, adv.

Arthrology *(arth-rol'-oj-i)* [G. arthron, joint; logos, discourse]. The science which deals with joints, their diseases and treatment.

مفصلیات۔ علم المفاصل : سائنس کی وہ شاخ جس میں جوڑ، ان کی بیماریوں اور علاج کا مطالعہ کیا جاتا ہے۔

Arthropathy *(arth-rop'-ath-i)* [G. arthron, joint; pathos, disease]. Any joint disease--arthropathic, adj.

مرض مفصل : یونانی الفاظ آرتھرون بمعنی جوڑ اور پیتھوس بمعنی مرض سے ماخوذ اصطلاح۔ جوڑ کی کوئی بیماری۔

Arthroplasty *(arth'-ro-plas-ti)* [G. arthron, joit; plassein, to form]. The formation of an artificial joint. **cup a.,** articular surface reconstructed and covered with a vitallium cup, **excision a.,** gap is filled with fibrous tissues as in Keller's operation. **replacement a.,** insertion of an inert prosthesis of similar shape. **Girdlestone a.,** excision arthroplasty of the hip. **McKee-Farrer a.,** stainless steel replacement of the head of femur and the acetabulum, the latter being comented into the bone--arthroplastic, adj.

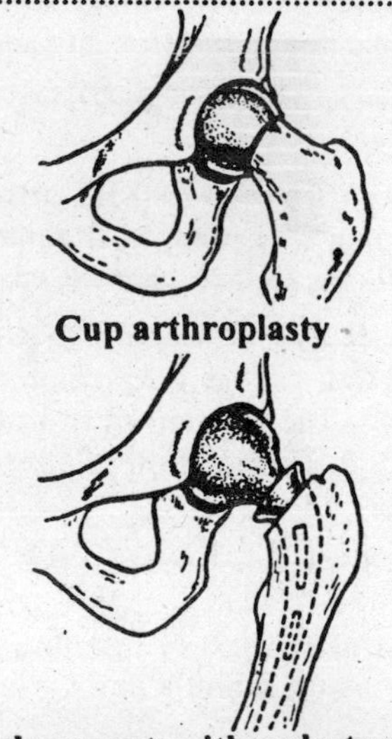
Cup arthroplasty

Replacement arithroplasty with metallic prothesis

تکوین مفصل : یونانی الفاظ آرتھرون بمعنی جوڑ اور پلیسین بمعنی بننا سے ماخوذ اصطلاح۔ ایک مصنوعی جوڑ کی بناوٹ

Arthroscope *(arth'-ro-skop)* [G. arthron, joint; skopein, to examine]. An instrument used for the visualization of the interior of the joint cavity. See ENDOSCOPE--arthroscopic, adj.

آرتھروسکوپ : یونانی الفاظ آرتھرون بمعنی جوڑ اور سکوپین بمعنی جانچنا سے ماخوذ اصطلاح۔ جوڑ کے کہفہ کے اندرونی جانب دیکھنے کے لئے استعمال ہونے والا ایک آلہ۔

Arthroscopy *(arth-ros'-kop-i)* [G. arthron, joint; skopein, to examine]. The act of visualizing the interior of the joint--arthroscopic, adj.

آرتھروسکوپی : یونانی الفاظ آرتھرون بمعنی جوڑ اور سکوپین بمعنی جانچنا سے ماخوذ اصطلاح۔ جوڑ کے اندرونی منظر کا عمل۔

Arthrosis *(ar-thro'-sis)* [G. arthron, joint; -osis, condition]. An articulation of joint; (Occasionally used to describe degeneration in a joint).

جوڑ بندی : یونانی الفاظ آرتھرون بمعنی جوڑ اور اوسس بمعنی حالت سے ماخوذ اصطلاح۔ ایک جوڑ۔ بعض اوقات جوڑ کے انحطاط کو بیان کرنے کے لئے یہ اصطلاح استعمال کی جاتی ہے۔ دو یا زائد ہڈیوں کے جوڑ کا مقام اتصال۔

Arthrotromy *(arth-rot-o-mi)* [G. arthron, joint; tome, a cutting]. Incision into a joint.

مفصل تراشی : یونانی الفاظ آرتھرون بمعنی جوڑ اور ٹوم بمعنی تراشہ سے ماخوذ اصطلاح۔ جوڑ میں قطع۔

Articular *(ar-tik'-u-lar)* [L. articulus, joint]. Pertaining to a joint or articulation. Applied to cartilage, surface, capsule, etc.

مفصلی : لاطینی لفظ آرٹیکولس بمعنی جوڑ سے ماخوذ اصطلاح۔ جوڑ سے متعلق۔

Articulation *(ar-tik-u-la'-shun)* [L. articulus, joint]. 1. The junction of two or more bones; a joint. 2. Enunciation of speech--articular, adj.

مفصل : دو یا زیادہ ہڈیوں کا جنکشن۔ ایک جوڑ۔ ایسی سطح جہاں دو ہڈیاں ملتی ہیں اور ایک قابل حرکت جوڑ بناتی ہیں۔

Artificial insemination Insertion of sperm into uterus using cannula and syringe instead of coitus.

مصنوعی غیر قدرتی : غیر قدرتی۔ آدمی کا بنایا ہوا یا ایجاد کردہ۔

Artosin *(ar'-tos-in)*. Tolbutamide, (q.v.).

Arvin *(ar'-vin)*. Ancrod (q.v.).

Asbestos *(as-bes'-tos)* [G. unquenchable]. A fibrous, mineral substance which does not conduct heat and is incombustible. It is used in making protective clothing for industry. Industrial workers may acquire hyperkeratotic papules on their hands--asbestos corns or warts.

اسبسطوس : ایک ریشہ دار، معدنی شے جو حرارت کے لئے غیر موصل ہے۔ انسانی صحت کے لئے مضر۔ سانس کے ذریعے اس کے ذرات جسم کے اندر جا سکتے ہیں۔ اس کے استعمال میں احتیاط لازمی ہے۔

Asbestosis *(as-bes-to'-sis)* [G. asbestos, unquenchable:-osis, condition]. Fibrosis of the lungs resulting from the inhalation of fine asbestos dust and fibris. Current research being done with radio-active gas to enable early detection. See PNEUMOCONIOSIS.

سمت اسبسطوس : پھیپھڑوں کی بیماری جو اسبسٹاس کے باریک گردے سے ہوتی ہے۔ کیونکہ وہ سانس کے ذریعے اندر جاتی ہے۔

Ascariasis *(as-kar-i'-a-sis)* [G. ask-karis, work in the intestines; N.L. -iasis, condition]. Infestation by the ascarides. The bowel is most commonly affected, but in the case of roundworm, infestation may spread to the stomach, liver and lungs.

صفاریت : یونانی لفظ اسکیرس بمعنی آنتوں میں کام اور نئی لاطینی زبان کے لفظ ایاسس بمعنی حالت سے مرکب اصطلاح۔ اسکیر ائیڈز کی وجہ سے آنت متاثر ہوتی ہے۔ پیٹ کے کیڑوں سے معدہ، جگر اور پھیپھڑے متاثر ہوتے ہیں۔

Ascaricide *(as-kar'-is-id)* [G. askaris, worm in the intestine; L. acaedere, to kill]. Lethal to ascarides--ascaricidal, adj.

صفارکش : یونانی لفظ اسکیرس بمعنی آنت میں کیڑا اور لاطینی لفظ سیڈ یئر بمعنی مارنا سے مرکب اصطلاح۔ اسکیر ائیڈز کے لئے مہلک۔

Ascraides *(as-kar'-i-dez)* [G. askaris, worm in the intestines]. Nematode worms of the family Ascaridae, to which belong the roundworm (Ascarislumbricoides) and the threadworm (Oxyuris vermicularis).

صفار : یونانی لفظ اسکیرس بمعنی آنتوں میں کیڑا سے ماخوذ اصطلاح۔ نیماٹوڈا کا ایک خاندان اس میں صفار ہے۔ جس کا سائنسی نام ایسکیرس لمبریکائیڈس ہے۔ یہ عام کرم ہیں۔ انتڑیوں میں پائے جاتے ہیں۔ وہاں سے نیم ہضم خوراک استعمال کرتے ہیں۔

Ascites *(as-si'-tez)* [G. askites, a kind of dropsy,

from askos, bag]. Free fluid in the peritoneal cavity. Syn., abdominal dropsy, hydroperitoneum--ascitic, adj.

استسقائے شکمی۔ پیٹ میں پانی : پیریٹونی کہفہ میں آزاد سیال۔ اگر پانی زیادہ ہو جائے تو ناف سے تقریباً ۴ انگل نیچے پیٹ میں ''ٹروکار اور کینولہ'' گھونپا جاتا ہے۔ٹروکار نکال لی جاتی ہے۔ پانی کینولہ کے راستے باہر آتا ہے۔ پیٹ کو سن کرنا چاہئے۔ اس کے لئے ایک گولی ہائیڈروکلور تھایا زائیڈ (ایسی ڈریکس) روزانہ ناشتہ کے بعد۔

Ascorbic acid *(a-askor'-bik)* Vitamin C. Used as dietary supplement in anaemia and to promote wound healing See VITAMIN C.

وٹامن سی۔ ایسکاربک ایسڈ : وٹامن سی۔ حیاتین ج۔ زخم ٹھیک کرنے اور قلت خون میں غذائی مد کے طور پر استعمال کیا جاتا ہے۔ سکروی کے علاج کے لئے ایسکاربک ایسڈ ۵۰۰ ملی گرام ایک گولی روزانہ۔ یہی خوراک برائے یرقان، پرپرا، فریکلز یعنی چھائیاں، ایری تھیما۔ ایک گولی صبح ایک شام برائے اکیوٹ گوؤٹ یا نقرس۔ اکوٹ ریوماٹائڈ ارتھرائی ٹس۔ کارنیل السر۔ ایک گولی صبح ایک دوپہر ایک شام برائے اکیوٹ ریومانزم۔

Asepsis *(a-sep'-sis)* [G. a-, not; sepsis, putrefaction]. The state of being free from living pathogenic organisms-asptic, adj.

عدم عفونت۔ پاکی : یونانی الفاظ اے بمعنی نہیں اور سپس بمعنی سڑانڈ سے ماخوذ اصطلاح۔ جاندار بیماری پیدا کرنے والے جسیموں سے آزاد ہونے کی حالت۔

Aseptic technique. A precautionary method used in any procedure where there is a possibility of introducing organisms into the patient's body. Every article used must have been sterilized.

دافع عفونت تکنیک : کسی طریق میں مستعمل ایک احتیاطی طریقہ جہاں مریض کے جسم میں جسیموں کے داخلے کا امکان ہے۔ ڈریسنگ کا یہ طریقہ بڑے ہسپتالوں میں ممکن ہے۔ جہاں ابالنے کا انتظام بہتر ہو۔

Aserbine *(as-er'-bin).* A desloughing cream, useful for burns, varicose and indolent ulcers. Emollient, contains benzonic acid, which is antinmycotic, and salicyclic acid.

ایسربن : ابلوں اور ناسوروں کے لئے کریم۔

Asilone *(as'-i-lon).* Polymethylsiloxane 250 mg and aluminium hydroxide 500 mg. Available in tablet, suspension and powder form to control non-specifidiarrhoea and flatulent distension of abdomen.

ایسی لون : دستوں وغیرہ میں مفید۔ اس میں ۲۵۰ ملی گرام پولی میتھائل سلوکسین اور ۵۰۰ ملی گرام ایلومینیم ہائیڈروکسائیڈ ہوتا ہے۔

ASO. Antistreptolysin O. See ANTISTREPTOLYSIN

Asparaginase *(as-par-a-jin'-as)* An enzyme derived from micro-organisms. Being tried in the treatment of asparagine-requiring cancers, especially the leukaemias--and especially acute lymphoblastic leukaemia.

اسپراجی نیز : خورد جسیموں سے ماخوذ ایک خامرہ۔ ایسے سرطان میں مفید ہے۔ اسپراجین کی ضرورت کا علاج ہو۔

Aspergillosis *(as-per'-ji-lo-sis)* [L. aspergere, to sprinkle; G. -osis, condition]. Any infection caused by any species of Aspergillus. More likely to occur in persons who handle grain or seeds. See BRONCHOMYCOSIS.

اسفرجلوسیت : لاطینی لفظ اسپرجیئر بمعنی چھڑکنا اور یونانی لفظ اوسس بمعنی حالت سے مرکب اصطلاح اسپرجلس کی ایک نوع سے پیدا ہونے والا مرض۔ یہ مرض ایسے اشخاص میں زیادہ پایا جاتا ہے۔ جو غلہ یا بیجوں کا کاروبار کرتے ہیں۔ ایک زرعی عارضہ۔ بھوسے سے ہونے والی بیماری۔

Aspergillus *(as'-per-jil'-us)* [L. aspergere, to sprinkle]. A genus of fungi, found in soil, manure and on various grains.

اسفرجلوس : لاطینی لفظ اسپرجیئر بمعنی چھڑکنا سے ماخوذ اصطلاح۔ سماروغ یا فنجائی کا ایک جنس جو مٹی، کھاد یا مختلف دانوں میں پایا جاتا ہے۔

Aspermia *(a-sper'-mi-a)* [G. a-, without; sperma, seed]. Lack of secretion of expulsion of semen--aspermic, adj.

بے منویت : یونانی الفاظ اے بمعنی بغیر اور سپرما بمعنی بیج سے ماخوذ اصطلاح۔ سیمن یا منی کے اخراج یا افراز کی کمی۔ منی میں سپرم نہ ہونا۔ اس کے لئے منی کا خوردبینی معائنہ منی کے اخراج کے دس منٹ کے اندر کیا جائے۔

Asphyxia *(as-fiks'-i-a)* [G. a-, not; sphyzein, to throb]. Suffocation; cessation of breathing. The O_2 content of the blood falls while the CO_2 rises and paralyses the respiratory centre, **blue a., a. livida,** deep blue appearance of the newborn baby. Good muscle tone. Responsive to stimuli. **white (pale) a., a. pallida.** more severe condition of new born. Pale, flaccid, unresponsive to stimuli.

اختناق : سانس کا گھٹنا۔ سانس بند ہونا۔ خون میں آکسیجن کی مقدار کم ہو جاتی ہے اور کاربن ڈائی آکسائیڈ زیادہ ہو جاتی ہے جس سے تنفسی مرکز بے کار ہو جاتا ہے۔ نظام تنفس کا مفلوج ہو جانا۔ موت کی وجوہات میں سے ایک۔

Aspiration *(as-pi-ra'-shun)* [L. aspirare, to breathe upon]. 1. The act of drawing in the breath; inspiration. 2. The withdrawal of fluids from a body cavity by means of a suction o siphonage apparatus. **a. pneumonia,** inflammation of lung from inhalation of foreign body, usually fluid or food particles--aspirate, v.t.

امتصاص ہواکشی: (۱) اندر کی طرف سانس لینا۔ سانس کھینچنا۔ (۲) جسمانی کھفہ سے سیالوں کا کھینچنا۔

Aspirator *(as'pi-ra-tor)* [L. aspirare, to breathe upon]. A negative pressure apparatus for withdrawing fluids from cavities.

ممصاص : کھفوں سے سیالوں کو کھینچنے کے لئے ایک منفی دباؤ کا سامان۔

Aspirin *(as'pir-in)*. Acetylsalicylic acid (q.v.).

اسپرین : دیکھئے ایسیٹائل سیلیسائیلک ایسڈ۔ دافع درد۔

Assimilation *(as-sim-i-la'-shun)* [L. assimilatio, similarity]. The process whereby the already digested foodstuffs are absorbed and utilized by the tissues. Syn., anabolism--assimilable, adj.; assimilate, v.t., v.i.

استحالہ : وہ عمل جس کے ذریعہ ہضم شدہ خوراک مادۂ حیات یا خمایہ میں تبدیل ہوتی ہے اور جزو بدن بنتی ہے۔

Association *(as-so-si-a'-shun)* [L. associare, to join to]. In psychology; **a. of ideas,** the principle by which ideas, emotions and movements are connected so that their succession in the mind occurs. **a. areas,** in the cerebral cortex the functions of which are known. **controlled a.,** ideas called up in consciousness in response to words spoken by the examiner. **free a.,** ideas arising spontaneously when censorship is removed.

ایسوسی ایشن۔ تلازم : لاطینی لفظ ایسوسی ایئر بمعنی شامل ہونا سے ماخوذ اصطلاح۔ نفسیات میں نظریات کی ایسوسی ایشن۔ اصول جس کے ذریعہ نظریات جذبات اور حرکات باہمی ربط پایا جاتا ہے۔ اس لئے ذہن میں ان کی ترتیب واقع ہوتی ہے۔

Asterognosis *(a-ste-ri-og-no'-sis)* [G. a-, not; stereos, solid; gnosis, knowledge]. Loss of power to recognize the shape and consistency of objects.

بے لمسی : اشیاء کی شکل وغیرہ کو پہچاننے کی قوت کا ضیاع۔

Asthenia *(as-the'-ni-a)* [G. asthenia, want of strength]. Weakness, debility. See KRETSCHMER--asthenic, adj.

ضعف : یونانی لفظ استھینیا بمعنی طاقت کی کمی سے ماخوذ اصطلاح۔ کمزوری۔

Asthenic type Physique with small trunk and long limbs sometimes associated with schizophrenia.

Asthenopia *(as-the-no'-pi-a)* [G. a-, not; stnenos, strength; ops, eye]. Poor vision--asthenopic, adj.; asthenope, n.

ضعف بصر : یونانی الفاظ اے بمعنی نہیں، ستھینوس بمعنی طاقت اور اوپس بمعنی آنکھ سے ماخوذ اصطلاح کمزور نگاہ۔

Asthma *(asth'ma)* [G. a panting]. Paroxysmal airways obstruction due to generalized narrowing of the bronchi which reverses either spontaneously or as the result of treatment. The extrinsic classification ranges from Atopic Type I allergy (reaction on skin testing is immediate) to Non-atopic Type III allergy (delayed reaction on skin testing). The intrinsic classification implies negative skin reactions; immunology unknown. **bronchial a.,** attack of breathlessness associated with bronchial obstruction or spasm. Characterized by expiratory wheeze. **cardiac a.,** nocturnal paroxysmal dyspnoea in left ventricular failure. **status asthmaticus,** repeated attacks of asthma without any period of freedom between spasms--asthmatic, adj.

دمہ : سانس میں دشواری کا حملہ۔ دائمی دمہ میں سانس مسلسل اکھڑا رہتا ہے۔

Astigmatism *(as-tig'-mat-izm)* [G. a-, not; sigma, a point]. Defective vision caused by inequality of one or more refractive surfaces, usually the corneal, so that the light rays do not converge to a point on the retina. May be congenital or acquired--astigmatic, astigmic, adj.

کج نظری : یونانی الفاظ اے بمعنی نہیں اور سٹگما بمعنی ایک نقطہ سے ماخوذ الفاظ۔ایک یا زیادہ انعطافی سطوح کی نابرابری کی وجہ سے ناقص نظر یا نگاہ۔ عموماً قرینہ کی سطح۔ ریٹنا پر روشنی کی شعاعیں ایک نقطہ پر مرکوز نہیں ہوتیں۔ آنکھوں کا نقص جو قرینہ میں خم ہونے کی وجہ سے ہوتا ہے۔اس کی وجہ سے چیزیں ٹیڑھی نظر آتی ہیں۔یہ نقص مرکب شیشوں کی عینک کے استعمال سے دور ہوسکتا ہے۔

Astringent *(as-trin'-jent)* [L. astringere, to bind together]. An agent which contracts organic tissue. thus lessening secretion--astringency, n.

قابض (دوا)۔خون بند (دوا) : لاطینی لفظ اسٹرنجیئر بمعنی اکٹھے باندھنا سے ماخوذ اصطلاح۔ایک ایجنٹ جو نامیاتی نسیج کو سکیڑتا ہے جس سے افراز میں کمی ہو جاتی ہے۔یہ جگہ کو خشک کر دیتے ہیں اور قابض ہوتے ہیں۔ مثلاً ٹینک ایسڈ۔

Astrocytoma *(as-tro-si-to'-ma)* [G. astron, a star; kytos, cell; -oma, tumour]. A slowly growing tumour of the glial tissue of brain and cord.

نجم خلوی سلعہ : یونانی الفاظ اسٹرون بمعنی ستارہ، کائیٹوس بمعنی خلیہ اور اوما بمعنی رسولی سے ماخوذ اصطلاح۔دماغ اور نخاع کی بافت میں آہستہ آہستہ بڑھنے والی رسولی۔

Asymmetry *(a-sim'-et-ri)* [G. a-, not; symmetria, symmetry]. Lack of similarity of the organs or parts on each side.

عدم تشاکل : ہر جانب اعضاء یا حصوں کی یکسانیت کی کمی۔دو برابر حصوں میں تقسیم نہ ہونے کی کیفیت۔

Asymptomatic *(a-simp-tom-at'-ik)* [G. a-, not; symptomatikos, from symptoma, symptom]. Symptomless.

بلا علامت : علامات کے بغیر۔

AT 10., Dihydrotachysterol (q.v.).

اے ٹی ۱۰ : تیل میں ڈائی ہائیڈروٹیکی سٹیرول کا محلول خون میں کیلیم زیادہ کرنے کے لئے مستعمل۔

Ataractic *(at-a-rak'-tk)* [G. ataraktos. cool, steady]. Drugs that, without drowsiness, help to relieve anxiety thus providing emotional equilibrium. Syn. tranquillizer, neuroleptic. Have reduced the incidence of leucotomy.

اٹیریکٹک : ادویہ جو نیند لائے بغیر پریشانی ختم کرنے میں مدد دیتی ہیں اس طرح جذباتی توازن قائم کرتی ہیں۔

Atactic *(a-tak'-tik)*. See ATAXIA.

Atarax: *(at'-a-raks)*. Hydroxazine. See ATARACTIC.

اٹیریکس : ہائیڈروکسازین۔

Atavism *(at'-a-vizm)* [L. atavas, ancestor]. The reappearance of an hereditary trait which has skipped one or more generations--atavic, atavistic, adj.

رجعت بسلف۔جدیت : لاطینی لفظ اٹاوس بمعنی جد امجد سے ماخوذ اصطلاح۔ایسی وراثتی خصوصیت جو ایک یا زیادہ نسلوں میں ظاہر نہ ہو، کا دوبارہ ظہور۔

Ataxia, ataxy *(a-taks'-i-a, a-taks'-i)* [G. ataxia, disorder]. Defective muscular control resulting in irregular and jerky movements. Staggering. **Friendreich's a.**, usually begins in childhood. Heredofamilial disease. Transmission occurs through both sexes, usually as a recessive gene, rarely a dominant one. Transmission from affected parent to child rare because adult sufferers are not as a rule able to procreate--ataxic, adj.

اختلال عضلات : ناقص عضلی کنٹرول جس کے نتیجہ میں بے قاعدہ اور جھٹکے دار حرکات ہوتی ہیں۔

Aterbin *(at'-e-brin)*. Mepacrine (q.v.).

Atelectasis *(at-el-ek'-ta-sis)* [G. ateles, imperfect; elitasis, extension]. No air in alveoli, lung solid. **congenital a.**, air has failed to enter lung immediately after birth--atelectatic, adj.

عدم تمدد (ریہ) : یونانی الفاظ اٹیلس بمعنی نامکمل اور اکٹاسس بمعنی بڑھاؤ سے ماخوذ اصطلاح۔ہوائی تھیلیوں میں ہوا نہ ہونا۔ٹھوس پھیپھڑا۔

Atherogenic *(ath-e-ro-jen'-ik)* [G. athere, porridge; genes, producing]. Capable of producing atheroma--atherogenesis, n.

اتھیروجینک : اتھیروما پیدا کرنے کا اہل۔نسوں کا عارضہ۔چربی زدہ مادہ ...ت سے پیدا ہوتا ہے جو نسوں کو سختی پیدا کر دیتا ہے۔

Atheroma *(ath-e-ro'-ma)* [G. athere, porridge; -oma, tumour]. Deposition of hard yellow plaques of lipoid material in the intimal layer of the arteries. May be related to high level of cholesterol in the blood, or excessive consumption of refined sugar. Of great importance in the coronary arteries in predisposing to cornoary thrombosis-- atheromatous, adj.

اتھروما۔سوزش شرائین : شریانوں میں لپائڈمادہ کا جمع ہونا۔

Atheorsclerosis *(ath'-e-ro-skle-ro'-sis)* [G. athere, porridge; sklerosis, a hardening]. Co-existing atheroma and arteriosclerosis--atherosclerotic, adj.

اتھیروسکلیروسس : اتھیروما اور آرٹیریوسکلیروسس دونوں کا ہونا۔

Athetosis *(ath-e-to'-sis)* [G. athetos, without position; -osis, condition]. A condition marked by purposeless movements of the hands and feet and generally due to a brain lesion--athetoid, athetotic, adj.

رعشہ اصابع : یونانی الفاظ اتھیٹوس بمعنی پوزیشن کے بغیر اور اوسس بمعنی حالت سے ماخوذ اصطلاح۔ ہاتھوں اور پیروں کی بے مقصد حرکات کی حالت۔اس کا سبب دماغ کا نقص ہے۔

Athlete's foot. See TINEA PEDIA.

Ativan *(at'-i-van).* Lorazep[am (q.v.).

atom [G. atomos, uncut, indivisible]. The smallest particle of the element capable of existing individually, or incombination with

Atom

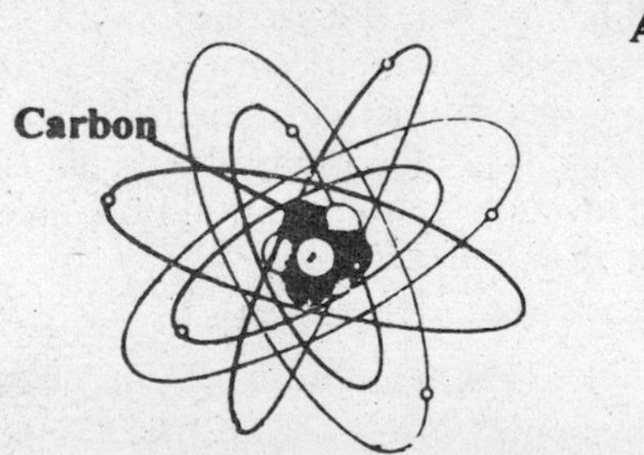

one or more atoms of the same or another element. **atomic weight,** the weight of an atom compared with that of an atom of hydrogen--atomic. adj.

ایٹم۔جوہر : یونانی لفظ ایٹموس بمعنی نا قابل تقسیم سے ماخوذ اصطلاح۔کسی عنصر کا سب سے چھوٹا ذرہ جو انفرادی طور پر وجود رکھتا ہے یا اسی یا دوسرے عنصر کے ایک یا زیادہ جوہر کے ساتھ مل کر رہ سکتا ہے۔جوہر میں پروٹون، نیوٹرون اور الیکٹرون پائے جاتے ہیں۔ایٹم بم میں توازنے پورے قابل انشقاق مادے کو توانائی اور تابکاری میں بدل دیتے ہیں۔جوہری کلاک وقت ناپنے کا آلہ ہے۔نیوکلیائی وزن کے بعد حاصل شدہ چھوٹے اجزاء کی کل قیمت، یورنیم کے مرکزہ کی کل کمیت سے کم ہوتی ہے۔اس طرح جو مادہ غائب ہوتا ہے، وہ توانائی میں تبدیل ہو جاتا ہے۔ایک سالمہ میں عنصر کے جوہروں کی تعداد کا تعین جوہریت کہلاتا ہے ایک عنصر کے تمام جوہر کا جوہری وزن یکساں ہوتا ہے۔ایک عنصر کے جوہر کا وزن دوسرے عنصر کے وزن سے مختلف ہوتا ہے۔کسی عنصر کا ایٹمی وزن اس کے ایٹم اور آکسیجن ایٹم کے وزن اور آکسیجن کے ایٹم کا وزن سولہ ایٹمی ماس اکائیاں تصور کیا جاتا ہے۔

Atomization *(at'-om-iz-a-shun)* . A mechanical process whereby a liquid is divided into a fine spray--atomizer, n.

Atomizer

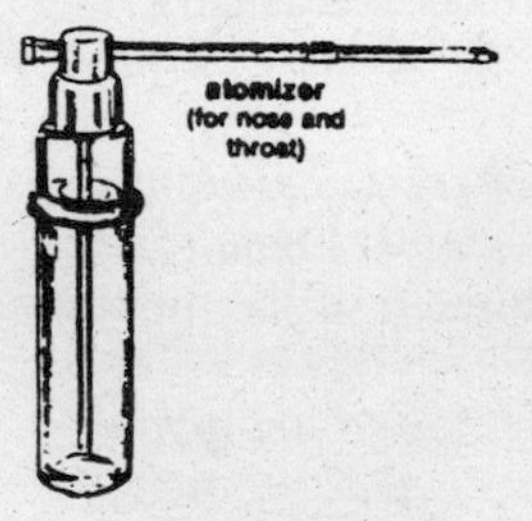

مائع پاشی۔عرق پاشی : ایک میکانکی طریق جس میں مائع کو ایک عمدہ سپرے میں تقسیم کیا جاتا ہے۔

Atonic *(a-ton'-ik)* [G. a-, not tonos, tone]. Without tone; **weak--atonia,** stony, atonicity. n.

نحیف : یونانی الفاظ اے بمعنی نہیں اور ٹونوس بمعنی آواز سے ماخوذ اصطلاح۔آواز کے بغیر کمزور۔

Atopy *(at'-op-i)* [G. a-, not; topos, place]. Familial allergy. Covers diseases such as hay fever, asthma, urticaria and eczema where there is a clear family history of these conditions--atopic, adj.

اٹوپی : الرجی کی قسم۔دمہ، خارش وغیرہ کی بیماریاں۔ایک موروثی بیماری۔

Atresia *(a-tre'-zi-a)* [G. a-, not; tresis, perforation]. Imperforation or closure of a normal opening or canal--atresic, atretic, adj.

رتق۔تنگی ثقبہ : کسی قنال یا سوراخ کی بندش یا سوراخوں کا نہ ہونا۔جسم کے کسی شگاف والے حصہ کا منہ بند ہونا۔

Atrial fibrillation *(a'-tri-al fib-rila'-shun).* Syn.

auricular fibrillation. Chaotic cardiac irregularity without any semblance of order. Commonly associated with mitral stenosis and nodular toxic goitre, but also with other diseases of the heart and sometimes in general toxic states.

اطاقی فائبرلیشن : آریکولر فائبرلیشن۔ واضح علامات کے بغیر عارضہ قلب۔

Atrial flutter *(a'-tri-al-flut'-er)*. Syn., auricular flutter. Rapid regular cardiac rhythm caused by irritable focus in atrial muscle and usually associated with organic heart disease. Speed of atrial beats between 260 and 340 per minute. Ventricles usually respond to every second beat, but may be slowed by carotid sinus pressure.

اطاقی فلٹر : تیز باقاعدہ کارڈیاک ردم۔ آریکولر فلٹر عارضہ قلب۔

Atrial septal defect Non-closure of foramen ovale at birth resulting in congenital heart defect.

Atrioventricular *(a'-tri-o-ven-trik'-u-lar)* [L. atrium; ventriculus, ventricle]. Perta- ining to the atria and the ventricles of the heart. Applied to a node, tract and valves. Syn. auriculoventricular.

اطاق بطینی : لاطینی زبان کے الفاظ ایٹریم بمعنی اذن یا ایٹریم اور وینٹریکوس بمعنی بطین یا وینٹریکل سے ماخوذ اصطلاح۔ دل کے ایٹریا اور وینٹریکلو کے متعلق۔ اس کا اطلاق نوڈ' ٹریکٹ اور ویلوز پر کیا جاتا ہے۔

Atrium *(a'-tri-um)* [L. atrium, chamber]. Cavity, entrance or passage. One of the two upper cavities of the heart. Also called 'auricle'.--artria, pl.; atrial, adj.

ایٹریم۔ اطاق : لاطینی لفظ ایٹریم بمعنی خانہ سے ماخوذ اصطلاح۔ کھفہ' جوف' داخل ہونے کا راستہ یا صرف راستہ۔ دل کے دو بالائی کھفوں میں سے ایک۔ اسے آریکل بھی کہتے ہیں۔

Atromid *(at'-ro-mid)*. Clofibrate (q.v.).

ایٹرومڈ : دیکھئے کلوفائیبریٹ۔ انجائنہ پیکٹورس یا دل کے درد اور فالج یا سر برل ہیمورج میں ایٹرومڈ ایس کے کیپسول ۳ تا چھ روزانہ۔

Atrophy *(at'-ro-fi)* (G. atrophia, want of food]. Wasting, emaciation, diminution in size and function. **acute yellow a.,** massive necrosis of liver associated with severe infection, toxaemia of pregnancy or ingested poisons. **progressive muscular a.,** syn., motor neurone disease. Disease of the motor neurones of unknown cause, characterized by loss of power and wasting in the upper limbs. May also have upper motor neurone involvement (spasticity) in lower limbs--**atrophied,** atrophic, adj.

لاغری۔ عدم نمو : یونانی لفظ اٹروفیا بمعنی قلت خوراک سے ماخوذ اصطلاح۔ سائز اور فعل میں کمی۔ طاقت میں کمی۔

Atrophine *(at' -or-pen)*. Principal alkaloid of belladonna. Has spasmolytic, mydriatic and central nervous system depressant properties. Given before anaesthetic to decrease secretion in bronchial and salivary systems and to prevent cardiac depression by depressing the vagus nerve thus quickening the heart beat. It can be given intravenously to produce tachycardia--(a) before giving Prostigmin; (b) when a patient has a very slow pulse. **a. methonitrate** is used in pylorospasm and in spray preparations for asthma and bronchospasm.

عرق مکو۔ ایٹروپین : برگ لفاح یا بیلاڈونا کا اہم الکلائڈ۔ اس کا ۱/۱۰ گرین کا ٹیکہ برائے کولی سس ٹائی ٹس ایک بے رنگ قلمی ناحل پذیر الکلائڈ۔ مفید برائے مرض کیسن' کارنیل آلسر یعنی آنکھ کا زخم اور آنکھ کی پتلی پھیلانے کے لئے۔ نقطۂ پگھلاؤ ۱۱۵س۔

ATS. Antitetanus serum. Contains tetanus antibodies. Produces artificial passive immunity. A test dose must be given first. Can cause anaphylaxis.

اے ٹی ایس : دافع تشنج سیرم۔ تشنج کی اینٹی باڈیز پر مشتمل۔

ATT. Antitetanus toxoid. Contains treated tetanus toxins. Produces artificial active immunity. Does not cause anaphylaxis.

اے ٹی ٹی : دافع تشنج ٹاکسائڈ۔ تشنج کی موثر دوائی۔

Attenuation *(at-ten-u-a'-shun)* [L. attenuare, to weaken]. A bacteriological process by which organisms are rendered less virulent by exposure to an unfavourable environment. They can then be used in the preparation of vaccines--attenuant, attenuated, adj. attenuate, v.t., v.i.

ترقیق۔تلطیف۔تخفیف۔تصغیف : لاطینی لفظ اٹینوایئر بمعنی کمزور کرنا سے ماخوذ اصطلاح۔ ایک جراثیمی طریق جس کے ذریعے جیسے کم زہریلے ہوجاتے ہیں کیونکہ انہیں نامساعد ماحول سے گزارا جاتا ہے۔

Atticotomy *(at-i-kct'-o-mi)*. Entry into the attic of the middle ear--that portion above the tympanic membrane (epitympanum) by removal of the outer attic wall to create a wide opening of the external auditory meatus into the attic.

علیہ تراشی : درمیانی کان کے ایٹک میں داخل۔

Attitude *(at'-ti-tud)* [F. attitude, from L. aptitudinem]. A settled mode of thinking.

رویہ۔اندازفکر۔وضع : سوچ کا مقررہ طریق۔رحم میں جنین کے بدن کے مختلف حصوں کے پڑے رہنے کی ترتیب۔وضع سے مراد ہے بچہ کا سر، گردن، پشت، بازو، ٹانگیں اور پاؤں کس انداز میں پڑے ہیں۔رحم میں جنین کی پشت کمان کی طرح خمدار ہوتی ہے۔گردن جھکی ہوئی اور سر جھک کر سینے سے لگا ہوا۔ ٹانگوں اور گھٹنوں کے جوڑ سمٹے ہوتے ہیں اور سینے کے ساتھ لگے ہوتے ہیں۔ بازو بھی سینے کے ساتھ لگے ہوتے ہیں۔

Atypical *(a-tip'-ik-al)*. Not typical; unusual, irregular; not conforming to type, e.g. atypical pneumonia.

غیرتمثیلی۔بےنمونہ : مثالی نہ ہونا۔غیرمعمولی۔معمول سے ہٹ کر۔ بے قاعدہ۔

Audiogram *(aw'-di-o-gram)* [L. audire, to hear; G. gramma, a letter]. A chart of hearing while using an audiometer. The acuity of hearing is plotted and a visual record obtained.

سمعی ترسیم : سماعت کا چارٹ جس میں سمع پیما استعمال ہوتا ہے۔

Audiology *(aw-di-ol'-o-ji)* [L. audire, to hear; G. logos, discourse]. The science dealing with hearing--audiological, adj.; audiologically, adv.

علم سماعت : سائنس جس میں سماعت کا مطالعہ کیا جاتا ہے۔

Audiometer *(aw-di-om'-et-er)* [L. audire, to hear; G. metron, a measure]. An apparatus for the clinical testing of hearing. It generates pure tones over a wide range of pitch and intensity--audiometric, adj.; audiometry, audiometrist, n.

سماعت پیما سمع پیا : لاطینی لفظ آڈایئر بمعنی سننا اور یونانی لفظ میٹرون بمعنی پیمائش سے مرکب اصطلاح۔سماعت جانچنے کا سامان۔

Auditory *(aw'-dit-o-ri)* [L. audire, to hear]. Pertaining to the sense of hearing. **a. area,** that portion of the temporal lobe of the cerebral cortex which interprets sound. **a. meatus,** the canal between the pinna and eardrum. **a. nerves,** the eight pair of cranial nerves. **a. ossiscles,** the three tiny bones--malleus, and stapes--stretching across the cavity of the middle ear.

سمعی۔سامعہ : لاطینی لفظ آڈایئر بمعنی سننا اور ماخوذ اصطلاح سماعت کی حس سے متعلق۔

Aura *(aw'-ra)* [G. breeze]. A premonition; a peculiar sensation or warning of an impending attack, such as occurs in epilepsy.

کپکپی۔مہک : ہونے والے حملے کا مخصوص احساس۔

Aural *(awr'-al)* [L. auris, ear]. Pertaining to the ear.

کان دیکھنے کے لئے ایک آلہ۔

Aurothiomalate *(awr-o-thi-om'-a-lat)*. Gold injection useful in chronic discoid lupus erythematosus and rheumatoid arthritis. Urine should be tested for albumen before each injection.

آروتھایوملیٹ : سونے کا انجکشن۔ہر انجکشن سے پہلے البومن کے لئے پیشاب ٹیسٹ کرنا چاہئے۔

Ausculation *(aws-kul-a'-shun)* [L. auscultare, to listen to]. A method of listening to the body sounds for diagnostic purposes, particularly the heart, lungs and fetal circulation. It may be; (1) immediate, by placing the ear directly against the body; (2) mediate, by the use of a stathoscope--auscultatory, adj.; auscult, auscultate, v.

استماع : لاطینی لفظ آسکلٹیر بمعنی سننا سے ماخوذ اصطلاح۔جسمانی آوازوں کو سننے کا طریقہ۔کان لگا کر یا سیتھسکوپ لگا کر آواز سننا۔

Australian lift Better described as shoulder lift. A method of lifting of heavy patient, whereby his weight is taken by the upper shoulder muscles of the two lifters, and the lift is achieved by straightening the lifters' flexed hips.

آسٹریلوی لفٹ : بھاری مریض کو اٹھانے کا طریقہ۔

Austism *(aw'tizm)* [G. autos, self]. Schizophrenic (q.v.) syndrome in childhood.

خودی۔معائنہ نفس : یونانی لفظ آٹوز بمعنی کود سے ماخوذ اصطلاح بچپن میں سنڈروم۔

Autistic *(aw-tis'-tik)* [G. autos, self]. Morbidly self-centred thinking, governed by the wishes of the individual; wishful thinking (phantasy), in contrast to reality thinking. Occurs in schizophrenia (q.v.)--autism,

خودفلری : یونانی لفظ آٹوز بمعنی کود سے ماخوذ اصطلاح۔

اذنی۔گوشی : لاطینی لفظ آرس بمعنی کان سے ماخوذ اصطلاح۔کان سے متعلق۔

Aureomycin *(aw-re-o-mi'-sin)* Chlortetracycline. SeeTETRACYCLINE.

اریومائی سین : ایک اینٹی بیاٹک جوکئی جسیموں کے خلاف استعمال کیا جاتا ہے۔

Auricle *(aw'-rik-l)* [L. auricula, the external ear]. 1. The pinna of the external ear. 2. An appendage to the cardiac atrium. 3. Commonly used mistakenly for atrium (q.v.)--auricular, adj.

اذین۔بیرونی کان۔لالہ گوش : لاطینی لفظ آریکولا بمعنی بیرونی کان سے ماخوذ اصطلاح۔بیرونی کان کا باہر والا حصہ پنا۔

Auricular fibrillation See ATRIAL F.

گوشی فائبرلیشن : دیکھئے ایٹریل فائبرلیشن۔واضح علامات کے بغیر عارضہ قلب۔

Auricular flutter. See ATRIAL F.

گوشی فلٹر : دیکھئے ایٹریل فلٹر۔تیز و باقاعدہ دھڑکن کے ساتھ عارضہ قلب۔

Auriculoventricular See ATRIOVENTRICULAR.

Auriscope *(aw'ris-kop)* [L. auris ear; G. skopein, to examine]. An instrument for examining the ear, usually incorporating both magnification and electric illumination.

گوش بین : لاطینی لفظ آرس بمعنی کان اور یونانی لفظ سکوپین بمعنی جانچنا سے مرکب اصطلاح۔

خودانہضام : یونانی لفظ آٹوز بمعنی خود اور لاطینی لفظ ڈائی جیریئر بمعنی ہضم کرنا سے مرکب اصطلاح۔جاندار جسم میں بافتوں کا اپنا انہضام۔

Autoeroticism *(aw-to-e-rot'-is-izm)* [G. autos, self; eros, love]. Self-gratification of the sex instinct. See MASTURBATION--autoerotic, adj.

خودشہوانیت : یونانی الفاظ آٹوز بمعنی محبت سے ماخوذ اصطلاح۔جنسی جبلت سے خودلذتی۔

Autogenous *(aw-toj'-e-nus)* [G. autos, self; genesthai, from gignesthai, to be produced]. Self-generated; endogenous. Applied to bone graft, skin graft, etc. **a. vaccine,** one prepared from bacteria obtained from the patient's own infection. Also AUTOGENETIC, AUTOGENIC.

خودزاد : آپ پیدا کیا ہوا۔مقامی۔جلدی پیوند یا استخوانی پیوند پر اس اصطلاح کا اطلاق کیا جاتا ہے۔

Autohaemotherapy *(aw-to-he-mo-ther'-a-pi)* [G. autos, self; haima, blood; therapeia, treatment]. Intramuscular injection of a patient using his own blood, e.g. in cases of recurring urtcaria.

خوددموی علاج : یونانی الفاظ آٹو بمعنی خود، ہیما بمعنی خون اور تھراپیا بمعنی علاج سے ماخوذ اصطلاح مریض کا اپنا خون استعمال کرتے ہوئے انجکشن۔

Autoimmunity *(aw-to-im-mun'-i-ti)* [G. autos, self; L. immunis, free from]. An abnormal immune reaction of unknown cause. In most cases it is directed against a constituent, often protein in nature, of the patient's own body. This constituent is regarded as a foreign body by the patient's own.

فردکی اپنی خواہشات کے مطابق سوچ

Antoantibody *(aw-to-an'ti-bod-i)* [G. autos, self; anti, against; A.S. bodig, body]. Substance produced in a reaction, something within the body acting as the stimulus (autoantigen):

ذاتی ضد جسم : یونانی الفاظ آٹوز بمعنی خود، اینٹی بمعنی خلاف اور اینگلوسکسن لفظ بوڈگ بمعنی جسم سے مرکب اصطلاح۔ردعمل میں

پیدا ہونے والی شے۔کوئی چیز جسم کے اندر ہی محرک طور پر کام کرتی ہے۔

Autoantigen *(aw-to-an'-ti-jen)* [G. autos, self; anti, against; genos, birth]. Something within the body capable of initiating the production of autoantibody.

آٹوانیٹی جن : یونانی الفاظ آٹوز بمعنی خود، اینٹی بمعنی خلاف اور جینوس بمعنی پیدائش سے ماخوذ اصطلاح۔آٹو اینٹی باڈی کی پیداوار شروع کرنے کے قابل جسم میں کوئی چیز۔

Autoclave *(aw'-to-klav)* [G. autos, self; L. clavis, key]. 1. An apparatus for high-pressure steam sterilization. 2. Sterilize in an autoclave.

آٹوکلیو۔ خودداب جوش دان : یونانی لفظ آٹوز بمعنی خود اور لاطینی لفظ کلیوس بمعنی چابی سے مرکب اصطلاح۔(۱) بھاپ کے ذریعہ پاک کرنے کا سامان۔(۲) آٹوکلیو میں پاک کرنا۔

Autodigestion *(aw-to-di-jest'-chun)* [G. autos, self; L. digerere, to digest]. Self-digestion of tissues within the living body. Autolysis (q.v.) faulty metabolic products elaborated within the body.

ذاتی تسمم : یونانی لفظ آٹوز بمعنی خود، لاطینی لفظ ان بمعنی میں اور یونانی لفظ ٹوکسیکون بمعنی زہر سے مرکب اصطلاح۔جسم میں ناقص حاصلات سے زہریلا پن۔

Autolysis *(aw-tol'-is-is)* [G. autos, self; tysis, a loosening]. Autodigestion (q.v.) which occurs if digestive ferments escape into surrounding tissues--autolytic, adj.

خودپاشی : اگر ہضمی خامرات اردگرد کی بافتوں میں چلے جائیں تو خود انہضام کا عمل ہوتا ہے۔اپنے ہی خامرات کے عمل کے نتیجہ میں حیاتی خلیوں کا موت کے بعد اپنے آپ کو تباہ کرنے کا عمل۔

Automatic *(aw-to-mat'-ik)* [G. automatos, seif-acting]. That which is performed without the influence of the will; spontaneous; non-volitional acts; involuntary acts.

خودکار۔خود : مرضی کے اثر کے بغیر کام کی ادائیگی۔غیر ارادی فعل۔

Automatism *(aw-tom'-at-izm)* [G. automatos, self-acting]. Performance of involuntary acts. Occurs in somnambulism, hysterical and epileptic states.

حرکت غیرارادی : غیر ارادی افعال کی ادائیگی۔

Autonomic *(aw-to-nom'-ik)* [G. autos, self; nomos, law]. Independent; self-governing. **a. nervous system** (ANS) is divided into parasympathetic and sympathetic portions. They are made up of nerve cells and fibres which cannot be controlled at will. They are concerned immune system which forms antibodies against the constituent as it would against any foreign invader.

خوداعفائیت : یونانی لفظ آٹوز بمعنی خود اور لاطینی لفظ امیونس بمعنی آزاد سے مرکب اصطلاح۔نامعلوم وجہ کا ایک خلاف معمول امیون ردعمل۔عموماء مریض کے اپنے جسم کے جزو کے خلاف ہوتا ہے اور یہ جزو اکثر پروٹین ہوتا ہے۔

Autoimmunization *(aw-to-im-mun-iz-a'-shun)* [G. autos, self; L. immunis, free from]. Sensitization of a person to a substance elaborated in his own body. Hashimoto's disease, myxoedema and Graves' disease are examples of autoimmune thyroid disease. Pernicious anaemia is another autoimmune disease.

خوداعفائیت : یونانی لفظ آٹوز بمعنی خود اور لاطینی لفظ امیونس بمعنی سے آزاد سے مرکب اصطلاح۔کسی شخص کا اپنے ہی جسم کے مادہ سے حساس ہونا۔

Autoinfection *(aw-to-in-fek'-shun)* [G. autos, self; L. inficere, to infect]. Infection arising from an organism within the body or transferred from one part of the body to another by fingers, etc.

ذاتی چھوت : جسم کے اندر ہی جیسے سے پیدا ہونے والی بیماری یا جسم کے ایک حصہ سے دوسرے حصہ میں انگلیوں وغیرہ سے بیماری منتقل ہوتی ہے۔

Autointoxication *(aw-to-in-toks-i-ka'-shun)* [G. autos, self; L. in-, in; G. toxikon, poison]. Poisoning from with reflex control of bodily functions.

خودزا۔جدا : یونانی الفاظ آٹوز بمعنی خود اور نوموس بمعنی قانون سے ماخوذ اصطلاح۔آزاد اپنے آپ کو کنٹرل کرنے والا۔

Autoplasty *(aw-to-plas'-ti)* [G. autos, self; plassein, to form]. Replacement of tissue by a graft of tissue from the same body--autoplastic, adj.; autoplast, n.

خود پیوندی : یونانی الفاظ آٹوز بمعنی خود اور پلیسین بمعنی بنانا سے ماخوذ اصطلاح۔ اسی جسم سے بافت کے پیوند کے ذریعہ بافت کا دوبارہ لگانا۔

Autopsy *(aw-top'-si)* [G. autopsia, seeing with one's own eyes]. The examination of a dead body for diagnostic purposes.

معائنہ لاش : یونانی لفظ آٹوپسیا بمعنی اپنی آنکھوں سے دیکھنا' سے ماخوذ اصطلاح۔ مردہ جسم کی پڑتال۔

Autosome *(aw'-to-som)* [G. autos, self; soma, body]. A chromosome other than a sex chromosome.

آٹوسوم۔ خودلونیہ : یونانی الفاظ آٹوز بمعنی خود اور سوما بمعنی جسم سے ماخوذ اصطلاح۔ عام کروموسوموں میں سے ایک جنسی اہمیت کے کروموسومز کو جنسی کروموسومز کہتے ہیں جو تعداد میں دو ہوتے ہیں۔ بقایا آٹو سوم ہوتے ہیں۔

Autosuggestion *(aw-to-su-jest'-yun)* [G. autos, self; L. suggestio, from suggerere, to suggest]. Self-suggestion; uncritical acceptance of ideas arising in the individual's own mind. Occurs in hysteria (q.v.).

خودایعاز : خود تجویز کرنا۔ فرد کے اپنے ذہن میں ابھرنے والے نظریات کی غیر تنقیدی قبولیت۔

Autotransfusion *(aw-to-trans-fuzhun)* [G. autos, self; L. transfusio, from transfundere, to pour off, transfer]. The infusion into a patient of the actual blood lost by haemorrhage, especially when it occurs into the abdominal cavity.

خودانتقال : مریض میں ضائع شدہ خون کے بدلے انتقال خون خصوصاً جب بطنی کہفہ میں خون ضائع ہونے کا عمل ہو۔

Avascular *(a-vas'-ku-lar)* [G. a-, not; L. vasculum, a small vessel]. Bloodless; not vascular, i.e. without blood vessels. **a. necrosis,** death of bone from deficient blood supply following injury or possibly through disease, often a precursor of osteoarthritis--avascularize, v.t., v.i.; avascularity, n.

بے رگ۔ غیر عروقی : یونانی لفظ اے بمعنی نہیں اور لاطینی لفظ واسکولم بمعنی چھوٹا برتن سے مرکب اصطلاح خون کے بغیر۔ خونی رگوں کے بغیر۔

A ventyl, Nortriptyline. Similar to amitriptyline (q.v.). See ANTIDEPRESSANT.

ایونٹائیل : نارٹرپٹائلین۔

Aversion *(a-ver'-zhun)*. A method of treatment by deconditioning. Effective in some forms of addiction and abnormal behaviour.

کراہت۔ نفرت : علاج کا ایک طریقہ۔ نشے اور خلاف معمول رویہ کی بعض اقسام میں موثر۔

Avertin *(av'er-tin)*. Bromethol (q.v.).

Avian *(a'-vi-an)* [L. avis, bird]. Pertaining to birds. **a. tubercle bacillus** resembles the other types of tubercle bacilli, but rarely causes disease in man.

طیوری : لاطینی لفظ ایوس بمعنی پرندہ سے ماخوذ اصطلاح پرندوں سے متعلق۔

Avidin *(av'-i-din)*. An antivitamin which interferes with the absorption of biotin (q.v.). Found in raw egg white.

ایویڈن : ضد حیاتین جو بایوٹن کے انجذاب میں مداخلت کرتا ہے۔ کچے انڈے کی سفیدی میں پایا جاتا ہے۔

Avirulent *(a-vir'-ul-ent)* [G. a-, not; L. virus, poison]. Without virulence (q.v.).

غیر قشمی : یونانی لفظ اے بمعنی نہیں اور لاطینی لفظ وائرس بمعنی زہر سے مرکب اصطلاح۔ زہریلے پن کے بغیر۔

Avitaminosis *(a-vit'-a-min-os-is)* [G. a-, not; L. vita, life; G. -osis, condition]. Any disease resulting from a deficiency of vitamins.

قلت حیاتین۔ بے وٹامنی : یونانی لفظ اے بمعنی نہیں' لاطینی لفظ وائیٹا بمعنی زندگی اور یونانی لفظ اوسس بمعنی حالت سے مرکب اصطلاح۔ حیاتین کی کمی سے واقع ہونے والا مرض۔

Avomine *(av'-o-men)*. An antiemetic drug with a powerful and prolonged action. Used in travel sickness, nausea and vomiting. Given 2 h before a journey, it will act for 6 to 12 h. Also has antihistamine properties, therefore useful in allergic conditions.

ایومین : متلی اور قے کے روکنے والی دوا۔ سفر سے دو گھنٹے پہلے دی جاتی ہے۔ اس کا اثر ۶ تا ۱۲ گھنٹے رہتا ہے۔ الرجی میں بھی مفید ہے۔ پرومیتھازین تھیوکلیٹ۔ قے روکنے کے لئے ایک گولی صبح ایک شام ہچکی روکنے کے لئے ایک گولی صبح ایک دوپہر ایک شام۔

Avulsion *(a-vul'-shun)* [L. avellere, to tear away]. A forcible wrenching away, as of a limb, nerve or polypus. **phrenic a.,** tearing of the phrenic nerve to paralyse one side of the diaphragm to rest a tuberculous base of lung.

قلع : زبردستی پرے ہٹانا۔ مثلاً کسی جارح یا لمب اور عصب کو۔

Axilla *(aks-il'-a)* [L.]. The armpit--axillary, adj., applied to nerves, blood and lymphatic vessels.

بغل۔ گوشہ : لاطینی لفظ۔ بغل۔

Axis *(aks'-is)* [L.]. 1. The second cervical vertebra. 2. An imaginary line passing through the centre; the median line of the body--axial, adj.

محوری مہرہ۔ محورہ۔ محور : (۱) گردن کا دوسرا مہرہ۔ (۲) مرکز میں سے گزرنے والی خیالی لکیر۔ جسم کی درمیانی لکیر۔

Axon *(aks'-on)* [G. axon, axis]. or axis cylinder. That process of a nerve cell conveying impulses away from the cell; the essential part of the nerve fibre and a direct prolongation of the nerve cell--axonal, adj.

محور جسم۔ محوریہ : یونانی لفظ ایکسون بمعنی محور سے ماخوذ اصطلاح۔ عصبی خلیے کا طریق یا زائدہ جس سے وہ خلیے سے دور امپلس بھیجتا ہے۔ عصبی ریشے کا لازمی حصہ اور عصبی خلیے کا براہ راست بڑھاؤ۔ فعلیات کی اکائی عصبی خلیہ یا نیورون ہے۔ اس میں نیوکلیس ہوتا ہے اس کے جسم سے پتلی پتلی شاخیں یا ڈینڈرائٹس نکلتی ہیں۔ سیل کی دوسری جانب ایک لمبا ریشہ ہوتا ہے جس کو ایکسون کہتے ہیں۔ ایکسون کا ایک سرا کسی عضو پر اور دوسرا کسی ایکسون کے ڈینڈرائٹس سے رابطہ قائم کر لیتا ہے۔ عصبی رو کی ایکسون میں نوعیت برقی لہر کی طرح ہوتی ہے مگر جب یہ لہر ایک عصبی خلیے سے دوسرے خلیے میں جاتی ہے تو اس کی نوعیت کیمیائی ہوتی ہے۔

Axonotemsis *(aks'-on-ot-mes'-is)* [G. axon, axis; tmesis, a cutting]. Peripheral degeneration as a result of damage to the axons of a nerve. The internal architecture is preserved and recovery depends upon regeneration of the axons, and may take many months (about 25.4 mm a month is the usual may result from pinching, crushing or-prolonged pressure.

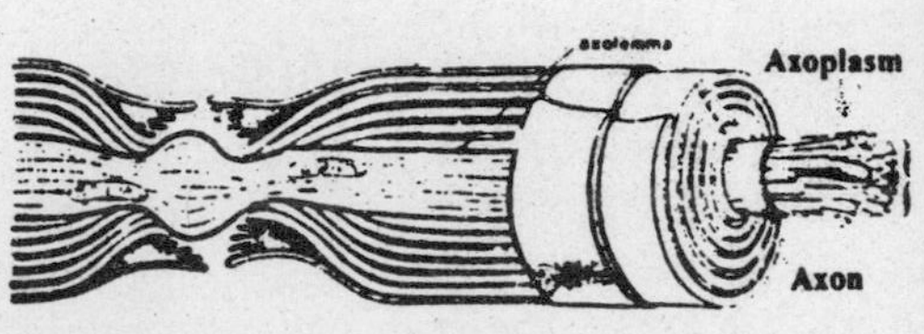

ایکسونوٹ میسس : عصب کے ایکسون کے نقصان کے نتیجہ میں جانبی تخفیف۔

Azacyclonal Frenquel. Tranquillizer.

ازاسائیکلونل : سکون پہنچانے والی دوائی۔

Azathioprine *(az-a-thi'-o-pren)*. Immuno-suppressive drug.

فقدان کرم منی : یونانی الفاظ اے بمعنی نہیں، زو بمعنی زندگی در سپرما بمعنی بیج سے ماخوذ اصطلاح نر کا بانجھ پن کیونکہ سپرمیٹوزوآ پیدا نہیں ہوتے۔

Azoospermia *(a-zo-o-sperm'-i-a)* [G. a-, not; zoe, life; sperma, seed]. Sterility of the male through non-production of spermatozoa.

خون میں موجودگی یوریا : یونانی الفاظ اے بمعنی نہیں، زوٹیکوس بمعنی زندگی محفوظ رکھنے کے لئے موزوں اور ہیما بمعنی خون سے ماخوذ اصطلاح۔ دیکھیے یوریمیا۔

Azotaemia *(az-ot-e'-mi-a)* [G. a-, not; zotikos fit for preserving life; haima, blood]. Syn. uraemia (q.v.)--azotaemic, adj.

Azathioprine *(az-a-thi'-o-pren)* Antimetabolite Work by competing against purine, ar essential metabolite for cell division.

ازاتھیوپرین : اینٹی میٹابولائیٹ۔ پیورین کے خلاف مقابلہ کر کے کام کرتا ہے۔

Azoturia *(az-ot-ur'-e-a)* [G. a-, not; zotikos, fi for preserving life; ouron, urine]. Pathologica excretion of urea in the urine--azoturic, adj.

ا جوروبولی : یونانی الفاظ اے بمعنی نہیں، زوٹیکوس بمعنی حفاظت زیست کے لئے موزوں اور اورون بمعنی پیشاب سے ماخوذ اصطلاح۔ پیشاب میں یوریا کا اخراج۔

Azygos *(az'-i-gos)* [G. a-, not; zygon, yoke] Occuring singly, not paired. **a. veins,** thre unpaired veins of the abdomen and thora which empty into the inferior vena cava -azygous, adj.

مجرد۔ بے جفت : جوڑا نہ بنانا۔ اکیلے ہونا۔ مجرد وریدیں بطن اور تھوریکس کی تین وریدیں ہیں۔ جو زیریں ورید اجوف میں کھلتی ہیں۔ ایک واحد۔

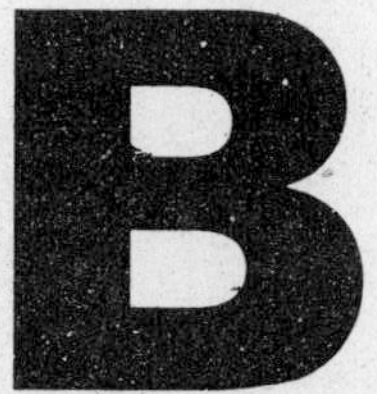

(be') Symbol for bel, boron, magnetic flux density.

بی: بورون، بیل اور مقناطیسی فلکس ڈینسٹی کی علامت۔

(beta) The second letter of the Greek alphabet. Symbol for the β-chain of haemoglobin.

بیٹا: یونانی حروف تہجی کا دوسرا حرف اور ہیموگلوبن کی زنجیر کا بیٹا حصہ۔

abin ski's reflex or sign *(ba'-bin-skez)* [Joseph Francois Felix Babinski, French neurologist, 1857-1932]. It is a movement disorder of big toe. When the sole of foot is touched, the toe move upwards (dorsiflexion) instead of downward (plantan flexion). It indicates that there is something wrong with upper motor neurons and present in organic not hysterical hemiplegio. Babies show dorsiflexion but after they start walking normal plantar flexion is exhibited.

بیبن سکائی ریفلیکس یا سائن: پاؤں کے انگوٹھے کی زیریں جانب کی بجائے بالائی جانب حرکت جو پاؤں کی ایڑی پر دباؤ پڑنے سے ہوتی ہے۔ یہ بالائی موٹر نیورانز کے زخمی ہونے کو یا بیماری کو ظاہر کرتی ہے۔ بچوں میں یہ حرکت پائی جاتی ہے لیکن جب وہ چلنا سیکھ لیتے ہیں تو یہ ختم ہو جاتی ہے۔ چھوٹے بچے میں یہ رجحان ہوتا ہے کہ جو چیز اس کے رکھی جائے، اسے پکڑنے کی کوشش کرتا ہے۔ جب بچہ دو سال کا ہو جاتا ہے تو یہ رجحان ختم ہو جاتا ہے۔

by *(ba'be')* An infant; a child not yet able to walk.

شیر خوار بچہ: وہ بچہ جو ابھی چلنے پھرنے کے قابل نہیں ہوتا۔

cillemia *(basi'le'-me-a)* [L. *bacillum,* stick; G. *heima,* blood]. The presence of bacilli in the blood.

عصیہ دمویت: لاطینی لفظ بیسلم بمعنی چھڑی اور یونانی لفظ ہیما بمعنی خون سے مرکب اصطلاح۔ خون میں سلاخ نما جراثیم کی موجودگی۔

Bacilluria *(bas-il-u'-ri-a)* [L. *bacillum,* stick; G. *ouron,* urine]. The presence of bacilli in the urine.

عصیہ بولی: لاطینی لفظ بیسلم بمعنی چھڑی اور یونانی لفظ اورون بمعنی پیشاب سے مرکب اصطلاح۔ پیشاب میں سلاخ نما جراثیم کی موجودگی۔

Bacillus *(bas-il'-us)* [L. *bacillum,* stick]. A term now restriced to a genus of bacteria consisting of aerobic, Grampositive, rod-shaped cells which produce endospores and the majority are motile by means of peritrichate flagella. These organisms are saprophytes and their spores are common in soil and dust of the air. Colloquially the word is still used to describe any rod-shaped micro-organism. *Bacillus anthracis* causes anthrax in man and in animals.

بیسلس، عصیہ: لاطینی لفظ بیسلم بمعنی چھڑی سے ماخوذ اصطلاح۔ جراثیم کا ایک جنس جو سلاخ نما ہوا بارش اور گرام مثبت پر مشتمل خلیے ہوتے ہیں۔ یہ بذرے بناتے ہیں۔ یہ گند خور ہیں۔ ان کے بذرے زمین اور ہوا کی گرد میں کثرت سے پائے جاتے ہیں۔ بیسلس انتھرے سس انسان اور جانوروں میں انتھرکس کی بیماری پیدا کرتا ہے۔ بے سلائی شکل میں لمبے ہوتے ہیں۔

Baclofen *(bak'-lo-fen).* Reduces spasticity of voluntary muscle; mode uncertain. Side effects include nausea, vomiting, diarrhoea, gastric discomfort, muscular inco-ordination, hytopnia, mental confusion, vertigo and drowsines. Particularly useful for multiple selerosis. Dosage needs to be 'titrated' to each individual, 100 mg being the maximum dose without hospital supervision.

Bacteraemia *(bak-te-rem'-i-a)* [G. rion, staff; haima, blood]. The presence of bacteria in the blood--bacterae- mic, adj.

جراثیم دمویت: یونانی الفاظ بیکٹیریوں بمعنی سٹاف سے اور ہیما بمعنی خون کا مجموعہ۔ خون میں جراثیم کی موجودگی۔

Bacteria *(bak-te'-ri-a)* [G. bakterion, staff]. A group of micro-organisms, also called the 'schizomycetes'. They are typically small cells of about 1 micron in transverse diameter. Structurally there is a protoplast, containing cytoplasmic and nuclear material (not seen by ordinary methods of microscopy) within a limiting cytoplasmic membrane, and a supporting cell wall. Other strucutures such as flagella, fimbriae and capsules may also be present. Individual cells may be spherical, straight or curved rods, or spirals; they may form chains or masses, and some show branching with mycelium formation. They may produce various pigments including chlorophyll. Some form endospores. Reproduction is chiefly by simple binary fission. They may be free living, saprophytic or parasitic; some are pathogenic to man, animals and plants--bacterium, sing.; bacterial, adj.

جراثیم: یونانی لفظ بیکٹیریوں بمعنی سٹاف سے ملغوز اصطلاح۔ خورد جسیموں کا ایک گروہ۔ انہیں شائزومائی سیٹس بھی کہا جاتا ہے۔ سب سے چھوٹے خلیے۔ بلغم کے خوردبینی امتحان میں جراثیم نظر نہیں آتے۔ کئی امراض ان کی وجہ سے ہوتے ہیں۔ شکل کے لحاظ سے یہ کاکسی' بے سلائی دیریو اور سپائرلا ہیں۔

Bactericide *(bak-ter'-i-sid)* [G. bakterion, staff; L. coedere, to kill]. Any agent which destroys bacteria--bactericidal, adj.; bactericidally, adv.

جراثیم کش دوا : یونانی لفظ بیکٹیریوں بمعنی سٹاف اور لاطینی لفظ سیڈیئر بمعنی مارنا سے مرکب اصطلاح۔ جراثیم کو تباہ کرنے والا ایجنٹ۔

Bactericidn *(bak-ter-i-sid'-in)* [G. bakterion, staff; L. coedere, to kill]. Antibody which kills bacteria.

بیکٹیریوسیڈن : یونانی لفظ بیکٹیریون بمعنی سٹاف اور لاطینی لفظ سیڈیئر بمعنی جان سے مارنا سے مرکب اصطلاح۔ جراثیم کو ختم کرنے

ی اینٹی باڈیز۔

Bacteriologist *(bak-ter-i-ol'-oj-ist)* [C bakterion, staff; logos, discourse]. One wh studies and is skilled in the science of bacte iology.

ثومیات دان۔ عالم جرثومیات :جراثیم کے علم کے ماہر۔

Bacteriology *(bak-te'-ri-ol'-oj-i)* [G. bakterio staff; logos, discourse]. The science and stuc of bacteria--bacteriological, adj.; bacteriolog cally, adv.

ثومیات۔ علم الجراثیم :یونانی الفاظ بیکٹیریون بمعنی سٹاف اور وس بمعنی بحث کا مجموعہ۔ جراثیم کا مطالعہ۔ جراثیم کی سائنس۔

Bacteriolysin *(bak-te-ri-o-li'-sin)* [G. bakterio staff; lysis, a lossening]. A specific antibo (q.v.) which causes dissolution of bacteria.

اثیم پاشین: ایک مخصوص اینٹی باڈی جراثیم کو ختم کرتی ہے۔

Bacteriolysis *(bak-ter'- i-ol'-is-is)* [G. bakterio staff; lysis, a lossening]. The disintegrati and dissolution of bacteria--bacteriolytic, adj

اثیم پاشی: جراثیم کا خاتمہ۔

Bacteriophage *(bak-ter'-i-o-faj)* [G. bakterio staff; phagein, to eat]. A virus parasitic bacteria. Some of these are used for typi staphylococci, etc.

ٹیریوفیج : یونانی الفاظ بیکٹیریون بمعنی سٹاف اور فیجین بمعنی کھانا کا عہ۔ جراثیم پر طفیلی وائرس جو فلٹر ہو جاتا ہے۔

Bacteriostasis *(bak-ter-i-o-sta'-sis)* [(bakterion, staff; stasis, a standing still]. Arre or hindrance of bacterial growth--bacterio atic, adj.

د جراثیم : یونانی الفاظ بیکٹیریون بمعنی سٹاف اور سٹیسس بمعنی سوش کھڑا ہونا کا مجموعہ۔ جراثیمی افزائش یا بڑھاؤ کی رکاوٹ یا اس تخفیف۔

Bacteriotherapy *(bak-ter'-i-o-ther'-ap-i)* [bakterion, staff; therapeia, treatment]. Tre ment of disease by introduction of bacte into the blood stream e.g. malaria in the tre ment of neurosyphilis--bacteriother- apeut adj.

ج کا مجموعہ۔ خون میں جراثیم داخل کر کے بیماری کا علاج کرنا۔

acteriuria *(bak-te-ri-u'-ri-a)* [G. bakterion, staff; ouron, urine]. The presence of bacteria in the urine (100,000 or more organisms per ml). Acute urinary tract infection may be preceded by, and active pyelonephritis may be associated with asymptomatic bacteriuria.

actrim *(bak'-trim)*. Trimethoprim (q.v.) and suphamethoxazole (q.v.). Useful for urinary tract infections and gonorrhoea.

aker's itch. Contact dermatitis (q.v.) resulting from flour or sugar.

جرب الخبازین۔ نابنائیوں کی خارش: آٹے یا شکر سے پیدا ہونے والی بیماری۔

AL. (British anti-lewisite). Dimercaprol (q.v.)

بی اے ایل: دیکھئے ڈائیمر کیپرول

alanitis *(bal-an-i-tis)* [L. balanus, acorn; G. -otis, inflammation]. Inflammation of the glans penis and prepuce.

سپاری کی سوجن۔ ورم حشفہ: عضو تناسل کی کھال کی سوزش۔

alanoposthitis *(bal-an-o-pos-thi'-tis)* [G. balanos, acorn; posthe, membrum virile; -itis, inflammation]. Inflammation of the glans penis and prepuce.

التہاب حشفہ قضیب وقلفہ: عضو تناسل کی کھال کی سوزش۔

alantidiasis *(bal-an-tid-i-a-sis)*. Infection with the ciliate Balantidium coli; uncommon parasite of man; may cause dysentery. Treated with full course of metronidazole.

بیلنٹی ڈایاسس: بیلنٹیڈیم کولی سے ہونے والی بیماری ۔ انسان پر طفیلی جس سے پیچش ہو جاتی ہے۔

alnus *(bal'-an-us)* [G. balanos, acorn]. The glans of the penis or clitoris.

حشفہ۔ سپاری: بظر یا عضو تناسل کی گلینز۔

alkan beam. Wooden beam attached to a hospital bed whereby a Thomas' bed splint can be slung up, with pulleys and weights attached, to allow movement and provide counterbalance to the weight of the splint and leg.

بلقانی جبیرہ: چوبی بیم جو ہسپتال میں بستر کے ساتھ ملحق ہوتی ہے۔

allottement *(bal-lot-mon(g))* [G. a shaking about]. Testing for a floating object, especially used to diagnose pregnancy. A finger is inserted into the vagina and the uterus is pushed forward; if a fetus is present it will fall back again, bouncing in its bath of fluid--ballottable, adj.

تہر۔ جنین کو ٹٹولنا: فرانسیسی لفظ جس کے معنی ہلانا ہیں۔ تیرنے والی شے کو ٹیسٹ کرنا۔ خصوصی طور پر وضع حمل کا پتہ چلایا جاتا ہے۔ ویجائنا میں انگلی داخل کی جاتی ہے اور یوٹرس کو آگے دھکیلا جاتا ہے ۔ اگر بچہ موجود ہو تو وہ واپس آجائے گی اور سیال لگا ہوگا۔

Balsam of peru *(bawl'-sam)*. A viscous aromatic liquid from the trunks of South American trees. Mild antiseptic used with zinc ointment for pressure sores.

پیرو کا مرہم: یک گاڑھا خوشبودار مائع جو جنوبی امریکہ کے درختوں کے تنوں سے حاصل کیا جاتا ہے۔ ہلکا دافع جراثیم جو جست کے مرہم کے ساتھ بستری ناسور کے لئے استعمال کیا جاتا ہے۔

Balsam of Tolu *(bwl'-sam of to-loo')*. Brown aromatic resin. Constituent of Friar's balsam. Used as syrup of Tolu in cough syrups.

تو بو کا شربت : کھانسی کے شربت میں مستعمل۔ بھوری خوشبو دار رال۔

Baltimore paste. See ALUMINIUM PASTE.

Bandage *(band'-aj)* [F. from bande, a strip] Traditionally a piece of cloth, calico, cotton, flannel. etc. of varying size and shape applied to some part of the body to retain a dressing or a splint; support, compress, immobilize; prevent or correct deformity. There are now several circular bandages that are applied with an applicator to almost any part of the body. Examples are Netalast, Tube-gauze, Tubigrip, **Capelline b.** [L. capella, a cap] or divergent spica, bandage covering head or amputation stump. **compression b.,** function is as name implies. Specially used to give support without constriction of vessels after an ankle sprain, by applying alternate layers of wool and bandage thrice. Compression bandage also used to shrink a part, as an amputation stump. **elastic b.** belongs to the preceding group, specially useful for varicose veins, after a sprain or removal of plaster. **Esmarch's b.,** made from elastic rubber; used to obtain a bloodless field in surgery of the limbs. **many-tailed b.,** composed of five narrow strips joined in their middle **triangular b.,** useful for arm slings, for securing splints, in first-aid work, and for inclusive dressings of a part, as a whole hand or foot. **Velpeau's b.,** the arm to chest bandage for a fractured clavicle. [Alfred Armond Louis Marie Velpeau, Parisian surgeon, 1795-1867.]

پٹی : فرانسیسی لفظ بینڈے بمعنی پٹی سے ماخوذ۔ کپڑے کا ایک ٹکڑا جو لمبائی کے رخ کٹا ہوتا ہے۔ کسی زخم وغیرہ پر باندھنے کے لئے استعمال ہوتا ہے۔

Bankhart's operation *(bak'-harts)*. For recurrent dislocation of shoulder joint; the decfect of the glenoid cavity is repaired. This is the modern procedure, augmented by reefing the joint capsule and pularissubsca muscle.

بینک ہیرٹ اپریشن : گلینائڈ کہفہ کے نقص کی مرمت کا طریقہ۔ شانے کی ہڈی اتر جائے تو اسے درست کرنے کا جدید طریقہ۔

Banocide *(ban'-o-sid)*. Diethylcarbamazide (q.v.).

بینوسائیڈ : دیکھئے ڈائی ایتھائل کاربامیزائڈ۔

Banti's disease Syn., splenic anaemia. Now regarded as a manifestation of portal hypertension (q.v.) with alimentary bleeding and splenomegaly causing leucopenia and thrombocytopenia. [Guido Banti, Italian physician, 1852-1925.]

مرض بنٹی۔ عظم الطحال: پورٹل وریدوں میں اضافی دباؤ۔ خون کی کمی اور آنتوں سے خون رسنا وغیرہ اس کی علامات ہیں۔

Barbados leg *(bar-ba-doz)*. Elephant leg. A tropical disease caused by a thread-like worm called 'Filaria'; lymphangitis, followed by sclerosis and fibrosis interferes with drainage of lymph, and oedema of the limb ensues. See ELEPHANTIASIS.

فیل پا: ایک مرض جو ایک کیڑے فلیریا سے ہوتا ہے۔

Barber's itch or rash See SYCOSIS.

حجامی خارش : دیکھئے سائیکوسس۔

Barbiturates *(bar-bit'-u-ratz)*. A widely used group of sedative drugs derived from barbituric acid (a combination of malonic acid ar urea). Small changes in the basic structu result in the formation of rapid-actin medium or long-acting barbiturates and wide range is now available. Continual u may result in addiction. Action potentiated presence of alcohol. Allergic skin reactio may occur in some patients. See also BU OBARBITONE PHENOBARBITONE. etc.

بیچوریٹ :باربیٹورک ایسڈ سے حاصل شدہ ادویات کا ایک گروہ۔ تار استعمال سے آدمی عادی ہو جاتا ہے۔ بعض اشخاص میں ان سے ر کی الرجی بھی ہوتی ہے۔ ممسک ادویات کا گروہ۔ خواب آور وں کا ایک گروہ جو سیکونل، نیم بیوٹل، لومینل، باربیٹل، سوڈیم، ایمیٹل ی دواؤں پر مشتمل ہے۔

Barbotage *(bar-bot-azh')* [F. from barboter, dabble]. Method of spinal anaesthesia; sma amount of solution from syringe injected in subarachnoid space. plunger partiall withdrawn allowing CSF to mix wit remaining solution in syringe. Part of th mixture then injected and plunger aga partially withdrawn. This process may b repeated several times before entire conten of syringe injected.

بوٹیج: سن کرنے کا ایک طریقہ جو انجکشن کے ذریعہ ہوتا ہے اور وہ ھ کی ہڈی پر لگایا جاتا ہے۔

Barium sulphate *(bar-i-um)*. Heavy insolub powder used as a contrast agent in X-r visualization of alimentary tract.

یم سلفیٹ: بھاری غیر حل پذیر سفوف۔

Barlow's disease syne., infantile scurvy (q.v [Thomas Barlow, English physicia 1845-1945.]

س بارلو : دیکھئے انفنٹائل سکروی۔

Barotrauma *(bar-o-traw'-ma)* [G. baro weight; trauma, wound]. Injury due to change in atmospheric or water pressure, e. ruptured eardrum.

وٹراما : یونانی الفاظ بیروس بمعنی وزن اور ٹراما بمعنی زخم کا مجموعہ۔ کی یا آبی دباؤ میں تبدیلی کی وجہ سے زخم مثلاً کان کا پردہ پھٹ

Barrier nursing A method of preventing t

spread of infection from an infectious patient to the other in an open-ward. It is achieved by 'isolation' technique.

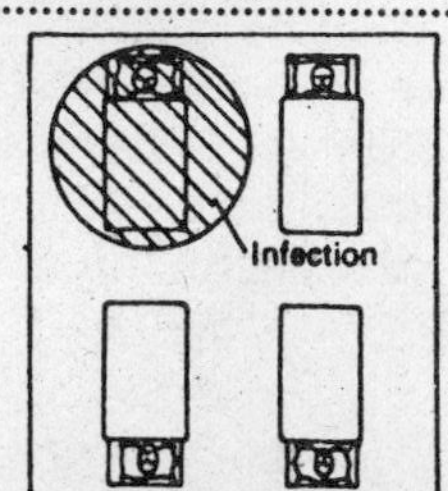

Barrier nursing

حاجز نرسنگ : کھلے وارڈ میں ایک مریض سے دوسرے مریض کو چھوت کی بیماری سے بچانے کا طریقہ۔ یہ علیحدگی کی تکنیک ہے۔

Bartholinitis *(bar-tol-in-i'-tis)* [after Caspar Bartholin; G. -itis, inflammation]. Inflammation of Bartholin's glands (q.v.).

التہاب غدہ برتولین : بارتھولن غدود کی سوزش۔

Bartholin's glands *(bar'-to-lin)*. Two small glands situated at each side of the external orifice of the vagina. Their ducts open just outside the hymen. [Caspar Bartholin, Danish anatomist, 1655-1748.]

شرمگاہ کے غدود۔ بصلتي الدهليز : اندام نہانی یا ویجانا کے بیرونی سوراخ کے ہر طرف واقع دو غدود۔ ان کی نالیاں پردۂ بکارت یا ہائیمن سے ذرا باہر کھلتی ہیں۔ ازدواجی ملاپ کے وقت ان غددوں سے پیلی پیلی چکنی رطوبت خارج ہوتی ہے اور ازدواجی فعل میں لطف اور سہولت پیدا کرتی ہے۔

Bartonella fever Non-protozoal haemolytic anaemia. Syn., Oroya fever.

بارٹونیلا بخار : خون کی کمی جس میں پروٹوزآ کا تعلق نہیں خون میں سرخ ذرات ہیموگلوبن کی کمی کی وجہ سے بخار۔

Basal ganglia *(ba'-sal-gan'-gli-a)* [G. basis, base; G. ganglion, a swelling]. Grey cells at the cerebral base. The lentiform nucleus, comprising globus pallidus and putamen, together with the caudate nucleus make up the corpus striatum, which with the claustrum is called the basal ganglia. Concerned with modifying and co-ordinating voluntary muscle movement. Site of degeneration in Parkinson's disease. See PARALYSIS.

اساسی عقود : سر برل اساس پر خاکی خلیے۔

Basal narcosis *(nar-ko'-sis)* [G. a benumbing]. The pre-anaesthetic administration of narcotic drugs which reduce fear and anxiety, induce sleep and thereby minimize postoperative shock.

بنیادی تنویم : نشے سے قبل خواب آور ادویات جن سے فکر اور پریشانی میں تخفیف ہو جاتی ہے اور وہ نیند لاتی ہیں۔اس لئے اپریشن کے بعد تکلیف میں کمی کرتی ہیں۔

Base *(bas)* [G. basis, base]. 1. The lowest part. 2. The main part of a compound. 3. In chemistry, the substance which combines with an acid to form a salt--basal, basic, basilar, adj.

اساس : یونانی لفظ بیسس بمعنی اساس یا بنیاد سے ماخوذ اصطلاح۔ (۱) سب سے زیریں حصہ۔ (۲) مرکب کا بڑا حصہ۔ (۳) کیمیاء میں وہ مادہ جو ترشہ کے ساتھ مل کر نمک بناتا ہے۔

Basilar-vertebral insufficiency. See VERTEBROBASILAR INSUFFICIENCY.

Basilic *(bas-il'-ik)*. [G. basilikos, royal]. Prominent. A vein on the inner side of the arm. The **median b.** at the bend of the elbow is generally chosen for venepuncture.

باسلیق : یونانی لفظ بیسلیکوز بمعنی شاہی سے ماخوذ اصطلاح۔ بہت نمایاں یا واضح۔ بازو کی اندرونی ایک ورید۔

Basophil *(ba'-zo-fil)* [G. basis, base; philein, to love]. Showing an affinity for basic dyes. Used in histology, e.g. basophilic; applied to some leucocytes (basophil polymorphonuclear).

Basophil

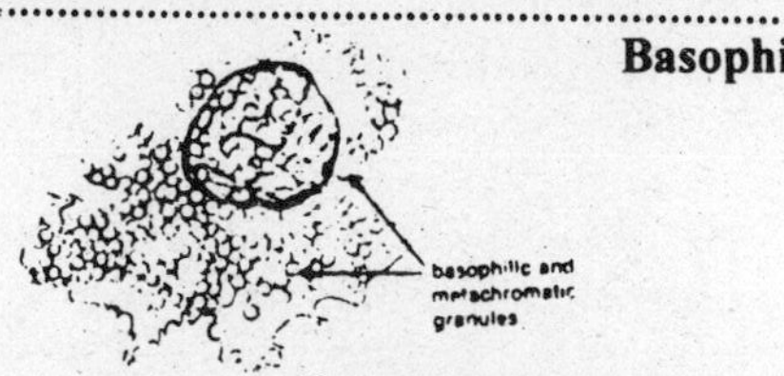

اساسی رنگ پسند۔ بے سوفل : یونانی الفاظ بیسس بمعنی بنیاد یا اساس اور فلین بمعنی محبت کرنا کا مجموعہ۔ اساسی رنگوں کے لئے کشش دکھانا۔ نسیجیات میں مستعمل خون میں ایک فیصد۔

Basophilia *(ba-zo-fil'-i-a)* [G. basis, base; philein, to love]. Increase of basophils in the blood: basophilic staining of red blood corpuscles.

سفید خلایتی دمویت : خون میں بیس فلز کی زیادتی۔ سرخ خونی۔ خلیوں کو بیسو فلک رنگنا۔

Batchelor plaster A type of double abduction plaster, with the legs encased from groins to ankles, in full abduction and medial rotation. The feet are then attached to a wooden pole or 'broomstick'. Alternative to frog plaster, but the hips are free

پلستر کی ایک قسم

Bath *(bath)* [A.S. boeth]. 1. The apparatus used for bathing. 2. The immersion of the body or any part of it into water or any fluid; or the application of spray, jet or vapour of such fluid to the body. The term is modified according to (a) temperature, e.g. cold, contrast, hot, tepid; (b) medium used, e.g.mud, sand, water, wax; (c) medicament added, e.g. Milton, potassium permanganate, saline, sulphur; (d) function of medicament, e.g. astringent, disinfectant; (e) part bathed, e.g. arm bath, sitz bath (f) environment, e.g. bed bath. See HYDROTHERAPY.

صحت گاہ۔ غسل۔ حمام : (۱) غسل کے لئے استعمال ہونے والا سامان۔ (۲) جسم یا اس کے کسی حصے کا پانی یا کسی سیال میں ڈوبنا یا سیال کے بخارات یا سپرے کا جسم پر اطلاق۔

Battered baby syndrome An infant who shows clinical or radiological evidence of lesions which are frequently multiple and involve mainly the head, soft tissues, or the long which cannot be unequivocally explained by natural disease or simple acc- ident. Described by Caffet in 1957. Widened to battered child syndrome by Kempe in 1961. Syne., 'abused child'; 'non-acidentally injured child'. All these terms reflect acc physical injuries done to child to exclusion of emotional problems of parents 'Child mishandling' therefore preferred by many people.

بیٹرڈ بے بی سنڈروم : دانت نکالنے والا بچہ جس کا جسم متورم ہو۔

Bauer's operation *(baw'-erz)*. Ligation o incompetent popliteal vein; useful when pai in calf is severe and foot is cyanosed.

Bazin's disease Erythema induratum. A chroni recurrent disorder, involving the skin of th legs of women. There are deep-seated nodule which later ulcerate. [Antoine Pierre Ernes Bazin, French dermatologist, 1807-78.]

زن مرض : خواتین کی ٹانگوں کی جلد کا نقص۔ گہرائی میں گرہیں پڑ جاتی ہیں جن سے السر بھی ہوسکتا ہے۔

BCG. *(Bacillus-Calmette-Guerin)*. A vaccin (q.v.) prepared from bovine tubercle bacill BCG vaccination by inhalation can be carrie out using an ultrasonic nebulizer for roomful of 500 people.

ی سی جی : جراثیم سے تیار شدہ ویکسین۔ تپ دق کے ٹیکے میں ستعمل دوا۔ اس ویکسین میں تپ دق کے کمزور لیکن زندہ جراثیم ہوتے ں۔ جہاں ٹیکہ لگتا ہے، وہاں پھنسی بن جاتی ہے۔

Bearing-down 1. A pseudonym for th expulsive pains in the second stage of labou 2. A feeling of weight and descent in th pelvis associated with uterine prolapse or pe vic tumours.

دزہ کا دوسرا درجہ : پیلوس میں وزن یا بوجھ کا احساس یا جھوٹا د۔ وضع حمل کے دوران ہونے والے درد جو وضع حمل کے دوسرے جہ میں ہوتے ہیں۔

Beat *(bet)* [A.S. beatan]. Pulsation of the bloo in the heart and blood vessels. **apex b.**, se APEX. **dropped b.** refers to the loss of a occasional ventricular beat as occurs in ext asystoles (q.v.) **premature b.**, an extrasystol

ڑکن : دل اور رگوں میں خون کی دھڑکن۔

Beaver-breather Intermittent positive pressu respirator, used in respiratory paralysis f short periods of artificial respiration.

صنوعی عمل تنفس : وقفوں سے مثبت دباؤ کے ساتھ سانس دینے ۔ مصنوعی تنفس میں مختصر وقفوں کے لئے تنفسی بے ہوشی میں مستعمل۔ ں میں ڈوبے شخص کو نکال کر دوبارہ تنفس جاری کرنے کا مصنوعی یقہ۔

Becosym *(be-kos'-im)*. Tablets, syrup ar

ampoules containing aneurine, riboflavine, nicotinamide and pyridoxine. Used in vitamin B deficiency.

بیکوسم : حیاتین ب کی کمی میں مستعمل۔ اینورین، ریبوفلیون، نکوٹینا مائڈ اور پیریڈوکسن پر مستعمل امپول، شربت یا گولیاں۔

Bedbug A blood-sucking insect belonging to the genus Cimex. Cimex lecturlarius is the most common species in temperate and C. hemipterus in tropical zones. They live and lay eggs in cracks and crevices of funiture and walls. They are nocturnal in habit and their bites leave a route for secondary infection.

کھٹمل : خون چوسنے والا کیڑا۔ یہ رات کے وقت باہر نکلتے ہیں۔ فرنیچر یا دیواروں کے شگافوں میں انڈے دیتے ہیں۔

Bedsore See PRESSURE SORE

ناسور پلنگ : پہلے پہل متاثر حصہ سرخ ہو جاتا ہے جو گرم و نرم ہو جاتا ہے۔ جلد پھٹ جاتی ہے اور ناسور ہو جاتا ہے۔

Beer's knife. Delicate instrument with triangular blade used in cataract operations for incision of cornea preparatory to removal of lens. [Georg Jospeh Beer, Austrian ophthalmologist, 1763-1821].

چاقو بیئر : ایک نازک اوزار جس میں تکونہ بلیڈ ہوتا ہے۔ اپریشن میں کام آتا ہے۔

Behaviour *(be-ha'-vur)*. In general sense, conduct. As a psychological term, means response of an organism to its situation in relation to its environment **b. therapy,** See AVERSION.

تاثر ۔ کردار ۔ عمل : کنڈکٹ۔ رویہ۔ ماحول کے تناسب سے کسی جیسے کا ردعمل۔

Behaviourism *(be-ha'-vur-izm)*. A psychological term which denotes an approach to psychology through the study of responses and reactions, i.e. behaviour.

کرداریت : ایک نفسیاتی اصطلاح جو عمل اور ردعمل کے مطالعہ کے ذریعہ نفسیات کو ظاہر کرتا ہے۔

Behcet's syndrome Described by Behcet in 1937. Stars with ulceration of mouth and/or genitalia with eye changes such as conjuunctiveitis, keratitis, or hypopyon iritis. One site may be affected months or years before the others. There may also be skin nodules. thrombophlebitis and arthfitis of one or more of the large joints. Pulmonary, gastrointestinal and neurological complications are being increasingly reported. Cause unknown; some favour virus, others an allergic vasculitis. No effective treatment apart from attempts to suppress worst phases with steroids. Blindness may result from ocular complications.

بہسیٹ سنڈروم : منہ یا اعضائے تولید کے ناسور شروع ہونے والی بیماری جو آنکھوں کو بھی متاثر کرتی ہے۔ کوئی موثر علاج نہیں۔ اندھا پن بھی واقع ہو سکتا ہے۔

Bejel *(bej'-el)*. Non-venereal syphilis.

بیجل : آتشک کی ایک قسم۔ بغیر جماع کا آتشک۔

Belladonna *(bel-a-don'-a)*. Dried leaves of deadly nightshade (Atropa belladonna). Powerful antispasmodic. Effects mainly due to the alkaloid atropine (q.v.).

بیلاڈونا۔ اٹروپین۔ بلاون : اٹرو یا بیلاڈونا کے خشک پتے۔ ان میں الکلائڈ ایٹروپین ہوتا ہے۔ ماہواری کے درد میں مفید۔ بے سلری پیچش میں ایک گولی صبح ایک دوپہر ایک شام۔ بستر پر پیشاب نکلنے کی صورت میں بچے کو نصف گولی سوتے وقت۔

Bellergal *(bel-erg'-al)*. Combination of phenobarbitone, belladonna alkaloids and ergotamine. Useful for menopausal syndrome, premenstrual tension and migraine.

Belle indifference' The incongruous lack of emotion despite incapacitating symptoms commonly shown by patients with hysteria. First noted by Janet in 1893. [Pierre Marie Felix Janet, French psychiatrist; 1859-1947.]

بیلے انڈفرنس : ہسٹریا کے مریضوں میں علامات جو جذبات کی کمی ظاہر کرتی ہیں۔

Bellocq's sound or cannual *(bel'-oks, kan'-u-la)*. A curved tube used for plugging the posterior nares.

بیکوکس ساؤنڈ یا کینولا : خلفی نتھنوں کے لئے مستعمل خمیدہ نلی۔

Bell's mania. Acute delirious mania. A severe psychosis combining delirium with the gross psychomotor activity of mania. Was almost invariably fatal before the introduction of electrotherapy.

بیلزمانیا : برقی تھراپی سے پہلے مہلک بیماری تھی۔ ہذیانی کیفیت۔ ذہنی انتشار کا آخری درجہ۔

Bell's palsy See PALSY.

Benactyzine *(ben-ak'-ti-zen)*. Tranquillizing drug with selective action, producing sense of detachment from environment. Used in anxiety and tension neuroses.

بینکٹیزین : ماحول سے الگ تھلگ رہنے کا احساس پیدا کرنے والی دوا۔ پریشانی میں استعمال کی جاتی ہے۔

Benadryl *(ben'-a-dril)*. Diphenhydramine (q.v.).

بیناڈرل : دیکھئے ڈائی فینائیڈرامین۔ بیش محسس دوائی کھانسی میں مفید۔

Bencard *(ben'-kard)*. See D-VAC ANTIGENS.

Bence-jones' protein. Protein bodies appearing in the urine of some patients with myelomatosis (q.v.). On heating the urine they are prescipitated out of solution at 50° to 60° c: they redissolve on further heating to boiling point and reprecipitate on cooling. [Henry Bence-Jones, London physician. 1814-73.]

بینس جونز پروٹین : استخوانی گودے کی بیماری میں، مبتلا اشخاص کے پیشاب میں لحمی اجسام کا ظہور۔ ہڈیوں کے گودے کی بیماری میں لحمی اجسام کا پیشاب میں آنا۔

Bendrofluazide *(bend-ro-flu'-a-zid)*. Diuretic that decreases reabsorption of sodium and chloride in kidney tubules. 10 mg daily orally, or intramuscularly on alternate days. Used with caution in renal or hepatic failure.

بنڈروفلوازائیڈ : ایپری نیکس۔ پیشاب آور۔ گردوں میں سوڈیم اور کلورائیڈ کے انجذاب کو کم کرتی ہے۔ بلڈ پریشر یا ہائپرٹنشن انلارجڈ پراسٹیٹ اور جگر کی سختی میں اس کی ایک گولی روزانہ ناشتہ کے بعد۔

Bends. See CAISSON DISEASE.

عوضی تشنج : دیکھئے کیسن مرض۔

Benedict's solution *(ben'-e-dikts sol-u'-shun)*. A solution of copper sulphate which is easily reduced, producing colour changes, Used to detect the presence of glucose. [Stanley R. Benedict, American chemist, 1884-1936.]

بنی ڈکٹس سلیوشن۔ بنی ڈکٹ محلول: نیلے تھوتھے کا محلول جس کی آسانی سے تخفیف یا تحویل ہو جاتی ہے اور رنگ تبدیل ہو جاتا ہے۔ گلوکوس یا انگوری شکر کی موجودگی کا پتہ چلانے کے لئے استعمال کیا جاتا ہے۔ امریکی کیمیا دان بینڈکٹ کے نام پر اس کا نام ہے جس کا دورحیات ۱۸۸۴ع تا ۱۹۳۶ع تھا۔

Benemid *(ben' i-mid)*. Probenecid (q.v.).

Benign *(be-nin')* [L. benigmus, kind]. Innocent. A term used to denote the opposite of malignant.

سلیم۔ معمولی مرض : لاطینی لفظ بنگنس بمعنی مہربان سے ماخوذ اصطلاح۔ معصوم۔

Benorylate *(ben-or'-i-lat)*. Esterified aspirin. Odourless. Tasteless. Well absorbed from gastrointestinal tract. Has anti-inflammatory, analgesic and antipyretic properties comparable with aspirin, and acts longer. Significantly less likely to cause hidden bleeding.

بینورائی لیت : ایسٹر شدہ اسپرین۔ بے بو اور بے ذائقہ۔ ہضمی قنال میں اچھی طرح جذب ہوجاتی ہے۔

Benuride *(ben'-u-rid)*. Phenylethylacetylurea (q.v.).

بینورائیڈ : دیکھئے فینائل ایتھائل ایسیٹائیلوریا۔

Benvil *(ben'-vil)*. Tybamate (q.v.).

بینول : دیکھئے ٹائیبامیٹ۔

Benzalkonium *(ben-zal-ko'-ni-um)*. Antiseptic with detergent action. Used as 1 per-cent solution for skin preparation, 1:20 000 to 1:40000 for irrigation. Incompatible with soap, with loss of activity.

بنزلکونیئم : دافع تعفن۔ جلد کے لئے اس کا ایک فیصد محلول استعمال کیا جاتا ہے۔

Benzedrine *(ben'-ze-drin)*. Amphetamine (q.v.).

بینزیڈرن : دیکھئے امفیٹامین۔

Benzene *(ben'-zen)*. A colourless inflammable liquid obtained from coal tar. Extensively used as a solvent. Its chief importance in the medical sphere is in industrial toxicology. Continued exposure to it results in leucopenia, anaemia and purpura.

بنزین :ایک بے رنگ مائع۔ آتش گیر۔ کولتار سے حاصل کیا جاتا

ہے۔ محلل کے طور پر مستعمل ہے۔ بنزول۔ نقطۂ جوش ۸۰ء۱ س' اس کے بخارات آنکھوں میں جلن پیدا کرتے ہیں۔

Benzhexol *(benz-heks'-ol)*. Antispasmodic used mainly for rigidity of Parkinsonism. Side effects include dryness of mouth, nausea and vertigo.

بینزہیکسول : دافع تشنج۔ اس سے منہ کی خشکی اور متلی بھی ہو سکتی ہے۔ آرٹین۔ اس کی ایک گولی صبح ایک دوپہر ایک شام برائے علاج پارکن سونزم یعنی رعشہ۔

Benzocaine *(ben'-zo-kan)*. Relatively non-toxic surface anaesthetic. Used as dusting powder (10 percent), ointment (10 percent), suppositories (5 g), lozenges (1½ g). Occasionally given orally in gastric carcinoma.

بنزوکین : نسبتاً غیر زہریلی' سطح کو سن کرنے والی دوا۔ سفوف۔ مرہم یا چوسنے والی گولی کے طور پر مستعمل۔

Benzodiazepine *(ben-zo-di-az'-e-pen)*. Tranquillizer; allays acute anxiety.

Benzoic acid *(ben-zo'-ik as'-id)*. Fungistatic and antiseptic. Used with salicylic acid in Whitfield's ointment (ung. acid. benz, co.) for ringworm. Rarely given orally owing to irritant effects.

لوبانی ترشہ : دافع تعفن اور سماروغ۔ رنگ ورم کے لئے مستعمل۔

Benzoin *(ben'-zo-in)*. Natural balsamic resin from Siam and Sumatra. Widely used as Friar's balsam by steam inhalation in bronchitis and other chest conditions.

لوبان۔ لبان جاوا۔ سلاجیت : قدرتی رال۔ چھاتی کے امراض میں مستعمل جاوا کا لوبان۔

Benzthiazide *(bens-thi'-az-id)*. Oral diuretic. See CHLOROTHIAZIDE.

بینز تھایازائیڈ : دیکھئے کلوروتھیازائیڈ۔

Benztropine methanesulphonate *(bens-trop-in-me-than-sul'-fon-at)*. Muscle relaxant. Anti-Parkinsonism.

بینزٹروپین۔ میتھین سلفونیٹ : اعضلات کو آرام پہنچانے والی دوا۔

Benzyl Benzoate *(ben'-zil ben'-zo-at)*. Aromatic liquid; has ascaricidal properties and used mainly in treatment of scabies though now replaced by Quella (q.v.). Occasionally given internally as an antispasmodic.

بینزائیل بنزوایٹ : ایک خوشبودار۔ مائع۔ خشکی یا کھجلی میں مستعمل۔

Benzyl penicillin *(ben'-zil)*. Penicillin (q.v.).

بنزائیل پنسلین : دیکھیے پنسلین۔

Beogex *(be'-o-jeks)*. Suppository that after insertion releases CO_2 which produces evacuation of bowel.

بیوجیکس : اس کے استعمال سے کاربن ڈائی آکسائیڈ خارج ہوتی ہے جس سے فضلہ خارج ہوتا ہے۔

Bephenium-hydroxynaphthoate *(bef-en'-i-um hi-droks-i-nat'-tho-at)*. Anthelmintic, effective against hookworm and roundworm. Given on an empty stomach at least one hour before food.

بفینیم ہائیڈروکسی نفتھوایٹ : ہک ورم اور راؤنڈ ورم کے خلاف موثر خوراک سے کم از کم ایک گھنٹہ پہلے خالی پیٹ دینی چاہیئے۔

Beri-beri *(ber'-e-ber'-e)* [Singhalese, beri, weakness]. A deficiency disease caused by lack of aneurine (vitamin B_1). Occurs mainly in those countries where the staple diet is polished rice. The symptoms are pain from neuritis, paralysis, muscular wasting, progressive oedema, mental deterioration and, finally, heart failure.

بیری بیری (مرض) : آنیورین یا حیاتین ب' کی کمی سے پیدا ہونے والی بیماری جو چاول کھانے والی اقوام میں ہوتی ہے۔

Berylloisis *(ber-il-i-o'-sis)*. Industrial disease; impaired lung function because of interstitial fibrosis from inhalation of beryllium. Steroids used in treatment.

Berkomine *(berk'-o-men)*. Imipramine (q.v.).

برکومین : دیکھئے امپرامین۔

Berkozide *(berk'-o-zid)*. Bendrofluazine (q.v.).

برکوزائید : دیکھئے بینڈروفلوآزین۔

Betadine *(bet'-a-den)*. Povidoneiodine. Antibacterial. Available as aerosol spray, surgical scrub, scalp lotion and ointment.

بیٹاڈین : جراثیم کو تباہ کرنے والی دوا۔ پوڈیڈون آیوڈین۔ گنجے پن

میں مستعمل۔

Betamethasone. *(bet-a-meth'-a-zon).* Slightly more potent than dexamethasone, q.v. Forty times more potent orally than cortisone. Less water retaining effects than prednisone. Exceptionally powerful anti-inflammatory action in skin disease when applied locally. Useful in chronic ulcerative colitis and Crohn's disease.

بیٹامیتھاسون : آتش گیر عمل کے خلاف موثر۔ بیٹنی لان۔ اس کی ایک ایک گولی دن میں ۳ دفعہ برائے سوزش گردہ مزمن' یوریمیا' سپرنگ کٹار' سورائے سز لیعنی چنبل۔

Betaptin *(bet-ap'-tin).* Alprenolol (q.v.).

بیٹیپٹن : دیکھیے الپرینولول۔

Betazole hydrochloride *(bet'-az-ol hi-dro-kl-or'-id).* Used to stimulate gastric juice in tests. Less reaction than histamine.

بیٹازول ہائیڈروکلورائیڈ : گیسٹرک جوس کوتحریک دینے کے لئے مستعمل۔

Bethanecol *(beth-an'-e-kol).* A compound resembling carbachol in activity, but is relatively non-toxic. Used in urinary retention, abdominal distension and myasthenia gravis.

بیتھینی کول : مرکب جو پیشاب کی بیماری اور بطنی پھیلاؤ میں مستعمل ہے۔

Bethanidine *(beth-an'-i-den).* Adrenergic blocking, antihypertensive drug. Interferes with transmission in sympathetic adrenergic nerves, especially sympathetically mediated vascular reflexes, thus can lead to postural and exercise hypotension.

بتھینی ڈین : ایک ضد بیش طنابی دوا۔

Betnesol *(bet'-nes'-ol).* Betamethasone (q.v.).

بیٹ نی سول : دیکھیے بیٹامیتھاسون۔ اس کے قطرے ناک' کان' آنکھ میں ڈالے جاتے ہیں۔ ورم اور خارش میں مفید۔

Betnovate *(bet'nov-at).* Cream containing fluorocortisone. More effective than those containing hydrocortisone (see COBADEX). but it can be absorbed through the skin and can produce local or systemic side effects.

بٹنوویٹ : دیکھیے بیٹامیتھاسون۔ زخموں پر لگانے کے لئے۔

Bicarbonate *(bi-kar'-bon-at).* A salt of carbonic acid. **blood b.,** that in the blood indicating the alkali reserve. Also called 'plasma bicarbonate'.

بائی کاربونیٹ : کاربانک ایسڈ کا نمک۔ کاربانک ایسڈ جس میں آدھی تیزابی ہائیڈروجن کی جگہ دھات لے لیتی ہے مثلاً سوڈیم بائی کاربونیٹ۔

Bicellular *(bi-sel'u-lar).* L. bis, twice; cella, stall, chamber]. Composed of two cells.

دوخلوی : لاطینی الفاظ بس بمعنی دگنا اور سیلا بمعنی خانہ کا مجموعہ۔ دو خلیوں پر مشتمل۔

Biconcave *(bi-kon'-kav)* [L. bis, twice; concavus, hollow]. Concave or hollow on both surfaces.

مقعر الطرفین : لاطینی الفاظ بس بمعنی دوگنا اور کنکیوس بمعنی کھوکھلا کا مجموعہ۔ دونوں سطوح پر کھوکھلا یا مقعر۔

Biconvex *(bi-kon-veks)* [L. bis, twice; convexus, convex]. Convex on both surfaces.

محدب الطرفین : لاطینی الفاظ بس بمعنی دوگنا اور کونیکسس بمعنی محدب کا مجموعہ۔ دونوں سطوح سے محدب۔

Bicornuate *(bi-korn'-u-at)* [L. bis, twice; conutus, horned]. Having two horns, generally applied to a double uterus or a single uterus possessing two horns.

والقرنین۔ دو قرنہ : دوسینگوں والا۔ ڈبل یا سنگل یوٹرس جس کے دو سینگ ہوں۔ دوہری بچہ دانی یا دو شاخوں والی۔

Bicuspid *(bi-kus'-pid)* [L. bis, twice cuspis point]. Having two cusps or points, **b. teeth** the premolars. **b valve,** the mitral valve between the left atrium and ventricle of the heart.

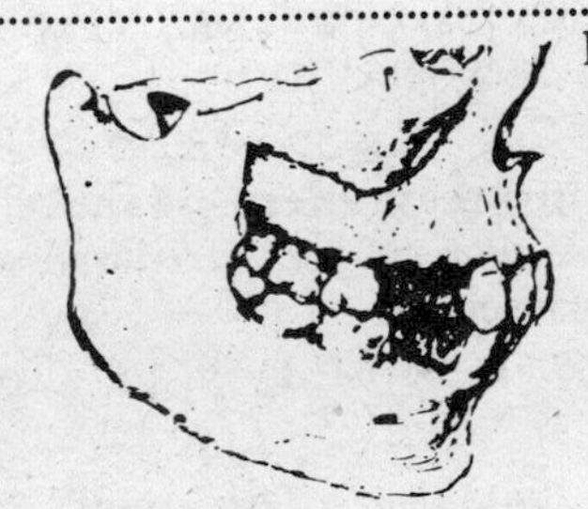

Bicuspids

دوشرفہ۔ دنکا : دولفظوں والا۔دو منہ ہونا۔

Bider *(bi'-da)*. Low-set, through-like basin in which the perineum can be immersed, whilst the legs are outside and the feet on the floor. Can have attachments for douching the vagina or rectum.

بیڈا : ایک بیسن جس میں پیرینیم رکھا جاتا ہے۔ جبکہ ٹانگیں باہر رہتی ہیں اور پاؤں فرش پر ہوتے ہیں۔ ڈوش دینے کا برتن۔ فرج یا مقعد کے لئے مستعمل آلہ۔

Bifid *(bi'-fid)* [L. bis, twice; finder, to cleave]. Divided into two parts. Cleft, Forked.

دوشاخہ۔ دو شگافہ : دوحصوں میں منقسم۔

Bifurcating *(bi'-gwan-ids)*. Oral antidiabetic agents. Useful for obese patients. Can be used with sulphonylureas. Syn., diaguanides.

Bilateral *(bi-lat'-er-al)* [L. bis, twice; lateralis, of the side]. Pertaining to both sides--bilaterally, adv.

دوجانبہ : دونوں اطراف سے متعلق۔

Bilateral

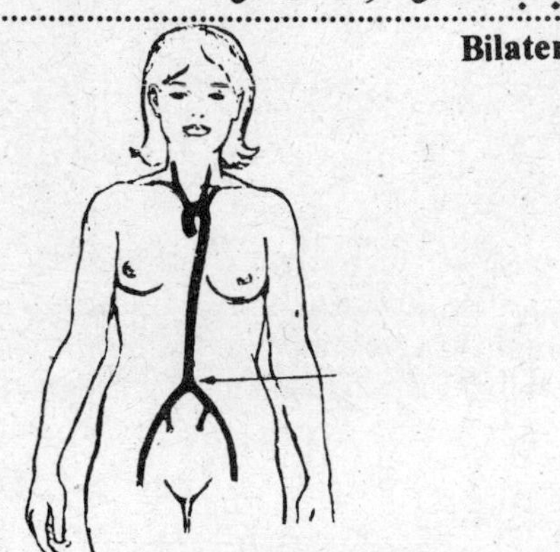

Bile *(bil)* [L. bilis]. A bitter, alkaline, viscid, greenish-yellow fluid secreted by the liver and stored in the gall-bladder. It contains water, mucin, lecithin, cholesterol, bile salts and the pigments bilirubin and biliverdin. **b. ducts,** the hepatic and cystic, which join to form the common bile duct. **b. salts,** emulsifying agents, sodium glycocholate and taurocholate--bilious, biliary, adj.

بائل۔ صفرا۔ پت : کڑوا، الکلائن، گاڑھا، سبزی مائل پیلا سیال جو جگر میں بنتا ہے اور پتے میں ذخیرہ ہوتا ہے۔

Bilhariza *(bil-har'-ze-a)*. Syn., Schistosoma (q.v.).

بل بارزیا : دیکھئے شسٹوسوما۔

Bilharziasis *(bil-har-zi'-a-sis)*. Syn., schistosomiasis (q.v.).

بل ہارزیائے سز : دیکھئے شسٹوسومیاسس۔ ٹریماٹوڈ قسم کے کیڑے جو انتڑیوں اور مثانے کی دیواروں پر لگے رہتے ہیں۔ ان کی انفیکشن عرب و افریقی ممالک میں زیادہ ہوتی ہے۔

Biliary *(bil'-i-ar-i)* [L. bilis, bile]. Pertaining to bile.-**b. colic,** paroxysmal pain in right upper guadrant of abdomen, due to smooth muscle spasm arising in the bile passages. **b- fistual,** an abnormal track conveying bile to the surface or to some other organ.

صفراوی : بائل سے متعلق۔

Bilious *(bil'-yus)* [L. bilis, bile]. 1. Pertaining to bile. 2. Pertaining to excess of bile. 3. A non-medical word signifying a digestive upset.

صفراوی : لاطینی لفظ بائلس بمعنی بائل سے ماخوذ اصطلاح۔ (۱) بائل سے متعلق۔ (۲) بائل کی زیادتی سے متعلق۔ (۳) نظام انہضام میں خرابی۔

Bilirubin *(bi-li-roo'-bin)* [L. bilis, bile; ruber, red]. A pigment largely derived from the breakdown of haemoglobin from red blood cells destroyed in the spleen. When it is released it is fat-soluble, gives an indirect reaction with Van den Bergh's test and is potentially harmful to metabolically active tissues in the body, particularly the basal nuclei of the immature brain. Indirect b. is transported to the blood attached to albumen to make it less likely to enter and damage brain cells. In the liver the enzyme glucuronyl transferase conjugates indirect fat-soluble b. with glucuronic acid to make it water-soluble, in which state it is relatively non-toxic, reacts directly with Van den Bergh's test and can be excreted instools and urine. See PHOTOTHERAPY.

سرخ صفرا۔ بلی روبن : لاطینی الفاظ بلس بمعنی بائل اور ربر بمعنی سرخ کا مجموعہ تلی میں تباہ شدہ سرخ خونی خلیوں سے ہیموگلوبن کی شکستی

سے اخذ شدہ پگمنٹ بڑی عمر کے بچوں اور بالغوں میں یہ مادہ جگر سے بڑی آنت میں خارج ہوتا ہے اور وہاں سے جسم سے باہر خارج ہو جاتا ہے۔ اس سے پہلے کہ بچے کا جگر کیمیائی عمل سے اس مادے سے فائدہ اٹھانے کی صلاحیت پیدا کر لے' یہ بچے کی خون ہی میں رہ جاتا ہے اور پیلے رنگ کا ہوجاتا ہے۔ ایسی حالت میں بچے کو چمکیلی روشنیوں میں رکھا جائے تاکہ یرقان کو کم کیا جا سکے۔

Biliuria *(bi-li-u'-ri-a)* [L. bilis, bile; G. ouron, urine]. The presence of bile pigments in the urine--biliuric, adj.

صفرابولی : لاطینی لفظ بلس بمعنی بائل اور یونانی لفظ اور ون بمعنی پیشاب سے مرکب اصطلاح پیشاب میں بائل پگمنٹس کی موجودگی۔

Biliverdin *(bi-li-ver'-din)* [L. bilis, bile; virens, green]. The green pigment of bile formed by oxidation of bilirubin.

سبز صفرا : لاطینی الفاظ بلس بمعنی بائل اور وائیرنز بمعنی سبز کا مجموعہ۔ بائل کا سبز پگمنٹ۔

Billorth's operation. Partial gastrectomy. B.O.I. Excision of the lower part of the stomach with anastomosis of the remaining part to the duodenum. B.O.II Resection of the distal end of the stomach with closure of the lines of section and gastrojejunostomy. [Christian Theodor Billroth, Austrian surgeon, 1829-94.]

بلراتھ اپریشن : معدہ کے زیریں حصے کا قطع

Billroth I operation

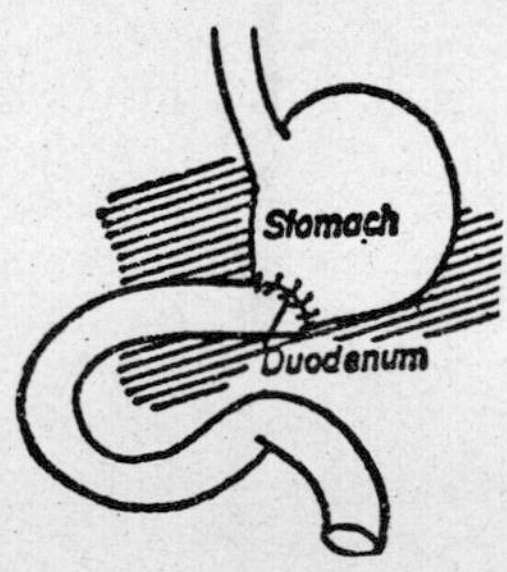

Bilobate *(bi-lo'-bat)* [L. bis, twice; G. lobos, rounded flap]. Having two lobes.

دو فضہ : دو لوبوں یا حصوں والا۔

bilobular *(bi-lob'-u-lar)* [L. bis, twice; G. lobos, lobe]. Having two little lobes or lobules.

دو لختکی : لاطینی لفظ بس بمعنی دوگنا اور یونانی لفظ لوبوس بمعنی لوب سے مرکب اصطلاح۔ دو چھوٹے لوبوں والا۔

bimanual *(bi-man'-u-al)* [L. bis, twice; manus, hand]. Performed with both hands. A method used in gynaecology where by the internal genital organs are examined between one hand on the abdomen and the other hand or finger within the vagina.

Biumanual method

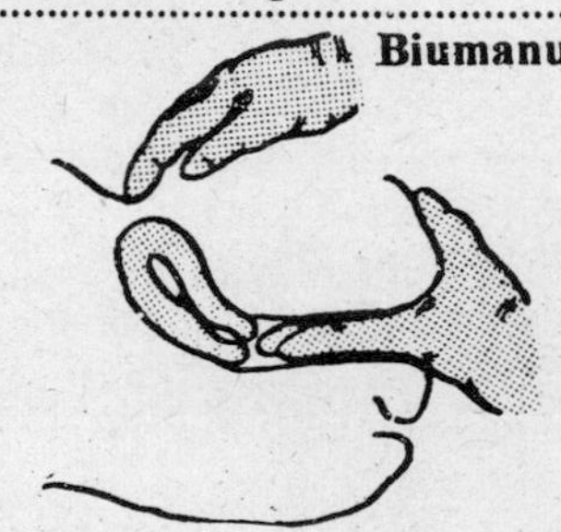

دو دستہ : لاطینی الفاظ بس بمعنی دوگنا اور مینس بمعنی ہاتھ کا مجموعہ۔ دونوں ہاتھوں سے کوئی کام کرنا۔ ایک ہاتھ پیٹ پر رکھا جاتا ہے اور دوسرا ہاتھ یا انگلی کو ویجائنا میں داخل کی جاتی ہے' اس طرح اندرونی اعضا کا مطالعہ کیا جاتا ہے۔

Binaural *(bin-aw'-ral)*. [L. bini, two by two; auris, ear]. Pertaining to, or having two ears. Applied to a type of stethoscope (q.v.).

دوگوشی : دوکان رکھنا یا دوکانوں سے متعلق۔ سٹیتھوسکوپ کی ایک قسم۔

Binet's test *(be'-na)*. Properly Binet-Simon scale. A series of graded intelligence tests in which an individual's intelligence level (mental age) is compared with his chronological age. [Alfred Binet, French psychologist, 1857-1911.]

بیناٹیسٹ : ذہنی آزمائشوں کا ایک سلسلہ۔ ذہنی صلاحیت معلوم کرنے کا طریقہ۔

Biniodide of mercury *(bin-i-o-did of mer'-kur-i)*. A solution of mercuric iodide in potassium iodide solution. It is less irritant and less toxic than mercuric chloride (perchloride, q.v.), and possibly less effective. Used as 1:2000 to 1:5000 solution for application to the skin: 1-10 000 for douches.

بینوڈائیڈ آف مرکری : پوٹاشیم آیوڈائڈ کے محلول میں مرکیورک ایوڈائیڈ کا محلول۔

Binocular *(bin-ok'-u-lar)* [L. bini, two by two; oculus, evy]. 1. The use of both eyes in vision. 2. An optical instrument requiring both eyes for its use.

دوچشمہ : (۱) مشاہدہ کے لئے دونوں آنکھوں کا استعمال۔ (۲) ایک الہ جس میں دونوں آنکھیں استعمال کی جاتی ہیں۔

Binovular *(bin-ov'-u-lar)* [L. bini, two by two; ovum, egg]. Derived from two separate ova. Binovular twins may be of different sexes. See UNIOVULAR.

دوبیضی : دو الگ بیضوں سے اخذ شدہ۔

Biochemistry *(bi-o-kem'-is-tri)* [G. bios, life; from chymos, juice]. Physiological chemistry--biochemical, adj.

حیاتی کیمیا۔ حیوی کیمیا : فزیالوجیکل کیمیا۔ جاندار اشیاء کی کیمیاء۔

Bioengineering *(bi'-o-en-jin-er'-ing)*. Designing sophisticated microelectronic or mechanical equipment for external use by patients, for attachment to patients, or placement inside patients.

بایوا انجینئرنگ : خود الیکٹرانی یا میکانکی سامان کی تیاری۔ طب سے متعلق انجینئرنگ کا شعبہ جو طبی معلومات کے لئے آلات ایجاد کرتا ہے۔ مثلاً ایکسرے مشین۔

Biogastrone *(bi-o-gas'-tron)*. Carbenoxolone sodium (q.v.).

بایوگیسٹرون : دیکھئے کاربنکسولون سوڈیم۔

Biology *(bi-ol'-oj-i)* [G. bios, life; logos, discourse]. The science of life, dealing with the structure, function and organization of all living things--biological, adj; biologically, adv.

حیاتیات۔ علم حیات : حیات یا زندگی کی سائنس جو تمام جاندار اشیاء کی بناوٹ، فعل اور تنظیم سے بحث کرتی ہے۔ علم کی وہ شاخ جس میں جان دار اشیاء کا مطالعہ کیا جاتا ہے۔ حیاتیات نیچرل سائنس کی سب سے اہم شاخ ہے۔ حیاتیات کی دو شاخیں ہیں علم الحیوانات یا حیوانیات اور علم النباتات یا نباتیات، حیوانیات جانوروں کے مطالعہ کا نام ہے اور نباتیات پودوں کے مطالعہ کا دراصل جانور اور پودے دونوں ہی جاندار ہیں۔ اس لئے حیاتیات دراصل مطالعہ زندگی ہے۔ زندگی کو مکمل طور پر سمجھنے کے لئے جانوروں کے ساتھ ساتھ پودوں کا مطالعہ بھی ضروری ہے۔ حیاتیات کی ایک اہم شاخ شکلیات ہے اسے علم ساخت بھی کہہ سکتے ہیں۔ علم کی یہ شاخ بیرونی و اندرونی ساخت یا بناوٹ کے متعلق بحث کرتی ہے اس کی دو شاخیں ہیں۔ بیرونی شکلیات میں جانور یا پودے کا بیرونی مطالعہ کیا جاتا ہے اور اندرونی شکلیات میں اندرونی مطالعہ، جانداروں کے اندرونی ساخت دو طرح سے مطالعہ کی جاتی ہے ایک تو صرف آنکھ سے اور دوسرے خوردبین سے اول الذکر کو تشریح الاعضاء یا علم تشریح کہتے ہیں اور موخرالذکر کو نسیجیات کہتے ہیں۔ خلیوں کا وسیع مطالعہ علم خلیات یا خلیاتیات کہلاتا ہے۔ فعلیات میں ہمیں یہ معلوم ہوتا ہے کہ جانداروں کے مختلف حصے کیا کام انجام دیتے ہیں۔ ماحولیات سے ہمیں یہ معلوم ہوتا ہے کہ جاندار اپنے اردگرد کے قدرتی حالت یا ماحول سے کیا اثر قبول کرتا ہے اور ان سے اس کے اندرونی و بیرونی ساخت میں کیا کیا تبدیلیاں پیدا ہوتی ہیں۔ جینیات میں ہم بھیکے میں بارودی اور جنین کے بڑھاؤ اور نمو کا حال شروع سے آخر تک معلوم کرتے ہیں۔ جماعت بندی میں ہم جانداروں کی زندگی کا حال اس لحاظ سے معلوم کرتے ہیں کہ وہ کس جماعت اور کس گروہ میں شامل کیے جاتے ہیں اور اس جماعت یا گروہ کی کیا خصوصیات ہیں۔

Biopsy *(bi-op'si)* [G. bios, life; opsis, version]. Observation of the living Excision of tissue from a living body for microscopic examination to establish diagnosis.

حیوی تشخیص۔ تشخیص نسیجی : جاندار کا مشاہدہ۔ تشخیص کی خاطر خوردبینی مشاہدہ کے لئے جاندار جسم سے بافت کا انقطاع۔

Biorhythmics *(bi-o-rith'-miks)* [G. bios, life; rhythmos, rhythm]. Modern study of the three main biological functions; physical, emotional and intellectual cycles.

Biotexin *(bi-o-teks'-in)*. Novobiocin (q.v.).

بایوٹیکسن : دیکھئے نوووبایوسن۔

Biothin *(bi'-ot-in)*. A member of vitamin B complex; also known as vitamin H and as co-enzyme R. Probably synthesized by intestinal flora. Lack of it may cause dermatitis in human beings.

بائیوٹین۔ وٹامن ح : حیاتین ب کمپلکس کا ایک رکن۔حیاتین ایچ اور مددگار خامرہ آر۔

Biparietal *(bi-par-i'-et-al)* [L. bis, twice; paries, wall]. Pertaining to both parietal bones.

جداریئی : دونوں پیرائٹل ہڈیوں سے متعلق۔

biparous *(bip'-ar-us)* [L. bis, twice; parere, to bring forth]. Producing two offspring at one birth.

توام زا : ایک پیدائش میں دو بچے پیدا کرنا۔ جڑواں بچے پیدا ہونا یا کرنے کی اہلیت۔

bipolar *(bi-po'-lar)* [L. bis, twice; polus, pole]. Having two poles.

دو قطبی : دوقطبوں والا۔

BIPP. A pasty mixture of bismuth subnitrate, iodoform, and liquid paraffin. Used as antiseptic dressing in acute osteitis.

بی آئی پی پی : بسمتھ سب نائٹریٹ' آیوڈوفارم اور مائع پیرافین کا پیسٹ۔

Birth The act of sxpelling the young from the mother's body; delivery; being born. **b. canal,** the cavity or canal of the pelvis through which the baby passes during labour. **b.certificate.** a legal document given on registration, within 42 days of a birth. **b. control,** prevention or regulation of conception by any means; contraception. **b. injury,** any injury occurring during parturition, e.g. fracture of a bone, subluxation of a joint, injury to peripheral nerve, intracranial haemorrhage. **b. mark,** naevus (q.v.). **premature b.,** one occurring after the 7th month of pregnancy, but before term.

پیدائش۔ جنم۔ ولادت : ماں کے پیٹ سے بچے کو باہر دھکیلنے کا عمل۔ پیدائش کا عمل۔

Bisacodyl *(bi-sa-ko'-dil).* Dulcolax (q.v.).

بائی سیکوڈل : دیکھئے ڈلکولیکس۔

Bisexual *(bi'-seks-u-al)* [L. bis, twice; sexus, sex]. Having the characteristics of both sexes; hermaphrodite--bisex-ually, adv.

دوزوجیہ۔ دونسلا : لاطینی الفاظ بس بمعنی دوگنا اور سیکسس بمعنی جنس یا سیکس کا مجموعہ۔ دونوں جنسوں کی خصوصیات رکھنا۔

bismuth *(biz'-muth).* A greyish metal. **b. carbonate,** a mild antacid, used with other alkalis in dyspepsia and peptic ulcer, **b. salicylate,** gastric sedative used in gastroenteritis, **b. sodium tartrate,** a soluble compound used occasionally by intramuscular injection in infective arthritis, **b. subgallate,** yellow insoluble powder. Used as dusting powder in eczema and in suppositories for haemorrhoids. Occasionally given orally as an astringent.

پھول کانسی۔ بسمت : ایک خاکستری دھات۔

Bisolvin *(bi-sol'-vin).* Bromhexine (q.v.)

Bistoury *(bis'-tu-ri)* [F. bistour]. A long narrow knife, straight or curved, used for cutting from within outwards in the opening of a hernial sac, an abscess, sinus or fistula.

نشتر : ایک طویل یا لمبا تنگ چاقو جو سیدھا یا خمیدہ ہوتا ہے جو سوراخ میں کاٹنے کے کام آتا ہے۔

Bitot's spots *(be-toz).* Collections of dried epithelium, flaky masses and micro-organisms at the sides of the cornea. A manifestation of vitamin A deficiency. Xerosis conjunctivae. [Pierre A. Bitot, Bordeaux physician 1822-88.]

بیٹوز سپاٹس : قورینہ کی اطراف پر خورد جسیموں' دوسرے مادوں یا خشک اپی تھیلیم کا جمع ہو جانا۔ حیاتین الف کی کمی کی وجہ سے ایسا ہوتا ہے۔

Bitters Substances, the extracts of which are used as stomachics (q.v.).

مریات : بھوک زیادہ کرنی والی اشیاء۔

Bivalve *(bi'-valv)* [L, bis, twice; valva, leaf of a door]. Having two blades such as in the vaginal speculum.l In orthopaedic work, to divide a plaster of Paris splint into two portions--an anterior and posterior half.

بائیوالو : دو بلیڈوں والا۔ پلاسٹر آف پیرس کو دو پورشنز میں تقسیم کرنا، ایک اوپر والا اور دوسرا نیچے والا۔

Blackwater fever *(bla'k-wa'ter-fi-ver)* A type of malaria fever.

سیاہ بولی بخار : ٹراپکس خصوصاً افریقہ میں ملیریا کی ایک بگڑی ہوئی صورت ۔ سرخ خونی خلیوں کی تباہی کی وجہ سے گہرے رنگ کا پیشاب آتا ہے۔

Bladder *(blad-ar')* [A.S. blaedre]. A membranous sac containing fluid or gas, **gall.b.**, a pear-shapped bag on the under surface of the liver; its function is to store and concentrate the bile, **ideal b.**, term used when ureters are transplanted into an isolated loop of small intestine, one end of which is made to open on the abdominal wall, See ILEOURETEROSTOMY **neurogenic b.**, interference with nerve contról gives rise to retention of urine, presenting as incontinence--or continuous dribbling without retention. Bladder emptied by manual pressure on anterior abdominal wall where necessary. **rectal b.**, term used when ureters are transplanted into the rectum in cases of severe disease of the urinary bladder, **urinary b.**, a muscular bag situated in the pelvis, a reservoir for urine.

مثانہ : سیال یا گیس پر مشتمل ایک جھلی دار تھیلی وہ تھیلی جس میں پیشاب جمع ہوتا ہے۔

Blalock-Hanlon operation Failing a successful Rashkind's septostomy (q.v.) a surgical opening is made between the right and left atrium.

Blalock's operation Anastomosis of the pulmonary artery (distal to a pulmonary stenosis) to a branch of the aorta. Most often performed for Fallot's tetralogy (q.v.). [Alfred Blalock, American surgeon, 1899-1964.]

بلے لاک اپریشن : ایورٹا کی شاخ کی طرف پلمونری شریان کا جال۔

Bland Mild, non-irritating, soothing.

ملطف : نرم ۔ سوزش نہ کرنے والا۔

Blastomyces *(blas'-to-mi-sez)* [G. blastos, germ; mykes, fungus]. A genus of yeast-like organisms--blastomycetic, adj.

نہوضی فطر : یونانی الفاظ بلاسٹوس بمعنی جرثومہ اور مائیکس بمعنی سماروغ کا مجموعہ۔ خمیر ایسے جسیموں کا جنس۔

Blastomycosis *(blas-to-mi-ko'-sis)* [G. blastos, germ; mykes, fungus; -osis, condition]. Granulomatous condition caused by budding, yeast-like organisms. May affect skin, viscera and bones--blastomycotic, adj.

نہوضی فطریت : یونانی الفاظ بلاسٹوس بمعنی جرثومہ، مائیکس بمعنی سماروغ اور اوسس بمعنی حالت کا مجموعہ۔ بڈنگ سے پیدا ہونے والی حالت۔

Blastula *(blas'-tu-la)* An early stage in development of the fertilized ovum when the morula becomes cystic and infolds to become the gastrula.

Bleb [A.S. bledan, to bleed]. One who is subject to frequent loss of blood, as one suffering from haemophilia (q.v.).

فصاد۔ نزیفی : اینگلوسیکسن زبان کے لفظ بلیڈن بمعنی خون سے بہنا سے ماخوذ اصطلاح۔ جس میں خون کا ضیاع ہو۔ مثلاً ہیموفلیا کا مریض۔

Bleeding time' *(bled'-ing tim).* The time required for the spontaneous arrest of bleeding from a skin puncture; under controlled conditions this forms a clinical test.

عرصۂ نزف : جلدی زخم سے خون کو روکنے کا دورانیہ۔

Blennophthalmia *(blen-of-thal'-mi-a)* [G. blenna, mucus; orphthalmia, ophthalmia]. Catarrhal conjunctivitis--blennophthalmic, adj.

بلینوفتھلمیا : ایک مرض۔

Blennorrhagia *(blen-o-raj'-i-a)* [G. blenna, mucus; rhegnynai, to burst]. 1. A copious mucous discharge. 2. Gonorrhoea.

سوزاک۔ جریان مخاط : (۱) میوکس کا اخراج۔ (۲) سوزاک۔

Blennorrhoea *(blen-or-e'-a)* [G. blenna, mucus; rheein, to flow]. Syn., blennorrhagia (q.v.)--blennorrhoeal, adj.

سوزاک۔ جریان مخاط : دیکھئے سوزاک یا مخاطی اخراج یا بلینورکیا۔

Blepharitis (blef-a-ri'-tis) [G. blepharon, eyelid; -itis, inflammation]. Inflammation of the eyelids, particularly the edges--blepharitic, adj.

سلاق۔ ورم اجفان : پپوٹوں کی سوزش۔ خصوصاً کناروں پر۔

Blepharon *(blef'-ar-on)* [G.]. The eyelid; palpebra--blephara, pl.

پپوٹا۔ جفن : آنکھ کا پپوٹا۔

Blepharoptosis *(blef-ar-op-to'-sis)* [G. blepharon, eyelid; plosis, a falling]. See PTOSIS--blepharoptotic, adj.

Blepharospasm *(blef'-a-ro-spazm)* [G. blepharon, eyelid; spasmos, spasm]. Spasm of the muscles in the eyelid, Excessive winking--blepharospastic, adj.

تشنج اجفان : پپوٹوں کا تشنج۔ آنکھوں کا زیادہ جھپکنا۔

Blind loop syndrome Resulting from intestinal obstruction or surgical anastomosis; there is stasis in the small intestine which encourages bacterial growth thus producing diarrhoea and salt deficiencies.

Blind spot. The spot at which the optic nerve leaves the retina. It is insensitive to light.

کورنقطہ۔ تاریک نقطہ : وہ جگہ جہاں اپٹک عصب ریٹنا کو چھوڑتی ہے۔ یہ روشنی کے لئے غیر حساس ہوتی ہے۔

Blsfer [O.N. blastr, a swelling]. Separation of the epidermis from the dermis by a collection of fluid, usually serum or blood. See VESICLE.

آبلہ۔ پھپھولا۔ چھالا : کسی سیال عموماً سیرم یا خون کے جمع ہونے سے ڈرمس سے اپی ڈرمس کی علیحدگی۔

Blistering Fluid Liquor epispasticus, a counterirritant.

منفط سیال : خارش ختم کرنے والا مائع۔

Blocadren *(blok'-a-dren)*. Timolol maleate (q.v.).

Blood [A.S. blod]. The red viscid fluid filling the heart and blood vessels. It consists of a colourless fluid, plasma, in which are suspended the red blood corpuscles, or erythrocytes, the white corpuscles, or leucocytes, and the platelets, or thrombocytes. The plasma (q.v.) contains a great many substances in solution including factors which enable the blood to clot, **b. bank,** a special refrigerator in which blood is kept after withdrwal from donors, until required for transfusion, **defibrinated b.,** that in which the fibrin is removed by agitation, **laked b.,** that in which the red cells are haemolysed. **occult b.,** that which is not visible. Its presence is determined by chemical tests.

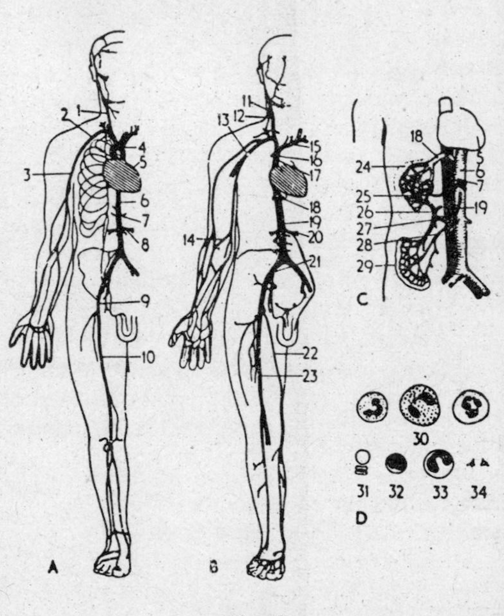

Blood

A. ARTERIAL SYSTEM. B. VENOUS SYSTEM. C. PORTAL SYSTEM. D. BLOOD CELLS OR CORPUSCLES

A. 1. Common carotid artery. 2. Right subclavian artery. 3. Brachial artery, 4. Arch of aorta. 5. Heart. 6. Aorta. 7. Coeliac artery. 8. Renal artery. 9. Exterior iliac artery. 10. Femoral artery. B. 11. External jugular vein. 12. Internal jugular vein. 13. Brachial vein. 14. Median basilic vein. 15. Innominate vein. 16. Vena azygos. 17. Superior vena cava. 18. Hepatic vein. 19. Inferior vena cava. 20. Renal vein. 21. Common ilic vein. 22. Long saphenous vein. 23. Femoral vein. C. 24. Liver. 25. Hepatic artery. 26. Portal vein. 27. Splenic vein. 28. Mesenteric artery. 29. Intestine. D. 30. Leucocytes. 31. Erythrocyte. 32. Lymphocyte. 33. Monocyte. 34. Platelets.

خون۔ دم۔ لہو : سرخ گاڑھا سیال جو دل اور خونی رگوں میں بھرا ہوتا ہے۔ انسانی جسم میں ۴ سیر خون ہوتا ہے۔ تقریباً ۵۰ لاکھ خونی سرخ ذرات ایک مکعب ملی میٹر خون میں موجود ہوتے ہیں۔خون کے ۴ گروپ اے، بی، اے بی اور او ہیں۔

Blood-brain barried. The membranes between the circulating blood and the brain. Some drugs can pass from the blood to the cerebrospinal fluid, through this barrier, others cannot, e.g. streptomycin.

بلڈ برین باریر : گردش کرنے والے خون اور دماغ کے درمیان جھلیاں۔

Blood casts. Casts of conglutinated red blood corpuscles, formed, in the renal tubules and found in the urine.

قوالب دمویہ۔ سبیکۂ دموی : پیشاب میں موجود اشیاء۔ خون کے سرخ ذرات جو منجمد ہو کر پیشاب میں شامل ہوتے ہیں۔

Blood clotting Primary phase; constriction of damaged vessel and adhesion of platelets to site of injury and to each other. Secondary phase in volves coagulation over and through the platelet mass. See table of plasma coagulation factors.

Factor Number	Synonyms
I	Fibrinogen
II	Prothrombin
III	Tissue thromboplastin
IV	Calcium ions
V	Proaccelerin
VI	Factor VII
VII	Antihaemophilic factor (AHF)
VIII	Christmas factor
IX	Stuart factor, Power factor
X	Plasma thromboplastin antecedent (PTA)
XI	Hageman factor
XII	Fibrin-Stabilizing factor

Blood count Calculation of the number of red or white cells per cubic millimetre of blood, using a haemocytometer, **differential b.c.** estimates the number of different types of white cell.

شمار الدم : خون کے فی کیوبک ملی میٹر میں سرخ یا سفید خلیوں کی تعداد۔

Blood culture After withdrawal of blood from a vein, it is incubated in a suitable medium, at an optimum temperature, so that any contained organisms can multiply and so be isolated and identified under the miscrocope. See BACTERAEMIA and SEPTICAEMIA.

خونی کلچر۔ کشت خون : ورید سے خون لے کر اس میں جراثیم کو پھلنے پھولنے کا موقعہ دیا جاتا ہے۔ اسے خونی کلچر کہتے ہیں۔

Blood formation See HAEMOPOIESIS

Blood groups. ABO system. There are four groups. A,B, AB and O. The cells of these groups contain the corresponding antigens. A.B. AB. except group O cells, which contain neither antigen A or B. For this reason group O blood can be given to any of the other groups and it is known as the universal donor. In the plasma there are agglutinins which will cause agglutination of any cell carrying the corresponding antigen, e.g. group A plasma contains anti-B agglutinins; group B plasma contains anti-A and anti-B aggultinins; group AB plasma contains no agglutinins.Group AB is therefore known as the universal recipient and can receive. A,B, and O blood, **rhesus b.g.,** the red cells contain four pairs of antigens which are known by the letters Cc, Dd, Ee and Ff. The letters denote allelomorphic genes which are present in all cells except the sex cells where a chromosome can carry C or c, but not both. In this way the rhesus genes and blood groups are derived equally from each parent. When the cells contain only the cde, groups, then the blood is said to be rhesus negative; when the cells contain C,D or E singly or in combination with cde, then the blood is rhesus positive.

These groups are antigenic, and can, under suitable conditions, produce the corresponding antibody in the serum. These antibodies are then used to detect the presence of Rh groups in cells. Antibodies to the Rh group are produced by (a) transfusion with Rh incompatible blood; (b) immunization during pregnancy by fetal cells containing the antigen entering the mother's circulation. This can cause erythroblastosis fetalis (q.v.).

دموی گروہ : خون کے چار گروہ ہیں۔ جن میں ان کے مطابق اینٹی جن پائے جاتے ہیں۔ البتہ ''او'' گروہ میں کوئی اینٹی جن نہیں ہوتا ہے۔ خون کی حلقہ بندی۔

Blood-letting Venesection (q.v.).

فصادی : دیکھئے وینی تراش۔ فصد کھولنا۔

Blood Plasma [G. plasma, from plassein, to form]. Liquid portion of blood. Composed of over 90 percent. water, the remainder being protein 6 to 8 percent, electrolytes, foodstuffs, waste products, clotting agents, antibodies and hormones.

خون مایہ : خون کا مائع حصہ۔ اس میں ۹۰ فیصد پانی ہوتا ہے اور اہم منحل لحمیات، نمکیات، شکر اور یوریا ہوتے ہیں۔

Blood pressure The pressure exerted by the blood on the vessel walls, measured in millimetres of mercury by the sphygmomanometer. The systolic pressure (when the heart muscle is at the maximum contraction) is recorded first, followed by the diastolic pressure (when the left ventricle is in a state of relaxation). e.g. 120 to 80 mm. See HYPERPIESIS and HYPOPIESIS.

بلڈ پریشر۔ فشار خون : رگوں کی دیواروں پر حون کا دباؤ۔

Blood sedimentation rate BSR. See ESR.

خون کی ترسپی شرح : دیکھئے ای ایس آر۔

Blood serum. The fluid which exudes when blood clots; it is plasma minus the clotting agents.

ماء الدم : خون جمتے ہوئے نکلنے والا سیال۔

Blood sugar The amount of glucose in the circulating blood; varies within the normal limits. See appendix. This level is controlled by various enzymes and hormones, the most important single factor being insulin (q.v.). See HYPERGLYCAEMIA and HYPOGLYCAEMIA.

دموی شکر : گردش کرنے والے خون میں گلوکوس کی مقدار جو کہ ۰٫۰۸ تا ۰٫۱۲ فیصد ہوتی ہے۔

Blood transfusion. The intravenous replacement of lost or destroyed blood by compatible citrated human blood. Also used for severe anaemia with deficient blood production. Fresh blood from a donor or stored blood from a blood bank may be used. It can be given 'whole'. or with some plasma removed ('packed-cell' transfusion). If incompatible blood is given severe reaction follows. See BLOOD GROUPS.

انتقال خون : ضائع شدہ یا تباہ شدہ خون کی جگہ نیا خون دینا۔ ہر ماہ ۲ بوتل خون برائے لیوکیمیا۔

Blood urea The amount of urea (the end product of protein metabolism) in the blood; varies within the normal range. See appendix. This is virtually unaffected by the amount of protein in the diet, when the kidneys which are the main organs of urea excretion are normal. When they are diseased the blood urea quickly rises. See URAEMIA.

دموی یوریا : خون میں یوریا کی مقدار۔

Blue baby. The appearance produced by some congenital heart defects. The appearance by contrast, of a newborn child suffering from temporary anoxia is described as 'blue asphyxia'.

کبود بچہ۔ مولودازرق : چند قلبی نقائص کی وجہ سے ظاہری شکل و صورت۔

Blue pus Bluish discharge from a wound infected with *Pseudomonas pyocyanea.*

blue stone. Copper sulphate (q.v.).

نیلا تھوتھا : دیکھئے کاپر سلفیٹ۔ قلمی کیوپرک سلفیٹ۔ بلیووٹریول۔

Bluxism *(bluks'-izm).* Teeth clenching which can cause headache from muscle fatigue.

BMR. See METABOLIC.

Body image *(bo'-di-im-aj).* The image in an individual's mind of his own body.

Distortions of this occur as a result of affective disorders, parietal lobe tumours or trauma.

جسمی عکس : کسی فرد کے ذہن میں اپنے ہی جسم کا امیج یا عکس۔

Boeck's disease *(beks)*. A form of sarcoidosis (q.v.).

مرض بیک : سارکائیڈوسس کی ایک قسم۔

Bohn's nodules; *(bonz)*. Tiny white nodules on the palate of the newly born.

boil [L. bullire, to bubble up]. A furuncle. An acute inflammatory condition, surrounding a hair follicle; caused by the Staphylococcus aureus. Usually attended by suppuration; it has one opening for drainage in contrast to a carbuncle (q.v.). See FURUNCULOSIS.

بال توڑ۔ پھوڑا۔ پھنسی : بال کے فولیکل کے گرد حالت۔ سٹے فائیلو کاکسی کی وجہ سے بالوں کی جڑ میں پھنسی بنتی ہے۔ پھر پیپ جمع ہو کر پھوڑا بن جاتا ہے۔ پلٹس سے پھوڑا نرم ہو کر پھوٹ جاتا ہے۔

Bolus *(bo'-lus)* [G. bolos, lump]. A soft, pulpy mass of masticated food.

نوالہ۔ لقمہ : نرم۔ چبائی ہوئی خوراک کا مادہ۔

Bone graft [A.S. ban, bone; O.F. greffe. from G. graphein, to write]. The transplantation of a piece of bone from one part of the body to another, or from one person to another. Used to repair bone defects, afford support, or to supply osteogrenic tissue.

استخوانی پیوند : ہڈی کے ٹکڑے کا پیوند۔ ہڈی کی قلمکاری۔ بدن کی یا کسی دوسرے شخص کی ہڈی کسی اور ہڈی سے جوڑنا۔

Bone

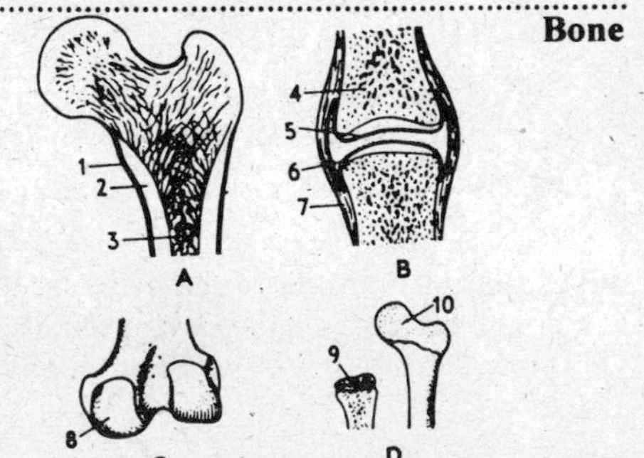

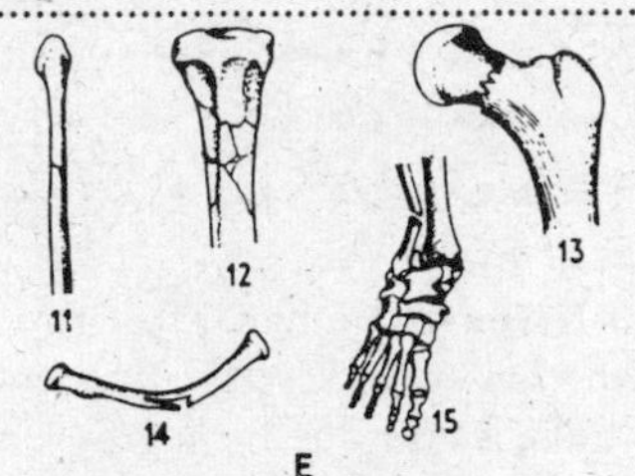

BONE: A. CROSS-SECTION OF HEAD OF FEMUR, B. CROSS-SECTION OF JOINT. C. ARTICULAR SURFACE. D. CHILD'S BONES. E. FRACTURES

A. 1. Periosteum. 2. Compact bone. 3. Marrow. B. 4. Bone. 5. Articular cartilage. 6. Synovial membrane. 7. Capsular ligament. C. 8. Condyle. D. 9. Epiphysis at head of child's ulna. 10. Cartilaginous head of child's femur, E. 11. Simple fracture. 12. Comminuted fracture. 13. Impacted fracture. 14. Greenstick fracture. 15. Pott's fracture.

Bonney's blue. Pig. tinctor, BNF. A solution of crystal violet and brilliant green in a mixture of methylated spirit and water. Used as a skin disinfectant.

بونیز بلیو : متھیلیٹڈ سپرٹ اور پانی کے آمیزہ میں کرسٹل وائلٹ اور شوخ سبز کا محلول۔ جلدی دافع کے طور پر استعمال کیا جاتا ہے۔

Borax *(bor'-aks)*. Mild antiseptic similar to boric acid. Used in alkaline mouthwashes. Glycerin of borax, and borax with honey are used as throat paints, but should be applied sparingly.

بوریکس۔ بورق۔ سہاگہ : الکلائن ماؤتھ واش میں مستعمل۔ بوریکس کی گلسرین اور شہد کے ساتھ بوریکس حلق میں لگاتے ہیں لیکن کبھی کبھار استعمال کرنا چاہیئے۔

Borborygmi *(bor-bor-ig'-mi)* [G. borborygmos, intestinal rumbling]. Rumbling noises caused by the movement of flatus in the intestines.

Boric acid *(bor'-ik-as'-id)*. Also known as **Boracic acid.** Mild antiseptic used mainly an eye lotions and ear drops. Dusting powders and lotions should not be applied to large raw areas, as there is a danger of boric poisoning.

بورک ایسڈ۔ سہاگے کا تیزاب : دافع جراثیم جو آنکھ کے لوشن یا کان کے ڈراپس کے طور پر استعمال کیا جاتا ہے۔ زیادہ استعمال نقصان دہ ہے۔ ایک سفید حل پذیر ٹھوس۔ آتش فشاں جگہوں پر قدرتی حالت میں پایا جاتا ہے۔ بوریکس سے بھی تیار کیا جاتا ہے۔

Bornbolm disease Named after the Danish island where it was described by Sylvest in 1934. Viral disease due to B group of Coxsackie viruses. Two to 14 days incubation. Symptoms include sudden onset of severe pain in lower chest or abdominal or lumbar muscles. Breathing may be difficult because of the pain, and fever is common. May last up to one week. There is no specific treatment.

بارن ہوم مرض : ۱۹۳۴ء میں سلویسٹ نے اس کی تشریح کی۔ وائرس کی بیماری۔ چھاتی کے نچلے حصے' یا بطنی یا لمبر عضلات میں شدید درد اٹھتا ہے۔ سانس لینا بھی دوبھر ہو جاتا ہے۔ اور بخار ہو جاتا ہے۔ ایک ہفتہ تک یہی حالت برقرار رہتی ہے۔

Botulism *(bot'-u-lizm)* [L. botulus, sausage]. An intoxication with the preformed exotoxin of Clostridium botulinum. Vomiting, constipation, ocular and pharyngeal paralysis and sometimes aphonia manifest within 24 to 72 h of eating food contaminated with the spores which require anaerobic conditions to produce the toxin. Hence the danger of home-tinned vegetables and meat.

کلمگی : جراثیم کی وجہ سے زہریلا پن۔ یہ جراثیم غیر ہوائی حالت میں ٹاکسن پیدا کرتے ہیں۔ اس لئے خوراک کے بند ڈبوں میں زہر پیدا ہو سکتا ہے۔

Bougie *(boo'-zhe)* [F. a candle]. A cylindrical instrument made of gum elastic, metal or other material. Used in varying sizes for dilating the anus, cardiac sphincter of stomach. oesophagus, urethra, etc.

بوجی۔ بتی : فرانسیسی زبان کا لفظ جس کے معنی موم بتی ہیں۔ کسی بھی چیز کا بنا ہوا ایک اسطوانی آلہ مقعد' یوریتھرا وغیرہ کو پھیلانے کے لئے استعمال کیا جاتا ہے۔

Bovine *(bo'-vin)* [L. bovinus, of a ox]. Pertaining to the cow or ox. The morphology and staining reactions of the bovine type of tubercle bacillus (Mycobacterium tuberculosis) are practically identical with those of the human type. The bovine type infects the bones, glands and joints in human beings.

بیل یا بھینس : گائے یا بیل سے متعلق۔ لاطینی لفظ بووینس بمعنی ''بیل کا'' سے ماخوذ اصطلاح۔ جراثیم کی یہ قسم ہڈیوں' غدود اور جوڑوں کو انسان میں متاثر کرتی ہے۔

Bowel *(bow'-el)*. [O. F.boel, from L. botulus, a sausage]. The intestine; the gut. See COLON.

معا : آنت۔ چھوٹی آنت اصل میں آنت کا ابتدائی حصہ ہے۔ جس کی لمبائی ۷ء۱۰ میٹر ہوتی ہے۔ اس کا پہلا حصہ ڈیوڈینم ہے جس کی لمبائی ۳ء۲۵ یا ۷ء۲۷ سم ہوتی ہے۔ اس کے بعد آنت کا

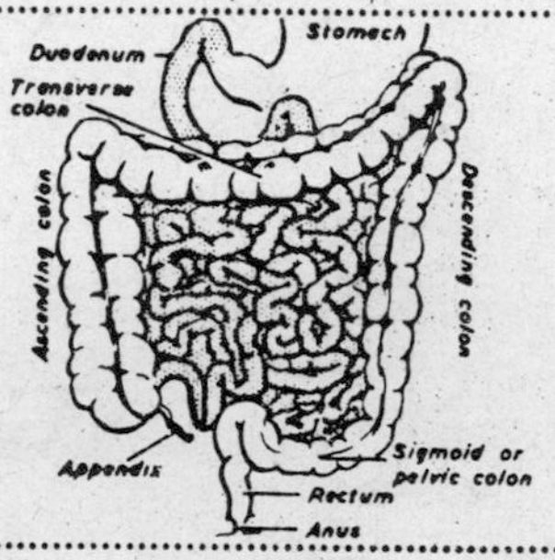

Bowel

دوسرا حصہ ہے اور بقایا الیئم ہے بڑی آنت ۸۲۸ء۱ میٹر لمبی ہوتی ہے۔ اس کی چوڑائی چھوٹی آنت کی چوڑائی سے زیادہ ہوتی ہے۔

Bow-leg *(bo'-leg)* [A.S. boga; O.N. leggr]. Syn., genu varum (q.v.).

Boyle's anaesthetic machine Apparatus by which chloroform, ether, nitrous oxide gas, and oxygen may be administered. Now adapted for use with cyclopropane. [Henry Edmund Gaskin Boyle, English surgeon, 1875-1941.]

بوائل کی بے ہوشی مشین : سامان جس سے کلوفارم' ایتھر' نائٹرس اکسائیڈ گیس اور آکسیجن دی جا سکے۔ اس کا نام انگریز سرجن ہنری ایڈمنڈ گیسکن بائل کے نام پر ہے۔ جس کا دور حیات ۱۸۷۵ء تا ۱۹۴۱ء ہے۔ بے ہوشی طاری کرنے یا آکسیجن وغیرہ دینے کی مشین۔

Boyle's law At any stated temperature, a given mass of gas varies in volume inversely as the pressure. [Robert Boyle, English physicist, 1627-91.]

کلیہ بائل : اس کا نام انگریز ماہر طبیعات رابرٹ بائل پر ہے جس

کا دور حیات ۱۶۲۷ع تا ۱۶۹۱ ع ہے۔ اس کے مطابق مستقل درجہ حرارت پر گیس کا حجم دباؤ کے بالعکس متناسب ہوتا ہے۔

Brachial *(bra'ki-al). Pertaining to the arm. Applied to vessels in this region and a nerve plexus at the root of the neck.*

بازوی۔ عضدی : بازو سے متعلق۔

Brachium *(bra'ki-um)* [L. bracchium, less correctly, brachium, arm]. The arm (especially from shoulder to elbow), or any arm-like appendage-brachina, pl.; brachial, adj.

بازو۔ عضد : بازو خصوصاً کندھے سے کہنی تک۔ بازو ایسا زائدہ۔

Bradford frame. A stretcher type of bed used for (1) immobilizing spine; (2) resting trunk and back muscles; (3) preventing deformity. It is tubular steel frame fitted with two canvas slings allowing a 101.6 to 152.4 mm gap to facilitate the use of a bedpan. [Edward H. Bradford, American orthopaedic surgeon, [1848-1926.]

بریڈفورڈ فریم : بستر کی سٹریچر والی قسم۔ امریکی سرجن بریڈ فورڈ کے نام پر ہے جس کا دور حیات ۱۸۴۸ء تا ۱۹۲۶ ع ہے۔ پشت کے عضلات ٹھیک کرنے کے لئے مستعمل ہے۔

بریڈوسول:

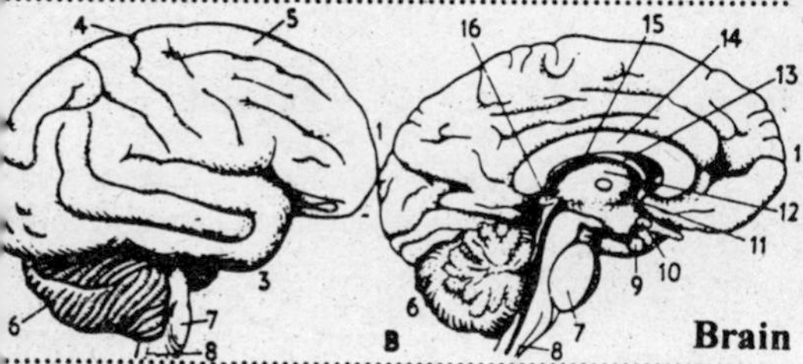

BRAIN; A. SIDE VIEW, B. LONGITUNIAL SECTION.

A. 1,2,3.Cerebrum (1. Frontal lobe. 2. Occipital lobe. 3. Temporal lobe). 4. Central sulcus. 5. Superior frontal gyrus. 6. Cerebellum. 7. Pons. 8. Medulla oblongata. B. 9. Pituitary gland or hypophysis. 10. Optic nerves. 11. Third ventricle. 12. Thalamus. 13. Fornix. 14. Corpus callosum. 15. Choroid plexus. 16. Pineal gland

Bradosol *(brad'-os-ol).* Domiphen (q.v.).

Bradycardia *(bra:di-kar'-di-a)* [G. bradys, slow; kardia, heart]. Slow rate of heart contraction, resulting in a slow pulse rate. In febrile states, for each degree rise in body temperature, the expected increase in pulse rate is ten beats per minute. When the latter does not occur, the term 'relative bradycardia' is used.

ضعف دل : یونانی الفاظ بریڈس بمعنی آہستہ اور کارڈیا بمعنی دل سے مرکب اصطلاح۔ دل سکڑنے کی کم شرح جس کی وجہ سے نبض کی رفتار بھی کم ہو جاتی ہے۔

Brain *(bran).* The encephalon; that part of the central nervous system contained in the cranial cavity. It consists of the cerebrum, cerebellum, pons varolii, midbrain (mesencephalon) and medulla oblongata. The last three divisions constitute the brain stem.

دماغ۔ مغز : یہ کھوپڑی میں ہوتا ہے۔ اس کے مختلف حصے ہیں۔ عصبی نظام کا مرکزی حصہ۔

Bran. The husk of grain. The coarse outer part of cereals, especially wheat, high in roughage and the vitamin B complex.

بھوسی۔ چھان : دانے کا چھلکا۔ کسی بھی غلے کا بیرونی حصہ خصوصاً گندم کا۔ اس میں وٹامن بی کمپلیکس پایا جاتا ہے۔

Branchial *(brang'-ki-al)* [G. bragchia, gills]. Pertaining to the fissures or clefts which occur on each side of the neck of the human embryo, and which enter into the development of the nose, ears and mouth. **b. cyst,** a swelling in the neck arising from such embryonic remnants.

خیشومی : ان شگافوں سے متعلق جو انسانی جنین میں گردن کی ہر جانب پائے جاتے ہیں اور وہ ناک، کان اور منہ کی تکمیل میں حصہ لیتے ہیں۔

Brandt Andrews technique Elevation of the uterus abdominally while holding the cord just taut--no traction. When the uterus is lifted the placenta will be in the cervix or upper vagina and is then expelled by suprapubic pressure directed below the fundus of the elevated uterus.

براانڈ اینڈ ریوز تکنیک : یوٹرس کا بطنی طور پر اوپر اٹھنا۔

Braun's frame. A metal frame, bandaged for use, and equally useful for drying a lower leg plaster, and for applying skeletal traction (Steinmann's pin or Kirschner wire inserted through the calcaneus) to a fractured tibia, after reduction

بران فریم : دھات کا بنا ہوا فریم۔

Braunula *(brawn -u-la)*. A plastic disposable cannula with metal needle for ease of insertion into vein.

Break-bone fever. See DENGUE.

ہڈی توڑ بخار :

Breast *(brest)* [A.S. breost]. The anterior upper part of the thorax; the mammary gland. **b.bone,** the sternum.

سینہ۔ چھاتی۔ پستان۔ چوچی۔ مرد(کی) : تھوریکس کا اگلا بالائی حصہ۔ پستانی غدود۔ عورت کی چھاتی۔

Breck feder a graduated glass tube of 28.3 g capacity, with a rubber bulb at one end and a teat at the other. Pressure on the bulb expels fluid through the teat. Used for feeding premature and weak babies.

بریک فیڈر : ایک درجہ دار شیشے کی نلی جس کے ایک سرے پر ربڑ کا بلب ہوتا ہے۔ جبکہ دوسرے پر نپل ہوتا ہے۔ بلب پر دباؤ سے سیال نپل سے خارج ہونے لگتا ہے۔ کمزور بچوں کو دودھ پلانے کے لئے استعمال کیا جاتا ہے۔

Breech (brech) [M.E. brech]. The buttocks (q.v.).

چوتڑ۔ سرین : دیکھئے بٹک۔

Bregma *(breg'-ma)* [G. front part of the head]. The junction of the coronal and sagittal sutures; the anterior fontanelle--bregmata, pl.; bregmatic, adj.

Bregma

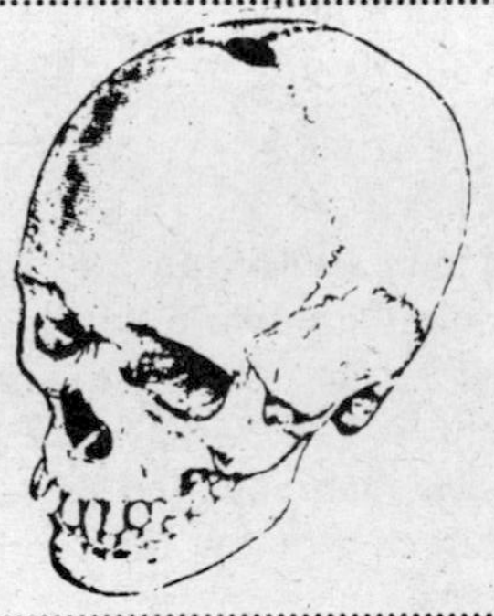

یما۔ نمغہ : یونانی زبان کا لفظ جس کا مطلب سر کا سامنے والا حصہ ۔ اگلا فونٹا نیلا۔

Bretylate *(bret'-i-lat)*. Acts by improving th way in which the natural electrical impulse that cause the heart to beat are conducted t the heart. In this way the heart, instead o slowing down, is actually speeded up.

Bretylium *(bret-il'-i-um)*. Adrenergic blocking antihypertensive drug.

ریٹائیلیم : دوائی کی ایک قسم۔ ڈریتھن۔

Brevidil *(brev'-i-dil)*. Suxamethonium (q.v.).

ریویڈل : دیکھئے سکسا میتھونیم۔

Brietal *(bri-et-al)*. Methohexitone sodium (q.v.)

Bright's disease Inflammation of the kidneys Nephritis (q.v.) [Richard Bright, Englis physician and clinician, 1789-1858.]

رض برائٹ۔ ضعف گردہ : گردوں کی سوزش۔ ایک انگریز زیشن رچرڈ برائٹ کے نام پر ہے۔ جس کا دور حیات ۱۷۸۹ء تا ۱۸۵۰ء رہا۔

Brilliant green. Antiseptic aniline dye. Used a lotion (1:1000), paint (1 percent), an ointment (2 per-cent).

چمکیلا ہرا : دافع تعفن اینلین رنگ۔ لوشن اور مرہم کے طور پر ستعمل ہے۔

Brinaldix *(brin'-al-dicks)*. Clopamide (q.v.).

ری نیل ڈکس : دیکھئے کلوپامائیڈ۔

Broadbent's sign Visible retraction of the lef side and back, in the region of the 11th an 12th ribs, synchronous with each heart bea and due to adhesions between the pericardiu and diaphragm. See PERICARDITIS[Willian Henry Broadbent, English physician 1835-1907.]

راڈبینٹ نشان : انگریز فزیسن ولیم ہنری براڈ بھینٹ کے نام پر ہے جس کا دور حیات ۱۸۳۵ء تا ۱۹۰۷ء ہے۔ بائیں جانب اور پیچھے کی طرف واضح کھچاؤ۔

Broad ligaments Lateral ligaments; double fol of parietal peritoneum which hands over th uterus and outstretched Fallopian tubes forming a lateral partition across the pelvi cavity.

چوڑے لگامنٹس : جانبی لگامنٹس۔

Broca's area *(brok'-a)*. The motor centre for speech; situated at the commencement of the Sylvian fissure in the left hemisphere of the cerebrum. Injury to this centre results in inability to speak. [Pierre Paul Broca, French surgeon and anthropologist, 1824-80.]

بروکی رقبہ۔ مرکز کلام : بولنے کا موثر مرکز۔ اسے نقصان پہنچنے کی صورت میں انسان بولنے سے معذور ہو جاتا ہے۔ یہ مرکز دماغ میں ہوتا ہے۔ فرانسیسی سرجن پیرے پال بروکا کے نام پر ہے جس کا دور حیات ۱۸۲۴ع تا ۱۸۸۰ء ہے۔

Brocillin *(bro-sil'-in)*. Propicillin (q.v.).

Brodie's adscess See ABSCESS. [Sir Benjamin Collins Brodie, English surgeon, 1783-1862.]

Bromethol *(brom'-eth-ol)*. A basalanaesthetic, used occasionally in surgery, in eclampsia and obstetric amnesia, and in tetanus. It is given as a freshly prepared 21/2 per-cent solution per rectum.

برامی تھال : بنیادی طور پر نشہ آور۔ بعض دفعہ سرجری میں مستعمل۔

Bromhexine *(brom'-hecks-en)*. Synthetic derivative of vasicine, an alkaloid derived from a plant. Mucolytic; taken orally; it loosens sputum prior to coughing. An intravenous preparation is available; useful in status asthmaticus.

برام ہیکسین : پودے سے اخذ شدہ الکلائڈ۔ بلغم پتلا کرنے کی دوائی۔

Bromides *(Bro'-midz)*. A small group of drugs, exemplified by potassium bromide, which have a mild depressant action on the central nervous system. Used extensively in epilepsy before phenobarbitone was introduced; now used in nervous insomnia and restlessness, often in association with chloral.

برومائیڈز : دوائیوں کا ایک گروہ مثلاً پوٹاشیم برومائیڈ۔ یہ ادویات مرکزی عصبی نظام کو متاثر کرتی ہیں۔ بے آرامی کی حالت میں دی جاتی ہے۔

Bromidrosis *(brom-i-dro'-sis)* [G. bromos, stench; hidros, sweat]. A profuse, foetid perspiration, especially associated with the feet--bromidrotic, adj.

بدبوئی پسینہ : پسینے کا آنا خصوصاً پاؤں پر۔

Bromisism *(bro'-mizm)*. Chronic poisoning due to continued or excessive used of bromides.

برومیت : برومائیڈز کے لگاتار یا زائد استعمال کی وجہ سے زہریلا پن۔

Bromocriptine *(bro-mo-krip'-ten)*. A dopamine receptor against useful in Parkinsonism.

Bromvaleton *(brom-val'-e-ton)*. Mild hypnotic and sedative similar to carbromal.

برام ویلی ٹون : ہلکی خواب آور دوائی۔

Bronchi *(brong'-ki)* [G. brogchos, windpipe]. The two tubes into which the trachea divides at its lower end--bronchus, sing.; bronchial, adj.

قصبی نالیاں۔ شعبات : یونانی الفاظ بروگکوس بمعنی ہوا کی نالی سے ماخوذ۔ دونلیاں جن میں ٹریکیا نچلے سرے پر منقسم ہوتی ہے۔

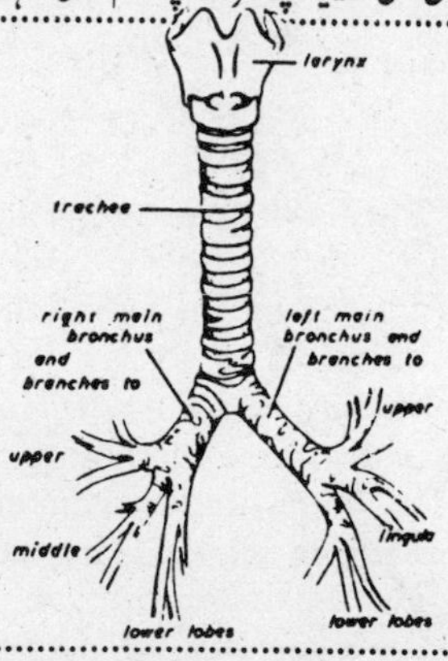

Bronchi

Bronchial tubes *(brong'-ke-al-tubz)* [G. brogchos, windpipe]. Subdivisions of the bronchi after they enter the lungs.

شعبی نالیاں : پھیپھڑوں میں داخل ہونے کے بعد برونکائی کی مزید تقسیم۔

Bronchectasis *(brong-ki-ek'-tas-is)* [G. brogchos, windpipe; ecktasis, extension]. Dilatation of the bronchial tubes following infection such as bronchopneumonia with lobular collapse (which may have occurred in infancy). Associated with profuse, foetid, purulent expectoration. May lead to greatly limited ventilatory capacity and recurrent infection of lungs, cerebral abscess or amyloid disease--bronchiectatic, adj.

تمدد۔ شعب : برونکیل نلیوں کا پھیلنا جو کسی بیماری کی وجہ سے ہوتا ہے۔ تمباکو نوشی سے پرانی کھانسی ہو جاتی ہے جس سے ہوا کی نالیاں پھیل جاتی ہیں۔

Bronchiole *(brong'-ki-ol)* [G. brogchos, windpipe]. One of the minute subdivisions of the bronchi which terminate in the alveoli or air sacs of the lungs bronchiolar, adj.

شعیب : یونانی لفظ برونکوس بمعنی ہوائی نالی سے ماخوذ۔ برونکائی کی مزید تقسیم سے بننے والی شاخ جو پھیپھڑوں کی ہوائی تھیلی پر ختم ہوتی ہے۔

Bronchiolitis *(brong-ke-ol-it'-is)* [G. brogchos, windpipe; -itis, inflammation]. Inflammation of the bronchioles, capillary bronchitis--bronchiolitic, adj.

ورم شعیبات : یونانی الفاظ برونکوس بمعنی ہوائی نالی اور الٹس بمعنی سوزش سے مرکب اصطلاح۔ برونکیولز کی سوزش۔

Bronchitis *(brong-ki-tis)* [G. brogchos, windpipe;-itis, inflammation]. Inflammation of the bronchi; may be primary or secondary, acute or chronic. The basic reaction in these stages is the same; excessive secretion of mucus following an overgrowth of the mucous glands, sometimes with an added infection. Symptoms are a productive cough, wheezy breathing and varying degrees of breathlessness. In **acute b.** all can return to normal but in even **simple chronic b.** the bronchial mucous glands are hypertrophied and are unlikely to return to normal. In **chronic obstructive b.** the glands have become so hypertrophied that the bronchial lumen is narrowed and this is exacerbated by the extra mucus produced. **acute b.** is currently defined as an illness with cough, sputum and wheezy breathing presenting in a patient who was previously well. **simple chronic b.** is defined as cough and sputum-for at least three months of the year, and occurring in at least two years; wheezing and shortness of breath are present either constantly or intermittently. **In chron obstructive b.** breathlessness is a more seve symptom; because of the narrowness of th bronchial airways it is more difficult both f oxygen to get into the lungs and for carb dioxide rises. Normally these two stimu increase breathing. In the patient with chron obstructive bronchitis and a raised bloc carbon dioxide, further elevation of carb dioxide fails to produce any response. The patients tend to respond in their breathi only to a lack of oxygen and not to exce carbon dioxide. Should such a patient given pure oxygen to breathe, he would robbed of his stimulus to breathing; h carbon dioxide would accumulate and cau coma and death; he may be given air enrich with oxygen but not pure oxygen. Chron bronchitis can cause right sided heart failu especially when associated with gro emphysema. See COR PULMONALE bronchitic, adj.

انسی۔ سعال۔ سرفہ۔ ورم شعب : یونانی الفاظ برونکوس ی ہوائی نالی اور الٹس بمعنی سوزش سے مرکب اصطلاح۔ برونکائی کی ش۔ اولیں یا ثانوی۔ سلفاڈایا زین ۲ گولیاں دن میں ۳ دفعہ۔ پچومائی سین پنسلین انجکشن (گرسٹا مائی سن انجکشن) روزانہ یا صبح و م۔ کھانسی کا مکسچر دن میں ۳ مرتبہ۔

Bronchoadenitis *(brong'-ko-ad-en-it'-is)* [brogchos, windpipe; aden, gland; -iti inflammation]. Inflammation of bronchi glands.

نکوایڈینی ٹس : یونانی اخذ برونکوس بمعنی ہوائی نالی' ایڈن بمعنی د اور الٹس بمعنی سوزش سے مرکب اصطلاح۔ برونکیل غدود کی ش۔

Bronchodilator *(brong'-ko-di-la'-tor)* [brogchos, trachea; L. dilatare, to dilate]. A agent which dilates the bronchi.

ع شعبات : یونانی لفظ برونکوس بمعنی ہوائی نالی اور لاطینی لفظ یٹر بمعنی پھیلنا سے مرکب اصطلاح۔ برونکائی کو پھیلانے والا ۔

Bronchogenic *(brong-ko-jen'-ik)* [G. brogch windpipe; genesthai, to be produced]. Arisi from a bronchus.

برانکوجنیک : برونکس سے ابھرنا۔

ronchogram *(brong'-ko-gram)* [G. brogchos, windpipe; gramma, letter]. Radiological picture of the bronchial tree rendered radio-opaque.

شعب نگارش۔ شعبی ارتسام : برونکیل شجر کی ریڈیولوجیکل پکچر۔

ronchography *(brong-kog'-raf-i)* [G. brogchos, windpipe; graphein, to write]. Preparation of X-ray film after introduction of radio-opaque substance into the bronchial tree-bronchographic, adj.; bronchographically, adv..

شعب نگاری : یونانی الفاظ برگکوس بمعنی ہوائی نالی اور گریفین بمعنی لکھنا کا مجموعہ۔ برونکیل شجر میں ریڈیوروک مادے کے تعارف کے بعد ایکسرے فلم کی تیاری۔

rronchomycosis *(brong'-ko-mi-ko'-sis)* [G. brogchos, windpipe; mykes, fungus; -osis, condition]. General term used to cover a variety of fungus infections of the bronchi and lungs, e.g. pulmonary moniliasis, aspergillosis (q.v.)--bronchomycotic, adj.

شعبی فطریت : یونانی الفاظ برونگکوس بمعنی ہوائی نالی، مائیکس بمعنی سماروغ اور اوسس بمعنی حالت کا مجموعہ۔ پھیپھڑوں اور برونکائی میں سماروغ لگنے کی عام اصطلاح۔

ronchophony *(brong-kof'-o-ni)* [G. brogchos, windpipe; phone, voice]. Abnormal transmission of voice sounds heard over consolidate lung or over a thin layer of pleural fluid.

برنکونی فونی : یونانی الفاظ برونگکوس بمعنی ہوائی نالی اور فون بمعنی آواز کا مجموعہ۔ پھیپھڑے پرسنی جانے والی آوازوں کی غیر معمولی ٹرانسمشن یعنی ترسیل۔ ہوا کی نالیوں میں آواز کی گونج۔

ronchopleural fistula *(brong-ko-ploo'-ral fis'-tul-a)* [G. brogchos, windpipe; pleura, rib; L. tube]. Pathological communication between the pleural cavity and a bronchus.

برانکوپلیورل فسٹولا : پلیورل کہفہ اور برونکس کے درمیان پیتھولوجیکل کمیونیکیشن۔

ronchopneumonia *(brong'-ko-nu-mo'-ni-a)* [G. brogchos, windpipe; pneumones, the lungs]. Small areas of the lungs are consolidated and coalesce, but do not have a lobular or lobar distribution; Complication of many medical conditions, especially measles and whooping cough. Relatively more common in infancy and old age-- bronchopneumonic. adj.

بونکو نمونیہ : یونانی الفاظ برونگکوس بمعنی ہوائی نالی اور نیومونز بمعنی پھیپھڑے کا مجموعہ۔ پھیپھڑوں کے مختصر حصے باہم مل جاتے ہیں لیکن لوبر تقسیم نہیں ہوئی۔

Bronchopulmonary *(brong'-ko-pul'-mon-ar-i)* [G. brogchos, windpipe; L. pulmo, lung]. Pertaining to the bronchi and the lungs--bronchopulmonic, adj.

شعبی ریوی : یونانی الفاظ برونگکوس بمعنی ہوائی نالی اور لاطینی لفظ پلمو بمعنی پھیپھڑا کا مجموعہ پھیپھڑوں اور برونکائی سے متعلق۔

Bronchorrhoea *(brong-ko-re'-a)* [G. brogchos, windpipe; rheein, to flow]. An excessive discharge of mucus from the bronchial mucous membrane--bronchorrhoeal, adj.

بلغمی کھانسی : یونانی الفاظ برونگکوس بمعنی ہوائی نالی اور رین بمعنی بہنا کا مجموعہ۔ برونکیل میوکس جھلی سے میوکس کا زائد اخراج ہوا کی نالیوں سے بلغم کا اخراج۔

Bronchoscope *(brong'-ko-skop)* [G. brogchos, windpipe; skopein, to examine]. A type of endoscope (q.v.) used for examining the interior of the bronchi, removal of a foreign body, biopsy, etc.--bronchoscopic, adj.; bronchoscopy, n.; bronchoscopically, adv.

شعبہ بین : یونانی الفاظ برونگکوس بمعنی ہوائی نالی اور سکوپین بمعنی جانچنا کا مجموعہ۔ برونکائی کی اندرونی حالت جانچنے کے لئے اینڈوسکوپ کی ایک قسم۔

Bronchospasm *(brong'-ko-spazm)* [G. brogchos, windpipe; spasm,]. Sudden constriction of the bronchial tubes due to contraction of involuntary plain muscle in their walls--bronchospastic, adj.

شعبی تشنج : دیواروں میں غیرارادی عضلے کے سکڑنے کی وجہ سے برونکیل نلیوں کی اچانک کنسٹرکشن۔

Bronchospirometer *(brong-ko-spi-rom'-et-er)* [G. brogchos, windpipe; L. spirare, to breathe; G. metron, a measure]. An instrument for measuring the capacity of one lung--bronchospirometric, adj.; bronchos- pirometry, n.

برونکوسپائیرومیٹر : پھیپھڑے کی اہلیت ناپنے کا ایک آلہ۔

Bronchostenosis *(brong-ko-sten-os'-is)* [G. brogchos, windpipe; stenos, narrow]. Narrowing of a bronchus--bronchostenotic, adj.

برانکوسٹینوسس : یونانی الفاظ بروگکوس بمعنی ہوائی نالی اور سٹینوس بمعنی تنگ کا مجموعہ۔ برونکس کا تنگ ہونا۔

Bronchotracheat *(brong-ko-trak-e'-al)* [G. brogchos, windpipe; trachus, rough]. Pertaining to bronchi and trachea.

شعبی قصبی :یونانی الفاظ بروگکوس بمعنی ہوائی نالی اور ٹریکس بمعنی رف کا مجموعہ۔

Brow [A.S. bru]. The forehead; the region of the supraorbital ridge.

جبین ۔ ابرو : پیشانی ماتھا۔ سپرا آربیٹل رج کا حصہ۔

Broxil *(broks'-il)*. Phenethicillin (q.v.).

Brucella *(broo-sel'-la)* [L. after David Bruce]. A genus of bacteria causing brucellosis (undulant fever in man; contagious abortion in cattle). Brucella abortus is the bovine strain, B. melitensis the goat strain, both transmissible to man via infected milk. [David Bruce, British pathologist and bacteriologist, 1855-1931.]

بروسیلا : لاطینی ڈیوڈبروس کے نام پر جراثیم کا ایک جنس۔ نہایت چھوٹے گرام منفی جراثیم۔ حرکت نہیں کرتے۔ سپورز نہیں بناتے۔ بکریوں کے دودھ میں ہوتے ہیں۔

Brucellosis *(broo-sel-lo'-sis)* [L. Brucella, after David Bruce: G. -osis, condition]. An infective reticulosis. A generalized infection in man resulting from one of the species of Brucella. There are recurrent attacks of fever and mental depression. The condition may last for months. Prescribed as an industrial disease under the National Insurance (Industrial Injuries) Act 1965 in relation to occupations involving contact with bovi[ne] animals infected by B. abortus, their carcass[es] or untreated products, or with laborato[ry] specimens containing B. abortus, by reason [of] employment as a farmworker, veterina[ry] worker, slaughterhouse worker, laborato[ry] worker or in any other work relating to t[he] care, treatment, examination or handling [of] such animals, carcasses or products.

[...]ا بخار : بروسیلا کی ایک نوع سے ہونے والی چھوت کی بیماری۔ [...] کے لگاتار حملے ہوتے ہیں۔ ایک صنعتی مرض۔

Brudzinski'ssign. immediate flexion of kne[es] and hips on raising head from pillow. Seen [in] meningitis [Josef von Brudzinski, Poli[sh] physician, 1874-1971.]

[...]ڈزنسکائی نشان : تکیے سے سراٹھانے پر جوڑوں اور گھٹنوں کو [...]ی جھٹکا۔

Brufen *(broo'-fen)*. Ibuprofen (q.v.).

bruise *(brooz)* [A.S. brysan, to crush]. [...] discolouration of the skin due to an extra[v]asation of blood into the underlying tissu[e] there is no abrasion of the skin. A contusion.

[...] : جلد کی رنگت اڑنا۔ رگڑ۔ خراش۔ جب کندآلے سے چوٹ [...] تو جلد نہیں پھٹتی' خون جلد کے نیچے جمع ہو جاتا ہے۔ شروع میں [...] کا رنگ سرخی مائل پھر سیاہی اور بعد میں بھورا ہو کر ختم ہو جاتا [...]

Bruit *(broo'-e)* [F.]. See MURMUR.

Bryani's gallows' traction. Skin traction (q.v.) is applied to the lower limbs, the legs are th[en] suspended vertically (from an overhe[ad] beam), so that the buttocks are lifted just cle[ar] of the bed. Used for fractures of the femur [in] children up to 4 years. [Sir Thomas Brya[nt] English surgeon, 1828-1914.]

[...]ئی اینٹ گیلوزٹریکشن : اس میں ٹانگیں عموی طور پر لٹک جاتی [...]۔ چار سال کی عمر تک کے بچوں میں فیمر کے فریکچر کے لئے [مست]عمل۔

BSR. Blood sedimentation rate. See ESR.

Bubo *(bu'-bo)* [G. boubon, groin]. Enlargeme[nt] of lymphatic glands, especially in the groin. [A] feature of soft sore (chancroid), lympho- gr[a]nuloma inguinable and plague--bubonic, adj.

گلٹی : لمفی غدود کا بڑھاؤ۔

ıccal *(buk'-al)* [L. bucca, cheek]. Pertaining to the cheek or mouth.

ذہنی رخساری۔ فمی : لاطینی لفظ بکا بمعنی رخسار سے ماخوذ۔ منہ یا رخسار سے متعلق۔

ıerger's disease *(ber'-gers).* Thromboangitis obliterans. Obliterative vascular disease of peripheral vessels. In an investigation, the incidence of HLA-A9 and HLA-B5 was significantly greater in those with Buerger's disease than in the controls. **B. exercises** were designed to treat this condition. The legs are placed alternately in elevation and dependence. [Leo Buerger, American physician, 1879-1943.]

مرض برگر : پرفرل رگوں کی بیماری۔ لیو برجر' ایک امریکی فزیشن کے نام پر جس کا دورحیات ۱۸۷۹ع تا ۱۹۴۳ع ہے۔

uffer 1. A chemical substance which, when present in a solution, causes resistance to pH (q.v.) change when acids or alkalis are added. 2. Anything used to reduce shock or jarring due to contact.

بفر : ایک کیمیائی مادہ جو محلول کی صورت میں پی ایچ میں تبدیلی کو مستقل رکھتا ہے جب ایسڈ یا الکلی کا اضافہ کیا جائے۔

ulbar [L. bulbus, onion]. Pertaining to the medulla oblongata. See PARALYSIS and POLIOMYELITIS.

بصلی نخاعی : لاطینی لفظ بلبس بمعنی پیاز سے ماخوذ اصطلاح میڈلا اوبلانگیٹا سے متعلق۔

ulbourethal *(bul-bo-ur-eth'-ral)* [L. bulbus, onion; G. ourethra, urethra]. Applied to two racemose glands (Cowper's) which open into the bulb of the male urethra.

بصلی مبالی : دو غدودوں پر اطلاق ہوتا ہے جو زیورتھرا کے بلب میں کھلتی ہیں۔

ulimia *(bu-lim'-i-a)* [G. bous, ox; limos, hunger]. Excessive appetite. See in some cerebral lesions, diabetes mellitus and psychotic states.

سعار۔ جوع البقر۔ (بھوک کا) ہوکا : یونانی الفاظ باؤس بمعنی بیل اور لیموس بمعنی بھوک کا مجموعہ۔ زائد بھوک۔ ذیابیطس وغیرہ

میں عموماً ایسے ہوتا ہے۔

Bulla *(bool'-la)* [L.] A large watery bister. In dermatology, bulla formation is characteristic of the pemphigus group of dermatoses, bu occurs sometimes in other disease of the skin, e.g. in impetigo, in dermatitis herpetiformis, etc.--bullae, pl.; bullate, bullous, adj.

آبلہ۔ چھالا : ایک بڑا آبی آبلہ۔ لاطینی لفظ۔

Bull's regime. A method of treating temporary uraemia by giving glucose and peanut oil via gastric drip.

مملکت بل : عارضی یوریمیا کے علاج کا طریقہ۔

Buller's shield. A watchglass enclosed within a frame of adhesive plaster, to protect one eye when the other is infected. [Frank Buller, Canadian oculist, 1844-1905.]

بلر شیلڈ : چپنے والا پلستر کے فریم میں بند واچ گلاس اس سے ایک آنکھ کی حفاظت ہوتی ہے۔ جبکہ دوسری خراب ہوتی ہے۔ کینیڈا کے فریک بلر کے نام پر ہے۔ جس کا دور حیات ۱۸۴۴ ع تا ۱۹۰۵ع ہے۔

Bumetanide *(bu-met'-an-id)* Potent diuretic. See ETHACRYNIC ACID.

Bunion *(bun'-yun)* [O.F. bugne, a swelling]. Syn., hallux valgus. A deformity on the head of the metatarsal bone at its junction with the great toe. Friction and pressure of shoes at this point cause a bursa to develop. The prominent bone, with its bursa, is known as a bunion.

Bunion

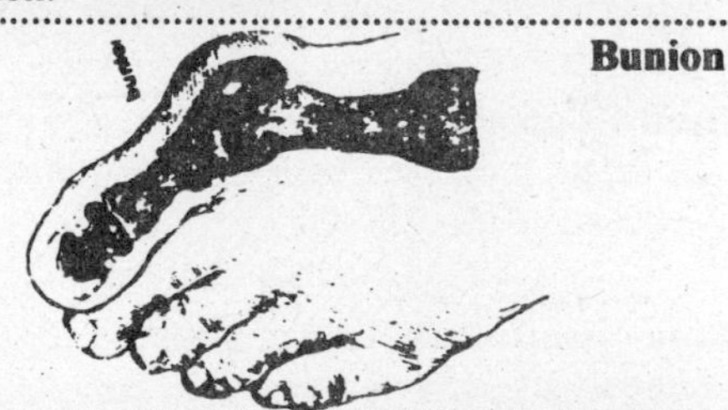

گٹا۔ شلجمیہ : پاؤں کے انگوٹھے کے ساتھ جنکشن پر میٹا ٹارسل ہڈی کے سر پر بدنمائی۔ اس نقطہ پر جوتے کے دباؤ اور رگڑ سے داغ پڑ جاتا ہے۔ اس ہڈی اور داغ کا نام۔

Buphthalmos *(buf-thal'-mos)* [G. bous, ox; ophthalmos, eye]. Oxeye. Congenital glaucoma (q.v.).

کبرالعین۔ کلاں چشمی : یونانی الفاظ باؤس بمعنی بیل اور اوفتھیلموس بمعنی آنکھ کا مجموعہ۔ بیل کی آنکھ۔ آنکھ کی بیماری۔

Bupivacaine *(bu-piv'-a-kan)*. One of the longer acting local anaesthetics. Synthetic; less toxic than cocaine. Suitable for obstetric analgesia by the caudal approach.

بیوپی وکین : نشہ آور دوا۔

Burimamide *(bu-rim'-a-mid)* A histamine H_2 receptorantagonist which is only active by injection. It has been superseded by cimetidine for the treatment of ulcers.

بریلے مائیڈ : ہسٹامین کی عمل کو زائل کرنے والی دوا۔ اس کا عمل یوٹرس، دل اور گیسٹرک جوس کے اخراج پر ہوتا ہے۔

Bukitt's lymphoma. Malignant lymphoma of the jaw and other sites in children previously infected with E B virus (q.v.). Occurs almost exclusively in Africa and New Guinea in area where malaria is endemic. [Denis Burkitt. Contemporary surgeon.]

برکت لمفوسارکوما : افریقی بچوں میں جبڑے کا مرض۔

Burn. A lesion of the tissues due to chemicals, dry heat, electricity, flame friction or radiation; classified in three degrees, viz, erythema, visiculation or deeper destruction.

داغ۔ چھالا : کسی وجہ سے بافتوں کا ابھار۔ مثلاً حرارت، بجلی، آگ، رگڑ، تابکاری یا کیمیائی مادے وغیرہ۔ اس طرح انسان جل یا جھلس جاتا ہے۔ علاج کے لئے فیوراسین، برلول، ٹینا فیس، جنشن وائلٹ، کوڈوپائرین مفید ہیں۔

Burow's operation. A flap operation for closing a defect in the lip. [Karl August Burow, German surgeon, 1809-74.]

بروآپریشن : ہونٹ میں نقص ختم کرنے کے لئے فلیپ آپریشن۔

Bursa *(bur'-sa)* [L. bursa, purse]. A fibrous sac lined with synovial membrane and containing a small quantity of synovial flouid. Bursae are found between (1) tendon and bone; (2) skin and bone; (3) muscle and muscle. Their function is to 'facilitate movement without friction between these surfaces--bursae, pl.

برسا۔ درجک : لاطینی لفظ برسا بمعنی پرس یا بٹوہ۔ ایک ریشہ دار
نہ۔ یہ عموماً ٹنڈان اور ہڈی کے درمیان یا جلد اور ہڈی کے درمیان یا
عضلے اور عضلے کے درمیان ہوتا ہے۔ ان کا کام رگڑ کے بغیر دو سطوح
کے درمیان حرکت پیدا کرتا ہے۔

Bursits *(bur-si'-tis)* [L. bursa, purse; G. -itis inflammation]. Inflammation of a bursa **olecranon b.**, miner's or student's elbow **prepatellar b.**, housemaid's knee. A blow results in haemorrhage into the bursa Infection may be super added, pyogenic tubercular or syphilitic.

رم درجک : لاطینی لفظ برسا بمعنی پرس اور یونانی لفظ ائس بمعنی سوزش سے مرکب اصطلاح۔ برسا کی سوزش۔

Buscopan *(bus-ko-pan)*. Hyoscine-N-buty bromide.

سکوپین : دردکا آرام پہنچانے والی دوا۔ خصوصاً درد زہ میں یوٹرس کے سکڑاؤ کے آرام اور سکون کے لئے مفید۔

Busuphan *(bu-sul'-fan)*. Cytotoxic, alkylatin drug used in chronic myeloid leukaemia an polycythaemia. Regular blood counts ar essential, as the compound is a powerful dep ressant of bone marrow.

بوسلفین : ایک دوائی سائیٹوٹاکسک۔ لیوکیمیا میں مستعمل۔

Butacaine *(bu'-ta-kan)*. Synthetic anaestheti similar to cocaine. Used in ophthalmology a 2 percent solution, which, unlike cocaine does not dilate the pupil.

بوٹاکین : کوکین کی طرح تالیفی نشہ آور۔ دو فیصد محلول میں مستعمل۔ پتلی کونہیں پھیلاتی۔

Butazolidine *(but-az-ol'-i-den)* Phenylbutazon (q.v.).

بوٹاز ولیڈین : دیکھئے فینائل بوٹازون۔ ایک مشہور دوائی اس کی ایک گولی صبح ایک دوپہر ایک شام برائے ایکوٹ گوٹ یا نقرس۔ آسٹیو آرتھرائی ٹس۔ اس کا ایک ٹیکہ روزانہ کولہے کے عضلات میں ۵ یوم تک برائے عرق النساء یا شیاٹیکا

Butobarbitone *(bu-to-barb'-i-ton)*. Hypnotic o medium rapidity and potency of action Soneryl.

بوٹوبارلی ٹون : درمیانہ درجہ کی خواب آور دوا۔ سونرل۔ سوتے وقت ایک گولی برائے بے خوابی۔

uttock *(but'-ok)* [M.E. but, end]. One of the two projections posterior to the hip joints. Formed mainly of the gluteal muscles.

چوتڑ۔ سرین : چوتڑ کے جوڑوں کے خلفی جانب دو ابھاروں میں سے ایک۔ گلوٹیل عضلات سے بنا ہوا۔ جنسی ملاپ کے انداز میں مرد عورت کے چوتڑوں کے نیچے ایک تکیہ رکھ دیتا ہے۔ اس سے مردانہ عضو اندام نہانی میں زیادہ گہرائی تک جا کر رحم کے منہ سے ٹکراتا ہے۔ اس طرح انزال کے وقت

مرد کا مادہ منویہ رحم کے منہ پر گرتا ہے اور سپرم آسانی سے رحم کے اندر جا سکتے ہیں۔ یہ طریقہ استقرار حمل کے لئے مفید ہے۔

utylaminobenzoate *(bu-til-am-in-o- ben'-z-o-at)* Local anaesthetic used as ointment (1 per-cent), suppositories (1 g), or dusting powder. A constituent of Proctocaine (q.v.).

بیوٹائیل امینوبنزوایٹ : مقامی طور پر سن کرنے کے لئے مرہم یا پوڈر کی صورت میں استعمال کیا جاتا ہے۔ پراکٹوکین کا ایک جزو۔

Butyn *(but'-in)*. Butacaine (q.v.).

بیوٹن : دیکھئے بوٹاکین۔

Byssinosis *(bis-in-o'-sis)* [G. byssos, flax; -osis, condition]. Form of pneumoconiosis due to inhalation of cotton or linen dust. Scheduled under the National Insurance (Industrial Injuries) Act.

لتانیت ریہ : کپاس یا لنن کے ذرات سانس کے ذریعے جسم کے اندر جانے کی وجہ سے نیوموکونیوسس کی قسم۔

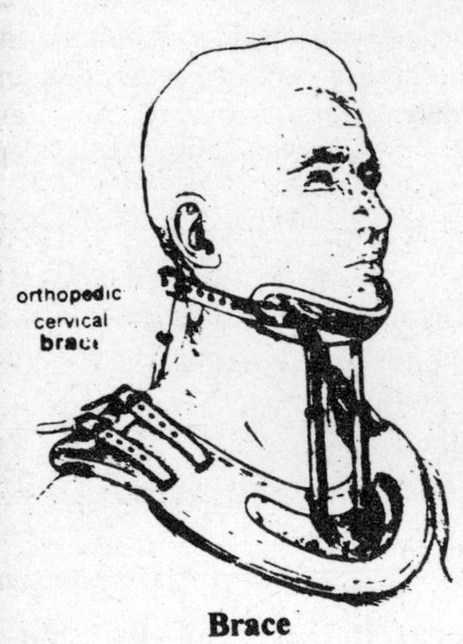

Brace

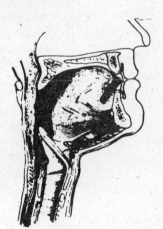

Bolus

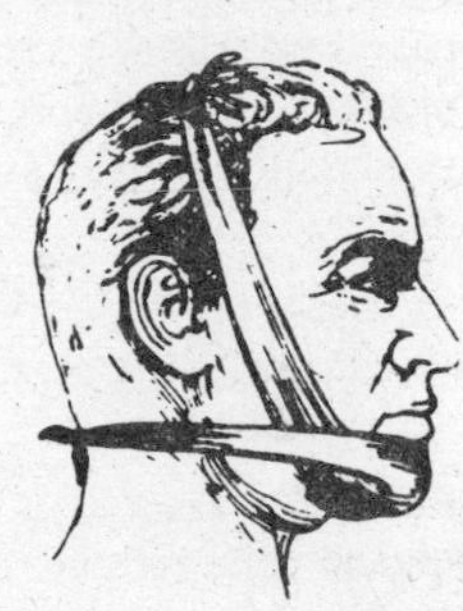

Barton's bandage

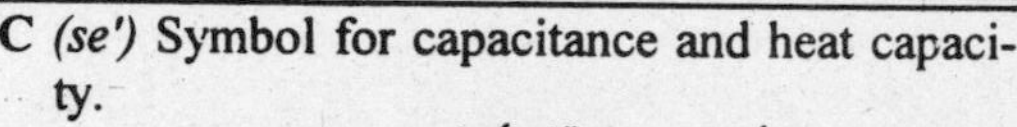

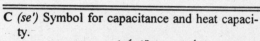

C *(se')* Symbol for capacitance and heat capacity.

سی: علامت ہے گنجائش کی اور حرارتی گنجائش کی۔

°C Symbol for degree celsius.

ڈگری سی: درجہ حرارت میں سیلیسس کی علامت۔

Cacao *(ka-ka-o)* It is the seed of theobroma cacao. Chocolate, cocoa and cacao butter is obtained from it. The butter does not vancid, so it melts at body temperature. Therefore, it is used as a base for suppositories, in ointments and as an emollient.

ککاؤ، نارجیل، کوکو: تھیو بروما کیکاؤ کے بیج جن سے چاکلیٹ، کوکو اور کیکاؤ مکھن تیار کئے جاتے ہیں۔ موخرالذکر جسمانی درجہ حرارت پر پگھل جاتا ہے۔ مرہم وغیرہ کی تیاری میں کام آتا ہے۔

Cacatory *(kak'-a-tor-e)* It is a condition which is marked by severe diarrhea.

پیچش لگنا: شدید قسم کے پیچش لگنے کی حالت۔

Cachet *(ka'sha')* [Fr.]. A disk-shaped wafer or capsule for enclosing a dose of medicine, for oral dose.

برشامہ: کیشے۔ کیسہ دوائیہ۔ چاول کے کاغذ سے بنا ہوا ایک چپٹا کیپسول جس میں کڑوی دوائی ہوتی ہے تاکہ اسے آسانی سے نگل سکیں۔

Cachexia *(ka-kek-se-a)* [G. *kakos,* bad; *hexis,* state, habit]. A profound and marked state of constitutional disorder, general ill health and malnutrition, emaciation of the body, sallow unhealthy skin and heavy lusterless eyes.

ضعفہ، فساد مزاج: یونانی الفاظ کیکوس بمعنی بری اور ہیکسس بمعنی حالت کا مجموعہ۔ ایک اصطلاح جو خراب حالت، غذائیت کی کمی اور عمومی خراب صحت کو ظاہر کرتی ہے۔

Cacomelia *(kako-mele-a)* [G. *kakos,* bad; *melos,* limbs]. Cogential deformity of a limb.

پیدائشی معذوری: ٹانگوں کی پیدائشی خرابی۔

Caecorectostomy *(se-ko-rek-tos-tom-e)* [L. *caecus,* blind; *rectus,* straight; G. *stoma,* mouth]. Cacecoproclostomy. Anestomesis between caecum and recturrm.

سیکوریکٹوسٹومی: لاطینی الفاظ سیکس بمعنی اندھا یا بند، ریکٹس بمعنی سیدھا اور یونانی لفظ سٹوما بمعنی منہ سے مرکب اصطلاح۔ سیکم اور ریٹم کے درمیان جال۔ آنت کے منہ پر جھلی آجانا یعنی آنت کا اندھا ہونا۔

Caecosigmoidostomy *(seko-sig-moid-os-to-mi)* [L. *caecus,* blind; G. *stoma,* mouth]. Surgical anastomosis between caecum and sigmoid flexure of colon.

سیکوسگمائڈوسٹومی: لاطینی لفظ سیکس بمعنی اندھا یا بند اور یونانی الفاظ حرف سگما اور سٹوما بمعنی منہ سے مرکب اصطلاح۔ سیکم اور کولون کے سگما نما فلیکسر کے درمیان سرجیکل جال۔

Caecum *(se-kam)* [L. *caecus,* blind]. A blind pouch-like commencement of the colon in the right iliac fossa. To it is attached the vermiform appendix; it is separated from the ileum by the ileocaecal valve.

اَعور، اندھی آنت: کولون کا بند اور تھیلی نما حصہ۔ اس کے زائد آنت جڑی ہوتی ہے۔

CaEDTA Abb. of Calcium disodium versanate. Used in lead poisoning and as eyedrops.

کیلشیمای ڈی ٹی اے: کیلشیم دسوڈیم ورسینیٹ۔ سیسے کے زہریلے پن کا استعمال کیا جاتا۔

Caesarean sectom *(se-zar'-i-an sek'-shun)*. Delivery of the fetus through an abdominal incision. It is said to be named after Caesar, who is supposed to have been born in this way. When delivery is accomplished extra-peritoneally, the term 'low cervical c.s.' is used.

قیصری تراش: پیٹ چیر کر بچے کی پیدائش۔ اس کا نام قیصر پر رکھا گیا ہے جس کے متعلق خیال ہے کہ وہ اسی طرح پیدا ہوا تھا۔

Caecium 137. A. radioactive substance which, when sealed in a container can be used for beam therapy instead of cobalt; when sealed in needles or tubes it can be used for local application instead of radium.

Caffeine *(kaf'-e-in)*. The central nervous system stimulant, present in tea and coffee. It has been given as a diuretic, but its main use is in analgesic preparations.

کیفین۔ قہوین۔ جوہر قہوہ: یہ مرکزی عصبی نظام کو تحریک دیتی ہے۔ چائے اور کافی میں موجود ہوتی ہے۔ پیشاب آور کے طور پر مستعمل۔ اے پی سی کی گولیوں میں ڈالی جاتی ہے۔ دافع درد ہے۔ تھمین۔ ایک سفید پیورین۔ نقطۂ پگھلاؤ ۲۳۷° س۔

Caisson disease *(ka'-son)* [F. caisse, from L. capsa, a box]. 'Decompression illness. The bends. It results from suddent reduction in atmospheric pressure, e.g. divers on return to surface, airmen ascending to great heights. Due to bubles of nitrogen which are released from solution in the blood; symptoms vary according to the site of these. The condition is largely preventable by proper and gradual decompression technique.

عوضی تشنج: فضائی دباؤ میں اچانک کمی کی وجہ سے یہ مرض لاحق ہوتا ہے' غوطہ خور کو کیسن سے فوراً باہر نہیں آنا چاہیے۔

Caladryl *(kal'-a-dril)*. Lotion and cream containing calamine and diphenhy-dramine (q.v.).

کیلاڈرل: کیلامین اور ڈائیفن ہائیڈرامین پر مشتمل کریم اور لوشن۔

Calamine *(kal'-a-min)*. Zinc carbonate tinted pink with ferric oxide. Widely employed in lotions and creams for its mild astringent action on the skin.

کیلامین۔ سلیمانی پتھر کچدھات جست: زنک کاربونیٹ۔ فیرک آکسائڈ کی ساتھ گلابی رنگ دیتا ہے۔ لوشن اور کریموں میں مستعمل ہے۔ کیلامین لوشن جلد کو تسکین دیتا ہے اور ایگزیما کے لئے مفید ہے۔

Calcareous *(kal-ka'-ri-us)* [L. calcarius from calx, lime]. Pertaining to or containing lime or calcium; of a chalky nature.

کلسیم دار: کیلسم یا چونے پر مستمل یا اس سے متعلق۔

Calciferol *(kal-sif'-e-rol)*. Synthetic vitamin D. This or natural vitamin D. is essential for the uptake and utilization of calcium. Given in rickets and to prevent hypocalcaemia in coeliac disease, and in parathyroid deficiency and lupus vulgaris.

کیلسی فیرول: تالیفی وٹامن ڈی۔ کیلیم کے استعمال کے لئے ضروری۔ جوڑوں کی بیماری میں مفید۔ ایک قلمی غیر سیر شدہ الکحل۔ نقطۂ پگھلاؤ ۱۵۵° س' یہ جسم میں کیلیم مرکبات کے جمع ہونے کو کنٹرول کرتا ہے۔ اس کی کمی سے رکٹس ہوتی ہے۔

Calcification *(kal-sif-i-ka'-shun)* [L. calx, lime; facere, to make]. The hardening of an organic substance by a deposite of calcium salts within it. May be normal as in bone or pathological as in arteries.

تکلس : لاطینی الفاظ کیلکس بمعنی چونا اور فیسئر بمعنی بنانا کا مجموعہ۔ کیلیم کے نمکیات جمع ہونے سے کسی نامیاتی مادے کا سخت ہونا۔

Calcitonin *(kal-si-ton'-in)* . Hormone produced in thyroid parafollicular or 'C' cells. Does not affect general metabolic progress. Role in normal physiology as yet uncertain. May link bone breakdown under special circumstances such as pregnancy. Now being used as drug therapy in Paget's disease.

کیلسی ٹونن : ایک ہارمون۔ عام افعال میں موثر نہیں۔

Calcium chloride *(kal'-si-um klor'-id)*. Deliquescent granules, very soluble in water. Occasionally given by injection in calcium deficiency, but, owing to its irritant propertieis, other calcium salts are preferred. Can be given by i.v. injection for cardiac resuscitation.

کیلسیم کلورائڈ : پانی میں حل پذیر دانے دار مرکب۔ بعض دفعہ کیلسیم کی کمی دور کرنے کے لئے انجکشن کے ذریعے دیا جاتا ہے۔ نقطہ پگھلاؤ ۷۷۲° س خشک اور محفوظ رکھنے کے لئے مستعمل۔

Calcium disodium versanate *(kal'-si-um di-so'-di-um ver'-san-at)* CaEDTA (q.v.).

کیلشیم ڈائی سوڈیم ورسینیٹ : دیکھئے کیلسیم ای ڈی ٹی اے۔

Calcium gluconate *(kal'-si-um gloo'-kon-at)*. A well tolerated and widely used salt of calcium. Indicated in all calcium deficiency states, in allergic conditions and in lead poisoning.

Calcium lactate *(kal'-si-um lak'-tat)*. A soluble salt of calcium, less irritating than calcium chloride. Used orally like calcium gluconate in all calcium deficiency states.

کیلسیم لیکٹیٹ : کیلسیم کا حل پذیر نمک۔ کیلسیم کلورائڈ سے کم سوزش والا۔ کیلسیم کی کمی کی حالتوں میں کیلسیم گلوکونیٹ کی طرح استعمال کیا جاتا ہے۔

Calculus *(kal'-ku-lus)* [L. small stone]. chiefly of mineral substances and formed in the passages which transmit secretions, or in the cavities which act as reservoirs for them--calculi, pl.; calculous, adj.

پتھری۔ سنگ گردہ : لاطینی زبان کا لفظ جس کا مطلب چھوٹا پتھر ہے۔ معدنی مادوں پر مشتمل پتھری جو کھفوں یا رطوبتوں کے راستے میں بنتی ہے۔

Calwell-Luc operation An opening is made above the upper canine tooth into the anterior wall of the maxillary antrum for drainage. [George Walter Caldwell, American surgeon, 1866-1946. Henri Luc, French laryngologist, 1855-1925].

کالڈویل لک اپریشن : میکسلری انٹرم کی اگلی دیوار میں بالائی کینائن دانت کے اوپر ایک سوراخ کیا جاتا ہے۔

Caliper *(kal'-ip-er)* [F. calibre, measurement]. 1. A two-pronged instrument for measuring the diameter of a round body. Used chiefly in pelvimetry (q.v.). 2.A two pronged instrument with sharp points which are inserted into the lower end of a fractured long bone. A weight is attached to the other end of the caliper, which maintains a steady pull on the distal end of the bone. 3. Thomas' walking caliper is similar to the Thomas' splint, but the W-shaped junction at the lower end is replaced by two small iron rods which slot into holes made in the heel of the boot. The ring should fit the groin perfectly, and all weight is then borne by the ischial tuberosity.

چاپ۔ سرل چاپ : فرانسیسی لفظ کلیبئر بمعنی پیمائش سے ماخوذ اصطلاح۔ (۱) کسی گول مجسم کے قطر کی پیمائش کے لئے الہ (۲) شکستہ طویل ہڈی کے لئے آلہ۔ (۳) تھامس متحرک کیلیپر۔

Callosity *(kal-os'-it-i)* [L. callosus, hard skinned]. A local hardening of the skin caused by pressure or friction. The epidermis becomes hypertrophied. Most commonly seen on the feet and palms of the hands.

صلابت جلد : لاطینی لفظ کیلوسس بمعنی سخت جلد والا سے ماخوذ اصطلاح۔ دباؤ یا رگڑ کی وجہ سے جلد کا مقامی طور سخت ہونا۔ عموماً پاؤں یا ہاتھ ہتھیلیوں پر ایسی حالت پائی جاتی ہے۔

Callus *(kal'-us)* [L. 1. A callosity (q.v.). 2. The partly calcified tissue which forms about the ends of a broken bone, which ultimately accomplishes repair of the fracture. When this is complete the bony thickening is known as 'permanent callus'--calous, adj.

صلابت جلد۔ پینہ : لاطینی لفظ۔ (۱) جلد کا سخت ہونا۔ (۲) ہڈی کا ابھار بننا۔

Calomel *(kal'-o-mel)*. Mercurous chloride (q.v.).

کیلومل۔ رسکپور : دیکھئے مرکیورس کلورائڈ۔ سارو غ کش ادویات مستعمل۔ سفید ناحل پذیر سفوف۔

Calor *(kal'-or)* [L.]. Heat; one of the classic local signs of inflammation.

کیلر۔ حرارت : لاطینی لفظ۔ حرارت۔ گرمی۔ سوزش کی مقامی علامات میں سے ایک۔

Calorie *(kal'-or-e)* [L. calor, heat]. A unit of head. Currently in scientific terms, energy, work, and quantity of hear are measured in the same units--the joule, (j), and it will replace calorie, the joule being approximately 1/4 calorie. The Small calorie is the amount of heat required to raise the temperature of 1 g of water 1^0 C; the **large calorie** used in the study of metabolism is the amount of heat required to raise the temperature of 1 kg of water 1^0 C, sometimes called a kilocalorie (kcal).

کیلوری۔ حرارہ : لاطینی لفظ کیلر بمعنی حرارت سے ماخوذ اصطلاح۔ حرارت کی اکائی۔ حرارت کی وہ مقدار جو ایک کلوگرام پانی کا درجہ حرارت ایک ڈگری یا درجہ سنٹی گریڈ زیادہ کرنے کے لئے درکار ہے۔ چھوٹی کیلوری حرارت کی وہ مقدار ہے جو ایک گرام پانی کا درجہ حرارت ایک درجہ سنٹی گریڈ زیادہ کرنے کے لئے درکار ہے۔ ایک کلوگرام پانی کا درجہ حرارت ایک درجہ سنٹی گریڈ بڑھانے کے لئے ۴۲۰۰ جول حرارت صرف ہوتی ہے۔ ایک حرارہ = ۴٫۲ جول۔

Calorific *(kal-or-if'-ik)* adj. [L. calor, heat; facere, to make]. Heat producing.

حراری (قیمت) : لاطینی الفاظ کیلر بمعنی حرارت اور فیسیئر بمعنی بنانا کا مجموعہ۔ حرارت پیدا کرنے والا۔ مختلف غذائی مادے مختلف کلوری کی مقدار مہیا کرتے ہیں۔ ایک گرام چربی ۹ کلوری پیدا کرتی ہے جبکہ ایک گرام پروٹین یا کاربوہائیڈریٹ ۴٫۱ کلوری پیدا کرتا ہے۔ حراری قیمت حرارت کی وہ مقدار ہے جو مکمل احتراق پر ایندھن کی دی ہوئی کمیت سے پیدا ہوتی ہے۔

Calvarium *(kal-va'-ri-um)* [L. calva, bald head]. The vault of the skull; the skull-cap.

کاسئہ سر : لاطینی لفظ کلوا بمعنی گنجا سر سے ماخوذ اصطلاح۔ کھوپڑی، کھوپڑی کا استخوانی ڈھانچہ۔

Camcolit *(kam'-ko-lit)*. Lithium carbonate (q.v.)

Camoquin *(kam'-o-kwin)*. Amodiaquine (q.v.).

کیموکوئن : دیکھئے اموڈیا کوئن۔ بچوں کو دینے کے ہلکی کونین۔

Camphor *(kam'-for)*. White solid with characteristic odour. Carminative and expectorant internally, and used as paregoric (q.v.) in cough mixtures. Applied externally in the form of camphorated oil as an analgesic and rubefacient--camphorated, adj.

کافور : مخصوص بو والا سفید ٹھوس۔ ہاضم۔ کھانسی کے شربتوں میں مستعمل۔ کیمفر لینمنٹ کی صبح و شام مالش برائے آسیٹوار تھرائی ٹس۔

Canaliculotomy *(kan-a-lik-ul-ot'-o-mi)* [L. canaliculus, small channel; G. tome, a cutting]. Excision of posterior wall of ophthalmic canaliculus and conversion of drain 'tube' into a channel.

قنالی کیولوٹومی : لاطینی لفظ کینا لیکولس بمعنی چھوٹی نالی اور یونانی لفظ بمعنی ایک تراشہ سے مرکب اصطلاح۔ افتھلمک کنالیکولس کی خلفی دیوار کاٹ کر نلی کو نالی میں تبدیل کرنا۔

Canaliculus *(kan-alik'-u-lus)* [L. small channel]. A minute capillary passage. Any small canal, such as the passage leading from the edge of the eyelid to the lacrimal sac, or one of the numerous small canals leading from the Haversian canals and terminating in the lacunae of bone--canaliculi, pl.; canalicular, adj.; canaliculization, n.

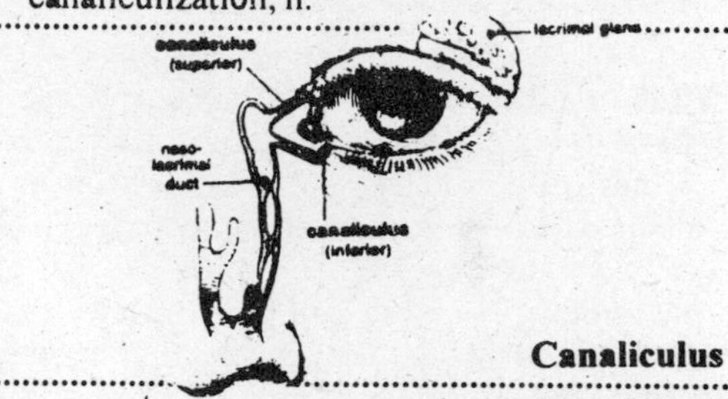

Canaliculus

قنات صغیر۔ قنالچہ : لاطینی لفظ جس کا مطلب ہے چھوٹی نالی۔ ایک باریک شعری راستہ۔ کوئی چھوٹی قنال۔

Cancellous *(kan'-sel-us)* [L. cancelli, lattice]. Resembling latticework; light and spongy; like a honeycomb.

اسفنجی۔ مسامدار : ہلکا اور اسفنجی۔ شہد کے چھتے کی طرح۔

Cancer *(kan'-ser)* [L. crab]. A general term which covers many malignant growths in many parts of the body. The growth is purposeless, parasitic, and flourishes at the expense of the human host. Characteristics are the tendancy to cause local destruction, to spread by metastasis, to recur after removal, and to cause toxaemia. Carcinoma refers to malignant tumours of skin or mucous membrane, sarcoma to tumours of connective tissue--cancerous, adj.

کینسر۔ سرطان : جسم کے مختلف حصوں میں بڑھاؤ کے لئے استعمال ہونے والی اصطلاح۔ یہ بڑھاؤ بے فائدہ، طفیلی اور فضول ہوتا ہے۔ کیکڑے۔ نما رسولیاں۔ سرطان جسم کے تقریباً ہر حصے میں ہوتا ہے۔ علاج کے لئے اپریسن، کلوریم بیوسل اور مرکیپٹوپیورین مفید ہیں۔

Cancerocidal *(kal-ser-o-sid'-al)* [L. cancer, crab; coedere, to kill]. Lethal to cancer.

سرطان کش : کینسر کے لئے مہلک۔

Cancerophobia *(kan-se-ro-fo-bi-a)* [L. cancer,

crab; G. phobos, fear]. Extreme fear of cancer.

سرطان تراشی : کینسر کا انتہائی خوف۔

Cancrumoris *(kan'-krum-or'-is)*. Gangrenous stomatitis of mouth in debilitated children. Often called 'noma.'

منہ کا ناسور : منہ کی بیماری جسے عموماً نوما کہا جاتا ہے۔ منہ کے اندر یا باہر آبلے پڑنا یا دانے نکلنا۔ بچوں میں پائی جانے والی بیماری۔

Candida *(kan'-di-da)*. A genus of fungi. Yeast-like cells that form some filaments. Widespread in nature. Candida (Monilia) albicans is a commensal of the mouth, throat, vagina, gut and skin of man. Becomes pathogenic in some physiological and pathological states. May produce infections such as thrush, vulvovaginitis, balanoposthitis and pulmonary disease. Infection can result from disturbed flora due to use of widesp-rectrum antibiotics, steroids, contraceptive pills, immunosuppressive and/or cytotoxic, drugs. Can also occur during pregnancy, secondary to debilitating general disease such as diabetes mellitus or Cushing's syndrome. Can be due to poor oral hygiene, including carious teeth and ill-fitting dentures.

مونیلیا : سماروغ کا ایک جنس۔ یہ آدمی میں جلد' منہ' گلا' آنت اور فرج یا ویجائنا میں بیماریاں پیدا کرتا ہے۔ کینڈیڈا ایلبی کینز یا مونیلیا پھپھوندی ہے جس سے تھرش (منہ پکنا) کا مرض ہوتا ہے۔

Candidiasis *(kan-did-i'-a-sis)*. Disease caused by infection with species of Candida (q.v.). Moniliasis (q.v.).

کین ڈی ڈیا سس : کنڈائڈ کی نوع سے پیدا ہونے والی چھوت کی بیماری۔ شدید سوزش اور خارش کا ہونا۔

Canitola fever *(kan-i-ko'-la)*. Infection (leptospirosis) of man by species of Leptospira from rats, dogs, pigs, (Leptospira canicola) foxes, mice, voles and possibly cats. There is high fever, headache, conjunctival congestion, jaundice, severe muscular pains, rigors and vomiting. As the fever abates in about one week, the jaundic disappears.

کینی کولا بخار : چوہوں' لومڑیوں وغیرہ سے لگنے والی بیماری۔ اس میں بخار' سر درد' یرقان' عضلی درد اور متلی وغیرہ ہو جاتے ہیں۔

Canine *(kan'-in)* [L. canis, dog]. Resembling a dog. **c. teeth,** four in all, two in each jaw, situated between the incisors and the prem-olars. Those in the upper jaw are popularly known as the 'eve teeth'.

کلبی : لاطینی لفظ کینس بمعنی کتا سے ماخوذ اصطلاح کتے سے مشابہ۔

Cannabis indica *(kan'-ab-is in'-dik-a)*. Indian hemp, a narcotic drug once used as a cerebral sedative in nervous disorders. Marijuana; 'pot'.

بھنگ : بھنگ۔ نشہ آور شے۔ پہلے ادویات میں استعمال کی جاتی تھی۔ اس کے استعمال سے مریض بولتا رہتا ہے۔ پاگل پن کی حرکات کرتا ہے پھر سو جاتا ہے۔ قے کرائی جائے یا معدہ دیا جائے۔ تیز چائے پلایئے۔ ایفی ڈرین اور کورامین کا ٹیکہ لگایئے اور سٹی ٹولنٹ مکسچر پلایئے۔

Cannula *(kan'-u-la)* [L. dim. canna, a reed]. A hollow tube for the introduction or **withdrawal** of fluid from the body. In some patterns the lumen is fitted with a sharp pointed trocar to facilitate insertion. It is withdrawn when the cannula is in situ--c-annulae, pl.

جراحی نلکی۔ قنولہ : سیال کو جسم میں داخل یا اس سے خارج کرنے کے لئے کھوکھلی نلی۔

Canthus *(kan'-thus)* [G. kanthos, corner of the eye]. The angle formed by the junction of the eye. The inner one is known as the **'nasal** canthus' and the outer as the 'temporal canthus'--canthal, adj.; canthi, pl.

Canthus

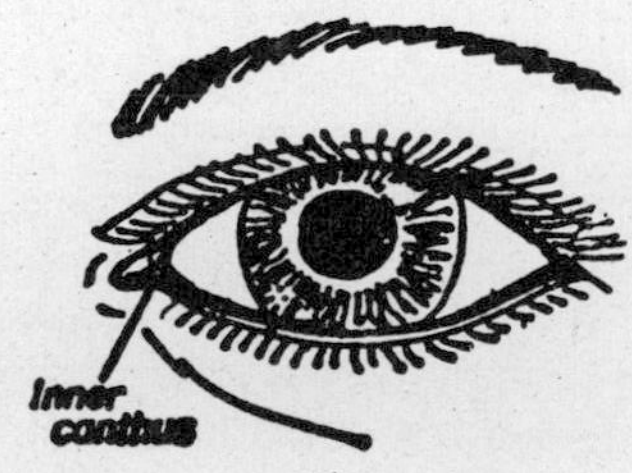

ماق۔ گوشہ چشم : یونانی لفظ کنتھوس بمعنی آنکھ کا کونا سے ماخوذ اصطلاح۔

پوٹوں کے جنکشن سے بننے والا زاویہ۔

Capastat *(kap'-a-stat)* . Capreomycin (q.v.).

کیپسٹیٹ : دیکھئے کیپریومائیسین۔ سماروغ سے حاصل شدہ اینٹی بایوٹک۔ تپ دق کے لئے مفید۔

Capillary *(kap-il'-a-ri)* [L. capillus, hair]. Hair-like. Any tiny thin-walled vessel forming part of a network which facilitates rapid exchange of substances between the contained fluid and the surrounding issues. **blue c.** begins in a space in the liver and joins others, eventually forming a bile duct. **blood c.** unites an arteriole and a venule. **c. fragility**, and expression of ease with which blood capillaries may rupture. **lymph c.** begins in the tissue spaces throughout the body and joins others, eventually forming a lymphatic vessel.

شعری۔ شعریہ : لاطینی لفظ کیپلس بمعنی بال سے ماخوذ اصطلاح بال نما۔ کوئی

Capillaries

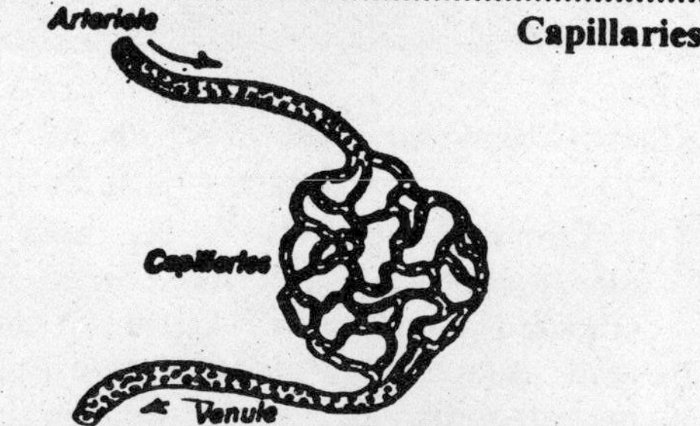

چھوٹی پتلی دیواروں والی رگ خون کی باریک نالیاں جو ہر عضو میں جال بناتی ہیں۔ یہ خوردبین سے دیکھی جاسکتی ہیں۔ ان میں خون کی آکسیجن، خوراک اور بیکار مادوں کا تبادلہ ہوتا ہے۔

Caplan's syndrome Rheumatoid pneumoconiosis. Occurs in coal or asbestos workers with pneumoconiosis, who have or may develop rheumatoid arthritis.

Capreomycin *(kap-re-o-mi'-sin)*. Peptide antibiotic derived from Streptomyces capreolus. Main indication is as a secondary drug in treating drug resistant tuberculosis.

کیپ ریومائی سین : ایک ضد جسیمہ یا اینٹی بیاٹک۔ سماروغ سے حاصل شدہ۔ تپ دق کے علاج کے لئے مفید دوائی۔

Capsicum *(kap'-si-kum)* . African pepper, used as a carminative and rubefacient.

لال مرچ : افریقی مرچ۔ ہاضم کے طور پر مستعمل۔

Capsule *(kap'-sul)* [L. capsula, small box]. 1. The ligaments which surround a joint. 2. A gelatinous or rice paper container for noxious drugs. 3. The outer membranous covering of certain organs, such as the kidney, liver, spleen, adrenals--capsular, adj.

کیپسول۔ غشائی کیسہ۔ درجک : لاطینی لفظ کیپسولا بمعنی چھوٹا بکس سے ماخوذ (۱) جوڑ کے گرد لگامنٹ۔ (۲) ایک جلاٹینی یا چاول کا کاغذ جس میں بدذائقہ دوائی بند کی جاتی ہے۔ (۳) بعض اعضاء کی بیرونی جھلی دار پرت۔ مثلاً گردہ، تلی، جگر وغیرہ۔

Capsulectomy *(kap-sul-ek'-to-mi)* [L. capsula, small box; G. ektome excision]. Surgical excision of a capsule. Refers to a joint or lens; less often to the kidny.

کیسہ براری : لاطینی لفظ کیپسولا بمعنی چھوٹا بکس اور یونانی لفظ ائس بمعنی سوزش سے مرکب اصطلاح۔ کیپسول کی سوزش۔ منجمد شانے کے لئے بھی اصطلاح استعمال کی جاتی ہے۔

Capsulitis *(kap-su-li'-tis)* [L. capsula, small box; G. -itis, inflammation]. Inflammation of a capsule. Sometimes used as a syn. for frozen shoulder (q.v.).

Capsulotomy *(kap-sul-ot'-om-i)* [L. capsula, small box; G. tome, a cutting]. Incision of a capsule, usually referring to that surrounding the cystalline lens of the eye.

Caput succedaneum *(kap'-ut-suk-se-da'-ne-um)* [G. caput, head; L. succedaneus, following]. A serious effusion overlying the scalp periostem on an infant's head. Due to pressure during labour.

سابیا : دردزہ کے دوران دباؤ کی وجہ سے بچے کے سر پر گولہ۔

Carbachol *(kar-ba-kol)*. Parasympathetic nervous system stimulant similar to acetylcholin (q.v.) but active orally, and has a sustained action by injection. Given in postoperative retention of urine and intestinal atony, and as eye drops for glaucom. Cholinergic agent.

کاربیکول : پیرا سمپتھیٹک عصبی نظام کو تحریک دینے والی دوا۔

Carbamates *(kar'-bam-atz)*. Tranquillizersm, For poisoning, see p. 337.

کربیمیٹز : سکون بخش دوا۔اس کا زیادہ استعمال صحت کے لئے مضر ہے۔

Carbamazepine *(kar-bam-az'-e-pen)*. Anticonvulsant; also relieves pain; especially useful in trigeminal neuralgia.

کاربیمے زیپن : بعض امراض مثلاً مرگی وغیرہ میں مفید دوا۔

Carbaminohaemoglobin *(karb-am-in'-o-he-m-o-glo'-bin)*. A compound formed between carbon dioxide and haemoglobin. Part of the carbon dioxide in the blood is carried in this form.

کاربامینوہیموگلوبن : کاربن ڈائی آکسائڈ اور ہیموگلوبن کے درمیان بننے والا مرکب۔کاربن ڈائی آکسائڈ کا ایک حصہ اس صورت میں کون لایا جاتا ہے۔

Carbaryl *(kar'-bar-il)*. Useful for treatment of head lice which are resistant to DDT and gammabenzenehexachloride.

Carbenicillin *(kar-ben-sil'-in)*. The only semisynthetic penicillin to show any reasonable activity against the antibiotic-resistant Pseudomonas aeruginosa. Unfortunately, even carbinicillin is not highly active against this organism. High concentrations can be achieved in the urine to destroy Pseudomonas there, but much larger does of the order of 30 to 40 g a day are required to achief sufficient concentration in the tissues. Such large does not only be given by intravenous infusion.

کیر بنی سلین : سوڈومونس ایروجینوسا کے خلاف استعمال ہونے والی نیم تالیفی پنسلین۔اس کی کافی مقدار جسم میں چاہئے۔اس لئے ۳۰ تا ۴۰ گرام روزانہ جسم میں داخل کی جاتی ہے جو انجکشن کے ذریعہ ہی ممکن ہے۔

Carbenoxolone *(kar-ben-orks'-o-lon)*. Extracted from liquorice. A relative of the corticosteroids. Specific healing effect on gastric but not doudenal ulcers. The method needs careful observation for the occurence of oedema and potassium depletion.

کاربینوکسولون : معدے کے ناسور کے لئے مخصوص اثر والی دوائی۔

Carbidopa *(kar-bi-do'-pa)*. When added to levodopa allows reduction of dose, decreases frequency of adverse reactions and improves control of symptoms.

Carbimazole *(kar-bim'-a-zol)*. An antithyroid drug that prevents combination of iodine and tyrosine. It is more potent and less toxic than methylthiouracil, and is the drug of choice in thyrotoxicosis.

Carbohydrate *(kar-bo-hi'-drat)* [L. carbo, coal; G. hydor, water]. An organic compound containing carbon, hydrogen adn oxygen. Formed in nature by photosynthesis in plants. Carbohydrates are heat producing; they include starches, sugars and cellulose, and are classified in three groups--monosaccharides, disaccharides and polysaccharides. See CALORIFIC.

کاربوہائیڈریٹ۔نشاستہ دار غذا : لاطینی لفظ کاربو بمعنی کوئلہ اور یونانی لفظ ہائیڈر بمعنی پانی سے مرکب اصطلاح۔کاربن ہائیڈروجن اور آکسیجن پر مشتمل ایک نامیاتی مرکب۔سبز پودوں میں ضیائی تالیف کے ذریعے یہ مرکب بنتا ہے۔یہ مرکبات حرارت پیدا کرتے ہیں۔ان میں نشاستہ، شکر اور سیلولوز شامل ہیں۔

Carbolic acid *(kar-bol'ik'as'-id)*. Phenol (q.v.).

کاربالک ایسڈ۔فینال : دیکھئے فینول۔

Carboluria *(kar-bol-u'-ri-a)* [L. carbo, coal; oleum, oil; G. ouron, urine]. Green or dark coloured urine due to excretion of carbolic acid, as occurs in carbolic acid poisoning--carboluric, adj.

کاربول بوئی : لاطینی الفاظ کاربو بمعنی کوئلہ اور اولیئم بمعنی تیل اور یونانی لفظ اورون بمعنی پیشاب سے مرکب اصطلاح۔کاربالک ایسڈ کے اخراج کی وجہ سے پیشاب کی سبز یا سیاہ رنگت۔ایسی رنگت کاربالک ایسڈ کے زہریلے اثرات کی وجہ سے ہوتی ہے۔

Carbon *(kar'-bon)*. A non-metallic element. **c. dioxide,** a gas; a waste product of many forms of combustion and metablosim, excreted via the lungs. When disolved in a fluid, carbonic acid is formed; a specific amount of this in the blood produces inspiration, in cases of insufficiency, inhalations of CO_2 ac-tas a respiratory stimulant. In its solid form--CO_2 snow--it is used in the removal of spider naevi, **c. monoxide,** a poisonous gas which forms a stable compound with haemoglobin, thus robbing the body of its oxygen-carrying mechanism; signs and symptoms of hypoxia ensue. **c. tetrachloride,** colourless liquid with an odour similar to chloroform. Used as an anthelmintic against hookworm and tapeworm, sometimes in combination with chenopodium oil. Previous fasting and subsequent purging is necessary.

Carbon

کاربن : ایک غیر دھاتی عنصر۔ کاربن ڈائی آکسائڈ ایک گیس ہے جو تنفس کے دوران پھیپھڑوں کے ذریعے جسم سے باہر آتی ہے۔ سیال میں حل ہوکر کاربالک ایسڈ بناتی ہے۔ کاربن مونو آکسائڈ ایک زہریلی گیس ہے جو ہیموگلوبن کے ساتھ پائدار مرکب بناتی ہے اس لئے آکسیجن لے جانے والی میکانیت کو ختم کر دیتی ہے۔ کاربن ٹیٹرا کلورائڈ ایک بے رنگ مائع ہے جس کی بو کلوروفامر ایسی ہوتی ہے۔ یہ مائع ہک ورم اور کدو کیڑے کے خلاف استعمال کیا جاتا ہے۔ کاربن کا جوہری عدد ۶ اور گرفت ۴ ہے۔ کاربن کی قلمی شکلیں ہیرا اور گریفائیٹ ہیں۔ کاربن عام نامیاتی مرکبات کا اہم جزو ہے۔

Carboxyhaemoglobin *(kar-boks'-i-hem-o-g-lo'-bin)* [L. carbo, coal; G. oxys, sharp; haima, blood; L. globus, globe]. A stable compound formed by the union of carbon monoxide and haemoglobin; the red blood cells thus lose their respiratory function.

کاربوکسی ہیموگلوبن : لاطینی لفظ کاربو بمعنی کوئلہ، یونانی الفاظ آکسس بمعنی تیز اور ہیما بمعنی خون اور لاطینی لفظ گلوبس بمعنی گلوب سے مرکب اصطلاح۔ کاربن مونو آکسائڈ اور ہیموگلوبن سے بننے والا ایک پائدار مرکب۔ اس کے بننے سے سرخ خونی خلیے اپنا تنفسی فعل سرانجام دینا ختم کر دیتے ہیں۔

Carboxyhaemoglobinaemia *(kar-boks'-i-hem-o-glo-bin-e'-mi-a).* Carboxyhaemoglobin in the blood--carboxyhaemoglobinaemic, adj.

کاربوکسی ہیموگلوبی نیمیا : خون میں کاربوکسی ہیموگلوبن۔

Carboxyhaemoglobinuria *(kar-boks'-i-hem-o-glo-bin-u'-ri-a).* Carboxyhaemxyhaemoglobinaemic. adj.

کاربوکسی ہیموگلوبی نیوریا : پیشاب میں کاربوکسی ہیموگلوبن کی موجودگی۔

Carbrital *(kar-brit-al).* Carbromal (q.v.).

کاربری ٹال: تفصیل کے لئے دیکھئے کاربرومل۔ ہلکی خواب آور دوائی۔

Carbromal *(kar-bro'-mal).* Mild non-barbituric sedative and hynotic. It may cause purpuric skin reactions in sensitive patients.

کاربرومل : ہلکا خواب آور۔ حساس مریضوں میں جلدی ردعمل ہوسکتا ہے۔

Carbuncle *(kar'-bung-kl).* An acute inflammation (usually caused by Staphylococcus) involving several hair follicles and surrounding subcutaneous tissue, forming an extensive slough with several discharging sinuses.

گحل۔ کاربنکل۔ شب چراغ: عموماً سٹیفائلوکاکسس کی وجہ سے انتہائی سوزش۔ اس میں بالوں کی جڑوں اور زیر جلد نسیج کا تعلق ہے۔ اس کی وجہ ذیابیطس شکری ہے۔ پیپ بن جائے تو چیرا دیجئے۔

Carcinogen *(kar-sin'-o-jen)* [G. karkinos, crab; genesthai, to be produced]. Any cancer-producing substances or agent--carcinogenic, adj.; carcinogenicity, n.

سرطان زا : کوئی بھی سرطان پیدا کرنے والا مادہ یا عامل۔

Carcinogenesis *(kar-sin-o-jen'-e-sis).* [G. karkinos, carb; genesis, production]. The production of cancer-- carcinogenetic, adj.

سرطانی تولید : سرطان کا پیدا ہونا۔

Carcinoid syndrome. Name given to a histologically malignant but clinically benign tumbour of the appendix that secretes serotomin, which stimulates smooth muscle causing diarrhoea, asthmatic spasm. flushing and other miserable symptoms.

کارسی نائڈ سنڈروم : آنت کا ناسور۔ بعض اوقات پھیپھڑے میں بھی ہوتا ہے۔

Carcinoma *(kar-sin-o'-ma).* [G. kakinos, crab; -oma, tumour]. Malignant growth of epidermal tissue (e.g. skin, mucous membrane) and derivatives such as glands. Cancer (q.v.) **e-in-situ,** asypmtomatic condition, also called **intraepithelial c.** of cervix. Cells closely resembling cancer cells grow from the cervical basal layer and eventually involve the whole epithelium so that its layers can no longer be recognized. Previously called pre-invasive c--carcinomatous, adj.; carcinomata, pl.

سرطان : سرطان کا مرض جس میں بالائی جلدی اور غدودی بافتیں اگتی ہیں۔ ختنہ نہ کرانے سے گندگی کی وجہ سے عضو تناسل کا یہ مرض ہوسکتا ہے۔

Carcinomatosis *(kar-sin-o-ma-to'-sis)*. A condition in which cancer is widespread throughout the body.

سرطانیت : سرطان کا سارے جسم میں پھیل جانا۔

Cardia *(kar'-di-a)* [G. kardia, heart]. The oesophageal opening into the stomac.

کارڈیا۔ قلب۔ دل فم معدہ : خوراک کی نالی کا سوراخ جس کے ذریعہ معدہ میں کھلتی ہے۔

Cardiac *(kar'-di-ak)*. [G. kardia, heart]. Pertaining to the heart, pertaining to the cardia. **c. arrest,** complete cessation of the heart's activity. Failure of the heart action to maintain an adequate cerebral circulation in the absence of a causative and irreversible disease (Milstein). The clinical picture of **cessation** of circulation in a patient who was not expected to die at the time. This naturally rules out the seriously ill patient who is dying slowly with an incurable disease, **c. asthma,** see ASTHMA. **c. bed,** one which can be manipulated so that the patient is supported in a sitting position. **c. catheterization,** a long plastic catheter or tubing is inserted into an arm vein and passed along to the right atrium, ventricle and pulmonary artery for (1) recording pressue in these areas; (2) introducing contrast medium prior to X-ray and high speed photography. Especially useful in the diagnosis of congenital heart defects. **c. oedema,** gravitational dropsy. Such patients excrete excessive aldosterone which increases excretion of potassium and conserves sodium and chloride. Antialdosterone drugs useful, e.g. spironala- ctone, triamterine. Both act as diuretics. **external c. message** done for cardiac arrest. With the patient of his back on a firm surface, the lower portion of sternum is depressed 37.2 to 50.8 mm each second. **c. tamponade,** compression of heart. Can occur in surgery and penetrating wounds or rupture of heart--from haemopericardium.

کارڈیک۔ قلبی : یونانی لفظ کارڈیا سے ماخوذ جس کے معانی دل میں۔ (۱) دل سے متعلق۔ (۲) کارڈیا سے متعلق۔

Cardialgis *(kar-di-al'-ji-a)* [G. kardia, heart; algos, pain]. Literally pain in the heart. Often used for heartburn.

دردفم معدہ۔ وجع الفواد : دل میں درد ہونا۔ دل میں جلن ہونا۔

Cardiazol *(kar-di'-a-zol)* Leptazol (q.v.).

کارڈیازال : دیکھئے لیپٹازول۔

Cardiogenic *(kar-di-o-jen'-ik)* [G. kardia, heart; genes, producing]. Of cardiac origin, such as the shock in coronary thrombosis.

قلب زاد : دل سے پیدا ہونے کے متعلق۔

Cardiogram *(kar'-di-o-gram)* [G. kardia heart; gramma, a drawing]. Recording traced by a cardiograph q.v.).

قلبی نگارش : کارڈیوگراف سے ٹریس شدہ ریکارڈنگ۔

Cardiograph *(kar'-di-o-graf)* [G. kardia, heart; graphein, to write]. An instrument for recording graphically the force and form of the heart beat--cardiographic, adj.; cardiographically, adv.

کارڈیوگراف۔ قلب نگار : یونانی الفاظ کارڈیا بمعنی دل اور گریفین بمعنی لکھنا کا مجموعہ۔ دل کی دھڑکن کی قوت اور قسم کو کاغذ پر ریکارڈ کرنے کا آلہ۔

Cardiologist *(kar-di-ol'-oj-ist)* [G. kardia, heart; logos, discourse]. A specialist in the study of cardiology.

ماہر قلبیات : کارڈیالوجی کا ماہر۔

Cardiology *(kar-di-ol'o-ji)* [G. kardia, heart; logos, discourse]. The science dealing with the heart and its functions.

کارڈیالوجی۔ قلبیات : سائنس کی شاخ جس میں دل اور اس کے افعال کا مطالعہ کیا جاتا ہے۔

Cardiomegaly *(kar-di-o-meg'-al-i)* [G. kardia, heart; megas, great]. Enlargement of the heart.

کلانی قلب : دل کا بڑھنا۔

ardiomyopathy *(kar-di-o-mi-op'-ath-i)* [G. kardia, heart; mys, muscle; pathos, disease]. An acute, subacute, or chronic disorder of heart muscle, of obscure aetiology, often with associated endocardial, or sometimes with pericardial involvement, but not atherosclerotic in origin--cardiomyopathic, adj.

کارڈیومایوپیتھی : قلبی عضلے کی تکلیف۔

ardiomyotomy *(kar'-di-o-mi-ot'-om-i)* [G. kardia, heart; sys, muscle; tome, a cutting]. Heller's operation (q.v.).

کارڈیوٹومی : دیکھئے ہیلرز اپریشن۔

ardiopathy *(kar-di-op'-ath-i)* [G. kardia, heart; pathos, disease]. Heart disease--cardiopathic, adj.

قلبی مرض : دل کی بیماری

ardiophone *(kar'-di-o-fon)*. Microphone strapped to patient allows audible and visual signal of heart sounds. By channeling pulse through an electrocardiograph, a graphic record can be made. Can be used for the fetus.

فلج القلب۔ مصوات القلب : مائیکروفون جس سے دل کی آوازیں سنی جا سکتی ہیں۔

ardioplasty *(kar-di-o-plas'-ti)* [G. kardia, heart; plassein, to form]. Plastic operation to the cardiac sphincter. See HELLER'S OPERATION--cardioplastic, adj.

ترقیع القلب : کارڈیک سفنکٹر کا پلاسٹک اپریشن۔

ardiopulmonary *(kar-di-o-pul'-mon-a-ri)* [g. kardia, heart; L. pulmo; lung]. Pertaining to the heart and lungs. **c. bypass,** used in open heart surgery. The heart and lungs are excluded from the circulation and replaced by a pump oxygenator--cardiopulmonic, adj.

قلبی شُشی : یونانی لفظ کارڈیا بمعنی دل اور لاطینی لفظ پلمو بمعنی پھیپھڑا سے مرکب اصطلاح۔ دل اور پھیپھڑوں سے متعلق۔

ardioquin *(kar'-di-o-qwin)*. Quinidine (q.v.).

کارڈیوکوئن : دیکھئے کونیڈین

ardiorator *(kar'-di-o-ra-tor)* Apparatus for visual recording of the heart beat.

کارڈیوریٹر : دل کی دھڑکن کی بصری ریکارڈنگ کا سامان۔

Cardioreal *(kar'-di-o-ra-tor)* [G. kardia, heart; L. renalis, of the kidney]. Pertaining to the heart and kidney.

قلبی کلوی : دل اور گردے سے متعلق۔

Cardiorespiratory *(kar-di-o-res-pir'-at-or-l)* [G. kardia, heart; L. respirare, breathe]. Pertaining to the heart and the respiratory system.

قلبی تنفّسی : یونانی لفظ کارڈیا بمعنی دل اور لاطینی لفظ ریسپیریئر بمعنی سانس لینا سے مرکب اصطلاح دل اور تنفّسی نظام سے متعلق۔

Cardiorraphy *(kar-di-or'-raf-i)* [G. kardia, heart; rhaphe, a suture]. Stitching of the heart wall. Usually reserved for traumatic surgery.

قلب دوزی : دل کی دیوار کو ٹانکے لگانا۔

Cardioscope *(kar'-di-o-skop)* [G. kardia, heart; skopein, to examine]. An instrument fitted with a lens and illumination, for examining the inside of the heart--cardioscopic, adj. cardioscopically, adv.

Cardiosocope

اصطلاح۔ دل کی اندرونی جانب جانچنے کے لئے ایک آلہ۔

Cardiospasm *(kar'-di-o-spazm)* [G. kardia, heart; spasmos, spasm] Spasm of the cardiac sphincter between the oesophagus and the stomach, causing retention within the oesophagus ('achalasia of the cardia'). Usually no local pathological change is found.

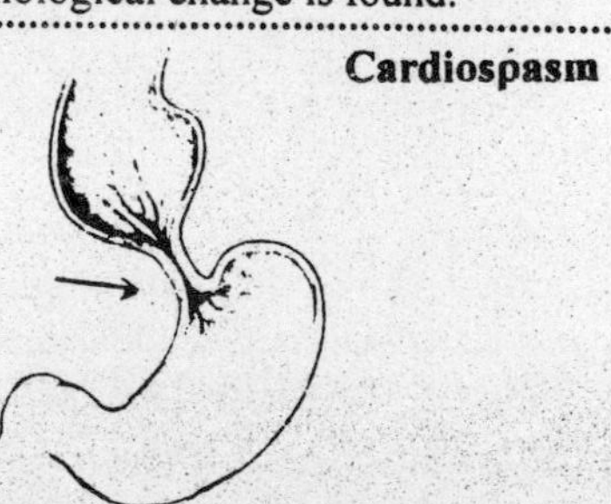

Cardiospasm

شنج الفواد : کارڈیک سفنکٹر کا سپازم۔

Cardiothoracic *(kar-di-o-thor-as'-ik)* [G. kardia heart; G. thorax]. Pertaining to the heart and thoracic cavity A specialized branch of surgery.

کارڈیوتھوراسک : دل اور تھوریکس کے کہفہ سے متعلق۔ سرجری کی ایک مخصوص شاخ۔

Cardiotocograph *(kar-di-o-to'-ko-grof)*. See CARDIOGRAPH and TOCOGRAPHY.

Cardiotocography *(kar-di-o-tok-og'-ra-fi)* Tocography and ECG. The fetal heart rate is measured either by an external microphone or by the application of an electrode to the fetal scalp, recording the fetal ECG and from it the fetal heart rate. Using either an internal catheter which is passed into the amniotic cavity, or an external transducer placed on the mother's abdomen, the maternal contractions can also be measured. Both measurments are fed through a monitor in such a way that extraneous sounds are excluded and both meassurements are recorded on heat-sensitive paper.

Cardiotomy syndrom *(kar-di-ot'-o-mi-sin'-d-rom)*. Pyrexia, pericarditis and pleural effusion following heart srugery.

Cardiovascular *(kar-di-o-vas'-kul-ar)* [G. kardia, heart; L. vasculum, a small vessel]. Pertaining to the heart and blood vessels.

قلبی عروقی : دل اور خونی رگوں سے متعلق۔

Cardioversion *(kar-di-o-ver'-shun)*. Use of electrical countershock for restoring heart rhythm to normal.

کاردیوورشن : دل کی دھڑکن کو معمول پر لانے کے لئے برقی جھٹکے کا استعمال۔

Carditis *(kar-di'-tis)*. [G. kardia, heart; -itis, inflammation]. Inflammation of the heart. A word seldom used without the corresponding prefix, e.g. endomyo-,pan-,peri-.

سوزش دل۔ ورم قلب : یونانی الفاظ کارڈیا بمعنی دل اور اٹس بمعنی سوزش سے مرکب اصطلاح۔ دل کی سوزش۔

Cardophyllin *(kar-dof'-il-in)*. Aminophyllir (q.v.).

ارڈوفلن : دیکھئے امینوفلن۔

Caries *(kar'-i-ez)* [L. decay]. Intlammator decay of bone of teeth, usually associate with pus formation spinal **c. Pott's** diseas (q.v.)--carious, adj.

سیدگی۔ کرم (خوردگی) دندان۔ کھوڑیں : لاطینی لفظ جس کے نی گلنا سڑنا ہے۔ ہڈی یا دانتوں کا سڑنا۔ عموماً پیپ بن جاتی ہے۔ دانت میں سوڑیں۔ رات کو سوتے وقت دانتوں کو اچھی طرح صاف کرنا چاہئے۔ موڑوں کو زنک آکسائیڈ یا چاندی سے بھروادیں۔ مریض کو کیلشیم اور وٹامن ی استعمال کرائیں۔ ہڈیوں کی ٹی بی۔

Carina *(kar-in'-a)* [L. keel]. Any keel-lik structure. Most frequently used for carir tracheae. a ridge across the base of the tra hea, where the two bronchi divide--carina adj.

رینا۔ زدرق : ایسی ساخت جو جہاز کے پیندے کی لکڑی کی طرح ۔ عموماً اس ٹریکیا (سانس کی نالی) کے لئے مستعمل ہے۔ جہاں دونوں نکائی کے اتصال کی جگہ ابھار ہوتا ہے۔

Carin

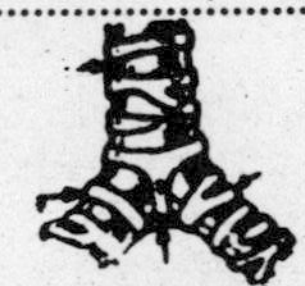

Carminative *(kar'-min-a-tiv)* [L. carminare, card; hence to cleanse]. Having the power relieve flatulence and associated colic. Th chief carminatives administered orally a aromatics, e.g. cinnamon, cloves, ginge nutmeg, peppermint, etc.

ں ریاح : آنتوں مین ریح یا بادی کو آرام دینے والا۔ ادرک وغیرہ ں میں شامل ہیں۔ آنتوں کا سنج ختم کرتا ہے۔ درد کم کرتا ہے، ہوا خارج کرتا بھوک اور قوت ہاضمہ کو زیادہ کرتا ہے۔

Carneous *(kar'-ni-us)* [L. caro, flesh]. Fleshy, **mole,** see MOLE.

ں : گودے دار۔ بھرا ہوا۔

Carotene *(kar'-o-ten)* [L. carota, carrot]. yellow pigment, which can be converted in vitamin A by the libver. A provitamin.

کیروٹین۔ جذرین : لاطینی لفظ کیروٹا بمعنی گاجر سے ماخوذ۔ ایک زرد پگمنٹ جسے جگر حیاتین الف میں تبدیل کرسکتا ہے۔

arotid *(kar-ot'-id)* [G. karotides, carotid arteries]. The principal artery on each side of the neck. At the bifurcation of the common carotid into the internal and external carotids there are; (1) the **c. bodies,** a collection of chemoreceptors, which, being sensitive to chemical changes in the blood, protect the body against lack of O_2; (2) the **c. sinus,** a collection of receptors sensitive to pressure changes; increased pressure causes slowing of the heart beat and lowering of blood pressure **c. compression tonography,** see TESTS.

Carotids

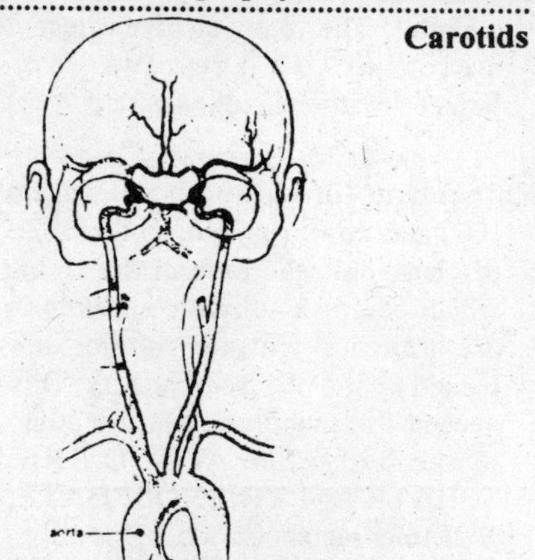

شاہرگ : یونانی لفظ کیروٹائیڈز بمعنی کرائنڈ شریانیں سے ماخوذ۔ گردن کی ہر جانب ایک بڑی شریان۔ مشترک کرائنڈ بیرونی واندرونی کرائنڈ میں منقسم ہو جاتی ہے۔

rpaltunnel syndrome Pain, numbness and tingling in the area of distribution of the median nerve in the hand. Due to compression as the nerve passes through the fascial band. Most common in middle-aged women. Noeturnal.

سخی سرنگ سنڈروم : ہاتھ کی میانی عصب کے تقسیم والے اریا میں درد اورسن ہونا۔ درمیانی عمر والی خواتین میں عام مرض رات کے وقت ہوتا ہے۔

rphology *(kar-fol'-o-ji)* [G. karphos, chips; legein, to collect]. Involuntary picking at the bedclothes as seen in exhaustive or febrile delirium.

بستر چینی : غیرارادی طور پر بستر کے کپڑے اٹھانا۔ ہذیانی کیفیت۔

Carpometacarpal *(kar'-po-met-a-kar'-pal)* [G. karpos, wrist; meta, beyong]. Pertaining to the carpal and metacarpal bones, the joints between them and the ligaments joining them.

ساعد بعد ساعد : کارپل اور میٹا کارپل ہڈیوں ان کے جوڑوں اور ان کے لگامنٹس سے متعلق۔

Carpopedal *(kar-po-pe'-dal)* [G. karpos, wrist; L. pes, foot]. Pertaining to the hands and feet, **c. spasm,** spasm of hands and feet in tetany, provoked by constriction of the limb. (Trousseau's sign.)

کارپوپیڈل : یونانی لفظ کارپوس بمعنی کلائی لاطینی لفظ پینس بمعنی پاؤں سے مخلوط اصطلاح۔ ہاتھوں اور پیروں سے متعلق۔

Carrier *(kar'-i-er).* A healthy animal or human host who harbours a pathogenic or potentially pathogenic micro organism and passes it to his environment.

حامل : ایک صحت مند جانور یا انسان جس میں مرض پیدا کرنے والے خورد جسیمے ہوں اور وہ انہیں اپنے ماحول کو دے دے۔

Cartilage *(ka'r-til-ayj)* A kind of soft bone.

Cartilages

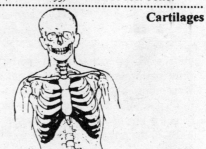

غضروف۔ کری : نرم ہڈی۔ چبنے والی ہڈی۔ اس کی کئی اقسام ہیں۔ بیرونی کان میں پائی جانے والی ہڈی ایسی ہی ہے۔

Caruncle *(ka-rung'kl)* [L. caruncula, small piece of flesh]. A red fleshy projection; that at the inner corner of eye being **lacrimal c. urethral c.** is a small bright red growth at the entrance to the urethra. It is very painful and bleeds readily on being touched. **carunculae myrtiformes,** the tag-like ends left after rupture of the hymen during coitus--caruncular, carunculate, carunculated, adj.

لحیمہ مبال : سرخ گودے دار ابھار۔ مثلاً آنکھ کے اندرونی کونے میں یا یورتھرا کے دخول پر چھوٹا سرخ ابھار۔ اسے چھونے پر درد ہوتا ہے اور خون بہنے لگتا ہے۔

Cascara *(kas-kar'a)*. Purgative bark, used as the dry extract in tablets and as liquid extract and elixir for chronic constipation.

کسکارا : دست آور چھال جو ادویات میں استعمال کی جاتی ہے۔

Caseation *(ka-zi-a'-shun)*. [L. caseus, cheese]. The formation of a soft, cheese like mass, as occurs in tuberculosis--caseous, adj.

جبنیت ۔ پنیراؤ : لاطینی لفظ کیسیس بمعنی پنیر سے ماخوذ۔ نرم پنیر نما مادے کا بننا۔ مثلاً تپ دق میں۔

Casein *(ka'-si-in)* [L. caseus, cheese]. A protein produced when a milk enters the stomach, Coagulation occurs and is due to the action of rennin upon the caseinogen in the milk, splitting it into two proteins, one being casein. The casein combines with calcium and a clot is formed. **c. hydrolysate,** predigested protein food derived from casein, easily added to other foods to increase the protein content.

کسین ۔ پنیری مادہ : لاطینی لفظ کیسیس بمعنی پنیر سے ماخوذ۔ معدہ میں دودھ جانے سے بننے والی پروٹین۔

Caseinogen *(ka-sin-in'-o-jen)* [L. caseus, cheese; G. genesthai, to be produced]. The principal protein in milk. It is not solube in water but is kept in solution in milk by inorganic salts. The propotion to lactalbumin is much higher in cows' milk than in human milk. In the presence of rennin it is converted into insoluble casein.

کسینوجن : دودھ میں موجود پروٹین۔ پانی میں ناحل پذیر لیکن غیر نامیاتی نمکیات سے دودھ میں محلول کی صورت میں رکھی جاتی ہے۔ رسوب بننے سے پیشتر کیسین کے لئے اصطلاح۔

Casilan *(kas'-e-lan)*. A proprietary powder containing 90- per cent protein. Useful for maintaining adequate protein intake when patient can only take fluids.

سفوف جس میں ۹۰ فیصد پروٹین ہوتی ہے۔

Cast Fibrous material and exudate which ha been moulded to the form of the cavity c tube in which it has collected, and this can b identified under the microscope. It is als classified according to its constitution, blooc epithelial, fatty, etc.

بیکہ ۔ لوچی چشم : ریشہ دار میٹریل۔

Castor oil *(kas'-tor)*. A purgative, of value i diarrhoea due to food poisoning. Also use with zinc ointment for napkin rash an pressure sores.

ںڈی کا تیل ۔ کیسٹر آئل : دست آور۔ خوراک کے زہریلے پن میں وثر۔

Castration *(kas-tra'-shun)* [L. castrare, t castrate]. The removal of the testicles in th male, or of the ovaries in th female--castrated, adj.; castrate, n. v.t.

ضا ۔ اختہ کاری : نر میں خصیے اور مادہ میں بیضہ دان ختم کرنا۔

Catabolism (or **katabolism**) *(ka-tab'-o-lizn* [G. kata, down; ballein, to throw]. The serie of chemical reactions in the living body i which complex substances, taken in as foo are broken down into simpler ones accon panied by the release of energy. This energy needed for anabolism and the other activiti of the body. See ADENOSINE DIPHC SPHATE and TRIPHOSPHATE, META BOLISM--catabolic, adj.

رق : زندہ جسم میں کیمیائی تعاملات کا سلسلہ جس میں خوراک سادہ اجزاء تقسیم ہو جاتی ہے اور توانائی حاصل ہوتی ہے۔

Castalase *(kat'al-az)*. An enzyme present most human cells.

Catalepsy *(kat'-a-lep-si)* [G. katalepsis, seizing]. Term used by psychiatrists describe sustained immobility (postur trace)--catalepic, adj.

د : غیر متحرک ہونا۔

Catalysis *(kat-al'-i-sis)* [G. kata, down; lysis, loosening]. An increase in the rate at which chemical action proceeds to equilibriu through the medium of a catalyst or catalys If there is retardation it is negative cat lysis--catalytic, adj.

عمل انگیزی : کیمیائی تعامل کی شرح کا بڑھنا۔ اس عمل میں عمل انگیز استعمال ہوتا ہے۔

Catalyst *(kat'-al-ist)* [G. kata, down; lysis, a loosening]. An agent which produces catalysis (q.v.). It does not undergo any change during the process. Syn. catalyser, enzyme, ferment.

عمل انگیز : عمل انگیزی پیدا کرنے والا عامل۔ کیمائی عمل میں کو دتبدیل نہیں ہوتا۔ خامرہ اس کا مترادف ہے۔

Cataplexy *(kat'-a-pleks-i)* [G. kataplexis, amazement]. A condition of muscular rigidity induced by severe mental shock or fear. The patient remains conscious--cataplectic, adj.

سکتہ جذباتی : ذہنی صدمہ یا خوف کی وجہ سے عضلاتی سختی کی حالت۔ اس میں مریض ہوش میں رہتا ہے۔

Catapres *(kat-a-pres)*. Clonidine (q.v.).

Cataract *(kat'-a-rakt)* [G. katarraktes, cataract]. An opacity of the crystalline lens or its capsule. It may be congenital, senile, traumatic or due to diabetes

Cataract

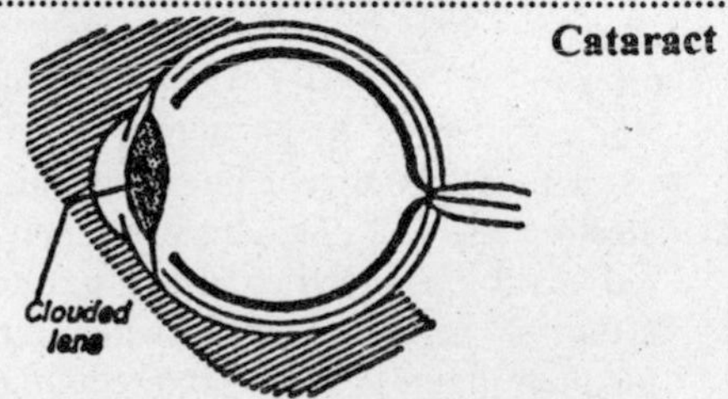

mellitus. **hard c.,** contains a hard nucleus, tends to be dark in colour and occurs in older people, **soft c.,** one without a hard nucleus, occurs at any age, but particularly in the young. Cataract usually develops slowly and when mature is called a 'ripe cataract'.

سفید موتیا۔ موتیابند : عدسے یا اس کے کیپسول کا غیر سفاف ہونا۔ سفید موتیابند۔

Catarrh *(kat-ar')* [G. katarrheein, to flow down]. Inflammation of a mucous membrane with constant flow of mucus--catarrhal, adj.

نزلہ : میوکس کے مستقل بہاؤ کے ساتھ میوکس جھلی کی سوزش۔ ناک کی جھلیوں میں سوزش رطوبت کا اخراج۔

Catcry syndrome. See 'CRI DU CHAT SYNDROME.

Catecholamines *(kat-e-ko'-la-mens)*. Adrenaline, noradrenaline and isoprenaline are the main catecholamines of pharmacological importance and they are all substances involved in the bio-chemical transmission of nerve impulses, particularly in the sympathetic system. Secreted by human tumours. Estimation of catecholamines in urine being carried out in research on hypertension and mental disorders. Experimental evidence suggests that catecholamines play an important role in mood regulation.

کیٹی کو لے مینز : ایڈرینالین، نارایڈرینالین اور آئیسو پرینالین۔ ان کا تعلق عصبی نظام سے ہے۔ انسانی ناسور سے خارج ہوتے ہیں۔ موڈ بنانے میں اہم کردار ادا کرتے ہیں۔

Catgut *(kat'-gut)*. A form of ligature and suture of varying thickness, strength and absorbability, prepared from sheep's intestines. After sterilization it is hermetically sealed in glass tubes in sizes 00000 to 8. The 'plain' variety is usually absorbed in 5 to 10 days. 'Chromicized' catgut and 'iodized' catgut will hold for 20 to 40 days.

تانت : بھیڑ کی انتوں سے تیار شدہ لگیچر اور سیوچر کی قسم۔ اس کی موٹائی اور مضبوطی مختلف ہوتی ہے۔ زخم کو سینے کے لئے مخصوص دھاگہ۔ اب مصنوعی پلاسٹک کا دھاگہ بھی استعمال کیا جاتا ہے۔

Catharsis *(ka-thar'-sis)* [G. kathersis, a cleansing]. In psychology, the outpouring from the patient's mind--cathartic, adj.

تنقیہ نفس : نفسیات میں مریض کے ذہن سے نکالنا۔ مریض سے گفتگو میں اس کے مرض کی معلومات حاصل کرنے کا طریقہ۔

Catheter *(kath'-e-ter)* [G. kathienai, to send down into]. A hollow tube of variable length and bore, usually having one fluted end and a tip of varying size and shape according to function. Catheters are made of many substances including soft and hard rubber, gum elastic, glass, silver, other metals and plastic materials, some of which are now radio-opaque. They have many uses, from insufflation of hollow tubes to introduction and withdrawal of fluid from body cavities. A recent innovation is the fibre-optic cardiac catheter which, when in situ, picks up pulses of light from which the oxygen saturation of the blood can be determined.

کتھیٹر۔(پیشاب کی) سلائی : مختلف لمبائی اور سوراخ کی ایک کھوکھلی نلی یا ٹیوب۔ یہ مختلف مادوں سے تیارہ کئے جاتے ہیں۔ مثلاً ربڑ' شیشہ' چاندی یا دوسری دھاتوں یا پلاسٹک سے۔ جسمی کہفوں میں سیال کو داخل کرنے یا خارج کرنے کے لئے استعمال کئے جاتے ہیں۔

Catheterization *(kath-e-te-ri-za'-shun)* [G. kathienai]. Insertion of a catheter, most usually into the urinary bladder, **cardiac c.,** fine polythene, or radio-opaque nylon tubing is passed via the median basilic vein at the elbow, into the heart; (1) to record pressures; (2) to introduce an opaque substance prior to X-ray; (3) to withdraw samples of blood-catheterize, v.t. See CATHETER.

سلائی گزارنا : کتھیٹر کا دخول عموماً مثانہ میں۔

Cathetron *(kath-e-tron)*. A high rate dose, remotely controlled, afterloading device for radiotherapy. Hollow steel catheters are placed in the desired position. They are then connected to a protective safe by hollow cables. The radioactive cobalt moves from the safe into the catheters. After delivery of the required dose, the cobalt returns to the safe, thus avoiding radiation hazard to staff.

کیتھیٹران : زیادہ شرح والی خوراک۔

Catghomycin *(kath'-o-mi'-sin)*. Novobiocin (q.v.).

Cat scratch fever; Atypical tularaemia (q.v.). Distinguished from tularaemia by a positive LGVCFT. Probably caused by a virus.

کیٹ سکریچ مرض : وائرس سے پیدا ہونے والا مرض۔

Cauda *(kaw'-da)* [L. cauda, tail]. A tail or tail-like appendage--caudal, caudate, adj.

دمچی : لاطینی لفظ کاڈا بمعنی دم۔ ایک دم یا دم نما زائدہ۔

Caudal block See EPIDURAL.

Caul *(kawl)* [F. cale]. The amnion, instead or rupturing as is usual to allow the baby through, persists and covers the baby's head at birth.

ف سر جنین : ایمنیان پھٹنے کے بجائے پیدائش کے وقت سر کو ڈھانپے ا ہے۔

Cauliflowergrowth *(kaw'-li-flour-groth)*. T proliferative free-growing type of canc which forms an excrescence on the affect surface.

ھی اگاؤ : سرطان کی ایک قسم۔

Causalgia *(kaws-al'-ji-a)* [G. kausis, heat; alg pain]. Excruciating neuralgic pain, resulti from physical trauma to a cutaneous nerv Also known as reflex sympathetic dystrophy

زشی درد۔ درد جلد : یونانی الفاظ کاسس بمعنی حرارت اور الگوس بمعنی درد مجموعہ۔ درد کی ایک قسم۔

Caustic *(kaws'-tik)* [G. kaustos, burnt Corrosive or destructive to organic tissue; t agents which produce such ganualation tissu warts or polypi. Carbolic acid, carbon dioxi snow and silver nitrate (lunar c.) are mo commonly employed.

سٹک۔ سوزندہ : نامیاتی تسیج کے لئے تباہ کن۔ ایسے نتائج کے حامل ل۔

Cautery *(kaw'-ter-i)* [G. kauterion, a brandi iron]. A caustic agent, **actual c.,** a hot ir used to apply direct heat. **galvanic c.** electrocautery, a platinum wire maintained red heat by an electric current. **paquelin's** a form of actual cautery in which the holl platinum point is kept at the required heat a current of benzene vapour which constantly pumped into it--cauterization, cauterize, v.t.

اۃ (آلہ) : کوئی کاسٹک عامل گرم لوہا جو براہ راست حرارت کے لئے مال کیا جاتا ہے۔

Caval infusion *(ka'-val in-fu'-zhun)*. A meth of treatment in acute renal failure with anur A radio-opaque nylon cardiac catheter passed via the femoral vein to lie near t opening of the renal veins or at the entran to the right atrium. A constant flow hypertonic fluid is thus possible.

ی انتقال : رینل خرابی کے علاج کا طریقہ۔

avamescenteric shunt *(ka-va-mes-en-ter'-ik)* [L. caverna, a hollow; G. mesos, middle; enteron; intestine]. After division of inferior vena cava the upper end is anastomosed to the superior mesenteric vein. Used in children when the portal vein is blocked.

کیوامسنٹرک شنٹ : لاطینی لفظ کیورنا بمعنی کھوکھلا' یونانی الفاظ میزوس بمعنی درمیان اور اینٹیر ان بمعنی آنت سے مرکب اصطلاح۔ پورٹل ورید کے بند ہونے پر بچوں میں استعمال کیا جاتا ہے۔

avernous *(kav-er-nus)* [L. caverna, a hollow]. Having hollow spaces, **c. sinus,** a channel for venous blood, on either side of the sphenoid bone. It drains blood from the lips, nose and orbits, Sepsis in these areas can cause c.s. thrombosis.

کہفی : جس میں کھوکھلی جگہیں ہوں۔

aved-S *(ka'-ved).* Liquorice compound for ulceration and inflammation of the upper intestinal tract.

avitation *(kav-i-ta'-shun)* [L. cavus, hollow]. The formation of a cavity as in pulmonary tuberculosis.

کہفیت ۔ جوف سازی : لاطینی لفظ کیوس بمعنی کھوکھلا سے ماخوذ۔ کہفہ کا بننا۔ مثلاً ششی تپ دق میں۔

avity *(kav'-i-ti)* [L. cavus, hollow]. A hollow; an enclosed area. **abdominal c.,** that below the diaphragm; the abdomen, **buccal c.,** the mouth. **cerebral c.,** the ventricles of the brain, **cranial c.,** the brain box formed by the bones of the cranium, **medulary c.,** the hollow centre of a long bone, containing yellow bone marrow or medulla, **nasal c.,** that in the nose, separated into right and left halves by the nasal septum. **oral c.,** buccal cavity, **pelvic c.,** that formed by the pelvic bones, more particularly the part below the iliopectineal line, **peritoneal c.,** a potential space between the parietal and visceral layers of the peritoneum. Similarly, the **pleural c.,** is the potential space between the pulmonary and parietal pleurae which in health are in contact in all phases of respiration. **synovial c.,** the potential space in a synovial joint. **uterine c.,** that of the uterus, the base extending between the orifices of the uterine tubes.

کہفہ ۔ جوف ۔ فراغ : لاطینی لفظ کیوس بمعنی کھوکھلا سے ماخوذ اصطلاح۔ ایک کھوکھلا' بند ایریا۔ بطنی کہفہ ڈایافرام کے نیچے ہوتا ہے۔ یعنی بطن یا شکم۔

Cavodil *(kav'-o-dil)* . Pheniprazine.

کیووڈل : فینی پرازین۔

CDH. Congenital dislocatiaon of the hip. Recognized in the neonate by limitation of hip abduction.

سی ڈی ایچ : جوڑ کا اپنی جگہ سے ہٹ جانا۔

Cedilanid *(sed-i-lan'-id)* Lanatoside C (q.v.).

سیڈی لے نڈ : دیکھئے لناٹو سائیڈ سی۔ کن جیسٹو ہارٹ فیلیوز میں اس کی ۲ گولیاں صبح ۲ دوپہر ۲ شام۔

Celbenin Sodium methicillin. Antibiotic, useful in resistant staphyl-ococcal infection.

سیلبینن : سوڈیم میتھی سلین۔ اینٹی بایوٹک۔ مدافعت کرنے والے سٹیفا ئلوکاکی کے خلاف مستعمل

Celevac *(sel'-e-vak).* Methycellulose. Gives bulk to intestinal contents and encourages peristalsis.

سیلیویک : میتھائل سیلولوز۔ آنتوں میں حرکت کو تیز کرتا ہے۔

Cell *(sel)* [L. cella, compartment]. A histological term for a minute mass of protoplasm containing a nucleus. Some cells, e.g. the erythrocytes, are non-

Cell

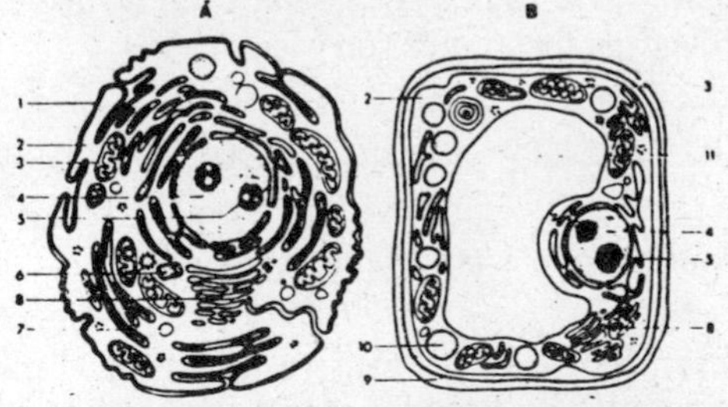

A. ANIMAL B. VEGETABLE
1,2. Cytoplasm (1. Ectoplasm, 2. Endoplasm). 3. Mitochondria. 4. Nucleus. 5. Nucleolus. 6. Centriole. 7. Oil droplet. 8. Golgi apparatus. 9. Cell wall. 10. Plastid.

11. Vacuole
nucleated; and others may be multinucleated--cellular, adj.

خلیہ : لاطینی لفظ سیلا بمعنی کمرہ سے ماخوذ۔ مرکزہ پر مشتمل مادۂ حیات یا نخرمایہ۔ بعض خلیوں میں مرکزہ نہیں ہوتا۔ بعض خلیوں میں کئی مرکزے ہوتے ہیں۔

Cellophane *(sel'-o-fan)* . Trade name for a brand of a transparent, impermeable derivative of cellulose. Used in face masks; to protect, and prevent evaporation from, surgical dressings.
سیلوفین : شفاف، ناقابل نفوذ سیلولوز کی ایک قسم۔ چہرہ ڈھانپنے کے لئے استعمال کیا جاتا ہے۔

Cellulitis *(sel-u-li'-tis)* [L. cellula, small cell; G. -itis, inflammation]. A diffuse inflammation of connective tissue, especially the loose subcutaneous tissue. When it involves the pelvictissues in the female it is called 'parametritis,' When it occurs in the floor of the mouth it is called 'Ludwig's angina.'
سیلولائی ٹس : لاطینی لفظ سیلولا بمعنی چھوٹا خلیہ اور ائٹس بمعنی سوزش ایک یونانی لفظ کا مرکب۔ اتصالی نسیج کی سوزش۔ جلد کے نیچے والے گوشت تک ورم اور چھوت۔

Cellulose *(sel'-u-loz)* [L. cellula, small cell]. A carbohydrate forming the outerwalls of plant and vegetable cells. A polysaccharide which cannot be digested by man but supplies roughage for stimulation of peristalsis.
سیلولوس : لاطینی لفظ سیلولا بمعنی چھوٹا خلیہ سے ماخوذ ایک کاربوہائیڈریٹ۔ نباتی خلیوں کی بیرونی دیوار بناتا ہے۔ ایک پولی سیکرائیڈ جو انسان میں ناقابل ہضم ہے۔

Celontin *(sel-on-tin)*. Methsuximide (q.v.).
سیلون ٹن : دیکھئے میتھ سکسی مائیڈ۔

Censor *(sen'-sor)* [L. censere, to value]. Term employed by Freud to define the resistance which prevents repressed material from readily re-entering the conscious mind from the subconscious (unconscious) mind.
سنسر۔ فوق شعور : مدافعت کی قسم۔ اس اصطلاح کو فرائڈ نے استعمال کیا۔

Centigrade *(sen'-ti-grad)*. [L. centum, hundred; gradus, a step]. Having one hundred divisior or degress. Usually applied to the thermon etric scale in which the freezing point o water is fixed at O^0 and the boiling point a 100°
ٹی گریڈ۔ مئی : سو درجے ہونا۔ عموماً تھرمامیٹر کے سکیل پر اس کا اطلاق کیا تا ہے جس میں پانی کا نقطۂ انجماد صفر اور نقطۂ جوش سو درجے ہوتا ہے۔

Centrifugal *(sen-trif'-u-gal)*. [G. kentron, centr of a circle; L. fugere, to flee]. Efferen Having a tendency to move outwards from th centre as the rash in smallpox.
رکز گریز : مرکز سے گریز کرنے والا۔ مرکز سے بیرونی جانب حرکت کرنے ر جحان۔

Centrifuge *(sen'-tri-fuj)* [G. kentron, centre of circle; L. fugere, to flee]. An appratus whic rotates, thereby increasing force of gravity s that substances of different densities ar separated. It is usually used to separate ('Spi down') particulate material from a suspendin liquid.
رکز گریزہ : ایسا سامان جو گھومتا ہے اور مختلف کثافتوں کے اجزاء علیحدہ ہو تے ہیں۔

Centripetal *(sen-trip'-et-al)* [G. kentron, centr of a circle; L. petere, to seek]., Afferent. Ha ing a tendancy to move towards the centre a the rash in chickenpox.
رکز جو : مرکز کی طرف حرکت کرنے کا رجحان۔

Centrosome *(sen'-tro-som)* [G. kentron centr of a circle; soma, body]. A minutes spot in th cytoplasm of animal cells supposed to b concerned with division of the nucleus.
نٹروسوم۔ مرکزی جسم : یونانی الفاظ کنٹران وسوما کا مجموعہ جن کے معانی ترتیب مرکز دائرہ اور جسم ہیں حیوانی خلیوں کے سائیٹو پلازم میں ایک چھوٹی خت جس کا تعلق تقسیم مرکزہ کے ساتھ سمجھا جاتا ہے۔

Centyl *(sen'til)*. Bendrofluazide (q.v.).

Cephalalgia *(kef-al-al'-ji-a)* [G. kephale, hea algos, pain]. Pain in the head. Headache.
دسر۔ صداع : سر میں درد۔ سر درد۔

Cephalexin *(kef-al-eks'-in)*. Cephalospori antibiotic, which unlike cephaloridine, is we absorbed when given orally. Useful fo urinary infections.

کیفالیکسن : سفیولوسپورن اینٹی بایوٹک۔ اگر یہ دوائی کھلائی جائے تو جذب ہو جاتی ہے۔ پیشاب کی بیماریوں میں مفید ہے۔

Cephalhaematoma *(kef-al-hem-a-to'-ma)* [G. kephale, head; haima, blood;-oma, tumour]. A collection of blood in the subperiosteal tissues of the scalp.

کیفل ہیماٹوما : یونانی الفاظ کفالے بمعنی سر، ہیما بمعنی خون اور اوما بمعنی ناسور کا مجموعہ۔ کھوپڑی میں خون کا جمع ہونا۔

Cephalic *(kef-al'-ik)* [G. kephale, head]. Pertaining to the head; near the head. **c. version,** an obstetric manoeuvre to change the fetal lie to a head presentation.

دافع دردسر : یونانی الفاظ کفالے بمعنی سر سے ماخوذ۔ سر سے متعلق۔ اگر بچہ رحم میں اس طرح ہو کہ اس کا لمبا رخ رحم کی لمبائی کے متوازن اور سر نیچے ہو تو یہ کفالک رخ ہے۔

Cephalocele *(kef'-al-o-sel)* [G. kephale, head; kele, tumour]. Hernia of the brain; protrusion of part of the brain through the skull.

فتق دماغ : دماغ کا ہرنیا۔ کھوپڑی میں سے دماغ کا ایک حصہ باہر آ جانا۔

Cephalohaematoma See CEPHALHAEMATOMA.

Cephalometry *(kef-al-om'et-ri)* [G. kephale, head; metron, a measure]. Measurement of the living human head.

سر پیمائی : زندہ انسانی سر کی پیمائش۔

Cephaloridine *(kef-al-or'-i-din)* Semispynthetic antibiotic derived from cephalosporin. Bactericidal against both penicillin sensitive and resistant strains of *Staphylococcus* aureus. Not active against *Pseudomonas pyocyanea.*

کیفالوریڈین : ایک اینٹی بایوٹک یا ضد حیاتیہ۔ جراثیم کش کیپوران۔ ایک ٹیکہ صبح ایک شام نمونیا کے لئے۔

Cephalothin *(kef-al-oth'-in).* Antibiotic (q.v.). See CEPHALEXIN.

Ceporin Cephaloridine (q.v.).

کیپورن : دیکھئے کفالورڈین۔ نمونیا کے لئے ایک ٹیکہ صبح وشام۔

Cerebellum *(ser-i-bel'-um)* [L.]. That part of the brain which lies behind and below the cerebrum. Its chief functions are the co-ordination of the fine voluntary movem ents and the control of posture--cerebellar, adj.

دمیغ۔ چھوٹا دماغ۔ مخیخ : لاطینی لفظ۔ دماغ کا وہ حصہ جو سربرم کے نیچے اور پیچھے واقع ہے۔ اس کے دو حصے ہیں سطح ناہموار لکیردار۔ سطح کے اوپر گرے میٹر اور اندر وہائیٹ میٹر ہوتا ہے۔ اس کے تین پیڈنکلز ہیں جن کے ذریعے اعصاب اندر و باہر گزرتے ہیں۔ یہ توازن اور تعاون برقرار رکھتا ہے۔

Cerebral *(ser'0i-bral)* [L. cerebrum, brain]. Pertaining to the cerebrum.

دماغی مخی : لاطینی لفظ سربرم بمعنی دماغ سے ماخوذ۔ سربرم سے متعلق۔

Cerebration *(ser-i-bra'-shun)* [L. cerebrum. brain]. Mental activity.

دماغی عمل : لاطینی لفظ سربرم بمعنی دماغ سے ماخوذ۔ ذہنی طور پر فعال ہونا۔

Cerebrospinal *(ser'-i-bro-spi'-nal)* [L. cerebrum, brain; spina, spine]. Pertaining to the brain and spinal cord, **c. fluid,** the clear fluid filling the ventricles of the brain and central canal of the spinal cord. Also found beneath the cranial and spinal meninges in the pia-arachnoid space. See MENINGITIS.

دماغی نخاعی : دماغ اور نخاع سے متعلق۔

Cerebrovascular *(ser'-i-bro-vas'-ku-lar)* [L. cerebrum, brain; vasculum, small vessel]. Pertaining to the blood vessels of the brain. **c. accident,** apoplexy caused by embolism, haemorrhage or thrombosis in brain.

دماغی عروقی : دماغ کی خونی رگوں سے متعلق۔

Cerebrum *(ser'-i-brum)* [L.] The largest and uppermost part of the brain; it does not include the cerebellum, pons and medulla. The longitudinal fissure divides it into two hemispheres, each containing a lateral ventricle. The internal substance is white, the outer convoluted cortex is grey--cerebral, adj.

سربرم۔ بڑا دماغ۔ مخ : لاطینی لفظ دماگ کا سب سے بڑا اور بالائی ترین حصہ۔ یہ دو نصف کروں میں منقسم ہے۔ یہ فرنٹل لوب، پیرائٹل لوب ٹمپورل لوب اور آکسی پٹل لوب پر مشتمل ہے۔ سربرم کے اندر وہائیٹ میٹر ہوتا ہے اس میں دو خلا لیٹرول وینٹریکل ہوتے ہیں جن کے درمیان ایک پتلا پردہ ہوتا ہے۔

Certified *(ser'-ti-fid).* A term used in relation to insanity, prior to the Mental Health Act, 1960. Those patients who cannot leave a mental hospital of their own accord are now referred to as 'detained' patients.

سند یافتہ : اصطلاح جو پاگل پن کے لئے مستعمل تھی۔

Cerumen *(ser-oo'-men)* [L. cera, wax]. A wax-like, brown secretion from special glands in the external auditory canal--ceruminous, adj.

کن میل : لاطینی لفظ سیرا بمعنی موم سے ماخوذ۔ بیرونی سمعی قنال میں مخصوص غدد سے موم ایسی، بھوری رطوبت کا افراز۔

Cervical *(ser-vi'-kal)* [L. cervix, neck]. Pertaining to; (1) the neck; (2) the cervix (neck of an organ. **c. canal,** the lumen of the cervix uteri, from the internal to the external os, **c. rib,** a supernumerary rib in cervical region, which may present no symptoms or it may press on nerves of the brachial plexus. Syn. thoracic inlet syndrome.

عنقی ۔ گردنی : لاطینی لفظ سروکس بمعنی گردن سے ماخوذ۔ گردن سے متعلق یا کسی عضو کی گردن سے متعلق۔ عضو تناسل کا سرطان یا سرویکل کینسر ختنہ کرانے سے نہیں ہوتا۔ سرویکل ورٹبری یا گردن کے مہرے تعداد میں سات ہوتے ہیں۔

Cervicectomy *(ser-vi-sek'-to-mi)* [L. cervix, neck; G. ektome, excision]. Amputation of cervix uteri.

ورم رحم براری : لاطینی لفظ سروکس بمعنی گردن اور یونانی لفظ ایکٹوم بمعنی قطع سے مرکب اصطلاح۔ سروکس یوٹرائی کا قطع و برید۔

Cervicitis *(ser-vis-i'-tis)* [L. cervix, neck; G. -itis, inflammation]. Inflammation of the cervix uteri.

ورم فتم رحم : لاطینی لفظ سروکس بمعنی گردن اور یونانی لفظ ائٹس بمعنی سوزش سے مرکب اصطلاح سروکس یوٹرائی کی سوزش۔

Cervix *(ser'-viks)* [L.]. A neck, **c. uteri,** the neck of the uterus--cervical, adj.

Cervix

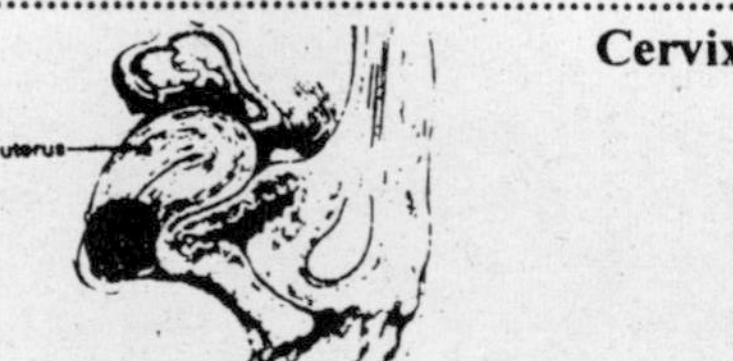

خم رحم۔ گردن رحم : لاطینی لفظ۔ گردن، سروکس یوٹرائی سے مراد یوٹرس کی گردن ہے۔ رحم یا یوٹرس کا زیریں حصہ جو فرج میں لٹکا رہتا ہے۔ اس میں غدود ہوتی ہیں جو مباشرت کے وقت رطوبت خارج کرتی ہیں۔ انزال کے بعد مادہ منویہ اس کے قریب جمع ہو جاتا ہے۔

Cestode *(ses'-tod)*. Tapeworm. See TAENIA.

Cetiprin *(set'-i-prin)*. Emepronium bromide (q.v.).

سیٹی پرن : دیکھئے امیپر ونیم برومائیڈ۔

Cetrihex *(set'-ri-neks)*. Mixture of cetrimide and Physohex.

سینٹری ہیکس : سٹری مائڈ اور فائزو ہیکس کا آمیزہ۔

Certrimide *(Set'-ri-mid)*. CTAB. Antiseptic with detergent properties, used as 1 per-cent solution for wound, burns and skin sterilization. Cetavlon is a proprietary preparation.

سیٹری مائیڈ : دافع تعفن۔ زخموں، آبلوں اور جلد کے لئے اس کا ایک فیصد محلول استعمال کیا جاتا ہے۔

CFT. Complement fixation test. See COMPLEMENT.

Chalazion *(kal-a'-zi-on)* [G.]. A cyst on the edge of the eyelid from retained secretion of the Meibomian glands.

Chalazion

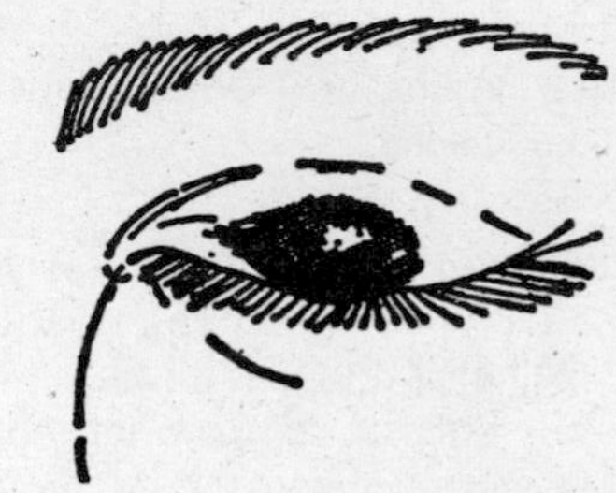

اولا۔ بردہ : یونانی لفظ۔ آنکھ کے پپوٹے کے کنارے پر سسٹ۔

Chalk *(chawk)*. Native calcium carbonate. Used with other antacide in peptic ulcer, and with astringents in diarrhoea.

چاک : کیلشیم کاربونیٹ۔ السر میں مستعمل۔ چھوٹے بحری جانداروں کے خول سے بنتا ہے۔ تختہ سیاہ پر لکھنے والا چاک کیلسیم سلفیٹ ہے۔

Chalone *(ka'-lon)*. A hormone which inhibits rather than stimulates, e.g. enterogastrone inhibits gastric secretions and motility.

کیلون۔ مسکن : کیمیائی روکنے والے جو حیوانات میں گلٹیوں کو روکتے

ہیں۔

Chancre *(shang'-ker)* [F. from L. *cancer,* crab]. The primary syphiliti ulcer associated with swelling of local lymph glands. The picture of chancer plus grgional adenitis constitutes 'primary syphilis.' The chancre is painless, indurated and highly infectious.

Chancre

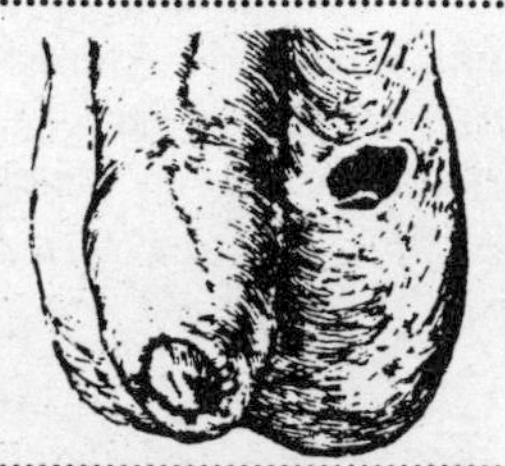

شینکر ۔ اکولہ : اولیں آتشک کا ناسور۔ مقامی لمف غدد متورم ہو جاتی ہیں۔

Chancroid *(shang'-kroid)* [L. *cancer,* crab; G. eldos, form]. Type of venereal disease prevalent in warmer climates. Also called 'soft sore'. Causes multiple, painful, ragged ulcers on the penis and vulva, often associated with bubo (q.v.) formation. Infection is by *Haemophilus* ducreyi.

Chancroid

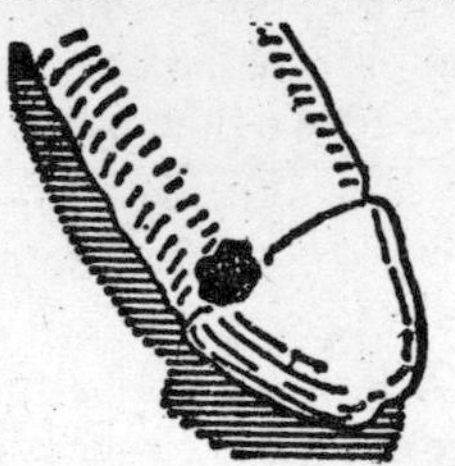

آتشک مجازی ۔ اکولہ نما : عضو تناسل اور شرمگاہ پر تکلیف دہ ناسور کا بننا یہ مرض گرم آب و ہوا میں ہوتا ہے۔

Character *(ka'-rak-ter).* The sum total of the known and predictable mental characteristics of an individual, particularly his conduct. c. **change,** denotes change in the form of conduct, to one foreign to the patient's naturaldisposition, e.g.indecent behaviour in a hitherto respectable person. Common in the psychoses.

امتیازی نشان ۔ خاصہ : کسی فرد کی معلوم ذہنی خصوصیات جن سے اس کے رویے کا پتہ چلتا ہے۔

Charcoal *(char'-kol).* The residue after burning organic substances at a high temperature in an enclosed vessel. Used in medicine for its adsorptive and deodorant properties.

لکڑی کا کوئلہ : کسی بند برتن میں زیادہ درجہ حرارت پر نامیاتی مادوں کو جلانے کے بعد بچ جانے والا مادہ ادویات میں استعمال کیا جاتا ہے۔

Charcoal's joint *(shar-kos joint)* Complete disorganization of a joint associated with syringomyelia or advanced cases of tabed dorsalis (Iocomotor ataxia). Condition is painless. c.**traid,** late manifestations of disseminated sclerosis nystagmus, intention tremor and staccato speech. [Jean Martin Charcot, French neurologist and clinician, 1825-93.]

شارکوس جوائنٹ یا جوڑ : کسی جوڑ کو مکمل طور پر کھول دینا۔

Cheilitis *(ki-li'-tis)* [G. *cheilos,* lip; itis, inflammation]. Inflammation]. Inflammation of the lip.

سوزش لب ۔ ورم لب : ہونٹ کی سوزش

Cheiloplasty *(ki-lo'-plas'-ti)* [G. *cheilos,* lip; plassein, to form]. Any plastic operation on the lip.

لب پیوندی : ہونٹ کا کوئی پلاسٹک اپریشن۔

Cheilosis *(ki-lo'-sis)* [G. *chellos,* lip; osis, condition]. Maceration at angles of mouth; fissures occur later. May be due to riboflavine deficiency.

کائی لوسس : ریبوفلیون کی کمی سے منہ کے زاویوں کا پھٹنا۔

Cheiropompholys *(ki-ro-pom'-fo-liks)* [G. *cheir,* hand; *pompholyx,* bubble]. Symmetrical eruption of skin of hands (especially fingers) characterized by the formation of tiny vesicles and associated with itching or burning. On the feet the condition is called podopompholyx.

ابلہ دستی : جلنے سے ننھے آبلوں کا انگلیوں پر بننا۔ ہاتھوں کی کھال کا اوپر ابھرنا۔

Chelating agents *(ke-la'-ting).* Soluble organic compounds that can fix certain metallic ions into their molecular structure. When given in cases of poisoning, the new complex so formed is excreted in the urine.

چنگالی عامل : حل پذیر نامیاتی مرکبات جو بعض دھاتوں آئنوں کو ان کی سالماتی ساخت میں فکس کر سکتے ہیں۔ یہ زہروں کے تریاقی کے طور پر استعمال کئے جاتے ہیں۔

Chemonucleolysis *(kem-o-nu-kle-ol'-i-sis).* Injection of an enzyme, usually into an invertbral disc, for dissolution of same--chemonucleolytic, adj.

Chemopallidectomy *(kem-o-pal-id-ek'-to-mi)* [Ar. *kumia;* L. pallidus, pale; G. *ektome,* excision]. The destruction of a prodetermined section of globus pallidus by chemicals.

کیموپیلی ڈیکٹومی : کیمکل کے ذریعے گلوبس پلیڈس کے پہلے سے متعین سیکشن کی تباہی۔

Chemoprophyiaxis *(ke'-mo-pro-fil-aks'-is)* [G. *prophylassein,* to guard against]. Prevention of disease (or recurrent attack) by admi nistration of chemicals--chemoprophylactic, adj.

کیموپروفائی لیکسس : کیمیائی مرکبات کھلا کر بیماری سے بچاؤ

Chemoreceptor *(kem-o-re-sep'-tor)* [Ar. kiia; L. *recipere,* to receive]. I. A chemical linkage in a living cell having an affinity for, and capable of combining with. certain other chemical substances. 2. A sensory end-organ capable of reacting to a chemical stimulus.

کیمیائی اخذ : زندہ خلیے میں کیمیائی لنیج جو دوسرے کیمیائی مادوں کے ساتھ کیمیائی الیف رکھتی ہے۔

Chemosis *(ke-mo'-sis).* An oedema or swelling of the bulbar conjunctiva--chemotic, adj.

تہیج ملتحمہ : بلبر جنکٹوا کا ورم۔

Chemosuppressvie *(ke-mo-sup-res'-iv).* Syn., chemoprophylactic. See CHEMOPROPH-YLAXIS.

کیموسپریسو : دیکھئے کیموپروفائیلیکس۔

Chemotaxis *(kem-o-taks'-is),* **chemotaxy** [Ar. kimia; taxis, arrangement]. Response of organisms to chemical stimuli; attraction towards a chemical being positive c, repulsion negative c.----chemotactic, adj.

کیمی ترتیب : جسیموں کا کیمیائی محرکات کی طرف ردعمل۔

Chemotherapy *(kem-o-ther'-ap-i)* [Ar. *kimia; therapeia,* treatment]. Use of a specific chemical agent to arrest the progress of , or eradicate, disease in the body without causing irreversible injury to healthy tissues, e.g. employment of sulpha drugs in lobar pneumonia, of arsenic in syphilis, of nitrogen mustard in Hodgkin's disease. Chemo-therapeutic agents are administered mainly by oral, intramuscular nd intravenous routed, and are distributed usually by the blood stream.

کیمیائی علاج : جسم میں بیماری کو روکنے کے لئے مخصوص کیمیائی عامل کا استعمال۔ کیمیائی اشیاء سے امراض کا علاج۔ ایسی کیمیائی اشیاء جراثیم وغیرہ کے لئے زہریلی ہوتی ہیں۔

Chendol *(ken'-dol).* Chenodeoxycholic acid, a detergent-like molecule normally present in bile. Being used to dissolve gall stones.

کینڈال : بائل میں موجود ہوتا ہے۔ پتے کی پتھری حل کرنے کے لئے استعمال کیا جاتا ہے۔

Cheyne-Stokes respiration See RESPIRA-TION.

Chiasm *(ki-azm)* [G. *chiasma,* cross]. An X-shaped crossing or decussation. **optic** c,or **chiasma opticum,** the meeting of the optic nerves; where the fibres from that medial or nasal half of each retina cross middle line to join the optic tract of the opposite side. Also **chiasma.**

صلیبیہ : یونانی لفظ کیازما بمعنی کراس سے ماخوذ x نما کراسنگ۔ بصری کائی زما بصری اعصاب کے ملاپ کی جگہ ہے۔

Chickenpox A mild, specific infection with vericella-zoster virus. Successive crops of vesicles appear first on the trunk; scab and heal without leaving scars. Syn., varicella.

کاکڑا لاکڑا : وائرس کے ذریعے لگنے والی بیماری۔

Chilblain *(chil'-blan).* Congestion and swelling attended with were severe itching and burning sensation in reaction to cold. Erythema pernio.

بوائی۔ خصرہ : ورم یا سوج۔ جلن محسوس ہوتی ہے۔ سردیوں میں ہاتھ پاؤں کی انگلیاں اور پاؤں کی ایڑیاں متورم ہو جاتی ہیں۔ ڈیلٹاسٹیب' پان سٹین' ایول اور آسٹوکیلشیم سے علاج کیجئے۔

Chimney sweepcancer. Scrotal epithelioma (q.v.)

خصیوں کا سرطان : دیکھئے سکروٹل اپی تھیلیوما۔

Chinese restaurant syndrome. Postprandial disturbance due to eating monosodium glutamate.

Chiniofon *(kin'-i-o-fen).* An amoebicide used in prophylaxis, and the treatment of acute and chronic amoebiasis, often in association with emetine.

کینوفن : ایباکش۔علاج میں مستعمل۔

Chiropodist *(ki-rip'-o-dist)* [G. *cheir,* hand; *pous,* foot]. One qualified in chiropody.

طبیب دست وپا : یونانی الفاظ چیئر بمعنی ہاتھ اور پاؤں بمعنی پاؤں کا مجموعہ۔کائیروپوڈی کا ماہر۔ہاتھ پاؤں کی بیماریوں کا معالج۔

Chiropody *(ki-rop'-o-di).* The treatment of callosities, corns, bunions and nail conditions.

کائیروپوڈی۔علاج دست وپا : ناخن وغیرہ کا علاج

Chiropractic *(ki-ro-prak'-tik).* Manual movement of the vertebrae to relieve the impingement of subluxated transverse processes on the nerve roots.

مہروں کی حرکت :

Chiropractor One who believes that many diseases are due to interference with nerve flow. Skilled in vertebral manipulation.

دستی معالج : ایسا شخص جو یقین رکھتا ہے کہ بہت سی بیماریاں عصبی بہاؤ میں مداخلت کی وجہ سے ہوتی ہیں۔

Chloasma *(klo-az'-ma).* Patchy brown discolouration of the skin, especially the face. Can appear during pregnancy.

Chloral hydrate *(klor'-al -hi-drat).* Rapid acting sedative and hypnotic of value in nervous insomnia.

کلورال ہائیڈریٹ : خواب آور دوا۔عموماً پوٹاشیم برومائیڈ کے ساتھ دیتے ہیں۔

Chlorambucil *(klor-am'-bu-sil).* An oral alkylating agent (q.v.) used in lymphoproliferative disorders (q.v.)

کلورم بیوسل : ایک کیمیائی مرکب۔لیوکی ران۔سرطان یا کینسر میں مفید۔

Chloramine *(klor'-am-en).* An organic compound that slowly liberates chlorine in solution. Has been used as a general surgical antiseptic as a 0.25 to 2 per cent solution.

کلورامین : ایک نامیاتی مرکب جو محلول میں آہستہ آہستہ کلورین چھوڑتا ہے۔

Chloramphenicol *(klor-am-fen'-ik-ol).* An orally effective wide range antibiotic. Drug of choice in typhoid and paratyphoid fevers, valuable in manuy infections resistant to other drugs. Used locally in eye and ear infections. Can cause aplastic anaemia.

کلورم فینی کال : ایک اینٹی بایوٹک دوائی۔۲۵۰ ملی گرام والے کیپسول دو ہر چھ گھنٹے بعد برائے ٹائیفائیڈ یا تپ محرقہ۔

Chlorcylizine *(klor-sik'-li-zen).* Longacting antihistamine with few side effects. Also used in travel sickkness.

کلورسائیکلیزین : سفر کی اکتاہٹ میں مستعمل۔۵۰تا۱۵۰ ملی گرام کی خوراک ہر چوتھے یا چھٹے گھنٹے برائے پتی اچھلنا' نوبتی زکام' تپ کاہی (ہے فیور) اور دمہ۔

Chlordiazepoxide *(klor-di-az-e-poks'-id).* A benzodiazepine drug. Relieves anxiety and tension. Very few side effects. Useful in temporal lobe (psychomotor) epilepsy.

کلورڈایازیپوکسائیڈ : پریشانی کا خاتمہ کرنے والی دوا۔لیبریم نامردی کے علاج کے لئے ایک گولی صبح ایک دوپہر ایک شام۔پاگل پن' خفقان اور پروسٹیٹوریا جریان کے علاج کے لئے بھی مذکورہ خوراکیں۔بے خوابی کے علاج کے لئے بھی۔

Chloretone *(klor'-e-ton).* Chlorbutol (q.v.)

کلوریٹون : دیکھئے کلوربوٹول۔دفع دردوائی۔

Chlorexolone *(klor-eks'-o-lon).* Thiazide diuretic. See CHLOROTHIAZIDE.

کلوریکسولون : دیکھئے کلوروتھیازائیڈ۔پیشاب آور اور خونی دباؤ کم کرنے والی دوا۔

Chlorhexidine *(klor-heks'-i-den).* An antiseptic effective against a wide range of bacteria. Used as 1:2000 solution as a general antiseptic, 1:5000 for douches and irrigation. Hand cream (1 per cent) is effective in reducing cross infecion. (Hibitane).

کلورہیکسی ڈین : جراثیم کے خلاف موثر دافع تعفن۔

Chlorine *(klor'-en).* A greenish-yellow,

irritating gaseous element. Powerful germicide, bleaching and deodorizing agent in the presence of moisture when nascent oxygen is liberated. Used chiefly as hypochlorites (eusol, Milton), chloramine or other compounds which slowly liberate active chlorine.

کلورین : ایک سبز زرد گیسی عنصر۔ جراثیم کش۔ رنگ کاٹ۔ جوہری عدد k' جوہری وزن ۳۵،۴۵۳' ناگوار بو' زہریلی گیس' تکسیدی عامل' حشرات کش۔

Chlormethizole *(klor-meth-i-a-zol)*. Hypno/sedative capsules. Effective in controling restless excitement with no Parkinsonian effects.

کلورمتھیازول : راحت بخش کیپسول' بے آرام جوش کو قابو کرنے میں موثر۔

Chlorocresol *(klor'-o-kre-sol)*. A bactericide widely used as a preservative for injections in multiple dose vials.

کلوروکریسول : جراثیم کش۔ ٹکول میں محفوظ کرنے کے لیے استعمال کیا جاتا ہے۔

Chlorodyne *(klor'-o-din)*. A solution of morphine, ether and chloroform in a mixture of liquorice, treacle and syrup. Widely used with kaolin as a gastric sedative as mist, kaolin et morph. BNF.

کلوروڈائن : کسی مکسچر یا شربت میں مارفین۔ ایتھر اور کلوروفارم کا محلول

Chloroform *(klor'-o-form)*. Heavy liquid, once used extensively as a general anaesthetic. Much used in the form of chloroform water as a flavouring and preservative in aqueous mixtures.

کلوروفارم : طیران پذیر بھاری مائع۔ سن کرنے کے لئے مستعمل۔ آبی مکسچروں میں بھی خوشبو وغیرہ کے لئے مستعمل ہے۔ مہروں اور چہرے و کھوپڑی کی ہڈیوں پر سبزی مائل زرد اگاؤ۔ اس سے بے ہوشی ہو جاتی ہے۔ اس میں مصنوعی سانس' سٹریکنین کا ٹیکہ' کورامین کا ٹیکہ' جسم کی مالش اور آکسیجن گیس سونگھانا مفید ہے۔

Chloroma *(klor'-o'-ma)* [G. *chloros,* pale green; *oma,* tumour]. a condition in which multiple greenish-yellow growths grow on periosteum of facial and cranial bones, and vertebrae. Very rare, in association with acute myloid leu kaemia.

Chloromycetin *(klor'-o-mi-se-tin)*. Chloramphenicol (q.v.)

کلورومائی سے ٹین : دیکھئے کلورم فینیکول۔ ایک معروف اینٹی بایوٹک دوا۔ ٹائی فائڈ کے لئے مفید

Chlorophyll *(klor'-o-fi)* [G. *chloros,* pale green; *phyllon,* lef]. The green colouring matter which assists in photosynthesis in plants. Now prepared medicinally and for external use as a deodorant.

کلوروفل' سبز مایہ' سبزینہ : یونانی الفاظ کلوروس بمعنی پیلا سبز اور فلن بمعنی پتا کا مجموعہ۔ سبز رنگ کا مادہ جو سبز پودوں میں ضیائی تالیف کے ذریعے خوراک بنانے میں مدد ہے۔ اب اسے دوائی کے طور پر تیار کیا جاتا ہے۔

Chloroquine *(klor'-o-kwin)*. A potent antimalarial effective in the treatment and suppression of hte disease . It is being added to the salt in some endemic areas. Also used in amoebic hepatitis and collagen diseases. Can cause ocular complications. Hs a mild anti-inflammatory effect and in the long term will lower the titre of the rheumatoid factor in the serum.

کلوروکوئن : ملیریا کے علاج کے لئے موثر دوا۔ پہلی خوراک چار گولیاں اور بارہ گھنٹے بعد دو گولیاں پانی یا مشروبات زیادہ استعمال کرنے چاہئیں۔ ایبائی بچس کے لئے ایک گولی صبح ایک شام ۲ اروز کے لئے۔

Chlorothiazide *(klor-o-thi-a-zid)*. Diuretic with a mild blood pressure lowering action which does not change much with posture and rerely gives rise to symptoms of hypotension.

کلوروتھیازائیڈ : پیشاب آور۔ خونی دباؤ کو کم کرتا ہے۔

Chlorotrianisene *(Klor-o-tri-an'-i-sen)*. Used as an alternative to stilbosestrol. Favoured by some for menopausal symptoms, because of its prolonged oestrogenic action by slow release, but this is not an advantage if side effects occur, as the effect of the hormone cannot be immediately discontinued.

کلوروٹرائی انی سین : سٹلبو ایسٹرول کے متبادل کے طور پر مستعمل بعض بندش حیض کے لئے استعمال کرتے ہیں۔ لیکن مضر اثرات بھی ہو سکتے ہیں۔

Chloroxylenol *(klor-oks'-i-len-ol)*. Antiseptic constituent of many non-caustic gerrhicides. Less effective than phenol against some organisms.

کلوریکسی لینول : غیر کاسٹک جراثیم کش ادویات کا دافع تعفن جزو۔ بعض جسیموں کے خلاف فینائل کی نسبت کم موثر۔

Chlorpheniramine *(klor-fen-i'-ra-men)*. Short-acting antihistamine.

کلورفنر امین : کم ایکشن والی اینٹی ہسٹامین۔ شرمگاہ کی خارش یا پروریٹس دلوی۔ زکام، سوزش، گردہ اور دمہ میں ایک گولی صبح ایک دوپہر ایک شام۔ السریٹوکولائی ٹس میں بھی مذکورہ خوراکیں۔

Chlorpromazine *(klor-pro'-ma-zen)*. A drug of exceptional pharmacological action, as it is a sedative, antiemetic, antispasmodic and hypotensive. It increases the effectiveness of hypnotics, anaesthetics, alcohol and analgesics. Valuable in psychiatric conditions and management of senile patients. May cause skin sensitization, leucopenia, Parkinsonism and jaundice.

کلور پرومازین : یہ خواب آور، نشہ آور، سن کرنے والی دوائی ہے اور الکحل کے اثر کو زیادہ کرتی ہے۔ مسکن دوا جو تے کو بھی روکتی ہے۔ دافع دردلار جیکٹل تے روکنے کے لئے ایک گولی صبح ایک دوپہر ایک شام۔ پاگل پن کے علاج کے لئے بھی مذکورہ خوراک۔

Chlorpropamide *(klor-pro'-pa-mid)*. One of the sulphonylureas. Antidiabetic agent.

کلور پروپیامائیڈ : ضد ذیابیطس عامل۔

Chlorprothixene *(klor-pro-thicks'-en)*. Tranquillizer. Useful in acute schizophrenic conditions, but is less effective as treatment is prolonged.

کلور پروتھکسین : راحت بخش دوا۔

Chlortetracycline *(klor-tet-ra-si-klin)*. Preparation of tetracycline (q.v.)

کلورٹیٹرا سائیکلین : ٹیٹرا سائیکلین سے تیارشدہ۔

Chlorthalidone *(klor-thal'- i-don)*. Oral diuretic given on alternate days. Action lasts up to 48 hours.

کلورتھیلیڈون : منہ سے کھائی جانے والی پیشاب آور دوا جو متبادل دنوں پر دی جاتی ہے۔ اس کا ۴۸ گھنٹوں تک برقرار رہتا ہے۔

Choana *(ko-a'-na)* [G. *choane,* funnel]. Funnel-shaped opening. The posterior nasal orifices or nares (q.v.)--choanae, pl,; choanal, adj.

نتھنا : یونانی لفظ کونے بمعنی قیف سے ماخوذ۔ قیف نما سوراخ۔ خلفی ناک کی سوراخ یا نتھنے۔

Choked disc *(or papilloedema)*. A blurring and obliteration of the cup or disc in the back of the eyeball (through which the optic nerve and vessels enter and leave the eye) by fluid distension, from whatever cause.

قرص مختنق : آنکھ کے گولے کی پشت میں پیالی یا تھالی کی رکاوٹ۔

Cholaemia *(kol-em'-i-a)* [G. *chole,* bile; *haima,* blood]. The presence of bile in the blood--cholaemic, adj.

صفرادمویت : یونانی الفاظ کول بمعنی بائل اور ہیما بمعنی خون کا مجموعہ۔ خون میں بائل کی موجودگی۔

Cholagogue *(kol'-a-gog)* [G. *chole,* bile; *agogos,* leading]. A drug which causes an increased flow of bile into the intestine.

کولاگگ۔ مدرصفرا : انت میں بائل کا بہاؤ زیادہ کرنے والی دوا۔

Cholangiogram *(kol-an'-ji-o-gram)* [G. chole, bile; aggeion, vessel; gramma. letter]. Film demonstrating hepatic, cystic and bile ducts.

کولنجیوگرام : جگری، سسٹک اور بائل نالیاں دکھانے والی فلم۔

Cholangiography *(kol-an-ji-og'-ra-fi)*. [G. chole, bile; aggeion, vessel; graphein, to write]. Radiographic examination of hepatic, cystic and bile ducts. Can be performed; (1) after oral or intravenous administration of radio-opaque substance; (2) at operation to detect any further stones in the ducts; (3) after operation by way of a T-tube in the common bile duct; (4) by means of an injection via the skin on the anterior abdominal wall and the liver. Percutaneious transhepatic c.--cholangiographic, adj.; cholangiograph, n.; cholangiographically, adv.

کولنجیوگرافی : جگری، سسٹک اور بائل نالیوں کا ریڈیوگرافک ٹیسٹ۔

Cholangiohepatitis *(kol-an'-ji-o-hep-a-ti-tis)* [G. chole, bile; aggeion, vessel, hepar, liver; -itis, inflammation]. Inflammation of the liver and bile ducts.

کولنجیو ہیپٹائی ٹس : جگراور بائل نالیوں کی سوزش۔

Cholangitis *(kol-an-ji'-tis)* [G. chole, bile; aggeion, vessel; -itis. inflammation]. Inflammation of bile ducts.

التہاب مرارہ۔ ورم قنوات صفرا : بائل نالیوں کی سوزش۔

Cholecystangiogram *(kol-e-sist-anj'-i-o-gram)* [G. chole, bile, kystis, bladder; aggeion, vessel; gramma, letter]. Film demonstrating gall-bladder, cystic and common bile ducts after administra-tion of opaque medium.

کول سٹینجیوگرام : غیر شفاف واسطہ کے بعد پتے، سسٹک اور مشترک بائل نالیاں دکھانے والی فلم۔

Cholecystangiography *(kol-e-sist-anj-i-og'-r-af-i)* [G. chole, bile; kystis, bladder; aggeion, vessel; graphein, to write]. Radiographic examination of the gall bladder, cystic and common bile ducts after administration of opaque medium--cholecyst- angiographic, adj.; cholecystangiographically, adv.; chole cystangiograph; n.

کول سٹینجیوگرافی : غیر شفاف واسطہ کے بعد پتے، سسٹک اور مشترک بائل نالیوں کا ریڈیوگرافک ٹیسٹ

Cholecystetomy *(kol-e-sis-tek'-to-mi)* [G. chole, bile; kystis, bladder; ektome, excision]. Surgical removal of the gall-bladder. Usually advised for stones, inflammation and occassionally for new growths.

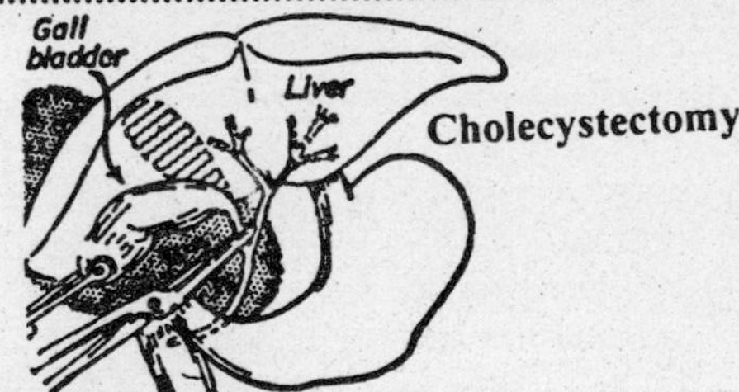

Cholecystectomy

مرارہ براری : پتے کو سرجری کے ذریعے نکالنا۔ پتھری یا سوزش کے لئے کرتے ہیں۔

Cholecystenterostomy *(kol-e-sist-en-te-r-os'-to-mi)* [G. chole, bile; kystis, bladder; enteron, intestine; stoma, mouth]. Literally, the establishment of an artifical opening (anastomosis) between the gall-bladder and the small intestine. Cholecystenterostomy

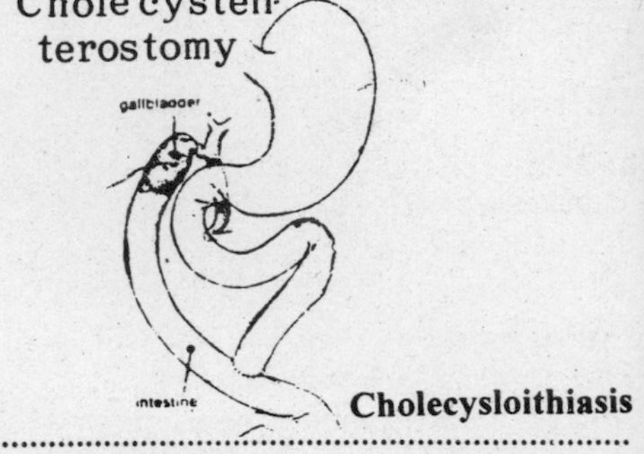

Cholecysloithiasis

Specific terminology more frequently used.

کولی سسٹینٹیرو سٹومی : یونانی الفاظ کول بمعنی بائل کسٹس بمعنی بلیڈر، انٹیران بمعنی آنت اور سٹوما بمعنی منہ کا مجموعہ۔ پتے اور چھوٹی آنت کے درمیان مصنوعی سوراخ کا قیام

Cholangitis *(kol-e-sis-ti'-tis)* [G. chole, bile; kystis, bladder; -itis, inflammation]. Infl-ammation of the gall-bladder.

Cholecystoduodenal *(kol-e-sis'-to-du-o-den'al)* [G. chole,l bile; kystis, bladder; L. duodeni, twelve at once; G. stoma mouth]. The esta-blishment of an anastomosis between the gall-bladder and the duodenum. Usually necessary in cases of stricture of common bile duct, which may be congenital, due to previous inflammation or operation.

مراری عفجی تفویہ : پتے اور ڈیوڈینم کے درمیان جال کا قیام۔

Cholecystogastrostomy *(kol-e-sis-to-gas-tr-os'-to-mi)* [G. chole, bile; kystis, bladder; gasterl, belly; stoma, mouth]. The establis-hment of an anastomosis between the gallbla-dder and the stomach; a palliative operation when the common bile duct is obstructed by an immovable growth.

مراری تفویہ : یونانی الفاظ کول بمعنی بوئل، کسٹس بمعنی بلیڈر، گیسٹر بمعنی پیٹ اور سٹوما بمعنی منہ کا مجموعہ۔ پتے اور معدے کے درمیان جال کا قیام۔ جب مشترک بائل نالی بند ہو جائے تو اپریشن ہوتا ہے۔

Cholecystogram *(ko-le-sis'-to-gram)* [G. chole, bile; kystis, bladder; gramma, letter]. Film demonstrating gall-bladder after administ-ra-tion of opaque medium.

مراری نگارش۔ مراری ترسیم : یونانی الفاظ کول بمعنی بائل، کسٹس بمعنی بلیڈر اور گریا بمعنی مکتوب کا مجموعہ۔ غیر شفاف واسطے کے بعد پتے کو دکھانے والی فلم۔

Cholecystography *(ko-le-sis-tog'-raf-i)* [G. chole, bile;kystis, bladder; graphein, to write]. Radiographic examination of the gall-bladder after administration of opaque medium--cholecystograp- hic, adj.; cholecystographically, adv.; cholecystograph, n.

پتے کا ایکسرے۔ : یونانی الفاظ کول بمعنی بائل، کسٹس بمعنی بلیڈر اور گرتیفین بمعنی لکھنا کا مجموعہ۔ غیر شفاف واسطے کے بعد پتے کا ریڈیوگرافی ٹیسٹ۔ مریض کو شام کے وقت چاول، چینی اور گھی کھانے کے لئے دیا جائے۔ پھر چھ اوپے کال کے کیپسول کھلائے جائیں۔ اگلے روز پتے کا ایکسرے کیا جائے۔

Cholecystojejunostomy *(kol-e-sis-to-je-jun-os'-tom-i)* [G. chole; bile; kystis, bladder; L. jejunus, empty; G. stoma, mouth]. an anastomosis between the gall-bladder and the jejunum. Performed for obstructive jaundice due to growth in head of pancreas.

مراری صائمی تفویہ : یونانی الفاظ کول بمعنی بائل، کسٹس بمعنی بلیڈر لاطینی لفظ جیجونس اور یونانی لفظ سٹوما بمعنی منہ سے مرکب اصطلاح۔ پتے اور جیجونم کے درمیان جال۔

Cholecystokinin *(kol-e-sis-to-ki'-nin)* [G. chole, bile; kystis, bladder, kinein, to move]. A hormone which contracts the gall-bladder. Secreted by the upper intestinal mucosa.

کولی سسٹوکائی نن : ہارمون جو کہ پتے کو سکیڑتا ہے۔

Cholecystolithiasis *(kol-e-sis-to-lith-i'-as-is)* [G. chole, bile; kystis, bladder; lithos, stone; N.L. -iasis, condition]. The presence of stone or stones in the gall-bladder.

کولی سسٹولتھیوسس : پتے میں پتھری کی موجودگی۔

Cholecystostomy *(kol-e-sis-tos'-to-mi)* [G. chole, bile; kystis. bladder, stoma, mouth]. A surgically established fistula between the gall-bladder and the abdominal surface; used to provide drainage, in empyema of the gall-bladder or after the removal of stones.

مراری تفویہ : سرجری کی وجہ سے شکم کی سطح اور پتے کی درمیان بنا ہوا

Cholecystotomy *(kol-e-sis-tot'-om-i)* [G. chole, bile; kystis, bladder; tome, a cutting]. Incision into the gall-bladder

پتاشگافی : پتے میں زخم۔

Choledochoduodenial *(kol-e-dok-o-du-o-d-en'-al)* [G. chole, bile; dechesthai, to receive; L. duodeni, twelve]. Pertaining to the bile ducts and duodenum, e.g. c. fistula.

کولی ڈاکوڈیوڈینل : بائیل کی نالیو اور ڈیوڈینم سے تعلق رکھنے والی۔

Choledochography *(kol-e-dok-og'-ra-fi)*. See CHOLANGIOGRAPHY.

ترسیم قناۃ مشترک صفراوی : جگری سسٹک اور بائل نالیوں کا ریڈیو گرافک ٹیسٹ۔

Choledocholithiasis *(kol-e-dok-o-lith-i'-as-is)* [G. chole, bile; dechesthai, to receive; lithos, stone; N.L. -iasis, condition]. The presence of a stone or stones in the bile ducts.

حصاتیت قنواۃ صفرا : بائیل نالیوں میں پتھری کی غیر موجودگی۔

Choledocholithotomy *(kol-e-dok-o-lith-o-t'-om-i)* [G.chole, bile; dechesthai, to receive; lithos, stone; tome, a cutting]. Surgical removal of a stone from the common bile duct.

حصاۃ براری از قناۃ مشترک صفراوی : سرجری کی مدد سے مشترک بائیل نالی سے پتھری کا نکالنا۔

Choledochostomy *(kol-e-dok-os'-to-mi)* [G. chole, bile; dechesthai, to receive; stoma, mouth]. Drainage of the common bile duct, usually after exploration for a stone.

تفویہ قناۃ صفرا : کسی پتھری کی تلاش کے بعد مشترک بائیل نالی کا نقصاص۔

Choledochotomy *(kol-e-dok-ot'-om-i)* [G. chole, bile; dechesthai, to receive; tome, a cutting]. Incesion into the common bile duct.

شگاف قناۃ صفرا : مشترک بائل نالی میں زخم۔

Choledyl *(ko'-le-dil)*. Choline theophyllinate (q.v.).

کولیڈل : کولین تھیوفیلیٹ۔ جو کہ امینوفیلین سے مشابہت رکھتی ہے۔

Cholelithiasis *(kol-e-lith-i'-a-sis)* [G. chole, bile; lithos, stone; N.L. -iasis, condition]. The presence of stones in the gall-bladder or bile ducts.

صفراوی حصاتیت : پتے یا بائل نالیوں میں پتھری کی موجودگی۔

Cholers *(kol'-e-ra)* [G.]. An acute epidemic disease, caused by Vibrio comma, occuring in the East. The måin symptoms are the evacuation of copious 'rice-water' stools accompanied by agonizing cramp and severe copllapse. Spread mainly by contaminated water, overcrowding and inanitary conditions. High mortality.

ہیضہ : وائبرو کوما کی وجہ سے بیماری۔ سفید پانی کی طرح دست آتے ہیں۔ زیادہ رش یا بھیڑ میں پھیلتا ہے۔ گندے پانی اور گندی غذا سے ہوتا ہے۔

Choleric temperament *(kol'-er-ik)*. One of the four classical types of temperament (q.v.), hasty and prone to emotional outbursts.

صفراوی مزاج : مزاجوں کی ایک قسم۔

Cholestasis *(kol-e-sta'-sis)* [G. chole, bile; stasis, a standing still]. Diminution or arrest of the flow of bile. **Intrahepatic c.,** syndrome comprising jaundice of an obstructive type, itching, pale stools and dark urine, but in which the main bile ducts outside the liver and patent--cholestatic, adj.

رکود صفرا : بائل کے بہاؤ میں کمی۔

Cholesteatoms *(kol-es'-te-a-to-ma)* [G. chole, bile; stear, fat; -oma, tumour]. A benign encysted tumour containing cholesterol. Mainly occurs in the middle ear--cholesteatomatous, adj.

شحمی سلعہ : ایک پھوڑا جس میں کولیسٹرول ہوتا ہے۔

Cholesterol *(kol-es'-te-rol)* [G. chole, bile; sterol, solid]. A crystalline substance of a fatty nature found in the brain, nerves, liver, blood and bile. It is not easily soluble and may crystallize in the gall-bladder and along arterial walls. When irradiated it forms vitamin D.

کولیسٹرول : دماغی خون، جگر وغیرہ میں قلمی مادہ۔

Cholesterosis *(ko-les-ter-o'-sis)* [G. chole, bile; stear, fat; -osis, condition]. Abnormal deposition of cholesterol.

کولیسٹرولیت : کولیسٹرول کا بے قاعدگی سے جمع ہونا۔

Cholestyramine *(kol-es-ti'-ra-men)*. A basic ion-exchange resin which combines with bile acids in the intestine to give a product which is unabsorbed. Not only is the digestion of dietary cholesterol inhibited, but the excretion of bile acids is very much increased. Since bile acids are made from cholesterol, this leads to a pronounced loss of cholesterol from the body resulting in hypocholesterolaemia.

کولی سٹیرامین : ذرے کے تبادلے کی ایک رال جو کہ آنت میں غیر جذب شدہ پیداوار دینے کے لئے بائل ایسڈز سے ملتی ہے۔

Choline *(ko'-len)*. A chemical found in animal tissues as a constituent of lecithin and acetylcholine. Thought to be part of the vitamin B complex, and is known to be a growth factor. Appears to be necessary for fat transportation in the body. Useful in preventing fat deposition in the liver in cirrhosis. Richest sources are dairy products. See CHOLEDYL..

کولین : ایک کیمیائی مرکب جو حیوانی بافتوں میں لیسیتھن اور ایسٹائل کولین کے جزو کے طور پر پایا جاتا ہے۔ اسے حیاتین ب کمپلکس کا حصہ تصور کیا جاتا ہے۔ نشوونما کے لئے ضروری۔ چکنائی کے انتقال کے لئے لازمی جگر کو چربی کی مانع ہونے سے بچاتا ہے۔ دودھ سے بنی چیزوں میں پایا جاتا ہے۔ بعض چکنائیوں اور انڈے کی زردی میں ہوتا ہے۔

Cholinergic *(kol-in-er'-jik)* [G. chole, bile; ergon, work]. Applied to parasympathetic nerves which liberate acetylcholine at their terminations. See ADRENERGIC.

کولی نرجک : یونانی الفاظ کول بمعنی ''بائل'' اور ارگن بمعنی ''کام'' کا مجموعہ۔ اس کا اطلاق پیراسیمپ تھیٹک اعصاب پر کیا جاتا ہے جو آخری سروں پر ایسٹائل کولین پیدا کرتے ہیں۔ یہ آنتوں کے درد اور مزور کا باعث بنتے ہیں۔ معدہ کے درد اور تھوک پیدا کرتے ہیں۔ ہوا، پیشاب اور پاخانہ خارج کرتے ہیں۔

Cholinesterase *(kol-in-es'-ter-az)*. An enzyme which hydrolyses acetylcholine into choline and acetic acid, at nerve endings.

کولین ایسٹریز : ایک خامرہ جو عصبی سروں پر ایسٹائل کولین کی آب پاشیدگی کر کے اسے کولین اور ایسٹک ایسڈ میں تبدیل کرتا ہے۔ شدید عضلاتی کمزوری میں اس کی زیادتی ہو جاتی ہے۔

Choline theophyllinate *(kol'-en the-of'-fil-at)*. This compound resembles aminophyline in its general effects, but is less erratic in action

The incidence of gastric irritation is much less, and the response more reliable.

holuria *(kol-ur'-i-a)* [G. chole, bile; ouron, urine]. The presence of bile in the urine--choluric, adj.

بول صفراوی : یونانی الفاظ کول بمعنی بائل اور اورون بمعنی پیشاب کا مجموعہ۔ پیشاب میں بائل کی موجودگی۔

hondritis *(kon-dri'-tis)* [G. chondros, cartilage; -itis, inflammation]. Inflammation of cartilage.

ورم کری : کری ہڈی یا کارٹیلج کی سوزش۔

ondrocostal *(kon'-dro-kos'-tal)* [G. chondros, cartilage; L. costa, rib]. Pertaining to the costal cartilages and ribs.

غضروفی ضلعی : کاسٹل کارٹیلجز اور پسلیوں سے متعلق۔

ondrodynia *(kon-dro-din'-i-a)* [G. chondros, cartilage; odyne, pain]. Pain in a cartilage.

دردی کری : کری ہدی یا کارٹیلج میں درد۔

ondrolysis *(kon-drol'-i-sis)* [G. chondros, cartilage; lysis, lossening]. Dissolution of cartilage--chondrolytic, adj.

غضروف پاشیدگی : کارٹیلج کا خاتمہ۔

ondroma *(kon-dro'-ma)* [G. chondros, cartilage; -oma, tumour]. A benign tumour of cartilage. Tends to recur after removal.

غضروف سلعہ : کری ہڈی یا کارٹیلج کی گلٹی یا رسولی جو انسانی جسم کے لئے مثبت پہلو رکھتی ہے۔

ondromalacia *(kon-dro-mal-a'-si-a)* [G. hondros, cartilage; malakia, softness]. oftening of cartilage.

لینت کری : کری ہڈی یا کارٹیلج کا نرم ہونا۔

ondrosarcoma *(kon-dro-sar-ko'-ma)* [G. hondros, cartilage; sarkoma, fleshy vergrowth]. Malignant neoplasm of cartilge--chondrosarcomatous, adj,; chondrosarco-nata, pl.

غضروفی لحمی سلعہ : کارٹیلج کا نیوپلازم۔

ondrosternal *(kon'-dro-ster'-nal)* [G. hondros, cartilage; sternon, breast]. Pertning to the rib cartilages and sternum.

غضروفی قصی : پسلیوں کی کارٹیلج اور سٹرنم سے متعلق۔

Chordee *(kor-de')* [G. corde, string]. Painful erection of the penis due to urethritis. Common in gonorrhoea.

سوزاک : عضو تناسل درد کے ساتھ سخت ہونا۔ سوزاک میں یہ حالت ہوتی ہے۔

Chorditis *(kor-di'-tis)* [G. chorde, string; -itis, inflammation]. Inflammation of the sprematic or vocal cords.

ورم حبل : یونانی الفاظ کارڈے بمعنی ڈوری اور ائٹس بمعنی سوزش کا مجموعہ۔ سپرمیٹک یا ووکل کارڈز کی سوزش۔

Chordotomy *(kor-dot'-o-mi)* [G. chorde, string, tome, a cutting]. Division of anterolateral nerve pathways in the spinal cord to give relief from the intense pain of advanced malignant disease. Temporary relief as for severe burns and shingles can be obtained by direct current electric c. under local anaesthesia. Also **cordotomy.**

حبل تراشی : شدید درد سے نجات دلانے کے لئے اگلی جانبی عصبی راہوں کو نخاع میں تقسیم کرنا۔

Chorea *(kawr-e'-a)* [G. choreia, dance]. Disease manifested by irregular and spasmodic movements, beyond the patient's control. Even voluntary movements are rendered jerky and ungainly. The childhood disease is often called 'rheumatic chorea' or 'St. Vitus's Dance'; the adult form is part of a cerebral degenerative process called 'Huntington's chorea'--choreal, choreic, adj.

کوریا۔ رقص۔ رقصہ : یونانی لفظ کوریا بمعنی رقص سے ماخوذ۔ مریض کے قابو سے باہر بے قاعدہ حرکات

Choreiform *(kawr-e'-i-form)* [g. choreia, dance; L. forma. form]. Resembling chorea.

رعشہ نما : یونانی لفظ کوریا بمعنی رقص اور لاطینی لفظ فارما بمعنی قسم سے مرکب اصطلاح۔ گوریا سے مشابہ۔

Choriocarcinoma *(kawr-i-o-kar-sin-o'-ma).* See CHORIONEPITHELIOMA.

سلوی سرطانی سلعہ : دیکھئے کوریونیپی تھیلی اوما۔ کوریانی خلیوں سے بننے والی گلٹی۔

Chorion *(kawr'-i-on)* [G. outer membrane]. The outer membrane forming the embryonic sac--chorial, chorionic, adj.

Chorion

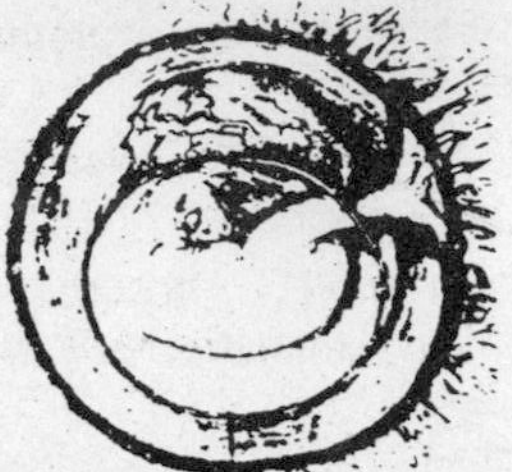

کوریان۔ سلیٰ : یونانی لفظ جس کا مطلب بیرونی جھلی ہے جنینی تھیلی بنانے والی بیرونی جھلی۔

Chorion epithelioma *(kawr-i-on-ep-i-the-l-i-o'-ma)* [G. chorion, outer membrane; -oma, tumour]. A highly maligant tumour arising from chorionic cells, usually after a hydatiform mole, but may follow abortion or even normal pregnancy, quickly metastasizing especially to the lungs. Cytotoxic drugs have improved the prognosis.

کوریونیپی تھیلی اوما : یونانی الفاظ کوریان بمعنی بیرونی جھلی اوراوما بمعنی گلٹی کا مجموعہ۔ کوریانی خلیوں س ے بننے والی گلٹی۔

Chorionic villi *(kawr-i-on'-ik-vil'-i)* [G. chorion, outer membrane; L. villus, shaggy hair]. Projections from the chorion from which the fetal part of the placenta is formed. Through the c.v. diffusion of gases, nutrient and waste products. occurs from the maternal to the fetal blood and vice versa.

سلوی ولائی : کوریان کے بڑھے ہوئے حصے۔

Chorioretinitis *(kawr-i-o-ret-in-it'-is)* [G. chorion, outer membrane; M.L. retina, from L. rete, net; G. -itis, inflammation]. Inflammation of the choroid and retina.

ورم مشیمیہ وشبکیہ : کورائڈ اورریٹنا کی سوزش۔

Choroid *(kawr'-oid)* [G. chorion, outer membrane, eidos, form]. The middle pigmented, vascular coat of the posterior five-sixths of the eyeball, continuous with the iris in front. It lies between the sclera externally and the retina internally, and prevents the passage of light rays--choroidal, adj.

کورائڈ۔ مشیمیہ : آنکھ میں موجود ایک تہہ۔

Choroiditis *(kawr-oid-i'-tis)* [G. chorion, oute membrane; eidos, form; -itis, inflammation] Inflammation of the choroid. **Tay's c.** degenerative change affecting the retin around the macula lutea. [Warren Tay English physician, 1843 1927].

رم مشیمیہ : کورائڈ کی سوزش۔

Choroidocyclitis *(kawr-oid-o-sik-li'-tis)* [G choroeides, choroid; kyklos, circle; -itis inflammation]. Inflammation of the choroi and ciliary body.

شیمیتی ہدبی التہاب : یونانی الفاظ کورائڈیز بمعنی کورائڈ' کالکلوس بمعنی ئرہ اوراٹس بمعنی سوزش کا مجموعہ۔ کورائڈ اور ہدبی جسم کی سوزش۔

Choroidoretinal *(kawr-oid-o-ret'-in-al)* [G choroeides, choroid; L. rete, net]. Pertainin to the choroid and the retina.

ورائیڈ وریٹینل : یونانی الفاظ کورائدیز بمعنی کورائڈ اور لاطینی لفظ ریٹے نی جال سے مرکب اصطلاح کورائد اور ریٹنا سے متعلق۔ آنکھ کے پردوں ے متعلق۔

choroidoretinitis Syn. chorioretinitis (q.v.).

یمیتی شبکیتی التہاب : دیکھئے کوریوریٹینٹس۔ کورائڈ اور ٹینا کی سوزش۔

Christims disease. Allied to haemophilia (q.v. Caused by hereditary deficiency of clottir Factor IX (plasma thromboplastin componer PTC).

س کرسمس : ہیموفلیا سے متحدہ۔ خون جمنے کے عامل کی توراثی کمی کے سبب یماری ہوتی ہے۔

Chromatogram *(kro'-ma-to-gram)* [G. chrom colour; gramma, letter]. Tracing produced chromatography.

رومیٹوگرام : یونانی لفظ کروما بمعنی رنگ اور گریما بمعنی مکتوب کا مجموعہ۔ ومیٹوگرافی سے پیدا ہونے والی ٹریسنگ۔ مختلف رنگوں اور مخصوص طریقوں ، تیار کردہ چارٹ۔ ساکن اور متحرک واسطوں کے ذریعے درمیانی فرق وم کرلیا جاتا ہے۔

Chromatography *(kro-ma-tog'-ra-fi)* [chroma, colour; graphein, to write]. Consi of the separation of substances on a chro atograph column. Such a column may constructed in various ways but alwa consists basically of two phases. One is stationary phase which may be solid, liquid or a mixtre of both, and is finely divided and fixed in place (e.g. paper, in paper chromatography). The second is the mobile phase which may be liquid or gaseous and fills the spaces of the stationary phase through which it flows. The stationary and mobile phases are so selected that compounds which are to be separated by the chromatogram have different distribution coefficients between the phases.

کرومیٹوگرافی۔لون نگاری : یونانی الفاظ کروما بمعنی رنگ اور گریفین بمعنی لکھنا کا مجموعہ۔ کرومیٹوگراف کالم پر اشیاء کی علیحدگی پر مشتمل

Chronic acid *(kro'-mik as'-id)* . In a 5 per-cent solution it is astringent, used in the preparation of chromicized catgut (q.v.); stronger solutions are caustic and can be painted on warts.

کرومی ترشہ : تیز محلول کاسٹک ہوتے ہیں اور آبلوں پر لگائے جاتے ہیں۔

Chromosome *(krom'-o-som)* [G. chroma, colour; soma, body]. Any one of the thread-like bodies into which the cell nucleus divides during mitosis, and which split longitudinally in that process. They carry hereditary factors (genes), the number being constant for each species--in man, 46 in each cell, except in the mature ovum and sperm where the number is halved as a result of reduction division. A set of 23 chromosomes is inherited from each parent--chromosomal, adj.

کروموسوم۔لونیہ : یونانی الفاظ کروما بمعنی رنگ اور سوما بمعنی جسم کا مجموعہ۔ ریشہ نما اجسام میں سے ایک جس میں مائیٹوسس کے دوران خلیے کا مرکزہ تقسیم ہوتا ہے اور اس میں وہ طوفانی طور پر تقسیم ہوتا ہے۔ ان پر جین ہوتے ہیں۔ ہر نوع میں کروموسوموں کی مقررہ تعداد ہوتی ہے۔ آدمی میں ۴۶ ہوتے ہیں۔ صرف بیضہ اور سپرم میں آدھے ہوتے ہیں۔ دو کروموسوم جنسی اہمیت کے حامل ہیں اس لئے انہیں جنسی کروموسوم کہتے ہیں' باقی آٹوسوم کہلاتے ہیں۔ جنسی کروموسوم عورت میں ڈبل ایکس اور مرد میں ایکس وائی ہوتے ہیں۔

Chronic *(kron'-ik)* [G. chronos, time]. Lingering, lasting, opposed to acute--chronically, adv.; chronicity, n.

کہنہ : یونانی لفظ کرونوس۔ بمعنی وقت سے ماخوذ برقرار۔ قائم۔ پرانی بیماری۔

Chvostek's sign *(shvos'-teks)*. Excessive twitching of the face on tapping the facial nerve. A sign of tetany [Franz Chvostek, Austrian surgeon, 1835-84].

شووس ٹیک علامت : تشنج کی علامت۔

Chyle *(kil)* [G. chylos, juice]. Digested fats which, as an alkaline milky fluid, pass from the small intestine via the lymphatics to the blood stream--chylous, adj.

کائل۔کیلوس : یونانی لفظ کائیلوس بمعنی رس سے ماخوذ۔ ہضم شدہ چکنائیاں جو بطور الکلائن دودھ یا سیال کے چھوٹی آنت سے لمفیٹکس کے ذریعے خون میں جاتی ہے۔

Chylothorax *(kil-o-thaw'-raks)* [G. chylos, juice; thorax, chest cavity]. Leakage of chyle from the thoracic duct into the pleural cavity.

کیلوس صدری : یونانی الفاظ کائیلوس بمعنی رس اور تھوریکس بمعنی چھاتی کا کہفہ کا مجموعہ۔ کائل کا تھوریک نلی سے پیورل کہفہ میں پہنچنا یا رسنا۔

Chyluria *(kil-ur'-i-a)* [G. chylos, juice; ouron, urine]. Chyle in the urine, which can occur in some nematode infestations, when either a fistulous communication is established between a lymphatic vessel and the urinary tract, or the distension of the urinary lymphatics causes them to rupture--chyluric, adj.

بول کیلوسی : یونانی الفاظ کائیلوس بمعنی رس اور اوزون بمعنی پیشاب کا مجموعہ۔ پیشاب میں کائل کی موجودگی۔

Chymar *(ki'-mar)*. Chymotrypsin (q.v.).

کائیمر : دیکھئے کائموٹرپسن۔ ایک خامرہ۔ وہائیٹ لیگ اور پلمونری ایمبولزم میں مفید۔

Chyme *(kim)* [G. chymos, juice]. Partially digested food which as an acid, creamy yellow, thick fluid, passes from the stomach to the duodenum. Its acidity controls the pylorus so that chyme is ejected at frequent intervals--chymous, adj.

کیموس : نیم ہضم شدہ خوراک جو معدہ سے ڈیوڈینم میں جاتی ہے۔

Chymopapain *(ki'-mo-pap-an')* A proteolytic enzyme obtained from the latex of hte pawpaw tree.

کائموٹرپس : ایک خامرہ۔ کائموورل۔ وہائیٹ لیگ کے مرض میں ایک گولی صبح ایک دوپہر ایک شام ۲ ہفتے تک۔ پلمونری ایمبولزم میں بھی مذکورہ خوراک۔

Chymoral *(ki'-mor-al)*. Enzymes trypsin and chymotrypsin.

Chymotrypsin *(ki-mo-trip'-sin)*. Proteolytic enzyme. Useful in debridment of necrotic tissue, etc. and for lossening secretions, e.g. in respiratory tract. Also facilitates lens extraction.

Cicatrin *(sik'-a-trin)*. Neomycin and bacitracin. Cicatrin aerosol spray is an amino acid antibiotic powder spray. It promotes healing of wounds under a light film. It is very convenient and time saving. Its best use is for superficial and shallow wounds. A two-second spray is all that is necessary at a distance of 20.32 to 30.48 cm from the wound. It has two disadvantages; if there is sensitivity to neomycin it must be stopped; it is expensive.

سکیٹرن : نیومائی سین اور میسٹراسین زخموں کے لئے مستعمل۔

Cicatrix *(sik'-a-triks)* [L. scar]. A scar; formed from connective tissue. See KELO- ID--cicatricial, adj.; cicatrization, n.; cicatrize, v.i.; v.t.

ندبہ : ایک نشان۔ اتصالی نسیج سی بنا ہوا۔ اندمال زخم کے بعد نشان۔

Cidex *(si-deks_*. Aqueous glutaraldehyde, a potent bactericidal agent useful for delicate surgical instruments and lenses.

سائی ڈیکس : آبی گلوٹرلڈیہائڈ اوزاروں اور عدسوں کے لئے جراثیم کش۔

Cidomycin *(sid-o-mi'-sin)*. Gentamicin sulphate (q.v.).

سائیڈومائی سن : دیکھئے جنٹامسن سلفیٹ۔

Cilia *(sil'-i-a)* [L.]. 1. The eyelashes. 2. Microscopic hair-like projections from certain epithelial cells. Membranes containing such cells are known as ciliated membranes, e.g. those lining the trachea and Fallopian tubes--cilium, sing,; ciliary, ciliated, cilial, adj.

اہداب۔ مژگانین : لاطینی لفظ۔ (۱) پلکیں (۲) بعض بیرونی یا سطحی خلیوں کے خوردبینی بال نما ابھار یا ساختیں ایسی جھلیوں کو ہدبی جھلیاں کہا جاتا ہے۔ ناک میں میوکس جھلی کی اپی تھیلیم میں باریک بال جو اپنی حرکت سے ناک کی گندی گرد آلود رطوبت یا بلغم کو لگاتار باہر نکالتے رہتے ہیں۔

Ciliary *(sil'-i-a-ri)* [L. cilium, eyelid]. Hair-like. **c.body,** a specialized structure in the eye connecting the anterior part of the choroid to the circumference of the iris; it is composed the ciliary muscles and processes. **c. muscle** fine hair-like muscle fibres arranged in circular manner to form a greyish-white ri immediately behind the corneoscler junction. **c. process,** about 70 in number, a projections on the undersurface of the choro which are attached to the **c. muscles.**

بی : لاطینی لفظ سلیم بمعنی پپوٹا سے ماخوذ۔ بال نما۔

Cimetidine *(sim-et'-i-din)* A histamine H receptor antagonist which inhibits bo resting and stimulated gastric acid secretio Useful for active duodenal and prepylor ulcers; should be taken after meals.

Cimex *(si'-meks)*. A genus of insects of th family cimicidae. Cimex lectularius is th common bedbug, parasitic to man; blood ucking.

ں کھٹل : حشرات کا ایک جنس۔ کھٹل بھی اس کی ایک نوع۔

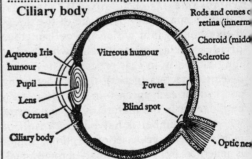

Ciliary body

Rods and cones c retina (innerm
Choroid (midd
Sclerotic
Vitreous humour
Aqueous humour
Iris
Pupil
Lens
Cornea
Ciliary body
Fovea
Blind spot
Optic ne

Cinchocaine *(sin'-ko-kan)*. Powerful loc anaesthetic used for surface anaesthetic (1 2 per-cent), infiltration (0.05 to 0.2 per-cen and spinal anaesthesia. Lozenges, supp sitories and ointment are available.

کین : طاقتور مقامی طور پر سن کرنے والی دوا۔

Cinchona *(sin-ko'-na)*. The bark from whi quinine (q.v.). is obtained. Occasionally us as a bitter tonic.

نا : چھال جس سے کونین حاصل کی جاتی ہے۔

Cinchonism *(sin-kon-ism)*. Quininism (q.v.).

نیت : دیکھئے کونینیزم۔

Cincophen *(sin'-ko-fen)*. Analgesic used in chronic gout and acute rheumatic fever. Toxic reactions such as nausea and jaundice may be severe.

سنکوفین : پرانے جوڑوں کے درد اور اس قسم کے بخار میں مستعمل۔ زہریلے ردعمل مثلاً متلی یرقان وغیرہ واقع ہوتے ہیں۔

Cineangiocardiography *(sin-e-an'-ji-o-kar-di-og'- ra-fi)* Motion picture of passage of contrast medium through the heart and blood vesells.

سائین اینجیو کارڈیوگرافی : دل اور خونی رگوں میں سے موازنی واسطے کے راستے کی موشن پکچر۔

Cineangiography *(sin-e-an-ji-og'-ra-fi)*. Motion picture angiography (q.v.).

سائین اینجیوگرافی : دیکھئے موشن پکچر انجیوگرافی۔

Cineradiography *(sin-e-ra-di-og'-ra-fi)*. [G. kineo, to move; L. radius, ray; G. graphein, to write]. Moving picture radiography, e.g. showing joints or heart in action.

سائن ریڈیوگرافی : یونانی لفظ کینو بمعنی حرکت کرنا' لاطینی لفظ ریڈیس بمعنی شعاع یا کرن اور یونانی لفظ گریفین بمعنی لکھنا سی مرکب اصطلاح۔ ریڈیوگرافی کی متحرک فلم۔ مثلاً جوڑوں اور دل کو ایکشن میں دکھانا۔

Cineradiology *(sin-e-ra-di-ol'-o-ji)*. Specialist interpretation of cineradiography.

سائن ریڈیالوجی : سائن ریڈیوگرافی کی وضاحت۔

Cinnamon *(sin'-a-mon)*. An aromatic bark with carminative and mildly astringent properties. Sometimes used with chalk and other carminatives in diarrhoea.

دارچینی : ایک خوشبودار چھال۔

Cinnarizines *(sin-a-ri'-zen)*. Antihistamine drug, useful in Meniere's disease; has powerful vestibular sedative effect without concomitant hypnotic effect.

ستاری زین : اینٹی ہسٹامن دوائی۔

Circadianrhythm Rhythm with a periodicity of 24 hours.

سرکیڈین ردم : ۲۴ گھنٹوں کے دورانیے کے ساتھ ردم۔

Circinate *(cur'-sin-at)* [L. circinare, to make round]. In the form of a circle or segment of a circle, e.g. the skin eruptions of late syphilis, ringworm, etc.

حلقوی : دائرے یا دائرے کے ایک حصے کی صورت میں۔

Circulation *(ser-ku-la'shun)*. [L. circulare, to form a circle]. Passage in a circle--circulatory, adj.; circulate, v.i. and v.t. **c of bile,** the passage of bile from the liver cells where it is formed via the gall-bladder and bile ducts ot the small intestine, where its constituents are partly reabsorbed into the blood and thus return to the liver. **c. of cerebrospinal fluid.** takes place from the ventricles of the brain to the cisterna megna, from whence the fluid bathes the surface of the brain, and cord, including its central canal. It is absorbed into the blood in the cerebral venous sinuses. **collateral c.,** that established through anastomotic communication channels, when there is interference with main blood supply. **coronary c.,** that of blood through the heart walls, **extracorporeal c.,** blood is taken from the body, directed through a machine ('heart-lung,' 'artifical kidney') and returned to the general circulation. **fetal c.,** that of blood through the fetus. umbilical cord and placenta. **lymph c.,** that of venous blood (collected from the intestines, pancreas, spleen and stomach) to the liver before return to the heart. **pulmonary c.,** deoxygenated blood leaves the right ventricle, flows through the lungs where it becomes oxygenated and returns to the left atrium of the heart. **systemic c.,** deoxygenated blood leaves the right ventricle, flows through the lungs where it becomes oxygenated and returns to the left atrium of the heart. **systemic c.,** oxygenated blood leaves the left ventricle and after flowing throughout the body, returns deoxygenated to the right atrium.

دوران۔ گردش : دائرے میں راستہ۔ انسانی جسم میں مختلف اقسام کی گردشیں۔

Circumcision *(ser-kum-sizh'-un)* [L. circumcisus, cut around]. Excision of the prepuce or foreskin.

ختنہ : عضو تناسل کی اگلی کھال کاٹنا۔ مسلمان مذہبی طور پر یہ فریضہ انجام

دیتے ہیں۔ختنہ بچے کے ایک ماہ کے اندر کرا دینا بہتر ہے۔گوشت چمٹی سے پکڑ کر کاٹ دیا جاتا ہے اور اندرونی گوشت کے چھلکے کو پیچھے ہٹا کر کٹے ہوئے گوشت کے ساتھ لگا دیا جاتا ہے۔روئی ٹنکچر بنزوین کو بھگو کر لگا دیں۔کورنیا کے گرد۔

Circumcorneal *(ser-kum-kor'-ni-al)* [L. circum, around; corneus, horny]. Around cornea.

تدویر :جوارح کے جھولنے کا عمل۔

Circumoral *(ser-kum-or'-al)* [L. circum, around; os, mouth]. Surrounding the mouth **c. palior,** a pale appearance of the skin around the mouth, in contrast to the flushed cheeks. A characteristic of scarler fever--circumorally, adv.

گرد دہنہ :منہ کے گرد۔

Circumvallate *(ser-kum-val'-lat)* [L. circumvallare, to surround with a wall]. Surrounded by a raised ring as the lingual papillae.

حائط :زبانی ابھاروں کے طور پر ابھرے ہوئے چھلے سے گھرا ہوا۔

Cirrhosis *(sir-o'-sis)* [G. kirrhos, orange-tawny; -osis. condition]. Applied almost exclusively to degenerative changes in the liver with resulting fibrosis **c. of liver** is increasing in prosperous countries. Damage to liver cells can be by virus, microbes or toxic substances, and dietary deficiencies interfering with the nutrition of liver cells--often the result of alcoholism. Associated developments are such as ascites (q.v.), obstruction of the circulation through the portal vein with haematemesis (q.v.). jaundice and enlargement of the spleen--cirhotic, adj.

تشمع۔سختی : کسی عضو کا سخت ہونا۔جگر میں خاتمے والی تبدیلیوں پر اس کا اطلاق ہوتا ہے۔جگری خلیوں کو جراثیم' وائرس یا زہریلے مادے نقصان پہنچاتے ہیں۔

Cirsoid *(sur'soid)* [G. kirsos, enlargement of a vein; eidos, form]. Resembling a tortuous, dilated vein (varix, q.v.). **c. aneurysm,** a tangled mass of pulsating blood vessels, appearing as a subcutaneous tumour, usually on the scalp.

دوالی نما : پھیلی ہوئی ورید سے مشابہ۔

Cisterna *(sis-ter'-na)* [L. cistern]. Any close space serving as a reservoir for a body flui **c. megna** is a subarachnoid space in the cle between the cerebellum and medull oblongata--cisternal, adj.

وض :جسمانی سیال کو جمع کرنے کے لئے بند جگر۔

Cisternal puncture See PUNCTURE.

Citanest *(sit'-a-nest)*. Prilocaine (q.v.).

ائیٹانیسٹ :دیکھئے پریلوکین۔

citric acid *(sit'-rik as'-id)*. The acid present i lemons. Widely used as potassium citrate; diuretic.

وں کا تیزاب :تیزاب جو لیموں میں موجود ہوتا ہے۔ پیشاب او پوٹاشیم سٹریٹ کے طور پر عام مستعمل ہے۔

Citrin *(sit'-rin)* Syn. vitamin P. Thought t enhance the action of vitamin C in th prevention of scurvy in human beings Capillary fragility is associated with lack this substance. It is found in rose hips, citru fruits and blackcurrants.

رن :حیاتین پی۔وٹامن سی ایکشن کو زیادہ کرتا ہے۔

Clap *(klap)*. A slang term for gonorrhoea.

وزاک :سوزاک کے لئے ایک اصلاح۔

Clauidication *(klaw-di-ka'-shun)* [L. clau dicatio, a limping]. Limping because there interference with the blood supply to the leg The cause may be spasm or disease of th vessels themselves. In 'intermittent claud ication' patient experiences severe pain in th calves when he is walking; after a short re he is able to continue.

روج : ٹانگوں میں خون کی سپلائی میں خلل کی وجہ سے لنگڑانا۔

Claustrophobia *(klaws-tro-fo'-bi-a)* [I clastrum, a confined space; G. phobos, fear A form of mental disturbance in which the is a morbid fear of enclosed spaces--claust ophobic, adj.

لت ترسی :ذہنی انتشار کی ایک قسم جس میں بند جگہ کا خوف ہوتا ہے۔

Clavicle *(klav'-ikl)* [L. clavicula, a small key The collar-bone--clavicular, adj.

لی :لاطینی لفظ کلیوبکولا بمعنی چھوٹی چابی سے ماخوذ۔کالر ہڈی۔ ہنسلی کی ی۔

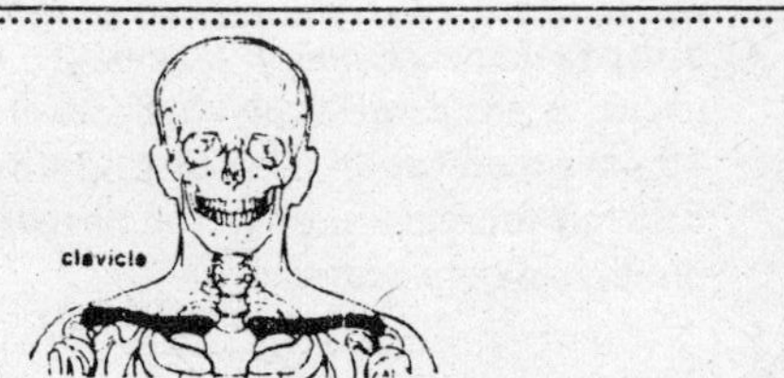

پتلی خمدار ہڈی جوشانہ کی ہڈی کی نوک سے سینہ کی ہڈی یا سٹرنم تک ہوتی ہے اور شانہ کی ہڈی کو اس کی جگہ پر رکھتی ہے۔ ہنسلی کی ہڈی کناروں پر سے موٹی اور درمیان سے پتلی ہوتی ہی جو کنارہ شانہ کی ہڈی سے جڑتا ہے، وہ دوسرے کنارے کے مقابلے میں زیادہ چوڑا ہوتا ہے۔ ہنسلی کی ہڈی سینہ کے جوف یا تھوریکس کے بالائی راستے کی حفاظت کرتی ہے۔

Clavus *(kla'-vus)* [L. nail, corn]. A corn, may be hard or soft.

گٹار : پاؤں یا پاؤں کے انگوٹھے پر گلٹی کا بننا جو سخت یا نرم ہوسکتی ہے۔

Claw-foot *(klaw-foot)*. A deformity where the longitudinal arch of the foot is increased in height and associated with clawing of the toes. It may be acquired or congenital in origin. syn., pes cavus.

چنگ پا : پاؤں کی طولانی قوس اونچائی میں بڑھ کر بدصورتی پیدا کرتی ہے۔

Claw-hand The hand is clawed and radially deviated, due to paralysis of the flexor carpi ulnaris, ulnar half of flexor digitorum longus, affecting the small muscles of the hand.

چنگ دست : ہاتھ جو پنجہ دار ہو۔

Cleft palate *(pal'-it)* [M.E. clift; L. palatum, pa late]. Congenital failure of fusion between the right and left palatal processes. Often associated with harelip.

حنک مشقوق : دائیں اور بائیں پیلیٹ کے زائدوں میں ملاپ نہ ہونا۔

Climacteric *(kli-mak'-te-rik)* [G. klimakter, rung of a ladder]. In the female, the menopause or 'change of life'. The end of the period of possible sexual reproduction, as evidenced by the cessation of menstrual periods. Other bodily and mental changes may occur. A corresponding period occurs in men and is called the **male c.**

بحرانی۔ سن یاس : یونانی لفظ کلائی میکٹر بمعنی سیڑھی کا ڈنڈا سے ماخوذ۔ مادہ میں مینو پاز یا تبدیلی۔ حیات۔ حیض بند ہو جاتے ہیں اور ممکن جنسی تولید کے عرصے کا خاتمہ ہو جاتا ہے۔

Clindamycin *(klin-da-mi'-sin)*. Derivative of lincomycin that is much more active than the parent compound.

کلنڈامائی سن : لنکومائی سن سے اخذ شدہ مرکب جو اس سے زیادہ عامل ہے۔

clinical *(klin'-ik-al)* [G. kline, bed]. Pertaining to a clinic. Practical observation and treatment of sick persons as opposed to theoretical study.

طبی : یونانی لفظ کلائن بمعنی بستر سے ماخوذ۔ کلینک سے متعلق۔

Clinimycin *(klin-i-mi'-sin)*. A brand of exytetracycline (q.v.).

کلینی مائی سن : آکسی ٹیٹرا سائیکلین کی ایک قسم۔

Clitoridectomy *(klit-or-i-dek'-to-mi)* [G. kleitoris, clitoris; ektome, excision]. Surgical removal of the clitoris.

تبظیر : یونانی الفاظ کلیٹورس بمعنی بظر اور اکٹومی بمعنی قطع کا مجموعہ۔ بظر کو اپریشن کے ذریعے قطع کرنے۔

Clitoriditis *(klit-or-id-i'-tis)* [G. kleitoris, clitoris; -itis, inflammation]. Inflammation of the clitoris.

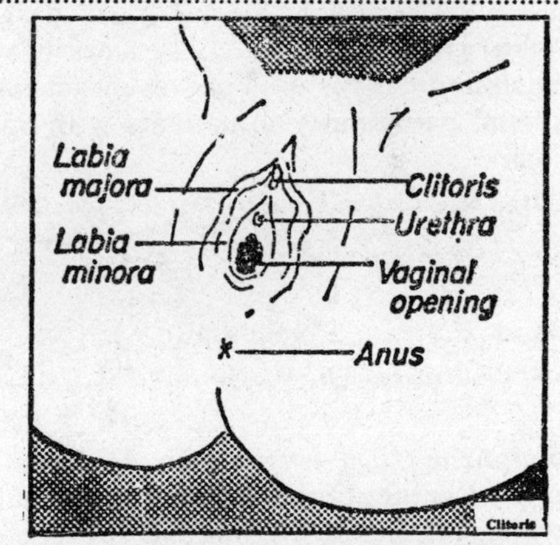

ورم بظر : یونانی الفاظ کلیٹورس بمعنی بظر اور اٹس بمعنی سوزش۔ بظر کی سوزش۔

Clitoris *(klit'-or-is)* [G. kleitoris]. A small erectile organ situated just below the mons veneris at the junction anteriorly of the labia minora.

بظر : یونانی لفظ کلیٹورس سے ماخوذ۔ چھوٹے لب کے آگے کی طرف جنکشن

پر واقع ایک چھوٹا ایستادہ عضو۔فرج کے اوپر ایک کونے مین مٹر کے دانے کی سکل کا۔اس میں کئی شریانیں اور اعصاب ہوتے ہیں۔جنسی ہیجان کے وقت یہ سخت اور واضح ہو جاتا ہے۔پیشاب کی نالی بظر اور فرج کے دہانہ کے درمیان کھلتی ہے۔انتہائی حساس جنسی عضو۔اگر اسے انگلی یا عضو تناسل کے حشفہ سے مسلا جائے تو عورت میں شدید جنسی ہیجان پیدا ہوتا ہے اور عورت مباشرت کے دوران جلد نقطۂ عروج پر پہنچی ہے۔اس کے نیچے اندام نہانی کا سوراخ ہے۔

Cloaca *(klo-a'-ka)* [L. sewer]. 1. The common opening of the intestinal and urogenital tract in fishes and birds and reptiles. 2. In osteomyelitis, the opening through the involucrum which discharges pus-cloacal, adj.

مخرج : آنت و بولی تولیدی راستوں کا مشترک سوراخ جو مچھلیوں، پرندوں اور رینگنے والے جانوروں میں پایا جاتا ہے۔

Clobetasol propionate *(klo-bet'-as-ol-pro-p-i-on-at)*. Soothing application for such skin conditions as eczema.

Clofazimine *(klo-faz'-i-men)*. Red dyegiven orally. Controls symptoms of erythema nodosum leprosum reaction in lepromatous leprosy better than prednisolone.

کلوفازمین : لال رنگ جو منہ کے ذریعے دیا جاتا ہے۔

Clofibrate *(klo-fib'-rat)*. Lowers blood cholesterol and is used to prevent fat embolism, particularly in patients with bone injury..

کلوفائی بریٹ : خون کی کولیسٹرول کو کم کرتا ہے۔انجائنہ پیک ٹورس یا درد دل مین ۳ تا ۶ گولیاں یا کیپسول روزانہ یہی خوراک برائے فالج یا سر برل ہیموریج۔

Clomid *(klo'-mid)*. Clomiphene (q.v.).

کلومڈ : دیکھیئے کلومیفین۔ماہواری کے پانچ دن ایک گولی روزانہ ۵ ایام تک برائے سیٹر یل ٹی یعنی ابتدائی بانجھ پن۔

Clomiphene *(klom'-i-fen)* (MRL. 41) 'Fertility pill". Synthetic non-steroidal compound which induces ovulation and subsequent menstruation in some otherwise anovulatory women. Consequently fertility is enhanced.

کلومی فین : تالیفی غیر سٹیرائڈ مرکب جس سے بیضہ بنتا ہے۔یہ زرخیزی یعنی بچے پیدا کرنے کی صلاحیت وک بڑھاتا ہے۔ماہواری کے پانچویں روز ایک گولی روزانہ ۵ دنوں تک، ہر ماہ چھ ماہ تک برائے ابتدائی بانجھ پن یا پرائمری سیٹر یلی ٹی۔

Clomipramine *(klom-ip'-ra-men)* One of the tricyclic antidepressants. Effective after 3 to 15 days medication. Can be given by slow i.v. drip, in increasing dose for obsessional and phobic anxiety states.

کلومی پرامین : پریشانی کی حالت میں دیا جاتا ہے۔

Clomocycline *(klo-mo-si'-klin)*. Modification of tetracycline (q.v.).

کلوموسائیکلین : ٹیٹراسائیکلین کی ترمیم شدہ صورت۔

Clonidine *(klon'-i-den)*. Similar to methyldopa, but causes less postural hypotension though it gives some patients a very dry mouth. Early results in the prvention of migraine are promising.

کلونیڈین : میتھائل ڈوپا سے مشابہ۔

Clonus *(klo'-nus)*. [G. klonos, violent). A series of intermittent muscular contractions and relaxations. Opp. tonic (q.v.)--clonic, adj.; clonicity, n.

جھٹکا : وقفوں کے ساتھ عضلات کا پھیلنا اور سکڑنا۔

Clopamide *(klo'-pa-mid)*. Thiazide diuretic. See CHLOROTHIAZIDE.

Clostridium *(klos-trid'-i-um)*. A bacterial genus. Clostridia are large Grampositive anaerobic bacilli found as commensals of the gut of animals and man, and as saprophytes in the soil. Endospores are produced which are widely distributed. Many species are pathogenic because of the exotoxins produced e.g. Clostridium telani (tetanus), C. botulinum (botulism); C. welchii (perfringens) (gas gangrene).

تکلیہ۔دوکیہ۔مغزلیہ : جراثیم کا ایک جنس۔بڑے گرام مثبت غیر ہوائی جراثیم۔آدمی کی آنت میں پائے جاتے ہیں۔زمین میں گندخور کے طور پر پائے جاتے ہیں۔بذرے پیدا کرتے ہیں۔اس کی کئی انواع بیماری پیدا کرتی ہیں۔اس کی انواع ٹیٹ نس، ویلشی اور بانولائینم ہیں۔

Clove oil *(klov)*. Has antiseptic, carminative and anodyne properties. Used to relieve toothache.

لونگ کا تیل : دافع تعفن۔دانت یا ڈاڑھ کے درد کو آرام پہنچاتا ہے۔

Cloxacillin *(kloks-a-sil'-lin)*. Semisynthetic penicillin active against penicillin-resistant staphylococci. Acid stable. Given orally or parenterally.

کلوکسا سلین : نیم تالیفی پنسلین جو پنسلین سے مدافعت کرنے والے سٹیفائلو کاکسی کے خلاف عمل کرتی ہے۔

Clubbed fingers. Swelling of the soft tissue at the extremities. Seen in heart and lung disease.

کلبڈ انگلیاں : سروں پر نرم نسیج کا ورم۔ دل اور پھیپھڑے کی بیماری میں ایسا ہوتا ہے۔

Club-foot [O.N. klubba; A.S. fot]. A congenital malformation, either unilateral or bilateral. See TALIPES.

Clubfoot

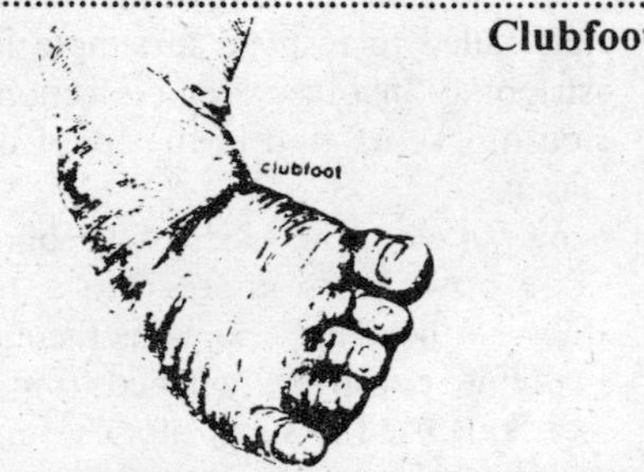

کج پائی : دیکھئے تلی پیز۔

Clumping See AGGLUTINATION.

Clutton's joints Symmetrical swelling of joints, usually painless,l the knees often being involved. Associated with congenital syphilis. [Henry Hugh Clutton, English surgeon, 1850-1909].

کلٹن کے جوڑ : جوڑوں کا ورم۔ عموماً درد نہیں ہوتا۔

Clysis *(kli' sis)* [G. klysis, a drenching by enema]. 1. The cleansing or washing out of a cavity. 2. Term used when administering fluids by other than the oral route; subcutaneously (hypodermoclysis); intravenously (venoclysis); rectally (proctoclysis).

حقنہ : (۱) کسی کہفے کو صاف کرنا یا دھونا۔ (۲) سیال کو منہ کے بجائے کسی دوسرے راستے سے داخل کرنا۔

Clysodrast *(kli'-so-drast)*. Specific enema in preparation for X-ray.

کلائیسوڈریسٹ : ایکس رے کی تیاری میں مخصوص انیما۔

Coagulase *(ko-ag'-u-las)*. An enzyme which clots plasma, e.g. thrombin, rennin. produced by some bacteria (e.g. Staphylococcus aureus). Use to type bacteria into c. negative and positive.

کوگولیس : خامرہ جو پلازما کو جماتا ہے۔ بعض جراثیم پیدا کرتے ہیں۔

Coagulum *(ko-ag'-u-lum)* [L.]. Any coagulated mass, Scab.

تکہ : لاطینی لفظ۔ کوئی جما ہوا مادہ۔

Coalesce *(ko-a-les')* [L. coalescere, to grow together]. To grow together; to unite into a mass. Often used to describe the development of a skin eruption, when discrete areas of affected skin coalesce to form sheets of a similar appearance, e.g. psoriasis. pityriasis rubra pilaris--coalescene, n.; coalescent, adj.

پیوستگی : اکٹھے اگنا۔ ایک مادہ میں متحدہ طور پر موجود ہونا۔

Coaltar The black substance obtained by the distillation of coal. Used in psoriasis and eczema. Liq. picis, carb. is an alcoholic solution of the soluble constituents of coal tar.

کولتار۔ تارکول : کوئلہ کی کشید سے حاصل شدہ کالا مادہ۔ خارش میں مستعمل۔

Coarctation *(ko-ark-ta'-shun)* [L. coarctare, to press together]. Contraction, stricture, narrowing; applied to a vessel or canal.

تقابل : سکڑاو یا تنگی۔ کسی کینال یا رگ پر اس کا اطلاق کیا جاتا ہے۔

Cobadex *(kob'-a-deks)*. Cream containing hydrocortisone which is not absorbed through the skin and so does not produce local or systemic side effects.

Cocain *(ko'-bawlt)*. A mineral element considered nutritionally essential in minute traces. Thought to be linked with iron and copper in prevention of anaemia. **Co 58,** used as tracer in study of cobalt metabolism **Co 60** super sedinp radium in radiotherapy **(Co bomb). Co edetate,** used in cyanide poiconing.

کوبالٹ : ایک معدنی عنصر جو قلیل مقدار میں لازمی ہے۔ خون کی کمی مفید ہے۔

Cobalt *(ko-kan')* . Powerful local anaesthetic obtained from coca leaves. It is toxic, especially to the brain. It may cause agitation, disorientation, and convulsions. It can induce addiction. It has vasoconstrictor properties, hence the blanching which occurs when it is applied to mucous membranes. It is now largely replaced by less toxic compounds such as procaine and lignocaine but is still used as eye drops, often with homatropine.

کوکین : کوکا کے پتوں سے حاصل شدہ نشہ آور دوا۔ دماغ کے لئے مضر۔ اس کی عادت پڑ جاتی ہے۔

Cocainism *(ko-kan'-izm)*. Mental and physical degeneracy caused by a morbid craving for, and excessive use of cocaine.

کوکینیت : کوکین کے زیادہ استعمال سے جسم وذہن کا متاثر ہونا۔

Coccus *(kok'-us)* [G. kokkos, berry]. A spherical, or nearly spherical bacterium--cocci, pl.; coccal, coccoid, adj.

کاکس۔ بنقہ : گول جرثومہ۔ گچھول کی شکل میں ہوں تو سٹے فیلو کا کسی' زنجیر کی صورت میں ہوں تو سٹر پٹو کا کسی اور دو اکٹھے ملے ہوں تو ڈپلو کا کسی کہلاتے ہیں۔

Coccydynia *(koks-e-din'-i-a)* [G. kokkyx, cuckoo, odyne, pain]. Pain in the region of the coccyx.

درد عصعص : دمچی کی ہڈی یا کاکسکس کا اپریشن کے ذریعے خاتمہ۔

Coccygectomy *(koks-e-je-kto'-mi)*. See *coccydynia*..

وجع العصعص۔ دمچی کی ہڈی کا درد : دیکھئے درد عصعص یا کاکسی ڈینا۔

Coccyx *(kok'-siks)* [G. kikkyx, cuckoo]. The last bone of the vertebral column. It is triangular in shape and curved slightly forward. It is composed of four rudimentary vertebrae, cartilaginous at birth, ossification being completed at about the 30th year--coccygeal, adj.

کاکسکس۔ عصعص۔ دمچی : ریڑھ کی ہڈی کی آخری ہڈی۔ یہ چار تخفیف شدہ مہروں پر مشتمل ہے جو سیکرم کے نیچے ایک چھوٹی نوکدار ہڈی بناتے ہیں۔ یہ ہڈی اکثر نامکمل ہوتی ہے اور اس تک حرام مغز نہیں پہنچتا۔

coccyx

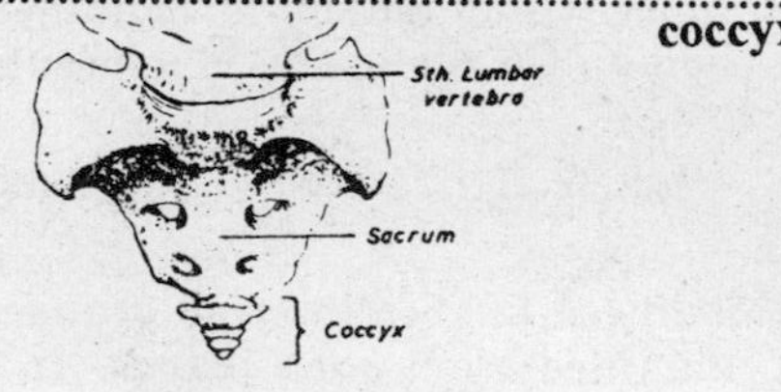

Cochlea *(kok'-le-a)* [L.snail]. A spiral canal resembling the interior of a snail shell, in the anterior part of the bony labyrinth of the ear--cochlear, adj.

قوقعہ : ایک پیچدار قنال جو کان میں ہوتی ہے۔ نالی تقریباً اڑھائی چکر لگاتی ہے۔ پہلا چکر بڑا دوسرا اس سے چھوٹا اور آخری آدھا سب سے چھوٹا ہوتا ہے۔ کاکلیا کا تعلق شنید سے ہے۔

Cockett's operation *(kok-ots)*. For recurrent varicose veins or impending ulceration which has failed to respond to simple ligation and stripping. Involves deep dissection; communicating veins tied at the level of the deep fascia.

Cocoa *(ko'-ko)*. The seeds of Theobroma cacao. The powder is made into a nourishing pleasant beverage. Contains theobromine and caffeine. **c. butter,** obtained from the roasted seeds; is used in suppositories, ointments and as an emolient.

کوکو : تھیوبروما کاؤ کے بیج۔ سفوف سے خوش گوار مشروب تیار کیا جاتا ہے۔ تھیوبرومین اور کیفین پر مشتمل۔

Codeine *(ko'-di-in)*. An alkaloid of opium. It has mild anagesic properties, and is used with aspirin and phenacetin in tab. codeine co. valuable as a cough sedative (linctus codeine) in dry and useless cough.

کوڈین۔ جوہر پوست : افیم کا الکلائڈ۔ خشک کھانسی میں مفید۔ کھانسی بند کرنے کے لئے کوڈین کف سیرپ (کوریکس) کا ایک چمچہ دن میں ۳ مرتبہ۔

Cod liver oil Contains vitamins A and D, and used on that account as a dietary supplement in mild deficiency. Can be applied as a dressing to promote healing.

کاڈ لور آئل۔ روغن ماہی : اس میں حیاتین اے اور ڈی سامل ہیں۔ اس کے ایملسن میں کاڈ لور آئل اڈرام' سفوف اکیسیا ۱۵ گرین اور ایکوا کلوروفارم ۱ اونس ہوتے ہیں۔ یہ سل دق اور رکٹس یا بچوں کی ہڈیوں کا ٹیڑھاپن کے لئے مفید۔

Coeliac *(se'-li-ak)* [g. koilia, belly]. Relating to the abdominal cavity. Applied to arteries, veins, nerves and a plexus. **c. syndrome,** now described as a number of separate and identifiable conditions of which the most important are cystic fibrosis (fibrocystic disease of the pancrease) and **c. disease** (gluten-induced enteropathy). Cystic fibrosis is largely an abnormality of the mucus-secreting glands. There is a definite excess of mucus and it appears to be thicker and more tenacious than normal. Histologically both the glands and the mucus appear normal. It usually affects the pancrease, small intestine and lungs. the mucus blocks the digestive juices, thus halting the digestion of food. As the disease progress the mucus-secreting glands are replaced by fibroid tissue and cysts. There is an increase of sodium and chloride in the sweat. Gluteninduced enteropathy is often called coeliac disease. It is due to intolerance to the protein gluten in wheat and rye, it being the gliadin fraction that is the harmful substance. Sensitivity occurs in the villi of the small intestine, and produces the malabsorption syndrome. Symptoms become apparent at three to six months, soon after the child is weaned on to cereals, as up to this time the digestion is not interferred with. On weaning the absorption of fats is impaired, and large amounts of split fats may be excreted in the stools. Se STEATORRHOEA.

شکمی ۔ معائی :یونانی لفظ کائلیا بمعنی پیٹ سے ماخوذ۔ بطنی کہفہ سے متعلق۔

Coelioscopy *(se-li-os'-ko-pi)* [G. *koilia,* belly; *skopein,* to view]. Syn., laparoscopy, peritoneoscopy (q.v.)

سیلیوسکوپی :دیکھئے پیری ٹونیوسکوپی۔

Co-enzyme *(ko-en'-zim)* [L.*cum,* with; G. *en,* in; *zyme,* leaven]. An enzyme activator; kinase. See BIOTIN.

معاون خمیر :خامرہ کے عمل کو تیز کرنے والا۔

Cogentin *(ko-jen'-tin).* Benztropine methanesulphonate (q.v.)

کوجنٹن :دیکھئے بینز ٹروپین میتھین سلفونیٹ۔

Cognition *(kog-ni'-shun)* [L.*cognitio,* recognition]. Awareness; one of the three aspects of mind, the others being affection (feeling or emotion), and conation (willing or desiring). They work as a whole but any one may dominate any mental process.

گیان ۔ تعقل :بیداری ۔ ذہن کی تین حالتوں میں سے ایک۔

Coitus *(ko'-it-us)* [L. from *coire,* to come together]. The act of sexual intercourse; copulation.

جماع :جنسی فعل کا عمل ۔ جماع کا عمل ۔ مباشرت۔

Colchicum *(kol'-chi-kum).* The dried corm of the autumn crocus. It contains colchicine, and is of value in the treatment of acute gout.

سورنجان :کچالو کا خشک کازم ۔ اس میں کولچیسین ہے جوڑوں کے درد کے لئے مفید۔

Colectomy *(ko-lek'-to-mi)* [G. *kolon; ektome,* excision]. Excision of part or the whole of the colon.

قولون براری :قولون یا اس کے ایک حصے کو قطع کرنا۔

Colic *(kol'-ik)* [G. *kolikos,* suffering in the colon]. Severe pain resulting from periodic spasm in an abdominal organ. **biliary c.,** spasm of smooth muscle in a bile duct caused by a gallstone. **intestinal c.,** abnormal peristalic movement of an irritated gut. **painter's (lead) c.,** spasm of intestine and constriction of mesenteric vessels. renal c., spasm of ureter due to a stone. uterine c., dysmenorrhoea (q.v.)--colicky, adj.

قولنج :بطنی عضو میں سخت درد۔

Coliform *(ko'-li-form)* [G. *kolon,* colon; *forma,* shape]. A word used to describe any bacterium of faecal origin which is morphologically similar to E.*coli.*

اغربالی :فضلے میں جرثومہ۔

Colistin *(kol'-is-in).* An antibiotic active against many Gram-negative organism. Useful in Pseudomonas pyocyanea infections. Less toxic than polymyxin B.

کولسٹن :ایک اینٹی بایوٹک جو گرام منفی جسیموں کے خلاف عمل کرتا ہے۔

Colitis *(ko-li'-tis)* [G. *kolon,* colon; itis, inflammation]. Inflammation of the colon.

May be acute or chronic, and may be accompanied by ulcerative lesions. **ulcerative c.**, an inflammatory and ulcerative condition of the colon. Aetiologically evidence is changing from psychosomatic factors to an immunological basis for the condition. Characteristically it affects young and early middle-aged adults, producing periodic bouts of diarrhoeal stools containing mucus and blood, and it may very in severity from a mild form with little constitutional uspet to a severe, dangerous and prostrating illness.

ورم قولون : قولون کی سوزش۔

Collagen *(kol'-a-jen)* [G. *kolla,* glue; *genesthai,* to be produced]. An albuminod substance arranged in bundles.It is the main constituent of white fibrous tissue. The collagen diseases are characterized by an inflammatory lesion of unkown aetiology affecting collagen and small blood vesse-ls,**c.diseases** said to be due to development of a hypersensitivity state. They inculde dermatomyositis. lupus erythemaosus, polyarteritis (periarteritis) nodosa, and scleroderma, and are almost in variably fatal--collagenic, collagenous,adj.

کولاجن : بنڈلوں میں مرتب البومن والا مادہ۔ سفید ریشہ دار نسیج کا بڑا جزو۔ جلد، ٹنڈان، لیگامنٹ اور ہڈی کا ریشہ دار جزو۔ پروٹین

Collagen proline hydroxylase *(kol'-a-jenpro'--len hi-droks'-i-las).* Enzyme necessary for wound healing, and vitamin C is necessary for this enzyme's maintenance and function. Reserch indicates that tissues which are rapidly synthesizing collagen (e.g. healing wounds) have high levels of this enzyme.

کولاجن پرولین ہائیڈروزائی لیز : خامرہ جو کہ زخم ٹھیک ہونے کے لئے ضروری ہے۔ اور اس کے لئے حیاتین ج ضروری ہے۔

Collapse *(kol-aps')* [L. *collapsus,* fallen togther]. I. Physical or nervous prostration.2. The falling in of a hollow organ or vessel, e.g. collapse of lung from change of air pressure inside or outside the organ.

نقاہت : کسی کھوکھلے عضو یا رگ ک متاثر ہونا۔ کسی شدید بیماری کے بعد ذہنی یا جسمانی نقاہت۔

Collar-bone [L. collum, neck; A.S. ban]. The clavicle.

ہنسلی : کلیویکل۔ ہنسلی کی ہڈی۔ گردن کی ہڈی۔

Collateral *(kol-lat'-er-I)* [L. *com,* with; *latera,* sides]. Accessory, secondary. c, circulation established by blood flowing in vessels alternative to the direct main one.

ہم بازو : زائد۔ ثانوی۔

Colles fracture. See FRACTURE.

Colles law. A mother may breastfeed a syphilitic baby without herself becoming infected, the explanation being that the mother had first acquired the disease and the fetus was thereafter infected in utero. The mother's apparent freedom form evidence of the infection implies that she is passing through the latent (hidden) phase of syphilis. [Abraham Colles, Irish surgeon, 1773-1843].

کولیز قانون : ماں اپنا دودھ آتشک زدہ بچے کو پلا سکتی ہے اور اس پر بیماری کا اثر نہیں ہوتا۔

Colliquative *(kol'-i-kwat-iv)* [L. *com,* with; *liquare,* to melt]. Profuse, excessive.

کثیر التعداد : زائد۔

Collodion *(ko-lo'-di-on).* A solution of pyroxylin with resin and castor oil. It forms a flexible film on the skin, and is used manly as a protective dressing.

کولوڈیان : رال کے ساتھ پائروکسلین اور کیسٹر ائل (ارنڈ کا تیل) کا محلول۔ یہ جلد پر حفاظتی تہہ بناتا ہے۔

Colloid *(kol'-oid)* [G. *kolla* glue; *eidos,* form]. A glue-like non-crystalline substance; diffusible but not solube in water; unable to pass through an animal membrane. Some drugs can be prepared in their colloidal form **c.goitre,** abnormal enlargement of the thyroid gland, due to the accumulation in if of viscid, iodine-containing colloid.

لسونت : ایک گاڑھا غیر قلمی مادہ۔ پانی میں ناحل پذیر لیکن قابل نفوذ۔ حیوانی جھلی میں سے ناقابل نفوذ۔

Coloboma *(kol-o-bo'-ma)* [G. *kolobos,* short-ened, mutilated]. A congenital fissure or gap in the eyeball or one of its parts, e.g., iri-dis--colobomata, pl.

شقاق : آنکھ کے گولے یا اس کے کسی حصے میں خلایا درز یا شگاف۔

Colocystoplasty *(kol-o-sis'-to-plas-ti)* [G. *kolon; kystis,* bladder; *plassein,* to form]. Operation to increase urinary bladder by using part of the colon--colocystoplastic, adj.

کولوسسٹو پلاسٹی : قولون کے حصے کے استعمال سے بولی مثانے کو بڑھانے کے لئے اپریشن۔

Colomycin Colistin (q.v.)

Colon *(ko'-lon)* [G. *kolon,* colon]. The large bowel extending from the caecum to the rectum. In its various parts it has appropriate names--ascending c., transversec., descending c., sigmoid c., spasmodic c., megacolon (q.v.)--colonic, adj.

قولون : سیکم سے ریکٹم تک کا حصہ۔

Colonoscopy *(ko-lon-os'-kop-i-).* Use of a tibreoptic colonoscope to view the inner membrane of the colon.

Colony *(kol'-on-i-)* [L. *colonia,* colony]. A mass of bacteria which is the result of multiplication of one

Colon

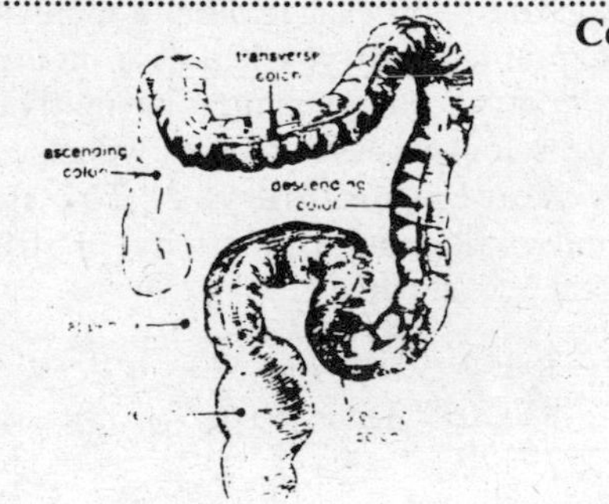

or more organisms. A colony may contain many millions of individual organisms and become macreoscopic (q.v.) its physical features are often characteristic of the species.

کالونی۔ جراثیمی نو آبادی : لاطینی لفظ کالونیا بمعنی کالونی سے ماخوذ۔ جراثیم کا جمگھاڑ جو تولید کے ذریعہ ہوتا ہے۔ لاکھوں کی تعداد میں ہوتے ہیں۔ اور نظر آنے لگتے ہیں۔

Colostomy *(kol-os'-tom)* [G. *kolon,* colon; *stoma,* mouth]. A surgically established fistula between the colon and the surface of the obdomen; this cacts as an artificial anus.

قولونی تفویہ : قولون اور بطن کی سطح کے درمیان اپریشن سے قائم شدہ سوراخ۔ مصنوعی مبرز یا مقعد۔

Colostrum *(kol-os'-trum)* [L.]. The relatively clear fluid secreted in the breasts during the first three days after parturition, before the formation of ture milk is established.

بوہلی کلوسٹرم : لاطینی لفظ۔ پہلے تین روز کی دوران چھاتیوں میں صاف سیال۔ اس کے بعد چھاتیوں میں دودھ آ جاتا ہے۔ نوزائیدہ بچے کے لئے بہترین غذا۔ بچے کے لئے مسہل یعنی بچے کے پیٹ کو صاف کر دیتا ہے۔ دودھ سے قدرے گاڑھا اور ہلکے پیلے رنگ کا۔ اس سے بچہ کئی امراض کے خلاف قوت مدافعت حاصل کرتا ہے۔ تیسرے یا چوتھے روز ماں کی چھاتیوں میں دودھ آ جاتا ہے۔

Colotomy *(kol-ot'-om-i)* [G. *kolon,* colon; *tome,* acutting]. Incision into the colon.

قولون شگافی : قولون میں شگاف ڈالنا۔

Colour blindness Achromatopsia (q.v.)

رنگ کوری : دیکھئے ایکرومیٹوپسیا یہ مرض وٹامن الف کی کمی سے ہوتا ہے۔ رنگوں کا اندھاپن۔ رنگ نظر نہ آنا۔

Colour index. A term formerly used to express the amount of heamoglobin in red blood cells. Replaced by MCHC.

لونی اشاریہ : کسی مریض کے سرخ خونی خلیوں میں ہیموگلوبن کی مقدار ظاہر کرنے کے لئے ایک اصطلاح۔

Colovesicoplasty *(kol-o-ves'-i-ko-plas-ti)* [G. *kolon,* colon; L. form]. Colocystoplasty (q.v.)

کولوویسیکو پلاسٹی : دیکھئے کولوسسٹو پلاسٹی۔

Colpitis *(kol-pi'-tis)* [G. *kolpos,* a hollow; *itis,* inflammation]. Inflammation of the vagina.

ورم مہبل : یونانی الفاظ کولپوس بمعنی کھوکھلا اور اٹس بمعنی سوزش۔ ویجائنا کی سوزش۔

Colpocentesis *(kol-po-sen-te'-sis)* [G. *kolpos,* a hollow; *kentesis,* puncture]. Withdrawal of fluid from the vagina, as in haematocolpos.

کولپوسنٹی سس : ویجائنا سے سیال کھینچنا۔

Colophysterectomy *(kol-po-his-ter-ek'-to-mi)* [G. *kolpos,* a hollow; *hystera,* womb; *ektome,* excision]. Removal of uterus through the vagina.

Coloperineorrhaphy *(kol-po-per-in-e-or'-af-i-)* [G. *kolpos,* as hollow; *perination,* space between the anus and scrotum; *rhaphe,* as suture]. The surgical repair of an injured vagina and deficient perineum.

رفوئے مہبل وعجان : زخمی ویجائنا اور تحیف شدہ پیرینیم کی اپریشن کے ذریعہ بحالی۔

Colophotography *(kol-po-fo-tog'-ra'-fi).* Filming the cervix using a camera and colposcope.

کولپوفوٹوگرافی : کیمرہ اور کولپوسکوپ استعمال کر کے سروکس کی فلم بنانا

Colporrhaphy *(kol-por'-af-i-)* [G. *kolpos,* a hollow; *rhaphe,* a suture]. Surgical repair of the vagina. Anterior c. for repair of cystocele (q.v.) and posterior c. for repair of a rectocele (q.v.)

مہبل دوزی : ویجائنا کی اپریشن کے ذریعے مرمت یا بحالی۔

Colposcope *(kol'-po-skop)* [G. *kolpos,* a hollow; *skopein,* to examine]. Culdoscope (q.v.)--colposcopically , adv.; colposcopy , n.

کولپوسکوپ۔مہبل بین : دیکھئے کلڈوسکوپ۔

Colpotomy *(kol-pot'-om-i)* [G. *kolpos,* a hollow; *tome,* a cutting]. Incision of the vaginal wall. Posterior c. to drain an abscess in the pouch of Douglas through the vagina.

مہبل شگافی : ویجائنا کی دیوار کا قطع کرنا۔

Coma *(ko'-ma)* [G. *koma,* deep sleep]. Complete loss of consciousness. Seen in alcoholism, diabetes, uraemia, and following an epileptic attack, etc.

کوما۔سحابیت۔بے ہوشی : ہوش کا مکمل ضیاع۔بے ہوشی کا تعلق دماغ کے فعل سے ہے۔اگر دماغ کا فعل کمزور ہو جائے تو بے ہوشی طاری ہو جاتی ہے۔پوری بے ہوشی کو قوما کہتے ہیں۔موت کی وجوہات میں سے ایک۔

Comatose *(kom'-a-toz)* [G. *koma,* deep sleep]. In a state of coma.

کومازدہ : کوما کی حالت میں بے ہوشی کے عالم میں۔

Comedo *(kom'-e-do)* [L. a glutton]. Blackhead. A worm-like cast formed of sebum which occupies the outlet of a sebaceous gland in the skin. Comedones have a black colour because of pigmentation; a feature of acnevulgaris.

چربی دانہ : مسا۔

Commensal *(kom-en'-sal)* [L. *cum,* with; *mensa,* table]. A parasitic microorganism adapted to grow on body surfaces of the host, forming part of the normal flora. Some commensals are potentially pathogenic.

ہم باش : طفیلی خورد جسمیہ جو میزبان کی جسمانی سطوح پر ہوتا ہے۔

Communicable *(kom-un'-ik-abl)* [L. *communicare,* to share, to impart]. Transmissible directly or indirectly from one person to another.

قابل اطلاع : ایک شخص سے دوسرے شخص تک پہنچنے کے قابل۔

Compatibility *(kom-pat-ib-il'-it-i-)* [L. *compati,* to suffer with one]. Suitability; congruity. The power of substance to mix with another without unfavourable results, e.g. two medicines, blood plasma and cells. See BLOOD GROUPS--compatible, adj.

موافقت : مناسب ہونا۔غیر موزوں نتائج کے بغیر ایک ادے کا دوسرے میں جانا۔

Compensation *(kom-pen-sa'-shun)* [L. *compensare,* to weigh against]. 1. A mental mechanism, employed by a person to cover up a weakness, by exaggerating a more socially acceptable quality. Used as c. neurosis in psychiatry to donte symptoms motivated by unconscious wish for monetary compensation for accident or injury. 2. The state of counterbalancing a functional or structural defect, e.g. **cardiac c.**

تعویض : (I) ذہنی میکانیت جسے ایک شخص کوئی کمزوری چھپانے کے لئے استعمال کرتا ہے۔(2) کسی نقص کو متوازن کرنے کی حالت۔وہ نقص ساختی یا فعلیاتی ہو سکتا ہے۔

Complan *(kom'-plan).* Powder, 100g of which contains 31g protein, 16g fat, 44g carbohydrate, and sufficient mineral salts and vitamins to maintain health.Can be taken orally or as liquid by tube.

کمپلان : سفوف کے ۱۰۰ گرام میں ۳۱ گرام لحمیات ۱۶ گرام چکنائی اور ۴۴ گرام کاربوہائیڈریٹ ہیں۔ان کے علاوہ معدنی نمکیات اور وٹامن ہیں یہ سب اشیا صحت کے لئے ضروری ہیں۔

Complement *(kom'-ple-ment)* [L. *complere,* to complete]. A normal constituent of plasma which is of great importacne in immunity mechanisms, as it combines with antigen-antibody complex (complement fixation), and this leads to the completion of reactions such as bacteriolysis and the killing of bacteria. Complement is thermolabile and non-specific and believed to consist of four fractions. **c.fixation test,** measures the amount of complement fixed by any given antigen-antibody complex.

تکملہ : پلازما کا عام جزو جوامیونٹی میں کافی اہم ہے کیونکہ یہ اینٹی جن اینٹی باڈی کمپلکس کے ساتھ ملتا ہے اوراس سے تعاملات کی تکمیل ہوتی ہے مثلاً اس سے جراثیم مرتے ہیں۔

Complex *(kom'-pleks)* [L. *complexus,* an encircling]. A series of emotionally charged ideas, repressed because they conflict with ideas acceptable to the individual, e.g. Oedipus c., a syndrome attributed to suppressed sexual desire of a son for his mother; **Electra c.,** of daughter for father.

پیچیدہ : پر جوش نظریات کا سلسلہ جو عام قابل قبول نظریات کی ضد ہوتے ہیں۔ دماغی الجھن۔ خود میں احساس کمتری' برتری یا محرومی' فرد کا ماحول کے خلاف جذباتی ردعمل

Complication *(Kom-plik-a'-shun)* [L. *complicare,* to fold together]. In medicine, an accident or second disease arising in the course of a primary disease; can be fatal.

پیچیدگی : اولیں بیماری کے دوران دوسری بیماری کا ابھرنا۔ بیماری کا پیچیدہ ہو جانا۔

Compos mentis *(kom'-pos-men'-tis)* [L.]. Of sound mind.

صحیح الدماغ ۔ سلیم العقل : صحت مند ذہن کے متعلق۔ اعلیٰ ذہنی صلاحیتوں کا حامل۔

Compound *(kom'-pownd)* [L. *componere,* to put together]. A substance composed of two or more elements, chemically combined in a definitive proportion to form a new substance with new properties.

مرکب : دو یا زیادہ عناصر کا کیمیائی طور پر مقررہ تناسب میں اس طرح ملنا کہ نئی چیز نئی خصوصیات کے ساتھ بن جائے۔

Comprehension *(kom-pre-hen'-shun)* [L. comprehensio]. Mental grasp of meaning and relationships.

ادراک : معانی وتعلقات ذہنی طور پر سمجھ جانا۔

Compress (kom'-pres). Usually refers to a wet dressing of several layers of lint. **cold c.** on the forehead relievfes **head-**ache. **glycerine** and **ichthyol c.** reduces inflammation. **lead** and **opium c.** relieves pain, swelling and bruises.

ترپٹی : لفٹ کی کئی تہوں کی گیلی ڈریسنگ

Compression *(kom-presh-un)* [L. *comprimere,* to press together]. The state of being compressed. The act of pressing or squeezing together. **cerebral c.,** arises from any space-occupying, intracranial lesion. **digital c.,** the pressure is applied by the fingers, usually to an artery to stop bleeding. **c. bandage,** see BANDAGE.

دباؤ : دبانے کی حالت۔ آپس میں دبانے یا نچوڑنے کا عمل۔ روانی خون کو دبا کر روکنا

Compromise *(kom-prom-iz)* [L. *compromissum,* mutual agreement]. A mental mechanism whereby a conflict (q.v.) is evaded by disguising the repressed wish to make it acceptable in consciousness.

مفاہمت : ایک ذہنی میکانیت جس میں جھگڑے سے بچا جاتا ہے

Conation *(ko-na-shun)* [L. *conari,* to try]. Willing or desiring. The conscious tendency to action. Oneof the three aspects of mind, the others being cognition (awareness, understanding) and affection (feeling or emotion).

طلب : چاہنا۔ خواہش کرنا۔ تیار۔ عمل کرنے کا رجحان۔ طبعی میلان کار

Concept *(kon-sept)* [L. *concipere,* to take in]. An abstract generalization resulting from the mental process of abstracting and recombining certain qualities or characteristics of a number of ideas, e.g. the individual's c. of honour, love, a rose, a house, etc.

تعقل : ایک ذہنی طریقہ جس میں کوئی اصول وضع کیا جاتا ہے۔ طرز فکر

Conception *(kon-sep-shun)* [L. *concipere,* to conceive]. 1. The act of becoming pregnant by the impregnation of the ovum by the spermatozoon. 2. an abstract mental idea of anything - conceptive, adj.

حمل، مفہوم :(۱) حاملہ ہونے کا عمل۔استقرارِ حمل۔عورت کا حاملہ ہو جانا
(۲) کسی چیز کا ذہنی نظریہ

Concordin *(kon-kor-din)* Protriptyline hydrochloride. Antidepressant (q.v.) In cases of insomnia, should not be administered later than mid-afternoon.

کنکورڈن :پروٹرپٹائلین ہائیڈروکلورائیڈ

Concretion *(kon-kre-shun)* [L. *concrescree,* to grow together]. A deposit of hard material; a calculus.

پتھری :سخت مادے کا جمع ہو جانا

Concussion *(kon-kush-un)* [L. *concussus* from *concutere,* to shake violently together]. A condition resulting from a violent jar or shock. **cerebral c.** characterized by loss of consciousnes, pallor, coldness and usually an increase in the pulse rate. There may be incontinence of urine and faeces.

صدمہ :دھماکے والے جار یا صدمے کے نتیجے میں حالت

Condensation *(kon-dens-ay-shun)* [L. *condensare,* to condense]. The process of becoming more compact, e.g. the changing of a gas to a liquid.

تکاثف :زیادہ گھنا ہونے کا طریقہ۔مثلاً گیس کا مائع میں تبدیل ہونا

Condom *(kon-dom)* A rubber sheath used as a male contraceptive.

رِفالہ :نر کے لئے ربڑ کی شیدیا غلاف۔فرنچ لیدر

Conduction *(kon-duk-shun)* [L. *conducere,* to conduct]. The transmission of heat, light or sound waves through suitable media; also the passage of electrical currents and nerve impulses through body tissues - conductivity, *n.*

ایصال :مناسب واسطوں میں سے حرارت نور یا آواز کی لہروں کی ترسیل۔
اسی طرح جسمانی بافتوں میں سے عصبی اور برقی لہروں کا گزر

Conductor *(kon-duk-ter)* [L. *conducere,* to conduct]. A substance or medium which transmits heat, light, sound, electric current, etc. **bad, good or non-c.,** designates degree of conductivity.

موصل، کنڈکٹر :کوئی مادہ یا واسطہ جو حرارت، نور، آواز یا برقی لہروں وغیرہ
کی ترسیل کرے۔

Condyloma *(kon-dil-o-ma)* [G. *kondylos,* knuckle; *-oma,* tumour]. Papiloma. Condylomata acuminta are acuminate (pointed) dry warts found under prepuce (male), on the vulva and vestibule (female)_, or on the skin of the perianal region. They are non-venereal. Condylomata lata are the highly infectious, moist, warty, excrescences found in moist areas of the body (vulva, anus, axilla, etc.) as a manifestation of late secondary syphilis - condylomatous *adj.* condylomata, *pl.*

آتشکی آبلہ :خشک آبلے نر میں عضو تناسل کی کھال کے نیچے اور مادہ میں
شرمگاہ اور دہلیز پر پائے جاتے ہیں۔

Condy's fluid *(kond-dez)* A proprietary preparation consisting of a solution of sodium permanganate (potassium permanganate is commonly substituted for it); ti is antiseptic; disintectant and deodorant.

کونڈی کا سیال :سوڈیم یا پوٹاشیم پرمینگنیٹ کا محلول جو دافع تعفن اور جراثیم
کش ہے

Confabulation *(kon-fab-u-la-shun)* [L. *confabulatio,* a talking together]. A smyptom common in confusional states when there is impairment of memory for recent events. The gaps in the patient's memory are filled in with fabrications of his own invention. Occurs in senile and toxic confusional states, cerebral trauma and Korsakoff's syndrome (q.v.)

سخن سازی :پریشانی کی حالت جس میں مریض تازہ ترین حالات بھی
بھول جاتا ہے اور خلا کو اپنی طرف سے پر کرتا ہے۔ذہنی خلجان۔خیالی دنیا میں
کھویا رہنا

Confection *(kon-fek-shun)* [L. *confectio,* a composing]. A preparation in which drugs are mixed with sugar, syrup and honey, e.g. c. of senna.

معجون :تیاری جس میں ادویات کو چینی، شربت اور شہد کے ساتھ ملایا جاتا
ہے

Conflict *(kon-flikt)* [L. *confligere,* to strike together]

. In psychiatry, presence in the unconscious o

two incompatible and contrasting wishes or emotions. When the conflict becomes intolerable, repression (q.v.) of one of the wishes may occur. Mental conflict and repression form the basic causes of many neuroses, especially hysteria.

onfluent *(kon-floo-ent)* [L. *confluere,* to flow together]. Becoming merged; flowing together; a uniting as a neighbouring pustules - confluence, *n.*

جڑواں :اکٹھے بہنا۔ باہم مل جانا۔ یکجا ہونا۔ دو پیپ دار پھوڑوں کا ایک ساتھ پھوٹنا

onfusion *(kon-fu-zhun)* [L. *confusio,* disorder]. Used to describe the mental state which is out of touch with reality and associated with a clouding of consciousness. Often present following epileptic fits, in cerebral arteriosclerosis, trauma, severe toxaemia.

اختلاط :ذہنی حالت جس کا حقیقت سے تعلق نہیں ہوتا۔ بوکھلاہٹ

ongenital *(kon-jen-it-al)* [L. *congenitus,* born together with]. Existing from birth or before. **c. dislocation of the hip** is due to faulty formation of the acetabulum. **c. heart disease,** developmental abnormalities in the anatomy of the heart, resulting postnatally in imperfect oxygenation of blood, inanifested by cyanois and breathlessness. Later there is clubbing of the fingers. See 'BLUE BABY'. **c. syphilis** is acquired by the fetusfrom the infected mother just after the 4th month of intrauterine life.

خلقی :پیدائش یا اس سے پہلے موجود۔ پیدائشی نقص یا مرض

ongestion *(kon-jest-yun)* [L. *congestio,* from *congerere,* to heap up]. Hyperemia. Passive congestion results from obstruction or slowing down of veous return, as in the lower limbs or the lungs - congest, *v.i., v.t.* congestive, *adj.*

اجتماعِ خون :ہائپر یمیا۔ وریدی خون کی واپسی میں رکاوٹ یا سست روی سے ہوجاتا ہے

ngestive heart failure A chronic inability of the heart to maintain an adequate output of blood from one or both ventricles resulting in manifest congestion and overdistension of certain veins and organs with blood, ans in an inadequate blood supply to the body tissues.

امتلائی دورۂ دل :دل وینٹریکل سے خون کی مناسب مقدار باہر نکالنے کی نااہلیت۔ اس سے جسمانی حصوں کو مناسب مقدار میں خون نہیں ملتا۔ علاج کے لئے سیڈی لے نڈیا ڈجاکس دو گولیاں صبح ۲ دوپہر ۲ شام۔ ہائیڈروکلور تھایازائیڈ (ایسی ڈریکس) ایک گولی روزانہ صبح ناشتہ کے بعد۔

Conization *(kon-iz-ay-shun)* [G. *konos,* cone]. Removal of a cone-shaped part of the cervix by the knife or cautery.

کونائیزیشن :یونانی لفظ کونوس بمعنی مخروط سے ماخوذ چاقو وغیرہ سے سروکس کے مخروط نما حصے کا خاتمہ

Conjugate *(kon-joo-gayt)* [L. *conjugare,* to yoke together]. A measurement of the bony pelvis. **diagonal c.,** the clinical measurement taken in pelvic assessment, from the lower border of the symphysis pubis to the sacral promontory=110.5 to 133.3 m.m. It is 18.9mm greater than obsterical conjugate. **obstetrical c.,** the available space for the fetal head, i.e. the distance from the sacral promontory to the posterior surface of the top of the symphysis pubis=107.9 to 114.2 mm. **true c.,** the distance from the sacral promontory to the summit of the symphysis pubis = 110.5mm.

مزدوج :ہڈی دار پلوس کی پیمائش

Conjunctiva *(kon-ungk-ti-va)* [L. *conjunctivus,* serving to connect]. The delicate transparent membrane which lines the inner surface of the eyelids (**palpebral c.**) and reflects over the front of the eyeball (**bulbar** or **ocular c.**)-conjunctival, *adj.*

کنجکٹیوا۔ آنکھ کی جھلی :نازک شفاف جھلی جو پپوٹوں کی اندرونی سطح پر ہوتی ہے اور آنکھ کے گولے کے سامنے منعکس کرتی ہے

Conjunctive

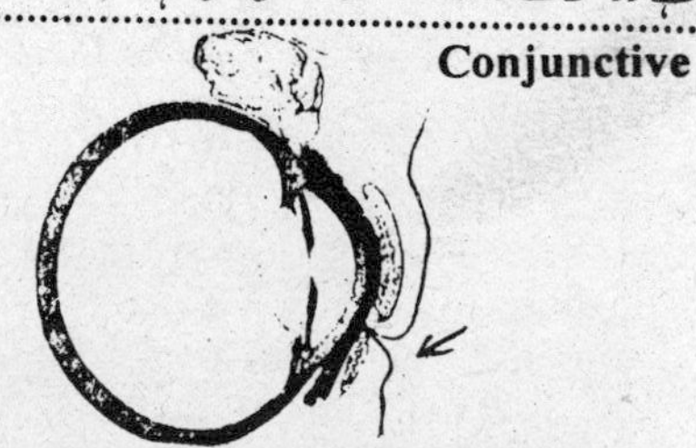

Conjunctivitis *(kon-jungk-ti-vi-tis)* [L. *conjunctivus*, serving to connect; *-itis*, inflammation]. Inflammation of the conjunctiva. **inclusion c.,** or inclusion blennorrhoea, occurs in countries with low standards of hygiene. The reservoir of infection is the urogenital tract. See TRIC AGENT.

آشوبِ چشم : کنجنکٹیوا کی سوزش

Conn'syndrome Too much aldosterone. Muscular weakness, hypertension, renal failure but no oedema. [J. Conn, American physician, 20th century].

Conotrane *(kon-o-tran)* A cream containing a silicone and penotrane (q.v.).

Consanguinity *(kon-sang-gwin-i-ti)* [L. *con*, with, *sanguis*, blood]. Blood relationship - consanguine- ous, *adj*.

قرابت : خونی رشتہ

Consolidation *(kon-sol-i-day-shun)* [L. *consolidare*, to make firm]. Becoming solid, as, for instance, the state of the lung due to exudation and organization in lobar pneumonia.

تجمد : ٹھوس ہونا۔ مثلاً نمونیہ میں پھیپھڑے کی حالت

Constipation *(kon-sti-pay-shun)* [L. *constipare*, to press closely together]. An implied chronic condition of infrequent and often difficult evacuation of faeces due to insuficient fod or fluid intake, or to sluggish or disordered action of the hbowel musculature or nerve supply, or to habitual failure to empty the rectum. Acute constipation signifies obstruction or paralysis of the gut of sudden onset.

قبض : فضلے کا مشکل سے باہر نکلنا۔ قبض ہونا۔ سبزی پھل زیادہ استعمال کیجئے۔ لیکوئڈ پرافین کے ۲ چھوٹے چمچے رات کو سوتے وقت پلایئے۔ کمپاؤنڈ افرودی سینٹ پاؤڈر (اینو، لیکسال) کے دو چھوٹے چمچے نصف گلاس پانی میں ملا کر صبح خالی پیٹ پندرہ بیس ایام تک پلایئے۔

Consumption *(kon-sum-shun)* [L. *consumere*, to consume]. 1. Act of consuming or using up. 2. Popular term of pulmonary tuberculosis (which 'consumed' the body) - consumptive, *adj*.

Contact *(kon-takt)* [L. *contactum*, from *con tingere*, to touch]. 1. Direct or indirec exposure to infection. 2. A person who ha been so exposed. **c. lens,** of glass or plastic worn under conjunctiva (in place of spec tacles) for therapeutic or cosmetic purposes.

رف۔ دِق : (۱) کسی شے کو استعمال میں لانے کا عمل (۲) پھیپھڑوں کے
پ دق کے لئے مشہور اصطلاح

Contagion *(kon-taj-un)* [L. *contagio*, to touch] Communication of disease from body to bod - contagious, *adj*. contagiousness, *n*.

نعدی مرض : ایک جسم سے دوسرے جسم میں بیماری کا پہنچنا

Contraceptive *(kon-tra-sep-tiv)* [L. *contra*, against; *conceptio*, conception]. An ager used to prevent conception, e.g. condon spermaticidal vaginal pessary or cream rubb cervical cap, intrauterine contraceptive devic (see IUCD), oral female medication contraception, *n*.

نع حمل : حمل روکنے کے لئے ایک عامل

Contract *(kon-trakt)* [L. *contractum*, fro *contrahere*, to draw together]. 1. Draw toge ther, shorten, decrease in size. 2. Acquire b contagion or infection.

ڑنا : (۱) سائز میں کم ہونا۔ مختصر ہونا۔ (۲) چھوت کے ذریعے حاصل کرنا

Contractile *(kon-trak-til)* [L. *contractum* Possesing the ability to shorten, usually whe stimulated, special property of muscle tissue contractility, *n*.

باضی : چھوٹا کرنے کی اہلیت رکھنا۔ عموماً جب اسے تحریک کیا جائے۔
لاتی نسیج کی مخصوص خاصیت

Contraction *(kon-trak-shun)* [from L. *contrahere*, to draw together] Shortenin especially applied to muscle fibres.

ضار : چھوٹا کرنا۔ اس اصطلاح کا اطلاق خصوصاً عضلاتی ریشوں پر ہوتا

Contracture *(kon-trak-ture)* [L. *contractus*, from *contrahere*, to draw togethe Shortening of muscle or scar tissue, prod cing deformity. **Dupuytren's c.,** painle chronic flexion of the digits, especially third and fourth, towards the palm; aetiology uncertain. some cases associated with hepatic cirrhosis. See VOLKMANN. [Guilame Dupuytren, French surgeon, 1777-1835].

انقباض : عضلے کا چھوٹا ہونا جس سے اس کی شکل بگڑ جاتی ہے

Contraindication *(kon-tra-in-dik-a-shun)* [L. *contra,* opposite to; *indicare,* to indicate]. A sign or symptom suggesting that a certain line of treatment (usually used for that disease) should be dis- continued or avoided.

عکسی علامت (مرض) : لاطینی الفاظ کنٹرا بمعنی خلاف اور انڈیکیٹر بمعنی ظاہر کرنا کا مجموعہ۔ علامت جس سے ظاہر ہوتا ہے کہ علاج کا یہ رخ کر دینا چاہئے۔

Contralateral *(kon-tra-lat-er-al)* [L. *contra,* opposite to; *latus,* side]. On the opposite side - contra- laterally, *adv.*

مقابل جانبی : مخالف سمت پر

Contre-coup *(kong-tr-koo)* [F.] Injury or damage at a point opposite the impact, resulting from transmitted force. More likely to occur in an organ or part containing fluid, as the skuli.

ضرب متقابل : فرانسیسی لفظ۔ ایک نقطے پر نقصان یا زخم

Controlled cord traction Used after the firm contraction of the uterus is felt follwing deliver and in response to an oxytocic. One hand holds the lower uterus with the index finger and exerts upward pressure on the corpus. Steady pressure downwards on the cord (using other hand) counteracts this upward pressure on the uterus and the placenta is usually delivered easily. Some people call this method a modified Brandit Andews Technique.

کنٹرولڈ کارڈ ٹرشن : بچے کی پیدائش کے بعد دباؤ ڈالنے کا طریقہ جس سے پلیسنٹا آسانی سے باہر آ جاتا ہے۔

Contusion *(kon-tu-zhun)* [L. *contusus,* crushed] A bruise; slight bleeding into tissues whilst the skin remains unbroken - contuse, *v.t.*

کوفتگی : بافتوں میں خون کا معمولی جاری ہونا۔ جبکہ کھال غیر شکستہ رہتی ہے۔ رگڑ خراش چوٹ اوپر لگتی ہے اور خون بہت نیچے جا کر جمع ہوتا ہے

Convection *(kon-vek-shun)* [L. *convectio,* from *convehere,* to carry together]. Transfer of heat from the hotter to the colder part; the heated substance (air or fluid), being less dense tends to rise. The colder portion, flowing in to be heated, rises in its turn, thus c. currents are set in motion.

حمل۔ ایصال حرارت : گرم حصے سے سرد حصے کی طرف حرارت کا انتقال

Conversion *(kon-ver-shun)* [L. *conversio,* turn round] Psychological conflict manifesting as a physical symptom.

عکس : نفسیاتی تضاد۔ نفسیاتی الجھنوں کا اظہار

Convolutions *(kon-vo-loo-shunz)* [L. *convolutum,* to roll together]. Folds, twists or coils as found in the intestine, renal tubules and surface of brain - convoluted, *adj.*

تلافیف : بل، جھیں یا چکر جیسا کہ آنتوں، بولی نلیوں اور دماغی سطح پر ہیں

Convulsions *(kon-vul-shunz)* [L. *convulsus,* from *convellere,* to rend]. Involuntary contractions of muscles resulting from abnormal cerebral stimulation from many causes. Occur with or without loss of consciousness, **clonic c.** show alternating contraction and relaxation of muscle groups. **tonic c.** reveal sustained rigidity - convulsive, *adj.*

تشنج : عضلات کا غیر ارادی طور پر سکڑنا۔ تشنج کے دورے جن میں اعضا اور جسم کے عضلات میں اینٹھن ہوتی ہے

Convulsive therapy *(kon-vul-siv-ther-a-pi)* Electroplexy; electrotherapy, electroconvulsive therapy (ECT). One of the most useful physical methods of treatment for mental disorders, notably depressive states, mania, stupor. Introduced in 1937 by Cerletti and Bini. Injections of cardiazol or metrazol also produce convulsions, and were introduced by Meduna in 1934 and widely used until the introduction of ECT.

تشنجی طریق علاج : ذہنی عارضہ کے علاج کا ایک طریقہ۔ مرض کا برقی علاج۔ مثلاً دماغی مرض

Cooley's anaemia Mediterranean anaemia or ṭhaiasaemia (q.v.) [Thomas Benton Cooley, American physician, 1871-1945].

کولی انیمیا : خون کی کمی کا مرض۔ بچوں میں ہوتا ہے اس کا علاج معلوم نہیں

Co-ordination *(ko-awr-din-ay-shun)* [L. *cum,* together; *ordinare,* to regulate]. Moving in harmony. **muscular c.,** the harmonious action of muscles, permitting free, smooth and efficient movements under perfect control.

ارتباط : اکٹھے ملکر حرکت کرنا

Copper, Present in traces in all animal tissues. Copper salts havẹ little use in medicine except the sulphate. This is used occasionlly as an astringent lotion, and in phosphorus poisoning. Copper sulphate is also used in Benedict'c and Fehling's solutions for testing urine for glucose.

تانبا : تمام حیوانی بافتوں میں قلیل مقدار میں موجود۔ کاپر سلفیٹ ادویات میں مستعمل ہے۔ پیشاب کے ٹیسٹ میں مستعمل۔

Coprolalia *(kop-ro-la'-li-a)* [G. *kopros,* dung; *ḷalia,* speech]. Filthy or obscene speech. Occurs as a symptom most commonly in cerebral deterioration or trauma affecting frontal lobes of the brain.

فحش کلامی : یونانی الفاظ کوپروس بمعنی گوبر اور لیلیہ بمعنی تقریر کا مجموعہ۔ گندگی یا فحش تقریر۔ دماغ کے اگلے لوب متاثر ہوتے ہیں۔

Coprolax *(kop'-ro-laks)* Dioctylsodium sulphosuccinate (q.v.).

کاپرولیکس : دیکھئے ڈائی آکٹائل سوڈیم سلفوسکسی نیٹ ایک دوائی۔

Coproporphyrin *(kop-ro-por-fi'-rin)* [G. *kopros,* dung; *porphyros,* purple]. Naturally occurring porphyrin in the faeces.

کوپروپورفائیرن : فضلے میں قدرتی طور پر پائی جانے والی پورفائیرن۔

Copulation *(kop-u-la'-shun)* [L. *copulare,* to bind together]. Sexual intercourse.

مباشرت : جنسی انٹرکورس۔ جماع۔

Coramine *(kor'-a-min).* Nikethamide (q.v.)

کورامین : دیکھئے نکیتھامائیڈ۔ مقوی قلب دوائی۔ دل گھٹنے اور بجلی سے جلنے پر ۲سی سی کا ٹیکہ۔ ایک ٹیکہ برائے سن سٹروک الرجی سٹوپر یا مدہوشی

Cord [G. *chorde* , string]. A thread-like structure. **spermatic c.,** that which suspends the testicles in the scrotum. **spinal c.,** a cord-like structure which lies in the spinal column, reaching from the formaen magnum to the first or second lumbar vertebra. It is a direct continuation of the medulla oblongata and is about 45.72 cm long in the adult. **umbilical c.,** the navel-string, attaching the fetus to the placenta. **vocal c.,** the membranous bands in the larynx, vibrations of which are responsible for the voice.

عصبہ۔ نخاع۔ ڈورا : دھاگہ نما ساخت۔

Cordilox *(kor'-dil-oks).* Verapamil (q.v.)

Cordotomy *(kor-dot-om-i-)* [G. *chorde,* string; *tome,* a cutting]. See CHORDOTOMY.

نخاع شگافی : دیکھئے کارڈوٹومی۔

Core *(kawr).* Central portion, usually applied to the slough in the centre of a boil.

قلب۔ مغز : مرکزی حصہ۔

Corlan *(kor'-lan).* Hydrocortisone (q.v.)

Corn *(kawrn)* [L. *cornu,* horn]. A coneshaped overgrowth and hardening of epidermis, with the point of the cone in the deeper layers; produced by friction or pressure, hard c. usually occurs over a toe joint. soft c., occurs between the toes.

عرن : اپی ڈرمس کا سخت ہونا اور مخروط نما زائد بڑھاؤ۔ مخروط کی نوک گہری تہوں میں ہوتی ہے۔

Cornea *(kor'-ni-a)* [L. *corneus,* horny]. The outwardly convex transparent membrane forming part of the anterior outer coat of the eye. It is situated in front of the iris and pupil and merges backwards into the sclera--corneal, adj.

قرنیہ : بیرونی محدب شفاف جھلی جو آنکھ کی اگلی بیرونی جوت کا حصہ بناتی ہے۔

Corneal graft *(kor'-ni-al)* [L. *corneus,* norny O.F. *greffe,* from G. *graphein,* to write] Corneal opacity excised and replaced by healthy, transparent, human cornea from a donor. Keratoplasty.

قرنی پیوند : قرنیہ کا غیر شفاف ہونا۔ ایسے قرنیہ کی جگہ دوسرا انسانی صحت مند قرنیہ لگانا۔

Corneoplasty *(kor-ni-o-plas'-ti)* [L. *corneus* horny; G. *plassein,* to from]. Synkeratoplasty See CORNEAL GRAFT.

کورنیو پلاسٹی : دیکھئے قرنی پیوند۔ کسی شخص کی تندرست آنکھ نابینا کو لگانا۔

Corneoscleral *(kor'-ni-o-skle'-ral)* [L. *corneus,* horny; G. *skleros,* hard]. Pertaining to the cornea and sclera, as the circular junction of these structures.

قرنیتی قرحی : قرنیہ اور سکلیرا سے متعلق۔

Coronary *(kor'-on-a-ri)* [L. *corona,* crown]. Crown-like; encircling, as of a vessel or nerve. **c.,arteries,** those supplying the heart, the first pair to be given off by the aorta as it leaves the left ventricle. Spasm or narrowing of these vessles produces angina pectoris. **c.,sinus,** channel receiving most cardiac veins and opening into the right atrium, **c.,thrombosis,** occlusion of a coronary vessel by a clot of blood.

اکلیلی : لاطینی لفظ' کردنا' بمعنی تاج سے ماخوذ۔تاج کی مانند۔کسی عصب یا رگ کے گرد گھیرا۔کاروزی تھرامبوسز یا ہارٹ اٹیک کی وجہ دل کو خون پہنچانے والی کسی شریان کا بند ہونا ہے۔

بدن : لاطینی لفظ۔ایک جسم۔

Corpuscle *(kor-pus'-l)* [L. *corpusculum,* small body]. A microscopic mass of protoplasm. There are many varieties but the term generally refers to the red and white blood cells. See ERYTHROCYTES and LEUCOCYTES--corpuscular, adj.

Coronary artery

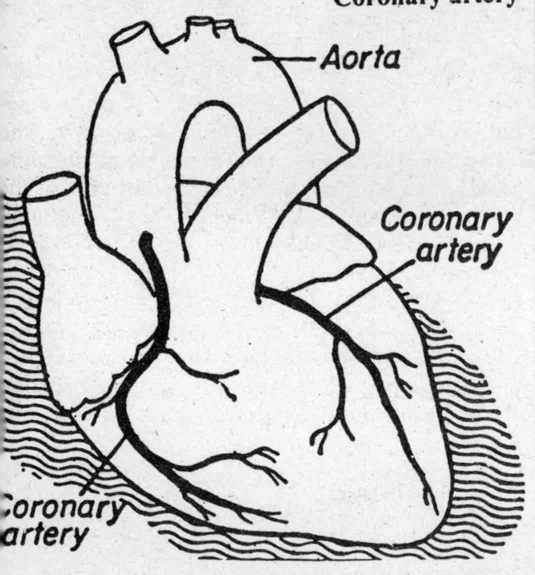

جسیمہ۔دانہ : لاطینی لفظ کارپسکولم۔بمعنی چھوٹا جسم۔مادہ حیات یا نخر مایا کا خوردبینی مادہ۔اس اصطلاح کا اطلاق عام طور پر سرخ و سفید خونی خلیوں پر ہوتا ہے۔خون کے سرخ دانے ہڈیوں میں پیدا ہوتے ہیں۔

Corective *(kor-ek'-tiv)* [L. *correctum,* from *corrigere,* to correct]. Changes, counteracts or modifies something harmful.

مصلح معدل : ضرررساں چیز میں تبدیلی یا ترمیم۔

Corigan's pulse. See PULSE.

Corrosive sublimate *(kor-ro'-ziv sub'-lim-at).* Perchloride of mercury (q.v.).

سلیمانی : مرکری پرکلورائیڈ۔

Cortex *(kor'-teks)* [L. rind or bark]. 1. The outer bark or covering of a plant.2. The outer layer of an organ beneath its capsule or membrane-cortices, pl; cortical, adj.

کارٹیکس۔پوست : لاطین لفظ بمعنی چھال۔(1) پودے کی بیرونی چھال۔ (2) کیپسول یا جھلی کے نیچے کسی عضو کی بیرونی پرت۔

Corticoid *(kor'-ti-koid).* A name for the several groups of natural hormones produced by the adrenal cortex and for synthetic compounds with similar actions. Examples of the three main groups are hydrocortisone, cortisone, prednisolone and prednisone in the first, deoxycortone acetate (DCA or DOCA) in the second, and the sex coronaviruses (kor-o-n-a-vi'-rus-es). A newly recognized group of viruses that can cause the common cold.

Corpulmonale *(kor-pul-mon-a-le')* [L. cor, heart; pulmo, lung]. Heart disease following on disease of lung (emphysema, silicosis, etc.) which strains the right ventricle.

کورپلمونالی : لاطینی لفظ کور بمعنی دل اور پلمو بمعنی پھیپھڑا کا مجموعہ۔پھیپھڑے کی بیماری کے بعد دل کی بیماری۔

Corpus *(kor'-pus)* [L.]. A body c., luteum, the yellow body formed in the ovary after rupture of a Graafian follicle and subsequent expulsion of the ovum. The false c.I. is formed in the non-pregnant state and persists for approximately one month, when it is reabsorbed. The true c.I. occurs in pregnancy and persists for 12 wks. See FOLLICLE--corpora, pl.homrmones in the third.

کارٹیکائڈ : ایڈرینل کارٹیکس سے تیار شدہ قدرتی ہارمونوں کے مختلف گروہوں کا نام۔ ایسے ہی تعاملات والے تالیفی مرکبات کا بھی نام۔

Corticosteroids *(kor-ti-ko-ster'-oids)*. Hormones which are steroids and produced by the adrenal cortex.

کارٹیکوسٹیرائڈز : ہارمون جو سٹیرائڈ ہوں اور ایڈرینل کارٹیکس سے پیدا ہوں۔

Corticotrophin *(kor-ti-ko-trof'-in)*. The hormone of the anterior pituitary gland which specifically stimulates the adrenal cortex to produce corticoids. Available commercially as a purified extract of animal anterior pituitary glands (ACTH). Only active by injection.

کارٹیکوٹروفن : اگلی پیچوایٹری گلینڈ کا رہامون جو خصوصی طور پر ایڈرینل کارٹیکس کو کارٹیکائڈز پیدا کرنے کی تحریک کرتا ہے۔

Cortisol *(kor'-ti-zol)*. Hydrocortisone , in adrenal cortical steroid essential to life. Increased in malignant phase hypertension but not in other forms of hypertension.

کارٹی زال : ہائیڈوکارٹیسون۔ ایک ایڈرینل کارٹیکل سٹیرائڈ جو زندگی کے لئے لازمی ہے۔

Cortisone *(kor'-ti-zon)*. One of the principal hormones of the adrenal gland. Converted into cortisol before use by the body. It has powerful anti-inflammatory properties, and is used in ophthalmic conditions, rheumatoid arthritis, pemphigus and Addison's disease. Side effects, such as salt and water retention, may limit therapy, and newer derivatives are now preferred for some conditions.

کارٹیسون : ایڈرینل گلینڈ کا ایک اہم ہارمون مختلف امراض کے لئے مفید۔ نقطۂ پگھلاؤ ۲۱۵° س' جوڑوں کے درد میں مفید۔

Corynebacterium *(kor-i-ne-bak-ter'-i-um)*. A bacterial genus. Gram-positive,rod-shaped bacteria averaging 3 microns in length, showing irregular staining in segments (metachromatic granules). Many strains are parasitic and some are pathogenic, e.g. *Corynebacterium diphtheriae*, producing a powerful exotoxin.

گزری جرثومہ : جراثیم کا ایک جنس۔ گرام مثبت۔ سلاخ نما جراثیم جن کی لمبائی تقریباً ۳ مائیکرون ہے۔ کئی طفیلی ہیں جبکہ بعض بیماریاں پیدا کرتے ہیں۔

Coryza *(kor-i-za)* [G. *koruza*, running at nose]. An acute upper respiratory infection of short duration; highly contagious; causative viruses include rhinoviruses, coronaviruses and adenoviruses (q.v.)

شدید زکام : وائرس کی وجہ سے تنفس کی بیماری۔ کم عرصہ رہتی ہے۔ اس کا زور ۳ ایام تک رہتا ہے۔ ناک میں کھجلی کے ساتھ پتلا پانی بہنے لگتا ہے۔ ہلکا بخار، سردرد۔ تیسرے دن بلغم گاڑھا ہو جاتا ہے۔

Cosmetic *(kos-met'-ik)* [G. *kosmesis*, an adorning]. That which is done to improve the appearance or prevent disfigurement.

حسن افروز : شکل وشباہت کو بہتر کرنے والا۔ اشیاء آرائش حسن۔ سنگھار کا سامان جو زیادہ تر خواتین استعمال کرتی ہیں۔

Costive *(kos'-tiv)* [O.F. costive, form L. constipare, to press together]. Lay term for constipation--costiveness, n.

قابض : قبض کے لئے ایک اصطلاح۔

Costoclavicular *(kos-to-klav-ik'-ul-ar)* [L. *cosia*, rib; *clavicula*, small key]. Pertaining to the ribs and the clavicle. c, **syndrome,** syn, for cervical rib syndrome. See CERVICAL.

ضلعی ترقوی : پسلیوں اور ہنسلی کی ہڈی سے متعلق۔

Co-trimoxazole *(ko-tri-moks'-a-zol)*. Active against most urinary pathogens.

Cotyledon *(kot-il-e'-don)* [G. *kotyledon* any cup-shaped hollow]. One of the subdivisions of the uterine surface of the placenta.

فلقہ جنین : پلیسنٹا کی یوٹری سطح کی تقسیموں میں سے ایک۔

Coumadin *(koo'-ma-din)*. A proprietary brand of warfarin. Derivative of discoumarol (q.v.)

کوماڈن : ڈائی کومارول سے اخذ شدہ۔

Counterextension *(kown'-ter-eks-ten'-shun)* [L. *contra*, against; *extendere*, to extend]. Traction upon the proximal extemity of a fractured limp opposing the pull of the extension apparatus on the distal extremity.

توسیع متقابل : ٹوٹے ہوئے بازو یا ٹانگ کے اگلے سرے پر کھچاؤ۔

Counterirritant *(kown-te-ir'-it-ant)* [L. *contra*, against; *irritar*, to irritate]. An agent, which , when applied to the skin, produces an inflammatory reaction (hyperaemia) relieving congestion in underlying organs--counterirrtation. n.

خراش آور : ایک عامل جو جلد پر لگانے کی صورت میں سوزش پیدا کرتا ہے ۔جلد کو سرخ کر دیتا ہے۔

:owper's glands *(kow'-perz)*. Bulbourethral glands. Two in number, lying lateral to the membranous urethra, below the prostrate gland, and deep to the perineal membrane. They open viashort ducts into the anterior (penile) uretha. [William Cowper, English surgeon. 1666-1709.]

غدہ ورمی : بلبو یوریتھرل غدود۔ ان کی تعداد دو ہے پراسٹریٹ غدود کے نیچے واقع ۔ ایک انگریز سرجن ولیم کاؤپر کے نام پر جس کا دور حیات ۱۶۶۶ء تا ۱۷۰۹ء۔

:oxa *(koks'-a)* [L.]. The hip joint . **c,valga,** an increase in the normal angle between neck and shaft of femur. **c.vara,** a decrease in the normal angle plus torsion of the neck, e.g. slipped femoral epiphysis--coxae, pl.

کو لہے کا جوڑ :لاطینی لفظ۔ چوتڑ کا جوڑ۔

:oxalgia *(koks-al'-ji-a)* [L. *coxa,* hip; G. *algos,* pain]. Literally pain in the hip joint. Often used as syn, for hip disease.

کو لہے کا درد : لاطینی لفظ کاکسا بمعنی چتون اور یونانی لفظ الگوس بمعنی درد سے مرکب اصطلاح چوتڑ کے جوڑ میں درد۔

:oxitis *(koks'-i-tis)* [L. *coxa,* hip; G. *itis,* inflammation]. Inflammation of the hip joint.

ورم لوض : لاطینی لفظ کاکسا بمعنی چتون اور یونانی لفظ ائس بمعنی سوزش سے مرکب اصطلاح چوتڑ کے جوڑ میں سوزش۔

:oxsackie viruses . First isolated at Coxsackie, N.Y. One of the three groups included in the family of enteroviruses. Divided into groups A and B. Many in groups A appear to be non-pathogenic. Others cause aseptic meningitis and herpangina. Those in group B also cause aseptic meningitis, Bornholm disease and myocarditis.

کاکس سیکی وائرس : انٹرووائرس کے خاندان میں تین گروہوں میں سے ایک۔

rab louse *(krab low)*. Pediculus pubis (q.v.)

جوں۔قمل موئے زہار : دیکھئے پیڈی کولس پیوبس۔

Cramp *(kramp)* [O.F. cramape]. Spasmodic contraction of a muscle or group of muscles, involuntary and painful; may result from fatigue. Occurs in tetany, food poisoning and cholera.**occupational c.** is such as occurs amongst miners and stokers.

اینٹھن : کسی عضلے یا عضلات کے گروہ کا سکڑنا جس سے درد ہوتا ہے۔ یہ تھکاوٹ سے ہوتا ہے ہیضہ اور زہریلی خوراک سے ہوتا ہے۔

Craniofacial *(kra-ni-o-fash'-al)* [G. *kranion,* skull; L. *facies,* face. external form]. Pertaining to the cranium and the face.

جمجمی وجہی : کھوپڑی اور چہرے سے متعلق۔

Craniometry *(kra-ni-om'-et-ri)* [G. *kranion,* skull; *metron,* a measure]. The science which deals with the measurement of skulls.

قحف پیمائی : کھوپڑیوں کی پیمائش سے متعلق سائنس۔

Craniopharyngioma *(kra-ni-o-far-in'-ji-o-ma)* [G. *kranion,* skull; *pharygx,* pharynx; *oma,* tumour]. A tumour which develops between the brain and the pituitary gland.

Cranioplasty *(kra-ni-o-plas'-ti)* [G. *kranion,* skull; *plasein,* to form]. Operative repair of a skull defect--cranioplastic, adj.

رفوئے جمجمہ : کھوپڑی کے نقص کی اپریشن کے ذریعے مرمت۔

Craniosacral *(kra-ni-o-sa'-kral)* [G. *kranion,* skull; L. *sacer* ,sacred]. Pertaining to the skull and sacrum. Applied to the parasympathetic nervous system.

جمجمی عجزی : کھوپڑی اور سکرم سے متعلق۔

Craniosynostosis *(kra'-ni-o-sin-os-to'-sis)* Premature ossification of skull bones with closure of suture lines, giving rise to facial deformities. See APERTS SYNDROME.

Craniotabes *(kra-ni-o-ta'-bez)* [G. *kranion,* skull; L. *tabes,* a wasting away]. A thinning or wasting of the cranial bones occurring in infancy. Can occur in rickets, syphilis and marasmus--craniotabetic, adj.

ہزال قحف : بچے میں کھوپڑی کی ہڈیوں کا پتلا رہ جانا۔

Craniotomy *(kra-ni-to'-om-i)* [G. *kranion,* skull; *tome,* a cutting]. A surgical opening of the skull in order to remove a growth, relieve pressure, evacusate blood clot or arrest haemorrhage. See LEUCOTOY.

قحف شگافی: سرجری کے ذریعے کھوپڑی کھولنا تا کہ زائد اگنے والی چیز ختم کی جاسکے۔ دباؤ کم کیا جائے یا جمے ہوئے خون کو صاف کیا جائے۔

Cranium *(kra-n'-i-um)* [G. *kranion,* skull]. The part of the skull enclosing the brain. It is composed of eight bones; the occipital, two parietals, frontal, two temporals, sphenoid and ethmoid--cranial, adj.

قحف۔ کاسئہ سر : کھوپڑی کا وہ حصہ جس میں دماغ ہے۔

Cranium

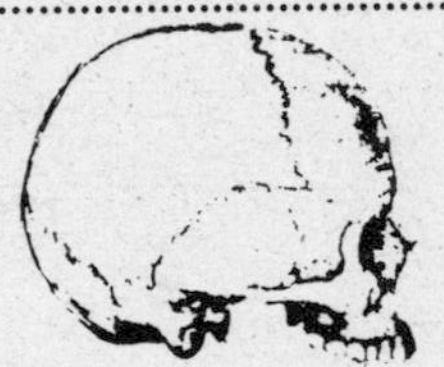

یہ آٹھ ہڈیوں پر مشتمل ہے۔ کاسئہ سر کے کنارے آری کے کنارے کی طرح دندانے دار ہوتے ہیں۔ ایک ہڈی کے دندانے دوسری ہڈی کے دندانوں میں پھنسے ہوتے ہیں۔ وہ ایک دوسرے کے ساتھ مضبوطی سے پیوست ہوتی ہیں۔ کاسئہ سر کی ہڈیاں ایک مضبوط بکس بناتی ہیں۔ اس میں دماغ ہوتا ہے۔ کاسئہ سر کی شکل ایسی ہے کہ چوٹ کا اثر بالائی ہڈیوں تک رہتا ہے۔ دماغ پر اثر نہیں ہوتا۔ کاسئہ سر کی بالائی ہڈیاں دو تہوں کی ہوتی ہیں جن کی وجہ سے چوٹ برداشت ہو جاتی ہے۔ کاسئہ سر کی ہڈیاں یہ ہیں' پیشانی کی ہڈی یا فرنٹل بون کھوپڑی کی بالائی ہڈیاں یا پیرائٹل بونز' کنپٹی کی ہڈیاں یا ٹیمپورل بونز' گدی کی ہڈی یا آکسیپیٹل بون' کھوپڑی کی تلی کی ہڈی یا سفینائڈ' جالی دار ہڈی یا اتھمائڈ بون۔

Crasnatin *(kras'-nat-in)* Asparaginase extracted from E.coli, Antileukaemic.

کراسناٹن : اسپراجینز۔

Creatine *(kre'-at-in)* [G. *kreas,* flesh]. A protein derivative found in muscle. The serum c. is raised in hyperthyroidism, values above 0.6 mg per 100ml of blood being suggestive.

لحمین : پروٹین سے اخذ شدہ جو عضلے میں پائی جاتی ہے۔

Creatinine *(kre-at'-in-en)* [G. *kreas,* flesh]. A waste product of protein (endogenous) metabolism found in normal urine. Probably derived from creatinine of muscle.

کریاٹینن : عام پیشاب میں پایا جانے والا پروٹین میٹابولزم کا فالتو مادہ۔

Creatinuria *(kre-at-in-u'-ri-a)* [G. *kreas,* flesh; *ouron,* urine]. Discovery of creatinine in the urine. Occurs in conditions in which muscle is rapidly broken down, e.g. acute fevers, starvation--creatinuric, adj.

کریٹینن بولی : پیشاب میں کریاٹینن کی دریافت۔

Crede's method *(kre'-dez).* A method of delivering the placenta by gently rubbing the fundus uteri until it contracts, and then, by squeezing the fundus, expressing the placenta into the vagina from whence it is expelled. [Karl Seigmund Franz Crede. German obstetrician, 1819-92]

کری ڈیز میتھڈ : پلیسنٹا کو ہل نکالنے کا طریقہ۔

Creosote *(kre'-o-sot).* A phenolic antiseptic obtained from beechwood. Occasionally used as a deodorant antiseptic and expectorant.

قطران : ضد تعفن۔

Crepitation *(krep-i-ta'-shun)* [L. *crepitare,* to *crackle*]. 1. Grating of bone ends in fracture. 2. Crackling sound in joints, e.g. in osteoarthritis.3. Crackling sound heard via stethoscope in lung infections. 4. Crackling sound elicited by pressure on emphysematous tissue.

کڑکڑاہٹ : جوڑوں میں کڑکڑ کی آواز۔

Cresol *(kre'-sol).* Principal constituent of lyso (q.v.)

کریسول : لائی سال کا اہم جزو۔ ہائیڈروکسی ٹالوین ایک مائع خوشبودار کیمیاتی مرکب جو کولتار سے حاصل کیا جاتا ہے۔ یہ پلاسٹک' آتش گیر' رنگ کی صنعتوں میں اور بطور دافع تعفن استعمال کیا جاتا ہے۔

Cretinism *(kret'-in-izm)* [F. *cretin*]. Due to congenital thyroid deficiency; results in a dull-looking child, underdeveloped mentally and physically, dwarfed, large head, thick legs, pug nose, dry skin, scanty hair, swollen eyelids, short neck, mute, short thick limbs clumsy uncoordinated gait--cretin, n.

بلہی : بدصورت بچے کا پیدا ہونا۔ ذہنی وجسمانی طور پر کمزور۔ قد چھوٹا' سر بڑا' موٹی ٹانگیں خشک کھال' متورم پپوٹے' چھوٹی گردن یہ علامات تھائیرائڈ ہارمون کی کمی سے پیدا ہوتی ہیں۔

Cribriform *(krib'-ri-form)* [L. *cribrum,* sieve

forma, shape]. Perforated , like a sieve, **c.plate,** that portion of ethmoid bone allowing passage of fibres of olfactory nerve.

سوراخ سوراخ : چھلنی کی طرح سوراخوں والی۔

Cricoid *(kri'-koid)* [G. *krikos,* ring; *eidos,* form]. Ring-shaped. Applied to the cartilage forming the inferior posterior part of larynx.

حلقوی : چھلانما۔ لیرنکس کا ایک حصہ۔

Cri du chat' suyndrome . Produced by partial loss of one of the number 5 chromosomes leading to mental subnormality. There are certain physical abnormalities and curious flat, toneless cat-like cry in infacny.

کرائی ڈو کیٹ سنڈروم : نمبر ۵ کروموسوموں میں سے ایک کے جزوی ضیاع کی وجہ سے ذہنی بگاڑ کا پیدا ہونا۔

Crisis *(kri'-sis)* [G. krysis, turning point]. 1. The turning point of a disease--as the point of defervescence in fever, the arrest of an anaemina. 2. Muscular spasm in tabed dorsalis referred to as visceral crisis (gastric, vesical, rectal, etc.). 3. Dietl's crises (q.v.) **oculogyric c.,** see OCULOGYRIC. **thyrotoxic c.,** sudden return of symptoms of thyrotoxicosis, due to shock,injury or thyroidectomy. **myasthenic c.,** sudden deterioration with weakness of respiratory muscles due to an increase in severity of myasthenia. **cholinergic c.,** respiratory failure resulting from over treatment with anticholinesterase drugs. The latter two crises are distinguished by 10 mg Tension i.v. Marked improvement confirms myasthenic c. Cholinergic c. needs 1 mg atropine sulphate i.v. and immediate mechanical respiration.

بحران۔ حرجہ : بیماری میں نمایاں تبدیلی

Crohn's disease See ILEITIS. [Burrill Bernard Crohn. American gastroenterologist, 1884].

مرض کروہن : نوعمر بالغ میں پایا جانے والا مرض۔

Cromoglycate. *(kro-mo-gli-kat).* Disodium cromoglycate (q.v.).

کروموگلائی کیٹ : دیکھئے ڈائی سوڈیم کروموگلائیکیٹ۔

Crosby capsule. Used for intestinal biopsy.

کراسبی کیپسول : آنتوں کی بیماری میں مستعمل۔

Crotamiton BP *(kro-ta-mit'-on).* Effective for scabies, especially in infants, as in kills the mite, and prevents itching. Is usually recognized.

کروٹامائی ٹن بی پی : خارش کے لئے موثر۔

Croup *(kroop).* Laryngeal obstruction. Croupy breathing in a child is often called 'stridulous, meaning noisy or harsh-sounding. Narrowing of the airway which gives rise to the typical attack with crowing inspiration may be the result of oedema or spasm, or both.

خناق : لیرنجیل رکاوٹ۔ بچے میں شور کے ساتھ سانس آنا۔ ہوا کی نالی تنگ ہو جاتی ہے۔ جس کی وجہ سے سانس اندر جاتے وقت آواز پیدا کرتا ہے۔

Cruciate *(kroo'-shi-at)* [L. crux, cross]. Shaped like a cross.

صلیب دار : کراس کی شکل جیسا۔

Crus *(kroos)* [L. leg]. Leg-like; root-like. Applied to various parts of body, e.g. crus of the diaphragm--crural, adj.; crura, pl.

ساق : بیخ نما۔ ٹانگ جیسا۔ جسم کے مختلف حصوں پر اس کا اطلاق ہوتا ہے۔

Crush' syndrome Traumatic uraemia. A condition resulting from damage to the renal tubules because their blood supply has been interfered with. Following an extensive trauma to muscle, there is a period of delay before the effects of renal damage manifest themselves. There is an increase of non-protein nitrogen of the blood, with oliguria, proteinuria and urinary excretion of myohaemoglobin. Loss of blood plasma to damaged area is marked. See TUBULAR NECROSIS.

کرش سنڈروم : بولی نالیوں کے نقصان سے ہونے والی حالت کیونکہ ان میں خون کی سپلائی متاثر ہوتی ہے۔

Crutch palsy Paralysis of extensor muscles of wrist, fingers and thumb from repea-ted pressure of a crutch upon the radial nerve in the axilla.

بیساکھی پالیسی : کلائی، انگلیوں اور انگوٹھے کی عضلات کا کام نہ کرنا۔

Cryoanalgesia *(kri-o-an-al-je-zi-a).* [G. kryos, cold; a not; algos, pain]. Relief of pain achieved by use of a cryosurgical probe to block peripheral nerve function.

Cryogenic *(kri-o-jen'-ik)* [G. kryos, cold; genos, origin]. Anything produced by low tempera ture. Also used to describe any means or apparatus involved in the production of low temperature.

بردزا : کم درجہ حرارت سے پیدا شدہ۔کم درجہ حرارت پیدا کرنے کے لئے سامان۔

Cryopexy *kri-o-peks'-i)* [G. kryos, cold; pexein, to clip]. Surgical fixation with freezing as replacement of a detached retina.

کرائیوپیکسی :اپریشن کے ذریعے جوڑنا۔

Cryophake *(kri-o-fak)* [G. kryos, cold; phagein, to eat]. Cataract extraction using freezing.

Cryoprecipitate therapy *(kri-o-pres-ip'-i-tat ther'-a-pi)* . Use of Factor VIII to prevent or treat bleeding in haemophilia. The term refers to the preparation of Factor VIII for injection. Sub-Arctic temperatures make it separate from plasma.

کرایو پریسی پیٹیٹ تھراپی :ہیموفلیا میں روانی خون کو روکنے کے لئے فیکٹر ۸ کا استعمال۔انجکشن کے لئے فیکٹر ۸ کی تیاری کے لئے بھی یہ اصطلاح استعمال ہوتی ہے۔

Cryoprobe *(kri'o-prob)* [G. kryos, cold; L. probo, to test]. Freezing probe. Can be used for biopsy. A flexible metal tube attached to liquid nitrogen equipment. The cryoprobe has tips of various sizes which can be cooled to a temperature of 180° C. Causes less tissue trauma and 'seeding' of malignant cells.

کرائیوپروب :فریزنگ پروب۔

Cryosurgery *(kri-o-sur'-je-ri)* [G. kryos, cold; kheirourgia, surgery]. The use of intense, controlled cold to remove or destroy diseased tissue. Instead of a knife or guillotine a cryoprobe is used.

کرائیوسرجری :غیر صحت مند نسیج کو ختم کرنے کیلئے سخت سردی کا استعمال۔

Cryothalamectomy *(kri-o-thal-am-ek'-to-mi)* [G. kryos, cold; thalamos, chambers, ektome, excision]. Freezing applied within the thalamus for Parkinson's disease and other hyperkinetic conditions.

کرائیوتھیلا میکٹومی : تھیلامس میں فریزنگ کا استعمال۔

Cryptococcus *(krip-to-kok'-us)* [G. kryptos, hidden; kokkos, berry]. A genus of fungi, Cryptococcus neoformans is pathogenic to man. It has a marked predilection for the central nervous system causing subacute or chronic disease.

کرپٹوجینک :وجہ معلوم نہ ہونا۔

Cryptomenorrhoea *(krip'-to-men-o-re'-a)* [G. kryptos, hidden; men, month; reheein, to flow]. Retention of the menses due to a congenital obstruction, such as an imperforate hymen or atresia of the vagina. Syn., haematocolpos.

طمث مخفی : حیض یا ماہواری کا بند ہو جانا۔

Cryptorchism *(kript-or'-kizm)* [G. kryptos, hidden; orchis, testis]. A developmental defect whereby the testes do not descend into the scrotum; they are retained within the abdomen or inguinal canal--cryptorchild, cryptorchis, n.

خفاء الخصیتین :ایک نقص جس میں خصیے سکروٹم میں نہیں اترتے۔پیدائشی طور پر خصیوں کا پیٹ کے اندر رہ جانا۔

Crystal violet *(kris'-tal vi'-o-let)*. Antiseptic dye, used as 0.5 percent solution for ulcers and skin infections.

کرسٹل وائلٹ :ایک واقع تعفن رنگ۔السر اور جلدی بیماریوں کے لئے ۰۰۵ فیصد محلول استعمال کیا جاتا ہے۔

Crystallin *(kris'-ta-lin)* [G. krystallos, ice]. A globulin, principal constitutent of lens of eye.

کرسٹلن :آنکھ کے عدسے کا اہم جز وگلوبولن۔

Crystalline *(kris'-tal-in)* [G. krystallos, ice]. Like a crystal; transparent. Applied to various structures. **c. lens** a biconvex body, oval in shape, which is suspended just behind the iris of the eye, and separates the aqueous from the vitreous humor. It is slightly less convex on its anterior surface and it refracts the light rays so that they focus directly on to the retina.

بلوری قلمی : قلم کی طرح۔شفاف۔

Crystalluria *(kris-tal-u'-ri-a)* [G. krystalios, ice; ouron, urine]. Excretion of crystals in the urine--crystalluric, adj.

کرسٹلوریا : پیشاب میں قلموں کا اخراج۔

CTAB. Cetrimide (q.v.).

سی ٹی اے بی : دیکھئے سٹریمائیڈ۔

CTG. Cardiotocorgraph.

Cubitus *(ku'-bi-tus)* [L]. The forearm; elbow--cubital, adj.

ساعد۔ پیش بازو : بازو کا اگلا حصہ۔ کہنی۔

Cuboid *(ku'-boid)* [G. kybos, cube; eidos, form]. Shaped like a cube.

مکعب نما : مکعب کی شکل کا۔ شش پہلو۔ ٹارسل ہڈیوں میں سے ایک۔

Cuirass *(kwir-as')* [F. cuirrasse, a breast-plate]. A mechanical apparatus fitted to the chest for artifical respiration.

جلد سینہ : مصنوعی تنفس کے لئے چھاتی کیس اتھ لگانے والا سامان۔

Culdocentesis *(kul-do-sen-te'-sis)* [F. culde-sax; kentesis, puncture]. Aspiration of the pouch of Douglas via the posterior vaginal wall.

کلڈوسینٹی سس : ڈگلس کی تھیلی کی ہوا کشی۔

Culdoscope*(kul'-do-skop)*. An endoscope used via the vaginal route.

کلڈوسکوپ : ویجائنا کے راستے میں استعمال ہونے والی اینڈوسکوپ۔ رحم کا معائنہ کرنے والا آلہ۔

Culdoscopy *(kul-dos'-ko-pi)* [F. cul-desax; G. skopein, to examine]. A form of peritoneoscopy, laparoscopy. Passage of a culdoscope through the posterior vaginal fornix, behind the uterus to enter the peritoneal

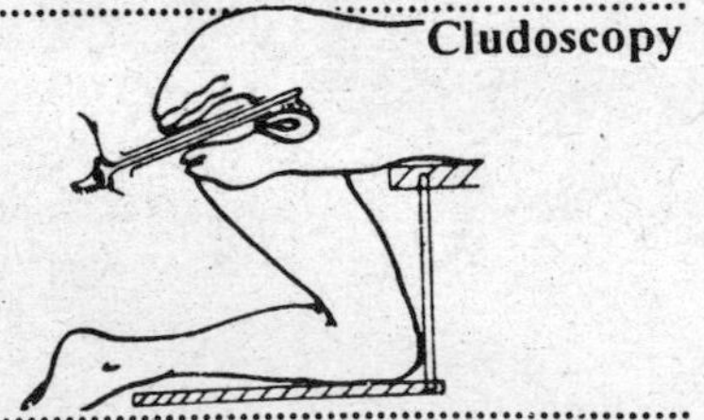

Cludoscopy

cavity, for viewing same--culdoscopic, adj.; culdoscopically, adv.

کلڈوسکوپی : خلفی ویجائنل فورنکس میں کلڈوسکوپ کا راستہ۔

Culture *(kul'-tur)* [L. cultura, colere, to till]. The development of micro-organisms on artifical media under ideal conditions for growth.

کشت : مصنوعی واسطوں پر خورد جسیموں کا بننا۔

Cumulative action *(ku-mu-la-tiv)*. If the dose of a slowly excreted drug is repeated too frequently, an increasing action is obtained. This can be dangerous as, if the drug accumulates in the system, toxic symptoms my occur, sometimes quite suddenly. Long acting barbiturates, strychnine, mercurial salts and digitalis are examples of drugs with a cumulative action.

مجموعی ایکشن : اگر آہستہ خارج ہونے والی دوائی وقفوں کے ساتھ زیادہ دفعہ دی جائے تو اس کا عمل زیادہ تیز ہو جاتا ہے۔ یہ خطرناک ہو سکتا ہے۔ کیونکہ دوائی اندر جمع رہتی ہے۔ اس لئے اچانک زہریلا پن پیدا ہو سکتا ہے۔

Cupping *(kup'-ping)*. [L. cupa, tub]. A method of counterirritation. A small bell-shaped glass (in which the air is expanded by heating, or exhausted by compression of an attached rubber bulb) is applied to the skin, resultant suction producing hyperaemia--dry c. When the skin is scarified before application of the cup it is termed 'wet c'.

سینگی کا سیت : خارش دور کرنے کا طریقہ۔

Curare *(ku-rar'-i)*. The crude extract from which tubocurarine is obtained.

کورارا۔ زہر مکو : ایک رس جس سے ٹیوبوکیورارین حاصل کیا جاتا ہے۔

Curettage *(ku-ret-azh')* [F.]. The scraping of unhealthy or exuberant tissue from a cavity. This may be treatment or may be done to establish a diagnosis.

جرف : فرانسیسی لفظ۔ کسی کہفہ میں سے غیر صحت مند نسیج کا کھرچنا۔

Curette *(ku-ret')* [F. curer, to cleanse]. A spoon-shaped instrument or a metal loop which may have sharp, and/or blunt edges for scraping out (curetting) cavities.

جراح کی چمچی : کہفوں کو کھرچنے کے لئے چمچ کی شکل کا آلہ۔

Curettings *(ku-ret'-ingz)*. The material obtained by scrapping of curetting and usually sent for examination in the pathology department.

کورینگز : کھرچنے سے حاصل ہونے والا مادہ۔

Cushingoid Used to describe the moon face and

central obesity common in people with elevated levels of plasma corticosteroid from whatever cause. See CUSHING'S DISEASE AND SYNDROME.

Cushing's disease. A rare disorder, mainly of females, characterized principally by virilism, obesity, hyperglycaemia, glycosuria and huypertension. Due to extrinisic and excessive hormone stimulation of the adrenal cortex by tumour, or by hyperplasia, of the anterior pituitary gland.

کشنگ مرض : ایک نسوانی مرض۔ پیچوئیٹری یا سپرارینل گلینڈ میں رسولی ہوتی ہے۔ مریض موٹا ہو جاتا ہے۔ رسولی کا اپریشن کرانا چاہیئے۔

Cushing' syndrome. A disorder clinically similar to Cushing's disease, but more common. It is due to eleva ted levels of plasma corticosteroid and is divided into two main groups dependent on exposure or non-exposure to excessive ACTH. 1. ACTH-dependent causes can be iatrogenic due to excessive doses; or the secretion of ACTH by non-endocrine tumours such as bronchial carcinoma. 2. Non ACTH-dependent causes can also be iatrogenic due to excessive doses of corticosteroids; or can be due to adenomas or carcinomas of the adrenal cortex.

کشنگ سنڈروم : ایڈرینل کارٹکس میں ہارمون کے زیادہ عمل کرنے کی وجہ سے مرض جس سے عورتوں میں مردانہ اور مردوں میں زنانہ خواص پیدا ہونے لگتے ہیں۔

Cusp *(kusp)* [L. cuspis, pointed end]. A projecting point, such as the edge of a tooth or the segment of a heart valve, The tricuspid valve has three, the mitral valve two cusps.

کنگرہ : ابھرا ہوا سرا۔ مثلاً دانت کا کنارہ یا دل کے ویلو کا ٹکڑا۔

Cutaneous *(ku-tan'-i-us).* [L. cutis, skin]. Relating to the skin. **c. ureterostomy,** the ureters are transplanted so that they open on to the skin of the abdominal wall. This may be done prior to a complete cystectomy.

جلدی : لاطینی لفظ کیوٹس بمعنی جلد سے ماخوذ جلد سے متعلق۔

Cuticle *(ku'-tik-l)* [L. cutis, skin]. The epidermis (q.v.); dead epidermis, as that which surrounds a nail--cuticular, adj.

برادمہ قشر : اپی ڈرمس۔ مردہ اپی ڈرمس جیسا کہ ناخن کے گرد ہوتی ہے۔

Cyanocobalamin *(si-an-o-ko-bal'-a-men).* Vitamin B_{12}. Present in food and absorbed from intestine only when gastric intrinsic factor present. Stored in liver. Deficiency results in megaloblastic erythropoiesis, e.g. pernicious anaemia which responds to intramuscular injection.

سیانوکوبالامن : حیاتین ب ۱۲۔ جگر میں موجود ہوتا ہے۔ خون کی کمی دور کرتا ہے۔ سائیٹامن۔ بجلی سے جلنے، انیمیا اور سپرد کے علاج میں مستعمل۔ درد دل یا انجائنہ پیکٹورس میں اس کا ایک سی سی کا ٹیکہ روزانہ لگایئے۔

Cyanosis *(si-an-o'-sis).* [G. kyanos, blue; -osis, condition]. A bluish tinge manifested by hypoxic tissue, observed most frequently under the nails, lips and skin. It is always due to lack of oxygen, and the causes of this are legion. **cnetral c.,** blueness seen on warm surfaces such as the oral mucosa and tongue. Increases with exertion--cyandoses, cyanotic, adj.

نیلا یرقان : نیلی رنگت جو عموماً ناخنوں، لبوں اور جلد کے نیچے ہوتی ہے۔ یہ ہمیشہ آکسیجن کی کمی سے ہوتی ہے۔

Cycle *(si-kl)* [G. kyklos, circle]. A regular series of movements or events; a sequence which recurs. **cardiac c.,** the series of movements through which the heart passes in performing one heart beat which corresponds to one pulse beat and takes-about one second. See DIASTOLE and SYSTOLE. **menstrual c.,** the periodically recurring series of changes in breasts, ovaries and uterus culminating in menstruation.

سائیکل : حرکات یا واقعات کا ایک باقاعدہ سلسلہ۔

Cyclical syndrome *(si'-klik-al-sin'-drom).* Currently used for premenstrual symptoms complex, to emphasize that these symptoms are due to normal physiological interaction between several endocrine glands under the cyclical control of the hypothalamus and pituitary.

حلقہ دار سنڈروم : حیض سے پہلے علامتی کمپلکس کے لئے مستعمل اصطلاح۔

Cyclical vomiting *(si'-klik-al vom'-it-ing)*. Periodic attacks of vomiting in children, associated with ketosis; no demonstrable pathological cause. Occurs in nervous children.

سائیکلیکل وامٹنگ : بچوں میں قے یا متلی کے باقاعدہ حملے۔

Cyclimorph 10 *(si'-kli-morf)*. Ampoules of 1 ml of solution for injection, containing morphine tartrate 10 mg and cyclizine tartrate (histamine, antiemetic) 50 mg. For relief of pain without cuasing nausea or vomiting.

سائکلی مارف ۱۰ : قے یا متلی کے بغیر درد کو آرام پہنچانے کے لئے۔ انجکشن کے لئے ایک ملی لیٹر محلول کے امپیول۔ مارفین ٹارٹریٹ ۱۰ ملی گرام اور سائیکلیزین ٹارٹریٹ ۵۰ ملی گرام۔

Cyclimorph 15. In each ampoule of 1 ml there is 15 mg morphine tartrate and 50 mg cyclizine tartrate.

سائکلی مارف ۱۵ : ۱۵ ملی گرام مارفین ٹارٹریٹ اور ۵۰ ملی گرام سائیکلیزین ٹارٹریٹ پر مشتمل ایک ملی لیٹر کا امپیول۔

Cyclitis *(si-kli'-tis)* [G. kyklos, circle; -itis, inflammation]. Inflammation of the ciliary body of the eye, shown by deposition of small collections of white cells on the posterior cornea called 'keratitic precipita tes' (KP). Often co-existent with inflammation of the iris. See IRIDOCYCLITIS.

ورم جسم هدبی : آنکھ کی ہدبی جسم کی سوزش۔

Cyclizine *(si'-kli-zen)*. See ANTHIHISTAMINES.

سائیکلی زین : دیکھئے اینٹی ہسٹامینز۔

Cyclobarbitone *(si-klo-bar'-bit-on)* . A short-acting barbiturate, useful when the onset of sleep is delayed. The general properties of these drugs are described under barbiturates (q.v.).

سائیکلو باربی ٹون : ایک مختصر عمل والی باربچوریٹ۔ دیر سے نیند آنے کی صورت میں مستعمل۔

Cyclodialysis *(si'-klo-di-al'-i-sis)*. [G. kyklos, circle; G., a separating]. Establishment of communication between anterior chamber and perichoroidal space to relieve intraocular pressure in glaucoma.

سائیکلوڈایالائی سس : کلاکوما میں دباؤ میں آرام کے لئے اگلے چیمبر اور پیری کورائڈل جگہ کے درمیان رابطہ کا قیام۔

Cyclodiathermy *(si-klo-di-a-ther'-mi)* [G. kyklos, circle; dia, through; therme, heart]. Destruction by diathermy of the ciliary body.

سائیکلوڈایاتھرمی : ہدبی جسم کی ڈایاتھرمی کے ذریعے تباہی۔

Cyclogyl *(si'-klo-jil)*. Cyclopentolate hydrochloride q.v.

سائیکلوجل : سائیکلو پینٹولیٹ ہائیڈروکلورائڈ۔ ایک تالیفی دوا۔ اس سے سائیکلوپلیجیا اور مڈریاسس ہوتا ہے۔

Cyclopenthiazide *(si-klo-pen-thi'-a-zid)*. Diuretic. Decreases reabsorption of sodium and chloride in kidney tubules. Effective orally.

سائیکلوپین تھیازائیڈ : پیشاب آور دوا۔ منہ کے ذریعے موثر۔ گردے کے ٹیوبیولز میں سوڈیم اور کلورائیڈ کے دوبارہ انجذاب کو کم کرتی ہے۔

Cyclopentolatge hydrochloride *(si-klo-pen'-t-ol-at hi-dro-klor'-id)*. A synthetic, spasmolytic drug. Causes cycloplegia and mydriasis.

Cyclophosphamide *(si-klo-fos'-fa-mid)*. Cytotoxic agent. A nitrogen mustard. Alkylating agent that interferes with synthesis of nucleic acid in cell chromosomes, particular in rapidly dividing cells such as those which occur in bone marrow, skin, gastrointestinal tract and fetal tissues. The main side effects therefore occur in these tissues causing anorexia, nausea, vomiting, diarrhoea, depression of bone marrow and alopecia. Main indications are disorders of lymphoid tissue.

سائیکلوفاسفامائڈ : سائیٹو ٹاکسک عامل۔ خلوی کروموسوموں میں نکلیک ایسڈ کی تالیف میں مخل ہوتا ہے۔ خصوصاً تیزی سے تقسیم ہونے والے خلیوں میں مثلاً ہڈی کے مغز، جلد وغیرہ میں۔ اس سے متلی بھی ہو جاتی ہے اور دست آتے ہیں۔ لمفائڈ بافت میں گڑبڑ پیدا ہوتی ہے۔

Cycloplegia *(si-klo-ple'-ji-a)* [G. kyklos, circle; plege, stroke]. Paralysis of the ciliary muscle of the eye--cycloplegic, adj.

سائیکلوپیجیا۔ سلل ہدبیہ : آنکھ کی ہدی عضلے کا سن ہو جانا۔ عضلات ہدبیہ کا استرخاء۔

Cycloplegics *(si-klo-ple'-jiks)* [G. kyklos, circle; plege, stroke]. Drugs which cause paralysis of the ciliary muscle, e.g. atropine, homatropine, scopolamine and lachesine.

مفلج الہدبیہ : ایسی ادویات جو ہدبی عضلے کو سن کرنے کا باعث بنتی ہیں۔ مثلاً ایٹروپین۔

Cyclopropane *(si'-klo-pro'-pan)*. A highly inflammable, gaseous anaesthetic, supplied in orange-coloured cylinders. Induction is rapid and recovery prompt. Used with closed circuit apparatus.

سائیکلو پروپین : زبردست آتش گیر۔ گیس کی صورت میں سلنڈروں میں مہیا کی جاتی ہے جو مالٹائی رنگ کی ہوتی ہے۔ سن کر دیتی ہے۔ فوری اثر والی اور اثر بھی فوراً ختم ہوتا ہے۔ چھوٹے سرکٹ میں سامان میں مستعمل۔

Cycloserine *(si-klo-ser'-in)*. antitubercular antibiotic. Given orally. Useful in some nontubercular urinary tract infections. Hepatotoxicity gaurded against by SGOT tests twice weekly. Can be epileptogenic. Can give rise to gastrointestinal side effects.

سائیکلوسرین : ضد تپ دق اینٹی بایوٹک۔ منہ کے ذریعے دی جانے والی دوا۔ اس کے استعمال سے پیٹ میں گڑبڑ بھی ہو سکتی ہے۔ بعض پیشاب کے راستے کی بیماریوں میں مفید۔ تپ دق میں ایک گولی یا کیپسول صبح دوپہر شام۔

Cyclospasmol *(si-klo-spas'-mol)*. Vasodilator used particularly for cerebral vascular disorders.

سائیکلو سپیسمول : سربرل واسکولر خرابیوں میں مستعمل۔

Cyclothymia *(si-klo-thi'-mi-a)* [G. kyklos, circle; thymos, mind]. A tendency to alternating mood swings between elation and depression such as occur in the manic-depressive psychoses.

جنون دوری : موڈ میں تبدیلی کا رجحان۔

Cyclotomy *(si-klot'-om-i)* [G. kyklos, circle; tome, a cutting]. A drianage operation for the relief of glaucoma, consisting of an incision through the ciliary body.

ہدبی عضلا تراشی : گلاکوما کے آرام کے لئے اپریشن جس میں ہدبی جسم میں شگاف ڈالا جاتا ہے۔

Cyesis *(si-e'-sis)*. [G. kyesis, conception]. Pregnancy. **pseudo c.,** signs and symptoms simulating those of early pregnancy occuring in a childless person with an overwhelmin desire to have a child.

ل : حالت حمل۔ جھوٹے حمل میں بغیر بچہ کے شخص میں بچے کی شدید اہش کے ساتھ ابتدائی حمل کو تحریک دینے والی علامات۔

Cyklokapron *(si-klo-kap'-ron)*. More powerf than Epsikapron (q.v.).

Cylindroma *(sil'-in-dro-ma)* [G. kylindro cylinder; -oma, tumour]. A tumour containin elongated twisted cords of hyaline materia found in malignancy of salivary flands, bas cell carcinomas and endotheliomas.

طوانی سلعہ : ہیالین مادہ کی بلوں والی طویل ڈوریوں پر مشتمل ناسور۔

Cyllin *(si'-lin)*. A disinfectant of the black-flu type. These products are solutions of coal-t acids in soap.

ین : سیاہ سیال قسم کا دافع تعفن۔ یہ حاصلات صابن میں کولتار ایسڈز کے ول ہوتے ہیں۔

Cynomel *(sin'-o-mel)*. A preparation of lioth yronine (q.v.), that has a standardized activit

ئینومل : لایوتھائرونین سے تیار شدہ۔

Cyst *(sist)* [G. kystis, bladder]. A sac wi membranous wall, enclosing fluid semisolid matter. **branchial c.,** in the nec region arising from anomalous developme of the embryonal branchial cleft(s). **chocola c.,** an endometrial cyst containing alter blood. the ovaries are the most usual sit **dermoid c.,** congenital in origin, usually the ovary, containing elements of hair, nai skin, teeth, etc. **hydatid c.,** is the envelope which Taenia echinococcus (tapewor produces its larvae--usually in the huma liver. **meibomian c.,** see CHALAZIO **ovarian c.,** ovarian new growth. Most a cystic, but some such as the fibroma are sol To be differentiated from a cystic ovary (q.v o.c. is enucleated from the ovary which conserved. **papilliferous c.,** an ovarian cyst which there are nipple-like (papillar outgrowths from the wall. May be benign malignant. **retention c.,** cause by blocking a duct, as a ranula (q.v.), **sebaceous** retention cyst of a sebaceous gland (we

thyroglossal c., cystic distension of thyroglossal duct near the hyoid bone, in the neck region.

سسٹ ۔سلعہ :یونانی لفظ کسٹس بمعنی بلیڈر سے ماخوذ اصلاح ۔جھلی دار دیوار والی ایک تھیلی جس میں سیال یا نیم ٹھوس مادہ ہوتا ہے۔

Cystadenoma *(sist-ad-en-o'-ma)*. [G. kystis, bladder; aden, gland; -oma, tumour]. An innocent cystic new growth of glandular tissue, Liable to occur in the female breast.

دویری غدی سلعہ :غدودی بافت نیا اگاؤ جو عورت کی چھاتی میں ہوتا ہے۔

Cystathioninuria *(sis-ta-thi-on-in-u'-ri-a)*. Inherited excessive excretion of thionine, an intermediate product in conversion of methionine to cysteine. Associated with mental subnormality.

سسٹا تھایونی نیوزیا :تھایونین کا زائد مقدار میں توراثی طور پر اخراج۔ متھیونین سے سسٹین کی تبدیلی میں ایک درمیانی حاصل ۔ ذہنی خرابی سے متعلق۔

Cystectomy *(sis-tek'-tom-i)* [G. kystis, bladder; ektome, excision]. Usually refers to the removal of part or the whole of the urinary bladder. this may involve the transplantation of one or both ureters--cutaneously or into the bowel.

سلعہ براری ۔مثانہ براری :بولی بلیڈر مکمل یا اس کے کسی حصے کو ختم کرنا۔

Cystic *(sis'-tik)* [G. kystis, bladder]. Pertaining to or resembling a cyst (q.v.). **c. duct,** the tube connecting the gall-bladder to the hepatic and common bile ducts. It conveys bile to and from the gall-bladder. **c. disease of lung,** fibrosis of pancreas, due to a recessive gene mutation. Affects about one child in 2500 live births. The control of pulmonary infection is the key to survival. See MUCOVISCIDOSIS.

مثانوی :یونانی لفظ کسٹس بمعنی بلیڈر سے ماخوذ ۔سسٹ سے مشابہ یا اس کے متعلق سسٹک نالی جگری اور مشترکہ بائل نالیوں کو پتے کیس اتھ ملاتی ہے۔ لبلبہ کی فائبروسس یا پھیپھڑے کی سسٹک بیماری ایک مغلوب جین میٹشن کی وجہ سے ہوتی ہے ۔اس سے اڑھائی ہزار نوزائیدہ بچوں میں سے ایک بچہ متاثر ہوتا ہے۔

Cysticerosis *(sis-ti-ko'-sis)* [G. kystis, bladder; -osis, condition]. Infection of man with cysticercus.

انسان ذنبیت :آدمی کو سسٹی سرکس کی بیماری لگنا۔

Cysticercus *(sis-ti-ser'-kus)* [G. kystis, bladder; kerkos, tail]. The larval form of tapeworms. After ingestion, the ova do not develop beyond this form in man, but form 'cysts' in subcutaneous tissues, skeletal muscles and the brain where they provoke epilepsv.

ذنبی کدودانہ : کدو کیڑوں کی لاروی صورت۔

Cystine *(sis'-ten)*. A sulphur-containing amino acid, produced by the breaking down of proteins during the digestive process.

سسٹین :امینوایسڈ پر مشتل گندھک جو عمل انہضام کے دوران لحمیات کی سکستگی سے بنتی ہے۔ ایک ناحل پزیر قلمی امینو ایسڈ۔ نقطہ پگھلاؤ ۲۴۷ تا ۲۴۹°س، تخفیف پر سسٹین بناتا ہے۔

Cystinosis *(sis-tin-o'-sis)*. [G. kystis, bladder; -osis, condition]. Metabolic disorder in which crystalline cystine is deposited in the body. Cystine and other aminoacids are excreted in the urine. Fanconi syndrome. See AMINOACIDURIA.

سسٹی نوسس :یونانی الفاظ کسٹس بمعنی بلیڈر اور اوسس بمعنی حالت کا مجموعہ۔ اس مرض کے دوران جسم میں سسٹین جمع ہو جاتی ہے۔ سسٹین اور دوسرے امینوایسڈز پیشاب میں خارج ہوتے ہیں۔

Cystinuria *(sis-tin-u'-ri-a)* [G. kystis, bladder; ouron, urine]. Metabolic disorder in which cystine appears in the urine. A cause of renal stones--cystinuric. adj.

سسٹین بولیت :یونانی الفاظ کسٹس بمعنی بلیڈر اور اورون بمعنی پیشاب کا مجموعہ۔ پیشاب میں سسٹین کا ظاہر ہونا۔ گردوں میں پتھری بننے کی وجہ۔

Cystitis *(sis-ti'-tis)*. [G. kystis, bladder; -itis, inflammation]. Inflammation of the urinary bladder, exciting cause usually bacterial. The condition may be acute or chronic, primary or secondary to stones, etc. More frequent in females as the urethra is short.

ورم مثانہ :یونانی الفاظ کسٹس بمعنی بلیڈر اور ائٹس بمعنی سوزش کا مجموعہ۔ بولی بلیڈر کی سوزش جو عموماً جراثیم کی وجہ سے ہوتی ہے۔ خواتین میں زیادہ ہوتی ہے کیونکہ ان میں یورتھرا مختصر ہوتا ہے۔ پیشاب بار بار آتا ہے۔ پیشاب لگ کے آتا ہے۔ پیشاب روکنا مشکل ہوتا ہے۔ پیٹ کے زیرین حصے اور فوطوں میں درد۔ علاج۔ کے لئے فینازو پیری ڈین، نائٹروفیورین ٹائن سٹرالکا اور ٹیٹرا

سائیکلین کلورم فینی کال۔

Cystitome *(sis'-ti-tom)*. Delicate ophthalmic instrument for incision of the lens capsule.

انبان تراش :عدسے کے کیپسول کے لئے نازک اوزار۔

Cystocele *(sis'-to-sel)* [G. kystis, bladder; kele, hernia]. Prolapse of the posterior wall of the urinary bladder into the anterior vaginal wall. See COLPORRHAPHY.

فتق مثانہ :بولی مثانہ کی دیوار کا اگلی ویجائنا کی دیوار میں دھنس جانا۔

Cystodiathermy *(sis'-to-di-ath-er'-mi)*. [G. kystis, bladder; dia, through; therme, heat]. The application of a cauterizing electrical current to the walls of the urinary bladder through a cystoscope, or by open operation.

سسٹوڈایاتھرمی :اپریشن کے ذریعے یا سسٹوسکوپ سے بولی مثانہ یعنی بلیڈر کی دیواروں پر برقی رو کا اطلاق۔

Cystogram *(sis'-to-gram)* [G. kystis, bladder; gramma, letter]., An X-ray film demonstrating the urinary bladder. **micturating c.**, taken during the act of passing urine.

سسٹوگرام :یونانی الفاظ کسٹس بمعنی بلیڈر یا مثانہ اور گریما بمعنی مکتوب کا مجموعہ۔ بولی مثانہ ظاہر کرنی والی ایکس رے فلم۔ پیشاب کرنے کے دوران لی گئی ایکسرے فلم۔

Cystography *(sis-tog'-ra-fi)*[G. kystis, bladder; graphein, to write]. Radiographic examination of the urinary bladder, after it has been rendered radio-opaque--cystographic, adj.; cystographically, adv.

سسٹوگرافی۔ مثانہ نگاری :یونانی الفاظ کسٹس بمعنی بلیڈر یا مثانہ اور گریفین بمعنی لکھنا کا مجموعہ۔ ریڈیو غیر شفاف کرنے کے بعد بولی مثانے کا ریڈیوگرافک ٹیسٹ

'ystolithiasis *(sis-to-lith-i'-as-is)* [G. kystis, bladder; lithos, stone; N.L. -iasis, condition]. The presence of a stone or stones in the urinary bladder.

حصاتیت مثانہ :بولی مثانے میں پتھری یا پتھروں کی موجودگی۔

Cystometrogram *(sis-to-met'-ro-gram)* [G. kystis, bladder; metron, a measure; gramma, letter]. A record of the changes in pressure within the urinary bladder under various conditions; used, in the study of certain disorders of paraplegia.

سسٹومیٹروگرام :مختلف حالتوں میں بولی مثانے میں دباؤ میں تبدیلیوں کا ریکارڈ۔

Cystometry *(sis-tom'-et-ri)* [G: kystis, bladder; metron, a measure]. The study of pressure changes within the urinary bladder--cystometric, adj.

مثانہ پیمائی :بولی مثانے میں دباؤ کی تبدیلیوں کا ریکارڈ۔

Cystometry *(sis-tom'-et-ri)* [G. kystis, bladder; pexy, fixation]. A 'siling' operation for stress incontinence whereby the blader neck is supported from the back of the symphysis pubis.

Cystoplasty *(sis'-to-plas-ti)* [G. kystis, bladder: plassein, to form]. Surgical repair of the bladder--cystoplastic, adj.

ترقیع مثانہ۔ تکوین مثانہ :بلیڈر کی سرجری کے ذریعے مرمت۔

Cystoscope

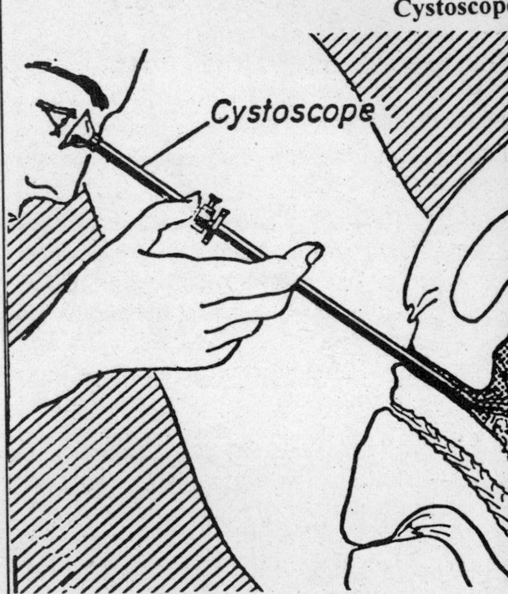

Cystoscope *(sis'-to-skop)* [G. kystis, bladde skopein, to examine]. An endoscope (q.v used in diagnosis and treatment of bladde ureter and kidney conditions--cystoscopy, n cystos-copic, adj.; cystoscopically, adv.

سسٹوسکوپ۔مثانہ بین :یونانی الفاظ کسٹس بمعنی بلیڈر اور سکوپین بمعنی جانچنا کا مجموعہ۔ بلیڈر، بولی نالی اور گردے کی حالت کی تشخیص اور علاج کے لئے استعمال ہونی والی اینڈوسکوپ۔

Cystostomy *(sis-tos'-to-mi)* [G. kystis, bladder; stoma, mouth]. The operation whereby a fistulous opening is made into the bladder via the abdominal wall. Usually the fistula can be allowed to heal when its purpose has been achieved.

مثانی تفویہ :یونانی الفاظ کسٹس بمعنی بلیڈر اور سٹوما بمعنی منہ کا مجموعہ۔ بطنی دیوار کے راستے بلیڈر میں اپریشن کے سوراخ کرنا۔

Cystotomy *(sis-tot'-o-mi)* [G. kystis, bladder; tome, a cutting]. Incision into the urinary bladder, often done to fulgurate a papilloma or to pass retrograde bougies. etc.

مثانہ شگافی :بولی مثانے میں شگاف۔

Cystourethritis *(sis-to-u-re-thri'-tis)* [G. kystis, bladder; ourethron, urethra; -itis, inflammation]. Inflammation of the urinary bladder and urethra.

مثانی مبالی التھاب :بولی مثانے اور یورتھرا کی سوزش۔

Cystourethrogram *(sis-to-u-re'-thro-gram)* [G. kystis, bladder; ourethra, urethra; gramma, letter]. An X-ray film demonstrating the urinary bladder and urethra.

سسٹو یورتھروگرام :بولی مثانے اور یورتھرا کو ظاہر کرنے والی ایکسرے فلم۔

Cystourethrography *(sis-to-u-re-throg'-ra-fi)* [G. kystis, bladder; ourethra, urethra; graphein, to write]. Radiographic examination of the urinary bladder and urethra, after they have been rendered radio-opaque--cystourethrographic, adj.; cystourethrographically, adv.

سسٹو یورتھروگرافی :ریڈیو غیر شفاف کرنے کے بعد بولی مثانے اور یوریتھرا کی ریڈیوگرافی جانچ۔

Cystourethropexy *(sis-to-ur-eth'-ro-peks-i)*. Forward fixation of the bladder and upper urethra in an attempt to combat incontinence of urine.

سسٹو یورتھروپیکسی :بالائی یوریتھرا اور بلیڈر کی فکسیسن۔

Cytamen *(sit'-a-men)*. Cyanocobalamin (q.v.).

سائی ٹامن :سیانوکوبالامن۔ حیاتین ب۱۲۔ یہ جگر میں پایا جاتا ہے۔ یہ خون کی کمی دور کرتا ہے۔ داد میں مستعمل۔ یہ انجکشن کے ذریعے دیا جاتا ہے۔ انیمیا، بجلی سے جلنے اور سپرہ کے علاج میں مستعمل۔ درد دل یا انجائنہ، پیکٹورس میں اس کا ایک سی سی کا ٹیکہ روزانہ لگایئے۔

Cytarabine *(si-ta'-ra-ben)*. See CYTOSINE ARABINOSIDE.

خلوی تشخیص :خلیوں کے خوردبینی مطالعہ کی تشخیص۔

Cytogenetics *(si-to-jen-et'-iks)*. Laboratory examination of a person's chromosomes by culture techniques, using either lymphocytes or a piece of tissue such as skin. Some abnormal chromosomes can be linked with physical and mental disorder--cytogenesis, n.

خلوی جینیات : کلچر تکنیک کے ذریعہ کسی شخص کے کروموسوموں کی تجربہ گاہی جانچ۔

Cytology *(si-tol'-oj-i)* [G. kytos, cell; logos, discourse]. Subdivision of biology, consisting of the microscopic study of the body cells, **exfoliative c.,** microscopic study of cells from the sruface of an organ or lesion after suitable staining.

خلویات :حیاتیات کی ایک شاخ جو جسمی خلیوں کے خوردبینی مطالعہ پر مشتمل ہے۔

Cytolysis *(si-tol'-i-sis)* [G. kytos, cell; tysts, a loosening]. The degeneration, destruction, disintegration or dissolution of cells--cytolytic, adj.

خلیہ پاشی :خلیوں کا خاتمہ یا تباہی۔

Cytomegalovirus *(si-to-meg'-al-o-vir'-us)* [G. kytos, cell; megas, large; L.]. Belongs to the same group of viruses as herpes simplex. Can cause latent and symptomless infection. Virus excreted in urine and saliva. Congenital infection is the most severe form of c. infection.

سائیٹو میگالووائرس :ہرپیز سمپلکس کے طور پر وائرس کے اسی گروہ کا۔ خوابیدہ اور بی علامتی مرض پیدا کر سکتا ہے۔ وائرس پیشاب اور سلائیوا میں خارج ہوتا ہے۔

Cytomegalovirus infection. Predominantly attects children and infants, but it has been found in adults undergoing open-heart surgery. Evidence of symptomless infection in pregnant women has also been described. It is characterized by the presence of intracellular inclusion bodies in the cells of many organs, so that the cells become grossly enlarged--hence the name a virus causing large cells. The respiratory tract, kidneys, adrenals, liver, gastrointestinal tract, blood, eyes and CNS--especially the brain--may be involved. In premature and neonatal infants the inclusion bodies are best seen in the kidneys. Virus may be present in saliva of patients for 4 weeks after infection and in urine for 2 years. It has also been recovered from normal infants. There is an increased incidence in children with mental or developmental retardation and blood disorders. It has been described in relation to Rh incompatibility and hepatitis in newborn infants and after intrauterine transfusions. Although in the majority of cases the condition is congenital the mode of transmission is uncertain, whether by blood or amnion. As a rule the mothers are not ill. Recovery of the virus from urine and cervix is more frequent in primipara than multipara. Affected infants are premature or below average weight and present with a large spleen and liver, jaundice, anaemia and purpura. Cerebral calcification, hydrocephalus and microcephaly and common. Pneumonitis and enterocolitis occur in older children. Outlook grave and fatality high. Permanent brain damage occurs in many survivors. Management of the infection is at present unsatisfactory due to lack of precise knowledge and virus-killing drugs.

سائیٹو میگالو وائرس انفیکشن : اس بیماری سے زیادہ تر بچے متاثر ہوتے ہیں یا وہ اشخاص جن کے دل کا اپریشن کیا جائے۔ بعض اوقات حاملہ عورتوں میں بھی ہوتا ہے۔ اس میں خلیے بڑھ جاتے ہیں۔ اس سے تنفسی راستہ، گردے، جگر، خون، آنتیں، آنکھیں وغیرہ متاثر ہوتی ہیں۔ بہت سے زندہ بچ جانے والوں میں دماغ کو نقصان پہنچتا ہے۔ اس کا مناسب علاج نہیں۔

Cytopathic *(si-to-path'-ik)* [G. kytos, cell; pathos, disease]. Pertaining to disease of the living cell.

سائیٹو پیتھک : یونانی الفاظ کائیٹوس بمعنی خلیہ اور پیتھوس بمعنی مرض کا مجموعہ۔ جاندار خلیے کی بیماری سے متعلق۔

Cytoplasm *(si-to-plazm)* [G. kytos, cell; plasma from plassein, to mould]. The living material of the cell external to the nucleus--cytoplasmic, adj.

خلیہ مار : مرکزہ سے باہر خلیے کا جاندار مادہ۔

Cytosar *(si-to-sar)* . See CYTOSINE ARABINOSIDE

Cytosine arabinosider *(sit'-o-sen ar-ab-i-n'-o-sid)*. Antimetabolite; used in acute leukaemia. Interrupts DNA synthesis. Also termed cytarabine, cytosar or Ara C.

سائیٹوسین اریبینو سائیڈ : اینٹی میٹابولائٹ۔ لیکومیا میں دی جانے والی دوائی۔ لنکلیو پروٹین کی تالیف میں مزاحمت کرتی ہے۔ یعنی ڈی این اے بننے نہیں دیتی۔

Cytostasis *(si-to-sta'-sis)*. [G. kytos, cell; stasis, a standing still]. Arrest or hin-drance of cell development--cytostatic, adj.

خلوی رکود : خلوی تکمیل کی رکاوٹ یا بندش۔

Cytotoxic *(si-to-toks'-ik)* [G. kytos, cell; toxikon, poison]. Any substance with is toxic to cells. Applied to the drugs used for the treatment of carcinomas and the reticuloses. Two main groups; (1) antimetabolites which block action of an enzyme system, e.g. methotrexate, fluouracil, mercaptopurine; (2) alkylating agents which poison cell directly, e.g. cyclophosphamide, mustine, Thiotepa.

خلیہ پاش : ایسا مادہ جو خلیوں کے زہریلا ہو۔ اس کا اطلاق بعض ادویات پر ہوتا ہے۔ اینٹی میٹابولائٹس خامرہ کے عمل کو روک دیتے ہیں جبکہ دوسرے خلیے کے لئے زہریلے ہیں۔

Cytotoxins *(si-to'-toks'-inz)* [G. kytos, cell; toxikon, poison]. See ANTIBODIES.

خلوی سم : یونانی الفاظ کائیٹوس بمعنی خلیہ اور ٹوکسیکون بمعنی زہر کا مجموعہ۔ لحمیات جو خون کے مائع حصے یا سیرم میں پائی جاتی ہیں۔ اینٹی جن کے ردعمل کے طور پر پیدا ہوتی ہیں۔

D

D, d Symbol for density and diameter.

ڈی: کثافت اور حجم کی علامت ہے۔

D860 Tolbutamide. An insuline enhancer.

ڈی ۸۶۰: ٹول بوٹامائڈ۔ آئی لیٹس آف لینگر ہانز کو تحریک کر کے انسولین زیادہ پیدا کرتا ہے۔ ذیابیطس کے علاج کے لئے کامیابی کے ساتھ زیر استعمال ہے۔ ذیابیطس کی شدت میں مفید نہیں۔

Da Costa's syndrome. [Jacob Mendes Da Costa, American surgeon, 1883-1900]. Cardiac neurosis. A state of excitement and anxiety where palpitations is the most prominant features.

نقرس راجع: پریشانی کی ایک حالت۔ دل کی دھڑکن میں شدت۔ اس بیماری کی نمایاں علامت ہے۔ الجھن کی کیفیت طاری ہونا۔

Dacry(o) adenitis *(dak-re-o-ade-ni-tis)* [G. *dacryo,* tear; *aden*, gland, *itis,* inflammation]. Inflammation of a lacrimal glands. It may be in mumps. It may be acute or chronic.

ورم غدہ دمعیہ: لکریمل غدود کی سوزش۔ کن پیڑوں کے دوران ہوتی ہے۔

Dacryocyst *(dak-ri-o-sist)* [G. *dakryon,* tear; *kystis,* bladder]. The lacrimal sac. It is an old term. The word is still used in its compound forms.

کیسۂ دمعی: یونانی الفاظ ڈکریان بمعنی آنسو اور کسٹس بمعنی بلیڈر کا مرکب۔ آنسو کی تھیلی کے لئے پرانی اصطلاح۔ آشوب چشم کی ایک قسم۔

Dacryocystectomy *(dak-ri-o-sis-tek'-to-mi)* [G. dakryon, tear; kystis, bladder, ektome, excision]. Excision of any part of the lacrimal sac.

ڈیک ریوسسٹیک ٹومی : یونانی الفاظ ڈکریان بمعنی آنسو، کسٹس بمعنی بلیڈر اور آکٹوم بمعنی قطع کا مجموعہ۔ لکریمل سیک یا آنسو کی تھیلی کا قطع۔

Dacryocystelgia *(dak'-reo-sist-aljia)* [G. *dacryo,* tear; *cyst,* sac; *algia,* pain]. Pain in the lacrimal sac.

غدۂ دمعیہ میں درد: غدہ دمعیہ میں درد ہو جانا۔ یونانی زبان کے لفظ ڈکریو بمعنی آنسو، سسٹ بمعنی تھیلی اور ایلجیا بمعنی درد سے ماخوذ ہے۔

Dacryocystitis *(dak-reo-sisti'tis)* [G. *dakryo,* tear; *cyst,* sac, *titis,* inflammation]. Inflammation of the lacorinal sac. This may result in absess formation and removal of tear duct, giving rise to epiphora.

Dacryocystoblennorrhea *(dak're-o-sis-to-blenorea)* A chronic catarrhal inflammation of the lacrimal sac with constriction of lacrimal duct.

سوزش غدۂ دمعیہ: آنسو کی تھیلی کی سوزش ہونا۔ اس سوزش کی وجہ جھلی ہو اور آنسو والی نالی بند ہو جائے۔

Dacryocystorhinostomy *(dak're-o-sis-to'ri-nosmi)* [G. *dacryo,* tear; *cyst,* sac; *rhino,* nose; *stomy,* mouth]. Surgical creation of a duct between lacrimal sac and nasal cavity. It is also called Toli's operation.

ڈیکریوسسٹورنوسٹومی: آنسو کی تھیلی سے ناک میں روانی برقرار رکھنے کے لئے آپریشن۔

Dacryolith *(dak-ri-o-lith)* [G. *dakryon,* tear; *lithos,* stone]. A concretion in the lacrimal sac orr duct.

حصات دمعی: اشکوں کی راہ میں رکاوٹ۔ آنسو کے راستے میں

سنگریزے۔

Dactyl *(dak'-til)* [G. daktylos, finger]. A digt, finger or toe--dactylar, dactylate, adj.

انگشت : انگلی۔ ہاتھ یا پیر کی انگلی۔

Dactylion *(dak-til'-i-on)*. Syndactyiy (q.v.).

انضمام اصابع : ہاتھوں یا پیروں کی انگلیوں کا جڑا ہونا۔

Dactylitis *(dak-til-i'-tis)*. [G. daktylos, finger; -itis, inflammation]. Inflammation of finger or tow. The digit becomes swollen due to periostitis. Met with in congenital syphilis, tuberculosis, sarcoid, etc.

ورم انگشت : ہاتھ یا پیر کی انگلی کی سوزش۔

Dactylogoy *(dak-til-ol'-o-ji)* [G. daktylos, finger; logos, discourse]. The finger sign method of communication with deaf and dumb people.

انگشتی اشاریات : بہرے اور گونگے لوگوں کے لئے اشاروں کی زبان یعنی انگلیوں سے اشارے کرنے کا طریقہ۔

Daltonism *(dawl'-ton-izm)*. Colour blindness, named after John Dalton, English chemist and physicist [1766-1844], who was afflicted with it.

رنگ کوری۔ ڈالٹینٹ : رنگ کی پہچان نہ ہونا۔ ایک انگریز سائنس دان جان ڈالٹن کے نام پر رنگوں کا اندھاپن۔

Dandruff *(dand'-ruff)*. The common scaly condition of the scalp. Called scurf. May be the diseases of the seborrhoeic type, such as flexural dermatitis.

سبوسہ : سر کی جلد پر سکیل بننا۔ خشکی ہونا۔ اس سے کئی جلدی امراض ہو سکتے ہیں۔

Dandy fever *(dan'-di fe'-ver)*. Dengue (q.v.).

ہڈی توڑ بخار : مشرق وسطیٰ کی بیماری۔ یہ بیماری مچھر کے کاٹنے سے ہوتی ہے جو ایک وائرس کو انسانی جسم میں منتقل کر دیتا ہے اس سے جوڑوں مین درد اور بخار ہو جاتا ہے۔

Dangerous Drugs Act. Replaced by the MISUSE OF DRUGS ACT (q.v.).

ادویہ خطرناک کا ایکٹ : قانون جس کے تحت نشہ آور ادویات کی تیاری، فروخت یا استعمال ممنوع ہے۔ یہ ادویات صرف ڈاکٹر دے سکتے ہیں۔ ان میں افیم، بھنگ، مارفین، کوکین وغیرہ شامل ہیں۔

Dantrium *(dan'-tri-um)*. Dantrolene sodium *(q.v.)*.

Dantrolene sodium (dan'-tro-len so'-di-um). *Antispasmodic.*

Daonil (da'-on-il). G.libenclamide (q.v.).

ڈاؤنل : گلبین کلیمائڈ۔

Dapsone *(dap'-son)*. A sulphone derivative used mainly in leprosy, but also valuable in dermatitis herpetiformis. Prolonged treatment may produce haemolytic anaemia with Heinz body formation, clinical signs of which are cyanosis of the lips; the patient is generally off-colour.

ڈیپسون : ایک سلفون حاصل جو خصوصاً کوڑھ کی بیماری میں استعمال کیا جاتا ہے۔

Daptazole *(dap'-taz-ol)*. Aminophenazole (q.v.).

ڈیپٹیزول : امینوفینازول۔ یہ دوا مرکز تنفس کو متاثر کرتی ہے۔

Darabdin *(dar'-ab-din)*. Given intramuscularly to encourage appetitie.

ڈریبڈن : یہ دوا بھوک تیز کرنے کے لئے انجکشن کے ذریعے دی جاتی ہے۔

Daranide *(dar'-a-nid)*. Dichlorphenamide (q.v.).

ڈیرانڈ : ڈائی کلورفنامائڈ۔ مختصر عرصہ کے لئے منہ کے ذریعے کھائی جانے والی پیشاب آور دوائی۔ کاربونک اینہائیڈریز کو روکنے والی۔ گلاکوما کے علاج کے لئے مستعمل۔

Daraprim *(da'-ra-prim)*. Pyrimethamine (q.v.).

دارا پرم : پائیری میتھامین۔ ملیریا سے بچنے کے لئے حفاظتی طور پر اسے استعمال کیا جاتا ہے۔ بچوں کو کھلانے کے لئے مناسب ہے۔ اس کی ایک گولی ہر ہفتے ۳ ماہ تک برائے ملیریا۔

Dartalan *(dar'-tal-an)*. Thiopropazate (q.v.).

ڈرٹیلان : تھایوپروپیزیٹ۔ سائیکو فیورونک حالتوں میں استعمال ہونے والی دوائی۔

Daunorubicin *(daw-no-roo'-bi-sin)*. Similar to adriamycin (q.v.). Antibiotic used in acute leukaemia. Believed to act by inhibiting DNA synthesis. Can cause severe bone marrow depression and toxicity of heart muscle.

ڈانوریوبیسن : ایڈریامائی سن سے مشابہ۔ اینٹی بایوٹک لیوکیمیا میں مفید۔ ڈی این اے کی تالیف میں رکاوٹ پیدا کرتی ہے۔ ہڈی کے گودے اور قلبی عضلے کے لئے ضرر رساں۔

Day hospital Patients attend daily. Recreaticnal and occupational therapy and physiotherapy often provided. Greatest use is in the geriatric and psychiatric fields.

روزستان ہسپتال: جہاں مریض روزانہ آتے ہوں۔

DBH. Dopamine-B-hydroxylase. an enzyme present in blood, increased in high blood pressure.

DBI. Phenformin (q.v.).

ڈی بی آئی: فینفارمن۔ ذیابیطس کے خلاف عامل دوا۔ یہ دوائی وزن کم کرتی ہے۔ یہ انسولین کی طرح عمل کرتی ہے۔ خلیوں کو زیادہ گلوکوس استعمال کرنے کیلئے تحریک کرتی ہے۔

DOS. Diaminodiphenyisslphone (q.v.).

ڈی ڈی ایس: ڈائی امینوڈائی فینائل سلفون۔ ملیریا کے مزاحمتی سٹرین کے خلاف استعمال ہونے والی ایک تالیفی دوائی۔ کوڑھ میں بھی مستعمل ہے۔

Deamination *(de-am-in-a'-shun)*. A process occurring in the liver whereby amino acids are broken down and urea formed.

ازالۂ امونیا۔ امینوربائی: جگر میں واقع ہونے والا عمل جس میں امینوایسڈز کی شکستگی ہوتی ہے اور یوریا بنتا ہے۔

Debendox *(deb'-en-docks)*. Dicyclomine hydrochloride (q.v.) with doxlamine (q.v.) and pyridoxine hydrochloride (q.v.). Useful for nausea and vomiting in pregnancy.

ڈائی بین ڈاکس: وضع حمل کے زمانہ میں متلی اور قے کے لئے مفید۔

Debridement *(da-bred'-mong)* [F]. In surgery, thorough cleansing of a wound with removal of all foreign matter and injured or infected tissue.

قطع ماؤفہ: فرانسیسی زبان کا لفظ۔ سرجری میں زخم کی مکمل صفائی۔

Debrisoquine *(deb-ris'-o-kwin)*. Hypotensive agent. Interferes with transmission in sympathetic adrenergic nerves, especially sympathetically mediated vascular reflexes, thus can lead to postural hypotension.

ڈیبریسوکوئن: اعصاب کو متاثر کرنے والی دوا۔

Deca-Durabolin *(dek'-a-du-ro-bol'-in)*. Synthetic androgen; anabolie. Given intramuscularly. Neutralizes oestrogen uptake by cancer cells.

ڈیکاڈیورو بولن: تالیفی اینڈروجن۔ یہ دوائی ٹیکے کے ذریعے دی جاتی ہے۔

Decalcification *(de-kal-si-fik-a'-shun)* [L. de-away; calx, lime; facere, to make]. Removal of mineral salts, as from teeth in dental caries, bone in disorders of calcium metabolism.

کلس ربائی: لاطینی الفاظ ڈی بمعنی دور، کلکس بمعنی چونا اور فیسیر بمعنی بنانا کا مجموعہ۔ معدنی نمکیات کا خاتمہ مثلاً دانتوں سے یا کیلیسم میٹابولزم کی خرابی میں ہڈی سے۔

Decannulation *(de-kan-u-ta'-shun)*. A term currently in use for the introduction of decreasingly smaller tubes to wean an infant from reliance on the original tracheostomy tube.

Decapsulation *(de-kap-su-la'-shun)*. [L. de-, away; capsula, little box]. Surgical removal of a capsule.

کیسہ ربائی: کیپسول کا سرجری سے خاتمہ۔

Decaspray *(dek'-a-spra)*. Aerosol containing dexamethasone and neomycin for topical application.

ڈیکا سپرے: ٹراپیکل اطلاق کے لئے ڈیکسامیتھاسون اور نیومائی سن پر مشتمل ایروسول۔

Decerebrate *(de-ser'-e-brat)*. [L. de-, away; cerebrum, brain]. Without cerebral function; a state of deep unconsciousness, **d. posture,** a condition of the unconscious patient in which all four limbs are spastic and which indicates severe damage to the cerebrum.

بے دماغ: لاطینی الفاظ ڈی بمعنی پرے اور سربرم بمعنی دماغ کا مجموعہ۔ سربرم کے فعل کے بغیر۔ گہری بیہوشی کی حالت۔

Decholin *(dek'-o-lin)*. Dehydrocholic acid. Cholagogue (q.v.).

ڈیکولن: ڈیہائیڈروکولک ایسڈ۔ آنت میں بائل کا بہاؤ زیادہ کرنے والی دوا کوہ گگ۔

Decicain *(des'-i-kan)*. Amethocaine (q.v.).

ڈیسی کین: امیتھوکین۔ امیتھوکین ہائیڈروکلورائڈ ایک تالیفی مادہ ہے جس کے کچھ خواص کوکین کے ہیں۔ سطحی دخول اور سپائن کو سن کرنے کیلئے مستعمل ہے۔ پروکین سے زیادہ زہریلا چوسنے والی گولیوں کی شکل میں دستیاب۔

Decidua *(de-sid'-u-a)* [L. deciduas, from decidere, to fall off]. The endometrial lining of the uterus thickened and altered for the reception of the fertilized ovum. It is shed when pregnancy terminates, **d. basalis,** that part which lies under the embedded ovum and forms the maternal part of the placenta. **d. capsularis,** that part that lies over the developing ovum. **d. vera,** the decidua lining the rest of the uterus--decidual, adj.

ڈیسیڈوا۔ غشائے ساقط: یوٹرس و بیز ہو جاتی ہے اور بازور بیضہ کو سنبھالنے کے لئے تبدیلی ہوتی ہے۔ جب حمل ختم ہوتا ہے تو یہ اندرونی تہہ جھڑ جاتی ہے۔ ڈیسیڈوا بسیلس وہ حصہ ہے جو دھنسے ہوئے بیضہ کے نیچے ہوتا ہے۔ ڈیسڈوا کیپسولیرس وہ حصہ ہے جو تکمیلی بیضہ کے اوپر ہوتا ہے اور پلیسنٹا کا ماروی حصہ بناتا ہے۔ ڈیسیڈوا ویرا بقایا یوٹرس کی اندرونی تہہ ہوتی ہے۔

Deciduoma malignum *(de-sid-u-o'-ma mal-ig'-num)* [L. deciduus, a falling off; G. -oma, tumour]. Chorionepithelioma (q.v.).

خبیث ریزینی سلعہ : کوریانی خلیوں سے بننے والی گلٹی۔

Declinax *(de-klin'-aks).* Debrisoquine (q.v.).

ڈیکلا ئینیکس : اعصاب کو متاثر کرنے والی دوا۔

Decompensation *(de-kom-pen-sa'-shun)* [L. de-, away; compensare, to compensate]. A failure of compensation in heart disease.

فشل تعویض: دل کی بیماری میں تلافی کرنے کی ناکامی۔

Decompression *(de-kom-presh'-un)* [L. de-, away; compressus, from comprimere, to compress]. Removal of pressure or a compressing force, **abdominal d.** currently being used in pregnancy and labour. Apparatus applied to anterior abdominal wall. Improves blood supply and results in shorter and less painful labour. Of value in pre-eclamptic toxaemia. **d. of brain** achieved by trephining the skull; **d. of bladder** in cases of chronic urinary retention, by7 continuous or intermittent drainage via catheter inserted per urethra. **d. chamber** used when returning deep-sea divers to the surface. See CAISSON DISEASE.

رفع دباؤ: دباؤ کا ہٹاؤ یا خاتمہ۔ بطنی وضع حمل اور دردزہ میں استعمال کی جاتا ہے۔ اگلی بطنی دیوار پر لگانے والا سامان۔ خون کی روانی کو درست کرتا ہے اور درد کے وقفوں کو کم یا مختصر کرتا ہے اور دردزہ کی شدت کو کم کرتا ہے۔

Decongestion *(de-kon-jest'-yun)* [L. de-, reversing, separating; congerere, to bring together]. Relief of congestion--decongestive, adj.

ڈی کنجیسٹیون: زیادتی سے آرام یا سکون۔

Decortication *(de-kort-ik-a'-shun)* [L. decorticare, to deprive of bark]. Surgical removal of cortex or outer covering of an organ **d. of lung** carried out when thickening of the visceral pleura prevents re-expansion of lung as may occur in chronic empyema. The visceral pleura is peeled off the lung, which is then re-expanded by positive pressure through an anaesthetic apparatus.

پوست اترنا: کسی عضو کے بیرونی غلاف یا کارٹیکس کو سرجری کے ذریعے ہٹانا یا ختم کرنا۔

Decubitus *(de-ku'-bit-us)* [L. from decumbere, to lie down]. The recumbent position; lying down. **d. ulcer,** pressure sore (q.v.)--decubital, adj; decubiti, pl.

تقاطع: کیازاما۔ اعصابی ریشوں کا کسی نقطے پر ایک دوسرے کو قطع کرنا۔

Defaecation *(de-fe-ka'-shun)* [L. de-, away; faeces, dregs, excrement]. Voiding of faeces per anus--defaecate, v.t.

پاخانہ کرانا: فضلے کا مبرز یا مقعد سے اخراج۔

Defervescence *(de-fer-ves'-ens)* [L. defervescere, to cease boiling]. The time during which a fever is declining. If the body temperature falls rapidly it is spoken of as 'crisis'; if it falls slowly the term 'lysis' is used.

تپ کی کمی: وہ وقفہ جس کے دوران بخار کم ہو رہا ہوتا ہے۔

Defibillation *(de-fib-ril-a'-shun)* [L. fibrilla, dim. of fibra, a fibre]. The arrest of fibrillation of the cardiac muscle (atrial or ventricular), and restoration of normal cycle--defibrillate, v.

ڈی فبریلیشن : قلبی عضلے میں ریشہ بندی ختم ہونا اور نارمل دور کا دوبارہ شروع ہونا۔

Defibrillator *(de-fib'-ril-a-tor).* Any agent, e.g. an electric shock, which arrests ventricular fibrillation and restores normal rhythm.

ڈی فبریلیٹر : کوئی عامل یا ایجنٹ مثلاً برقی صدمہ جو قلبی ریشہ بندی کو ختم کر کے نارمل ردم شروع کرتا ہے۔

Defibrinated *(de-fi'-brin-at-ed)* [L. de-, away; fibra, fibre]. Rendered free from fibrin (q.v.).

A necessary process in the preparation of serum (q.v.)--defibrinate, v.

ڈی فبر ینیٹڈ : لاطینی لفظ ڈی بمعنی دور اور فائبرا بمعنی دھاگہ یا ریشہ کا مجموعہ۔ فائبرن سے آزاد کرنا۔ سیرم کی تیاری میں ایک ضروری عمل۔

eficiency disease Disease resulting from dietary deficiency of any substance essential for good health, especially the vitamins.

مرض قلت (وٹامنی) : خوراک میں کسی لازمی شے خصوصاً حیاتین کی کمی سے پیدا ہونے والا مرض۔

egeneration *(de-jen-er-a'-shun)* [L. degenerare, to depart from]. Deterioration in quality or function. Regression from more specialized to less specialized type of tissue. **afferent d.,** degeneration spreading up sensory nerves. **amyloid d.,** a wax-like tissue resulting from atrophy in a tuberculoma or gumma. **colloid d.,** mucoid degeneration of tumours. **fatty d.,** inwhich droplets of fat occur in atrophic tissue, as in the myocardium. **hyaline d.,** affecting connective tissue, especially of blood vessels, in which the tissue takes on a homogeneous or formless appearance. **senile d.** is the clinical picture of old age in which the acuity of thought and performance is blunted. **subacute combined d.,** of the spinal cord, heralded by paraesthesis (q.v.)., is a complication of untreated pernicious anaemia--degenerative, adj; degenerate, v.i.

انحطاط : کوالٹی یا فعل میں معیار کا کم ہونا۔ کسی بافت میں تخصیص گھٹنا۔

eglutition *(de-gloo-tish'-un)* [L. deglutire, to swallow down]. The process of swallowing, partly voluntary, partly involuntary.

نگلنا : نگلنے کا عمل جو جزوی طور پر ارادی اور جزوی طور پر غیر ارادی ہو۔

egranol *(de-gran'-ol)*. Mannomustine (q.v.).

ڈیگرانول : مینومسٹین۔ اینٹی مائیوٹک عامل۔ کینسر یا سرطان میں مفید۔

hiscence *(de-his'-ens)* [Ldehiscere, to gape]. The process of splitting or bursting open, as of a wound.

شگفتگی : پھٹنے یا کھلنے کا عمل مثلاً زخم کا کھلنا۔

hydration *(de-hid-ra'-shun)* [L. *deaway;* G. *hydor,* water]. Loss or removal of fluid. In the body this condition arises when the fluid intake fails to replace fluid loss. This is liable to occur when there is bleeding, diarrhoea, excessive exudation from a raw area, excessive sweating, polyuria or vomiting, and usually upsets the body's electroyte balance. If suitable fluid replacement cannot be achieved orally then parenteral administration must be instituted--dehydrate, *v.t.*

نابیدگی۔ آب ربائی : لاطینی لفظ ڈی بمعنی دور اور ہائیڈر بمعنی پانی کا مجموعہ۔ کسی سیال کا ضایع یا ہٹاؤ۔ جسم میں یہ حال اس وقت ہوتا ہے جب ضائع شدہ سیال کی جگہ مزید سیال آنے میں ناکام رہے مثلاً روانی خون، پیچس یا دست، قے یا پسینے کی زیادتی۔

Dehydrocholic acid *(de-hid-ro-kol'-ik-as'-id)*. Cholagogue (q.v.)

ڈی ہائیڈروکلورک ایسڈ : کولاگگ۔ بائل کے بہاؤ میں اضافہ کرنے والی دوا۔

Deja vu phenomenon [F. seen before]. Occurs in epilepsy involving temporal lobers of the brain and in certain epileptic dream states. An intense feeling of familiarity as if everything had happened before.

ڈیجا دو فینا مینا : یہ احساس کہ ہر شے پہلے سے جانی پہچانی ہے۔ یہ کوڑھ کی بیماری میں دماغ کے ٹمپورل لوبوں کی وجہ سے ہوتا ہے۔

Deladroxate *(del-a-droks'-at)*. Contains hormones, similar to those in the once-daily contrceptive pills. Given as monthly injection.

ڈیلاڈروکسٹ : ہارموز پر مشتمل۔ روزانہ ایک مانع حمل گولیوں سے مشابہ۔ ماہانہ ٹیکہ کے ذریعے دیا جاتا ہے۔

Delhi boil See ORIENTAL SORE.

دہلی دمل : جلد یا کھال پر ابھار۔ استوائی اور نیم استوائی خطوں کی بیماری۔

Deliuescent *(del-i-kwes'-ent)*. Capable of absorption, thus becoming fluid.

آب گیر : انجذاب کے اہل اس لئے سیال بن جاتا ہے۔

Delirium *(de-lir'-i-um)* [L.]. Abnormal mental condition based on hallucinations or illusion. May occur in high fever, in mental disease, or be toxic in origin. **d. tremens** results from alcoholic intoxication and is represented by a picture of confusion, terror, restlessness and hallucinations--delirious, adj.

ڈلیریم ۔ ہزیان ۔ سرسام: ذہنی حالت خلاف معمول ہونا۔ کسی ذہنی بیماری۔ زیادہ بخار یا زہریلے پن کی وجہ سے ایسا ہوسکتا ہے۔ ڈلیریم ٹریمنز زیادہ الکحل پینے سے ہوتا ہے۔ جس سے خون' بے آرامی اور پریشانی ہوتی ہے۔

Delta-Cortef *(del'-ta-kawr'-tef)*. Prednisolone (q.v.)

ڈیلٹا کارٹیف: پریڈنیسولون۔ ایک تالیفی ہارمون جو خواص میں کورٹیسون کے مشابہ ہے لیکن اس سے جانبی اثرات کم ہوتے ہیں۔

Delta-Cortelan *(del'-ta-kawr'-te-lan)*. Prednisone (q.v.)

ڈیلٹا کارٹی لان: پریڈنیسون۔ کورٹیسون سے اخذ شدہ لیکن کم خوراک میں اثر زیادہ کرتا ہے۔ عمل' استعمال اور خوراک میں پریڈنیسولون سے مشابہ۔

Deltacortone *(del'-ta-kawr'-ton)*. Prednisone (q.v.)

ڈیلٹا کارٹون: کورٹیسون سے حاصل شدہ لیکن اس کی خوراک کم دی جاتی ہے۔ کیونکہ زیادہ موثر ہے۔

Deltoid *(del'-toid)* [G. *delta,* fourth letter of the G. alphabet ; *eidos,* form]. Triangular,d. muscle, base lies over shoulder region, apex inserted into midshaft of humerus.

ڈیلٹائڈ۔ مثلثی۔ عضلہ دالیہ: تکون نما۔ مثلث نما۔ ڈیلٹائڈ عضلہ کا

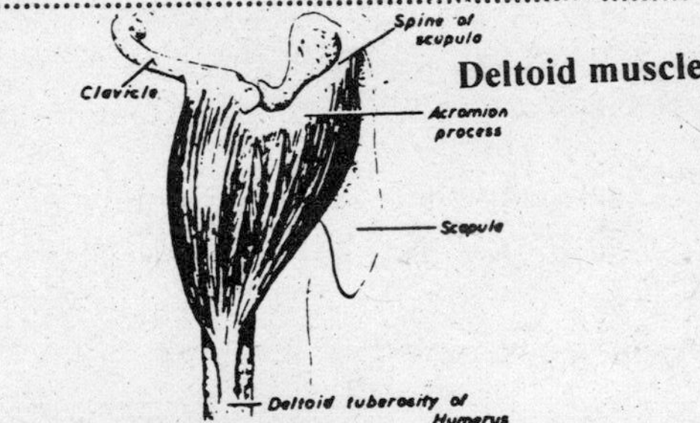

Deltoid muscle

اساس شانے کے حصے کے اوپر رہوتا ہے اور راس ہیومرس کے مڈشافٹ میں ہوتا ہے بازو کا عضلہ جو انٹرا اسکولر انجکشن یا عضلاتی ٹیکہ کے لئے مناسب ہے۔

Delusion *(de-lu'-zhun)* [L. *delusum,* from *deludere,* to deceive]. A false belief which cannot be altered by argument or reasoning. Found as a psychotic symptom in several types of insanity, notably schizophrenia, paraphrenia, paranoia, senile psychoses, mania and depressive states including involutional melancholia.

ہم: غلط عقیدہ جسے کسی دلیل سے تبدیل نہیں کیا جا سکتا۔ پاگل پن کی مختلف ...سام میں نفسیاتی نظام کے طور پر پایا جاتا ہے۔

Demarcation *(de-mar-ka'-shun)*. An outlinin of the junction of diseased and healthy tissu and usually referring to gangrene.

...د بندی: بیمار اور صحت مند بافت کے ملاپ کی بیرونی سطح۔

Dementia *(de-men'-shi-a)* [L. being out of one mind]. Irreversible organic deterioratioin mental faculties. **d. paralytica,** gener paralysis of the insane. See GENERAL **praecox,** see SCHIZOPHRENIA. **preseni d.,** Alzheimer's disease. Dementia occurrrin in the under fifties. Due to hyalin degeneration of medium and smaller cerebr blood vessels. [Alois Alzheimer, Germa physician, 1864-1915.]

...ا ہٹ: ذہنی جبلتوں کا انحطاط۔

Demethylchlortetracycline *(de-meth'-il-k awr-tet-ra- si'-klin)*. One of the tetracyclin (q.v.)

...بتھائل کلورٹیٹرا سائیکلین: ایک ٹیٹرا سائیکلین ۔ اینٹی بایوٹک۔ ... کا ایک کیپسول صبح ایک دوپہر ایک شام برائے ورم دماغ یا این کیف لائی ... مفید برائے آسٹیومائی لائی ٹس یعنی گھمبیرا کیوٹ اینڈے سائی ٹس۔

Demography *(dem-og'-ra-fi)* [G. *demos,* th people; *graphein,* to write]. Social scierc including vital statistics.

...دم نگاری: یونانی الفاظ ڈیمس بمعنی لوگ ور گریفین بمعنی لکھنا کا مجموعہ۔ ...ل سائنس بشمول شماریات۔ مردم شماری کا علم۔ اعداد و شمار مرتب کرنا۔

Demulcent *(de-mul'-sent)* [L. *demulcere,* stroke down]. A slippery, mucilaginous flu which allays irritation and soothes inflar mation, especially of mucous membranes.

...لمن: ایک پھسلنے والا سیال جو سوزش یا جلن کو آرام کرتا ہے۔ خصوصا میوکس ...وں کی۔ گلیسرین وغیرہ۔

Demyelinization *(de-mi-el-in-iz-a'-shun)*. destructi of the myelin sheaths surrounding ner fibres; occurs in multiple sclerosis, S SCLEROSIS.

Dendrite or **Dendron** *(den'drit; den'-dron)* [*dendron,* tree]. One of the branched filame which are given off from the body of a ne cell. That part of a neurone which transm an impulse to the nerve cell-dendritic, adj.

شجر یہ: یونانی لفظ ڈینڈران بمعنی درخت۔شاخ دار ریشوں میں سے ایک جو عصبی خلیے کی باڈی سے ابھرتے ہیں۔نیورون کا وہ حصہ جو عصبی خلیے کو تحریک کرتا ہے۔

endritic ulcer Linear corneal ulcer that sends out tree-like branches. Caused by herpes simplex, See IDOXURIDINE.

شجرینی ناسور: سرطان کی ایک قسم جس میں شجر نما شاخیں بنتی ہیں۔ یہ داد سے ہوتا ہے۔

enervation *(de-ner-va'-shun)*. The means by which a nerve supply is cut off. Usually refers to incision, excision or blocking of a nerve.

عصب ربائی۔عصب بندی: وہ ذرائع جن کی وجہ سے عصبی سپلائی منقطع ہو جاتی ہے۔عموماً عصب کا بند یا قطع ہونا۔

engue *(deng'-ga)*. Disease of the tropics. Causative agent is an arbovirus conveyed by a mosquito. Characterized by rheumatic pains, fever and a skin eruption, Sometimes called 'break-bone fever'.

لال بخار: مشرق وسطی کی بیماری۔ مچھر کے کاٹنے سے ایک وائرس انسانی جسم میں داخل ہو جاتا ہے۔اس بیماری میں بخار اور جوڑوں کا درد ہوتا ہے۔اور جلد پھٹ جاتی ہے۔اسے ہڈی توڑ بخار بھی کہا جاتا ہے۔

ennis Browne splints, Splints used to correct congenital talipes equinovarus.The splints are of metal, padded with felt, with a joining bar , to which the baby's feet are strapped. [Dennis Browne, British surgeon, 1892-1967.]

ڈینس براؤن تختیاں: دھاتی تختیاں جن کے نتیجے نرم پیڈ لگے ہوتے ہیں ۔ایک سلاخ انہیں ملاتی ہے۔اس میں بچے کے پاؤں اڑاتے ہیں۔ برطانوی سرجن ڈینس براؤن کے نام پر ہے جس کا دور حیات ۱۸۹۲ع تا ۱۹۶۷ع ہے۔

entine *(den'-ten)* [L. *dens,* tooth]. The calcified tissue enclosing the pulp cavity of a tooth.

دنتین: لاطینی لفظ ڈینس بمعنی دانت سے ماخوذ۔دانت کے پلپ کہفہ کے گرد کلسی بافت۔

entition *(den-tish'-un)* [L. *dentition,* from *dentire,* to teethe]. Teething. **primary d.,** eruption of the deciduous, 'milk' or temporary teeth. **secondary d.,** eruption of the 'adult' or permanent teeth.

دندانیت: دانتوں کا اگنا۔ عارضی یا دودھ کے دانتوں کا اگنا پرائمری اور مستقل دانتوں کا اگنا ثانوی کہلاتا ہے۔

Deodorant *(de-od'-or-an)* [L. *de*-away; odor, smell]. Any substance which destroys or masks an (unpleasnat) odour. Potassium permanganate and hydrogen peroxide are deodorants by their powerful oxidizing action; chlorophyll has some reputation as a deodorant for foul-smelling wounds, but its value in masking other odours is doubtful--deodorize, v.t.

دافع بدبو: ایسی شے جو ناخوشگوار بو کو ختم کر دے۔ مثلاً پوٹاشیم پرمینگنیٹ' ہائیڈروجن پر آکسائیڈ کلوروفل۔

Deoxycortone *(de-oks-i-kor'-ton)*. An important hormone of the adrenal cortex, controlling the metabolism of sodium and potassium. Used mainly in the management of Addison's disease. DOCA.

ڈی آکسی کارٹون: ایڈرینل کارٹیکس کا ایک اہم ہارمون۔سوڈیم و پوٹاشیم کے میٹابولزم کو کنٹرول کرتا ہے۔چوتھے یا ساتویں روز ایک ٹیکہ برائے امراض ایڈیشن۔مفید برائے انلارجڈ پراسٹیٹ۔

Deoxygenation *(de-oks-i'-jen-a-shun)* [L. *de*-away; G. *oxys,* sharp; *genesthai,* to be produced]. The removal of oxygen--deoxygenated, adj.

آکسیجن ربائی: آکسیجن کا ہٹاؤ یا خاتمہ۔

Deoxyribonucleic acid *(de-oks-i-ri-bon-uk'-li-ik)*. DNA. The natural carbohydrate consituent of cell nuclei. In conjunction with deoxyribonucleoprotein it makes up the autoreproducing component of chromosomes and many viruses. Together they are fundamental components of living tissue.

ڈی آکسی ریبونکلیک ایسڈ: ڈی این اے۔خلیوں کے مرکزوں کا کاربوہائیڈریٹ والا جزو۔کروموسوموں اور کئی وائرسوں میں ڈی آکسی ریبو نکلیو پروٹین کے ساتھ مل کر خود تولیدی جزو بناتا ہے۔وہ جاندار بافت کے لئے بنیادی اجزاء ہیں۔یہ وراثت میں اہم کردار ادا کرتا ہے۔ایک نسل سے دوسری نسل میں منتقل ہو جاتا ہے۔ ہر نوع کا ڈی این اے مختلف ہوتا ہے۔ڈی این اے ایک دوہرے طویل ریشے کی مانند ہے۔ریشے کی دونوں لڑیوں نے ایک دوسرے کے گرد بل کھائے ہوئے ہیں۔اور ایک دوسرے کے ساتھ ملی ہوتی

ہیں۔ ان لڑیوں کو نکلیوٹائیڈز کہا جاتا ہے۔ نیا کروموسوم بنتے وقت اس میں موجود ڈی این اے کی نقل تیار ہوتی ہے جو پرانے ڈی این اے کے عین مطابق ہوتی ہے۔

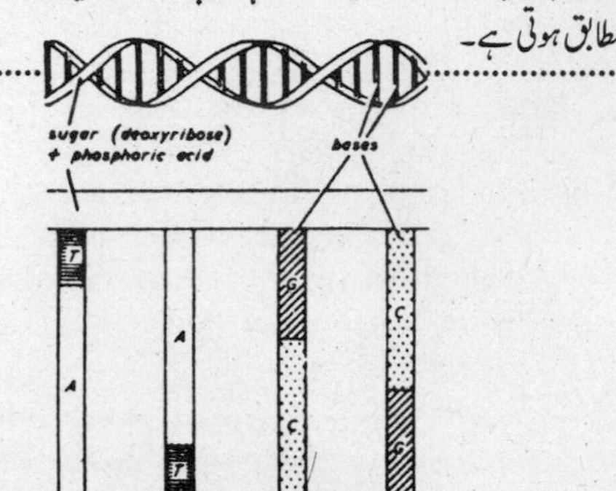

Deoxyribonucleic acid
T = Thymine
A = Adenine
G = Guanine
C = Cytosine

ان دونوں میں سے ایک پرانے کروموسوم میں اور دوسری نقل نئے کروموسوم میں چلی جاتی ہے۔ اس طرح نیا کروموسوم ہو بہو پرانے کروموسوم کی نقل ہوتا ہے۔ جب یہ کسی نئے خلیے میں جاتا ہے تو اس میں اور پرانے خلیہ میں کروموسوم کے لحاظ سے کوئی فرق نہیں ہوتا اس طرح ڈی این اے جانداروں میں ایک خلیہ سے دوسرے خلیہ میں اور ایک نسل سے دوسری نسل میں منتقل ہوتا رہتا ہے۔ ہر نکلیوٹائیڈ میں حسب ذیل چار نائٹروجنی اساسوں میں سے ایک ہوتا ہے۔ ایڈنین، سائیٹوسین، گوانین اور تھائمین۔ تین اساس ایک امینوایسڈ کے کوڈ کو ظاہر کرتے ہیں۔ ڈی این اے کے سالمے کی ساخت ایک بٹے ہوئے رسے کی سیڑھی کی مانند ہے جس کی دونوں اطراف شوگر فاسفیٹ زنجیروں پر مشتمل ہیں۔ سیڑھی کے ڈنڈے نائٹروجنی اساسوں پر مشتمل ہیں۔ ڈنڈے تکمیلی اساسی جوڑوں پر مشتمل ہیں جو ہائیڈروجن بانڈز کے ذریعے ملے ہوئے ہیں۔

Depersonalization *(de-per-son-al-i-za'-shun).* A subjective feeling of having lost one's personality, sometimes that one no longer exists. Occurs in schizophrenia and more rarely in depressive stantes.

عدم شخصیت: اپنی شخصیت کے ضیاع کا احساس۔

Depilate *(dep'-il-at)* [L. *de*, away ; *pilus*, hair]. To remove hair from--depilatory, adj. n; **depilation, n.**

ر بائی: لاطینی الفاظ ڈی بمعنی پرے اور پائلس بمعنی بال کا مجموعہ۔ کسی جگہ بال صاف کرنا۔

Depilation electric

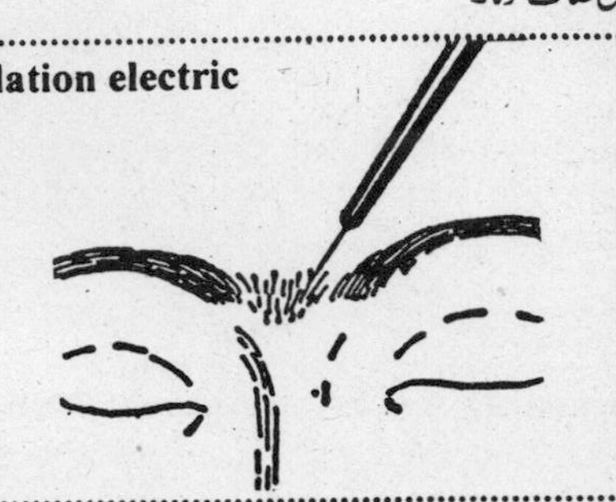

Depilatories *(de-pil'-at-or-iz).* Substanc usually made in pastes (e.g. barium sulphid which remove excess hair only temporari they do not act on the papillae, consequent the hair grows again. See EPILATION.

صفا (دوائیں): اشیاء جو عموماً پیسٹ کی صورت میں تیار کی جاتی۔ مثلاً بیریم سلفائیڈ جو فالتو بالوں کو عارضی طور پر صاف کرتی ہیں۔ چونکہ وہ کی جڑوں تک عمل نہیں کرتیں اس لئے بال دوبارہ اگ آتے ہیں۔

Depo-Provera *(dep'-o-pro-ver-a)* Medroxy rogesterone acetate (q.v.)

Depression *(de-presh'-un)* [L. *depressus,* fro *deprimere,* to depress]. 1. A hollow place indentation.2. Diminution of power or activi 3. A low condition, either mentl or physic In psychiatry, emotional disorder. Of tv distinct types, neurotic and psychotic. T neurotic type,**reactive d.,** occurs as a reacti to stress. The psychotic type, **endogenous** occurs as a reaction to stress. The psycho type, **endogenous d.,** arises spontaneously the mind. the symptoms are almost the sa in both conditions and vary from mild to fa and are: insomnia, headaches, exhaustic anorexia, irritability, emotionalism or loss attect, loss of interest, impaired concentrati feelings that life is not worth living, a suicidal thoughts. **involution d.,** that occuri at the climacteric.

کی کمی۔ مالی خولیا: (۱) ایک کھوکھلی جگہ۔ (۲) طاقت یا عاملیت کی ۔ (۳) ذہنی یا جسمانی حالت میں کمی۔ بھوک اور بات چیت میں کمی۔

پریشانی کی حالت۔

privation syndrome Usually the result of parental rejection of offspring. Includes dwarfism, malnutrition with potbelly, gluttonous appetite, superficial affectionate attachment to any adult, old healed sores on buttocks, chilblain scars on fingers and toes, very thin hair.

سلبی سنڈروم: اولاد کی پدری عدم مقبولیت کا نتیجہ۔ اس کی مختلف علامات میں بوناپن، زیادہ بھوک کسی بڑے کے ساتھ رہنا، چوتڑوں پر۔ پرانے ٹھیک ہوئے ناسور، انگلیوں اور انگوٹھوں پر نشانات اور باریک بال شامل ہیں۔

ptropin citrate *(dep-tro'-pen sit'-rat)* Tablets and injection for bronchor-rhoea, bronchial asthma, vasomotor rhinitis and maintenance therapy in bronchitis.

ڈیپٹروپین: دمہ کے لئے گولیاں اور ٹیکے۔

rbyshire neck *(dar'-bi-sher)*. Goitre (q.v.).

گلہڑ: گھینگا۔ تھائیرائڈ غدود کا بڑھنا۔

realization *(de-re-al-iz-a'-shun)*. [L. de-, away from; res, thing]. Feelings of unreality, such as occur to normal people during dreams. A symptom often found in schizohrenia and depressive states.

خیالی احساس: ناحقیقت کے احساسات۔ جیسا کہ خوابوں کے دوران عام لوگوں کے ساتھ واقع ہوتا ہے۔

reistic *(de-re-is'-tik)*. Thinking not adapted to reality. Autistic thinking.

ڈیریسٹک: حقیقت کے مطابق نہ ہونے کا سوچنا۔

rmatitis *(der-ma-ti'-tis)*. [G. derma, skin; -itis, inflammation]. Inflammation of the skin (by custom limited to an eczematous reaction), **d. herpetiformis,** an intensely itchy skin eruption of unknown cause, most commonly characterized by vesicles, bullae and pustules on urticarial plaques, which remit and relapse. When occuring in pregnancy it is known as 'hydroagravidarum, **juvenile d. herpetiformis,** recurrent bullous eruption on genitalia, lower abdomen, buttocks and face, mainly in children under 5 boys being affected more often than girls. In Great Britain the incidence is higher in northern parts of country. Treatment is dapsone possibly until puberty; maintenance dose that prevents new lesions appearing. **industrial d.** is a term used in the National Insurance (Industrial Injuries). Act, to cover occupational skin conditions '.....due to dust or liquids'.

ورم جلد: یونانی الفاظ ڈرما بمعنی جلد اور ائٹس بمعنی سوزش کا مجموعہ۔ جلد یا کھال کی سوزش جلد اپنی پوری موٹائی تک متورم ہو جاتی ہے۔ جلد کی رنگت سرخ، درد، بخار، چھالے اور زخم ہو جاتے ہیں۔ مقامی طور پر زنک بورک ایسڈ مرہم لگائیے۔ کرسٹامائی سین کا ایک ٹیکہ صبح ایک شام لگائیے۔

Dermatoglyphics *(der-mat-o-gli'-fiks)* [G. derma, skin; glyphos carved]. Study of the ridge patterns of the skin of the fingertrips, palms and soles to discover developmental anomalies.

ڈرمیٹوگلائی فکس: تکمیلی خرابیاں معلوم کرنے کے لئے ایڑیوں، ہتھیلیوں اور انگلیوں کے راس کا مطالعہ۔

Dermatographia *(der-mat-o-graf-i-a)*. See DERMOGRAPHIA.

Dermatologist *(der-mat-ol'-oj-ist)* [G. derma, skin; logos, discourse]. One who studies skin diseases and is skilled in their treatment. A skin specialist.

ماہر امراض جلد: جلد کا ماہر۔ جلد کی بیماریوں کا مطالعہ کرنے والا اور ان کی علاج میں ماہر۔

Dermatology *(der-mat-ol'-o-ji)* [G. derma, skin; logos, discourse]. The science which deals with the skin, its structure, functions, diseases and their treatment--dermatological, adj.; dermatologically, adv.

علم امراض جلد: سائنس جس میں جلد یا کھال، اس کی ساخت، افعال، امراض اور ان کے علاج کا مطالعہ کیا جاتا ہے۔

Dermatome *(der'-mat-om)* [G. derma, skin; tome, a cutting]. A instrument for cutting slices of skin of varying thickness, usually for grafting.

جلد شگاف: عموماً پیوندکاری کے لئے مختلف دبازت کی جلد کی قاشیں کاٹنے کا آلہ۔

Dermatomycosis *(der-mat-o-mi-ko'-sis)* [G. derma, skin; mykes, fungus; -osis, condition]. Fungal infection of the skin--dermatomycotic, adj.

جلدی فطریت: یونانی الفاظ ڈرما بمعنی جلد' مائیکس بمعنی سماروغ اور اوسس بمعنی حالت کا مجموعہ۔ جلد کا سماروغی بیماری۔

Dermatomyositis *(der'-mat-o-mi-os-it'-is)* [G. derma, skin; mys, muscle; -itis, inflammation]. An acute inflammation of the skin and muscles which presents with oedema and muscle weakness. May result in the atrophic changes of sclerodema (q.v.). See COLLAGEN.

سوزش جلد و عضلات: جلد اور عضلات کی سوزش۔

Dermatophytes *(der-mat-o-fitz')* [G. derma, skin; phyton, a plant]. A group of fungi which invade the superfical skin.

جلد پودا: یونانی الفاظ ڈرما بمعنی کھال' فائیٹون بمعنی پودا یا نبات کا مجموعہ۔ سماروغ کا ایک گروہ جو سطحی جلد پر حملہ آور ہوتا ہے۔

Dermatophytosis *(der'-mat-o-fi-to'-sis)* [G. derma, skin; phyton, a plant; -osis, condition]. Syn. athlete's foot. See TINEA PEDIS.

ڈرمیٹوفائی ٹوسس: یونانی الفاظ ڈرما بمعنی کھال' فائیٹون بمعنی پودا اور اوسس بمعنی حالت کا مجموعہ۔ اتھلیٹ کا پاؤں۔ پاؤں کا رنگ ورم۔ ٹینا پیڈس

Dermatosis *(der-mat-os'-is)* [G. derma, skin; -osis, condition]. Generic term for skin disease--dermatoses, pl.

مرض جلد: یونانی الفاظ ڈرما بمع نی کھال اور اوسس بمعنی حالت کا مجموعہ۔ جلدی بیماری کے لئے جنسی اصطلاح۔

Dermis *(der'-mis)* [G. derma, skin]. The true skin; the cutis vera; the layer below the epidermis.

جلد حقیقی: یونانی لف ظ ڈرما بمعنی جلد کے سے ماخوذ۔ اصلی کھال یا جلد۔ کیوٹس ویرا۔ اپی ڈرمس کی نچلی تہہ۔

Dermographia *(der-mo-graf'-i-a)* [G. derma, skin; graphein, to write]. A condition in which weals occur on the skin after a blunt instrument or fingernail has been lightly drawn over it. Seen in vasomotor instability and urticaria.

جلدی نگاری: یونانی الفاظ ڈرما بمعنی جلد اور گریفین بمعنی لکھنا کا مجموعہ۔ ناخن یا کسی کند اوزار سے جلد پر نشانات پڑ جانا۔

Dermoid *(der'-moid)* [G. derma, skin; eidos, form]. Pertaining to or resembling skin. See CYST.

ی: کھال سے مشابہ یا اس کے متعلق۔

Dermo-jet *(der'-mo'-jet)* Apparatus for delive of fluid under pressure into the dermis. It is painless method, twice as fast as need injection and free from the danger of hepati transmission.

موجیٹ: ڈرمس میں دباؤ کے تحت سیال پہنچانے کا سامان۔ اس طریقے ں درد نہیں ہوتا۔ سوئی سے ٹیکہ لگانے سے دوگنا تیز۔

Dermovate *(der'-mo-vat)*. Clobetasol propiona (q.v.).

Desensitization *(de-sen-sit-iz-a'-shun)*. Th neutralization of acquired hypersensitivene to some agent acting on the skin or internal used in asthma and for treatment of peop who have become allergic to drugs such penicillin and streptomycin, **systematic d.,** phobic patient using i.v. methohexito sodium to achieve psychólogical relaxatio In this state the phobic situation is imagin without fear and the patient 'unlearns' h irrational fear-- densensitize, v.t.

یت ربائی: اندرونی طور پر یا جلد پر عمل کرنے والی کسی عامل کی حسیت کرنا۔ دمہ اور ایسے لوگوں کے علاج جو اینٹی بایوٹک ادویات مثلاً پنسلین، پٹومائی سین وغیرہ سے الرجک ہوگئے ہوں' کے لئے مستعمل۔

Deseril *(des'-er-il)*. Methysergide (q.v.).

یرل: میتھائی سرجائڈ۔ مائیگرین کے لئے مستعمل۔

Desferrioxamine *(des-fer-ri-oks'-a-men)*. Us in iron poisoning and haemosiderosis (q. (p. 137).

ں فیری آکس امائین: لوہے کے زہریلے پن میں مستعمل۔

Desipra mine See ANTIDEPRESSANT

ی پریمائین: اضمحلال کم کرنے والی دوائی۔

deslanoside *(des-lan'-o-sid)*. Natural glycosi Cardiac therapeutic agent.

Desmopressin *(des-mo-press'-in)*. Antidiuret See VASOPRESSIN.

Desoxycorticosterone Deoxycortone (q.v.).

ں آکسی کارٹیکوسٹیرون: ڈی آکسی کورٹون۔

Desquamation *(des-kwa-ma'-shun)* [desquamare, to scale off]. Shedding; flak off; casting off--desquammate, v.i., v.t.

تقشہ : جھڑنا۔گرنا۔

etergent *(de-ter'-jent)*. [L. detergere, to wipe off]. A cleansing agent. Is often applied to drugs of the cetrimide type, which have both antiseptic and cleaning properties, and so are valuable in removing grease, dirt, etc., from skin and wounds, and scabs and crusts from skin lesions. **d. application,** useful for removing greasy ointments from the skin; contains arachis oil, emulsifying wax and water.

مصفی: صفائی کرنے والا عامل۔ چونکہ دافع تعفن بھی ہوتا ہے اس لئے زخم دھونے کے لئے استعمال کیا جاتا ہے۔

etoxication *(de-toks-e-ka'-shun)* [L. de-, away; G. toxikon, poison]. The process of removing the poisonous property of a substance--detoxicant, adj., n.; detoxicate, v.

سم ربائی: کسی شے کی زہریلی خاصیت ختم کرنے کا طریقہ۔

etritus *(det-ri'-tus)* [L. detritum, from deterere, to wear away]. Matter produced by detrition; waste matter from disintegration.

چورا: فضول مادے کا بننا۔

etrusor *(de-troo'-ser)* [L. detrudere, to thrust from]. The muscle of the urinary bladder.

ڈی ٹروسر: مثانے کا عضلہ۔

ettol. A non-caustic antiseptic of the chloroxylenol type.

ڈیٹول: ایک غیر کاسٹک دافع تعفن۔

examethasone Thirty times as active as cortisone in suppressing inflammation. Less like to precipitate diabetes than the other steroids. Sometimes given to unconscious patients to prevent cerebral oedema.

ڈیکسا میتھاسون: سوزش کو کم کرنے والی دوائی۔ شرمگاہ کی خارش یا پردریش دلوی کے علاج کے لئے' سوزش گردہ مزمن اور دمہ میں ڈیکسا میتھاسون گولیاں ایک صبح ایک دوپہر ایک شام۔ یہی خوراک برائے ایکزیمہ۔

examphetamine *(deks-am-fet'-a-men)*. Central stimulant similar to amphetamine (q.v.) and used for similar purposes. Sometimes used as an appetite depressant in obesity.

ڈیکس ایمفیٹامین: امفیٹامین کی طرح مرکزی محرک اور انہی مقاصد کے لئے مستعمل ہے۔ بھوک کو کم کرتی ہے۔

Dexedrine. Dexamphetamine (q.v.).

ڈکسٹرین۔ نشاستین: یہ دوائی بھوک کو کم کرتی ہے۔ امفیٹامین کی طرح مرکزی محرک اور انہی مقاصد کیلئے مستعمل۔

Dextran *(deks'-tran)*. A blood plasma substitute, obtained by the action of a specific bacterium on sugar solutions. Used as a 6 or 10 percent solution in haemorrhage, shock, etc.

ڈکسٹران: خونی پلازما جو شربت پر مخصوص جرثومہ کے عمل سے حاصل کیا جاتا ہے۔ صدمہ کی صورت میں ۶ تا ۱۰ فیصد محلول استعمال کیا جاتا ہے۔

Dextranase *(deks'-tran-as)*. An enzyme that stops sugar from leaving the sticky deposit which sets free the acid that eats into tooth enamel and cannot be brushed away. Made from a mould brushed away. Made from a mould related to that producing penicillin.

ڈکسٹرانیز: ایک خامرہ جو دانتوں کی خرابی کا باعث ہے۔

Dextrin *(deks'-trin)*. A soluble polysac-charide formed during the hydrolysis of starch.

ڈکسٹرین۔ نشاستین: نشاستہ کی آب پاشیدگی کے دوران بننے والا ایک حل پذیر پولی سیکرائیڈ۔

Dextrocardia

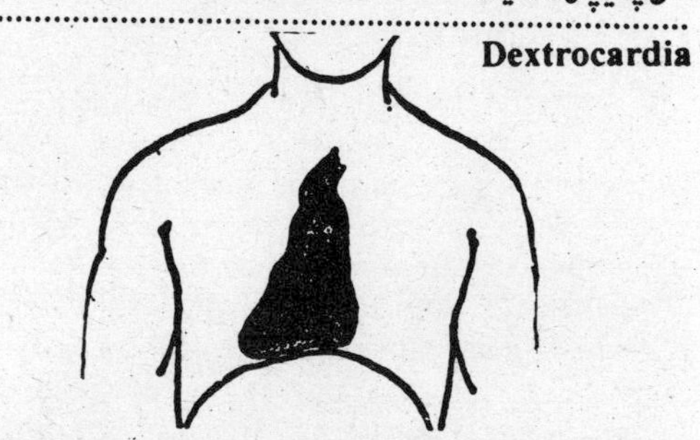

Dextrocardia *(deks-tro-kar'-di-a)*. [L. dexter, right; G. kardia, heart]. Transposition of the heart to the right side of the thorax--dextrocardial, adj.

یمین قلبی۔ راست دلی: دل کو تھوریکس کے دائیں طرف تبدیل کرنا۔

Dextromoramide *(deks-tro-mor'-a-mid)*. Substitute for morphine. Can cause drug dependence.

ڈکسٹرومورامائیڈ: مارفین کا متبادل۔ اس کی عادت بھی پڑ جاتی ہے۔

Dextropropoxyphene *(deks'-tro-pro-po- ks'-i -fen)*. Milder type of analgesic used as

morphine substitute.
ڈکسٹروپروپوکسی فین: مارفین کی جگہ مستعمل۔ تاثیر میں ہلکی۔

Dextrose *(deks'-tros)*. Glucose, a soluble carbohydrate (monosaccharide) widely used by intravenous infusion in dehydration, shock and postoperatively. Also given orally as a readily absorbed sugar in acidosis and other nutritional disturbances.
شکرانگور۔ ڈیکسٹروس: گلوکوس۔ انگوری شکر۔ مونوسیکرائیڈ۔ ایک حل پذیر کاربوہائیڈریٹ۔ پانی کی کمی میں مستعمل۔ خوراک کی کمی صورت میں بھی دیا جاتا ہے۔

DFP. Dyflos (q.v.).
ڈی ایف پی: فلورین کا اخذ شدہ۔

DF 118. Dihydrocodeine tartrate (q.v.).
ڈی ایف ۱۸۸: ڈائی ہائیڈروکوڈینون۔ اس کی عادت نہیں پڑتی۔ درد' مُدوائفری' کھانسی اور سانس کی بیماریوں میں مفید۔ یہ دوا منہ یا ٹیکے کے ذریعے دی جاتی ہے۔

Dhobie itch *(do'-be)*. Tinea cruris (q.v.). Derived from belief that ringworm of the groin originated from infection of the Indian laundryman (dhobie).
مرض دھوبی: دھوبی سے لگنے والی بیماری۔ کپڑوں کی چھوت سے آیا ہوا جلدی مرض۔

Diabetes *(di-a-be'-tez)* [G. diabainein, to cross through]. A disease characterized by polyuria. Used without qualification it means **d. mellitus, d. innocens,** renal glycosuria, where there is unusual permeability of the kidneys to glucose, the concentration in the blood remaining within normal limits. **d. insipidus, a** disease (congenital or following injury or infection) of the posterior pituitary gland or its adnexa. There is a dehydration, polydipsia, polyuria, urine being pale and of low specific gravity. **nephrogenic d. insipdus,** brought to medical attention 25 years ago, is, like haemophilia, inherited through females but appears only in males. Afflicted persons known as 'water drinkers' Characterized by polydipsia and polyuria but there is normal secretion of antidiuretic hormone. **d. mellitus,** a condition characterized by hyperglycaemia due to deficiency or diminished effectivenes of insulin. The hyperglycaemia leads t glycosuria, which in turn causes polyuria an polydipsia. Sever dehydration, sometime sufficient to cause unconsciousnes (hyperosmolar non-ketoacidotic, diabeti coma). my occur. Impaired utilization o carbohydrate is associated with increase secretion of antistorage hormones such a glucagon and growth hormone in an attemp to provide alternative metabolic substrate Glycogenolysis, gluconeogenesis an lipolysis are all increased. The latter results i excessive formation of ketone bodies whic in turn leads to acidosis. If untereated this wi eventually cause coma (ketoacidotic diabeti coma) and death. Two main clinical types ar recognized; **Juvenile-onset diabetes** usuall develops before the age of 40 and i characterized by complete lack of insulin Such patients require treatment with insulin **Maturity-onset diabetes** usually appears i middle-aged or elderly patients who are ofte obese. They have a variable, although les than normal amount of plasma insulin and ca usually be controlled by dietary means alone or by an oral hypoglycaemic drug. Potentia diabetics have a normal glucose tolerance tes but are at increased risk of developin diabetes for genetic reasons. Latent diabetic have a normal glucose tolerance test but ar known to have had an abnormal test unde conditions imposing a burden on th pancreatic beta cells, e.g. during infection c pregnancy. In the latter instance the terr gestational diabetes is commonly used.
یابیطس: پیشاب میں گلوکوس کا اخراج۔ لبلبہ سے انسولین کی مقدار کم ہو تی ہے۔ اس میں انسولین سادہ یا گلائیبین کلامائیڈ کی گولیاں دی جاتی ہیں۔ ور پروپامائیڈ کی گولیاں بھی مفید ہیں۔

Diabetic *(di-ab-et'-ik)*. Pertaining to diabetes.
یابیطسی: ذیابیطس سے متعلق۔

Diabetogenic *(di-a-bet-o-jen'-ik)* [G. diabainei to cross throgh; gignesthai, to be produced 1. Causing diabetes. 2. Applied to an anteric pituitary hormone.

ذیابیطس زا: (۱) ذیابیطس پیدا کرنا۔ (۲) اگلے پچوائیٹری ہارمون پر اطلاق۔

Diabinese *(di'-ab-in-ez)*. Chlorpropamide (q.v.).

ڈایابینیز: کلور پروپامائیڈ۔ ضد ذیابیطس عامل۔ ایک دو گولیاں ناشتہ کے بعد دیجئے۔

Diacetic acid *(di-a-se'-tik as'-id)*. Syn., acetoacetic acid (q.v.).

ڈائی ایسیٹک ایسڈ: ایسیٹو ایسی ٹک ایسڈ۔ ایک اساسی کیٹوتیزاب۔ انسانی جسم میں چکنائیوں کی تکسید سے پیدا ہوتا ہے۔ ذیابیطس کی بیماری میں خون میں اس کی مقدار زیادہ ہو جاتی ہے اور پیشاب کے ذریعے خارج ہوتا ہے۔ اگر پیشاب کو ساکن رکھا جائے تو یہ ایسیٹون میں تبدیل ہو جاتا ہے۔ خون میں تیزاب کی زیادتی بیہوشی بھی کر سکتی ہے۔

Diaginol *(di-aj'-in-ol)*. Sodium acetrizoate (q.v.).

ڈائی ایجینال: سوڈیم اسٹریزوایٹ۔ ایک نامیاتی آیوڈینی مرکب۔

Diagnosis *(di-ag-no'-sis)* [G. dia, through; gnosis, recognizing]. The art of act of distinguishing one disease from another. **differential d.,** arriving at a correct decision between diseases presenting a similar clinical picture--diagnose, v.t.; diagnosis, pl.; See CYTODIAGNOSIS.

تشخیص: ایک بیماری کو دوسری بیماری سے ممیز کرنے کا فن۔ تشخیص کے لئے نظری معائنہ، دستی معائنہ، ٹھونک کر دیکھنا۔ آسکل ٹیشن اور دوسرے ٹیسٹ ضروری ہیں۔

Diagnostic *(di-ag-no'-tik)*. [G. dia, through; gnosis, recognizing]. 1. Pertaining to diagnosis. 2. Serving as evidence in diagnosis--diagnostician, n.

تشخیصی: (۱) تشخیص سے متعلق۔ (۲) تشخیص کے لئے ثبوت۔

Diaguanides *(di'-a-gwan-ids)*. See BIGUANIDES.

Dial *(di'-al)* Allobarbitone (q.v.).

ڈائل: الوباربیٹون۔ اثر کا دورانیہ اور شدت کا درمیانہ ہونا۔

Dialysis *(di-al'-i-sis)*[G. a separating]. Separation of substances in solution by taking advantage of their differing diffusability through a porous membrane as in the artifical kidney. **peritoneal d.,** a method of irrigating the peritoneum; urea and other waste products are exuded into the irrigation fluid and withdrawn from the abdominal cavity--dialyse, v.t./; dialyses, pl. See HAEMODIALYSIS.

تفرق: محلول میں اشیاء کی علیحدگی جو کسی سام دار جھلی میں سے ان کے مختلف نفوذ کی وجہ سے ہوتی ہے۔ مثلاً مصنوعی گردے میں۔

Diaminodiphenylsulphone Synthetic drug for use against resistant strains of malaria; and for leprosy.

ڈائی ایمائینوڈائی فینائل سلفون: ملیریا کے مدافعتی سٹرین کے خلاف استعمال ہونے والی تالیفی دوا۔

Diamorphine *(di-a-mor'-fen)*. Heroin, a derivative of morphine, but liable to cause addiction. Valuable in severe pain, and as a cough depressant in useless cough.

ڈایامارفین: ہیروئن۔ مارفین سے اخذ شدہ۔ اس کا استعمال عادی بنا دیتا ہے۔ شدید درد اور کھانسی کو دبانے کے لئے مفید۔

Diamox *(di'-a-moks)*. Acetazolamide (q.v./).

ڈایاموکس: ایسیٹازولامیڈ۔ یہ مرکب کاربونک این ہائیڈرس کے عمل کو روکتا ہے۔ امراض مرگی میں مفید۔ الکلائن پیشاب کی زائد مقدار کو خارج کرتا ہے۔

Dianabol *(di-an'-a-bol)*. Methandienone (q.v.).

ڈائی اینابال: متھنڈی اینون۔ تخریبی افعال کے خلاف عامل۔ عضلہ کے ضیاع میں مفید۔ قلبی بے قاعدگی اور مسکولر ڈس ٹرافی میں ایک گولی صبح شام۔ بیماری کے بعد کمزوری، نقاہت اور وزن کی کمی کے لئے مفید۔

Diandrone *(di'-an-dron)*. Dehydroisoandrosterone. Endocrine useful in psychoneurosis, neurasthenia and schizophrenia.

ڈائی اینڈرون: کئی امراض میں مفید۔

Diapedesis *(di-a-pe-de'-sis)*. [G. dia, through; pedesis, springing]. The passage of blood cells through the vessel walls into the tissues--diapedetic, adj.

خلیات خون: بافتوں میں رگوں کی دیواروں میں سے خونی خلیوں کا گزرنا۔

Diaphoresis *(di-at0-or-e'-sis)* [G.dia, through; phorein, to carry]. Perspiration.

عرقیت: پسینہ۔

Diaphoretic *(di-af-or-et'-ik)*. [G. dia, through; phorein, to carry]. An agent which induces diaphoresis.

پسینہ آور: ایسا عامل جس سے پسینہ آتا ہے۔ بخار اتارنے کے لئے مفید۔

Diaphragm *(di'-a-farm)* [G. diaphragma, partition]. 1. The dome-shaped muscular partition between the thorax above and the abdomen belwo. 2. Any partitioning membrane or septum--diaphragmatic, adj.

ڈایافرام ۔ پردۂ شکم ۔ پیٹ کی جھلی: (۱) اوپر تھوریکس اور نیچے پیٹن کے درمیان عضلی تقسیم کرنے والا جسمانی حصہ۔ (۲) علیحدہ کرنے والی جھلی یا پردہ۔

Diaphysis *(di-af'-i-sis)* [G. a growing through]. The shaft of a long bone--diaphyseal, adj.; diaphyses, pl.

درنامیہ: لمبی ہڈی کا شافٹ۔

Diaplacental *(di-a-pla-sen'-tal)* [G. dia, through; L. placenta, cake]. Through the placenta.

ڈایاپلیسنٹل: پلیسنٹا میں سے۔

Diarrhoea *(di-a-re'-a)* [G. diarrhoia, a flowing throgh]. Deviation from established bowel rhythm characterized by an increase in frequency and fluidity of the stools. Epidemic diarrhoea of the newborn is a highly contagious infection of maternity hospitals. The gastroenteritis is probably the result of virus infection.

اسہال ۔ دست: دستوں کا آنا۔ اسہال کی صورت میں بچوں کو پانی کی جگہ او آر ایس کا محلول دیا جاتا ہے۔ سکسے تائیل سلفا تھایازول (سلفا ںکسی ڈین) یا فیورازولے دین (فیورکسون) ۲ گولیاں صبح ۲ دوپہر ۲ شام۔ آکسی ٹیٹرا سائیکلین ہائیڈروکلورائڈ (ٹیرامائی سین) یا پروکسی کوٹنولین کمپاؤنڈ (ان ٹسٹوپین فورٹ) ایک کیپسول دن میں چار مرتبہ۔ کلورم فینی کال سٹرپٹو مائی سین ۲ کیپسول ہر ۶ گھنٹے بعد۔

Diarthrosis *(di-ar-thro'-sis)* [G. articulation]. A synovial, freely movable joint--diarthrodial, adj.; diarthroses, pl.

سہل الحرکت جوڑ: آسانی سے گھومنے والا جوڑ۔

Diasonograph *(di-a-son'-o-graf)*. Ultrasound machine used to show position of organs inside body.

Diastase *(di'-as-tas)* [G. diastasis, a separation]. An amylase produced by animal, plant and bacterial cells, **pancreatic d.** is excreted in the urine (and saliva) and therefore estimation of urinary diastase may be used as a test of pancreatic function.

خمیرۂ جو: حیوانی، نباتی و جراثیمی خلیوں سے پیدا ہونی والا امائی لیز۔ اولیں دریافت شدہ کامرہ۔

Diastasis *(di-as'-tas-is)* [G. separation]. A separa tion of bones without fracture; dislocation.

تصال برنامیہ: شکستگی کے بغیر ہڈیوں کی علیحدگی۔

Diastole *(di-as'-to-li)* [G. diastole, difference] The relaxation period of the cardiac cycle, as opposed to systole--diastolic, adj.

انبساط (قلب): قلبی دور کے پھیلاؤ کا دورانیہ۔ سسٹول کے برعکس۔

Diathermy *(di-a-ther'-mi)*. [G. dia through therme, heat]. The passage of a high frequency electric current through the tissues whereby heat is produced. When both electrodes are large, the heat is diffused over a wide area according to the electrical resistance of the tissues. In this form it is widely used in the treatment of inflammation especially when deeply seated (e.g. sinusitis pelvic cellulitis). When one electrode is very small the heat is concentrated in this area and becomes great enough to destroy tissue. In this form (surgical diathermy) it is used to stcp bleeding at operation by coagulation of blood, or to cut through tissue in operation for malignant disease.

ـقی حریت: بافتوں میں سے زیادہ فریکوینسی کی برقی رو کا گزر جس سے ـرارت پیدا ہوتی ہے۔ سوزش کے لئے مستعمل۔ مفید برائے آسٹیو آرتھرائی ـں۔

Diazepam *(di-az'-e-pam)*. Tranquillosedativ with muscle relaxant properties. Useful in i.v infusion for status epilepticus and tetanus.

ـیازپام: سکون بخش دوا۔ عضلات کا آرام پہنچاتی ہے۔ ویلیم ہارٹ اٹیک ـں ۲ تا ۵ ملی گرام۔

Diazoxide *(di-az-oks'-id)*. Supresses activity o insulin-producing beta cells, therefore usef in hypoglycaemia from pancreatic tumour. I main use is as a hypotensive agent by rap i.v. injection in hypertensive emergencies.

ـی ایزوکسائیڈ: یہ دوا انسولین پیدا کرنے والے بیٹا خلیوں کی عاملیت کو ـرتی ہے۔

Dibenyline *(di-ben'-il-in)*. Phenoxybenzamine (q.v.).

ڈائی بنی لن : فینا کسی بینزامین۔ ایک دوا۔

Dibistine This is a mixture of antazoline and tripelennamine, A ntiallergic.

ڈائی بسٹن : الرجی ختم کرنے والی دوا۔ انٹازولین اور ٹرائی پیلینا مین کا آمیزہ یا مکسچر۔

Dibotin *(dib'-o-tin)*. phenformin (q.v.).

ڈبوٹن : فنفارمن۔ ذیابیطس کے خلاف عامل۔ وزن کو کم کرتا ہے۔ خلیوں کو گلوکوس جذب کرنے میں تحریک کرتا ہے۔

Dibromonannitol *(di-bro-mo-man'-it-ol)*. Oral drug which has an action similar to busulphan and may be effective when busulphan has been used previously.

ڈائی برومامینی ٹول : منہ سے کھائی جانے والی دوا۔

Dicephalous *(di-kef'-a-lus)*. Two-headed.

دوراسہ : دوسروں والا۔

Dichloraphenazone *(di-klor-al-fen'-a-zon)*. Causes less gastric irritation than chloral hydrate. Hypnotic of the chloral group. Particularly suitable for children.

ڈائی کلورایفنازون : بچوں کے لئے مناسب دوا۔ اس سے معدی سوزش کم ہوتی ہے۔

Dichlorophen *(di-klor'-o-fen)*. Synthetic anthelmintic effective against tape-worm. Preliminary fasting and purging as with filix mas, is unnecessary.

ڈائی کلوروفین : مختصر دورانیہ کی پیشاب اور دوا جو منہ کے ذریعے دی جاتی ہے۔

Dichuchwa Term for non-venereal syphilis used in Bechuanaland.

آتشک : آتشک کے لئے اصطلاح۔

Dicloxacillin *(di-cloks-a-sil'-in)*. See FLUCLOXACILLIN.

ڈائی کلاکساسلین : پنسلین کی ایک قسم جو سٹیفائلوکاکسس اریس کے پنسلینز پیدا کرنی والے سٹرین کے خلاف عمل کرتی ہے۔ انسان میں جذب ہو جاتی ہے۔

Diconal *(di-kon'-al)*. Dipipanone hydrochloride (q.v.). and cyclizine (q.v.).

Dicophane *(di'-ko-fan)*. Dichlorodiphenyltrichloroethane (DDT). Well known insecticide, used against pediculosis capitis and other body parasites as lotion or dusting powder.

ڈائیکوفین : ڈی ڈی ٹی۔ مشہور زمانہ حشرات کش محلول یا سفوف کی صورت میں مستعمل۔

dicoumarol *(di-koo'-mar-ol)*. Early orally effective anticoagulant. Now largely replaced by more controllahble drugs.

ڈائیکومیرول : منہ کے ذریعے کھائی جانے والی دوا۔ موثر طور پر خون جمنے نہیں دیتی۔

Dicrotic *(di-kro'-ik)*. [G. dikrotos, double beating]. Pertaining to, or having a double beat, as indicated by a second expansion of the artery during diastole. **d. wave,** the second rise in the tracing of a dicrotic pulse.

دوضربی۔ ضرب مکرر۔ ضرب ثنیٰ : شریان کے پھیلاؤ کے دوران دوہری دھڑکن ہونا یا اس سے متعلق۔

Dicyclomine *(di-si'-klo-men)*. An antispasmodic resembling atropine, but less potent. Used in pylorospasm and gastric hypermotility.

ڈائی سائیکلومین : ایٹروپین سے مشابہ۔

Dicynene *(di'-sin-en)*. Ethamsylate (q.v.).

Dienoestrol *(di-ne'-strol)*. A synthetic oestrogen similar to stilboestrol, but less active.

ڈائی نیسٹرول : ایک تالیفی دوا۔ سٹلبوایسٹرول سے مشابہ لیکن کم عامل۔

Dietetics *(di-e-tet'-iks)* [G. diata, mode of living, from diatoein, to support life]. The interpretation and application of the scientific principles of nutrition to feeding in health and disease.

علم الاغذیہ۔ غذائیات : صحت اور بیماری میں خوراک کھانے کے سائنسی اصولوں کا اطلاق اور ان کی وضاحت۔

diethazine *(di-eth'-a-zen)*. Synthetic anti-Parkinson drug.

ڈائی ایتھازین : ایک تالیفی دوا۔

Diethylcarbamazine *(di-eth'-il-kar-bam-ez-en)*. Oral filaricide especially active agaisnt young worms. Call kill roundworms.

ڈائی ایتھائیل کاربیمازین : نوعمر کیڑوں کے خلاف خصوصی طور پر عامل۔ منہ سے کھائی جانے والی دوا۔ اس دوا سے راؤنڈ ورم مر جاتے ہیں۔ ۲ گولیاں صبح ۲ دوپہر ۲ شام برائے فائی لیری اے سس۔

Diethylpropion hydrochloride *(di-eth'-il-p-ro-pi-on- hi-dro-klor-id)* CNS stimulant used as an appeute suppressant.

ڈائی ایتھائیل پروپیون ہائیڈروکلورائیڈ: سی این ایس محرک۔

Dietitian *(di-e-tish'-un)*. One who applies the principlēs of nutrition to the feeding of an individual or a group of individuals in a haterogeneous setting of economics or health, e.g. in schools, hospitals, institutions, restaurants, hotels, food factories, and in the World Health Organization.

غذائیات دان: خوراک کھانے کے اصولوں کا اطلاق کرنیوالا۔

Diet's crisis *(det'-lzkri'siz)*. A complication of 'floating kidney' (nephroptosis). Kinking of the ureter is throught to be responsible for the severe colic produced in the lumbar region. [Jozef Dietl, Polish physician, 1804-78].

ڈیٹلز کرائیسز : گردے کی پیچیدگی۔

Differential blood count The estimation of the relative proportions of the dıfferent leucocyte cells in the blood. The normal differential count is: polymorphs, 65 to 70 percent; lymphocytes, 20 to 25 percent; monocytes, 5 percent; eosinophils, 0 to 3 percent; basophils, 0 to 0.5 percent. In childhood the proportion of lymphocytes is higher.

تفریقی خون سماری: خون میں مختلف لیوکوسائیٹ خلیوں کے تقابلی تناسب کا اندازہ یا تخمینہ۔

Diffusion *(dif-fu'-zhun)* [L. diffundere, to pour]. 1. The process whereby ga ses and liquids of different denisities intermingle when brought into contact, until the density is equal throughout. 2. Dialysis.

نفوذ : لاطینی زبان کے لفظ ڈفنڈیئر بمعنی انڈیلنا سے ماخوذ اصطلاح۔ گیسوں کے سالمات آزادانہ حرکت کرتے ہیں اور جس برتن میں گیس ہوتی ہے' اس میں مساوی طور پر تقسیم ہونے کا رجحان رکھتے ہیں۔ گراہم کا کلیۂ نفوذ کے مطابق ''گیسوں کے نفوذ کی رفتاریں ان کی کثافتوں کے جذر کے بالعکس متناسب ہوتی ہے۔'' جبکہ ساری پیمائش یکساں حالات دباؤ اور تپش پر عمل میں لائی جائیں۔ اگر محلولوں کا نفوذ ہو تو منحل کے آئن یا سالمات محلل میں سے آزادانہ حرکت کرتے ہیں جبکہ محلول ارتکاز میں یکساں ہوتا ہے۔

Digestion *(di-jest'-chun)* [L. digestio, distribution]. The process by which food is rendered absorbable--digestible, digestive, adj.; digestibility, n.; digest, v.t., v.i.

ہضم : ہضم سے مراد ناحل پذیر مادوں کا حل پذیر ہونا ہے۔ یہ عمل ہضمی خامروں کی مدد سے ہوتا ہے۔

Digit *(dij'-it)* [L. digitus, finger]. A finger or toe-digital, adj.

انگلی: لاطینی لفظ ڈیجیٹس بمعنی انگشت سے ماخوذ ہاتھ یا پیر کی انگلی۔

Digitaline *(dij-it-al'-en)* . Digitoxin.

ڈجٹلین : ڈیجی ٹاکسن۔

Digitalis *(dij-it-a'-lis)*. Leaf of the common fox-glove. Powerful cardiac tonic, widely used in congestive heart failure and atrial fibrillation. Large initial doses are sometimes given.

ڈیجی ٹیلس۔ زہرالکشاتبین: ایک پودے کا پتا جو دل کو طاقت دیتا ہے۔ شروع میں زیادہ خوراک دی جاتی ہے۔

Digitalization *(dij-it-al-i-za'-shun)*. Physiological saturation with digitalis, to obtain optimum therapeutic effect.

ڈیجی ٹیکس کے زیر اثر لانا: ڈیجی ٹیکس کا فزیالوجیکل ارتکاز۔

Digitoxin *(dij-it-oks'-in)*. Giycoside of digitalis.

ڈیجی ٹاکسن : ڈیجی ٹیکس کا گلوئیکوسائیڈ۔

Digoxin *(dij-oks'-in)* Glycoside of digitalis.

ڈجاکسن : ڈیجی ٹیس کا گلائیکوسائیڈ۔ کن جیسٹو ہارٹ فیلیور میں اس کی ۲ گولیاں صبح ۲ دوپہر ۲ شام' دل کی رفتار آہستہ ہونے پر ایک گولی صبح ایک شام۔ سی طرح دمہ قلبی' بیری کارڈائی ٹس اور اختلاج القلب نوبتی میں دیکھئے۔

Diguanides *(di'-gwan-ids)*. Oral hypoglycaemic agents, thought to function as such by increasing glucose uptake in muscle and skin.

ائی گوانائیڈز: جلد اور عضلے میں گلوکوس کے انجذاب کو بڑھاتا ہے۔

Diguanil *(di'-gwan-il)*. Metformin (q.v.).

ائی گوانل: ضد ذیابیطس عامل۔

Dihydrocodeine tartate *(di-hi-dro-ko'-den ta r'-trat)*. Non-habit forming analygesic, usefu for suppression of cough, respiratory infect ions and painful wounds. Can be given orall or by injection.

Dihydromorphinone *(di-hi'-dro-mor'-fin-on)* A morphine-like analgesic of high potenc but short action. It has little hypnotic effec

Ocassionally used as a dedpressant in severe cough. Considered less habit-forming than morphine.

ڈائی ہائیڈرو مارفیون : مارفین ایسی دوائی۔ کھانسی کو دبانے میں موثر خواب آور کم۔

Dihydrostreptomycin *(di-hi'-dro-str- ep'-t-o-mi-sin)*. A derivative of streptomycin and used for similar purposes. A mixture of both antibiotics is sometimes employed to reduce any neurotoxic effects.

ڈائی ہائیڈروسٹر۔پٹو مائی سین: سٹرپٹو مائی سین سے حاصل شدہ۔

Dihydrotachysterol *(di-hi-dro-tak-is-te'-rol)*. Prepared in oil; used to raise the blood calcium, especially in parathyroid tetany.

Diiodohydroxyquinoline *(di-i-o'-do-hi-droks'-i-kwin'-o-lin)*. Used chiefly in amoebic dysentery in association with emetine.

ڈائی آئیوڈوہائیڈروکسی کیولولین : امیبی پیچش میں مستعمل۔ ایمے کوئن۔ڈائی اوڈوکوئن۔ امیبائی پیچش کے لئے ایک گولی صبح ایک دوپہر ایک شام۔

Dilatation *(di-la-ta'-shun)* [L. dilatare, to spread out]. Stretching or enlargement. May occur physiologically, pathologically or be induced artificially.

انبساط۔اتساع: پھیلنا یا بڑا ہونا۔

Dilaudid *(di-law'-did)*. Dihydromorphinone (q.v.).

ڈائی لاوڈ : مارفین کی نسبت اس کی عادت کم پڑتی ہے۔ ڈائی ہائیڈرو مارفینون۔

Dill water Aqua anethi, Popular preparation of a volatile oil used as a carminative for infants to relax muscular tone in digestive colic or flatulence.

اجوائن کا پانی: بچوں کو نظام ہضم کی درستگی کے لئے یہ دوا دی جاتی ہے۔

Diloxanide furoated *(dil-oks'-an-id-fu'-ro-at)*. For amoebic dysentery.

ڈلوکسینائیڈ فیوروایٹ: امیبی پیچس کے لئے۔

Dimelor *(dim-e'-lor)*. Acetohexamide (q.v.).

ڈائم لر: ایسیٹو ہیکسامائڈ۔دافع ذیابیطس عامل۔

Dimenhydrinate *(di-men-hid'-rin-at)*. Powerful antiemetic for travel sickness, vomiting of pregnancy and vertigo.

ڈائی مین ہائیڈری نیٹ: وضع حمل کی وجہ سے متلی میں مفید سفر کی پریشانی میں بھی مفید ہے۔ڈرامامین قے روکنے کے لئے ایک گولی صبح ایک دوپہر ایک شام سفر شروع کرنے سے پہلے کھائے۔

Dimercaprol *(dimer'-ka-prol)*. an organic compound used as an antidote for poisoning by arsenic and gold. Also useful in mercury poisoning if treatment is prompt, but it is not suitable for lead poisioning. It forms soluble compounds with the metals, which are then rapidly excreted. Syn., BAL.

ڈائی مرکیپرل: ایک نامیاتی مرکب جو سونے اور سنکھیا کے زہریلے اثرات کو ختم کرتا ہے۔ پارے کے زہر کے لئے بھی تریاق لیکن سیسے کے زہر کے لئے غیر موثر۔ یہ دھاتوں کے ساتھ حل پذیر مرکبات بناتا ہے۔ اس طرح انہیں فوراً جسم سے خارج کر دیتا ہے۔

Dindevan *(din'-de-van)*. Phenindione (q.v.).

ڈنڈی وین: فینڈیون۔منہ سے کھائی جانے والی دوا۔ کارونری تھرامبوسنز یا ہارٹ اٹیک میں اس کی گولی صبح ایک شام ایک ماہ تک۔

Dioctyl-Medo *(di-ok'-til-med-o)*. Dioctyl sodium sulphosuccinate (q.v.).

ڈائی آکٹل میڈو: ترکرنے والا عامل۔

Dioctylsodium sulphosucinate *(di-ok'-til-so'-d-i-um sul-fo-suks'-in-at)*. Wetting agent helpful in prevention of faecal impaction. Should be taken regularly for this purpose.

ڈائی آکٹل سوڈیم سلفوسکسی نیٹ : تر رکھنے والا عامل۔ اجابت کے لئے مفید۔

Diodone *(di'-o-don)*. Organic oidine compound used as X-ray contrast agent in intravenous pyelography.

ڈائی اوڈون: نامیاتی ایوڈینی مرکب۔

Diodoquin *(di-od'-o-kwin)*. Di-iodohydroxy-quinoline (q.v.).

ڈائی اوڈوکوئن : امبی پچس میں مستعمل۔ ایک گولی صبح ایک دوپہر ایک شام۔ ڈی آئیوڈوہائیڈروکسی کوئنولین۔ ایمے کوئن۔

Dioptre *(di-op'-ter)* [G. dioptra, an optical instrument]. A unit of measurement in refraction. A lens of one dioptre has a focal length of 1 metre.

بصریہ: انعطاف میں پیمائش کی ایک اکائی۔

Dioxide *(di-oks'-id)*. Oxide formed by combination of two atoms of oxygen with one of metal or non-metal.

ڈائی آکسائیڈ: دھات یا ادھات کے ایک ایٹم کے ساتھ آکسیجن کے دو ایٹموں کے ملاپ سے بننے والا آکسائیڈ۔

Diparcol *(di-par'-kol)*. Diethazine (q.v.).

ڈائی پرکول: ایک تالیفی دوا۔

Diphenhydramine *(di-fen-hid'-ra-min)*. One of the first antihistamines (q.v.). Widely used in allergic conditions and travel sickness. Also has sedative action.

ڈائی فین ہائیڈرامین: سفر کی پریشانی اور الرجی میں مفید۔

Diphenoxylate *(di-fen-oks'-i-lat)*. Prescribed for acute and chronic diarrhoea, and gastrointestinal upsets. It has some morphine-like actions: 1. It depresses the respiratory centre: 2. It acts as a cortical depressant: 3. It reduces intestinal mobility. Atropine is included to provide dryness of the mouth should patient take an overdose.

ڈائی فناکسی لیٹ: پیٹ میں گڑبڑ اور دستوں یا اسہال میں مفید۔ یہ دوا مارفین کی طرح عمل کرتی ہے۔

Dihenylhydantion *(di-fen-il-hid'-an-tion)*. Used in digitalis poisoning. See p.344.

ڈائی فنائل ہائیڈن ٹائن: زہریلے پن میں مفید۔

Diphtheria *(dif-the'-ri-a)* [G. diphthera, leather, membrane]. An actue, specific, infectious, notifiable disease caused by Corynebacterium diptheriae. Characterized by a grey, adherent, false membrane growing on a mucous surface, usually that of the upper respiratory tract. Locally there is pain, swelling and may be suffocation. Systemically the toxins attack the heart muscle and nerves--diphtheritic, adj.

خناق: اس مرض میں تنفسی راستے متاثر ہوتے ہیں۔ اس میں زہریلے مادے آخرکار قلبی عضلے اور اعصاب پر حملہ آور ہوتے ہیں۔ کارینے بیکٹیریم ڈفتھری سے ہونے والی چھوت کی بیماری۔

Diphtheroid *(dif'-ther-oid)* [G. diphthera, leather; eidos, form]. Any bacterium morphologically and culturally resembling Corynebacterium diphtheriae.

خناق نما عصیہ: کارینے بیکٹیریم ڈفتھری سے مشابہ کوئی جرثومہ۔

Dipipanone *(di-pi-pan'-on)*. Synthetic morphine substitute with both sedative and pain relieving properties.

ڈائی پی پینون: تالیفی طور پر تیار کردہ مارفین کا متبادل جو درد کو آرام کرتا ہے۔

Diplegia *(di-ple'-ji-a)* [G. dis, twice; plege, a stroke]. Symmetrical paralysis of legs, usually associated with cerebral damage--diplegic, adj. [Cf. p[araplegia.).

دوطرف فالج: ٹانگوں کا سن ہونا۔

Diplococcus *(dip-lo-kok'-us)* [G. diploose, double; kokkos, grain]. A coccal bacterium characteristically occuring in pairs. Diplococcus may be used in a binominal to describe a characteristically paired coccus e.g. Diplococcus pneumoniae=pneumococcus.

ڈپلوکاکس۔ جفت بنقہ: یونانی الفاظ ڈپلولوس بمعنی ڈبل اور کاکس بمعنی دانہ کا مجموعہ۔ کاکس جرثومہ۔ جو جوڑے کی صورت میں ہوتا ہے۔ خصوصی طور پر جوڑے والے کاکس کے لئے یہ نام استعمال کیا جاتا ہے۔ مثلاً ڈپلوکاکس نمونی یا نموکاکس۔

Diplopia *(dip-lo'-pi-a)* [G. diploos, double; opsis, vision]. Double vision.

ذوبینی۔ دونظری: دوہرا ویژن۔

Diprophylline *(di-prof-i-lin)*. Diuretic. Xanthine derivative. Can be given orally, intravenously and as a suppository.

ڈائی پروفلین: پیشاب آور۔ زینتھین سے حاصل کردہ۔

Dipsomania *(dip-so-ma'-ni-a)* [G. dipsa, thirst, mania, madness]. Alcoholism in which the drinking occurs in bouts, often with long periods of sobriety between--dipsomaniac, adj., n.

جنون خمر۔ ے مانیا: یونانی الفاظ ڈپسا بمعنی پیاس اور میپیا بمعنی پاگل پن کا مجموعہ۔ الکلوم کی ایک قسم۔

Dipyridamole *(di-pir-id'-a-mol)*. Inhibits platelet thrombus formation on dialyser membranes and reduces the frequency of embolic complications in patients with prosthetic heart valves.

Direma *(dir-e'-ma)*. Hydrochlorothiazide (q.v.).

ریما: ہائیڈروکلوروتھیازائڈ۔ کلوروتھیازائڈ سے زیادہ طاقتور پیشاب آور دوا۔

Disablement Resettlement Office Appointed by the Department of Employment to ensure the local operation of the Disabled Persons Employment Acts, 1944 and 1958.

افسر بحالیٔ معذوراں: شعبہ روزگار کا مقرر کردہ اہلکار تاکہ معذور اشخاص کے روزگار ایکٹ ۱۹۴۴ اور ۱۹۵۸ پر عمل کرائے۔

Disaccharide *(di-sak'-ar-id)*. A sugar (carbohydrate, e.g. lactose, maltose, sucrose) which yields two molecules of monosaccharide on hydrolysis.

ڈائی سیکرائد: ایک شکر جو آب پاشیدگی پر مانوسیکرائڈ کے دو سالمات دیتی ہے۔ جیسا کہ کاربوہائیڈریٹ مثلاً لیکٹوز، مالٹوز، سکروز۔

Disalcid *(di-sal'-sid)*. An ester of salicylic acid which is insoluble in gastric juice therefore less likely than aspirin to cause gastric irritation and erosion.

Disarticulation *(dis-art-ik-u-la'-shun)* [L. dis, asunder; articulus, joint]. Amputation at a joint.

بتر مفصلی: جوڑ کھل جانا۔

Discectomy *(dis-sek'-to-mi)* Surgical removal of a disc, usually an intervertebral disc.

Discission *(dis-si'-shun)* [L. discissum, from discindere, to tear]. Rupturing of lens capsule to allow absorption of lens substance in the condition of cataract. Syn., needling.

تابیر: عدسہ کے کیپسول کا پھٹنا تاکہ عدسے کے کا انجذاب ہو سکے۔

Discogenic *(dis-ko-jen'-ik)*. Arising in or produced by a disc, usually an intervertebral disc.

Discogram *(dis'-ko-gram)*. See DISCOGRAPHY.

Discography *(dis-kog'-ra-fi)* [G. diskos, disc; gra phein, to write]. X-ray of an intervertebral disc after it has been rendered radio-opaque. Normal disc accepts not more than 0.5 ml; damaged disc may accept 2 to 3 ml. Injection frequently reproduces pain -discographic, adj.; discographically, adv.; discograph, n.

رکاڈنامہ: یونانی الفاظ ڈسکوس بمعنی تھالی اور گریفین بمعنی لکھنا کا مجموعہ۔ ریڈیائی غیر شفاف ہونے کے بعد انٹرورٹبرل ڈسک کا ایکس رے۔

Disinfectants *(dis-in-fek'-tants)* [L. dis, the reverse of; infestare, to infest]. Germicides which are too corrosive or toxic to be applied to tissues, but whoich are suitable for application in inanimate objects.

دافع عفونت: جراثیم کش ادویات جو زہریلی ہوتی ہیں۔ اس لئے جانداروں پر نہ چھڑکی جائیں۔ صرف بے جان اشیاء پر چھڑکی جائیں۔

Disinfection *(dis-in-fek'-shun)* [F. desinfecter]. The destruction of all micro-organisms, except spores, and can refer to the action of antiseptics as well as disinfectants.

دافع چھوت: بذروں کے سوا تمام خورد جسیموں کی تباہی۔

Disinfecstation *(dis-in-fes-ta-shun)* [L. dis, the reverse of; infestare, to infest]. Extermination of infesting agents, especially lice. Delousing.

کرم کشی: جوؤں وغیرہ کا خاتمہ۔

Disipal *(di'-si-pal)*. Orphenadrine (q.v.).

ڈیسپیل: سکون بخش ادویات سے پیدا ہونیوالی پارکنسنزم کو زائل کرنے والی گولیاں۔

Disipidin *(di-sip'-i-din)*. Posterior pituitary snuff. Useful in enuresis, diabetes insipidus and nocturnal frequency in the aged.

ڈائی سی پی ڈن: کئی امراض میں مفید۔

Dislocation *(dis-lo-ka'-shun)* [L. dis, separation; locare, to place]. A displacement of organs or articular surfaces, so that all apposition between them is lost. It may be congenital, spontaneous, traumatic, or recurrent. Syn., luxaction--dislocated. adj.; dislocate, v.t.

جوڑ اکھڑنا۔ ہڈی کا اترنا: کسی عضو یا گھومنے والی سطح کو اپنی جگہ سے ہٹانا تاکہ رکاوٹ نہ رہے۔ جب ہڈی اترتی ہے تو وہ اپنی جگہ سے ہٹ کر اوپر یا نیچے ہو جاتی ہے۔ درد ہوتا ہے اور سوج ہو جاتی ہے۔ ہڈی پوری ہٹ گئی ہو تو مکمل، پوری نہ اتری ہو تو نامکمل، ہڈی اترنے کے ساتھ زخم بھی ہو تو مرکب اور زخم نہ ہو تو سادہ ہڈی اترنا کہتے ہیں۔

Disobliteration *(dis-ob-lit-er-a'-shun)*. Rebore, Removal of that which blocks a vessel, most often intimal plaques in an artery, when it is called endarterect tomy (q.v.).

اختتام رکاوٹ: رگ میں موجود رکاوٹ کو دور کرنا۔

Disodium cromoglycate *(di-sod'-i-um-kro-mo-gli'-cat)*. Useful in allergic airway disease. It is not anti-inflammatory, nor is it a bronchodilator. It inhibits the effects of some specific types of reaginic antibody-antigen reactions. Gives relief of bronchospasm in asthma.

ڈائی سوڈیم کروموگلائی کیٹ: الرجی والی ہوائی بیماری میں مفید دمہ میں کبھی آرام پہنچاتی ہے۔

Disorientation *(dis-or-i-en-ta'-shun)* [L. dis, separation; oriens. East]. Loss of orientation (q.v.)

ماحول ناشناسی: لاطینی الفاظ ڈس بمعنی علیحدگی اور اوری انز بمعنی مشرق کا مجموعہ۔ مشرقیت کا ضیاع۔

Dissection *(dis-sek'-shun)* [L. dis-secare, to cut in pieces]. Separation of tissues by cutting. **block d. of glands,** the total excision of a group of lymph nodes, usually part of the treatment of carcinoma.

چیر پھاڑ: لاطینی لفظ ڈائی سیکیئر بمعنی ٹکڑوں میں کاٹنا سے ماخوذ۔ کاٹ کر بافتوں کی علیحدگی۔

Disseminated sclerosis *(dis-em'-in-at'-ed-skler-o'-sis)* See. SCLEROSIS.

Dissociation *(dis-so-shi-a'-shun)* [L. dissociare, to separate from fellowship]. In psychiatry an abnormal mental process by which the mind achieves non-recognition and isolation of certain unpalatable facts. This involves the actual splitting off from consciousness of all the unpalatable ideas so that the individual is no longer aware of them. Dissociation is a common symptom in hysteria but is seen in its most exaggerated form in delusional psychoses, e.g. a woman who, being deluded, believes she is a Queen cheerfully scrubbing the ward floor. Her royal status and the fact that she is charring are competely separated or dissociated in her mind and she does not recognize the incongruity.

احتباس: خلاف معمول ذہنی حالت ہسٹریا کی علامات مثلاً کسی خاتون کا خود کو ملکہ سمجھنا۔

Distal *(dis'tal)* [L. distare, to be distant]. Farthest from the head or source--distally, adv.

بعیدی: سر یا منبع سے دور۔

Distalgesic *(dis-tal-jez'-ik)* Dextropropoxyphene with paracetamol. Useful analgesic, especially for chronic conditions.

Distaquaine *(dis'-ta-qwan)*. Various prepara tions of penicillin (q.v.).

ڈسٹا کوائن: پنسلین سے تیار کردہ مختلف ادویات۔

Distichiasis *(dis-tik-i'-as-is)* [G. dis, twice; stichos, row]. An extra row of eyelashes at the inner lid border, which is turned inward against the eye.

جفت اہدابی: یونانی الفاظ ڈس بمعنی دگنا اور سٹیکوس بمعنی قطار کا مجموعہ۔ پلکوں کی ایک زائد قطار جو پپوٹوں کی اندرونی جانب کنارے پر ہوتی ہیں۔ یہ اندر کی طرف مڑی ہوتی ہیں۔

distractibility *(dis-trak-tib-il'-i-ti)* [L. distractus, from distrahere, to draw apart]. A psychiatric term applied to a disorder of the power of attention when it can only be applied momentarily.

انتشار توجہ: توجہ کی طاقت میں گڑبڑ جب اس کا اطلاق عارضی ہو۔

Disulfiram *(di-sul'-ir-am)* . A sulphur compound that in the presence of alcohol causes nausea and vomiting. Hence used in alcoholism.

ڈائی سلفی ریم: گندھک کا ایک مرکب جو الکحل کی موجودگی میں متلی اور قے کی وجہ بنتا ہے۔ اس لئے الکحلزم میں مستعمل۔

Dithranol *(di-thra'-nol)*. Similar to chrysarobin (q.v.), but more powerful. Sensitivity tests necessary before treatment begins.

ڈائی تھرانول: کرائی سارو بن سے مشابہ لیکن زیادہ طاقتور۔ اس کے مرہم میں اس کا ایک گرام اور پیلا نرم پیرافین ۹۹۹ گرام ملاتے ہیں جو چنبل، داد رنگ ورم اور دھوبی حارش کے لئے مفید ہے۔

Diuresis *(di-u-re'-sis)* [G. diourein, to pass urine]. Increased secretion of urine, **forced d.,** term used when diuresis is part of intensive therapy, particularly in poisoning.

درار (بول): پیشاب کا زائد اخراج۔

Diuretic *(di-u-ret'-ik)*. [G. diouretikos, diuretic] 1. Increasing the flow of urine. 2. An agent which increases the flow of urine.

پیشاب آور: (۱) پیساب کا بہاؤ بڑھاؤ۔ (۲) عامل جو پیشاب کا بہاؤ بڑھاتا ہے۔

Divaricator *(di-var'-i-ka -tor)* [L. divaricare, to spread asunder]. A hingedx wooden splint permitting various degrees of divarica tion in congenital dislocation of the hip.

منشعب : ایک مڑنے والی چوبی پھٹی جو چوتڑے کے جوڑ کو صحیح کرنے کے لئے استعمال کی جاتی ہے۔

Diverticulitis *(di-var-tik-u-li'-tis)* [L. diverticulum, a bypath; -itis, inflammation]. Inflammation of a diverticulum.

ورم عطفات قولون : تھیلی یا موڑ کی سوزش۔ بڑی آنت کی دیوار کا ورم۔ بہت الٹیاں آنا، بخار، پیٹ میں درد اور پیٹ پھولنا علامات ہیں۔ بستر پر آرام ضروری ہے۔ فینن کاربامائڈ کمپاؤنڈ (سپازموڈال درون) اور میٹا میزال کمپاؤنڈ (برلگین) ایک گولی صبح ایک دوپہر ایک شام پین کریاٹن بائیل سالٹس (این زار) ایک گولی صبح ایک دوپہر ایک شام۔ ٹیٹرا سائیکلین کیپسول ہر چھ گھنٹے بعد ایک۔

Diverticulosis *(di-ver-tik-u-lo'-sis)* [L. diverticulum, a bypath; -osis, condition]. A condition in which there are many diverticula, especially in the intestines.

عطفیت : آنتوں میں کئی تھیلیوں یا موڑوں کی موجودگی۔

Diverticulum *(di-ver-tik'-u-lum)* [L.]. A pouch or sac protruding from the wall of a tube or hollow organ. May be congenital or acquired--diverticula, pl.

diverticulum

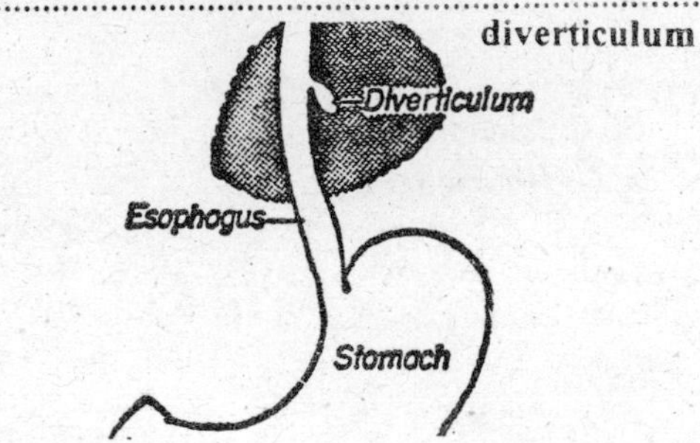

عطفہ : لاطینی لفظ کو کھلے عضو یا نلی کی دیوار سے ابھرنے والی تھیلی۔

Dixarit *(diks'-ar-it)*. Clonidine (q.v.).

ڈکسیرٹ : کلونیڈین۔ میتھائل ڈوپا سے مشابہ۔

DNA. Deoxyribonucleic acid (q.v.).

ڈی این اے۔ ڈن ا : ڈی آکسی ریبونکلیک ایسڈ۔ خلیوں کے مرکزوں کا کاربوہائیڈریٹ والا جزو۔ یہ وراثت میں اہم کردار ادا کرتا ہے۔ ایک نسل سے دوسری میں منتقل ہوتا ہے۔ ہر نوع کا ڈی این اے مختلف ہوتا ہے۔ ڈی این اے ایک دوہرے طویل ریشے کی مانند ہے۔ ریشے کی دونوں لڑیوں نے ایک دوسرے کے گرد بل کھائے ہوئے ہیں اور ایک دوسرے کے ساتھ ملی ہوتی ہیں۔ ان لڑیوں کو نکلیوٹائیڈز کہا جاتا ہے۔ دوسرے الفاظ میں ڈی این اے کے سالمے کی ساخت ایک بٹے رسے کی سیڑھی کی مانند ہے جس کی دونوں اطراف شوگر فاسفیٹ زنجیروں پر مشتمل ہیں۔ سیڑھی کے ڈنڈے نائٹروجنی اساسوں پر مستمل ہیں جو ہائیڈروجن بانڈز کے ذریعے ملے ہوئے ہیں۔ ایڈنین، سائیٹوسین، گوانین اور تھائی مین۔ تین اساس ایک امینوایسڈ کے کوڈ کو ظاہر کرتے ہیں۔ نیا کروموسوم بنتے وقت اس میں موجود ڈی این اے کی نقل تیار ہوتی ہے جو پرانے ڈی این اے کے عین مطابق ہوتی ہے۔ ان دونوں میں سے ایک نقل نئی کروموسوم میں چلی جاتی ہے۔ اس طرح نیا کروموسوم ہو بہو پرانے کروموسوم کی نقل ہوتا ہے جب یہ کسی نئے خلیہ میں کروموسوم کے لحاظ سے کوئی فرق نہیں ہوتا۔ اس طرح ڈی این اے جانداروں میں ایک خلیہ سے دوسرے خلیہ میں ایک نسل سے دوسری نسل میں منتقل ہوتا رہتا ہے۔

Dobutamine *(do-bu-ta-men)*. A directly acting stimulant of heart muscle which augments myocardial contractility in severe cardiac failure and shock syndrome, e.g. after myocardial infarction.

Dobutrex. Doubutamine (q.v.).

DOCA Deoxycortone (q.v.).

ڈی او سی اے : ڈی آکسی کورٹون۔ ایڈرینل کارٹیکس کا ایک اہم ہارمون۔ سوڈیم اور پوٹاشیم کے میٹابولزم کو کنٹرول کرتا ہے۔ چوتھے یا ساتویں روز ایک ٹیکہ برائے مرض ایڈیسن۔

Doderlein's bacillus Lactobacillus acidophilus). Gram-positive rod bacterium which produces acid; occurs in the normal vagina , and the pH of the vaginal secretions is largely due to the growth of the organism. Also found in the intestine and the bacilli are especially numberous if the diet is rich in milk or milk products. Non-pathogenic. [Albert Doderlein, German obstetrician and gynaecologist, 1860-1941].

ڈوڈرلینز بے سلس : گرام مثبت سلاخ جراثیم جو تیزاب پیدا کرتے ہیں۔ وہ عام ویجائنا میں پائے جاتے ہیں۔ آنت میں بھی پائے جاتے ہیں۔ اگر خوراک دودھ اور دودھ بننے والی اشیاء پر مشتمل ہو تو آنت میں کثرت سے پائے جاتے ہیں۔ یہ جرثومہ کوئی مرض پیدا نہیں کرتا۔

Dogger Bank itch. Sensitization dermatitis due to Alcyonidium (seaweed family). Clinical features include a papular and vesicular rash on hands and forearms with facial erythema and oedema.

ڈاگر بینک اچ: السی اونیڈیم کی وجہ سے بیماری۔

Dolor *(do'-lor)* [L.]. Pain.

درد: لاطینی لفظ۔ دکھ؛ درد۔

Doloxene *(dol'-oks-en)*. Dextropropoxyphene (q.v.).

ڈولوکسین: ڈکسٹروپروپوکسی فین۔ مارفین کی جگہ مستعمل لیکن تاثیر میں کم۔

Dominant *(dom'-in-ant)* [L. dominans, ruling]. A character possessed by one parent, which, in the offspring, masks the corresponding alternative character derived from the other parent. Opp. recessive. See MENDEL'S LAW.

غالب۔ نمایاں: والدین میں سے ایک کی خاصیت جو اولاد میں والدین میں سے دوسرے کی خاصیت کو ڈھانپ لیتی ہے۔

Domiphen bromide *(dom'-ifen bro'-mid)*. White, uncoated lozenges for mouth and throat infections.

ڈومی فین برومائیڈ: منہ اور گلے کی بیماری کے لئے چوسنے والی سفید گولیاں جن پر کسی اور شے کی تہہ جمی ہوئی نہیں ہوتی۔

Donovan's bodies See LEISHMANDONOVAN.

ڈولوونیز باڈیز: مریضوں میں پائے جانے والے پروٹوزوا آلشمانیا کی گول اقسام۔

Dopamine *(dop'-a-min)* A catecholamine neurotrasmitter, closely related to adrenaline and noradrenaline. Increases cardiac output and renal blood flow but does not produce peripheral vasoconstriction. Most valuable in hypotension and shock of caridac origin. Normally present in high concentration in those regions of the brain which are selectively damaged in Parkinsonism.

ڈوپیمن: یہ دوائی دل کی کارکردگی کو بہتر بناتی ہے۔

Doptone *(dop'-ton)*. Instrument using echo-sounder principles to detect fetal heart a very early stage.

ڈاپٹون: آلہ جو دل کی حالت بتاتا ہے۔

Dorbanex *(dor'-ban-eks)*. Contains faecal-softening agent and laxative for constipation. Available as capsules and in two strengths of highly palatable liquid.

ڈاربے نیکس: فضلے کو نرم کرتا ہے اور اجابت کو آسان بناتا ہے۔ کیپسولوں اور مائع کی صورت میں مہیا ہے۔

Doriden *(do'-ri-den)*. Glutethemide (q.v.).

ڈوری ڈین: گلوٹھیمائڈ۔ درمیانہ درجہ کی خواب آور دوا۔ سوتے وقت ایک گولی برائے بے خوابی۔

Dorsal *(dor'sal)* [L. dorsum, back]. Pertaining to the back, or the posterior part of an organ.

ظہری۔ پشتی: لاطینی لفظ ڈارسم بمعنی پشت سے ماخوذ۔ پشت سے متعلق یا کسی عضو کا خلفی حصہ ڈارسل ورٹبری یا پشت کے مہرے تعداد میں بارہ ہوتے ہیں اور ان سے پسلیوں کے بارہ جوڑے جڑے ہوتے ہیں۔

Dorsal root

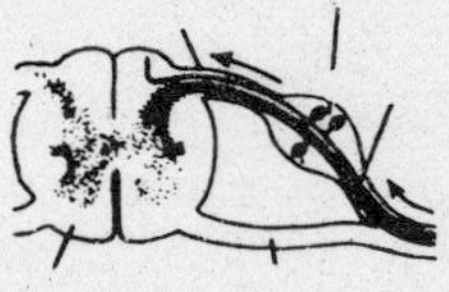

Dorsiflexion *(dor-si-flek'-shun)* [L. dorsum, back; flectere, to bend]. Bending backwards In the case of great toe--upwards. See BABINSKI'S REFLEX.

ظہری خمیدگی: پچھلی جانب جھکنا۔ پاؤں کے انگوٹھے کی صورت میں اوپر کی طرف۔

Dorsocentral *(dor-so-sen'-tral)* [L. dorsum, back; G. kentron, centre of a circle]. At the back and in the centre.

ظہر مرکزی: پشت پر اور مرکز میں۔

Dorsolumbar *(dor-so-lum'-bar)* [L. dorsum, back; lumbus, loin]. The lumbar region of the back.

ظہری بدنی: پشت کا لمبر حصہ۔

Douche *(doosh)* [F.]. A stream of fluid directed agaisnt the body externally or into a body cavity.

ڈوش۔ آبریزش: فرانسیسی لفظ۔ جسمی کہفہ میں یا جسم کے باہر سیال کا بہاؤ۔

Dover's powder A time-honoured remedy containing 10 percent of opium and ipecacuanha. Once used extensively as a diaphoretic, but is now prescribed less often. [Thomas Dover, English physician, 1660-1742].

سفوف ڈوور : یہ دوا پہلے زیادہ مستعمل تھی' اب اس کا استعمال کم کر دیا گیا ہے۔اس میں افیم ہوتی ہے۔انگریز فزیشن تھامس ڈور پر اس کا نام رکھا گیا ہے جس کا دور حیات ۱۶۶۰ع تا ۱۷۴۲ع ہے۔

own's syndrome Mongol (q.v.).

ڈاؤن سنڈروم : منگول۔ بچہ ذہنی طور پر کمزور ہوتا ہے۔شکل سے منگول ریس یا نسل کا لگتا ہے۔اسے لیوکیمیا آسانی سے ہوسکتا ہے۔اس میں کروموسوم نمبر ۲۱ صحیح نہیں ہوتا۔کروموسوم نمبر ۲۱ کی تقسیم میں ناکامی کی وجہ سے ایک زائد کروموسوم ہوتا ہے۔بچے میں ۴۷ کروموسوم ہوتے ہیں۔عموماً ایسے بچے زیادہ عمر کی ماؤں کے پیدا ہوتے ہیں۔کروموسوم ۴۶ بھی ہو سکتے ہیں لیکن ایکسوان کروموسوم صحیح نہیں ہوتا۔دوسری صورت نوجوان ماؤں کے ہاں پیدا ہونیوالے بچوں میں ہوسکتی ہے۔

oxepin *(doks'-e-pin)*. One of the tricyclic antidepressants. Effective after 3 to 15 days medication.

ڈاکسیپین : پریشانی کم کرنے والی دوا۔اس کا اثر ۳ تا ۱۵ روز علاج کرنے سے ہوتا ہے۔

oxycycline *(doks-i-si'-klin)*. New, rapidly excreted tetracycline.

-penicillamine *(pen-i-sel'-a-men)*. Drug of first choice in 'rheumatoid factor positive' rheumatoid arthritis. See PENICILLAMINE

Dracon'iasis *(dra-kon-ti'-a-sis)*. Infestation with Dracunculus medinensis (Guinea worm). a nematode parasite which infests man from contaminated drinking water. From the patient's intestine the adult female migrates to the skin surface to deposit her larvae, producing a cord-like thickening which ulcerates. Common in India and Africa.

مرض نارووا: یہ بیماری ایسا پانی پینے سے ہوتی ہے جس میں نیما ٹوڈ ورم' گنی ورم ہوتا ہے۔یہ مرض بھارت وافریقہ میں عام ہے۔مادہ کے لاردے مریض کی آنت سے جلد میں منتقل ہو جاتے ہیں اور وہاں ڈوری نما دبازت پیدا کرتے ہیں۔

Dracunculus medinensis Nematode parasite responsible for dracontiasis (q.v.).

ناروا۔نارو: نیماٹوڈ طفیلی جو مذکورہ بالا مرض پیدا کرتا ہے۔

Dramamine *(dram'-a-men)*. Dimenhydrinate (q.v.).

ڈرامامین : ڈائمن ہائیڈرینیٹ۔وضع حمل کی وجہ سے متلی میں مفید۔سفر کی شروع کرنے سے پہلے کھائیے۔

DRO. Disablement Resettlement Officer (q.v.).

ڈی آر او : شعبۂ روزگار کا مقرر کردہ اہلکار جو معذور اشخاص کے روزگار ایکٹ ۱۹۴۴ع اور ۱۹۵۸ع پر عمل کراتا ہے۔

Droleptan *(dro-lep'-tan)*. Droneridol (q.v.).

ڈروپیپٹین : ایک دوا۔ڈروپیری ڈول۔

Dromoran *(drom'-or-an)*. Levorphanol (q.v.).

ڈرامورین: لیورفینول۔مارفین کا متبادل لیکن مارفین سے کم خواب آور۔

Drop attacks Periodic falling because of suddent loss of postural control of the lower limbs, without vertigo or loss of consciousness. Usually followed by suddent return of normal muscle tone, allowing the person to rise, in uninjured. See VERTEBROBASILAR INSUFFICIENCY.

Droperidol *(drop-er'-i-dol)*. A butyrophenone compound. Neuroleptic agent. Can be used as a preoperative premedication. Induces state of mental detachment without loss of consciousness or effect upon respiratory system.

ڈورپیری ڈول: سکون بخش دوا۔

Dropsy *(drop'-si)* [G. hydrops, from hydor, water]. See ANASARCA, ASCITES and OEDEMA--dropsical, adj.

استسقا: استسقالحمی۔خلوی بافتوں کا دخول۔

Drostanolone *(dros-tan'-o-lon)*. Anabolic agent. Has less virilizing effect than Durabolin or deca-Durabolin.

ڈراسٹینولون: انابولک ایجنٹ۔

Drug dependence A normal jont state arising from repeated administration of a drug on a periodic or continuous basis (WHO, 1964). Drug depe- ndence now a preferable turm to d addiction and d. habituation.

دواخوئی: کسی دوا کے بار بار استعمال سے یہ حالت ہوتی ہے کسی دوا کا عادی ہو جانا۔ایسی دوا جس کی وجہ سے فعلیاتی یا جذباتی انحصار ہو جائے۔

Drug fast. A term used to describe resistance of microbial cells to the action of anti-microbial drugs.

ڈرگ فاسٹ : خودجسمی خلیوں کی مدافعت واضح کرنے کے لئے ایک اصطلاح۔

Ducrey's bacilus *(haemophilus ducreyi) (du-cra'-i).* Gram-negative rod. The causative organism of soft chancre (chancroid). a venereal disease, [Augosto Ducrey, Italian dermatologist, 1860-1940].

جرثومہ آتشک: چھوٹے گرام منفی سلاخ والے جراثیم۔

Ductless glands *(dukt'-les).* See ENDOCRINE GLANDS.

بے قنات غدود: اینڈوکرائن گلینڈز۔ جسم میں بغیر نلی والی غدود۔

Ductus arteriosus *(duk'-tus ar-te-ri-o'-sus).* A blood vessel connecting the left pulmonary artery to the aorta, to bypass the lungs, in the fetal circulation.**patient d. a.** is a form of congenital heart defect wherein this 'shunt' remains open.

جنین کی وریدی نالی: بائیں ششی شریان کو ایورٹا سے ملانے والی۔

Duhamel's operation. For Hirschsprung's disease (q.v.).

ڈہامیل اپریشن: ہرس شپرنگ بیماری کے لئے۔

Dulcolax *(dul-ko-laks).* A synthetic laxative that is effective without griping. Bisacodyl.

ڈلکولیکس: تالیفی ہاضمی والی دوا۔

Dumping syndrome The name given to the symptoms which often follow a partial gastrectomy, bilious vomiting and a feeling of faintness and weakness after meals.

ڈمپنگ سنڈروم: ایسی علامات کا نام مثلاً متلی ہونا' کھانے کے بعد کمزوری محسوس کرنا وغیرہ۔

Duodenitis *(du-o-den-i'-tis)* [L. *duodeni,* twelve; *-itis* inflammation]. Inflammation of the duodenum.

ورم عفج: ڈیوڈینم کی سوزش۔

Duodenojejunal *(du-o-de-no-je-joo'-nql)* [L. duodeni, twelve; jejunus, empty]. Pertaining to the duodenum and jejunum.

عفجی صائمی: ڈیوڈینم اور ججونم سے متعلق۔

Duodenopancreatectomy *(du-o-de'-no-pan-k-re- at-ek'-to-mi)* [L. duodeni, twelve; G. pankreas, pancreas; ektome, excision]. Surgical excision of the duodenum and part of the pancreas, carried out in cases of cancer arising in the region of the head of the pancreas (e.g. lower end of common bi duct).

ع ولبلبہ براری: لبلبہ کا حصہ اور ڈیوڈینم کا اپریشن کی ذریعے قطع۔ یہ لبلبہ ے سر کے حصہ میں سرطان کی وجہ سے کیا جاتا ہے۔

Duodenostomy *(du-o-de-nos'-to-mi)* [L. duodeni, twelve; G. stoma, mouth]. surgically made fistula between the duod enum and another cavity, e.g. cholecys toduodenostomy, a fistula between the gal bladder and duodenum made to relieve jaun dice in inoperable cancer of the head of th pancreas.

فجی تفویہ: لاطینی لفظ ''ڈیوڈینی'' بمعنی ''بارہ'' اور یونانی لفظ ''سٹوما'' بمعنی 'منہ' سے ماخوذ ڈیوڈینم اور ایک اور کہفہ کے درمیان سرجری کے ذریعہ ئے گئے ناسور کا نام۔

Duodenum *(du-o-de'-num)* [L. duodeni twelve]. The fixed, curved, first portion of th small intestine, connecting the stomach abov to the jejnum below--duodenal, adj.

فج۔ اثناعشر: لاطینی لفظ 'ڈیوڈینی' بمعنی 'بارہ' سے ماخوذ۔ چھوٹی آنت کا پہلا حصہ جو کہ معدے اور جیوجینم کو آپس میں ملاتا ہے۔

Duogastrone *(du-o-gas'-tron).* Carbenoxolone Capsules for duodenal ulcer Swell to twice their size in stomach and 'pop' to release drug

واوگیسٹرون: عفجی ناسور کے لئے کیسہ۔

Dupuyren's contraction *(du'-pwi-terns).* Contracture of the palmar fascia, which bends and fixes one or more fingers.

Dupuytren's contraction

Durabolin *(dur'-a-bol-in)* An agent with testosterone- like activity. Useful for secondary cancer deposits in bone. Metabolically a protein sparer; used where there is extensive tissue damage, e.g. burns and scalds.

ڈیورابولین: ایسا عامل جو 'ٹیسٹوسٹی رون' جیسا عمل کرتا ہے۔ اس کا ایک ٹیکہ صبح ایک شام برائے یوریمیا۔ مفید برائے انلارجڈ پراسٹیٹ کمزوری' گردے

کی بیماری' وزن کی کمی اور عضلاتی کمزوری۔

ıuvadilan *(du-va-dil'-an)*. Isoxuprine hydrochloride (q.v.).

·Vac antigens *(an'-ti-jens)*. Used for desenstization in conditions of allergy.

ڈی ویک اینٹی جنز: الرجی کی صورت میں استعمال کئے جانے والی ''انٹی جن''۔

VT. Deep vein thrombosis (q.v.). See THROMBOSPHLEBITIS.

warf *(dwawrf)* [A.S. dweorg]. Person of stunted growth. Condition is found in achondroplasia, hypothyroidism (cretinism). congenital heart disease, etc. Two types due to underactivity of anterior pituitary gland. **Lorain d.** delayed skeletal growth; retarded sexual development; alert; intelligent. **Frolich's d,** stunted growth; obesity; arrested sexual development; lethargic; somnolent; mentally subnormal--dwarfism, n.

بونا۔ پست قد: ایسا شخص جس میں بڑھنے کا عمل انتہائی کم ہو۔ یہ پچوٹری گلینڈ کے زیر عمل ہوتا ہے۔ لورین ڈوارف اور فلورک ڈوارف اس کی دو اقسام ہیں۔ کوئی نقص ہو تو بچپن میں علاج کرنا چاہئے۔ ہارمونوں کی کمی دور کرنی چاہئے۔

·yflos *(dif'-los)*. A fluorine derivative with an action similar to that of eserine and neostigmine. Used mostly as a 0.1 per-cent solution in oil for glaucoma, when a very long action is required. As an organophosphorous compound, it is used as an insecticide in agriculture. Powerful and irreversible anticholinesterase action. Potentially dangerous to man for this reason.

ڈفلاس: آرگینو فاسفورس مرکب کے طور پر زراعت مین کیڑے مار دوا کے طور پر استعمال کیا جاتا ہے۔ طاقتور اینٹی کولین ایسٹریز عمل کی وجہ سے انسان کے لئے خطرناک۔

)ynamic psychology *(di-nam'-ik si-kol'-o-ji)* [G. dynamis, strength; psyche, soul; logos, study]. A psychological theory which stresses the element of energy in mental process.

حرکیاتی نفسیات: یونانی لفظ ''ڈائنامس'' بمعنی ''طاقت'' ''سائیکی'' بمعنی ''روح'' اور لاکوس بمعنی ''مطالعہ'' سے ماخوذ۔ وہ نفسیاتی مطالعہ جس میں ذہنی عمل میں ''انرجی'' کے عنصر پر زور دیا جائے۔

Dynamometer *(di-nam-om'-e-ter)* [G. dynamis, strength; metron, measure]. Apparatus to test the strength of grip.

انقباض عضلہ پیما: گرفت کی طاقت جانچنے کا سامان۔

Dysaesthesia *(dis-es-thez'-i-a)*. [G. dys-, difficult; aisthesis, sensation]. Impairment of touch sensation.

بے حسی: چھونے کی قوت میں کمی واقع ہونا۔

Dysarthria *(dis-arth'-ri-a)* [G. dys-, difficult; arthron, joint]. Impairment of articulation. Stammering.

لکنت: جوڑ کی جگہ سے گھمانے میں دقت۔

Dysarthosis *(dis-ar-thro'-sis)* [G. dys-, difficult; arthron, joint; -osis, condition]., Any joint condition limiting movement.

مفصل کاذب: جوڑ کی ایسی حالت جس سے حرکت محدود ہو جائے۔

Dychezia *(dis-ke'-zi-a)* [G. dys-, difficult; chezein, to go to stool]. Difficult or painful defaecation.

قبض شدید: فضلہ کا تکلیف سے آنا۔

Dyschondroplasia *(dis-kon-dro-pla'-zi-a)* [G. dys, difficult; chondros, cartilage; plassein, to form]. Normal trunk, short arms and legs.

ڈس کانڈروپلیزیا: دھڑ نارمل لیکن بازو اور ٹانگیں چھوٹی۔

Dyscoria *(dis-kor'-e-a)* [G. dys-, abnormal kor; pupil]. Abnormality of the pupil.

ڈسکوریا: پتلی کا نارمل نہ ہونا۔

Dyscrasi *(dis-kra-zi-a)* [G. dys-, difficult; krasis, mixing]. A morbid general state resulting from the presence of toxic materials in the blood. **blood d.,** usually refers to abnormality of the blood cells.

خون کی خرابی: خون میں زہریلے مادوں کی موجودگی کی وجہ سے حالت۔

Dysentery *(dis'-en-ter-i)* [G. dys-, difficult; enteron, intestine]. Inflamation of the bowel with evacuation of blood and mucus, accompanied by tenesmus and colic. **amoebic d.** is caused by the protozoon Entamoeba histolytica. **bacillary d.** is caused by bacillus of Shiga, Flexner or Sonne. Disease results from poor sanita tion and the house-fly carries the infection from faeces to food. See AMOEBIASIS--dysenteric, adj.

پیچش: خون اور میوکس کا آنا۔ ایبای پیچش ایبا ہسٹولائیٹیکا کی وجہ سے ہوتی ہے۔ یہ بیماری مکھی کے ذریعے پھیلتی ہے۔

Dysfunction *(dis-fungk'-shun)* [G. dys-, abnormal; L. functus, from fungi, to perform]. Abnormal functioning of any organ or part.

فسادفعل۔فتورفعل: کسی عضو یا حصے کا صحیح طور پر کام نہ کرنا۔

Dysgammaglobulinaemia *(dis-gam'-m-a-gl-ob'-u- lin-e'-mi-a)*. Syn., antibody deficiency syndrome. Disturbance of gammaglobulin production. Can be transient, congenital or acquired. Normally there is transfer of IgG from mother to baby, the amount so transferred gradually falls. This can lead to transient hypogammagl -obulinaemia with repeated respiratory infections. Injections of gammaglobulin are given until normal levels occur. Congenital agammaglobulinaemia is a sex-linked recessive genetic variety and is the commonest type of total deficiency. The lymph nodes and spleen are abnormal. Males are solely affected, females being carries of the abnormal gane. As yet there is no means of detecting carriers. The disease usually presents in the second or third years as severe, recurrent bacterial infections with high fever. Virus infections are handled well, becausc the defence mechanism is different. Acquired agammaglobuli- naemia occurs at any age and in either sex. Cause unknown. Secondary agammaglobulinaemia may occur in lymphoma, leukaemia and myeloma, especially after chemotherapy or radiation. It may also be found in bullous skin disorders such as pemphigus and eczema and after burns when it is due to excessive loss of protein in the exuded fluid.

ڈسگیما گلوبولینیمیا: اینٹی باڈی کی کمی کا سنڈروم۔ موروثی مرض

Dysgenesis *(dis-jen'-es-is)* [G. dys-, abnormal; genesis, descent]. Malformation during embryonic development dysgenetic, adj.; dysgenetically, adv.

[...]ر تناسل: جینی تکمیل کے دوران بگڑی ہوئی صورت۔

Dysgerminoma *(dis-jer-min-o'-ma)*. [G. dys[...] abnormal; L. germen germ; G. -oma, tumou[...] A tumour of the ovary of low grac[...] malignancy. It is not hormone secreting, as [...] is developed from cells which date back to t[...] undifferentiated state of gonad[...] development, i.e. before the cells have eith[...] male or female attributes.

[...]س جرمی نوما: بیضہ دان کا ناسور۔

Dyshidrosis *(dis-hid-ro'-sis)* [G. dys-, abnorma[...] hidrosis, sweating]. A vesicular skin eruptio[...] thought to be caused by blockage of the swe[...] ducts at their orifice

[...]بلہ دستی: جلدی ابھار۔ خیال ہے کہ ایسا پسینے کی نلیوں کے سوراخ بند ہونے [...] وجہ سے ہوتا ہے۔

Dyskaryosis *(dis-kar-i-o'-sis)*. Term used for th[...] first stage of abnormality in a cervical smea[...] Follow-up test may revert to normal, but som[...] may become positive and demand biopsy.

[...]س کیریوسس: سرویکل سمیئر کا اولیں مرحلہ۔

Dyskinesia *(dis-ki-ne'-zi-a)* [G. dys-, difficult[...] kinesis, motion]. Impairment of voluntar[...] movement--dyskinetic, adj.

[...]ترحرکیت: ارادی حرکت میں تخفیف۔

Dyslalia *(dis-la'-li-a)* [G. dys-, difficult; lalein[...] to talk]. Difficulty in taking due to defect o[...] speech organs. Immature articulatio[...] -dyslalic, adj.

[...]لکنت: تقریر اعضاء میں نقص کی وجہ سے بولنے میں دقت۔

Dyslexia *(dis-leks'-i-a)* [G. dys-, difficult; lexis[...] word]. Impairment of reading ability. Th[...] child usually has difficulty with groups o[...] letters, but intelligence is unimpaired. Ofte[...] associated with miror-writing--dyslexic, adj.

[...]سر القراۃ: پڑھنے کی اہلیت میں کمی۔

Dysmaturity *(dis-mat-ur'-it-i)* [G. dys-difficult; L. maturare, to make ripe]. Sign and symptoms of growth retardation at birth 'Small for dates'.

[...]س میٹوریٹی: پیدائش کے وقت نشو ونما میں کمی کے آثار۔

ysmelia *(dis-mel'-i-a)* [G. dys-, difficult; melos, limb]. Limb deficiency.

ڈس میلیا: جوارح میں کمی۔

ysmenorrhoea *(dis-men-o-re'-a)* [G. dys-, difficult; men, month; rheein, to flow]. Painful menstruation, **spasmodic d.,** comes on during the first day of a period, often with an hour or two of the start of bleeding. It comes in spasms of acute colicky pain in the lower part of the abdomen, and sometimes in the back and inner parts of the thighs. The spasms can be bad enough to cause fainting and vomiting. The victims, with some exceptions, are immature shy girls, with small breasts, pale nipples and not much pubic hair, **congestive d.,** caused not by too little oestrogen, but by too little progesterone. Sufferers known several days in advance that their period is coming, because they have a dull aching pain in the lower abdomen, increasing heaviness, perhaps constipation, nausea and lack of appetite. There may also be breast tenderness, headache and backache. The sufferers, again with exceptions, tend to have rounded, feminine hips, large breasts with dark nipples, ample pubic hair, with a marked maternal instinct and the wish for a large family (though each pregnancy seems to make the dysmenorrhoea get worse, not better). Fluid retention at this time leads to typical oedema and weight gain; this can be helped by the use of diuretics but the principal treatment is with progesterone.

عسر الطمث ۔ ماہواری کا درد: ماہواری درد سے انا۔ پیلوک بیماری کی وجہ سے بھی ایسا ہوتا ہے۔ حیض کا مشکل سے آنا۔ اس مرض میں حیض یا تو ابتداء سے نہیں آتا یا کچھ مدت آ کر بند ہو جاتا ہے یا مقررہ مقدار سے کم آتا ہے۔ یا تھوڑا تھوڑا رک رک کر درد کے ساتھ آتا ہے۔ حیض میں اعضاء شکنی اور بے چینی ہوتی ہے۔ پیڑو کے مقام پر گرائی کمر، کولہے اور رانوں میں درد ہوتا ہے۔ جسم میں کمزوری، سستی و کاہلی ہو جاتی ہے۔

Dysmorphogenic *(dis-mor-fo-jen'-ik)* [G. dys, difficult; morphe, form; gignesthai, to be produced]. Now preferred to teratogenic (q.v.) when applied to drugs taken during pregnancy.

ڈس کارفوجینک: ہونے والے بچے پر برے اثرات مرتب کرنے والی اسیاء۔ مثلاً وہ ادویات جو حمل کے دوران استعمال کی جاتی ہیں۔

Dysopia *(dis-o'-pi-a)* [G. dys-, difficult; opsis, vision]., Painful or defective vision.

ضعف بصارت: ناقص بینائی۔ بصارت جس سے درد ہو۔

Dysorexia *(dis-o'-reks'-i-a)* [G. dys-, abnormal orexis, appetitie]. An abnormal or unnatural appetite.

نقص اشتہا: غیر معمولی یا غیر قدرتی بھوک۔

Dyspareunia *(dis-par-u'-ni-a)* [G. dys-, difficult; pareunos, lying beside]. Painful or difficult coitus.

عسر مجامعت: جماع کے دوران عورت کو درد ہونا۔

Dyspagia *(dis-pep'-si-a)* [G. dys-, difficult; peptein, pessein, to cook]. Indigestion--dyspeptic, adj.

ڈس پپن سیا: ہاضمہ کی خرابی۔

Dyspepsia *(dis-fa'-ji-a)* [G. dys-, difficult; phagein, to eat]. Difficulty in swallowing---dysphagic, adj.

عسر البلع: نگلنے میں دشواری۔

Dysphasia *(dis-fa'-zi-a)* [G. dys-, difficulty; phasis, speech]. Incomplete language function. **motor d.,** patient is aware of what is said, knows what he wants to reply, but is unable to assemble the symbols of language (speech) in any coherent order, thus giving the impression that he does not understand. In **receiptive d.,** patient unable to put any meaning to the words he hears though he may well be able to understand other forms of communication, such as miming, drawing and writing--dysphasic, adj.

نقص تکلم ۔ فتور نطق: بولنے میں دقت۔

Dysplasia *(dis-plaz'-i-a)* [G. dys-, difficult; plasis, a moulding]. Formation of abnormal tissue--dysplastic, adj.

غیر طبعی نمو: غیر معمولی بافت کا بننا۔

Dyspnoea *(dis-ne'-a)* [G. dys-, difficult; pnoia, breath]. Difficulty in, or laboured breathing; can be mainly of an inspiratory or expiratory nature--dyspnoeic. adj.

دم کشی: سانس میں دشواری۔

Dysrhythmia *(dis-rith'-mi-a)* [G. dys-, abnormal; rhythmos, rhythm]. Disordered rhythm--dysrhthmic, adj.

خلل توازن: غیر مرتب ردم۔

Distaxia *(dis-taks'-i-a)* [G. dys-, difficult; taxis, arrangement]. Difficulty in controlling voluntary movements--dys-taxic, adj.

جزوی بے نسقی ۔ عدم نسق حرکت : ارادی حرکات کو قابو کرنے میں دشواری۔

Dystocia *(dis-tos'-i-a)* [G. dys-, difficult; tokos, birth]. Difficult or slow labour.

عسر ولادت: بچے کی پیدائش کے وقت دردوں کا آہستہ ہونا۔

Dystonic reaction. Refers to 'mental' drugs. Disorder of tissue tonicity. May be above or below normal.

Dystrophy *(dis'-tro-fi)* [G. dys-, faulty; trophe, nourishment]. Defective nutrition. **muscular d.,** genetically determined primary degenerative myopathy--dystrophic, adj.

نقص خوراک: ناقص تغذیہ۔خوراک کی کمی۔

Dysuria *(dis-u'-ri-a)* [G. dys-, difficult; ouron, urine]. Diffiuclt or painful micturition--dysuric, adj.

سر بول: پیشاب تکلیف کے ساتھ آنا۔اس مرض میں پیشاب مشکل سے
تا ہے یا رک جاتا ہے۔ پیشاب کی نالی میں کسی رکاوٹ، سوزاک بدگوشت
ری اور عورت میں رحم یا خصیۃ الرحم کے کسی مرض یا ایام حمل میں بعض دفعہ
تناق الرحم کی شکایت میں پیشاب رک رک کر مشکل سے آتا ہے۔ یا بند ہو
تا ہے۔ پہلے بار بار پیشاب کی حاجت ہوتی ہے پھر پیشاب رک رک کر آتا
ہے اور پیشاب کی دھار باریک ہو جاتی ہے۔ کبھی پیشاب بالکل رک جاتا
ہے۔

Dytac *(di tak).* Triamterene (q.v.).

ائی ٹک: دیکھئے ترائی امٹرین۔

Dytide *(di'-tid).* Triamterene (q.v.) 50 mg an benzthiazide (q.v.) 25 mg.

ائی ٹائیڈ: ٹرائی امٹرین ۵۰ ملی گرام اور بنتھیازائیڈ ۲۵ ملی گرام۔

Dystransin *(di-tran'-sin).* Mild anti-inflam matory agent. No gastro-intestinal irritatio which continued use. A few cases of hepati toxicity have been reported. Occasiona SGOT estimations advised. Useful for th chronic rheumatic disorders.

یٹرنیس: ہلکا آتش گیر یا سوزشی عامل۔ متواتر استعمال سے آنتوں میں
وزش نہیں ہوتی۔ پرانے جوڑوں کے درد میں مفید۔

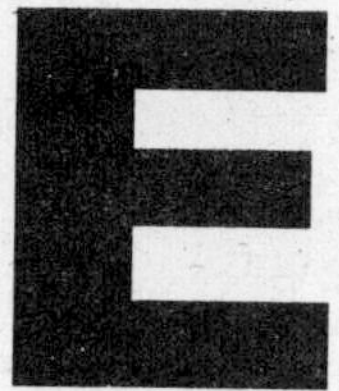

Symbol for elastance, energy, expectancy, elctromotive force, electric intensity and redox potential.

ای: علامت ہے لچک، قوت، توقع، برقی رو کی قوت، برقی شدت اور ریڈاکس پوٹینشل کی۔

Estradiol.

ای2: ایسٹراڈائی اول۔عورتوں کا ایک خاص ہارمون ہے۔

onation *(e-bon-a'-shan)* [L. *e,* out; *bona,* bone]. The removal of bone fragments from a wound.

ہڈی نکال: زخم میں سے ہڈی کا ٹکڑا یا چھوٹا ذرہ نکالنا۔

bolic *(ek-bol-ik)* [G. *ekbolikos,* throwing out]. Oxytacic. Any agent which stimulates the contraction of uterus and expulsion of its contents.

واضح حمل (دوا): ایسا عامل جو گریوڈیوٹرس کے سکڑنے کو تحریک دیتا ہے اور اس میں موجود مواد کو باہر دھکیلنے میں تیزی پیدا کرتا ہے۔حمل کو ساقط کرنے والا۔مثلاً ارگٹ، پچوٹری ایکسٹریک وغیرہ۔

chondroma *(ek'-on-dro-ma)* [G. *ek,* out; *chond,* cartilage, *rome,* tumor]. A hyperplastic growth of the cartilage tissue developing on the surface of a cartilage or projecting under the peri-osteum of a bone.

سلعہ غُضرُوف: ناسور کی ایک قسم جو ہڈی کی سطح پر پایا جاتا ہے۔

hymosis *(ek'-i-mo'sis)* [G. *ek,* out of; *chymos,* juice; *osis,* condition]. A small hemorrhagic spot, larger than a petechia in the skin or mucus membrane forming a non-elevated, rounded or irregular, blue or purplish patch.

طرفہ۔کدمہ: چھوٹا خون رسنے سے بننے والا جلد کے نیچے نشان جو نقطے سے بڑا ہو۔جلد یا جھلی پر ابھار پیدا نہ کرے۔گول یا بے شکل قسم کا نیلا یا بنفشی رنگ کا نشان یا داغ۔

ECG Electrocardiogram.

ای سی جی: الیکٹروکارڈیوگرام۔برقی قوت سے حرکاتِ قلب کا گراف تیار کرنا۔

Echinococcus *(e-ki'-no-kok-as)* [G. *echinos,* hedgehog]. A genus of small tapeworms of the family taentidae. The adults worms infest the primary host i.e. dog while the eneysled larvae infest the secondary host i.e. man and cause hydrated disease.

شوکی نبقہ: کدو کیڑے کی ایک جنس۔

Echo-cardiography *(ek'-o-kahr-de-og-rafe)* [G. *echo,* sound (arcturned); *cardios,* heart; *graphein,* to record]. A method of graphically recording the position andmotion of the heart walls or the internal structures of the heart and the neighbouring tissues by the echo obtained from beams of ultrasonic waves directed through the chest wall.

ایکو کارڈیوگرافی: گراف کے اوپر دل کی دیواروں یا دوسری بافتوں کی حرکات ریکارڈ کرنا۔اس میں الٹراسانک شعاعیں سینے کی دیوار پر ڈالی جاتی ہیں اور ان کی بازگشت کے ذریعے اندرونی اعضاء کی پوزیشن اور حرکات نوٹ کی جاتی ہیں۔

Echolalia *(ek-o-la-lea)* [G. *echo,* speech; *lalie,* babble]. Stereotyped repitition of some other's phrases or words.

لفظی رٹ: سنے ہوئے الفاظ کا فوری طور پر اعادہ۔معصوم بچوں میں پائی جانے والی خصوصیت شائزوفرینیا میں بھی ایسا ہوتا ہے۔

E3. Lachesine (q.v.).

ای ۳ : دیکھئے لیکسین۔

EACA. Epsilon Aminocaproic acid (q.v.).

ای اے سی اے : دیکھئے اپسیلان ایمائنوکیپرائک ایسڈ۔

Eaton agent Isolated in 1944 from pleural secretions of patients with non-bacterial pneumonia. In 1962 identified as PPLO (q.v.), already assigned the generic name Mycoplasma. Mycoplasma pneumoniae, proposed as alternative to E. a.

ایٹن ایجنٹ : اس کا متبادل نام مائیکو پلازما نمونی تجویز کیا گیا ہے۔

EBI. ***Emetine bismuth oidide.***

ای بی آئی : امیٹن بسمتھ ایوڈائڈ۔

EB virus. *(vi-rus)*. See EPSTEIN BARRVIRUS.

ای بی وائرس : دیکھئے اپسٹائین بیروائرس۔

ECBOLIC *(ek-bol'-ik)* [G. ekbole, a throwing out]. Any agent which stimulates contraction of the gravid uterus and hastens expulsion of its contents.

واضع حمل (دوا) : ایسا عامل جو گریو ڈیوٹرس کے سکڑنے کو تحریک دیتا ہے اور اس میں موجود مواد کو باہر دھکیلنے میں تیزی پیدا کرتا ہے۔ حمل کو ساقط کرنے والا۔ مثلاً ارگٹ، پیچوئیٹری ایکسٹریکٹ وغیرہ۔

Ecchondroma *(ek-kon-dro'-ma)* [G. ek, out of; chondros, cartilage; -oma, tumour]. A benign tumour composed of cartilage which protrudes from the surface of the bone in which it arises--ecchondromata, pl.

سلعۂ غضروف : ناسور کی ایک قسم جو ہڈی کی سطح پر پایا جاتا ہے۔

Ecchymosis *(ek-i-mo'-sis)* [g. ek, out of; chymos, juice; -osis, condition]. An extravasation of blood under the skin. Syn., bruise--ecchymoses, pl.

طرفہ کدمہ : جلد کے نیچے خون کا جمع ہونا۔

EGG. Electrocardiogram. See ELECTROCARDIOGRAPH.

ای سی جی: الیکٹرو کارڈیوگرام۔ برقی قوت سے حرکات قلب کا گراف تیار کرنا۔

Echinococcus *(ek-i'-no-kok'-us)* [G. echinos, hedgehog]. A genus of tape worms, the adults infesting a prima ry host, e.g. a dog. In man (secondary host) the encysted larvae cause 'hydatid disease'.

نوکی بنقہ : کدو کیڑے کی ایک جنس۔

Echoencephalographgy *(ek-o-en-kef-al-o g'-ra-fi)* [G. echo; egkephalos, brain graphein, to write]. Passage of penetratin sound waves across the head. Can detec abscess, blood clot, injury or tumour withi brain.

یکوانیکفالوگرافی : سر کے آر پار صوتی لہروں کا گزر۔

Echolalia *(ek-o-la'-li-a)* [G. echo; lalia, talk Repetition, almost automatically of words o phrases heard. Occurs most commonly i schizophrenia and dementia; sometimes i toxic delirious, states. A characteristic of a infants' speech--echolalic, adj.

فظی رٹ : سنے ہوئے الفاظ کا فوری طور پر اعادہ۔ معصوم بچوں ں پائی جانے والی خصوصیت شائزوفرینیا میں بھی ایسا ہوتا ہے۔

Echophony *(ek-of'-o-ni)* [G. echo, echo; phone voice]. The echo of a vocal sound hear during ausculation of the chest.

یکوفونی : چھاتی کے معائنہ کے دوران گلے کی آواز کی بازگشت۔

Echopraxia *(ek-o-prak'-si-a)* [G. echo; praxis action]. Involuntary mimicking of another' movements.

Echoviruses Enteric Cytopathic Human Orphar This name was given because these viruse were originally found in the stools c diseaseless children. They have cause meningitis and mild respiratory infection i children. At least 30 types.

Eclampsia *(ek-lamp'-si-a)* [G. eklampsis, shining forth]. 1. A severe manifestation c toxaemia of pregnancy, associated with fi and coma. 2. A suddent convulsiv attack--eclamptic, adj.

شناج : وضع حمل کے دوران بے ہوشی کے دورے۔ حمل کی یت۔

Ecmnesia *(ek-ne'-zi-a)* [G. ek, out of; amnesi forgetfulness]. Impaired memory for rece events with normal memory of remote one Common in old age and in early cerebral det rioration.

ض نسیان : یادداشت کا کم ہو جانا۔ بڑھاپے میں یادداشت کم ہو

جاتی ہے۔ مریض کو ماضی قریب یا زمانہ حال کے واقعات یاد نہیں رہتے لیکن ماضی بعید کے واقعات یاد رہتے ہیں۔

conomycin *(ek-on-o-mi'-sin)*. Tetracycline(q.v.).

ایکانو مائی سین : دیکھئے ٹیٹرا سائیکلین۔

craseur *(a-kra-zer)* [F.]. An instrument with a wire loop that can be tightened round the pedicle of a new growth to sever it.

مخفقہ : ایک الہ۔

CT. Electroconvulsive thereapy. See ELECTROTHERAPY.

ای سی ٹی : الیکٹروکنولسوتھراپی۔

cthyma *(ek-thi'-ma)* [G. ekthyma, pustule]. A crusted eruption of impetigo contagiosa on the legs, producing necrosis of the skin, which heals with scarring. A similar condition occurs in syphilis.

چھالے۔ آبلے : ٹانگوں پر کھرنڈ والے ابھار۔

ctoderm *(ek'-to-derm)* [G. ektos, without; derma, skin]. The external primitive germ layer of the embryo. From it are developed the skin structures, the nervous system, organs of special sense, pineal gland and part of the pituitary and adrenal glands--ectodermal, adj.

ایکٹوڈرم۔ بیرونی جلد : جنین کی بیرونی اولیں جنینی پرت۔ اس سے بیرونی جلد، اعصابی نظام اور چند غدود بنتے ہیں۔

ctodermosis *(ek-to-derm-o-'sis)* [G. ektos, outside; derma, skin; osis, condition]. Disease of any organ or tissue derived from the ectoderm

ایکٹوڈرموسس : ایکٹوڈرم سے ماخوذ نسیج یا عضو کی بیماری۔

ctogenous *(ek-toj'-en-us)* . Originating outside the organism. Opp. to endogenous.

ctoparasite *(ek-to-par'-a-sit)* [G. ektos, outside; parasitos, parasite]. A parasite that lives on the exterior surface of its host-ectoparasitic, adj.

برون طفیلی : ایسا طفیلی جو اپنے میزبان سے باہر رہ کر خوراک حاصل کرے۔

topia *(ek-to'-pi-a)* [G. ektopos, away form a place]. Malposition of an organ or structure, usually congenital. **e. vesicae,** an abnormally placed urinary bladder which protrudes through or opens on to the abdominal wall--ectopic, adj.

بے جائی : کسی عضو یا ساخت کا غلط جگہ پر ہونا۔

Ectopic pregnancy *(ek-top'-ik preg'-nan-si)* Extrauterine gestation, the Fallopian tube being the most common site. At about the 6th week the tube tuptures, constituting a 'surgical emergency'.

ایکٹاپک پریگننسی : جنین کا غلط جگہ قائم ہونا۔ بعض دفعہ حمل بچہ دانی کے بجائے فیلوپین نلی میں ہو جاتا ہے۔ تیسرے ماہ نلی پھٹ جاتی ہے۔ خون جاری ہو جاتا ہے۔ درد ہوتا ہے۔ اپریشن سے حمل ضائع کر دیجئے۔

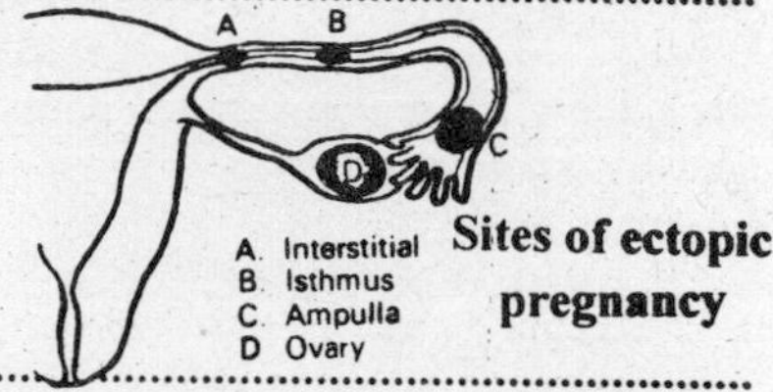

Sites of ectopic pregnancy

Ectozoa *(ek-to-zo'a)* [G. ektos, outside; zoon animal]. External parasites.

برون طفیلی : بیرونی طفیلی

Ectrodactylia *(ek-tro-dak-til'-i-a)* [G. ektrosis, miscarriage; daktylos, finger]. Congenital absence of one or more fingers or toes or parts of them.

بے انگشتی : ہاتھ یا پاؤں کی انگلیوں یا ان کے حصوں کا کم ہونا۔

Ectropion *(ek-tro'-pi-on)* [G. ek, out of; trepein, to turn]. An eversion or turning outwards,

Ectropion

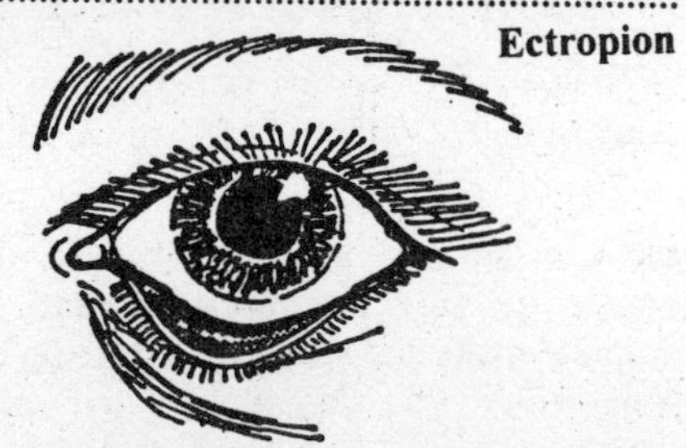

especially of the lower eyelid or of an unyhealed lesion of the cervix uteri

شترۂ خارجی : کسی چیز کا الٹ جانا یعنی باہر کی طرف ہو جانا مثلاً انکھ کا زیریں پوٹا وغیرہ۔

Eczema *(ek'-ze-ma)* [G. ek, out; zeo, boil]. Precise meaning has not been agreed upon. Some medical men use the term as synonymous with 'dermatitis' (q.v.). Others regard it as one form of dermatitis, decribing it as the 'eczema reaction' to an irritant on an already susceptible skin. The reaction begins with erythema, then vesicles appear. These rupture, forming crusts or leaving pits which ooze serum. This is the exudative or weeping stage. In the process of healing, the area becomes scaly. Some authorities limit term 'eczema' to the cases with internal causes while those caused by external contact factors are called dermatitis.

A. Internal causes:
1. Atopic
2. Seborrhoeic
3. Discoid
4. Gravitational.

B. External causes:
5. Contact
   a) by primary irritation
   b) by allergic sensitization.

ایکزیما۔ چنبل۔ چھاجن : جلد پر خارش ہونا اور ابلے پڑ جانا۔ جسم کے متاثرہ حصے پر خارش ہوتی ہے اور ابھار بنتا ہے جس میں دائرے کی صورت میں دانے نکلتے ہیں۔ بیچ میں گڑھے بن جاتے ہیں۔ اس میں سے سفید پانی جیسا لعاب یا سیرم نکلنے لگتا ہے۔ اسے ایکزیما کا رونے والا مرحلہ کہتے ہیں۔ یہ چھوت کا مرض ہے اور ایک دوسرے کو لگتا ہے۔ علاج کے لئے اسٹوکیلیم، پری ٹون، ڈیکسامیتھاسون بیٹنو ویٹ این کریم۔

atopic e. is an inflammatory skin condition in which the skin becomes red and small vesicles, crusts and scales may develop on the skin surface. The skin is very itchy causing scratching, usually at night. It is found mostly on the face and in the flexor areas of the arms and legs, usually does not occur under 6 months of age. **infantile e.**, an allergic eczema of infants aged between 2 months and 2 years, often limited to the cheeks and forehead and which is very irritating. Such infants should not be vaccinated or inoculated with a foreign serum. May be followed by **flexural e.**, (Besnier's prurigo) in childhood. **seborrhoeic e.**, is confined to the napkin area and the face. This form is not itchy but the skin looks very dry. The prognosis is very good as the condition clears in a relatively short time. **e. asthma syndrome,** affected infants begin with infantile eczema and in childhood develop asthma as the eczema remits; frequently the asthma remits at puberty--eczematous, adj.

EDD. Expected date of delivery (q.v.).

Edecrin *(ed'-e-krin).* Ethacrynic acid (q.v.).

ایڈیکرن : دیکھئے ایتھاکرینک ایسڈ۔

Edentulous *(ed-ent'-u-lus).* Without teeth.

بے دانت: دانتوں کے بغیر۔

Edosol *(ed'-os-ol).* Salt-free dried milk.

ایڈوسال : بغیر نمک کے خشک دودھ۔

Edward's syndrome. Autosomal trisomy associated with mental subnormality. The cells have 47 chromosomes. Sometimes called trisomy E.

ایڈورڈ عارضہ : ایک کروموسوم زائد ہوتا ہے یعنی چھیالیس کے بجائے ۴۷ کروموسوم پائے جاتے ہیں۔ ایسا فرد ذہنی طور پر متاثر ہوتا ہے۔

EEG Electroencephalogram. See ELECTROENCEPHALOGRAPH.

ای ای جی : ایکٹرو انسفالوگرام۔

Efcortesol *(ef-kor'-ti-sol).* Hydrocortisone phosphate in stabilized solution for intravenous use.

ایفکار ٹیسول : متوازن محلول میں ہائیڈرو کارٹیسون فاسفیٹ ایڈرینل کی میں مستعمل۔

Effector *(e-fek'-tor)* [L. efficere, to carry out]. A motor or secretory nerve ending in a muscle, gland or organ.

موثر : عضو، گلینڈ یا عضلے میں ختم ہونیوالی موٹر یا رطوبتی عصب۔

Efferent *(ef'-er'-ent)* [L. effere, to carry away].

Carrying, conveying, conducting away from a centre. Opposite to afferent (q.v.).

برآور : مرکز سے دور لے جانے والی۔ برآور اعصاب یا موٹر نرو پیغام سے باہر کی طرف لے جاتے ہیں۔

Effort syndrome *(ef'-fort sin'-drom)*. A form of anxiety neurosis, manifesting itself in a variety of cardiac symptoms including precordial pain, for which no pathological explanation can be discovered.

جھد عارضہ : پریشانی کی ایک قسم۔

Effusion *(ef-fu'-zhun)* [L. effundere, to pour out]. Extravasation of fluid into body tissues or cavities.

انصباب۔ ریزش : جسمانی بافتوں یا کھفوں میں سیال کا بہاؤ۔

Ego *(eg'-o)* [L. I]. Refers to the unconscious self, the T, that party of personality that deals with reality and is influenced by social forces. It modifies behaviour by unconscious compromise between the primitive instinctual urges (the id) and the conscience.

خودی۔ نفس : خودی سے متعلق ۔ اپنے آپ سے متعلق انانیت۔ ۔

Ehrlich's theory of immunity, Postulated that tissue cells received molecules of antigen by means of receptors. Under certain conditions these receptors were overproduced and released into the body-fluids. The free receptor groups became the antibodies and were capable of combining specifically with antigen molecules. **E's diazo reagent,** used for the detection of urobilinogen in urine **E's '606'** Salvarsan, discovered in 1909 as a result of the 606th experiment. See NEOARSPHENAMINE [Paul Ehrlich, German bacteriologist and pathologist, 1854-1915].

اہرلک کا نظریہ مزاحمت : خلیے ریسپٹرز کے ذریعے اینٹی جن کے سالمات حاصل کرتے ہیں۔ بعض حالات میں ریسپٹرز زیادہ تعداد میں پیدا ہونے کی وجہ سے جسمانی سیالوں میں آجاتے ہیں۔ آزاد ریسپٹر گروہ اینٹی باڈیز بن جاتے ہیں اور اینٹی جن کے سالمات کے ساتھ ملنے کے اہل ہوتے ہیں۔

Ejaculation *(e-ja k-u-la'-shun)* [L. ex, from; jaculatus, thrown out]. A suddent emission of semen.

انزال : سیمن یا منی کا اچانک اخراج۔

Ejaculatory duct *(e-jak'-u-tat-or-i-dukts)*. Two fine tubes, one on either side, commencing at the union of the seminal vesicle with the vas deferens, and termina ting at their union with the prostatic urethra.

انزالی نالیاں : دو باریک نالیاں۔

Else ointment A cleansing agent used in the debridement of necrotic debris and purulent exudates from wounds.

الیس مرہم : صاف کرنے والا عامل۔ زخموں کی صفائی کرنے کے لئے ایک مرہم۔

Elastoplast *(e-las'-to-plast)*. Elastic cotton cloth without rubber threads, with porous adhesive and non-fray edges. **E. bandages are applied** firmly in the ambulatory treatment of varicose ulcers and after injection treatment of veins; the compression reduces oedema and pain and promotes healing. Removal of the bandages should be carefully carried out by cutting with special flatbladed scissors. **E.derssings are** elastic, porous, adhesive dressings for surgical purposes, with a central pad impregnated with Domiphen Bromide BPC (0.15 percent) on an elastic cotton cloth, and spread with porous adhesive. **E. extension plaster,** 2.743 m length of elastic cotton cloth spread with porous adhesive in which the stretch is across the width; rigid lengthwise for skin traction in orthopaedic conditions.

لچکدار پٹی : اس کی پٹیاں استعمال کی جاتی ہیں۔

Electra complex. Excessive emotional attachment of daughter to father. The name is derived from Greek mythology.

Electrocardiograph *(e-lek-tro-kar'-di-o-graf)* [G. electron, amber; cardia, heart; graphein, to write]. An instrument containing a string galvanometer through which passes the electrical current produced by the heart's contraction. A permanent record (electrocardiogram, ECG) of these oscillations is made on a moving drum of graph paper -electrocardiographic, adj.; electrocardiographically, adv.

An electrocardiogram (ECG) tracing

الیکٹروکارڈیوگراف : برقی قلب نگار۔ ایک آلہ۔ قلب کے امراض مد۔قلبی عضلے۔کے سکڑنے سے متعلق رو اور وولٹیج موج قسموں کو ریکارڈ کرنے کے لئے ایک الہ۔

Electrocoagulation *(e-lek-tro-ko-ag-u-l-a'-shun).* Technique of surgical diathermy. Coagulation, especially of bleeding points, by means of electrodes.

برقی انجماد : سرجری کی ایک تکنیک۔ برقی لہروں سے بہتے خون کا انجماد۔

Electrocochleography *(e-lek-tro-kok-le-o-q'-ra-fi).* ECoG. Direct recording of movement in the fluid in the internal ear.

Electrocorticography *(e-lek-tro-kor-ti-k-og'-ra-fi).* Direct recording from the cerebral cortex during operation -electrocortic- ographic, adj.; electrocorticographically, adv.

الیکٹروکارٹیکوگرافی : اپریشن کے دوران سربرل کارٹیکس سے براہ راست ریکارڈنگ۔

Electrode *(e-lek'-trod)* [G. electron, amber; hodos, path]. A conductor in the form of a pad or plate, whereby electricity enters or leaves the body in electrotherapy.

الیکٹروڈ۔ برقیرہ : پیٹ یا پیڈ کی صورت میں کنڈکٹر علاج بالبرق میں استعمال ہونے والی اصلاح۔

Electrodessication *(e-lek-tro-des-i-ka'-shun).* Technique of surgica' diathermy. There is drying and subsequent removal of tissue, e.g. papillomata.

برقی خشکاؤ : سرجیکل ڈایا تھرامی کی تکنیک۔ بجلی سے کسی نسیج کو خشک کرنا اور اپریشن کر کے ختم کرنا۔

Electrodiagnosis *(e-lek'-tro-di-ag-no'-sis).* The use of graphic recording of electrical irritability of tissues in diagnosis--electrod- iagnc stic, adj.

.قی تشخیص : تشخیص میں بافتوں کی برقی ناحسیت کی گرافک یکارڈنگ کا استعمال۔ بجلی کے ذریعہ امراض کی تشخیص۔

Electroencephalograph *(e-lek'-tro-en-ke f'-al-ograt).* [G. electron, amber; egkephalo brain; graphein, to write]. An instrument b which electrical impulses derived from th brain can be amplified and recorded on pape in a fashion similar to that of th electrocardiograph. The record is an electrc encephalogram (EEG)--electroencephalog raphic, adj.; electroencephalographically, adv

ائی برق نگار : ایک آلہ جس سے دماغ سے برقی تحریکوں کو کاغذ . ریکارڈ کیا جاتا ہے۔

Electrolysis *(e-lek-trol'-is-is)* [G. electron amber; luein, to loose]. 1. Chemical decompc sition by electricity. 2. Destruction o individual hairs (epilation); eradication o moles, spider naevi, etc,. using electricity.

ق پاشی : (۱) بجلی کے ذریعے کیمیائی بوسیدگی۔ (۲) بجلی کی تعمال سیانفرادی بالوں کی تباہی اور مسوں کا خاتمہ۔

Electrolyte *(e-lek'-tro-lit)* A liquid or solution c a substance which is capable of conductin electricity. On passing an electric curren through the substance a chemical change always takes place. The change is 'electrolysi (q.v.). **e. balance,** a normal state in which th action and reaction of two or mor electrolytes is of normally balanced propor ions--electrolytic, adj.

ق پاش : محلول یا مائع جس میں سے بجلی گزر سکتی ہو۔

Electromyography *(el-ek-tro-mi-og'-ra-fi)* [C electron, amber; myos, muscle; graphein, t write]. Graphic recording of electrica currents generated in active muscle. EMG electromyogram, n.; electromyogr- aphica adj.; electromyorgraphically, adv.

ھلی برق نگاری : عامل عضلے میں پیدا ہونے والی برقی لہروں ں گرافک ریکارڈنگ۔

Electro-oculogram *(e-lek-tro-ok'-u-lo-gram* Graphic record of eye position and move ment, and potential difference between fron and back of eyeball using electrodes placed on skin near socket. Can be used as an electrod-iagnostic test.

الیکٹرو آکولوگرام : آنکھ کی حرکت اور حالت کی گرافک ریکارڈنگ۔

Electrolplexy *(e-lek-tro-pleks'-i)* [G. electron, amber; plassein, to form]. See ELECTROTH-ERAPY.

برقی علاج : دیکھئے الیکٹروتھراپی

Electropyrexia *(e-lek'-tro-pi-rek'-si-a)* [G. electron, amber; pur, fire]. A high body temperature produced by an electrical apparatus. (Keltering cabinet or inductotherm.)

الیکٹروپائیریکسیا : برقی سامان کی وجہ سے جسم کے درجہ حرات کا زیادہ ہونا۔

Electroretinogram *(e-lek-tro-ret'-in-o-gram)* [G. electron, amber; L. rete, net; G. gramma, letter]. ERG. Graphic record of electrical curr-ents generated in active retina.

الیکٹروریٹنوگرام : عامل ریٹنا میں پیدا ہونے والی برقی لہروں کا گرافک ریکارڈ۔

Electrosection *(e-lek-tro-sek'-shun)*. Technique of surgical diathermy for cutting the skin o* parting soft tissues.

برقی تراشہ : سرجیکل ڈایا تھرمی کی تکنیک۔

Electrotherapy *(e-lek-tro-ther'-a-pi)* [G. elektron, amber; therapeia, treatment]. Electrical treatment. Syn., ECT, electroplexy, electroshock. A form of physical treatment widely used by psychiatrists in the treatment of depression, acute mania and toxic confusional states. Also used in cases of stupor and certain types of schizophrenia. an apparatus is used which delivers a definate voltage for a precise fraction of a second to electrodes placed on the head, producing a convulsion **modified e.,** the convulsion is modified with an intravenous anaesthetic and a muscle relaxant, e.g. scoline. **unilateral** **ECT** is probably in the dominant cerebral hemisphere which is the left in practically all people. ECT is therefore applied to the right hemisphere to minimize memory disturbance. See CONVULSIVE THERAPY.

الیکٹروتھراپی۔ برقی علاج : برقی علاج۔ طبیعی علاج کی ایک قسم جو ماہر نفسیات استعمال کرتے ہیں۔

Element *9el'-e-ment)* One of the constitutents of a compound. The elements are the primary substances which in pure form, or combined into compounds, constitute all matterr.

عنصر : مرکب کے اجزاء میں سے ایک۔ اناصر مادہ بناتے ہیں۔

Elephantiasis *(el-ef-an-ti'-a-sis)* [G. elephas, elephant; -iasis, condition]. The swelling of a limb, usually a leg, as a result of lymphatic obstruction (lymphoedema), and subcuta-neous tissues. A complication of filariasis in tropical countries, but by no means rare in Britain as a result of syphilis or recurring streptococcal infection (e. nostras). See BARBADOS LEG.

فیل : کسی جارح عموماً ٹانگ کا متورم ہو جانا۔

Elixir *(e-liks'-er)*. A sweetened, aromatic solution of a drug, often containing an appreciable amount of alcohol. Elixirs differ from syrups in containing very little sugar, and in requiring dilution before use.

اکسیر : کسی دوا کا شیریں، خوشبو دار محلول جس میں عموماً الکحل بھی ہوتا ہے۔

Elliptocytosis *(el-ip-to-si-to'-sis)*. Anaemia in which the red blood cells are oval.

الپٹوسائی ٹوسس : خون کی کمی جس میں سرخ خونی خلیے بیضوی ہوتے ہیں۔

Eltroxin *(el-troks'-in)*. A preparation of thyr-oxine (q.v.) that has a standardized activity.

الٹراکسن : تھائیراکسن تیار شدہ۔

Emaciation *(e-ma-shi-a'-shun)* [L. macies, thinness]. Excessive leanness, or wasting of body tissue--emaciate, v.t.

اختہ گری : مردانہ تولیدی قوت ختم کرنا۔

Embequin *(em'-be-quin)*. Di-iodohydroxy-quinoline (q.v.).

ایمبے کوئن : ڈائی اوڈوکوئن۔ دیکھئے ڈائی ہائیڈروکسی کیونولین۔ ایمائی پیچش کے لئے ایک گولی صبح ایک دوپہر ایک شام۔

Embolectomy *(em-bol-ek'-to-mi)* [G. embolos, plug; ektome, excision]. Surgical removal of an embolus.

سدابراری : اریشن کے ذریعے امبولس کا انقطاع۔

Embolic *(em-bol'-ik)* [G. embolos, plug]. Pertaining to an embolism or an embolus.

سدادی : امبولس سے متعلق۔

Embolism *(em'-bol-ism)* [G. embolos, plug]. Obstruction of a blood vessel by the impaction of a solid body (e.g. thrombi, fat globules, tumour cells) or an air bubble.

سدایت۔انجماد خون شریان : کسی ٹھوس شے یا ہوائی بلبے کی وجہ سے خونی رگ میں رکاوٹ۔

Embolism

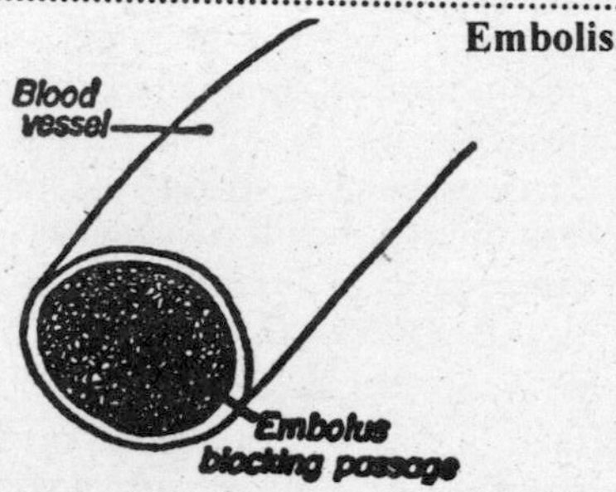

Embologenic *9em-bol-o-jen'-ik)* [G. embolos, plug; genesis, descent]. Capable of producing an embolus.

امبولوجینک : امبولس پیدا کرنے کا اہل۔

Embolus *(em'-bol-us)* [G. embolos, plug]. Solid body or air bubble transported in the circulation. See EMBOLISM--emboli, pl.

امبولس۔ سداد : خونی گردش میں کوئی ٹھوس شے یا ہوائی بلبلہ۔

Embryo *(em'-bri-o)* [G. embruon, embryo]. The term applied to the developing ovum during the early months of gestaiton--embryonic, adj.

جنین : وضع حمل کے ابتدائی دنوں بیضے کا ارتقاء حمل کے تین ہفتوں سے آٹھ ہفتوں تک کا جنین۔ اگر پہلے ماہ جنین کو شروع سے آخر تک ناپا جائے تو یہ تقریباً چوتھائی انچ لمبا ہوتا ہے۔ ریڑھ کی ہڈی کے ایکسرے پر سر بہت نمایاں ہوتا ہے۔ اس مرحلہ پروہ نلی جو بعد میں دل میں تبدیل ہوئی ہے، بن چکی ہوتی ہے اور جسم کی دیوار پر ایک گول ابھار بناتی ہے۔ اس ابتدائی دور میں بھی یہ ابھار باقاعدہ دھڑکتا ہے۔ لمبی پتلی نلی منہ سے لے کر کشادگی تک جاتی ہے جو آگے چل کر معدہ بن جاتی ہے۔ بازوں اور ٹانگیں بھی چھوٹی کلیوں کی شکل میں ظاہر ہوتی ہیں۔ دوسرے ماہ جنین انسانی شکل اختیار کرنا شروع کر دیتا ہے۔ ب اس کا چہرہ واضح طور پر انسانی ہوتا ہے اس کے بازو، ٹانگیں، وں اور پیروں کی انگلیاں، کہنیاں اور گھٹنے بھی واضح ہو جاتے ہیں۔ ضائے جنس بھی نمودار ہو جاتے ہیں لیکن نر اور مادہ میں تمیز کرنا مشکل تا ہے۔

Egg
18 days
24 days
26 days
5 wks.
8 wks.
2½ months

Embryo: stages of developmen

Embryology *(em-bri-ol'-oj-i)* [G. embruon, embryo, discourse]. Study of the developmen of an organism from fertilization to extgrauterine life--embryological, adj.; embryologically, adv.

Embryoma *(em-bri-o'-ma)* [G. enbruon, embryo; -oma, tumour]. Teratoma (q.v.).

مضغی سلعہ : دیکھئے ٹراٹوما۔

Embryopathy *(em-bri-op'-ath-i)* [G. embruon, embryo; pathos, disease]. Disease or abnormality in the embryo More serious if it occurs in the first three months. Includes the 'rubella syn-drome'--embryopathic, adj.; embryopathically, adv.

ایمبر یوپیتھی : جنین میں مرض۔

Embryotomy *(em-bri-ot'-o-mi)* [G. embruon, embryo; tome, a cutting]. Mutilation of the fetus to tacilitate removal from womb, when natural birth is impossible.

جنین تراشی : بطن سے جنین کو علیحدہ کرنا۔

Emepronium bromide *(em-e-pro'-ni-um_ bro-mid)*. Atropine-like drug with inhibitory influence on bladder contraction. Reduces nocturnal frequency of micturition.

ایمی پرونیم برومائیڈ : ایک دوا جو بلیڈر کو سکڑنے سے روکتی ہے۔

Emesis *(em'-i-sis)* [G.]. Vomiting.

استفراغ : قے کرنا۔ قے آنا۔

Emetic *(e-met'-ik)* [G. emetikos, provoking sickness]. Used in amoebic dysentery, often in association with other amoebicides.

ایمے ٹین : ایک الکلائڈ۔ امیبائی پیچش میں مستعمل نصف گرین کا ٹیکہ سات ایام تک۔ مریض لیٹا رہے۔ ایک گرین کا ٹیکہ روزانہ چھ ایام تک برائے جگر کا پھوڑا۔

EMI scan Non-invasive technique which produces a pictorial print-out reveling the density of tissues, thereby demonstrating the presence or absence of a tumour.

Emission *(e-mish'-un)* [L.]. An ejaculation or sending forth. An involuntary ejaculation of semen.

انزال : اخراج مادہ تولید یا منی کا اچانک اخراج۔ خروج منی۔

Emmetropia *(em-met-rop'i-a)* [G. emmetros, in measure; ops, eye]. Normal or perfect vision--emmetropic, adj.

بصارت طبعی : مکمل بصارت۔

Emollient *(e-mol'-i-ent)* [L. emollire, to soften]. An agent which softens and soothes skin or mucous membrane.

ملائم کنندہ : جلد یا میوکس جھلی کو نرم کرنے والا عامل۔ یہ جلد کی خراش اور سوزش کو ختم کرنے میں ممد ہوتے ہیں۔ مثلاً ویزلین، تیل وغیرہ۔

Emotion *(e-mo'-shun)* [L. *emovere* to stir up]. The tone of feeling recognlized in ourselves by certain bodily changes, and in others by tendencies to certain characteristic behaviour. Aroused usually by ideas or concepts.

جوش ۔ ہیجان : تبدیلیوں کی وجہ سے اندرونی احساس۔

Emotional *(e-mo'-shun-al)*. Characteristic of or caused by emotion. e, bias, tendency of e. attitude to affect logical judgement. e, state, effect of emotions on normal mood, e.g. agitation.

جذباتی : جذبات کی وجہ سے پیدا ہونے کی خصوصیت ۔

Empathy *(em'-pa-thi)* [G. *empatheia*, passion]. Identifying oneself with another person or the actions of another person.

ہم گذاری ۔دراحساسی : دوسرے شخص سے اپنے آپ کو ممیز کرنا۔

Emphysema *(em-fi-se'-ma)* [G. inflation]. Gaseous distension of the tissues.**pulmonary e.,** alveolar distension; (1) generalized--often accompanying chronic bronchitis; (2) localized--either distal to partial obstruction of a bronchus or bronchiole (obstructive e.) or in alveoli adjacent ot segment of collapsed lung (compensatory e.). **surgical e.**, air in the subcutaneous tissue planes following trauma of surgery or injury emphysematous, adj.

ہوائی چھالا : بافتوں میں گیس ہونا ۔

Empirical *(em-pir'-ik-al)* [G. *empeirikos*, experience]. Based on observation and experience and not on scientific reasonting.

عملی ۔ تجربی : سائنسی توضیح کے بجائے مشاہدہ اور تجربہ پر بنیاد ہونا۔

Empyema *(em-pi-e'-ma)*. [G. *empuos*, discharging matter]. A collection of pus in a cavity, hollow organ or space.

پیپ سینہ : کہفہ، کھوکھلے عضو یا جگہ میں پیپ کا جمع ہونا ۔

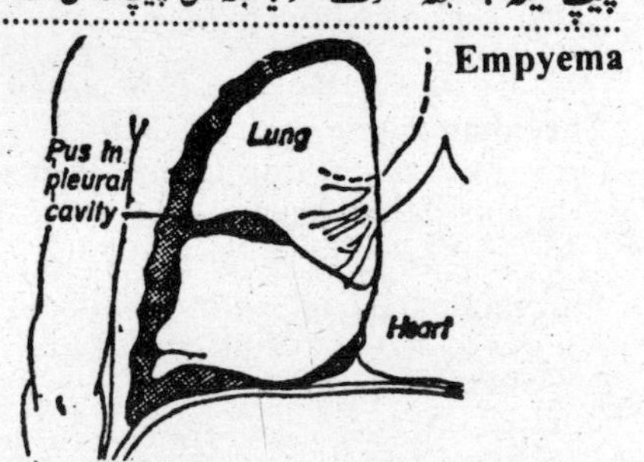

Emulsion *(e-mul'-shun)* [L. *emulgere*, to milk out]. A uniform suspension of fat or oil particles in an aqueous continuous phase (O/W emulsion) or aqueous droplets in an oily continuous phase (W/O emulsion).

ایملشن ۔ شیرہ : چکنائی یا تیل کے ذرات پر مشتمل سیال جو دودھیا سفید ہوتا ہے ۔ تیل اور پانی کے ملاپ سے بنائے جاتے ہیں، کیکر کا گوند بھی شامل کرتے ہیں ۔

Emylcamate Striatran. Tranquilizer.

ایمائل کامیٹ : سٹر یا ٹران ۔ سکون بخش دوا ۔

Enamel *(e-nam'-el).* The hard external covering of the crown of a tooth.

مینا : دانت کے کراؤن کا سخت بیرونی غلاف ۔

Encapsulation *(en-kap-su-la'-shun)* [G. *en,* in; capsula, small box]. Enclosure within a capsule.

کیسہ بندی : کیپسول کے اندر ہی خانہ ۔

Encephalitis *(en-kef-a-li'-tis)* [G. *egkephalos,* brain; itis, inflammation]. Inflammation of the brain.

ورم دماغ : دماغ کی سوزش ۔ وائرس کی بیماری ۔

Encephalocele *(en-kef'-al-o-sel)* [G. *egkaphalos,* brain; *kele* , hernial]. Protrusion of brain substance through the skull. Often associated with hydrocephalus when the protrusion occurs at a suture line.

فتق دماغ : کھوپڑی میں دماغی مادے کا باہر نکل آنا ۔

Encephalogram *(en-kef'-al-o-gram)* [G. *egkephalos,* brain; *gramma,* letter]. See PNEUMOENCEP-HALOGRAPHY.

انکفالوگرام ۔ تصویر دماغ : دیکھئے نیوموانکفالوگرافی ۔

Encephalography *(en-kef-al-og'-ra-fi)* [G. *egkephalos,* brain; *graphein,* to write]. See PNEUMOENCEPHALOGRAPHY.

انکفالوگرافی ۔ دماغ نگاری : دیکھئے نیوموانکفالوگرافی ۔

Encephaloma *(en-kef-al-o'-ma)* [G. *egkephalos,* brain; *oma,* tumour]. A tumour of the brain--encephalomata, pl.

دماغی پھوڑا : دماغ کا ایک ناسور ۔

Encephalomalacia *(en-kef'-al-o-mal-as-i-a)* [G. *egkephalos,* brain; *malakia,* softness]. Softening of the brain.

لینت دماغ : دماغ کا نرم ہونا ۔

Encephalomyelitis *(en-kef'-al-o-mi-e-li'-tis)* [G. *egkephalos,* brain; *myelos,* marrow; *itis,* inflammation]. Inflammation of the brain and spinal cord.

دماغی نخاعی التہاب : دماغ اور شوکی ڈورا کی سوزش ۔

Encephalomyelopathy *(en-kef-al-o-mi-el-op'-ath-i)* [G. *egkephalos,* brain; *myelos* marrow; *pathos,* disease]. Disease affecting both brain and spinal cord--encephalomyelopathic, adj.

مرض دماغ و نخاع : دماغ اور شوکی ڈورا دونوں کو متاثر کرنے والا مرض ۔

Encephalon *(en-kef'-a-lon)* [G. *egkephalos*] The brain.

Encephalopathy *(en-kef-al-op'-a-thi)* [G. *egkephalos,* brain; *pathos,* disease]. Any disease of the brain--encephalopathic, adj.

مرض دماغی : دماغ کا کوئی مرض ۔

Enchondroma *(en-kon-dro'-ma)* [G. *en,* in *chondros,* cartilage; *oma,* tumour]. A cartilaginous tumour--enchondromata, pl.

غضروفی سلعہ : کارٹیلج والا ناسور ۔

Encopresis *(en-ko-pre'-sis)* [G. *en,* in; *kopros* dung]. Involuntary passage of faces-encopretic, adj. n.

این کوپ ریسس : فضلے کا غیر ارادی گذر ۔

Endamoeba *(en-da-me'-ba)* [G. *endon,* within *amoibe,* change]. Syn., Entamoeba.

اینڈ امیبا : پروٹوزوا کے طفیلیوں کا ایک جنس ۔

Endarterectomy *(end-art-e-rek'-to-mi)* [G. *endon,* within, *arteria,* artery; *ektome* excision]. Surgical removal of an atheromatous core from an artery. Disobliteration or 'rebore.' **gas e.,** or carbo-dissection, the use of carbon dioxide gas to separate the occlusive core

Endarterectom

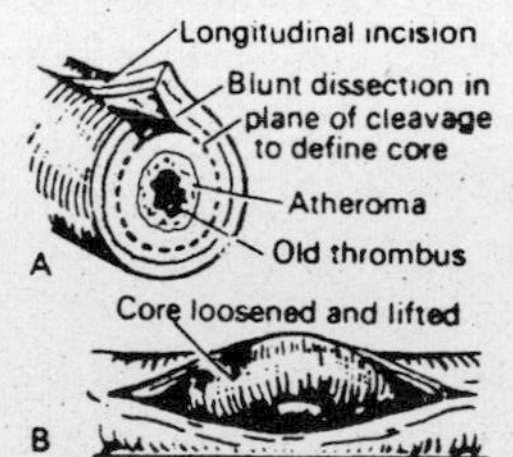

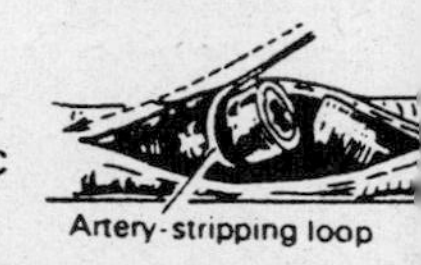

اینڈ آرٹی ریکٹومی : شریان کا اپریشن۔

Endarteritis *(end-art-e-ri'-tis)* [G. *endon,* within; *arteria,* artery; *-itis,* inflammation]. Inflammation of the intima or lining coat of an artery. **e, obliterans,** the new intimal connective tissue obliterates the lumen.

ورم درشریان : شریان کی پرت سوزش۔

Endaural *(end-awr'-al)* [G. endon, within; L. auris, ear]. Pertaining to the inner portion of the external auditory canal.

اینڈ آرل : بیرونی سمعی قنال کے اندرونی حصے سے متعلق۔

Endemic *(en-dem-ik).* [G. endemos, dwelling in a place].Recurring in a locality, (Cf. epidemic).

مقامی : کسی خاص جگہ کے ساتھ مخصوص۔

Endemiology *(en-dem-i-ol'-o-ji)* [G. endemos, dwelling in a place; logos, discourse]. The special study of endemic diseases.

مقامی امراضیات : انڈیمک امراض کا مخصوص مطالعہ۔

Endocarditis *(en-do-,kar-di-tis).* [G. endon, within; kardia, heart; -itis, inflamation]. Inflammation of the inner lining of the heart (endocardium) most commonly due to rheumatic fever. **valvular e.,** when one or more heart valves are affected. See SUBACUTE.

ورم درون قلب : دل کی اندرونی پرت کی سوزش۔

Endocardium *(en-do-kar'-di-um)* [G. endon, within; kardia, heart]. The lining membrane of the heart, which covers the valves.

درون قلب : دل کی اندرونی جھلی جو ویلوؤں کو ڈھکتی ہے۔

Endocervical *(en-do-ser-vi'-kal)* [G. endon, within; L. cervix, neck]. Pertaining to the inside of the cervix uteri.

دروں عنقی التہاب : سروکس یوٹری کی اندرونی میوکس جھلی کی سوزش۔

Endocrine *(en'-do-krin)* [G. endon, within; krinein, to separate]. Secreting internally, **e. glands,** the ductless glands of the body; those which make an internal secretion or hormone which passes into the blood stream and has an important influence on general metabolic processes; e.g. the pineal, pituitary, thyroid, parathyrods, thymus, adrenals, overaies, testes and pancreas. The last- mentioned has both an internal and external secretion. Opp, to exocrine--endocrinal, adj.

درون افرازی : اندرونی طور پر رطوبت کا اخراج۔ اینڈوکرائن گلینڈ بلا نالی گلینڈ میں۔ مثلاً تھائیرائڈ' لبلبہ' پھیپھڑے' بیضہ دان وغیرہ۔

Endocrinology *(en-do-krin-ol'-o-ji)* [G. endon, within; krinein, to separate; logos, discourse]. The study of the ductless glands and their internal secretions.

درافرازیات : بلانالی گلینڈز اور ان کی اندرونی رطوبتوں کا مطالعہ۔

Endocrinopathy *(en-do-krin-op-ath-i)* [G. endon, within; krinein, to separate; pathos, disease]. Abnormality of one or more of the endocrine glands or their secretions.

بے نالی غدہ کے فعل میں خرابی سے مرض : بلانالی گلینڈز یا ان کی رطوبتوں میں سے کسی کا نارمل نہ ہونا یعنی ان کا مرض۔

Endogenous *(en-doj'-en-us)* [G. endon, within; genesthai, to be produced]. Originating within the organism. Opp. to ectogenous.

درون لمف : اندرونی کان کی جھلی دار لیبی رنتھ میں سیال

Endolymphatic shun *(en-do-lim-fat'-ik).* Drainage of excess endolymph from the semicircular canals to the subarachnoid space where it flows to join the cerebrospinal fluid. Performed for patients with Meniere's disease.

اینڈولائی سن : مادہ جو اندر پہنچنے والے جراثیم کو تباہی سے ہمکنار کرتا ہے۔

Endolysin *(en-do-li'-sin)* [G. endon, within; lysis, a lossening]. An intracellural, leucocytic substance which destroys engulfed bacteria.

درون رحمی سلعہ : ایک ناسور۔

Endometrioma *(en-do-me-tri-o'-ma).* [G. endon, within; metra, womb; -oma tumour]. A tumour of misplaced endometrium. Adenomyoma (q.v.). See CYST (chocolate)--endometriomata, pl.

درون رحمیت : غیر معمولی جگہوں پر اینڈومیٹریم کی موجودگی۔

Endometriosis *(en-do-met-ri-os'-is)* [G. endon, within; metra, womb; -osis, condition]. The presence of endometrium in abnormal sites.

See CYST (chocolate).

ورم درون رحم : اینڈومیٹریم کی سوزش۔

Endometritis *(en-do-me-tri'-tis).* [G. endon, within; metra, womb; -itis, inflammation]. Inflammation of the endometrium.

اینڈومیٹریم۔ درون رحمہ : یوٹرس کے اندرونی موکوسا۔ اگر حمل نہ ٹھہرے تو رحم کی تہہ ٹوٹ پھوٹ جاتی ہے۔ اس تہہ کو اینڈ میٹریم کہا جاتا ہے۔ اس صورت میں رحم سے خون جاری ہو جاتا ہے اور وہ بیضہ جو زرخیز یا بارودنہیں ہو پاتا اسی کون میں بہ جاتا ہے۔ اس میں چار پانچ روز صرف ہوتے ہیں۔ اسے انحطاطی حالت کہا جاتا ہے۔

Endometrium *(en-do-met'-ri-um)* [G. endon, within; metra, womb]. The lining mucosa of the uterus--endometrial, adj.

Endumyocardium *(en-do-mi-o-kar'-di-um)* [G. endon, within; mys, muscle; kardia, heart]. Relating to the endocardum and myocardium--endomyocardial, adj.

اینڈو مایو کارڈیم : اینڈوکاردیم اور مایو کارڈیم سے متعلق۔

Endoneurium *(en-do-nu'-ri-um)* [G. endon within; neuron, nerve]. The delicate, inner connective tissue surrounding the nerve fibres.

درون عصبہ : عصبی ریشوں کے گرد نرم اندرونی رابطی بافت۔

Endoparasite *(en'-do-par'-a-sit)* [G. endon, within; parasitos, parasite]. Any parasite living within its host--endo-parasitic, adj

درون طفیلی : میزبان کے اندر رہنے والا طفیلی۔

Endophlebitis *(en-do-fle-bi'-tis).* [G. endon, within; phleps, vein; -itis, inflammation]. Inflammation of internal lining of vein. Can occur after prolonged intravenous infusion.

درون وریدی ورم : ورید کی اندرونی پرت کی سوزش۔

Endophthalmitis *(en-dof-thal-mi'-tis).* [G. endon, within; ophthalmos, eye, -itis, inflammation]. Internal infection of eye globe, usually as a result of a perforting injury.

ورم درون چشم : آنکھ کے گولے کی اندرونی سوزش۔

Endoscope *(en'-do-skop).* [G. endon, within; skopein, to examine]. An instrument for visualization of body cavities or organs. If of the fibre-optic variety, light is transmitted by means of very fine glass fibres along a flexible tube. It can permit examinatic photography and biopsy of the cavities organs of a relaxed conscious person. S PHOTOENDOSCOPE--endoscopic *aa* endoscopy, *n.*

ن بین : جسمانی کھفوں یا اعضاء کو دیکھنے کا آلہ۔

Endospore *(en'-do-spor)* [G. endon, withi sporos, seed]. A bacterial spore which has purely vegetative function. It is formed by t loss of water and probable rearrangement the protein of the cell, so that metabolism minimal and resistance to environment conditions, especially high temperatur desiccation and antibacterial drugs, high. T only genera which includes pathogen species that form spores are Bacillus a Clostridium.

ون بذرہ : جراثیمی بذرہ۔ اس میں قوت مدافعت زیادہ ہوتی ۔ زیادہ درجہ حرارت کو برداشت کرتا ہے۔

Endothelioid*(en-do-the'-li-oid)* [G. endo within; thele, nipple; eidos, form]. Rese bling endothelium.

ڈوتھیلی انڈ : اینڈوتھیلیم سے مشابہہ۔

Endothelioma *(en-do-the-li-o'-ma)* [G. endo within; thele, nipple, -oma tumour]. A mali nant tumour derived from endothelial cells.

لمی سلعہ : ایک ناسور۔

Endothelium *(en-do-the'-li-um)* [G. endo within; thele, nipple]. The lining membrane serous cavities, heart, blood and lymph ves els-- endothelial, adj.

ڈوتھیلیم۔ درحلمہ : سیرس کھفوں، دل، لمفی اور خونی رگوں کی رونی جھلی۔

Endotoxin *(en-do-toks'-in)* [G. endon, withi toxikon, poison]. A toxic product of bacter which is associated with the structure of t cell, and can only be obtained by destructi of the cell-endotoxic, adj. Opp. to exotoxin.

م داخلی : خلیے کی تباہی سے حاصل ہونے والا جراثیم کا زہریلا ۔

Endotracheal *()en-do-trak-e'-al)* [G. endo within; trachus, rough]. Wtihin the trachea.

اینڈوٹریکیل : ٹریکیا کے اندر۔

ıdoxana *(en-doks-an'-a)* Cyclophos. phamide (q.v.).

اینڈآکسانا : دیکھئے سائیکلو فاسفامائیڈ۔

ıduron *(en'-dur-on)*. Methyclothiazide. See CHLOROTHIAZIDE.

ıduronyl *(en-dur'-on-il)*. Methyclo- thiazide. See CHOROTHIAZIDE.

ıema *(en'-e-ma)* [G. injection]. The injection of a liquid into the rectum, to be returned or retained. It can be further designated according to the function of the fluid--A small bowel enema can be given after duodenal intubation (q.v.). Followed by radiography of the small and, if necessary, the large bowel--enemas, enemata, pl.

Technique of giving enema

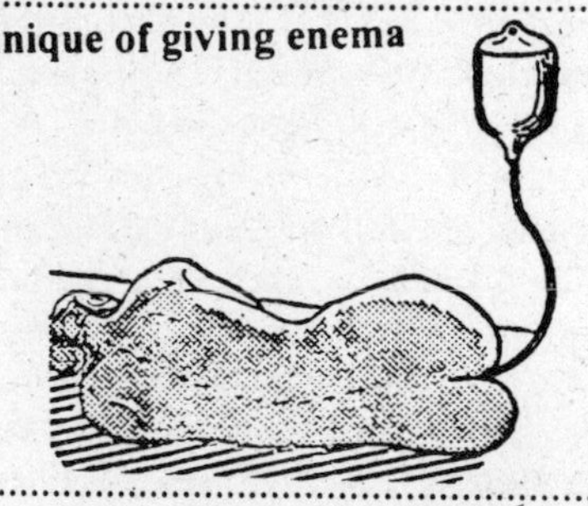

انیما۔ حقنہ : ریکٹم کی مائع داخل کرنا۔ پچکاری کے ذریعے مقعد میں داخل کرنا۔ عموماً رفع حاجت کے لئے کیا جاتا ہے۔

ıglate *(eng'-lat)*. Theophlline sodium glycinate. See THEOPHYLLINE.

اینگیٹ : دیکھئے تھیوفلین۔ بچوں کے لئے چائے والا۔ چھوٹا ایک چمچہ صبح دوپہر شام، دمہ، نمونیا اور برونکائی ٹس میں سانس کی رکاوٹ کے لئے مستعمل۔

ıophthalmos *(en-of-thal'-mos)* [G. enin; opthalmos, eye]. A bony growth within the medulary canal of a bone. See EXOSTOSIS.

درتعظم : ہڈی کی میڈلری کینال میں استخوانی اگاؤ۔

ıpac *(en'-pak)*. Antidiarrhoeal.

اینپیک : دافع اسہال۔

ısiform *(en'-si-form)*[L. ensis, sword; forma, shape]. Sword shaped; xiphoid.

سیفی۔ خنجری : تلوار کی طرح۔

Entamoeba *(en-ta-me'-ba)*. A genus of protozoon parasites, three species infesting man; Entamoeba coli, non-pathogenic, infesting intestinal tract; E. gingivalis non-pathogenic, infesting mouth; E. hystolyica, pathogenic causing amoebic dysentery (q.v.). Syn., Endamoeba (q.v.).

درون امیبا : دیکھئے اینڈ امیبا۔

Enteral *(en'-ter-al)* [G. enteron, intestine]. Within gastrointestinal tract.

معائی : معدی آنت کے راستے کے اندر۔

Enteric *(en-ter'-ik)* [G. enteron, intestine]. Pertaining to the intestine, **e. fever** includes typhoid and paratyphoid fever (q.v.).

معائی : آنت سے متعلق۔

Enteritis *(en-te-ri'-tis)* [G. *enteron,* intestine, *-itis,* inflammation]. Inflammation of the intestines. **regional e.,** currently preferred term to Crohn's disease (q.v.).

ورم امعا : آنتوں کی سوزش۔ آنتوں کی سوجن۔

Entero-anastomosis *(en'-te-ro-an-as-to-m-o'-sis)* [G. enteron, intestine; anastomosis, opening]. Intestinal anastomosis.

معائی تفویہ : آنت کا سوراخ۔

Enterobiasis *(en-ter-o-bi'-as-is)*. Infestation with threadworms.

Enterobius vermicularis *(en-ter-o'-bi-us-v-er-mik- u-lar'-is)* [G. enteron, intestine; bios, life; L. vemiculus, little worm]. A nematode which infests the small and large intestine. Threadworm. Because of autoinfective life-cycle, treatment aims at complete elimination. Each member of household given three single does treatments at weekly intervals of either piperazine citrate, 75 mg per kg, or viprymium embonate (Vanquin) 5 mg per kg. Latter gives red stools. Hygiene measures necessary to prevent, re-infestation during treatment.

معاباش : ایک نیا ٹوڈ جو چھوٹی اور بڑی آنت کو متاثر کرتا ہے۔ جرنے یا چبونے۔

Enterocele *(en'-ter-o-sel)* [G. enteron, intestine; kele, tumour]. Prolapse of intestine. Can be into the upper third of vagina.

فتق آمعا : آنت کا ناسور۔ فیجائنا میں بالائی تہائی میں ہو سکتا ہے۔

Enterocylsis *(en-te-ro-kli'-sis)* [G. enteron, intestine; klysis, a drenching]. The introduction of fluid into the rectum. Syn., proctoclysis.

اشراب معوی۔ حقنہ کرنا : ریکٹم میں سیال کا دخول۔

Enterococcus *(en-te-ro-koks-us)* [G. enteron, intestine; kokkos, seed. A Gram-positive coccus which occurs in short chains and is relatively resistant to heat. Enterococci being to Lancefield's group D, and occur as commensals in human and warm-blooded animal intestines, and sometimes as pathogens in infections of the urinary tract, ear and wounds and, more rarely, in endocarditis.

معائی بنقہ : گرام مثبت کاکس جو چھوٹی زنجیروں کی شکل میں ہوتا ہے اور حرارت سے متاثر نہیں ہوتا۔ آنت میں پایا جاتا ہے۔

Enterocolitis *(en-ter-o-kol-i-tis).* [G. enteron, intestine; kolon, colon; -itis, inflammation]. Inflammation of the small intestine and colon.

معائی انزیم : آنت کے رس میں پایا جانے والا خامرہ۔ یہ غیر عامل ٹرپسینوجن کو عامل ٹرپسن میں تبدیل کرتا ہے۔

Enterolith *(en'-te-ro-lith)* [G. enteron, intestine; lithos, stone]. An intestinal concretion.

سنگ معا : آنت کی پتھری۔

Enterolithiasis *(en-te-ro-lith-i'-a-sis)* [G. enteron, intestine; lithos, stone; N.L -iasis, condition]. The presence of intestinal concretions.

حصاتیت امعا : آنت میں پتھریوں کی موجودگی۔

Enteron *(en'-te-ron)* [G. intestine]. The gut.

معا : آنت۔ قنات ہاضمہ۔

Enterostomy *(en-te-ros'-to-mi)* [G. enteron, intestine; stoma, mouth]. A surgically established fistula between the small intestine and some other surface, **gastro-e.,** a fistula between stomach and jejunum, sometimes made in treatment of doudenal ulcer. See DOUDENOSTOMY, ILEOSTOMY, JEJUNOSTOMY--enterostomal, adj.

عائی تفویہ : چھوٹی آنت اور کسی دوسرے سطح کے درمیان اپریشن کے ذریعے قائم کردہ فسٹولا۔

Enterotomy *(en-te-rot'-o-mi)* [TG. enteron intestine; tome, a cutting]. An incision int the small intestine.

معائی تفویہ : چھوٹی آنت میں شگاف۔ چھوٹی آنت میں عمل جراحی کے ذریعہ ردوبدل کرنے کا عمل۔

Enterotribe *(en'-te-ro-trib)* [G. enteron intestine; tribein, to crush]. A metal clam which causes necrosis of the epur of th double-barrelled colostomy, as a preliminar to its closure.

ینٹیر وٹرائیپ : دھات کا بنوا ہوا شکنجہ۔

Entero-vioform *(en-te-ro-vi'-o-form)* A antidiarrhoeal which was promoted fo traveller diarrhoea but is now restricted due t its association with SMON, a disease whic occurs particularly in Japan.

نٹراوایوفارم : اسہال یا دستوں کو بند کرنے والی دوا۔

Enteroviruses *(en'-te-ro-vi'-rus-es)* [G. enteron intestine; L. virus, poison]. Enter the body b the alimentary tract. Comprise the polio myelitis, Coxsackie and ECHO groups o viruses. They tend to invade the centra nervous system. Enteroviruses, together wit rhinoviruses, are now to be called picorna viruses.

نٹرو وائرسیس : جسم میں انتوں کے راستے داخل ہونے والے ائرس وہ مرکزی عصبی نظام پر حملہ آور ہوتے ہیں۔

Enteroviruse

Enteroviruses
Poliovirus (3 types)
Coxsackie virus
Echovirus (30 types)
Group A (23 types)
Group B (6 types)

Enteroviruses

Enerozoa *(en-te-ro-zo'-a)* [G. enteron, intestine zoion, living being]. Any animal parasite infesting the intestines--enterozoon, sing.

عائی حونیات : آنتوں میں رہنے والے حیوانی طفیلی۔

Entonox *(en'-to-noks).* Inhalant analgesic Mixture of 50 percent nitrous oxide and 5 per-cent oxygen.

انٹانا کس : پچاس فیصد نائٹرس آکسائیڈ اور پچاس فیصد آکسیجن کا آمیزہ

Entropion *(en-tro'-pi-on)* [G. en, in; tre-pein, to turn]. Inversion of an eyelid so that the lashes are in contact with the globe of the eye.

شترہٴ داخلی : آنکھ کے پپوٹے کا الٹنا۔ اس طرح پلکیں آنکھ کے گولے کو اس کے خانے سے نکالنا۔

Entropion

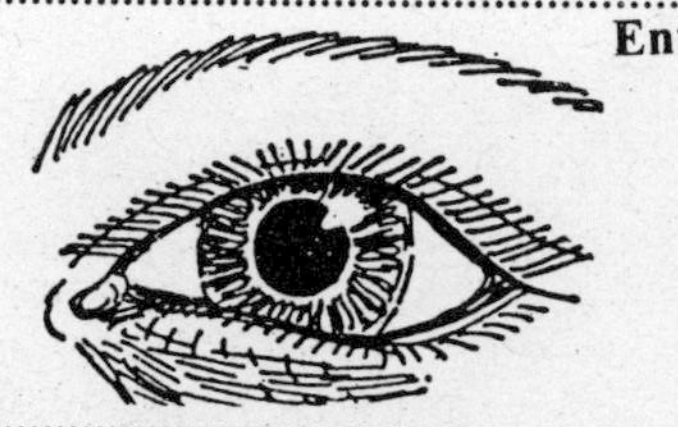

Enucleation *(e-nu-kle-a'-shun)* [L. e, out of; nucleus, kernel]. The removal of an organ or tumour in its entirety, as of an eyeball from its socket.

انقاف : کسی ناسور یا عضو کو اپنی جگہ سے نکالنا۔ مثلاً انکھ کے گولے کو اس کے خانے سے نکالنا۔

Enuresis *(en-u-re'-sis)*. [G. enourein, to make water in]. Incontinence of urine, especially bed-wetting.

بول بستری : پیشاب میں ضعف ضبط ہوتا ہے۔ خصوصاً بستر پر پیشاب نکل جانا۔

Envacar *(en'-va-kar)* Guanoxan sulphate (q.v.).

اینویکیر : گوانکسان سلفیٹ۔

Environment *(en-vi'-ron-ment)* [F. environ, about]. External surroundings. Environmental factors are conditions influencing an individual from without.

ماحول : باہر سے اثر انداز ہونے والے عوامل۔

Enzyme *(en'-zim)* [G. en, in; zyme, leaven]. Soluble colloidal protein produced by living cells. See CATALYST.

خامرہ : یہ پروٹینی ہوتے ہیں۔ کیمیائی تعاملات کی رفتار تیز کرتے ہیں۔ ان کی قلیل مقدار کافی رہتی ہے۔ یہ بذات خود تبدیل نہیں ہوتے لیکن دوسری اشیاء میں تبدیلی پیدا کرتے ہیں۔ اگر انہیں ۱۰۰ درجے سنٹی گریڈ تک گرم کیا جائے تو بیکار ہو جاتے ہیں۔ محرک کار۔ کیمیائی خمیر۔

Enzymology *(en'-zim-ol'-oj-i)* [G. en, in; zyme, leaven; logos, discourse]. The science dealing with the structure and function of enzymes--enzymological, adj.; enzymologically, adv.

علم خامرات : خامرات کی ساخت اور فعل سے متعلق سائنس۔

Eosin *(e'-o-sin)* [G. eos, dawn]. A red staining agent used in histology and laboratory diagnostic procedures.

ایوسین : ایک سرخ رنگنے والا عامل جو نسیجیات اور تجربہ گاہی تشخیصی طریقوں میں استعمال کیا جاتا ہے۔

Eosinophil *(e-o-sin'-o-fil)* [G. eos, dawn; philein, to love]. 1. Cells having an affinity for eosin. 2. A type of polymorphonuclear leucocyte containing eosinstaining granules--eosinophilic, adj.

ایوسینوفل : (۱) ایوسین کے لئے کشش رکھنے والے خلیے۔ (۲) سفید خونی خلیے کی قسم۔ خون میں ۲ فیصد۔

Eosinophilia *(e-o-sin-o-fil'-i-a)* [G. cos, dawn; philein, to lve]. Increased eosinophils in the blood.

ایوسین افزونی : خون میں ایوسینوفلز کی بڑھتی ہوئی مقدار۔

Epanutin *(ep-a-nu'-tin)*. Phenytoin (q.v.).

Ependymoma *(ep-end-im-o'-ma)* [G. ependyma, an upper garment; -oma, tumour]. Neoplasm arising in the lining of the cerebral ventricles or central canal of spinal cord. Occurs in all age groups.

گبر غلفی سلعہ : نخاعی ڈوری کی مرکزی قنال یا سربرل وینٹریکلز کی دیواروں سے ابھرنے والا نیوپلازم۔

Ephedrine *(ef-ed-rin)*. Widely used in asthma and bronchial spasm for its relaxant action on bronchioles, raises blood pressure by peripheral vasoconstriction. Useful in hay fever.

ایفیڈرین : دمہ میں مستعمل عام دوا۔ اس سے بلڈ پریشر زیادہ ہوتا ہے۔ فیور میں مفید۔ سفید رنگ کی گولیاں جو دمہ اور تنفسی امراض میں استعمال کی جاتی ہیں۔ مفید برائے شدید عضلاتی کمزوری، ہیٹ سٹروک، باسٹو پر یا مدہوشی شاک۔

Ephelides *(e-fe'-lids)* [G. ephelis]. Freckless--ephelis, sing.

ایلفیلائیڈز : فریکلز۔ چہرے پر داغ دھبے عموماً خواتین کے چہرے

پر نکل آتے ہیں۔

Epicanthus *(ep-i-kan'-tus)* [G. epi, on; kanthos, corner of the eye]. The congenital occurence of a fold of skin obscurring the inner canthus of the eye--epicanthal, adj.

برماق: آنکھ کے اندرونی کونے میں جلدی تہہ۔

Epicardium *(ep-i-kar-di-um)* [G. epi, on; kardia, heart]. The visceral layer of the pericardium--epicardial, adj

برقلب : پیری کارڈیم کی دسرل تہہ۔

Epicritic *(ep-i-krit'-ik)* [G. epi, on; krin- ein, to separate]. The term applied to the finer sensations of heat, touch, etc. As opposed to protopathic (q.v.).

سریع الحس : ایک اصطلاح جس کا اطلاق حرارت، چھونے وغیرہ کی حس پر ہوتا ہے۔

Epidemic *(ep-i-dem'-ik)* [G. epi, on; demos, people]. Simultaneously affecting many people in an area. (Cf. endemic).

وبا : کسی علاقے میں جمہوریہ بیک وقت اثر انداز ہوتا۔ آبادی کے بیشتر افراد کو متاثر کرنے والا مرض۔

Epidemiology *(ep-i-dem'-i-ol'-o-ji)* [G. epi, on; demos, people; logos, discourse]. The scientific study of the distribution of disease--epidemiological, adj.; epidemiologically, adv.

وبائیات : امراض کی تقسیم کا سائنسی مطالعہ۔

Epidermis *(ep-i-der'-mis)* [G. epi, on; derma, skin]. The external non-vascular layer of the skin; the cuticle. Also known as the 'scarf-skin--epidermal, adj.

اپی ڈرمس : جلد کا بیرونی غیروعائی پرت۔ کیوٹیکل۔

Epidermophyton *(ep-i-der-mo'-fi-ton)* [G. epi, on; derma, skin; phyton, plant]. A genus of fungi which affects the skin and nails.

اپی ڈرموفائٹن : سمارغ کا ایک جنس جو جلد اور ناخنوں پر اثر انداز ہوتا ہے۔

Epidermophytosis *(ep-i-der-mo-fi-to'-sis)* [G. epi, on; d3erma, skin; phyton, plant; -osis, condition]. Infection with fungi of the genus epidermophyton.

برادی فطریت : سماروغ کے جنس اپی ڈرموفائٹن کے ساتھ مرض۔

Epididymis *(ep-i-did-i-mek'-to-mi)* [G. epi, on; didumoi twins, ektome, excision]. Surgical removal of the epididymis.

برنج براری : اپیڈ ایڈائمس کو اپریشن کے ذریعے ختم کرنا۔

Epididymis *(ep-i-did-i-mis)* [G. epi, on; didumoi, twins]. A small oblong body attached to the posterior surface of the testes. It consists of the tubules which convey the spermatozoa from the testes to the vas diferens.

برنج : خصیوں کی خلفی سطح سے ملحق جسم۔ یہ ٹیوبولز پر مشتمل ہے۔ شکل میں مستطیل کا۔

Epididymitis *(ep-i-did-i-mi'-tis)* [G. *epididymis; -itis,* inflammation]. Inflammation of the epididymis (q.v.).

ورم برنج : ایپڈیڈائمس کی سوزش۔

Eipdidymo-orchitis *(ep-i-did'-i-mo-o-r-ki'-tis)* [G. *epididymis;* orchis, testis; *-itis,* inflammation]. Inflammation of the epididymis and the testis.

التہاب برنج وخصیہ : خصیے اور ایپڈ ایڈائمس کی سوزش۔

Epidural *(ep-i-dur'-al)* [G. epi, on; L. durus, hard]. Upon external to the dura, **e. block,** injection of local anaesthetic, usually in the lumbar or caudal region prior to rectal examination and surgery, a forceps delivery or Caesarean section. Currently used for crush injuries to chest: the analgesia can be maintained for a week or more.

برجانی : ڈیورا کے اوپر یا بیرونی۔

Epidurography *(ep-i-dur-og'-ra-fi)* [G. epi, on; L. durus, hard; G. graphein, to write]. Radiographs taken after epidual injection of contrast medium.

اپی ڈیوروگرافی : تضاد واسطے کے اپی ڈرمس انجکشن کے بعد لئے گئے ریڈیوگرافس۔

Epigastrium *(ep-i-gas'-tri-um)* [G. epi, on; gaster, stomach]. The abdominal region lying directly over the stomach--epigastric, adj.

برمعدہ : معدہ کے اوپر براہ راست بطنی حصہ۔

Epiglottis *(ep-i-glot'-is)* [G. epi, on; glottis]. The thin leaf-shaped flap of cartilarge behind the tongue which, during the act of swallowing, covers the opening leading into the larynx.

برمزمار : زبان کی پیچھے کا لیتھ کا پتلا پتے نما فلیپ جو نگلنے کی دوران لیرنکس کی طرف جانے والے سوراخ وک ڈھکتا ہے۔

Epiglottitis *(ep-i-glot-i'-tis)* [G. epi, on; glottis; -itis, inflammation]. Inflammation of the epiglottis.

التہاب ملکی : اپی گلاٹس کی سوزش۔

Epilation *(ep-il-a'-shun)* [L. e, out; pilus, hair]. Extraction or destruction of hair roots, e.g. by coagulation necrosis, electrolysis or forceps--epilate, v.t.

تعلیع : بالوں کی جڑوں کی تباہی۔

Epilatory *(ep-il'-a-tor-i)* [L. e, out; pilus, hair]. An agent which produces epilation.

بال صفا (دوا) : بالوں کی جڑوں کو تباہ کرنے والا عامل۔

Epilepsy *(ep-i-lep'-si)* [G. epilepsis, seizure]. Correctly called the epilepsies. Result from disordered electrical activity of brain. The 'fit' is caused by an abnormal electrical discharge that disturbs cerebration and usually results in loss of consciousness. **major e.** (grandmal), loss of consciousness with generalized convulsions. When p[atient does not regain consciousness between attacks the term status epilepticus is used; **focal e. (Jacksonian),** motor seizure begins in one part of body, can spread to other muscle groups so that the fit is similar to clonic stage of major epilepsy. Fits can be sensory, i.e. abnormal feeling in one part, which spread to other parts. **psychomotor e., temporal lobe e., limbic disorder,** 'psychic' warning of fit consists of feelings of unreality, deja-vu, auditory, visual gustatory or olfactory hallucinations. Jerking not as severe as in major epilepsy. **minor e.** (petit mal), characterized by transitory interruption of consciousness without convulsions. Chararacteristic spike and wave pattern on EEG. Any seizure not conforming to this definition is not petit mal. The term is widely misused. All except petit mal can be symptomatic or idiopathic, but focal and temporal lobe epilepsy carry a higher incidence of symptomatic causes. Petit mal is always idiopathic. See AKINETIC--epileptic, adj.

مرگی۔ صرع : دماغ کی غیر منظم برقی عاملیت کا نتیجہ۔

Epileptic *(ep-i-lep'-tik)*. Pertaining to epilepsy. **e. aura,** premonitory subjective phenomena (tingling in the hand or visual or auditory sensation) which precede an attack of grand mal. **e. cry,** the croak or shout heard from the epileptic person as the falls unconscious.

صرعی : صرع کے متعلق۔

Epileptogenic *(ep-il-ep-to-jen'-ik)* [G. epilepsis, szizure; genesis, production]. Agent capable of causing epilepsy.

صرع آور صرع انگیز : ایسا عامل جو مرگی پیدا کرنی کا اہل ہو۔

Epileptiform *(ep-i-lep'-ti-form)*. Resembling epilepsy.

مرگی یا سرع نما : مرگی سے مشابہ۔

Epiloia *(ep'-il-oi-a)*. An inherited abnormality of brain tissue, resulting in mental defect. May be associated with epilepsy. Also known as 'tuberose sclerosis'.

صرعیت : دماغی بیج میں خلل جو توراث میں چلتا ہے اس سے ذہنی نقص پیدا ہوتا ہے۔

Epimenorrhoea *(ep-i-men-or-re'-a)* [G. epi, on; men, month; rheein, to flow]. Reduction of the length of the menstrual cycle.

تعدد طمث : حیض کے سائیکل کی طوالت میں تخفیف

Epinephrine *(ep-i-nef'-rin)*. Adrenaline (q.v.).

برگردی مادہ : ایڈرینالین

Epiphora *(e-pif'-o-ra)* [G. epi, on; pherein, to carry]. Pathological overflow of tears on to the cheek.

ڈھلکا : آنسوؤں کا رخساروں پر بہنا۔

Epiphysis *(e-pif'-i-sis)* [G.epi, on; phyein, to grow]. The growing part of a bone, especially long bones., Separated from the main shaft (diaphysis) by a plate of cartilage (epiphyseal plate) which disappears due to ossification when growth ceases, **slipped e.,** displacement of an epiphysis, especially the upper femoral--epiphyses, pl.; epiphyseal, adj.

برنامیہ : کسی ہڈی، خصوصاً طویل ہڈیوں کا بڑھنے والا حصہ۔

Epiphysis

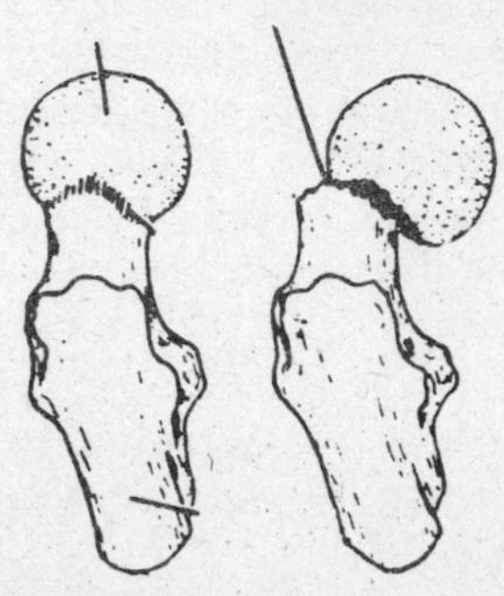

Epiphysitis *(e-pif-i-si'-tis)* [G. epi, on; phyein, to grow; -itis, inflammation]. Inflammation of an epiphysis.

ورم برنامیہ : اپی فائسس کی سوزش۔

Epiploon *(ep-i-plo'-on)* [G.]. The grea tomentum (q.v.)--epiploic, adj.

ثرب : بڑا اومینٹم۔

Episclera *(ep-i-skle'-ra)* [G. epi, on; skleros, hard]. Loose connective tissue between the sclera and conjunctiva--episcleral, adj.

برصلبیہ : سکلیرا اور کنجیکٹوا کے درمیان پایا جانے والا ڈھیلا اتصالی نسیج۔

Episcleritis *(ep-i-skle-ri'-tis)*. Inflammation of hte episclera.

التہاب برصلبیہ : اپیس کلیرا کی سوزش۔ آنکھ کے سفید پردے کی بافت کی سوج۔

Episiorrhaphy *(e-pes-i-or'-raf-i)* [G. epision, public region; raphe, a suture]. Surgical repair of a lacerated perineum.

Episiotomy *(e-pes-i-ot'-o-mi)* [G. epision, public region; tome a cutting]. A perineal incision made during the birth of a child when the vaginal orifice does not stretch sufficiently.

فرج شگافی : بچے کی پیدائش کے وقت جگہ کھلی نہ ہو تو ویجائنا کے شگاف میں چیر دیا جاتا ہے تاکہ بچے کی پیدائش کے لئے جگہ کھل جائے۔ گھر پر پیدائش میں یہ عمل مڈوائف قینچی سے بھی کر سکتی ہے اس

ے بعد سلائی کر دی جاتی ہے۔

Epispadias *(ep-i-spa' di'as)* [G. epi, on; spaei to draw]. A congenital opening of the urethr on the anterior (upper side) of the penis. (C hypospadias).

ق مبالیت : عضو تناسل کی بالائی جانب یورتھرا کا سوراخ۔

Epispastic *(ep-i-spas'-tik)* [G. epi, on; spaein, draw].A blistering agent.

بلہ ریز : آبلہ ڈالنے والا عامل۔

Epistaxis *(ep-i-staks'-is)* [G. epi, on; stazein, drip]. Bleeding from the nose--epistaxes, pl.

سیر : ناک سے خون کا بہنا۔

Epithelioma *(ep-i-thel-i-o'-ma)* [G. *epi,* o *thele,* nipple; *-oma,* tumour]. A maligna growth arising in epithelial tissue, usually th skin; a squamous cell carcinoma.

رطان لب : اپی تھیلیل بافت خصوصاً جلد میں ابھار۔

Epithelialization *(ep-i-the-li-al-i-za'-shun)*. Th growth of epithelium over a raw area; th final stage of healing.

وئے اپی تھیلیم یا برحلہ : خام ایریا پر اپی تھیلیم کا اگنا یا ھنا۔ صحت مند ہونے کا آخری مرحلہ۔

Epithelium *(ep-i-thel'-i-um)* [G. epi, on; thel nipple]. The surface layer of cells coverir cutaneous. mucous and serous surfaces. It classified according to the arrangement ar shape of the cells it contains--epithelial, adj.

لمہ : خلیوں کی سطحی تہہ۔

Epodyl *(ep'-o-dil)*. Ethoglucid (q.v.).

Epontol *(ep'-on-tol)*. Intravenous anaesthet agent; in about 5s causes unconsciousne which is maintained for 3 to 5 min. Patei awakens quickly without nausea ar vomiting.

یدی مخدر : سن کرنے والا عامل۔ یہ سیکنڈ میں بے ہوشی طاری کر ے ہے جو ۳ تا ۵ منٹ رہتی ہے۔

Eppy *(ep'-i)* Neutral adrenaline eye drops f use in open angle glaucoma.

Epsikapron *(ep-si-kap'-ron)*. Epsilon amino aproic acid (q.v.).

ی کیپران : اپسیلون امینوکیپرونک ایسڈ۔ روانی خون کو روکتا

ہے۔

Epsilon aminocaproic acid *(ep'-sil-on-a-m-in'-o- kap-ro-ik as'-id)*. EACA Prevents formation of fibrinolysin (q.v.), hence used in attempts to arrest bleeding.

اپسیلون امینوکیپرونک ایسڈ : خون کی روانی کو روکتا ہے۔

Epsom salts. Magnesium sulphate (q.v.).

نمک اپسم : میگنیسم سلفیٹ۔

Epstein Barr virus *(ep'-stin bar vi'rus)*. Causative agent of infections mononucleosis (q.v.). A verstile herpes virus which infects many people throughout the world; does not always produce symptoms. Cancer research workers have discovered EBV genome in the malignant cells of Burkitt's lymphoma and nasopharyngeal carcinoma.

ایپ سٹائین بیروائرس : برکٹ لمفو سارکوما سے متعلق۔

Epulis *(ep'-u-lis)* [G. epi, on; oulon, gum]. A tumour growing on or from the gums.

جبڑے کی رسولی : مسوڑھوں پر یا ان سے اگنے والا ناسور۔

Equagesic *(e-kwa-jez'-ik)*. Ethoheptazine (q.v.); meprobamate (q.v.); aspirin (q.v.); and calcium carbonate. A nalgesic and relaxant; useful for musculoskeletal disorders.

Equanil *(e-kwan'-il)*. Meprobamate (q.v.).

ایکوانل : میٹربامیٹ

Eraldin *(er'-al-din)*. Practolol (q.v.). Now restricted to emergency i.v. use only, due to the occurence of a serious adverse reaction syndrome following long-term oral use.

ابرلڈن : پریکٹولول۔

Erb's palsy. See PALSY.

Errectile *(e-rek'-til)* [L. erigere; to raise up]. Upright; capable of being elevated, **e. tissue,** highly vascular tissue, which, under stimulus, becomes rigid and erect from hyperaemia.

نعوظی : سیدھا بلند ہونے کا اہل۔

Erection *(e-rek'-shun)*. The state achieved when erectile tissue is hyperaemic.

نعوظ۔ خیزش : ایتادہ نسیج کی حالت۔ گرم مصالحہ جات خیزش کو زیادہ کرتے ہیں یعنی خواہش جماع کو بڑھاتے ہیں۔

Erector *(e-rek'-tor)*. A muscle which achieves erection of a part.

عضلہ نعوظی : ایسا عضلہ جس کا کوئی حصہ ایستادہ ہو جائے۔

Erepsin *(e-rep'-sin)*. A proteolytic enzyme in succus entericus.

ارپشن : ایک خامرہ۔

Ergodryl Antimigraine.

ارگوڈرل : ضد مائیگرین۔

ERG. Electroretinogram (q.v.).

ای آر جی : الیکٹرورٹینوگرام۔

Ergography *(er-gog'-ra-fi)* [G. ergon, work; graphein, to write]. A method of measuring and recording the state of muscle by its output of effort to an electrical stimulus.

Ergometrine *(er-go-met'-rin)*. Main alkaloid of ergot (q.v.). Widely used in obstetrics to reduce haemorrhage and improve contraction of uterus.

آرگومیٹری : ارگٹ کا الکلائڈ۔ یوٹرس کو سکیڑنے کے لئے مستعمل ہے۔ رحم کے کم سکڑنے میں ایک گولی صبح ایک دوپہر ایک شام۔

Ergometry *(er-gom'-et-ri)* [G. ergon, work; metron, measure]. Measurement of work done by muscles--ergometric, adj.

فعل پیمائی : عضلات کے ذریعے کام کی پیمائش۔

Ergonomics *(er-go-nom'-iks)*. The applica tion of various biologica l disciplines in relation to man and his working environment.

کاری ماحولیات : انسان اور اس کے ماحول کے تعلق میں مختلف حیاتی ضابطوں کا اطلاق۔

Ergosterol *(er-gos'-ter-ol)*. A provitamin present in the subcutaneous fat of man and animals. On irradiation it is converted into vitamin D_2 which has antirachitic properties.

آرگوسٹیرول : آدمیوں اور جانوروں کی جلدی چربی میں پرووٹامن موجود ہوتا ہے جو دھوپ میں وٹامن ڈی ۲ میں تبدیل ہو جاتا ہے۔ سفید قلمی سٹیرول۔ نقطہ پگھلاؤ۔

Ergot *(er'-got)*. A fungus found on rye. Widely used as ergomtrine for postpartum haemorrhage.

ارگٹ : رائی پر پایا جانے والا سماروغ۔

Ergotamine *(er-got'-a-min)*. An alkaloid of

ergot used in the treatment of migraine. Early e. treatment of an attack is more effective, especially when combined with antiemetics.

آرگوٹامین : ارگٹ کا ایک الکلائڈ جو مائیگرین کے علاج میں مستعمل ہے۔ کثرت حیض یا مینوریجیا میں علاج کے لئے ارگوٹامین یا گائی زجین کی گولیاں ایک صبح ایک دوپہر ایک شام۔

Ergotism *(er'-got-izm)*. Poisoning by ergot.

ارگٹیت : ارگٹ سے زیادہ زہریلاپن۔

Ergotrate *(er'-go-trat)*. Ergometrine (q.v.).

ارگوٹریٹ : آرگومٹرین۔ رحم کے کم سکڑنے یا سب انوولیوشن آف یورٹرس میں ایک گولی صبح ایک دوپہر ایک شام۔

Eructation *(e-ruk-ta'-shun)* [L. eructare, to belch forth]. Noisy, oral expulsion of gas from the stomach.

ڈکار : معدہ سے گیس کا پرشور اخراج۔

Erysipelas *(e-ri-sip'-e-las)* [Etym. dub. G. erythros, red; L. pellis, skin]. An acute, specific, infectious disease, in which there is a spreading, streptococcal inflammation of the skin and subcutaneous tissues, accompanied by fever and constitutional disturbances.

سرخباده : چھوت کی مخصوص بیماری۔ اس میں بخار ہو جاتا ہے۔ جلدی مرض۔

Erysipeloid *(e-ri-sip'-e-loid)*. A skin condition resembling erysiopelas. It occurs in butchers, fishmongers or cooks. The infecting organism is the Erysipelothrix of swine erysipelas.

سرخباد نما (مرض) : جلا کی حالت، قصابوں، مچلی کے شائقین اور خانساماؤں میں ہوتی ہے۔

Erythema *(e-ri-the'-ma)* [G.]. Reddening of the skin--erythematous, adj. **e. induratum** is Bazin's disease (q.v.). **e. multiforme** is a form of toxic or allergic skin eruption which breaks out suddenly and lasts for days; the lesions are in form of violet-pink papules or plaques and suggest urticarial weals. Severe form called Stevens-Johnson syndrome (q.v.). **e. nodosum** is an eruption of painful red nodules on the front of the legs. It occurs in young women, and is generally accompanied by rheumaticky pains. It may be a symptom of many disease including tuberculosis, acute rheumatism, gonococcal septicaemia, etc. **e. pernio,** chilblain (q.v.).

حمرۃ الجلاء : جلاء کی سرخ رنگت، زیادہ تر ہاتھوں اور بازوؤں پر دھبے۔

Erythraemia *(e-rith-re'-mi-a)* [G. erythros, red; haima, blood]. See ERYTHROCYT- HAEMIA.

سرخ دمویت : یونانی زبان ارتھروس بمعنی سرخ اور ہیما بمعنی خون کا مجموعہ۔

Erythroblast *(e-rith'-ro-blast)* [G. erythros, red; blastos, germ]. A nucleated red blood cell found in the red bone marrow and from which the erythrocytes are derived--erythroblastic, adj.

احمر نہوض : ہڈی کے سرخ گودے میں پایا جانے والا مرکزے والا سرخ خونی خلیہ۔

Erythroblastosis fetalis *(e-rith-ro-blasto'-sis-fe-ta'-lis)* [G. erythros, red; blastos, germ; L. fetus, offspring]. A pathological condition in the newborn child due to rhesus incompatibility between the child's blood and that of its mother. Red blood cell destruction occurs with anaemia, often jaundice and an excess of erythroblasts or primitive red blood cells in the circulating blood. Immunization of women at risk, using gammaglobulin containing a high titre of anti-D, prevents EF.

ارتھروبلاسٹوسس فیٹیلس : نوزائیدہ بچے اور ماں کے خون میں فرق کی وجہ سے بچے کی حالت۔ سرخ خونی، خلیے ختم ہو جاتے ہیں اور عموماً یرقان ہو جاتا ہے۔

Erythrocin *(e-rith'-ro-sin)*. Erythromycin (q.v.).

اریتھروسین : ارتھرومائی سین۔ منہ سے کھائی جانے والی دوائی ہے تک دوائی ہے۔ پنسلین کی طرح عمل کرتی ہے جب دوسری اینٹی بایوٹک دوائیاں غیر موثر ہو جائیں تو یہ دوائی دی جاتی ہے۔

Erythrocyanosis frigida *(e-rith-ro-si-an-o'-sis frig'id-a)* [G. erythros, red; kyanos, blue; -osis, condition; L. frigus, cold]. Vasospastic disease with hypertrophy of arteriolar muscular coat--erythrocyanotic, adj.

حمراری زراق : ایک مرض۔

Erythrocytes *(e-rith'-ro-sitz)* [G. erythros, red; kytos, cell]. The normal non-nucleated red cells of the circulating blood; the red blood corpuscles-- erythrocytic, adj.

سرخ خلیے : گردشی خون کے نارمل غیر مرکزائی سرخ خلیے خون کے وہ خلیے جن میں ہیموگلوبن ہوتا ہے۔ اور ان کا کام جسم کے تمام حصوں میں آکسیجن پہنچانا ہے۔

Eurax *(u'-raks)*. Crotaminton (q.v.).

Erythrocythaemia *(e-rith-ro-si-the'-mi-a)* [G. erythros, red; kytos, cell; haima, blood]. Overproduction of red cells. 1. This may be a physiological response to a low atmospheric oxygen tension (high altitudes), or to the need for greater oxygenation of the tissues (congenital heart disease) and is then referred to as erythrocytosis. 2. The idiopathic condition is polycythaemia vera (erythraemia)--erythrocythaemic, adj.

سرخ خلیہ دمویت : سرخ خلیوں کی زیادہ پیداوار۔

Erythrocytopenia *(e-rith-ro-si-to-pe'-ni-a)* [G. erythros, red; kytos, cell; penia, want]. Deficiency in the number of red blood cells--erythrocytopenic, adj.

ارتھروسائیٹوپنیا : سرخ خونی خلیوں کی تعداد میں کمی۔

Erythrocytosis *(e-rith-ro-si-to'-sis)* [G. *erythros,* red; *kytos,* cell; *-osis,* condition] See DERYTHROCYTHAQEMIA.

افراط خلیات سرخ : یونانی الفاظ ارتھروس بمعنی سرخ' کائیٹوس بمعنی خلیہ اور اوسس بمعنی حالت کا مجموعہ۔

Erythroedema polyneuritis *(e-rith-re-de'-ma pol-i-nu-ri'-tis)* [G. *erythros,* red; *oidema,* swelling; *polys,* many; *neuron,* tendon; *-itis,* inflammation]. A disease of infancy characterized by red swollen extremities. Nervous irritability is extreme, leading to anorexia and wasting. Syn., pink disease. Swift.s disease.

مرض گلابی : معصوم بچوں کی بیماری جس میں سرے سرخ اور متورم ہو جاتے ہیں۔

Erythrodema *(e-rith-ro-derma)* [G. erythros, red; derma, skin]. Excessive redness of the skin.

سرخی جلد۔ احمرار الجلد : جلد کا زائد سرخ ہونا۔

Erythrogenic *(e-rith-ro-jen'-ik)* [G. erythros, red; genesis, production]. 1. Producing or causing a rash. 2. Producing red blood cells.

اریتھروجینک : سرخ خونی خلیے پیدا کرنا۔

Erythromycin *(e-rith-ro-mi'-sin)*. An orally active antibiotic, similar to penicillin in its range of action. Best reserved for use against organisms resistant to other antibiotics. Risk of jaundice, particularly with e. estolate.

اریتھرومائی سین : آریتھروسین: منہ کے ذریعے کھائی جانے والی اینٹی بایوٹک دو جو عمل میں پنسلین کی طرح ہے۔ جب دوسری دوائیں عمل نہ کریں تو یہ دوا موثر ہوتی ہے۔ ٹانسی لائی ٹس اور سوزش گردہ مزمن میں ایک گولی ہر چھ گھنٹے بعد۔ یہ دوائی ایکٹینو مائیسیٹ پھپھوندی سے پیدا ہوتی ہے۔

Erythropoiesis *(e-rith'-ro-poi-e-sis)*[G. erythros, red; poiesis, production]. The production of red blood cells. See HAEMOPOIESIS.

خلیات سرخ سازی : سرخ خونی خلیوں کی پیداوار۔

Esbach's albuminometer *(es'-baks al-bu-min-om'-et-er)*. A graduated glass tube in which albumin in urine is precipitated in 24 hours by the addition of **E.'s reagent.** See APPENDIX ON URINE TESTING [George H. Esbach, Paris physician, 1843-90].

Esbatall *(es'-bat-al)*. Bethanidine (q.v.).

اسبیٹل : بتھانیڈین

Eschar *(es'-kar)* [G. eschara, scab]. A slough, as results from a burn, application of caustics, diathermy, etc.

کھرنڈ : کسی آبلے کا کھرنڈ۔

Escharotic *(es-kar-ot'-ik)* [G. eschara, scab]. Any agent capable of producing an eschar.

کاوی (عامل) : کھرنڈ پیدا کرنے کا اہل عامل۔

Escherichia *(esh-er-ik'-i-a)*. A genus of bacteria. Motile, Gram-negative rod bacteria which are widely distributed in nature, especially in the intestinal tract of vertebrates. Some stains are pathogenic to man, causing enteritis, peritonitis, pyelitis, cystitis and wound infections. The type species is E. coli.

ایشیر کیا : جراثیم کا ایک جنس۔ متحرک ۔ گرام۔ منفی۔ سلاخی جراثیم جو کثرت سے پائے جاتے ہیں۔ خصوصی طور پر مھریوں کی آنتوں میں ہوتے ہیں۔

Eserine *(es'-e-ren)*. Physostigmine (q.v.).

ایسیرین : فائیسوسٹگمین۔

Esidrex. Hydrochlorothiazide (q.v.).

ایسی ڈریکس : ہائیڈروکلورو-تھازائیڈ۔ ہائپرٹنشن یا بلڈ پریشر میں اس کی ایک گولی صبح ایک دوپہر ایک شام۔ سوزش گردہ مزمن سوزش گردہ، پیٹ میں پانی، گن جیسٹو ہارٹ فیلیور اور دمہ قلبی میں ایک گولی روزانہ ناشتے کے بعد ۔ دن میں ۳ گولیاں برائے مرض میٹیر پیشاب آور۔ حمل کے دوران پاؤں پر ورم آجائے تو یہ دوا دی جا سکتی ہے۔

Esmarch's bandage A rubber roller bandage used to procure a bloodless operative field in the limbs. [Johann Friedrich August von Esmarch, Germany military surgeon, 1823-1908].

ربڑ کی پٹی : ربڑ کی پٹی جو جوارح میں بے خون اپریشن کے لئے مستعمل ہے۔

Esmodil *(es'-mo-dil)*. Antispasmodic drug similar to carbachol.

ایموڈل : ضد تشنجی دوا۔

ESN. Educationally subnormal. May attend a special school, or a special class in an ordinary school

ای ایس این : تعلیمی طور پر کم۔ عام سکول میں مخصوص جماعت یا مخصوص سکول میں حاضری دی جا سکتی ہے۔

Espundia *(es-pun'-de-a)*. South American mucocutaneous leishmaniasis (q.v.). Causes ulceration of the legs with later involvement of nose and throat.

ایسپنڈیا : ایک مرض جس سے ٹانگوں میں ناسور ہو جاتا ہے۔ آخر میں ناک اور گلاب خراب ہو جاتے ہیں۔

ESR. Erythrocyte sedimentation rate. Citrated blood is placed in a narrow tube. The red cells fall, leaving a column of clear supernatant serum, which is measured a t the end of an hour and reported in millimetres. Tissue destruction and inflammatory conditions cause an increase in the ESR.

ای ایس آر : ارتھروسائیٹ ترسیب کی شرح۔ خون کا ایک امتحان۔

ای ایس آر سٹینڈ پر تقریباً چھ ای ایس آر ٹیو بیں بیک وقت رکھی جا سکتی ہیں۔ ای ایس آر پیٹ تقریباً اڑھائی ملی میٹر بور کی جاتی ہے اور اوپر سے نیچے کی طرف صفر سے ۲۰۰ ملی میٹر تک نشان لگے ہوتے ہیں۔

Essence *(es'-ens)*. A solution of a volatile oil in rectified spirit.

ست ۔ روح۔ جوہر : مصفی سپرٹ میں طیران پذیر تیل کا محلول۔

Estigyn *(es'-ti-jin)*. Ethinyloestradiol (q.v.).

ایسٹی جن : اتھینائلواسٹراڈیول

Estopen *(es-to-pen')*. A penicillin and iodine compound, with a selective affinity for lung tissue.

ایسٹپین : پنسلین اور آیوڈین کا مرکب جو پھیپھڑوں کے نسیج کے لئے الف رکھتا ہے۔

Estrovis *(es-tro-vis')*. Quinestrol (q.v.).

Ethacrynic acid *(eth-a-krin'ik)*. Diuretic with a wider range of effectiveness than the thiazide group. Called a 'loop' diuretic because it prevents the concentration of urine by an action on the loop of Henle.

ایتھا کرینک ایسڈ : پیشاب آور۔ زیادہ اثر دو گھنٹوں کے بعد ہوتا ہے اور آٹھ گھنٹوں تک اثر رہتا ہے۔

Ethamsylate *(eth-am'-sil-at)*. Systemic haemostatic agent.

Ethambutol *(eth-am-but'-ol)* Synthetic antituberculosis drug. Oral, Highly effective when used with isoniazid for tuberculosis. A lmost non-toxic, but occasionally its toxic effect is retrobulbar neuritis.

ای تھیمبوٹال : تپ دق کے خلاف ایک تالیفی دوا جو غیر زہریلی ہے لیکن بعض دفعہ زہریلا اثر ہو جاتا ہے۔ مائی ایمبوٹال۔ تپ دق میں صبح ناشتے کے بعد اکٹھی ۵ گولیاں روزانہ۔

Ethanolamine oleate *(eth'-an-ol-a-min-o-l'-e-at)*. A sclerosing agent used in varicose vein therapy.

اتھانولامن اولسی ریٹ : ورید کے علاج میں مستعمل عامل۔

Ether *(e'ther)* [G. aither, pure air]. Inflammable liquid; one of the oldest volatile anaesthetics and less toxic than chloroform. Occasionally used orally for its carminative action.

ایتھر : آتش گیر مائع۔ کلوروفارم سے کم زہریلا۔ بعض دفعہ ہاضمے کے لئے منہ کے ذریعے دیا جاتا ہے۔

thiazide *(eth'-i-a-zid)*. See CHLOROTHIA-ZIDE.

اِیتھیازائیڈ : کلوروتھیازائیڈ۔

thics *(eth'-iks)* [G. ethos, custom]. A code of moral principles derived from a system of values and beliefs. **nursing e.,** the code governing a nurse's behaviour, especially to her patients, visitors and colleagues. Ethics apply to national groups and to smaller ones, e.g., professional and business.

اخلاقیات : عقائد اور اقدار کے نظام سے ماخوذ اخلاقی اصولوں کا ضابطہ۔

thinamate *(eth-in'-am-at)*. Tranquilizer. One of the carbamates. For poisoning see p.337.

اِیتھینامیٹ : سکون بخش دوا۔ کاربامیٹس میں سے ایک۔

thinloestradiol *(eth-in-il'-es-tra-di-ol)*. Powerful orally effective oestrogen, usually well tolerated.

اِیتھی نائیل ایسٹراڈائی اول : منہ کے ذریعے کھائی جانے والی اسٹروجن عورت کے بانجھ پن کے علاج کے لئے ۵ ملی گرام کی ایک گولی روزانہ زبان کے نیچے رکھیں۔ ۲۰ دن دیں۔ ماہواری سے ۵ دن پہلے اور ماہواری کے ایام میں ناغہ۔ چھ ماہ تک دیں۔

thionamide *(eth-i-on'-a-mid)*. Expensive synthetic antitubercular compound. Oral. Hepatotoxicity guarded against by twice weekly SGOT tests. Like isoniazid, e. can be neurotoxic. It can produce gastrointestinal side effects.

اِیتھوناماِئیڈ : تپ دق کے خلاف استعمال کیا جانے والا ایک مہنگا تالیفی مرکب۔

histerone *(eth-i-ste'-ron)*. An orally active compound with progesterone-like propertieis. The average dose is six times that of progesterone by injection.

اِیتھی سٹیرون : پروجسٹرون کی خصوصیات والا مرکب ثانوی امینوریا یعنی ماہواری بند ہونے کی مرض میں مفید۔

hmoid *(eth'-moid)* [G. ethmos, sieve; eidos, form]. A spongy bone forming the lateral walls of the nose and the upper portion of the bony nasal septum.

غربالی ہڈی : ناک کی جانبی دیواریں اور استخوانی ناک کے پردے کا بالائی حصہ بنانے والی اسفنجی ہڈی جو چھلنی کی مانند اور کاغذی ہوتی ہے کھوپڑی کی تلی کے سامنے کا حصہ بناتی ہے۔ دونوں حلقوں کی درمیانی جگہ کو پر کرتی ہے اور ناک کا بڑا حصہ بناتی ہے۔ اس کے سوراخوں میں سے سونگھنے کے اعصاب دماغ سے ناک تک پہنچتے ہیں۔

Ethmoidectomy *(eth'-moid-ek'-to-mi)* [G. ethmos, sieve; eidos, form; ektome, a cutting]. Surgical removal of a part of the ethmoid bone, usually that forming the lateral nasal walls.

مصفات براری : اتھمائڈ ہڈی کے ایک حصے کا آپریشن کے ذریعہ خاتمہ۔ عموماً وہ حصہ جو ناک کی جانبی دیواریں بناتا ہے۔

Ethoglucid *(eth-o-g!oo'-sid)*. Intraarterial, anticancer, neurotoxic agent.

Ethoheptazine *(e-tho-hep'-ta-zen)*. Analgestic that relieves muscle spasm. Related to pethidine. Zactirin.

ایتھوہیپٹازین : پیتھیڈین سے متعلق۔ دافع درد یہ دو عضلاتی اینٹھن کو آرام پہنچاتی ہے۔

Ethopropazine *(e-tho-pro'-pa-zen)*. An antispasmodic used chiefly in rigidity of Parkinsonism. May have more side effects than other drugs.

ایتھوپروپیزین : ایک دافع تشنج دوا۔ عموماً پارکنسونزم کی سختی میں استعمال کی جاتی ہے۔ دوسری دواؤں کی نسبت زیادہ اطرافی اثرات پیدا کرتی ہے۔

Ethosuximide *(eth-o-toin)*. For major, focal and psychomotor epilepsy.

ایتھوٹائن : مرض مرگی میں مفید ہے۔

Ethyl biscoumacetate *(eth'-il bis-koom-a-s'-e-tat)*. A blood anticoagulant of the dicoumarol type, but with a more rapid and controllable action.

ایتھائل بسکوم ایسی ٹیٹ : خون کو جمنے نہ دینے والا عامل۔

Ethyl carbamate *(eth'-il-kar'-bam-at)*. urethane (q.v.).

ایتھائل کاربیمیٹ : یوریتھین۔ ایک سفید قلمی ٹھوس مرکب۔ نقطۂ پگھلاؤ ۴۸ س، پگھلی ہوئی صورت میں بطور محلول مستعمل۔ بطور انٹرمیڈیٹ رالوں اور دوائیوں کی تیاری میں مستعمل۔

Ethyl chloride *(eth'-il-klor'-id)*. A volatile general anaesthetic for short operations, and a local anaesthetic by reason of the intense cold produced when applied to the skin; useful in sprains.

ایتھائل کلورائیڈ : مختصر اپریشن کے لئے ایک طیران پذیر سن کرنے والی دوا۔ جلد پر لگانے سے انتہائی ٹھنڈک پیدا کر کے سن کر دیتی ہے۔

Ethyloestrenol *(eth-il-es'-tren-ol)*. An anaboiic steroid; useful for treating severe weight loss, debility and osteoporosis.

اتھیولول امین اولی ایٹ : تصلب زدہ عامل

Ethyloleamine oleate *(eth-il-ol'-a-men ol-e-at)*. Sclerosing agent.

Ethyl pyrophosphate *(eth'-il pi-ro-fos'-fat)*. Organo-phosphorous compound used as insecticide in agriculture. Powerful and irreversible anticholinesterase action. Potentially dangerous to man for this reason.

طا-یتھائیل پائیر وفاسفیٹ : زراعت میں استعمال ہونے والا کرم کش مرکب انسان کے لئے خطرناک ہے۔

Ethynodiol diacetate *(eth-in-o'-di-ol di-as'-a-s'-e-tat)*. Controls uterine bleeding.

Etiology *(e-ti-ol'-o-ji)*. See AETIOLOGY.

علم الاسباب : سائنس کی ایک شاخ جو امراض کے متعلق بحث کرتی ہے۔

Etophylate *(et-o-fil'-at)*. Theophyline (q.v.).

ایٹوفائیلیٹ : تھیوفائیلین۔

EUA. Examination (of the uterus) under anaesthetic.

Eucalyptus oil *(u-ka-lip'-tus)*. Has mild antiseptic properties, and is sometimes used in nasal drops for catarrh.

یوکلپٹس آئل : معمولی دافع تعفن خصوصیات کا حامل۔

Eucortone *(u-kor'-ton)*. Adrenal cortex extract.

یوکارٹون : ایڈرینل کارٹیکس کا عرق۔

Eudemine *(u'-de-men)*. Diazoxide (q.v.).

یوڈیمائین: ڈائی ازوکسائیڈ

Euflavine *(u-fla'-ven)*. See ACRIFLAVINE.

یوفلیوین : ایکریفلیون۔

Eugenics *(u-jen'-iks)* [G. eu, well; genos, birth]., The science dealing with those factors which improvesuccessive generations of the human race-- eugenic, adj.

Euglucon *(u-gi'-kon)*. Glibenclamide (q.v.).

گلوکون : گلبین کلامائیڈ۔

Eugynon *(u-gi'-non)*. Low oestrogen ora contraceptive.

Eumydrin *(u'-mid-rin)*. Atropine methonitrat (q.v.). Specially useful in pylorospasm

میڈرین : ایٹروپین میتھونائیٹریٹ۔ معدے کے نچلے حصے کی ٹھن میں مفید۔

Eunuch *(u'-nuk)*. [G. eunouchos, guarding th couch]. A human male from whom the teste have been removed; a castrated male.

صی، ہیجڑا : ایسا آدمی جس کے خصیے کاٹ دیئے گئے ہوں۔

Eupepsia *(u-pep'-si-a)* [G. eu, well; peptein, t digest]. Normal disgestion.

دہ ہاضمہ : نارمل انہضام۔

Euphoria *(u-for'-e-a)* [G. eu, well; pherestha to turn out]. In psychology an exaggerate sense of well-being--euphoric, adj.

حت، جنونی بشاشت : نفسیات میں بہتری کی لئے مبالغہ آ ری۔

Eurhythmics *(u-rith'-miks)* [G. euruthmia, goc rhythm]. Harmonious bodily movements pe formed to music.

نمکس : موسیقی کے انداس میں جسمانی حرکات۔

Eusol *(u'-sol)*. Antiseptic solution prepared fro chloride of lime and boric acid. Effectiv when freshy prepared, but solutions lo strength rapidly.

سال : کیلشیم کلورائیڈ اور بورک ایسڈ سے تیار شدہ واقع تعفن ل۔ تازہ بنا ہوا۔ محلول موثر ہوتا ہے۔

Eustachian *(u-sta'-ki-an)*. A cana l, partly bon partly cartilaginous, measuring 38.0 to 50 mm in length, connecting the pharynix wi the tympanic cavity. It allows air to pass in the middle ear, so that the air pressure is ke evven on both sides of the eardrum. **catheter,** an instrument used for dilating t Eustachian tube when it becomes blocke [Bartolommeo Eustachius, Italian anatomi 1520-74].

ناخی : ایک قنال یا نالی جو فیرنکس کو ٹمپنگ کہفہ سے ملاتی ہے۔

اس کے ذریعے درمیانی کان میں ہوا جاتی ہے اور دونوں طرف ہوا کا دباؤ یکساں رہتا ہے۔

Euthanasia *(u-than-a'-zi-a)* [G. eu, well; thanatos, death]. 1. A good, inferring a painless, death. 2. Frequently interpreted as the painless killing of a person suffering from an incurable disease.

موت راحت : (۱) دکھ کے بغیر موت ۔ (۲) لاعلاج مریض کو بغیر تکلیف مارنا۔

Euthyroid state *(u-thi'roid stat)*. Denoting normal thyroid function.

یوتھایئرائڈ سٹیٹ : نارمل تھائیرائیڈ عمل۔

Eutocia *(u-to'-si-a)* [G. eu, well; tokos, childbirth]. A natural and normal labour without any complications.

سہل ولادت : پیچیدگیوں کے بغیر قدرتی دردزہ

Eutonyl. MAOI (q.v.).

یوٹونل : ایم اے اور آئی۔

EVA. Evacuation (of the uterus) under anaesthetic.

Evacuant *(e-vak'-u-ant)* [L. evacuare, to empty out]. An agent which causes an evacuation, particularly of the bowel. **e. enema** fluid injected into the rectum, to be returned, as distinct from retained.

قے آور : مقی قبض کشا عامل۔

Evacuation *(e-vak' u-ant)* [L. evacuare, to empty out]. The act of empting a cavity; generally referred to the discharge of faecal matter from the rectum.

انخلاء : کسی کہفہ کو خالی کرنے کا عمل۔ ریکٹم سے فضلے کے اخراج کے لئے عموماً یہ اصطلاح مستعمل۔

Evacuator *(e-vak'-u-a-tor)* [L. evacuare, to empty out[. An instrument for procuring evacuation, e.g. the removal from the bladder of a stone, crushed by a lithotrite.

تبخیر ہونا : حرارت کے ذریعے مائع کو گیسی حالت میں تبدیل کرنا۔

Evaporating lotion *(e-vap'-o-rat-ing lo'-shun)*. One which, applied as a compress, absorbs heat in order to evaporate, and so cools the skin.

تبخیر والا لوشن : یہ حرارت کو جذب کر کے بخارات بناتا ہے۔ اس طرح جلد کو ٹھنڈا رکھتا ہے۔

Eversion *(e-ver'-shun)* [L. evertere, to turn out]. A turning outwards, as of the upper eyelid to expose the conjunctival sac.

برگردانی : باہر کی جانب الٹنا۔

Evisceration *(e-vis-e-ra'-shun)*. [L. eviscerare, to disembowel]. Removal of internal organs.

احشابراری : اندرونی عضاء کو نکالنا۔

Evulsion *(e-vul'-shun)* [L. evulsus from evellere, to tear out]. Forcible tearing away of a structure.

قلع : کسی ساخت کو زبردستی ختم کرنا۔

Ewing's tumour. Sarcoma involving shaft of long bone before twentieth year. Current view holds that it is a secondary bone deposit from a malignant neuroblastoma of the adrenal gland. [James Ewing, American pathologist, 1866-1943].

ایوئنگ سلعہ : ثانوی استخوانی ذخیرہ۔

Exacerbation *(eks-as-er-ba'-shun)* [L. exacerbare, to irritate]. Increased severity, as of symptoms.

شدت مرض : علامات کا شدید ہونا۔

Exanthema *(eks-an-them'-a)* [g. eruption]. A skin eruption--exanthemata, pl.; exanthematous, adj.

قوبار بثور : جلد کا پھٹنا۔

Ethinyloestradiol *(eth-in-ilo'-es-tra-di-ol)*. Powerful orally effective oestrogen, usually well tolerated.

قطع : کسی حصے کو کاٹ کر اس کی جگہ سے ہٹانا۔

Excitability *(ek-sit-a-bil'-i-ti)* [L. excitare, to arouse]. Rapid response to stimuli; a state of being easily irritated--excitable, adj.

تحریک پذیری : آسانی سے حساس ہونے کی حالت۔

Excitation *(ek-si-ta'-shun)* [L. excitare, to arouse]. The act of stimulating an organ or tissue.

تحرک : کسی عضو یا بافت کو تحریک دینے کا عمل۔

Excoriation *(eks-kor-i-a'-shun)* [L. ex, from; corium, hide; so excoriare, to fray]. See ABRASION.

پوست تراشی : جلد یا میوکس جھلی پر سطحی کے زخم جو عموماً رگڑ سے آجاتا ہے۔

Excrement *(eks'-kre-ment).* Faeces (q.v.).

فضلہ۔ براز : غیر ہضم شدہ خوراک جو جسم سے باہر نکل جاتی ہے۔

Excresence *(eks-kres'-ens)* [L. excrescere, to grow out]. An abnormal protuberance or growth of the tissues.

فضلہ۔ پھنسی، پھوڑے : بافتوں کا اگاؤ یا غیر معمولی ابھار۔

Excreta *(eks-kre'-ta).* The waste matter which is normally discharged from the body, particularly urine and faeces.

براز۔ فضلات : جسم سے خارج ہونے والا فضول مادہ خصوصاً پیشاب اور فضلہ۔

Excretion *(eks-kre'-shun).* The elimination of waste material from the body, and also the matter so discharged--excretory, adj., n.; excrete, v.t.

جسم سے فضول مادے کا اخراج

Exenteration *(eks-en-te-ra'-shun)* [L. extenterare,k from G. ex; out of ; enteron, intestine]. Removal of the viscerea. **pelvic e.**, a radical operation for advanced cancer of the pelvic organs.

اسعابراری : وسرا کا خاتمہ۔

Exfoliation *(eks-fo-li-a'-shun)* [L. exfoliare, to strip off leaves]. The scaling off of tissues in layers-- exfoliative, adj. See CYTOLOGY.

پرت ریزی : بافتوں کی تہوں کی صورت میں اتارنا۔

Exhibitionism *(eks-i-bish'-un-izm)* [L. exhibere, to hold forth]. Any kind of 'showing off; extravagant behaviour to attract attention including such perverted behaviour as indecent exposure-- exhjbitionist, n.

نمائش اعضائے تناسل۔ نمود و نمائش : نمائش کی کوئی قسم۔ دوسروں کی توجہ حاصل کرنے کے لئے غیر معمولی سلوک۔

Exocrine *(eks'-o-krin)* [G. exo, outside; krinein, to separate]. Glands from which the secretion passes via a duct. Secreting externally. Opp. of endocrine--exocrinal, adj.

برون افراز (غدود) : مخالف اینڈ کرائن۔ نالی والی غدود۔

Exogenous *(eks-oj'-en-us)* [G. exo, outside; genes, producing]. Of external origin.

برون زاد : بیرونی ماخذ کا۔

Exolan *(eks'-o-lan).* Non-staining, non-burning form of dithranol.

ایکسولین : ڈتھرانول کی بے دھبہ و بے آبلہ قسم۔

Exomphalos *(eks-om'-fal-os)* [G. ex, out; omphalos, navel]. A condition present at birth and due to failure of development of the abdominal wall. The intestines protrude through a gap in the umbilical region, covered only by a thin membrane.

بروزسرہ : پیدائش کے وقت ایک حالت۔ بطنی دیوار کی تکمیل کی ناکامی کی صورت میں آنتیں بڑھ کر ناف والے حصہ میں پہنچ جاتی ہے۔

Exophthalmos *(eks-of-thal'-mos)* [G. ex, out; opthalmos, eye]. Protrusion of the eyeball. See GOITRE--expohthalmic, adj.

خروج چشم : آنکھ کے گولے کا باہر آنا۔

Exophthalmos

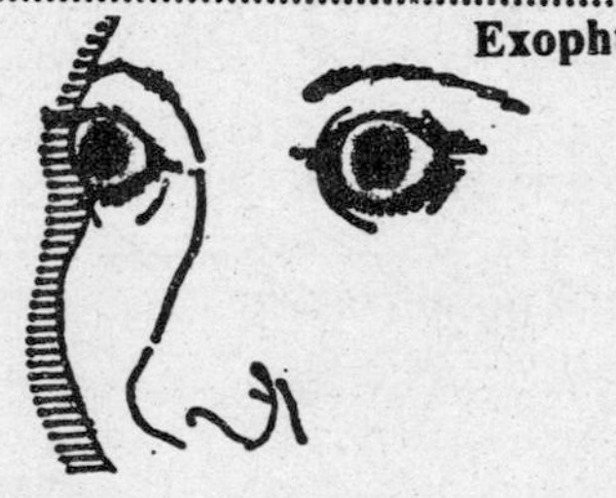

Exostosis *(eks-os-to' sis)* [G. ex, out; osteon, bone; -osis, condition]. An overgrowth of bone tissue forming a tumour.

Exostosis

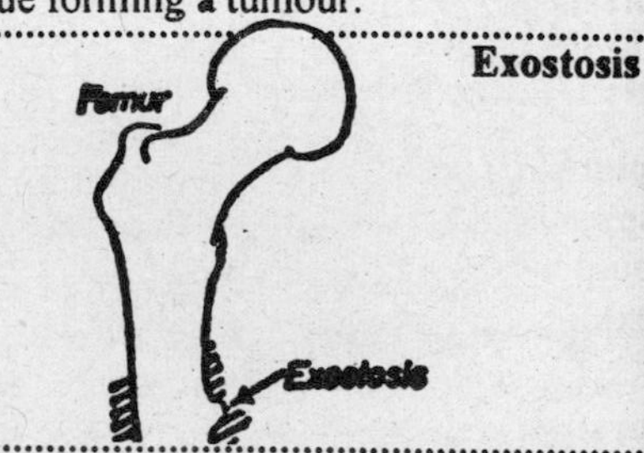

برون تعظم : استخوانی نسیج کا بڑھاؤ۔ جس سے ناسور بن جاتا ہے۔

Exotoxin *(eks-o-toks'-in)* [G. exo, outside;

toxikon, poison]. A toxic product of bacteria which is passed into the environment of the cell during growth. Opp. to endotoxin--exotoxic, adj.

سم خارجی : جراثیم سے بننے والا زہریلا مادہ۔

pected date of delivery Usually dated from the first day of the last normal menstrual period, even though for the next 14 days there is really no pregnancy.

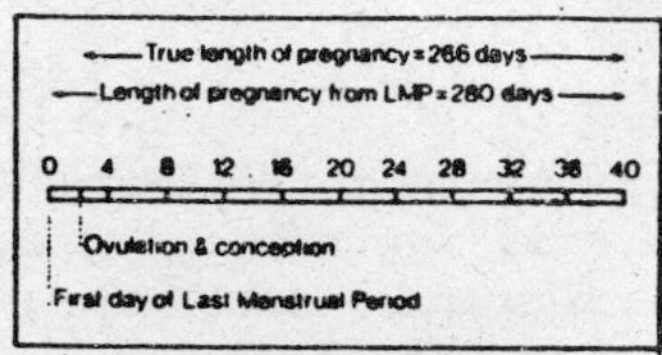

Expected date of delivery chart

pectorant *(eks-pek'-to-rant)* [L. expectorare, to drive from the breast]. A drug which promotes or increases expectoration.

دافع بلغم : رطوبت کو روکنے والی دوائی ۔ بلغم خارج کرنے میں مد لیکن زیادہ مقدار میں آور۔ مثلاً امونیم کاربونیٹ۔ ٹنکچراپی کیک۔ ٹنکچر سلا۔

pectoration *(eks-pek-tor-a'-shun)* [L. expectorare, to drive from the breast]. 1. The elimination of secretion from the respiratory tract by coughing. 2. Sputum (q.v.)--expectorate, v.t.

دفع بلغم : کھانسی کی وجہ سے تنفسی راہ میں حائل رطوبت کا خاتمہ یا اخراج۔

pira tion *(eks-pi-ra-shun)* [L. expirare, to breathe out]. The act of breathing out air from the lungs--expire, v.t., v.i.; expiratory, adj.

سانس نکالنا : پھیپھڑوں سے ہوا کو خارج کرنے کا عمل۔

ploration *(eks-plor-a'-shun)* [L. explorare, to spy out]. The act of exploring for diagnostic purposes, particularly in the srugical field--exploratory, adj.

استقصار : تشخیص کرنے کے لئے معلومات حاصل کرنے کا عمل۔

pranolol *(eks-pran'-o-lol)*. Propranolol (q.v.).

ایکس پرینولول : پراپرینولول۔

pression *(eks-presh'-un)* [L. ex, out; premere, p[ress]. 1. Expulsion by force as of the placenta from the uterus; milk from the breast, etc. 2. Facial disclosure of feelings, mood, etc.

اظہار : (۱) طاقت کے ذریعے اخراج مثلاً یوٹرس سے پلیسنٹا کا اخراج۔ چھاتی سے دودھ کھینچنا وغیرہ۔ (۲) موڈیا احساسات کا چہرہ سے اظہار۔

Exsanguination *(eks-sang-gwin-a'-shun)* [L. exsanguis, deprived of blood]. The process of rendering bloodless--exsanguinate, v.t.

دفع الدم : بے خون بنانے کا طریقہ کار۔

Extension *(eks-ten'-shun)* [L. extendere, to stretch out]. 1. Traction upon a fractured or dislocated limb. 2. The straightening of a flexexd limb or part.

راستی : جوارح یا ان کے حصوں کو سیدھا کرنا۔

Extensor *(eks-ten'-sor)* [L. from extendere, to stretch out]. A muscle which on contraction extends or straightens a part. Opp. to flexor.

باسطہ (عضلہ) : ایسا عضلہ جو سکڑنے پر جسم کے کسی حصے کو سیدھا کرتا ہے۔

Extirpation *(eks-ter-pa'-shun)* [L. exstirpare, to pluck out]. Complete removal or destruction of a part.

بیخنی : کسی حصے کا مکمل خاتمہ۔

Extra-capsular *(eks-tra-kap'-su-lar)* [L. extra, outside of; capsula, small box]. Outside the capsule.

Extra-articular *(eks-tra-ar-tik'-u-lar)* [L. extra, outside of; articulus, dim. of aitus, joint]. Outside a joint.

خارج المفصل : جوڑ سے باہر۔

Extracardiac *(eks-tra-kar'-di-ak)* [L. extra, outside of: G. kardia, heart]. Outside the heart.

برون قلبی : دل سے باہر۔

Extracellular *(eks-tra-sel'-u-lar)* [L. extra, outside of; cellula, little cell]. Occuring outside the cell.

بدرکیسی : کیپسول سے باہر۔

Extracorporeal *(eks-tra-kor-por'-ri-al)* [L. extra, outside; corporeus, bodily, material].

Outside the body. See CIRCULATION.

برون جسمی : جسم سے باہر۔

Extract *(eks'-trakt)* [L. extrahere, to draw out]. A preparation obtained by evaporating a solution of a drug.

ست عصارہ : کسی دوا کو محلول سے بخارات میں تبدیل کر کے حاصل شدہ عرق۔

Extraction *(eks-trak'-shun)* [L. extrahere, to draw out]. The act of drawing out, **e. of lens,** surgical removal of the lens. **extracapsular e.,** the capsule is ruptured prior to delivery of the lens. **intracapsular e.,** the lens is removed within its capsule.

ست نکالنا : نکالنے کا عمل۔ آپریشن کے ذریعہ عدسہ نکالنا۔

Extradural *(eks-tra-dur'-al)* [L. extra, outside of; durus, hard]. External to the dura mater.

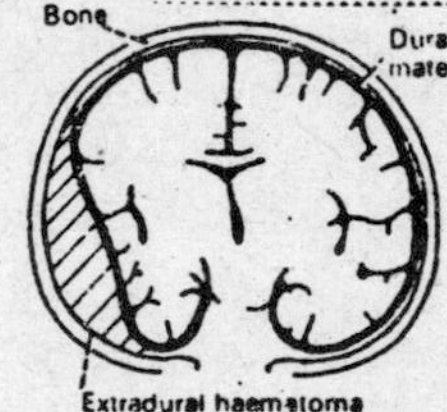

برون جامیہ : ڈیورامیٹر سے باہر۔

Extragenital *(eks-tra-jen'-it-al)* [L. extra, outside of; genitalis, genital]. On areas of the body apart from genital organs, **e. chancre** is the primary ulcer of syphilis occuring on the finger, the lip, the breast, etc.

برون اعضائے تناسل : تولیدی اعضا سے الگ جسم کے حصوں پر۔

Extrahepatic *(eks-tra-hep-at'-ik)* [L. extra, outside of; G. hepar, liver]. Outside the liver.

برون کبدی : جگر سے باہر۔

Extramural *(eks-tra-mur'-al)* [L. extra, outside of; murus, wall]. Outside the wall of a vessel or organ--extramurally, adv.

برون جامعہ برون دیوار : عضو یارگ کی دیوار سے باہر۔

Extraperitoneal *(eks-tra-per-it-on-e'-al)* [L. extra,

Thenar eminence

outside of; G. peri, round; teinein, to stretch]. Outside the perition-eum--extraperitoneal adv.

ن پیری ٹونیئم : پیری ٹونیم سے باہر۔

Extrapleural *(eks-tra-ploo'-ral)* [L. ext outside, of; G. pleura, side]. Outside the p ura, i.e. between the parietal pleura and t chest wall. See PLOMBAGE.

ن پلیورائی : پلیورا سے باہر۔

Extrarenal *(eks-tra-re'-nal)* [L. extra, outsi of; renalis, of the kidney]. Outside the kidne

ردہ سے باہر۔ :

Extrasystole *(eks-tra-sis'-to-li)* [L. extr outside of; G. systole, a drawing together].] emature beats in the pulse rhythm; the cardi impulse is intiated in some focus apart fr the sinoatrial node.

ں انقباض قلب : نبض کچی چلنا۔

Extrathoracic *(eks-tra-thor-as'-ik)* [L. ext outside of; G. thorax]. Outside the thorac cavity.

ن صدری : تھوراسک کہفہ سے باہر۔

Extrauterine *(eks-tra-u'-ter-in)* [L. extr outside of; uterus, womb]. Outside the uter See ECTOPIC PREGNANCY.

ٹرس سے باہر

Extravasation *(eks-trav-a-sa'-shun)* [L. extr outside of; vas, vessel]. An escape of flu from its normal enclosure into the surr unding tissues.

بدری : سیال کا نزدیکی بافتوں میں بہہ نکلنا۔

Extravenous *(eks'-tra-ven'-us)* [L. extr outside; vena, vein]. Outside a vein.

ل وریدی : ورید سے باہر

Extrinsic *(eks-trin'-sik)* [L. extrinsecus, on t outside]. Developing or having its origin from

without; not internal, **e. factor,** vitamin B (cyanocobalamin), which is normally prese in the diet and absorbed from the gut; it essential for normal haemopoiesis.

نی (عضلہ) : اندرونی نہ ہونا۔

Extroversion *(eks-tro-ver'-shun)* [L. extra, o side of; vertere, to turn]. Turning inside o **e. of the bladder,** ectopia vesicae (q.v.).

psychology, the direction of thoughts to the external world.

برون گردانی : اندر سے بیرونی جانب الٹ جانا۔ نفسیات میں خیالات بیرونی دنیا کی طرف ہونا۔

trovert *(eks'-tro-vert)* [L. extra, outside; vertere, to turn]. Sometimes **extravert.** Used by Jung to describe one extreme of personality dimension. The person described as e. regulates his behaviour in response to other people's attitude to him.

غیر باطنی : جو شخص اپنا رویہ دوسروں کا رویہ دیکھ کر تبدیل کرے۔

Exudate *(eks'-u-dat).* [L. exudare, to sweat out]. The product of exudation.

رشحہ : خارج ہونے والا مادہ۔

Exudation *(eks-u-da'shun)* [L. exudare, to sweat out]. The zing out of fluid through the capillary walls, or of sweat through the pores of the skin--exudate, n.; exude, v.t., v.i.

ارتشاح : جلد کے مساموں سے پسینے کا بہنا شعری دیواروں میں سے سیال کا بہنا۔

Eye-teeth. The canine teeth in the upper jaw.

بالائی تالاب : بالائی جبڑوں کے سوئے یعنی نوکیلے دانت۔

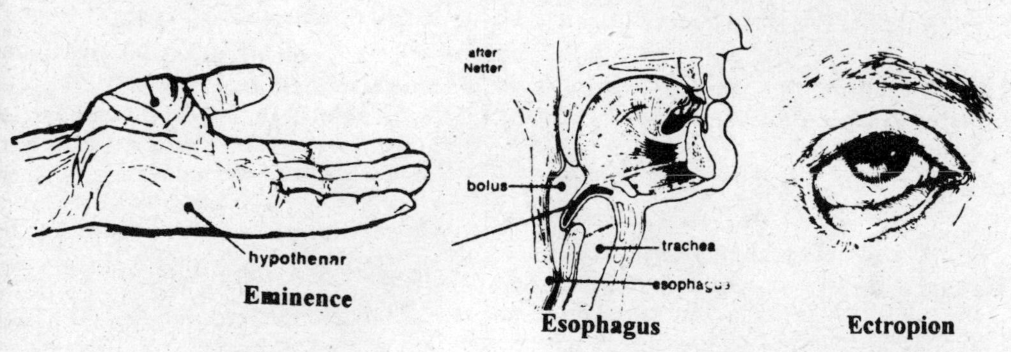

Eminence

Esophagus

Ectropion

F

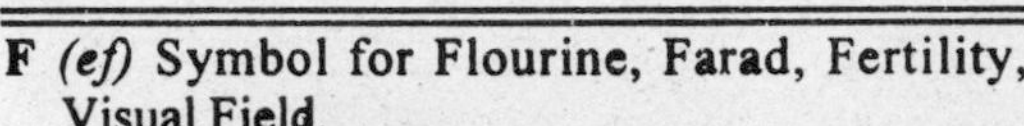

F *(ef)* Symbol for Flourine, Farad, Fertility, Visual Field.

الیف: علامت ہے فلورین، فیراڈ، فرٹیلٹی اور دیکھنے کی وسعت کی۔

°F Symbol for Degree Fahrenheit.

الیف°۔ الیف ڈگری: درجہ حرارت کی پیمائش کے نظام ڈگری فارن ہائیٹ کی علامت۔

Faber's syndrom *(fah'-barz sin-drom)* (Knud Helge Faber, Danish physician 1862-1956) Hypochronic anemia.

فیبر زسنڈروم: نوڈ ہیلیج فیبر ایک ڈنمارک کا طبیب تھا۔ اس کے نام پر اس بیماری کا نام رکھا گیا ہے۔ اس میں آئرن کی کمی کی وجہ سے خون کے ذرات اندر سے خالی ہو جاتے ہیں۔ اس طرح خون کی بھی کمی واقع ہو جاتی ہے۔

Face *(fa's)* [L. *facies,* appearance]. The anterior ventral part of the head starting from forehead and tasting at chin. Any presenting aspect or surface.

چہرہ: سر کا اگلا اور اوپر کا حصہ جو ماتھے سے شروع ہو کر ٹھوڑی پر ختم ہوتا ہے۔ کسی بھی چیز کا سامنے والا حصہ یا سطح۔

Facet *(fas'-et)* [F. *facette,* little face].. A small, plane surface on a hard body as on a bone.

Facioplegia *(fa'she-o-ple-ja)* [G. *plege,* stroke]. Facial paralysis or stroke of the face.

چہرہ کا فالج: چہرے پر اثر انداز ہونے والا فالج۔

Facultative *(fak-al-ta'tiv)* Not obligatory, capable of adaptation to different conditions. In bacteriology, a bacterium that can grow aerobically or anaerobically.

مطابقت پذیری: کوئی حالت مخصوص نہ ہونا۔ کسی بھی حالت میں یا ماحول میں اپنے آپ کو ڈھال لینا۔ بیکٹیریالوجی میں اس بیکٹیریا کو کہتے ہیں جو ہوایا

والے اگ سکتا ہے۔

Faeces *(fa-sez)* [L. *faeces,* during]. The wa matter excreted from the bowel. It is the ju of indigestible cellulose, indigested fo intestinal secretion and bacteria.

فضلہ: انتڑیوں سے خارج ہونے والا فضول مادہ۔

Fahrenheit Scale *(fah'renhi't ska'l)* [Gabr Danial Fahrenheit, a German physicist 16 1736]. It is a temperature measuring sc formulated by German physicist. Accordi to it, the freezing point of water is taken 32° while the boiling point is noted at 212°.

ن ہائیٹ سکیل: یہ درجہ حرارت ماپنے کا ایک پیمانہ ہے جس کے مطابق کا نقطہ جماؤ °32 فارن ہائیٹ اور پانی کا نقطہ کھولاؤ °212 فارن ہائیٹ مانا ہے۔

Failure *(fa'-lu'r)* Inability to perform. Car failure means heart attack or heart failure.

می: کسی کام کے کرنے میں ناکام ہو جانا۔ مثلاً دل کا دورہ جس میں دل کنے میں اور خون پہنچانے میں ناکام ہو جاتا ہے اور اس طرح موت بھی ہو سکتی ہے۔

Faint *(fa'nt)* Syncope. A temporary condition unconsciousness.

ی۔ بیہوشی: بے ہوشی کی عارضی حالت۔

Fairbank splint It is a supporting chip of wo used for treatment in Erb's palsy. The arms made immobilized in abduction and shoul is also kept at one place by placing the ar elbow at 90°C.

بینک تختی: فالج کے علاج میں مستعمل۔

Fllopiam tubes *(fal-lo'-pi-am)*. Two tubes opening out of the upper part of the uterus. Each measures 10.16 cm and the distal end is fimbriated and lies near the ovary. Their function is to convey in the ova into the uterus. [Gabriel Fallopius, Italian anatomist, 1523-63].

بیض نالیاں : یورٹرس کے بالائی حصے پر کھلنے والی دونلیاں۔ ان کا کام بیضوں کو یورٹرس میں پہنچانا ہے۔

Fallot's tetralogy *(fal'-os tet-ral'-o-ji)* Congenital heart defect comprising interventricular septal defect, pulmonary stenosis, right ventricular hypertrophy and malposition of the aorta. [Etienne L. A. Fallot, French physician, 1850-1911].

فیلوس ٹیٹرالوجی : دل کا نقص۔

Falx *(fal-ks)* [L. sickle]. A sickle-shaped structure, **f. cerebri,** that portion of the dura master separating the two cerebral hemispheres.

منجل : درانتی نما ساخت۔

Fallot's tetralogy

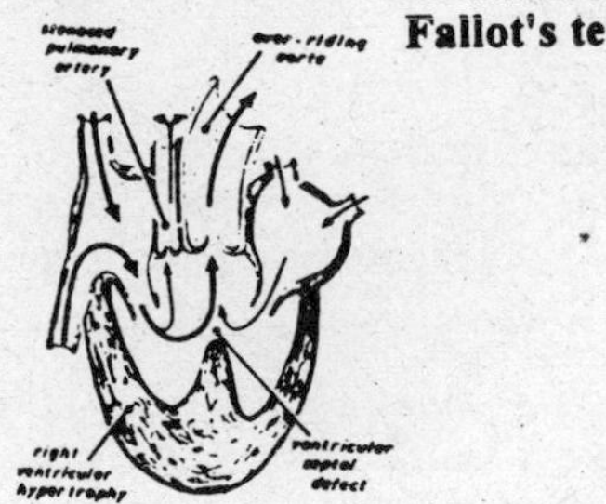

Familial *(fam-il'-i-al)* [L. familia, household]. Pertaining to the family, as of a disease affecting several members of the same family.

خاندانی : خاندان سے متعلق۔ خاندان کے مختلف اراکین کو ایک ہی مرض ہونا۔

Fanconi syndrome. See AMINOACIDURIA. [Guido Fanconi, Swiss Paediatrician, 1892].

فینکونی سنڈروم : سوئٹزرلینڈ کے فنکونی کے نام پر

Fang The root of a tooth.

ناب۔ : سخ دانت کی جڑ۔

Fantasy *(fan'-ta-si)* [G. phantasia]. Imagination, where images or chains of images are directed by the desire or pleasure of the thinker, normally accompanied by a feeling of unreality. Occurs pathologically in schizophrenia.

قوت متخیلہ : تصور یا تخیل جس میں سوچنے والے کی مسرت یا خواہش کے مطابق عکس یا ان کی زنجیر بنتی چلی جاتی ہے۔

fecundation *(fe-kun-da'-shun)* [L. fecun dus, fertile]. Impregnation. Fertilization.

Farmer's lung A form of pneumoconiosis arising from the dust of mouldy hay or other mouldy vegetable produce. Recognized as an industrial disease.

فارمرز لنگ : ایک صنعتی مرض۔

Fascia *(fash'-i-a)* [L. band]. A connective tissue sheath consisting of fibrous tissue and fat which unites the skin to the underlying tissues. it also surrounds and separates many of the muscles, and, in some cases, holds them together--fascial, adj.

نسیجی غلاف : ایک واصل بافتی تہہ جو ریشہ دار بافت اور چکنائی پر مشتمل ہوتی ہے۔ یہ جلد کو زیریں حصوں کے ساتھ متحد کرتی ہے۔ بعض عضلات کو جدا کرتی ہے اور بعض کو اکٹھا رکھتی ہے۔

Fasciculation *(fas-ik-u-la•shun)*. Visible flickering of muscle; can occur in the upper and lower eyelids.

Fasciculus *(fas-sik'-u-lus)* [L. small bundle]., A little bundle, as of muscle or nerve--fascicular, adj.; fasciculi, pl.

حزیمہ : ایک چھوٹا بنڈل مثلاً عضلے یا عصب کا۔

Fasciotomy *(fash-i-ot'-om-i)* [L. fascia, band; G. tome, a cutting]. Incision of a fascia.

فیشیوٹومی : بندھن کا انقطاع۔

Fastigium *(fas-tij'-i-um)* [L. summit]. The highest point of a fever; the period of full development of a disease.

اوج بخار : بخار کا نقطۂ عروج۔ بیماری کی مکمل تکمیل کا عرصہ۔

Fat An oil which may be of animal or vegetable origin, and may be either solid or liquid f. soluble vitamins A, D, E and K. See CALOR-

IFIC--fatty, adj.

چربی۔ شحم : تیل جو حیوانات یا نباتات سے حاصل کیا جاتا ہے۔ ٹھوس یا مائع فلسڈ تیل جو عام درجہ حرارت پر منجمد ہو جاتا ہے۔

Fatigue *(fa-teg')* [L. fatigare, to tire]. Weariness. Term used in physiological experiments on muscle to denote diminishing reaction to stimulus applied--fatigability, n.

تکان : تھکاوٹ عضلے پر فعلیاتی تجربات میں ردعمل کی کمی۔

Fatty degeneration Degeneration (q.v.). of tissues which results in appearance of fatty droplets in the cytoplasm; found especially in disease of liver, kidney and heart.

شحمی انحطاط : بافتوں کا ختم یا معدوم ہو جانا۔ اس سے سائیٹو پلازم میں چربیلے ذرات نمودار ہوتے ہیں۔ خصوصاً جگر۔ گردے اور دل کی بیماری میں۔

Fauces *(faw'-sez)* [L. throat]. The opening from the mouth into the pharynx, bounded above by the soft palate, below by the tongue. Pillars of the f., anterior and posterior, lie laterally and enclose the tonsil--faucial, adj.

حلقوم : منہ سے فیرنکس کی طرف سوراخ۔

Favism *(fa'-vism)* [from It fava, bean]. Reduced amount of enzyme G6PD (glucose-6-phosphate dehydrogenase) in red blood cells. Afficted people develop a severe haemolytic anaemia when they eat fava beans.

فیوزم : سرخ خونی خلیوں میں خامرہ گلوکوس۔٦۔ فاسفیٹ ڈی ہائیڈروجینز کی خفیف مقدار۔

Favus *(fa'-vus)* [L. honeycomb]. A type of rignworm not common in Britain; caused by Trichophyton schoenleini. Yellow cup-shaped crusts (scutula) develop especially on the scalp.

تپ تپش : بخار ہو جانا۔

Fecundation *(fe-kun-da'-shun)* [L. fecundus, fertile]. Impregnation. Fertilization.

بارورسازی : باروری۔ استقرار حمل۔

Fecundity *(fe-kun'-di-ti)* [L. fecundus, fertile]. The power of reproduction; fertility.

حمل : تولید کی طاقت۔ زرخیزی۔

Fehling's solution *(fa'-loings)*. An alkaline, copper solution used for the detection and estimation of amount of sugars. [Herman vor Fehling, German chemist, 1812-85].

فی لنگ کا محلول۔ فحلنگ سلوشن : ایک الکلائن تانبے کا محلول جو شکروں کی مقدار معلوم کرنے اور تخمینہ کرنے کے لئے استعمال کیا جاتا ہے۔ ٦٢ء٣٤ کاپر سلفیٹ ٣٠٠ سی سی آب مقطر میں حل کر کے مزید آب مقطر سے ٥٠٠ سی سی کر لیجئے۔ ١٨٠ گرام سوڈیم پوٹاشیم ٹارٹریٹ کرسٹلائن ٣٠٠ سی سی گرام آب مقطر میں حل کر کے فلٹر کر لیجئے اور ٧٠ گرام خالص کاسٹک سوڈا ١٠٠ گرام کاسٹک پوٹاش ملا کر ٹھنڈا کیجئے اور فلٹر کیجئے مزید آب براں ڈال کر ٥٠٠ سی سی کر لیجئے۔ بوقت ضرورت دونوں محلول ملا لیجئے۔ یہ غلنگ محلول ہے۔

Felty's syndrome Enlargement of liver, spleen and lymph nodes as a complication of rheum atoid arthritis. [Augustus Roi Felty, American physician, 1895].

فیلٹی سنڈروم : ورم مفصل۔

Felypressin *(fel-i-pres'-in)*. Vasoconstrictor Related to posterior pituitary hormone vasop-ressin. Sometimes combined with local anaes thetic.

فیلی پریسن : قابض شرائین۔

Femergin *(fem'-er-gin)*. Ergotamine tartrate (q.v.).

فیمرجن : ارگٹامین ٹارٹریٹ۔

Femoropoliteal *(fem-or-o-pop-lit-e'-al)* [L femur, thigh bone; poles, ham]. Usually referring to the femoral and popliteal vessels.

فیمروپاپ لیٹیل : عموماً فیمورل اور پوپلٹیل رگوں سے متعلق۔

Femur *(fe'-mur)* [L.]. The thighbone; the longest and strongest bone in the body--femoral, adj., femora, pl.

Femur

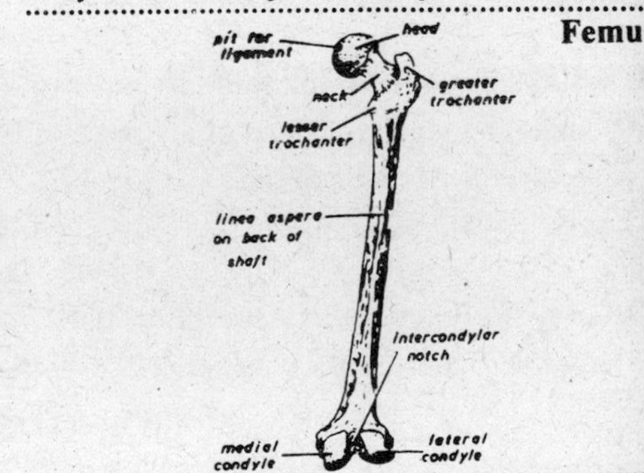

عظم الفخذ ۔ فیمر : ران کی ہڈی جسم کی طویل ترین و مضبوط ترین ہڈی۔ اس کا بالائی کنارہ گول اور چکنا ہوتا ہے جو کولھے کی ہڈی کے جوف یا ایسی ٹیبولم میں رہتا ہے اور ایک مضبوط رباط سے بندھا ہوتا ہے۔ فیمر کا گول سر ہڈی کی لمبائی سے ایک ترچھے ٹکڑے سے جڑا ہوتا ہی جسے فیمر کی گردن کہا جاتا ہے۔

enestra *(fen-es'-tra)* [L. window]. A window-like opening. **f. ovalls,** an oval opening between the middle and internal ear. Below it lies the **f. rotunda,** a round opening.

روزنہ : ایک کھڑکی نما سوراخ۔ مثلاً درمیانی و اندرونی کان کے درمیان بیضوی سوراخ۔

enestration *(fen-es-tra'-shun)*. [L. fenestra, window]. 1. The surgical creation of an opening (or fenestra) in the inner ear for the relief of deafness in otosclerosis. 2. A type of walking seen in such nervous diseases as paralysis against, when patient trots along in little bursts, getting faster and faster until he has to stop and then start off again, otherwise he would fall over.

نافذیت : (۱) بہرے پن کے آرام کے لئے اندرونی کان میں اپریشن کے ذریعے سوراخ کرنا۔ (۲) چلنے کی قسم۔ یہ عصبی بیماریوں میں دیکھنے میں آتی ہے۔

enfluramine hydrochloride *(fen-flu'-ra-men)* Appetite depressant. Free from the disadvantages of the amphetamines.

فینفلیورامین ہائیڈروکلورائیڈ : بھوک کم کرنے والا عامل۔

entazine, Perphenazine (q.v.). Closely allied to chlorpromazine (q.v.).

فینٹازین : پرفینٹازین۔ کلورپرومازین سے مشابہ۔

rement *(fer'-ment)* See CATALYST.

خمیر : عمل انگیزی پیدا کرنے والا عامل۔

ermentation *(fer-men-ta'-shun)* [L. fermentum, ferment]. The chemical changes brought about by the action of ferments, usually accompanied by liberation of heat and gas. Excellent examples are the making of bread, cheese and wine.

تخمیر : عمل انگیزوں کے عمل سے لائی جانے والی کیمیائی تبدیلیاں۔ ڈبل روٹی۔ پنیر اور شراب اس کی مثال ہیں۔

erric *(fer'-ik)* [L. ferrum, iron]. Pertaining to trivalent iron, as of its salts and compounds.

فیرک ۔ آہنی : سہ گرفتہ لوہے سے متعلق۔ اس کے نمکیات و مرکبات۔

Ferrivenin *(fer-ri-ven'-in)*. A solution of saccharated iron oxide, used by intravenous injection for severe iron deficiency anaemia.

فیری وینن : لوہے کی کمی سے خون کی کمی کے لئے ائرن آکسائیڈ کا محلول۔

Ferrous *(fer'-rus)* [L. ferrum, iron]. Pertaining to divalent iron, as of its salts and compounds. Ferrous carbonate, f. fumarate, f. gluconate, f. succinate and f. sulphate are oral preparations for iron-deficiency anaemias.

فیرس ۔ آہنی : دو گرفتہ لوہے سے متعلق۔ اس کے نمکیات و مرکبات۔ فیرس فیومریٹ کئی ادویہ پر مشتمل۔

Fertilization *(fer-til-i-za'-shun)* [L. fertilis, fertile]. The impregnation of an ovum by a spermatozoon.

جفتہ سازی ۔ بارودی : زخم کا بیضے سے ملاپ۔ سپرم کو نوک دار سر اور گردن رحم کے بیضہ کے مرکزے میں داخل ہوتا ہے۔ پھر اس کی دم ضائع ہو اجتی ہے اور باقی حصہ یعنی سر، گردن اور جسم باقی رہ جاتا ہے۔ اس عمل کو عمل زرخیزی یا بارودی بھی کہتے ہیں۔

Fester *(fes-tin-a'-shun)* [L. festinare, to hasten]. An involuntary hastening in gait as seen in paralysis agitans.

تندقدمی : چال میں ارادی طور پر تیزی۔

Fetishism *(fet'-ish-izm)*. A condition in which a particular object is regarded with an irrational fear or a strong emotional attachment.

Fetor *(fe'-tor)* [L. offensive smell]. Offensive odour, stench, **f. oris,** bad breath. Also foetor.

بدبو : ناخوشگوار بو۔

Fetus *(fe'-tus)* [T.]. An unborn child. **f. papyraceous,** a dead fetus, one of a twin which has become flattened and mummified--fetal, adj.

جنین : بطن میں موجود بچہ جو آٹھ ہفتوں سے خاتمہ حمل تک ہوتا ہے۔ تیسرے ماہ جنین کی لمبائی تین انچ سے کچھ زیادہ ہوتی ہے۔ ہاتھ اور پیر کی انگلیوں کے ناخن باریک جھلیوں کی صورت میں۔ دودھ کے دانتوں کی کونپلیں اگ آتی ہیں۔ ایک ابتدائی گردہ بن جاتا ہے۔ چوتھے ماہ جنین سر سے پیر کی انگلیوں تک ساڑھے چھ انچ لمبا ہوتا ہے۔ جلد پر نہایت باریک بال یا رواں اگ آتے ہیں۔ اس ماہ کے آخر میں جنین کی خفیف حرکات حاملہ کو محسوس ہونے

لگتی ہیں۔ پانچویں ماہ جنین کی لمبائی تقریباً دس انچ ہو جاتی ہے۔ ڈاکٹر عموماً پہلی بار جنین کے دل کی آواز سن سکتی ہے۔ حاملہ جنین کی حرکات محسوس کرتی ہے۔ چھٹے ماہ میں جنین کی لمبائی ۱۲ انچ ہو جاتی ہے اور ایک چھوٹے بچے کے مشابہ ہوتا ہے۔ ساتویں ماہ میں لمبائی تقریباً پندرہ انچ ہوتی ہے اور وزن تقریباً اڑھائی پونڈ۔ آٹھویں ماہ جنین کی لمبائی ساڑھے سولہ انچ اور وزن تقریباً پانچ پونڈ ہوتا ہے۔ بچے کے زندہ رہنے کے زیادہ امکانات ہوتے ہیں۔ نویں ماہ میں جنین تقریباً پورا بچہ بن جاتا ہے۔ اس کی لمبائی تقریباً ۱۹ انچ اور وزن تقریباً چھ پونڈ ہوتا ہے۔ دسویں ماہ میں مدت پوری ہو جاتی ہے۔ لمبائی تقریباً ۲۰ انچ ہوتی ہے۔ جلد سفید یا گلابی ہوتی ہے۔ انگلیوں کے ناخن مضبوط ہو جاتے ہیں۔

Fever *(fe'-ver)* [L. febris, fever]. An elevation of body temperature above normal. Syn., pyrexia. Designates some infectious conditions, e.g. **paratyphoid f., scarlet f., typhoid f.,** etc.

بخار : جسم کا نارمل سے زیادہ درجہ حرارت پی یو او بخار ایک جسمانی ردعمل ہے۔ علامات میں سردرد، بھوک میں کمی۔ متلی سردی لگنا گھبراہٹ کمزوری، پسینہ آنا، بے خوابی وغیرہ ہیں۔

Fibogel *(fi'-bo-jel)* A hydrophyllic gel which is a mucilaginous polysaccharide.

Fibre *(fi'-ber)* [L. fibra, fibre]. A threadlike structure--fibrous, adj.

ریشہ : ایک دھاگہ نما ساخت۔

Fibril *(fi'-bril)* [L. fibra, fibre]. A component filament of a fibre. A small fibre.

ریشک : چھوٹا ریشہ۔

Fibrillation *(fi-bril-a '-shun)*. Uncoordinated quivering contraction of muscle; referring usually to atrial (auricular) f. in the myocardium whrin the atria (auricles) beat very rapidly and are not synchronized with the ventricular beat. The result is a total irregularity of the pulse.

ریشہ سازی : عضلے کا سکڑاؤ۔

Fibrin *(fi'-brin)*. The matrix on which a blood clot is formed. The substance is formed from solube fibrinogen of the blood by the catalytic (enzymatic) action of thrombin--fibrinous, adj.

فائبرن : میٹرکس جس پر خون کا دھبہ جمتا ہے۔

Fibrin foam. A white, dry, spongy materia made from fibrinogen. It is used i conjunction with thrombin as a haemostatic i brain and lung survery.

فبین جھاگ : فائبرینوجن سے بننے والا سفید، خشک، اسفنجی مادہ۔

Fibrinogen *(fi-brin'-o-jen)*. A soluble protein o the blood from which is produced th insoluble protein called fibrin (q.v.). essentia to blood coagulation.

ائبرینوجن۔ فائبرن افزا : خون کی حل پزیر پروتین جس سے ناحل یر پروٹین فائبرن پیدا ہوتی ہے۔ یہ تھرومبین کے عمل سے خون کو جماتی ہے س کے نتیجہ میں فائبرن بنتی ہے۔

Fibrinogenopenia *(fi-brin-o-jen-o-pe'-ni-a)* [L fibra, fibre; G. genesthai, to be produced penia, poverty]. Lack of blood plasm fibrinogen. Can be congenital or due to live disease. Fibrinopenia. Hypofibrinogenaemia.

قلت فائبرینوجن : خونی پلازما فائبرینوجن کی کمی۔

Fibrinolysin *(fi-brin-o-lis'-in)* [L. fibra, fibre G. lysis, a loosening]. Blood stream enzym thought to dissolve fibrin occuring after mino inuries. Has been administered intraven- ousl in thrombosis.

ائبرینولائی سن : خون میں موجود خامرہ۔

Fibrinolysis *(fi-brin-ol'-i-sis)* [L. fibra, fibre; G lysis, a loosening]. The dissolution o fibrin--fibrinolytic, adj.

ائبرینولائی سس : فائبرن کا خاتمہ۔

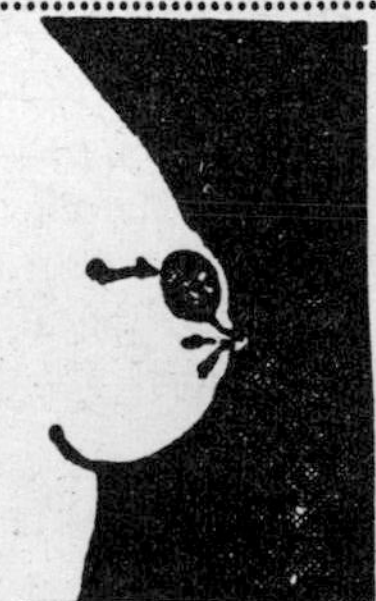

Fibroadenoma of breas

لیفی غدی سلعہ : ریشہ دار اور غدود یہ بافت پر مشتمل ناسور۔

Fibroblast *(fi'-bro-blast)* [L. fibra, fibre; G. blastos, germ]. A cell which gives rise to connective tissue. Syn., fibrocyte--fibroblastic, adj.

لیفی نہوض : خلیہ جس سے واصل یا رابطی نسیج بنتا ہے۔

Fibrocartilage *(fi-bro-kar'-til-aj)* [L. fibra, fibre; cartilago, cartilage]. Cartilage containing fibrous tissue--fibro-cartilaginous, adj.

ریشی کری : ریسہ دار نسیج پر مشتمل کارٹیلج۔

Fibrocaseous *(fi-bro-ka'-se-us)* [L. fibra, fibre; caseus, cheese]. A soft, cheesy mass infiltrated by fibrous tissue, formed by fibroblasts.

فائبروکیسیس : ایک نرم، پنیری مادہ جس میں ریسہ دار نسیج بھی ہوتا ہے۔

Fibrochondritis *(fi-bro-kon-dri'-tis)* [L. fibra, fibre: G. chondros, cartilage, -itis, inflammation]. Inflammation of fibro-cartilage.

ورم غضروف لیفی : فائبروکارٹیلج کی سوزش۔

Fibrocyst *(fi'-bro-sist)* [L. fibra, fibre; G. kystis, bladder]. A fibroma which has undergone cystic degenration--fibro-cystic, adj.

فائبروسسٹ : فائبروما جس کا سسٹک اختتام ہو چکا ہو۔

Fibrocystic *(fi-bro-sis'-tik)*. Pertaining to fibrocyst. **f. disease of bone,** cysts may be solitary or generalized. The latter condition, when accompanied by decalcification of bone, is due to hyperparathyroidism. **f. disease of breast,** see MASTITIS. **f. disease of pancreas,** see MUCOVISCIDOSIS.

فائبروسسٹک : فائبروسسٹ سے متعلق۔

Fibrocyte *(fi'-bro-sit)* [L. fibra, fibre; G. kytos, cell]. See FIBROBLAST--fibrocytic, adj.

لیفی خلیہ : خلیہ جس سے رابطی بافت بنتی ہے۔

Fibroid *(fi'-broid)* L. fibra, fibre, G. eidos, form]. A fibromuscular benign tumour usually found in the uterus. An interstitial uterine f. is embedded in the wall of the uterus (intramural)--if extended to the outer surface it becomes subperitoneal (subserous), if to the inner or endometrial surface it become submucous or even a f. polypus.

Uterine fibroids

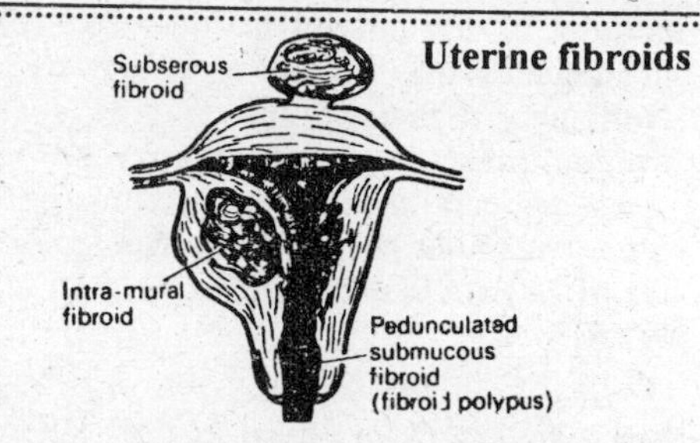

ریشہ دار : عموماً یوٹرس میں پایا جانے والا ریشہ دار، عضلاتی ناسور۔ فائبرائڈ یوٹرس رحم کی عضلاتی رسولی ہوتی ہے۔

Fibroma *(fi-bro'-ma)* [L. fibra, fibre; G. -oma, tumour]. A benign tumour composed of fibrous tissue--fibromatous, adj.; fibromata, pl.

فائبروما۔ ریشکی رسولی: ریشہ دار بافت سے بنا ہوا ناسور جو عموماً گوشت کے ساتھ ملحق ہوتا ہے۔ اسے شروع میں ہی نکال دینا چاہئے۔

Fibromuscular *(fi-bro-m,us'-ku-lar)* [L. fibra, fibre; musculus, muscle]. Pertaining to fibrous and muscle tissue.

لیفی عضلی : ریشہ دار اور عضلاتی بافت سے متعلق۔

Fibromyoma *(fi-bro-mi-o'-ma)* [L. fibra, fibre; G. mys, muscle; -oma, tumour]. A benign tumour consisting of fibrous fibromyomatous, adj.

لیفی عضلی سلعہ : ریشہ دار اور عضلاتی بافت پر مشتمل ناسور۔

Fibrosarcoma *(fi-bro-sar-ko'-ma)*. [L. fibra, fibre; G. sarx, flesh; -oma, tumour]. A form of sarcoma. A malignant tumour derived from fibroblastic (fibrocytic) cells--fibrosarcomata, pl.; fibrosarcomatous, adj.

لیفی لحمی سلعہ : سارکوما کی ایک قسم۔

Fibrosis *(fi-bro'-sis)* [L. fibra, fibre; G. -osis, condition]. The forma tion of excessive fibrous tissue in a structure--fibrotic, adj.

لیفیت : کسی ساخت میں زائد ریشہ دار بافت کا بننا۔

Fibrositis *(fi-bro-si'-tis)* [L. fibra, fibre; G. -itis, inflammation]. Pain of uncertain origin which affects the soft tissues of the limbs and trunk. It is generally associated with muscular stiffness and local tender points--fibrositic nodules. Cause unknown; some disturbance in immunity may be factor, as may be gout. Non-specific factors include chill, postural trauma, muscular strain and psychological stress especially in tense, anxious people. Syn., muscular rheumatism. See BORNHOLM DISEASE, LUMBAGO, PLEURODYNIA.

ریشکی ورم : درد جو جوارح اور ڈھڑ کے نرم حصوں کو متاثر کرتا ہے۔

Fibrovascular *(fi-bro-vas'-ku-lar)* [L. fibra, fibre; vasculum, small vessel]. Pertaining to fibrous tissue, which is well supplied with blood vessels.

فائبرو اسکولر: ایسی ریشہ دار بافت کے متعلق جس میں خونی رگوں کی کثرت ہو۔

Fibula *(fib'-u-la)* [L. clasp]. One of the longest and thinnest bones of the body; situated on the outer side of the leg and articulating at the upper end with the lateral condyle of the tibia and at the lower end with the lateral surface of the talus (astragalus) and tibia--fibular, adj.

پنڈلی کی بیرونی ہڈی۔ فبولا : جسم کی طویل ترین اور سب سے پتلی ہڈی ہڈیوں میں سے ایک ٹانگ کے بیرونی جانب واقع۔ ٹبیا کے متوازی۔ بالائی کنارہ سے گھٹنے کے نیچے جڑا ہوتا ہے۔ پھیلا ہوا زیریں کنارہ ٹخنے کی ہڈی اسٹرا گیلس کے ساتھ ٹخنے کا جوڑ بناتا ہے۔

Field of vision The area in which objects can be seen by the fixed eye.

میدان بصر : وہ ایرا جس میں ساکن آنکھ سے اشیاء کو دیکھا جا سکتا ہو۔

Filaria *(fil-a'-ri-a)* Parasitic, thread-like worms, found mainly in the tropics and subtropics. The adults of Filaria bancrofti and Brugia malayi live in the lymphatics, connective tissues or mesentery, where they may cause obstruction, but the embryos migrate to the blood stream. Completion of the life-cycle is dependent upon passage through a mosquito--filarial, adj.

فلیریا۔ خیطیہ : طفیلی، دھاگہ نما کیڑے۔ دور حیات کی تکمیل کا انحصار مچھر میں سے گزرنے پر ہے۔

Filariasis *(fil-er-i'-a-sis)* infestation with Filaria. See ELEPHANTIASIS.

خیطیت۔ فیل پا : خیطیہ یا فلیریا کی وجہ سے بیماری۔ اس کے پھیلانے کا سبب مچھر ہیں۔ ان کیڑوں کی نشو و نما مچھر اور انسان میں ہوتی ہے۔ ٹانگ یا فوطوں کا ورم۔ رات کے وقت ٹانگوں میں درد۔ علاج کے لئے ڈائی ایتھائل کا ربیمازین۔

Filaricide *(fil-er'-i-sid)* [L. filum, thread; coedere, to kill]. An agent which destroys Filaria.

خیطیہ کش : لاطینی لفظ۔ فائلم بمعنی دھاگہ اور سیڈیز بمعنی قتل کرنا کا مجموعہ۔ فلیریا کو تباہ کرنے والا عامل۔

Filiform *(fi'-li-form)* [L. filum, thread; forma, shape]. Threadlike. **f. papillae,** small projections ending in several minute processes; found on the tongue.

خیطی : دھاگے کی طرح۔

Filipuncture *(fi-li-pungk'-tur)* [L. fihum, thread; punctura, puncture]. Insertion of wire thread, etc into an aneurysm to produce coagulation of contained blood.

وخز انورسمائی : تار والے دھاگے کے ذریعے خون کو جمانا۔ انورسما میں تار ڈال کر علاج کرنا۔

Filixmas *(fi'-liks mas)*. Male fern extract, used to expel tapeworm.

سرخس۔ قرقس۔ کیل داور : کدو کیڑے کو نکالنے کے لئے مستعمل زفون کا عرق۔

Filtrate *(fil'-trat)*. That part of the substance which passes through the filter.

مقطر : مادے کا وہ حصہ جو فلٹر میں سے گزر جائے۔

Filtration *(fil-tra'-shun)*. The process of straining through a filter. The act of passing fluid through a porous medium. **f. under pressure** occurs in the kidneys, due to the pressure of blood in the glomeruli.

تقطیر : فلٹر میں گزارنے کا طریقہ۔

Filum *(fi'-lum)* [L. thread]. Any filamentous or thread-like structure. **f. terminale,** a strong fine cord blending with the spinal cord above and the periosteum of the sacral canal below.

خیط : کوئی ریشہ دار یا دھاگہ نما ساخت۔

Fimbria *(fim'-bri-a)* [L. finge]. A fringe or frond; resembling the fronds of a fern; e.g. the fimbrae of the Fallopian tubes--fimbrial, fimbriated, adj.; fimbriae, pl.

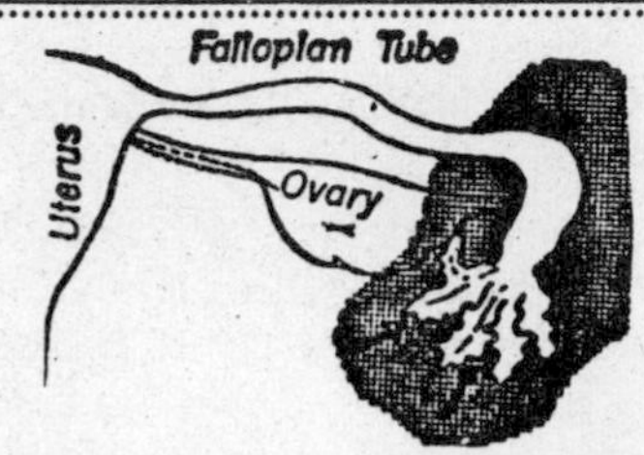

Fimbria of the fallopian tube

جھالر : فرن کے پتوں سے مشابہ۔

Finger *(fing'-ger)*. A digit, **clubbed f.,** swelling of terminal phalanx which occurs in many lung and heart disease.

انگلی۔انگشت : ہاتھ یا پیر کی انگلی۔

Fission *(fish'un)* [L. fissus, from findere, to split]. A method of reproduction common among the bacteria and protozoa.

انشقاق : پروٹوزوآ اور جراثیم میں پایا جانے والا تولید کا عام طریقہ۔

Fissure *(fish'-ur)* [L. fissura, cleft]. A split or cleft. **anal f.,** a linear ulcer on the margin of the anus, **palpebral f.,** the opening between the eyelids.

شقاق : شگاف۔علیحدہ ہونے والی جگہ۔

Fistula *(fis'-tu-la)* [L. tube]. An abnormal communication between two body surfaces or cavities, e.g. gastrocolic f., between the stomach and colon; colos-tomy, between the colon and the abdominal surface--fistular, fistulous, adj.; fistulae, pl.

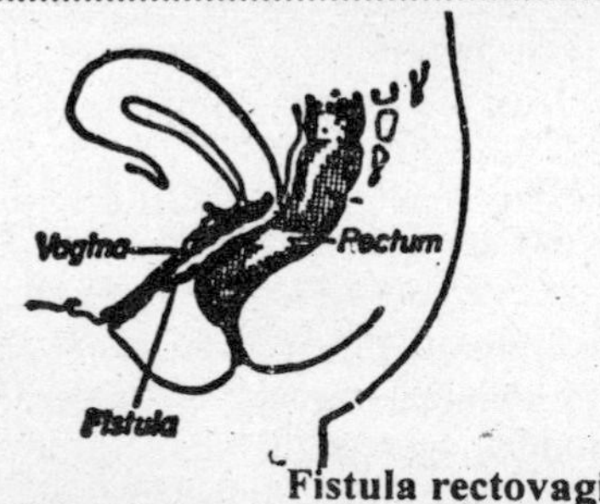

Fistula rectovaginal

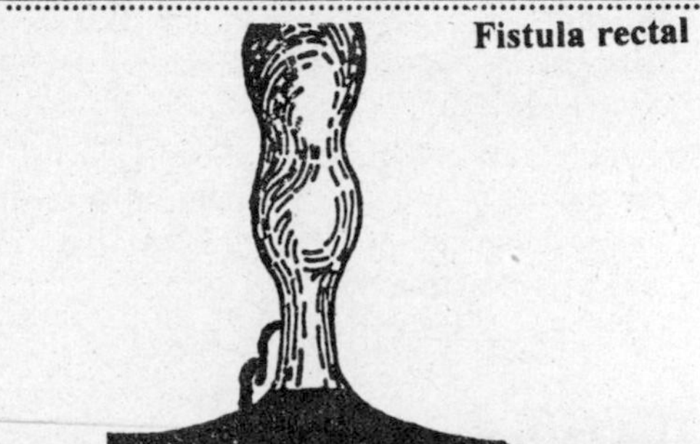

Fistula rectal

ناسور۔نالی: دوجسمانی سطحوں یا کھفوں کے درمیان غیر معمولی رابطہ۔

Fits Convulsions. See EPILEPSY.

غش۔دورے : بے ہوشی کے دورے۔

Fixation *(fiks-a'-shun)* [L. fixus, from figere, to fix]. In optics, the direct focusing of one or both eyes on an object so that the image falls on the retinal disc. As a psychoanalytical term, an emoparent, causing difficulty in forming new attachments later in life. **complement f.,** when antigen and homologous antibody unite to form a complex, complement may unite with such a complex, and this is referred to as fixation.

قبثیت : کسی شے پر ایک یا دونوں آنکھوں سے براہ راست فوکس تاکہ عکس ریٹنا کی ڈسک پر پڑے جذباتی وابستگی۔

Flaccid *(flak'-sid)* [L. flacus, flabby]. Soft, flabby, not firm. See PARALYSIS--flaccidity, n.

لچلچا : نرم۔

Flagellum *(fla-jel'-um)* [L.]. A fine, hair-like appendage capable of lashing movement. Characteristic of spermatozoa, certain bacteria and protozoa--flagella, pl.

سوطہ : ایک باریک، بال نما ساخت، حرکت کی اہل، پروٹوزوا بعض جراثیم اور سپرمیٹوزورآ میں موجود۔

Flagyl. Metronidazole (q.v.).

فلیجل : میٹرونڈازول۔امیبائی پیچش میں ۲ گولیاں صبح ۲ دوپہر ۲ شام دس ایام تک۔یہی خوراک برائے جگر کی امیبی پھوڑا۔

Flail chest Unstable thoracic cage due to fracture. See RESPIRATION.

زائدالحرکت چھاتی : فریکچر کی وجہ سے ناپائیدار تھوریکس کا پنجرہ۔

Flat-foot. A congenital or acquired deformity marked by depression of arches of the feet. See TALIPES.

چپٹا پا۔ پائے سطح: ایک نقص جو پاؤں میں پایا جاتا ہے۔

Flat pelvis. A pelvis in which the anteroposterior diameter of the brim is reduced, causing pelvic contraction.

چپٹا پیٹرو : پیڑو جس میں کنارے کا امامی خلفی قطر کم کر دیا جاتا ہے جس سے پیڑو میں سکڑاؤ ہوتا ہے۔

Flatulence *(flat'-u-lens)* [L. flatus, a blowing]. Gastric and intestinal distension with gas--flatulent, adj.

اپھراؤ۔ ریاح : گیس سے معدے اور آنتوں کا پھیلاؤ۔ نفخ شکم۔ انیزائیم وٹامن کمپاؤنڈ کیپسول ایک صبح ایک دوپہر ایک شام ۔ آکسی ٹیٹرا سائیکلین (ٹیرامائی سین) کیپسول دن میں چار مرتبہ۔

Flatus *(fla'-tus)*. [L.]. Gas in the stomach or intestines.

ریح : معدے یا آنتوں میں گیس۔

Flavine *(fla'-ven)*. See ACRIFLAVINE

فلیون۔ زرد رنگ : ایکریفلیون۔

Flavoxate *(flav-oks'-at)*. Oral urinary antiseptic.

Flaxedil *(flaks'-e-dil)*. Gallamine (q.v.).

Flea *(fle)*. A blood-sucking wingless insect of the order Siphonaptera; it acts as a host and transmits disease. Its bite leaves a portal of entry for infection **human f.,** Pulex irritans. **rat f.,** Xenopsylla cheopis, transmitter of plague (q.v.).

پسو: خون چوسنے والا بے پر حشرہ۔ میزبان کے طور پر کام کرتا ہے اور بیماری پیدا کرتا ہے۔ طاعون پھیلاتا ہے۔

Flex, Bend.

خم : جھکاؤ۔ موڑ۔ جھکنے کا عمل۔

Flexbilitas cerea *(fleks-ib-il'-it-as as'-re-a)*. Literally waxy flexibility. A condition of generalized hypertonia of muscles found in catatonic schizophrenia. When fully developed, the patient's limbs retain positions in which they are placed, remaining immobile for hours at a time. Occasionally occurs in hysteria as hysterical rigidity.

مومی خم پذیری: لغوی طور پر موم دار جھکاؤ یا لچک۔ عضلات کی ایک حالت ۔ انسانی جوارح جہاں پڑے ہوں، وہیں رہ جاتے ہیں، ان میں ہلنے کی سکت نہیں ہوتی۔

Flexion *(flek'-shun)* [L. flexus, bent]. The act of bending.

خمیدگی : مڑنے کا عمل۔

Flexner's bacillus (Shigella flexneri). A pathogenic, Gram-negative rod bacterium, which is the most common cause of bacillary dysentery epidemics, and sometimes infantile gastroenteritis. It is found in the faeces of cases of dysentery and carriers, from whence it may pollute food and water supplies, or be transferred by contact. [Simon Flexner, Americal pathologist, 1863-1946].

فلیکسنر بیسلس : مرض پیدا کرنے والا گرام منفی سلاخی جرثومہ جس سے پیچش پھیلتی ہے۔ پیچش کے مریضوں کے فضلے سے خوراک میں پہنچتا ہے۔

Flexor *(fleks'-or)* [L. flexus, bent]. A muscle which on contraction flexes or bends a part. Opp. to extensor.

قابضہ : عضلہ جو سکڑنے پر کسی حصے کو جھکاتا ہے۔

Flexure *(fleks'-ur)* [L. flexura, a bending]. A bend left colic or **splenic f.** is situated at the junction of the transverse and descending parts of the colon. It lies at a higher level than the **right colic** or **hepatic f.,** the bend between the ascending and transverse colon, beneath the liver, **sigmoid f.,** the S-shaped bend at the lower end of the descending colon. It is continuous with the rectum below--flexural, adj.

خماؤ۔ انحنا : جھکاؤ۔

Floaters *(flo'-ters)* Floating bodies in the vireous humour (of the eye) which are visible to the person.

Floating kidney Abnormally mobile kidney. See NEPHROPEXY.

Flooding A popular term to describe excessive bieedintg from the uterus.

افراط حیض : یوٹرس سے زیادہ خون بہنا۔

Flocculation *(flok-ul-a'-shun)*. The coalescence of colloidal particles in suspension resulting in their aggregation into large discrete masses which are often visible to the naked eye.

گالاسازی : معلق ذرات باہم مل کر محلول میں نظر آنے لگتے ہیں۔

'**loppy infant** (benign congenital hypotonia). Usually no demonstrable muscular neural pathology is present.

lorid *(flor'-id)* [L. floridus, flowery]. **Flushed,** high coloured.

بھڑکیلا : تیز شوخ رنگ والا۔

'**lowmeter.** A measuring instrument for flowing gas or liquid.

loxapen *(flok'-sa-pen)*. Flucloxacillin (q.v.).

فلوکساپین : پنسلین کی ایک قسم۔

'**lucloxacillin** *(floo-cloks-a-sil'-lin)*. An isoxazole penicillin, active against penicillinase-producing strains of Staphylococcus aureus. Well absorbed in man after oral and intramuscular administration. The chlorine of cloxacillin has been replaced with fluorine.

فلوکلاکس ایسلین : یہ پنسلین ایسے جراثیم کے خلاف کام کرتا ہے جو پنسلین کو ختم کرنے والا خامرہ پیدا کرتے ہیں۔

'**luctuation** *(fluk-tu-a'-shun)*. [L. fluctuare, to move as a wave]. A wave-like motion felt on digital examination of a fluid-containing tumour, e.g. abscess--fluctuant, adj.

تورم جسم : موج کی طرح حرکت جو سیال پر مشتمل ناسور دیکھتے وقت انگلیوں پر محسوس ہوتی ہے۔

'**ludrocortisone** *(floo-dro-kor'-ti-zon)*. Sodium-retaining tablets. Useful in some cases of Addison's disease.

فلڈروکاٹیسون : سوڈیم والی گولیاں۔ایڈیسن کی بیماری میں مفید ہے۔

lufenamic acid *(floo-fen'-a-mik)*. Non-steroidal, anti-inflammatory, antipyretic anagesic, especially useful for disorders of the musculoskeletal system. Does not interfere with uricosuric action of sulphinpyrazone, therefore useful in gout.

فلوفینیمک ایسڈ : عضلاتی استخوانی نظام میں گڑبڑ کے لئے مفید۔سکون بخش دوا۔جوڑوں کے درد میں مفید۔

luke *(flook)*. A trematode worm of the order Digenea. The European or sheep f. (Fasciola hepatica) usually ingested from water-cress. There is fever, malaise, a large tender liver and eosinophilia. No satisfactory treatment though chloroquine helps. The Chinese f. (Clonorchis sinesis) is usually ingested with raw fish. The adult fluke lives in the bile ducts and while it may produce cholangitis, hepatitis and jaundice, it may be asymptomatic, or be blamed for vague disgestive symptoms. lung f. (Paragonimus) usually ingested with raw crab in China and Far East.

کرم جگر۔وشیعہ۔فلوک : ایک ٹریماٹوڈ ورم۔ایک نوع بھیڑ بکریوں کے جگر پر پایا جاتا ہے۔کلوروکوئن کے سوا کوئی تسلی بخش علاج نہیں۔

Fluocinolone *(floo-o-sin'-o-lon)*. Cortisone derivative for topical application.

فلواسینولون : کارٹیسون حاصل

Flouocortolone *(floo-o-kor'-to-lon)*. Topical corticosteroid.

فلواکارٹولون : ٹاپیکل کارٹیکوسٹرائیڈ

Fluorescein *(floo-or-es'-in)*. Red substance that forms green fluorescent solution. Used as eye drops to detect corneal lesions, which stain green.

فلوریسین : سرخ مادہ جو سبز محلول بناتا ہے۔قلمی نامیاتی مرکب۔نقطۂ پگھلاؤ ۳۱۴ مس رنگوں میں مستعمل۔

Fluoridation *(floo-or-id-a'-shun)*. The addition of fluorine. When added to water to prevent dental caries, it is used in a 1:1000 000 dilution.

فلوریڈیشن : فلورین کا اضافہ۔بڑھتے ہوئے بچوں کے دانتوں میں کیریز سے حفاظت کے لئے پینے کے پانی میں فلورائیڈز کی معمولی مقدار کا اضافہ۔

Fluoride *(floo-or-id)*. A salt sometimes present in water. It prevents caries but in gross excess causes mottling of the teeth.

5-Fluorocystosine *(floo-or-o-si'-to-sen)*. Antifungal agent.

۵۔فلورسائیٹوسین : سماروغ کو تباہ کرنے والا عامل۔

Fluorohydrocortisone *(floo-or-o-hi-dro-kor'-ti-zon)*. 125 times as active as cortisol in causing sodium retention, therefore useful in Addison's disease.

فلورہائیڈروکاٹیون : مرض ایڈیسن میں مفید۔

Fluoroscopy *(floo-or-os'-ko-pi)* [L. fluere, to flow: G. skopein, to examine]. X-ray examination by means of fluorescent screen commonly called 'screening'.

فلوریت بینی : ایکس رے کے ذریعے جانچنا سکرینگ۔

Fluorouracil, 5-FU *(floo-o-ro-u'-ra-sil)*. Antimetabolic cytotoxic agent.

فلوروراسل : اینٹی میٹابولک سائٹوٹاکسک عامل۔

Fluothane *(floo'-o-than)*. Halothane (q.v.).

فلواوتھین : ہیلوتھین۔

Fluphenazine enanthate *(floo-fen'-a-zen en'-an-that)*. Used in psychiatry. Can be given as a depot injection. A newer preparation is **f. deconoate.**

فلوفینازین اینتھیٹ : طب دماغی میں مستعمل۔ڈپوانجکشن کے طور پر دیا جاسکتا ہے۔

Flkupenthixol

f deconoate/enanthate *(floo-pen-thiks'-ol dek-on- o-at/en'-an-that)*. Less likely than fluphenazine d. and e. to produce extrapyramidal side effects to produce extrapyramidal side effects and has a mile antidepressant action.

Flurbiprofen *(flurb-i-pro'-fen)*. A non-steroidal anti-inflammatory agent.

Flux *(fluks)* [L. fluxum, from fluere, to flow]. Any excessive flow of any of the body excretions.

اسہال شدید : کسی جسمانی فضول مادے کا زائد بہاؤ۔

Foetor *(fe'-tor)*. See FETOR.

بد مادے دہن : ناخوشگوار بو۔

Foetus *(fe'-tus)* [L.]. See FETUS.

جنین : بچہ جو ابھی بطن میں ہو۔

Foelling's disease. Phenylpyruvic oligophrenia [Asbjorn Foelling. Contemporary Norwegian Professor.].

مرض فوئانگ : فضائل پائیروک اولیگوفرینیا

Folic acid *(fo'-lik-as'-id)* [L. folium, leaf]. A member of the vitamin B complex abundant in green vegetables, yest and liver. Absorbed from small intestine and an essential factor for normal haemopoiesis and cell division generally. Used in treatment of megaloblastic anaemias (q.v.). other than those due to vitamin B_{12} deficiency.

لک ایسڈ : وٹامن بی کمپلکس کا ایک رکن خون کی کمی میں بعض دفعہ کون
اکرنے کی لئے مستعمل جگر۔خمیر۔گردوں اور سبز پتوں والی سبزیوں میں
ثرت سے پایا جاتا ہے۔۵ ملی گرام کی ایک ایک گولی صبح دوپہر شام برائے
سیا اسے حیاتین م بھی کہتے ہیں۔

Folicin *(fo'-lis-in)* Folic acid and antianaem compound especially for prevention of ana mia in pregnancy.

لیسین : فولک ایسڈ اور خون کی کمی دور کرنے والے مرکبات جو خصوصاء
ح حمل میں خون کی کمی کے لئے استعمال ہوتے ہیں۔

Folie a deux. A rare psychiatric syndrome, i which one member of a close pair has a psy hosis and imposes his delusions on the other

لی اے ڈیوکس : نفسی عارضہ جو دو قریبی افراد پر اثر ہوتا ہے۔

Follicle *(fol'-ikl)* [L. folliculus, small sac]. 1. small secreting sac. 2. A simple tubular glan **follicle stimulating hormone** (FSH), sec eted in the anterior pituitary gland; it trophic to the ovaries in the female, where develops the ovum-containing (Graafia follicles; and to the testes in the male, whe it is responsible for sperm productio **Graafian f.,** minute vesicles contained in t stroma of an ovary, each containing a sing ovum. When an ovum is extruded from a G. each month, the corpus luteum is forme under the influence of luteotrophin from t anterior pituitary gland. If fertilization occu the corpus luteum persists for 12 weeks, if n it only persists for 12 to 14 days, **hair f.,** t sheath in which a hair grows-- follicular, adj.

اب (بال کا) غدہ : (۱) ایک چھوٹی رطوبت خارج کرنے والی
لی۔(۲) ایک سادہ نلی نما غدہ۔

Folliculitis *(fol-ik-ul-i'-tis)* [L. folliculus, sma sac; G. -itis, inflammation]. Inflammation follicles, such as the hair folicles.

Folliculosis *(fol-ik-ul-o-sis)* [L. folliculus, sma sac; G. -osis, condition]. Hypertrophy folicles. **conjunctival f.,** overgrowth conjunctival follicles.

Fomentation *(fo-men-ta'-shun)* [L. fomentu poultice]. A hot, wet application to produ hyperaemia. When the skin is intact, stri cleanlines is observed (medical f); when the skin is broken aseptic technique is used (surgical f.). **fomite** (fo'-mit) [L. formes, touchwood]. Any article which has been in contact with infection and is capable of transmitting same.

نکور : گرم وتر اطلاق۔

Fomitte *(fo-mit)* [L. fomes, touchwood]. Any article which has been in contact with infertion and is capable of transmitting same.

حامل العدوی : ایسی چیز جو بیماری سے لگ کر اسے آگے پھیلائے۔

Fontanelle *(fon-ta-nel')* [F. a little fountion]. A membranous space between the cranial bones. The diamond-shaped anterior f. (bregma) is at the junction of the frontal and two parietal bones. It ossifies during the second year of life. The triangular posterior f. (lambda) is a t the junction of the occipital and two parietal bones. It ossifies within a few weeks of birth.

نافوخ : کھوپڑیوں کی ہڈیوں کی درمیان ایک جھلی دار جگہ۔ دودھ پیتے بچوں میں گر کی مختلف ہڈیاں آپس میں اچھی طرح جڑی نہیں ہوتیں بلکہ درمیان میں کئی جگہ پر ہڈی نہیں ہوتی۔ انہیں فانٹے نیلز کہا جاتا ہے۔ دواڑھائی برسوں میں آسیفیکیشن ہونے پر یہ بند ہو جاتے ہیں۔ دو فانٹے نیلز ایک کر کے اگلی طرف اور ایک پچھلی طرف زیادہ دیکھے جاسکتے ہیں۔

Food poisoning Vomiting, with or without diarrhoea, resulting from eating food contaminated with chemical poison, preformed bacterial toxin, or live bacteria; or poisonous natural vegetation, e.g. berries, toad stools (fungi).

تسمم غذا : دستوں کے ساتھ یا دستوں کے بغیر الٹی یا قے آنا۔ یہ ایسی خوراک کھانے سے ہوتا ہے جس میں کیمیائی زہر۔ جراثیمی زہر یا جراثیم ہوں۔ بعض زہریلی سماروغ وغیرہ کی وجہ سے بھی ایسا ہوتا ہے۔

Foot. That portion of the lower limb below the ankle.**athlete's foot,** tinea pedis (q.v.). **foot drop,** inability to dorsiflex foot, as in severe sciatica and nervous dīsease affecting lower lumbar regions of the cord. **madura f.,** mycetoma (q.v.). **trench f.,** immersion f., occurs in frost-bite or other conditions of exposure where there is local deprivation of blood supply.

پا۔ پاؤں۔ پیر : ٹانگ کا ٹخنے سے نچلا حصہ۔

Foramen *(for-a'-men)* [L.]. A hole or opening. Generally used with reference to bones. **foramen magnum,** the opening in the occipital bone through which the spinal cord passes. **obturator f.,** found in the anterior portion of the innominate bone, **foramen ovale,** a fetal cardiac, interatrial communication. Closes at birth--foramina, pl.

منفذ : ایک سوراخ۔ ہڈیوں کے حوالے سے استعمال کیا جاتا ہے۔

Forceps *(for'-seps)* [L. pincers]. Surgical instruments with two opposing blades which are used to grasp or compress tissues, swabs, needles and many other surgical appliances. The two blades are controlled by direct pressure on them (tong-like), or by handles (scissor-like).

چمٹی : اپریشن کے لئے الات جس میں دو مخالف بلیڈ لگے ہوتے ہیں۔ جو بافتوں، سوئیوں وغیرہ کو پکڑنے یا دبانے کے کام آتے ہیں۔

Forensic medicine Also called 'legal m.' The applicatiaon of medical knowledge to questions of law.

طب قانونی : قانونی سوالات پر میڈیکل علم کا اطلاق۔

Foreskin *(for'-skin)*. The prepuce or skin covering the glans penis.

قلفہ : عضو تناسل کے سرے کو ڈھانپنے والی کھال جسے ختنہ میں کاٹ دیا جاتا ہے۔

Formaldehyde *(for-mal'-de-hid)*. Powerful germicide. Formalin is a 40 per-cent solution; used mainly for room disinfection and the preservation of pathological specimens.

فارمل ڈیہائیڈ : ایک طاقتور جراثیم کش دوائی۔ فارملین ۴۰ فیصد محلول کی صورت میں ہوتی ہے۔ کمرے کے تعفن کو ختم کرنے کیلئے استعمال کی جاتی ہے۔

Formication *(for-mi-ka'-shun)* [L. formica, ant]. A sensation as of ants running over the skin. Occurs in nerve lesions, particularly in the regenerative phase.

حس نملی : جلد پر چیونٹیاں رینگتی ہوئی محسوس ہوتی ہیں۔

Formula *(form'-u-la)* [L. small pattern]. A prescription. A series of symbols denoting the chemical composition of a substance--formulae, formulas, pl.

فارمولا۔نسخہ : تجویز کردہ نسخہ۔علامات کا سلسلہ جو کسی شے کی کیمیائی ترکیب کو ظاہر کرتا ہے۔

Formulary *(form'-u-la-ri)*. A collection of formulas. The **British National F.** is produced by the Joint Formulary Committee.

دستورالعمل : کلیوں کا مجموعہ۔

Fornix *(for'-niks)* [L. arch]. An arch; particularly referred to the vagina, i.e. the space between the vaginal wall and the cervix of the uterus, **conjunctival f.,** the line of reflection of the conjunctiva from the eyelids on to the eyeball--fornices, pl.

قوسیہ : محراب۔خصوصاً ویجائنا کے لئے مستعمل۔

Fortral *(for'-tral)*. Pentazocine (q.v.).

فارٹریل : پینٹازوسین۔

Fossa *(fos'-sa)* [L. ditch]. A depression or furrow-- fossae, pl.

حضرہ : ایک زیریں جگہ۔

Fothergill's operation. Anterior colporrhaphy, amputation of part of the cervix and posterior colpoperineorrhaphy performed for genital prolapse. [William Edward Fothergil, English gynae-cologist, 1865-1926].

اپریشن فودرگل : ایک اپریشن۔انگریز ایڈورڈ گل کے نام پر اس کا نام ہے۔

Fouadin*(fu'-a-din)*. Stibophen (q.v.).

فواڈن : سٹیبوفن۔

Fourchette *(foor'-shet)*. [F.]. A membranous fold connecting the posterior ends of the labia minora.

قیدالشفرتین : لیبیا مائینورا کے خلفی سروں کو ملانے والی جھلی دار تہہ۔

Foves *(fo'-vi-a)* [L. a small pit]. A small depression or fossa; particularly the fovea centralis retinae, the site of most diustinct vision.

جوف۔قعر: ایک چھوٹی سی زیریں جگہ یا فوسا۔

FPL 670. *Disodium cromoglycate (q.v.).*

ایف پی ایل ۶۷۰: ڈائی سوڈیم کروموگلائی گیٹ

Fracture *(frak'-tur)* [L. fractura]. Breach in continuity of a bone. **Bennett's f.,** of proximal end of first metacarpalinvolving the articular surface. Simulates a dislocated thumb. **closed (simple) f.,** there is no communication with external air. **Colles'f.,** of th lower end of radius giving typical 'dinner fork deformity. **comminuted f.,** the bone is broken in to several pieces. **complicated f.,** there i injury to surrounding organs and strucutures **compression f.,** usually of lumbar or dorsa region

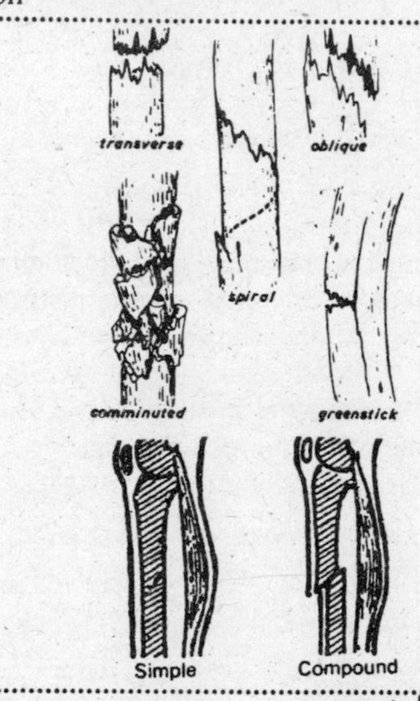

کسر۔ہڈی ٹوٹنا

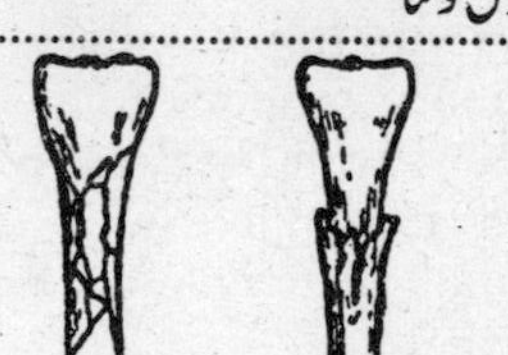

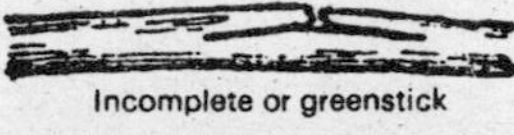

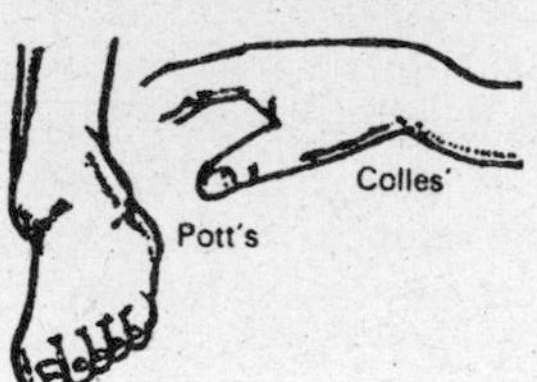

Types of fracture

due to hyperflexion of spine; the anterior vertebral bodies are crushed together, **depressed f.,** the broken bone presses on an underlying structure, such as brain or lung. **impacted f.,** one end of the broken bone is driven into the other, **incomplete f.,** the bone is only cracked or fissured--called '**greenstick f.**' when it occurs in children. open (compound) f., there is a wound permitting communication of broken bone end with air. **pathological f.,** one caused by local disease of bone. **Pott's f.,** occurs at the lower end of the fibula; often accompanied by dislocation of the tarsal bones and injury to the ligaments. **spontaneous f.,** one occurring without appreciable violence; may be synonymous with pathological f.

ہڈی ٹوٹ جانا : کمپاؤنڈ فریکچر کو مرکب کسر یا کسر مع زخم کہا جاتا ہے۔ فریکچر ڈسلوکیشن کو کسر وضع کہتے ہیں۔ ٹوٹی ہوئی (ہڈی) کو مکسور کہا جاتا ہے۔ ہڈی ٹوٹنے کی پہچان یہ ہے کہ عضو میں۔

raenotomy *(fren-ot'-om-i)* [L. frenum, bridle; G. tome, a cutting]. Surgical severance of a fraenum, particularly for tongue-tie. Also FRENOTOMY.

فرینوٹومی : بندیا فرینم کو اپریشن کے ذریعے ختم کرنا۔

raenum *(fre'-num)* [L. a bridle]. A fold of membrane which checks or limits the movement of an organ, e.g. **f. linguae,** from the undersurface of the tongue to the floor of the mouth. Also frenum.

فرینم۔ بند : جھلی کی ایک تہہ جو کسی عضو کی حرکت کو محدود کرتی ہے یا روکتی ہے۔

ragilitas *(fraj-il'-i-tas)* [l.]. Brittleness, **fragilitas** ossium, congenital disease characterized by abnormal fragility of bone, multiple fractures and a china blue colouring of the sclera.

تقصف : نازک۔ جلد ٹوٹنے والی شے۔

amboesia *(fram-be'-zi-a)*. [F. framboise, raspberry]. Yaws (q.v.).

یاز : ایک مرض۔

amycetin *(fra-mi-set'-in)*. Closely related to neomycin. Used as a local application or orally for its effect on the bowel flora.

فریمائسٹن : نیومائی سین سے مشابہ۔

Franol *(fra'-nol)*. Ephedrine hydrochloride, theophyline and phenobarbitone. For chronic bronchitis and asthma.

Franol plus, F. plus an antibistamine.

Franol expect., F. plus a mucolytic expectorant.

فرینول : دمہ کے لئے مفید۔ تھیوفائیلین کمپاؤنڈ فورٹ۔ ایک گولی ہر ۳ گھنٹے بعد۔ یہ دوا عارضی طور پر سانس ٹھیک کر دیتی ہے۔

Freamine *(fre'-a-men)*. Mainly synthetic preparation of those amino acids normally ingested as protein in egg, meat and fish.

Freiberg's disease. Osteochondritis of the second metatarsat head. [Albert Henry Freiberg. American orthopaedic surgeon, 18-68-1940].

مرض فری برگ : امریکی سرجن فریبرگ کے نام پر ایک مرض

French chalk Tale (q.v.).

فرانسیسی : کھریا ٹالکم پوڈر۔

Frenkel's exercises Exercises for tabes dorsalis to teach muscle and joint sense. [Heinrich Frenkel, Swiss neurologist, 1860-1931].

لجام تراشی : بندیا فرینم کو اپریشن کے ذریعے ختم کرنا۔

Frenquel. Azacyclonal (q.v.).

فرینکوئل : ازسائیکلونل۔

Frenulum *(fren'-u-lum)* [L. frenum, a bridle]. A small fraenum (q.v.).

لجیم : ایک چھوٹا فرینم۔

Frenum See FRAENUM.

فرینم۔ لجام۔ بند : کسی عضو کی حرکت کو روکنے یا محدود کرنے والی جھلی کی تہہ۔

Freud *(froid)*. The originator of psycho-analysis and the psychoanalytical theory of the causation of neuroses. He first described the existence of the unconscious mind, censor, repression, the theory of infantile sexuality, and worked out in detail many mental mechanisms of the unconscious which modify normal, and account for abnormal human behaviour. [Sigmund Freud, Austrian psychiatrist, 1856-1939].

فروئڈ : نفسیاتی تجزیہ کی تھیوری کا خالق۔ آسٹریا کا رہنے والا تھا۔ اس کے مطابق انسانی لاشعور میں جنسی خواہشات اور عقل میں ذہنی چپقلش رہتی ہے۔ جس سے نظام عقل درہم برہم ہو جاتا ہے۔

Freyer's operation. Suprapubic transvesical type of prostatectomy (q.v.). [Peter Johnston Freyer, English surgeon, 1851-1921].

اپریشن فیئر : اپریشن کی ایک قسم جس کا نام انگریز سرجن کے نام پر ہے۔

Friable *(fri-abl)* [L. friare, to break into small pieces.]. Easily crumbled; readily pulverized.

بھربھرا : آسانی سے ٹوٹ جانے والا۔

Friar's balsam *(fri'ars bawl'-sam)*. Ancient remedy for bronchitis. Contains benzoin, storax, aloes and balsam of Tolu, dissolved in alcohol. It is added to hot water and the vapour is inhaled. Of dubious value.

فرایئر یا بسم : برونکائیٹس کا پرانا علاج۔

Friction *(frik'-shun)* [L. fricere, to rub]. Rubbing. **friction murmur,** heard through the stethoscope when two rough or dry surfaces rub together, as in pleurisy and pericarditis.

رگڑ: چیزوں کو آپس میں رگڑنا۔

Friediander's bacillus *(Klebsiella pneumoniae)*. A large Gram-negative rod bacterium occasionally found in the upper respitaory tract, of which it can cause inflammation. Pneumonia so caused (less than 1 per-cent of all cases) is severe, with tissue necrosis andabscess formation. [Carl Friedlander, German pathologist, 1847-87].

فریڈلینڈرز بے سلس : ایک بڑا گرام منفی سلاخ جرثومہ۔ بعض دفعہ بالائی۔ تنفسی راہ میں پایا جاتا ہے اور اس سے نمونیہ بھی ہوسکتا ہے۔ تنفسی راہ میں سوزش پیدا کرتا ہے۔ ۵۵ درجے سینٹی گریڈ پر نصف گھنٹے تک رکھنے سے مر جاتے ہیں۔ پنسلین اور سلفاڈرگز ان کے لئے بے ضرر ہیں۔ سٹرپٹومائی سین موثر ہے۔

Friedreich's ataxia, A progressive familial disease of childhoo, in which there develops a selerosis of the sensory and motor columns in the spinal cord, with consequent muscular weakness and staggering (ataxia). [Nikolaus Friedreich, German neurologist, 1825-82].

موروثی لڑکھڑاہٹ : بچپن میں ہونے والی بیماری۔ اس میں عضلاتی کمزوری اور ہلکا پن پیدا ہو جاتے ہیں۔

Frigidity *(frij-id'-it-i)* [L. frigus, cold]. Lack of normal sexual desire. Used mainly in relation to the female.

جمعہ دزن۔ سرد مہری : عام جنسی خواہش کی کمی۔ مادہ کے متعلق مذکورہ اصطلاح مستعمل ہے۔ عورتوں میں خواہش کی کمی۔

Frog plaster Conservative treatment of congenital dislocation of the hip, whereby t[he] dislocation is reduced by gentle manipulati[on] and both hips are immobilized in plaster [of] Paris, botn limbs abducted to 80 degrees.

[فرا]گ پلستر: چوتڑ کا جوڑ کھل جانے کا قدیم علاج۔

Frohlich's syndrome or **dystrophia adiposo[g]enitalis** Uncommon but recognized syndro[me] resulting from anterior pituitary insufficien[cy] secondary to hypothalamic neoplas[m]. Characterized by obesity, stunted growt[h], arrested sexual development and knoc[k] knees. [Alfred Frohlich, Vienna neurologi[st], 1871-1953].

[فرو]حلیک سنڈروم: سنڈروم کی ایک قسم۔ پیدائش مرض۔ امامی پچوٹری [گلی]نڈ کے ہارمون کی کمی سے بچہ قد میں چھوٹا بہت موٹا اور جنسی طور پر کمزور۔

Frontal *(fron'-tal)* [L. frons, forehead]. Pertaining to the front of a structure; the bo[ne] of the forehead. **frontal sines,** a cavity at t[he] inner aspect of each orbital ridge on t[he] frontal bone.

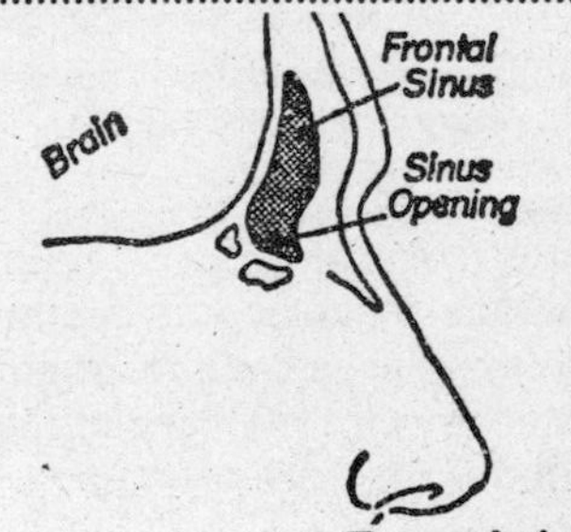

Frontal sinuses

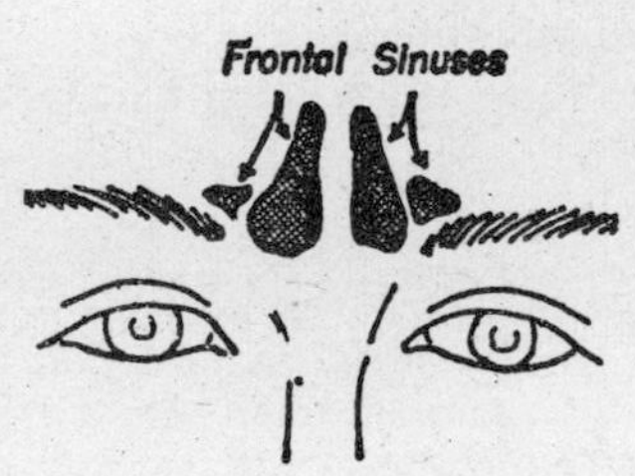

Frontal sinuse

جبہی : ساخت کے سامنے والے حصہ کے متعلق پیشانی کی ہڈی جو پرچ نما خمدار ہوتی ہے اس کی گہری سطح اندر کی طرف ہوتی ہے۔ بیرونی ابھری ہوئی سطح۔ پیشانی اور پہلو کنپٹی کا کچھ حصہ بناتے ہیں۔

ost-bite *(frost'-bit)*. Freezing of the skin and superficial tissues resulting from exposure to extreme cold. The lesion is similar to a burn and may become gangrenous.

پالا مار: انتہائی سردی کی وجہ سے جلد اور سطحی بافتوں کا جم جانا۔ بعض جسمانی خصوں میں دوران خون بند ہو جاتا ہے۔

ozen shoulder Cause unknown. Initial pain followed by stiffness, lasting several months. As pain subsides, exercises are intensified until full recovery is gained.

منجمند شانہ: پہلے درد ہوتا ہے پھر سختی آ جاتی ہے جو کئی ماہ تک رہتی ہے۔

uctose *(frunk'-tos)* [L. fructus, fruit]. A monosaccharide found with glucose in plants. It is the sugar in honey and is a constituent of cane sugar. Syn., laevulose.

قندمیوہ: ایک مونوسیکرائڈ جو پودوں میں گلوکوس کے ساتھ پایا جاتا ہے۔ شہد اور گنے کی شکر کا جزو۔

usemide *(fru'-se-mid)*. Produces prompt and effective diuresis. Lasts approximately 4 h after oral administration, and 2 h after parenteral administration. Valuable in pulmonary and cerebral oedema, and in congestive heart failure when the response to other diuretics is inadequate. Acts by inhibition of active chloride transport in the thick limb of the loop of Henle. It has been reported to cause a fall in glomerular filtration rate during diuresis. In consequence, handling of drugs which are removed from the body predominantly by glomerular filtration may be altered by coincidental frusemide therapy. Potassium supplements are given routinely in prolonged f. therapy.

فرد سے مائیڈ: موثر تے آور دوا۔ لازکس۔ ہائی بلڈ پریشر میں اس کی ایک تا دو گولیاں روزانہ۔

SH. Follicle stimulating hormone. See FOLLICLE.

ایف ایس ایچ: فولیکل کو تحریک دینے والا ہارمون۔

icidin *(fu'-i-din)*. Sodium salt of fusidic acid. A steroid antibiotic with high activity against Staphylococcus. Can be given intravenously, orally or locally.

فیوسیڈن : فیوسیڈک ایسڈ کا سوڈیم نمک۔ سٹرائیڈ اینٹی بیاٹک جو سٹیفائلوکاکس کے خلاف کام کرتا ہے۔

Fugue *(fug)* [L. fuga, a fleeing from]. An attempt to escape from reality. A period of loss of memory.

فرار: حقیقت سے بھاگنے کی کوشش۔ یادداشت ضائع ہونے کا عرصہ۔

Fulguration *(ful-gur-a'-shun)*. [L. fulgur, lightening]. Destruction of tissue by diathermy.

لمعان۔ برقی خشکاؤ: نسیج کی تباہی۔

Full term. Mature--when pregnancy has lasted 40 weeks.

فل ٹرم: جب حمل کو چالیس ہفتے ہو جائیں۔

Fulminant *(ful'-min-ant)*; fluminating (ful'-min-a-ting) [L. fulminare, to thunder and lighten]. Developing quickly and with an equally rapid termination.

Fumigation *(fu-mi-ga'-shun)* [L. fumigare, to smoke]. Disinfection by exposure to the fumes of a vaporized disinfectant.

دھونی: دافع تعفن کے بخارات سے تعفن دور کرنا۔

Function *(fung'-shun)* [L. functio, performance]. The special work performed by an organ or structure in its normal state.

فعل : مخصوص کام جو کوئی عضو یا ساخت اپنی نارمل حالت میں انجام دیتی ہے۔

Functional *(fungk'-shun-al)*. In general sense, pertaining to function. Disorder of the function but not the structure of an organ. As psychiatric term, of neurotic origin, i.e. psychogenic, without primary organic disease.

فعلی۔ تفاعلی: کام یا فعل سے متعلق۔ کام کا صحیح نہ ہونا۔ لیکن عضو کی ساخت صحیح ہوتی ہے۔

Fundus *(fun'-dus)* [L. bottom]. The basal portion of a hollow structure; the part which is distal to the opening--fundi, pl.; fundal, adj.

قاعہ : کسی کھوکھلی ساخت کا اساسی حصہ۔ سوراخ سے دور حصہ۔

Fungicide *(fun'-ji-sid)* [L. fungus, mushroom; coedere, to kill]. An agent which is lethal to fungi--fungicidal, adj.

فطرکش: سماروغ کے لئے مہلک عامل۔

Fungiform *(fun'-ji-form)* [L. fugus, mushroom; forma, form]. Resembling a mushroom.

فطرنما: کھمبی سے مشابہ۔

Fungilin *(fun'-ji-lin)*. Amphotericin B (q.v.).

فنجیلن : ایمفوٹیری سن۔

Fungistatic *(fun-ji-stat'-ik)* [L. fungus, mushroom; G. staikos, causing to stand]. An agent which inhibits the growth of fungi.

مانع نموئے فطر: سماروغ کی نشوونما کو روکنے والا عامل۔

Fungizone *(fung'-i-zon)*. Amphotericin B (q.v.).

Fungus *(fung'-gus)* [L. mushroom]. A low form of vegetable life including many microscopic organisms capable of producing superficial and systemic disease in man. **ray f.**, the original term for the Actinomyces genus, descriptive of the radial arrangement of the filaments which make up the 'sulphur granules' or colonies of the organism in pus. See ACTINOMYCOSIS. RINGWORM--fungi, pl.; fungal, adj.

فطر۔ سماروغ۔ حرام گوشت۔: نباتی حیات کی ایک زیریں قسم۔ جس میں کئی خوردبینی جسیمے بھی شامل ہیں۔ بہت سے انسان میں بیماریاں پیدا کرنے کے اہل۔ ان میں کھوروفل نہیں ہوتا۔ اس لئے اپنی خوراک بنانے کے ناقابل۔ طفیلی یا گندخور بذرے بہت زیادہ تعداد میں بناتے ہیں۔

Funiculitis *(fu-nik-u-li'-tis)* [L. funis, a cord; G. -itis, inflammation]. Inflammation of the spermatic cord.

ورم حبل منی: منوی ڈوری کی سوزش۔

Funiculus *(fu-nik'-u-lus)*. [L.]. A cord-like structure.

ناڑ۔ بندناف: ایک ڈوری نما ساخت۔

Funnel chest, A congenital deformity in which the breast-bone is depressed towards the spine. (Pectus excavatum).

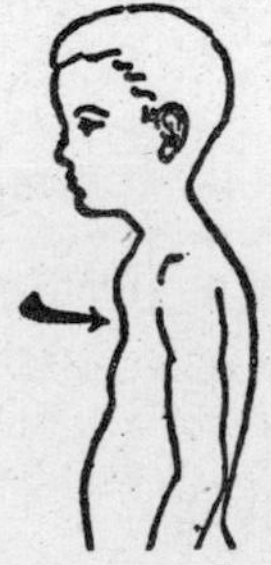

Funnel chest in rickets

فی چھاتی : ایک نقص کی ہدی جس میں چھاتی کی ہڈی سپائن کی طرف ب جاتی ہے۔

Furacin *(fu'-ra-sin)*. Nitrofurazone (q.v.). Available as dressings or ointment.

وراسین: نائٹروفیورازون۔ ڈریسنگ یا مرہم کی صورت میں ملتی ہے اگر گ سے جل کر پیپ پڑ جائے تو یہ مرہم لگائیے۔ الیکٹرک برن میں زخم پر لگا کر پٹی باندھئے۔ مفید برائے اپسے ٹائیگو

Furadantin *(fu-ra-dan'-tin)*. Nitrofurantio (q.v.).

وراڈینٹین : نائٹروفیورنٹائن۔ گردے اور مثانہ کی انفیکشن میں مفید وائی۔

Furamide *(fu'-ra-mid)* Diloxanide furoat (q.v.).

ورامائیڈ: ڈائی لوکسانائیڈ فیوروایٹ

Furazolidone *(fu-ra-zol'-i-don)*. Used fo non-specific diarrhoeas, bacillary dysenter and bacterial food poisoning.

ورازولیڈون: غیر مخصوص اسہال کے لئے مستعمل۔ جراثیمی پیچش اور راثیمی خوراک کے زہریلے پن میں بھی استعمال ہوتی ہے۔ فیوروکسن۔

Furor *(fur-or')* [L.]. Fury, madness, range.

نون۔ شور۔ غیظ: غصہ۔ پاگل پن۔ لاطینی لفظ ہے۔

Furoxone *(fu-roks'-on)*. Furazolidone (q.v.).

ورکسون: فیورازولیڈون۔ غیر مخصوص اسہال، جراثیمی پیچش اور جراثیمی وراک کے زہریلے پن میں مستعمل۔ دست روکنے کے لئے ۲ گولیاں۔

Furuncle *(fur'-ung-kl)* [L. furunculus, boil]. Se BOIL.

ل: آبلہ یا چھالا۔

Furunculosis *(fur-ung-ku-lo'-sis)* [L. *furunculus,* boil; G. *-osis,* condition]. A conditio of affliction due to boils.

ملیت: آبلوں کی وجہ سے تکلیف کی حالت۔

Furunculus orientalis *(fur-un'-ku-lus o-ri-en-ta'-lis)*. Oriental sore (q.v.).

ل: مشرق کا پھوڑا۔

Fusiform *(fu'-zi-form)* [L. fusus, a spindle forma, shape]. Resembling a spindle.

کلہ نما: تکلا سے مشابہ۔

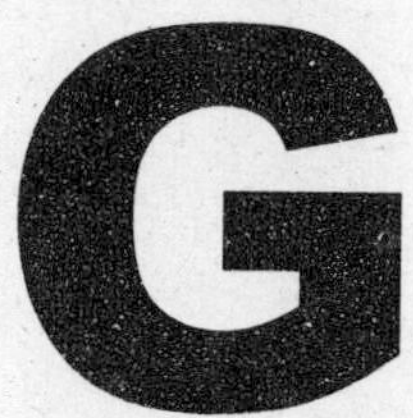

Symbol for Gravitational Constant, Gibbs free energy and Gravitational Force.

جی: علامت ہے تجاذبی مستقل، گبز فری توانائی اور تجاذبی قوت کی۔

Symbol ffor gram, standard gravity.

جی: علامت ہے گرام کی اور معیاری کثافت کی۔

(gamma) The third letter of the Greek alphabet and is a symbol for heavy chain of aminoglobin and the γ chain of fetal hemoglobin also symbol for microgram (μg).

گیما: یونانی حروف تہجی کا تیسرا حرف۔ امینوگلوبن کی بھاری زنجیر کا جزو اور فیٹل ہیموگلوبن کا گیما چین۔ مائیکروگرام کی علامت۔

ag *(gag)* A surgical device for holding the mouth open, to velch, to vomit.

کف گیر: منہ کھلا رکھنے کے لئے دانتوں کے درمیان رکھنے والا آلہ۔

ait *(ga't)* The manner or style of walking **atom g.** an unsteady, uncoordinated walk, like staggering cerebellar gait. **scissor g.** a gait in which one foot is passed in front of the other, producing a cross legged progression. **spastic g.** paraplegic spasltic gait.

چال: چلنے کا انداز۔ کسی کے چلنے کا مخصوص طریقہ۔

alactacrasia *(ga-lak'ta-kra-sha)* [G. *galact,* milk; *a,* neg.; *krasis,* mixture]. Abnormal condition of the breast milk.

خراب شیر: شیر یا دودھ کی خراب حالت یا ملاوٹ والا دودھ۔

alactagogue *(ga-la'k-ta-gog)* [G. *agogue,* enhance]. Promoting the flo of milk. An agent that enhances the flow of milk.

شیر افزا: عامل جس سے دودھ کا بہاؤ شروع یا تیز ہوتا ہے۔

Galectischia *(ga-lak-tis-kea)* [G. *ischein,* to suppress]. Suppression of the secretion of milk.

رکاوٹ سیلان شیر: دودھ کے بہاؤ میں یا خارج ہونے میں کمی ہو جائے یا رک جائے۔

Galactocele *(ga-lak-to-sel)* [G. *kele',* tumor]. Cystic enlargement of the mammary gland, containing milk. A hydrocele filled with a milky fluid.

شیری قیلہ: دودھ یا دودھ سے مشابہ سیال پر مشتمل سسٹ۔

Galactometer *(ga-lak-tom-e'-ter)* An instrument for measuring the specific gravity of milk.

گلیکٹو میٹر: دودھ کی کثافت اضافی ماپنے کے لئے آلہ۔

Galactophoritis *(ga-lak'-to-for-i-tis)* [G. *phorein,* to milk; *itis,* inflammation]. Inflammation of the milk ducts.

سوزش نالی دودھ: دودھ کی نالیوں کی سوزش ہو جانا۔

Galactorrhoea *(ga-lak-to-re-a)* [G. *rhoia,* flow] Excessive or spontaneous flow of milk, persistant secretion of milk irrespecttive of nursing.

سیلانِ شیر: دودھ کا زائد بہاؤ۔

Galactosaemia *(ga-lak-to-se-mia)* Excess of galactose in the blood. Normally laktase present in small intestine converts lactose into glucose and galactose into glucose. In absence of these enzymes galactose is not converted to glucose. It is a congeniter defect.

گلیکٹو سیمیا: خون میں گلیکٹوز کی زیادتی۔ چھوٹی آنت میں لیکٹیز لیکٹوز کو گلوکوز اور گلیکٹوز میں تبدیل کر دیتا ہے۔

Gallie's operation *(gal'-es)*. The use of fascial strips from the thigh for radical cure after reduction of a hernia . [William Edward Gallie, surgeon of Toronto, Canada, 1882-1959].

اپریشن گیلی: ہرنیا میں تخفیف کے بعد علاج کے لئی ران سے سٹرپ کا استعمال۔ کینیڈا کے سرجن ایڈورڈ گیلی پر اس کا نام رکھا گیا ہے۔

Gallipot *(gal'-i-pot)*. A small vessel for lotions.

مرتبان: لوشن کے لئے ایک چھوٹا برتن۔

Galls *(gawls')* . The excrescences which form on certain oak trees, and from which tannic acid (q.v.). is obtained. Ung. Gallae c Opio is an astringent cintment used mainly for haemorrhoids.

گالس: شاہ بلوط کے بعض درختوں سے خارج ہونی والا مادہ جس سے ٹینک ایسڈ حاصل کیا جاتا ہے۔

Galvanocauterization *(gal-van'-o-kaw-ter-i-za'-shun)*. The use of a wire heated by galvanic current to desroy tissue.

گلوینو کاٹیرائیزیشن: نسیج تباہ کرنے کے لئے گرم تار کا استعمال۔

Galvanometer *(gal-van-om'-et-er)*. An instrument for measuring an electrical current.

برقی روپیما: بجلی کی پیائش کے لئے ایک آلہ۔

Gamete *(ga'-met)* [G. gamein, to marry]. A male or female reproductive cell. See OVA. SPERMATAZOON.

گیمجی : جاذب کا ایک برانڈ۔ گاز میں سفید کپاس۔

Gamma-benzene hexachloride *(gam'-a ben'-zen heks-a-klor'-id)* Used as shampoo for treatment of head lice. Less irritant than benzyl benzoate for scabies; requires only one application.

Gamma-encephalography *(gam-ma-en-ke-f-al-og'- ra-fi)* [gamma, G. third letter of alphabet; egkephalos, brain]. A small dose of isotope is given. It is concentrated in many cerebral tumours. The pattern of radioactivity is then measured.

گیما اینکیفالوگرافی: آئی سوٹوپ کی تھوڑی سی خوراک دی جاتی ہے۔ پھر سربرل ناسوروں میں تابکاری کی پیمائش کی جاتی ہے۔

Gammaglobulin *(gam-ma-glob'-u-lin)*. One of the several protein globulins (A. D,E, G and M). Often referred to as immunoglobulins, abbreviated to IgA, etc. They take part in various immune responses of the body to antigens, which can be bacteria, when we speak of immunity; a foreign substance, when we speak of allergy; a substance produced by the body, when we speak of autoimmunity. When the substance produced by the body is in response to transposed tissue, e.g. organ transplant, we speak of rejection. **anti-D g.** (anti-Rh_0) clears injected Rh-positive cells from the recipient's circulation. Used to prevent formation of antibodies in an Rh-negative mother delivered of an Rh-positive baby.

گیما گلوبولن: مختلف پروٹین گلوبولنز میں سے ایک (اے۔ ڈی۔ ای۔ جی اور ایم)

Gammexane *(gam'-eks-an)*. A powerful insecticide similar to DDT. but not so toxic.

گیمیکسین : ایک کرم کش دوا جو طاقتور ہوتی ہے لیکن ڈی ڈی ٹی ایس زہریلی نہیں ہوتی۔

Ganglion *(gang'-li-on)* [G. a swelling]. 1. A mass of nerve tissue forming a subsidiary nerve centre which receives and sends out nerve fibres, e.g. the ganglionic masses forming the sympathetic nervous system. 2. Localized cyst-like swelling near a tendon, sheath or joint. Contains a clear, tredansparent gelatinous or colloid substance; sometimes occurs on the back of the wrist due to strain such as excessive practice on the piano. 3. An enlargement on the course of a nerve such as is found on the receptor nerves before they enter the spinal cord. 4. an enlarged lymphatic gland. **Gasserian g.,** deeply situated within the skull, on the sensory root of the fifth cranial nerve. It is involved in trigeminal neuralgia--ganglia, pl.; ganglionic, adj. [Johann Leurentus Gasser, Professor of Anatomy in Vienna, 1723-63].

عقدہ۔ غدہ غصب : برآمدگی (۱) عصبی نسیج کا اکٹھ۔ (۲) ایک سسٹک سور۔ (۳) عصب کا بڑھا ہوا حصہ۔ (۴) بڑھی ہوئی لمفیٹک گلینڈ۔

anglionectomy *(gang-li-on-ek'-tom-i)* [G. ganglion, swelling; ektome, a cutting]. Surgical excision of a ganglion.

گینگلیان ایکٹومی: ابھار کو اپریشن کے ذریعے کاٹنا۔

angliosidosis *(gang-li-o-sid-o'-sis)*. See TAY-SACHS' DISEASE.

angrene *(gang'-gren)* [G. gag-graina]. Death of part of the tissues of the body. Usually the result of inadequate blood supply, but occasionally due to direct injury (traumatic g.) or infection (e.g. gas g.). Deficient blood supply may result from pressure on blood vessels (e.g. tourniquets, tight bandages and swelling of a limb), from obstruction within healthy vessels (e.g. arterial embolism; frost-bite, where the capillaries become blocked), from spasm of the vessel wall (e.g. ergot poisoning), or from thrombosis due to disease of he vessel wall (e.g. arteriosclerosis in arteries; phlebitis in veins). **dry g.,** occurs when the drainage of blood from the affected part is adequate; the tissues become shrunken and black. **moist g.** occurs when venous drainage is inadequate so that the tissues are wollen with fluid--gangrenous, adj.

خورہ: جسمانی بافتوں کے حصے کی موت۔ گوشت کا مردہ ہو جانا۔ خشک۔ تر گیس گینگرین ہوتا ہے۔ مردہ عضو میں دوران خون بند ہوتا قوت حسن ناپید گوشت کی رنگت میں تبدیلی اور حرکت سے محروی ہو جاتی ہے اور وہ عضو ٹھنڈا ہو جاتا ہے۔

nser state *(gan'-ser)*. A hysterical ondition--simulating dementia, approximate nswers to questions are given which show at the correct answers are known.

trisin *(gan'-tri-sin)*. Sulphafurazoir (q.v.).

denal *(gar'-den-al)*. Phenobarbitone (q.v.).

گارڈی نال: فینوباربیٹون۔ لیمی نال۔ اس کی ایک گولی دن میں ۳ دفعہ برائے مرگی یا اپی لیسی۔

gle *(gar'-gl)*. The act of washing the throat. solution used for washing the throat.

غرغرہ۔ غرارہ: گلا دھونے کا طریقہ۔ گلا دھونے کے لئے مستعمل ایک محلول۔

goylism *(gar-goul-izm)* [L. gurgulio, gullet]. ongenital mucopolysaccharide disorder of metabolism with recessive or sex-linked inheritance. The polysaccharides chondroitin sulphate 'B' and heparitin sulphate are excreted in the urine. Characterized by skeletal abnormalities, coarse features, enlarged liver and spleen, mental subnormality. ACTH useful. Hunter-Hurler syndrome.

گیرگائلزم: پیشاب میں وپلی سیکرائیڈز کونڈرائٹن سلفیٹ بی اور ہیپریٹین سلفیٹ خارج ہوتے ہیں۔ جنس سے ملحقہ وراثت میں چلنے والی بیماری۔ جگر اور تلی بڑھ جاتے ہیں۔ دماغ کمزور ہوتا ہے۔ خدو خال بھدے ہوتے ہیں۔ ہڈیوں کا ڈھانچہ نارمل نہیں ہوتا۔ اے سی ٹی ایچ مفید ہے۔

Garoin. Phenytoin sodium and phenobarbitone sodium. For grand-mal epilepsy, psychomotor seizures.

گیروئن: فنائٹائن سوڈیم اور فینوباربیٹون سوڈیم۔

Gartner's bacillus *(Salmonella enteritidis)*. A motile Gram-negative rod bacterium, widely distributed in domestic and wild animals, particularly rodents, and sporadic in man as a cause of food poisoning [August Gartner, German bacteriologist, 1848-1934].

گارٹنرس بیلس: ایک متحرک گرام منفی سلاخی جرثومہ جو خوراک کو زہریلا کرتا ہے۔

Gas One of the three states of matter. It retains neither shape nor volume when, released. **gas and air analgesia,** an authorized inhalation to lessen the pain of uterine contraction in labour. **laughing g.,** nitrous oxide (q.v.). **marsh g.,** methane, liberated in the activated sludge method of sewage disposal and converted into electricity--gaseous adj.

گیس۔ غار: مادہ کی تین حالتوں میں سبس ے ایک۔ اس کی کوئی شکل نہیں ہوتی۔

Gas gangrene A wound is infected by anaerobic organisms, especially Clostridium welchii, normally found in the intestine of man and animals, consequently there are many sources from which infection can arise, including operation on the intestine. See GANGRENE.

Gasserectomy *(gas-er-ek'-to-mi)*. Surgical excision of the Gasserian ganglion (q.v.).

گیسری عقدہ براری: گیسرین کو ابھار کر بذریعہ اپریشن کاٹنا۔

Gastralgia *(gas-tral'-ji-a)* [G. gaster, belly; algos, pain]. Pain in the stomach.

دردمعدہ: معدہ میں درد۔

Gastrectomy *(gas-trek'-to-mi)* [G. gaster, belly; ektome, excision]. Removal of a part or the whole of the stomach. **billroth I** is a partial g., least commonly performed and usually reserved for ulcer on the lesser curvature. **polyapartial g.** (known in America as **billroth II**) is the most commonly performed g. Used for doudenal ulcer and as a palliative procedure for gastric cancer. Transverse colon and its mesentery intervene between stomach and jejunum. A hole can be made

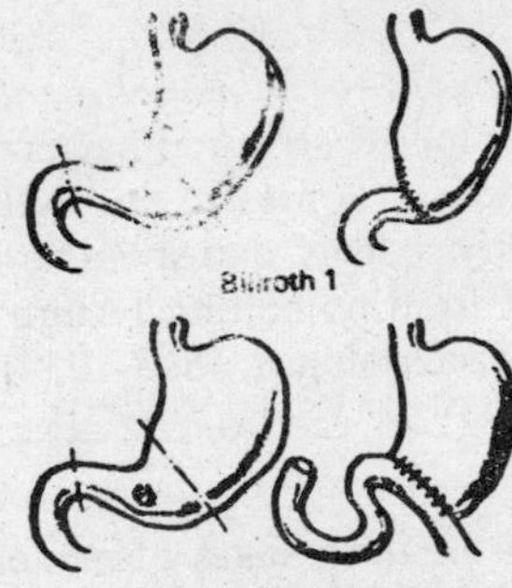

Types of gastrectomy

in the mesentery so that the anastomosis lies behind the transverse colon, **retrocolic g.**; or the loop of jejunum can be lifted up anterior to the transverse colon, **antecolic g. total g.**, is carried out only for cancer of the stomach. See ROUX-EN-Y OPERATION.

معدہ براری: سارا معدہ یا اس کا ایک حصہ ختم کرنا۔

Gastric *(gas'-trik)* [G. gaster, belly]. Pertaining to the stomach. **gastric crisis,** see CRISIS. **gastric juice** is acid in reaction and contains two proteolytic enzymes. **gastric influenza,** a term used when gastrointestinal symptoms predominate.**gastric suction,** may be intermittent or continuous to keep the stomach empty after some abdominal operations .**gastric ulcer,** see ULCER.

Gast

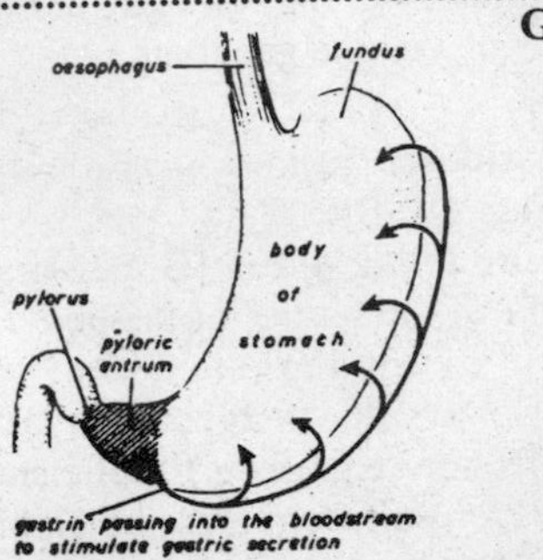

سٹرین: ایک ہارمون جس سے گیسٹرک جوس کے بہاؤ میں اضافہ ہوتا

Gastritis *(gas-tri'-tis)* [G. gaster, belly; -i inflammation]. Inflammation of the stoma especially the mucous membrane lining.

ش معدہ: معدہ کی سوزش۔

Gastrocnemius *(gas-trok-ne'-mi-us)* [G. gas belly; kneme, tibia]. The large two-hea muscle of the calf.

ساق: بچھڑے کا دوسر والا بڑا عضلہ۔ پنڈلی کا مضبوط عضلہ جو چلنے م آتا ہے۔

Gastrocolic *(gas-tro-kol'-ik)* [G. gaster, be kolon, colon]. Pertaining to the stomach the colon **gastrocolic refex,** sensory stim arising on entry of food into stomach, r lting in strong peristaltic waves in the colo

قولونی: معدہ اور قولون سے متعلق۔

Gastroduodenal *(gas-tro-du-o-den'-al)* gaster, belly; L. duodeni, twelve at on Pertaining to the stomach and duodenum.

اثنا عشری: معدہ اور ڈیوڈینیم سے متعلق۔

Gastroduodenostomy *(gas-tro-du- en-os'-to-mi)* [G. gaster, belly; L. duoc twelve at once; G. stoma, mouth]. A sur anastomosis between the stomach anc duodenum.

عجی تفویہ: معدہ اور ڈیوڈینیم کے درمیان بذریعہ اپریشن منہ بنانا۔

Gastrodynia *(gas-tro-din'-i-a)* [G. gaster, b odyne, pain]. Pain in the stomach.

درد معدہ: معدہ میں درد یا تکلیف۔

astroenteritis *(gas-tro-en-ter-i'-tis)* [G. gaster, belly; enteron, intestine; -itis, inflammation]. Inflammation of mucous membranes of stomach and small intestine; although sometimes the result of dietetic error, the cause is usually a bacterial infection.

ورم معدہ یا امعا: معدہ اور چھوٹی آنت کی میوکس جھلی کی سوزش۔ جس کی وجہ عموماً جراثیم ہوتے ہیں۔

astroenterology *(gas-tro-en-ter-ol'-o-ji)* [G. gaster, belly; enteron, intestine; logos, discourse]. Study of the stomach and intestines and their diseases-- gastroenterological, adj.; gastroenterologically, adv.

گیسٹر وانٹر الوجی: معدہ، آنتوں اور ان کی بیماریوں کا مطالعہ۔

astroenteropathy *(gas-tro-en-te-rop'-a-thi)* [G. gaster, belly; enteron, intestine; pathos, disease]. Disease of the stomach and intestine--gastroent- eropathic, adj.

گیسٹر وانٹر وپیتھی: معدہ اور آنت کی بیماری۔

astroenteroscope *(gas-tro-en'-ter-o-skop)* [G. gaster, belly; enteron, intestine; skopein, to examine]. An endoscope (q.v.). for visualization of stomach and intestine--gestroenteroscopic, adj.; gastroenteroscopically, adv.

گیسٹر وانٹر وسکوپ: معدہ اور آنت کے لئے اینڈوسکوپ۔

astroenterostomy *(gas-tro-en-ter-os'-to-mi)* [G. gaster, belly; enteron, intestine; stoma, mouth]. A surgical anastomosis between the stomach and small intestine.

معدی معوی تفویہ: معدہ اور چھوٹی آنت کے درمیان بذریعہ آپریشن منہ بنانا۔

strografin *(gas-tro-gra'-fin)*. Sodium and meglumine diatrizoates Can be used ealry in patients with haematemesis. Its detergent and purgative effects are used in meconium ileus, when it is given as an enema.

گیسٹر وگریفن: ایکسرے سے پہلے پانی میں حل پذیر تابکاری سے غیر شفاف آیوڈین دی جاتی ہے۔

strointestinal *(gas-tro-in-tes-tin'-al)* [G. gaster, belly; L. intestinum, intestine]. Pertaining to the stomach and intestine.

معدی معوی: معدہ اور آنت سے متعلق۔

Gastrojejunostomy *(gas-tro-je-joon-os'-to-mi)* [G. gaster, belly; L. jejunus, empty; stoma, mouth]. A surgical anastomosis between the stomach and the jejunum.

معدی صائمی تفویہ: معدہ اور جیجونم کے درمیان بذریعہ اپریشن منہ بنانا۔

Gastro-oesophageal *(gas-tro-e-sof'-a-jel)* [G. gaster, belly; oisophagos, gullet]. Pertaining to the stomach and oesophagus as g. reflux in heartburn.

گیسٹر وایسوفیجیل: معدہ اور ایسوفیگس سے متعلق۔

Gastropathy *(gas-troip'-ath-i)* [G. gaster, belly; pathos, disease]. Any disease of the stomach.

مرض معدہ: معدہ کی کوئی بھی بیماری۔

Gastropexy *(gas-tro-peks'-i)* [G. gaster, belly; pexein, to clip fix]. Surgical fixation of a displaced stomach.

معدی بطنی تثبیت: متبادل معدہ بذریعہ اپریشن لگانا۔

Gastrophrenic *(gas-tro-fren'-ik)* [G. gaster, belly; phren, midriff]. Pertaining to the stomach and diaphragm.

معدی حجابی: معدہ اور ڈایافرام سے متعلق۔

Gastroplasty *(gas'-tro-plas-ti)* [G. gaster, belly; plassein, to form]. Any plastic operation on the stomach. Currently used for reconstruction of the cardiac orifice of the stomach, where fibrosis prevents replacement below the diaphragm in cases of hiatus hernia.

معدہ پیوندی: معدہ کا کوئی پلاسٹک اپریشن۔

Gastroplication *(gas-tro-plik-a'-shun)* [G. gaster, belly; L. plicare, to fold]. An operation for the cure of dilated stomach by pleating the wall.

معدی تثنیت: پھیلے ہوئے معدے کے علاج کے لئے اپریشن۔

Gastroptosis *(gas-trop-to'-sis)* [G. gaster, belly; ptosis, a falling]. Downward displacement of the stomach.

سقوط معدہ: معدے کا زیریں جانب تبادلہ۔

Gastropylorectomy *(gas-tro-pi-lor-e-k'-to-mi)*[G. gaster, belly; pylouros, gate keeper; ektome, excision]. Excision of the pyloric end of the stomach.

تواب براری: معدہ کا پائیلورک سرا کاٹنا۔

Gastroscope *(gas'-tro-skop)* [G. gaster, belly; skopein, to examine]. See ENDOSCOPE--gastroscopic, adj.; gastroscopy, n.

معدہ بین: اینڈوسکوپ۔

Gastroistomy *(gas-tros'-to-mi)* [G. gaster, belly; stoma, mouth]. A surgically established fistula between the stomach and the exterior abdominal wall; usually for artificial feeding.

معدہ تفویہ: مصنوعی طریقے سے خوراک کھلانے کے لئے معدہ اور بیرونی بطنی دیوار کے ذریعے بذریعہ اپریشن قائم کیا گیا فسٹولا۔

Gastrotomy *(gas-trot'-o-mi)* [G. gaster, belly; tome, a cutting]. Incision into the stomach.

معدہ شگافی: معدہ میں شگاف لگانا۔

Gastrula *(gas'-troo-la)*. Next stage after blastula in embryonic development

Gaucher's disease *(go'-sha)*. A rare familial disorder mainly in Jewish children, characterized by a disordered lipoid metabolism (lipid reticulosis) and usually accompanied by very marked enlargement of the spleen. Diagnosis follows sternal marrow puncture and the finding of typical Gaucher cells (distended with lipoid). [Phillippe Charles Ernest Gaucher, French physician, 1854-1918].

قلت الامِ طحالی: اس بیماری میں تلی بڑھ جاتی ہے۔

Gauze *(gawz)*. A thin open-meshed material used in all surgical procedures.

گاز۔ جالی: تمام اپریشنوں میں مستعمل۔

Gee's linctus *(jez ling'-tus)* [L. linctus, a licking]. A cough suppressant containing camphorated tincture of opium, squill and syrup of Tolu balsam. [Samuel Gee, British physician, 1839-1911].

جیز لنکٹس: کھانسی دبانے والی دوا۔

Gefarnate *(gef'-ar-nat)*. Heals gastric ulcer.

Gefarnil *(gef'-ar-nil)*. Gefarnate (q.v.).

عداد ججر رطلر: تابکاری معلوم کرنے اور اس کا اندراج کرنے کا آلہ۔

Gelatine *(e) (jel'-a-ten)* [L. gelare, to freeze]. The protein-containing, glue-like substance obtained by boiling bones, skins and other animal tissues. Used as a base for pessaries as the adhesive constituent of Unna's paste and in jellies and pastilles--gelatinous, adj.

لاٹین: پروٹین پر مشتمل مادہ جو ہڈیوں۔ کھال اور دوسری حیوانی بافتوں کو ل کر حاصل کیا جاتا ہے۔

Gene *(jen)* [G. genesis, decent]. A factor in the chromosome responsible for transmission c hereditary characteristics. **dominant g.,** capable of transmitting its characteristic irrespective of the genes from the other paren t, **recessive g.,** can transmit characteristic only if they are present in a similar recessiv g. from the other parent.

ن۔ مورثہ: کروموسوم میں ایک فیکٹر جو توراثی خصوصیت کا انتقال کا ذمہ ہے۔

Geneal paralysis of the insane; (GPI). Involv ment of the brain by syphrilitic infection wi consequent dementia. The onset may be slo or rapid; loss of memory is an early sign a there is disintegration of the personality. S BACTERIOTHERAPY. MALARIA THERAPY.

شکی شلل: ایک دماغی مرض۔ اولین نشانی یادداشت کا ضیاع ہے۔ پھر یت ٹوٹ پھوٹ جاتی ہے۔

Generative *(jen'-er-at-iv)* [L. generare, beget]. Pertaining to reproduction.

یدی: تولید سے متعلق۔

Genetic code *(jen-et'-ik kod)*. Name given arrangement of genetic material stored in DNA molecule of the chromosome.

Genetics *(jen-et'-iks)* [G. genesis, descen Study of the part played by nuclear a extranuclear cellular structures in hum heredity.

یات، علم تکوین، تکوینیات: انسانی توارث میں مرکزائی اور بروں ائی خلوی ساختوں کے حصے یعنی ان کی شرکت کا مطالعہ۔

Genital *(jen-it-al)* [G. genesis, descer Pertaining to the organs of generation.

ل: نسل کے اعضاء سے متعلق۔

Genitalia *(jen-it-a'-li-a)* [G.]. The organs generation.

ائے تناسل: نسل کے اعضاء۔

enitocrural *(jen-it-o-kroo'-ral)*[L. genitalis, from gignere, to beget; crus, leg]. Pertaining to the genital area and the leg.

تناسلی بولی: تولیدی وبولی اعضاء سے متعلق۔

enome *(jen'-om)* [G. genos, birth]. A complete set of chromosomes derived from one parent.

enophylin *(jen-of'-il-in)*. Aminophylline (q.v.).

جینوفلن: امینوسیلن۔

enotype *(jen'-o-tip)* . The inherent endowment of the individual.

نسلی نوع: فرد کی توارثی خصوصیات۔

entamicin *(jen'-ta-mi-sin)* Antibiotic produced by Micromonospora purpurea. Antibacterial, especially against Pseudomonas and staphylococci resistant to other antibiotics. Given intramuscularly and as eye and ear drops. Ototoxis and dangerous in renal failure.

جینٹامائی سین: اینٹی بایوٹک۔ جراثیم کے لئے تباہ کن انکھوں اور کانوں کے ڈراپس یا قطروں کی صورت میں مستعمل۔

entian violet *(jen'-shun)*. A brilliant violet-coloured, antiseptic, aniline dye. Syn., crystal violet (q.v.).

enticin *(jen'-tis-in)*. Gentamicin (q.v.).

جینٹیئین: جینٹامن۔

enu *(jen'-u)* [L.]. The knee. genu valgum, knock- knee. genu varum, bowleg.

زانو: گھٹنا۔

enus *(je'-nus)* [L race]. A classification ranking between the family (higher) and the species (lower).

جنس: خاندان اور نوع کے درمیان جماعت بندی میں ایک درجہ۔ قریبی انواع ایک ہی جنس میں رکھی جاتی ہیں۔ مثلاً شیر ببر، سیر، بلی کو ایک ہی جنس میں رکھا گیا ہے جو فیلس ہے اسی طرح سرسوں، شلجم اور گوبھی کو ایک ہی جنس براسیکا میں رکھا گیا ہے کئی جنس مل کر ایک خاندان بناتے ہیں۔

riatrician *(jer-i-at-rish'n)* [G. geras, old age]. One who specializes in geriatrics.

جیری ایٹریشن: بڑھاپے اور بڑھاپے کی بیماریوں کا ماہر۔

riatrics *(jer-i-at'-riks)* [G. geras, old age; iatrikos, healing]. The branch of medical science dealing with old age and its diseases.

بوڑھوں کا معالجہ، طبیہ: میڈیکل سائنس کی وہ شاخ جو بڑھاپے اور اس کی بیماری سے بحث کرتی ہے۔

Germ *(jerm)* [L. germen bud]. A unicellular micro-organism, especially used for a pathogen.

جرم۔ جرثومہ: ایک ایک خلوی خورد جسیمہ۔

German measles See RUBELLA.

جرمن خسرہ۔ چھوٹا خسرہ۔ روبیلا: خسرہ کی ایک قسم۔

Germicide *(jer'-mi-sid)* [L. germen, bud; coedere, to kill]. An agent which kills germs--germicidal, adj.

جراثیم کش: جراثیم کو ہلاک کرنے والا عامل۔

Gerontology *(jer-on-tol'-oj-i)* [G. geron, old man; logos, discourse]. The scientific study of aging-- gerontological, adj.

علم پیراں: بڑھاپے کا سائنسی مطالعہ۔

Gestation *(jes-ta'-shun)* [L. gestare, to carry]. Pregnancy--gestational, adj. ectopic g., extrauterine pregnancy, usually in the Fallopian tube.

حمل: حمل یا وضع حمل۔

Gestyl *(jes'-til)*. Serum gonadotrophin.

جیسٹل: سیرم گونیڈوٹرافن۔

Ghon focus. Primary lesion of tuberculosis in lung. [Anton Ghon, Austrian pathologist, 1866-1936].

گونز فوکس: پھیپھڑے میں تپ دق کا اولین زخم۔

GH-RIH. Growth-hormone-release-inhibiting hormone. See SOMATOSTATIN.

Giant cell arteritis See ARTERITIS.

Giardiasis *(ji-ar-di'-a-sis)*. Infection with the flagellate Giardia intestinalis. Often symptomless, especially in adults. Can cause diarrhoea with steatorrhoea, Treatment is mepacrine hydrochloride or metronidazole orally. Syn. lambliasis.

گیاردیت: جیارڈیا انٹسٹائیفیلس کی وجہ سے مرض عموماً بغیر علامات خصوصاً بالغوں میں اسہال میں مبتلا کر سکتا ہے۔ علاج کے لئے منہ کے ذریعے میپا کرائن ہائیڈروکلورائڈ یا میٹرونیڈازول دیا جائے۔

Gigantism *(ji-gan'-tizm)*[G. gigas, giant]. An abnormal overgrowth, especially in height. May be associated with anterior pituitary tumour if the tumour develops before fusion of the epiphyses.

عفریتیت : غیر معمولی بڑھاؤ خصوصاً قد میں۔

Gilliam's operation. A method of correcting retroversion by shortening the round ligaments of the uterus. [David Tod Gilliam, American gynaecologist, 1844-1923].

اپریشن گلیلیم : رحم کے الٹ جانے کو ٹھیک کرنے کا طریقہ۔

Ginger *(jin'-jer)*. An aromatic root with carminative properties. Used as syrup or tincture for flavouring purposes.

ادراک : ایک خوشبودار زیر زمین تنہ۔اس میں ہاضمے کی خصوصیات پائی جاتی ہیں۔شربت یا ٹنکچر کے طور پر خوشبو کے لئے مستعمل ہے۔

Gingiva *(jin-ji'-va)* [L.]. The gum; the vascular tissue surrounding necks of the teeth.

مسوڑا : مسوڑھا۔جبڑا۔دانتوں کی گردنوں کے گرد واسکولر بافت۔

Gingivectomy *(jin-jiv-ek'-to-mi)* [L. gingiva, gum; G. ektome, excision]. Excision of a portion of the gum, usually for pyorrhoea.

لثہ براری : مسوڑے یا جبڑے کا ایک حصہ نکالنا عموماً پائیوریا کے لئے کیا جاتا ہے۔

Gingivitis *(jin-ji-vi'-tis)*. [L. gingiva, gum; G. -itis, inflmmation]. Inflammation of the gums. pregnancy g. occurs due to hormonal changes.

ورم لثہ : مسوڑھوں کی سوزش یا سوج۔

Giovannetti diet Used for patients with chronic renal failure; protein intake lowered to 20g per day which although less than the recommended intake, can achieve normal balance. This is because the 20g is chosen from proteins containing the essential amino acids, and uraemic patients can synthesize more non-essential amino acids (utilizing ammonia split from urea in the gut) than normal people. Urea production from exogenous protein can be kept at a minimum and a little of the excess urea is used up synthesizing the non-essential amino acids.

Girdle *(ger'-dl)*. A belt, **g. pain,** a constricting pain round the waist region, occurring in tabetic persons, **pelvic g.,** comprises the two innominate bones, sacrum and coccyx, **shoulder g.,** comprises the two clavicles and scapular.

چپنی : پٹی۔کمر والے حصے کے گرد عموماً درد ہو جاتا ہے۔

Girdlestone's operation Pseudoarthrosis of hi[p] for osteoarthritis. Part of the acetabulum an[d] the femoral head and neck are removed. A muscle mass is stitched between the bon[e] ends. [Gathorne Robert Girdlestone, Englis[h] surgeon, 1881-1950].

[ا]پریشن گرڈل سٹون : اپریشن کی ایک قسم۔انگریز سرجن گرڈل سٹون کے نام پر اپریشن کا نام ہے۔

Gland [L. glans, an acorn]. An organ o[r] structure capable of making an internal o[r] external secretion. **lympathic g.,** (node)doe[s] not secrete, but is concerned with filtration o[f] the lymph. See ENDOCRINE--glandular, adj.

[اند]رونی یا بیرونی رطوبت بنانے کا اہل عضو یا ساخت

Glanders *(glan'-derz)*. A contagious, febril[e] ulcerative disease communicable from horse[s] mules and asses to man.

[خ]نار: انسان کو گھوڑوں، گدھوں اور خچروں سے لگنے والی بیماری۔

Glandular fever syndrome *(gland'-u-lar fe'-ve[r] sin'-drom)*. A contagious self limiting disea[se] almost certainly due to infection with th[e] Epstein-Barr virus. Most common in childre[n] and adolescents. Characterized by fever, so[re] throad, enlarge of superfical lymph nodes an[d] appearance of atypical lymphocytes in th[e] blood. Agglutination tests, Paul-Bunnell an[d] monospot slide test are useful in diagnosis. Syn., infectious monoucleosis.

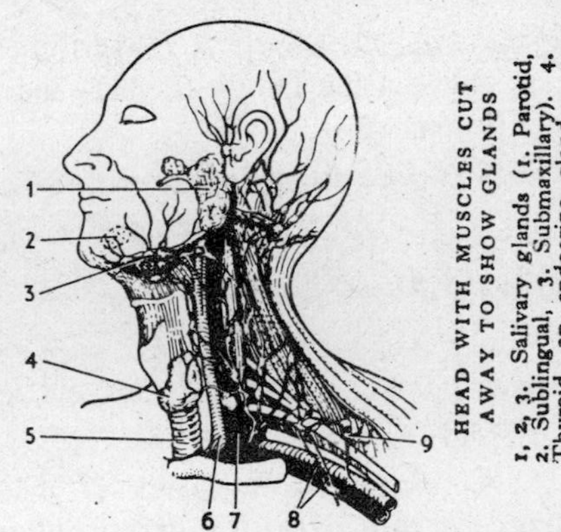

1
2
3
4
5
6
7
8
9
HEAD WITH MUSCLES CUT AWAY TO SHOW GLANDS
1, 2, 3. Salivary glands (1. Parotid, 2. Sublingual, 3. Submaxillary). 4. Thyroid, an endocrine gland. 5. Trachea. 6. Common carotid artery. 7. Jugular vein. 8. Lymphatic ducts.

Head with muscles cut away to show glands

تپ غدودی: چھوت کی بیماری۔ بو سے والی بیماری۔ ۳ تا ۵ اور ۱۵ تا ۲۵ سالوں کے درمیان ہوتی ہے۔ بخار ہوتا ہے اور گلینڈ بڑھ جاتی ہے۔ عموماً کھال پھٹ جاتی ہے۔

ans *(glanz)*. [L.]. The bulbous termination of the clitoris and penis.

گھینگا۔ حشفہ: عضو تناسل یا بظر کا پھولا ہوا سرا۔ اس کی چوٹی پر پیشاب کی نالی کا سوراخ ہوتا ہے۔ اس کے کنارے اور گردن پر چھوٹے چھوٹے غدود ہوتے ہیں جن سے ایک قسم کی بدبودار سفید رطوبت پیدا ہو کر خصیوں کو تر رکھتی ہے۔ حشفہ کے اوپر کھال کو غلفہ کہتے ہیں۔ سارا حشفہ اسفنجی ہوتا ہے۔

auber's salts *(glaw'-bers)*. Sodium sulphate (q.v.).

گلابری نمک: سوڈیم سلفیٹ۔

aucoma *(glaw-ko'-ma)* [G. glaukos, blue-green]. A condition where the intraocular pressure is raised. In the acute stage the pain is severe--glaucomatous, adj.

سبز موتیا۔ کالا موتیا: اس مرض میں سخت درد ہوتا ہے۔ آنکھ کے اگلے حصے میں پانی کے دباؤ کی زیادتی اس مرض کا اپریشن ہے۔

enohumeral *(gle-no-hu'-mer-al)*. [G. glene, socket; L. humerus]. Pertaining to the glenoid cavity of scapula and the humerus.

وقبی ذراعی: ہیومرس اور سکیپولا کے گلینائڈ کہفہ سے متعلق۔

enoid *(gle'-noid)* [G. glene, socket; eidos, form]. A cavity on the scapula into which the head of the humerus fits to form the shoulder joint.

وقبی: سکیپولا پر کہفہ جس میں ہیومرس گلائیڈ ہو کر شانے کا جوڑ بناتا ہے۔

ia *(gli'-a)*. [G. glue]. Neuroglia (q.v.)--glial, adj.

(عصبی) سریش: نیوروگلیا۔

ibenclamide *(gli-ben'-kla-mid)* Potent oral hypoglycaemic agent.

گلائبین کلیمائیڈ: ہائپوگلائی سیمک عامل۔

ioblastoma multiforme *(gli-o-blass-to'-ma mul-ti-form)* [G. glia, glue; blastos, germ; -oma, tumour; L. mulus, many; forma, form]. A highly malignant brain tumour.

لاصقی یا ھضی سلعہ: دماغ کا ناسور۔

ioma *(gli-o'-ma)* [G. glia, glue; -oma, tumour]. A malignant growth which does not give rise to secondary deposits. It arises from neuroglia. One form occurring in the retina is hereditary--gliomata, pl.

لاصقی سلعہ: بڑھاؤ جس میں ثانوی طور پر کچھ جمع نہیں ہوتا۔

Gliomyoma *(gli-o-mi-o'-ma)* [G. glia, glue; mys, muscle; -oma, tumour]. A tumour of nerve and muscle tissue--gliomyomata, pl.

لاصقی عضلی سلعہ: عصبی و عضلی نسیج کا ناسور۔

Globin *(glo'-bin)* [L. globus, ball]. A protein which combines with haematin to form haemoglobin.

گلوبن: ایک پروٹین جو ہیماٹن کے ساتھ مل کر ہیموگلوبن بناتی ہے۔

Globulin *(glob'-u-lin)* [L. globulus, little ball]. A fraction of serum or plasma protein from which antibody is formed. There are several varieties designated by the letters A, D, E, G and M. See GAMMAGLOBULIN.

گلوبولن: سیرم یا پلازما پروٹین کا حصہ جس سے اینٹی باڈی بنتی ہے اس کی مختلف اقسام کو حروف اے۔ ڈی ای جی اور ایم سے ظاہر کیا جاتا ہے۔

Globulinuria *(glob-ul-in-u'-ri-a)* [L. globulus, little ball; G. ouron, urine]. The presence of globulin in the urine.

گلوبولین بولیت: پیشاب میں گلوبولن کی موجودگی۔

Globus hystericus *(glo'-bus his-ter'-ik-us)*. Subjective feeling of neurotic origin of a lump in the throat. Can also include difficulty in swallowing and is due to tension of muscles of deglutition. Occurs in hysteria, anxiety states and depression. Sometimes follows slight trauma to throat, e.g. scratch by foreign body.

باؤ گولہ: گلے کی تکلیف جس سے نگلنے میں بھی دشواری ہوتی ہے۔ ہسٹریا، پریشانی اور فکر میں ایسا ہوتا ہے۔

Glomerulitis *(glom-er-u-li'-tis)* [L. glomus, ball; G, -itis, inflammation]. Acute suppurative inflammation of the glomeruli of the kidney.

قنبلکی التہاب: گردے کے گلومیرولائی میں سوزش۔

Glomerulonephritis *(glom-er-u-lo-nef-ri-tis)* [L. glomus, ball; G. nephros, kidney; -itis, inflammation]. A term used in bilateral , non-suppurative inflammation of the glomeruli of the kidneys. Preceded by streptococcal infection of the skin and throat in the majority of cases.

قنبلکی کلوی التہاب: گردوں کی گلومرولائی میں سوزش' اندھاپن ہوسکتا ہے۔جلداور گلے میں تکلیف ہوتی ہے۔

Glomerulosclerosis *(glom-er-u-lo-skler-o'sis)* Fibrosis of the glomeruli of the kidney, the result of inflammation. **intercapillary g.** is a common pathological finding in diabetics. See NEPHROTIC SYNDROME--glomerulosclerotic, adj.

گلومیرولوسکلیروسس: سوزش کے نتیجے مین گردے کے گولومرولائی کی فائبروسس۔

Glomerulus *(glom-er'-u-lus)*. A coil of minute arterial capillaries held together by scanty connective tissue. It invaginates the entrance of the uriniferious tubules in the kidney cortex-- glomerular, adj., glomeruli, pl.

عروق: باریک شریانی نسوں کا گچھا۔جس میں رباطی نسیج کم ہوتا ہے۔

Glossa *(glos'-a)* [G.]. The tongue--glossal, adj.

لسان: زبان۔

Glossectomy *(glos-ek'-to-mi)* [G. glossa, tongue; ektome, excission]. Excision of the tongue.

لسان براری: زبان کاٹنا۔

Glossitis *(glos'-i-tis)* [G. glossa, tongue; -itis, inflammation]. Inflammation of the tongue.

ورم زبان: زبان کی سوزش۔

Glossodynia *(glos-o-din'-i-a)* [G. glossa, tongue; odyne, pain]. Name used for painful tongue when there is no visible change.

Glossopharyngeal *(glos-o-far-in'-ji-al)* [G. glossa, tongue; pharynx, throat]. Pertaining to the tongue and pharynx. The ninth pair of cranial nerves.

لسانی بلعومی: زبان اور فیرنکس سے متعلق۔کرینیل اعصاب۔کانواں جوڑ جومیڈلا آبلانگیٹا سے شروع ہوتا ہے اور ذائقہ کی خبر دیتا ہے۔

Glossoplegia *(glos-o-ple'-ji-a)*[G. glossa, tongue; plege, stroke]. Paralysis of the tongue.

فالج زبان: زبان کارعشہ۔

Glottis *(glot'-is)* [G.]. The part of the larynx associated with voice production.

rimaglottidis, the opening between the fr margins of the vocal cords--glottic, adj.

خلق: لیرنکس کاوہ حصہ جس کاتعلق آواز پیدا کرنے سے ہے۔

Glucagon *(gloo'-ka-gon)*. Hormone produced alpha cells of pancreatic islets of Langerhan Causes breakdown of glycogen into glucos thus preventing blood sugar from falling to low during fasting. Can now be obtaine commercially from the pancreas of animal Given to accelerate breakdown of glycogen the liver and raise blood sugar rapidly. As it a polypedtide hormone, it must be given b injection.

وکاگون: لبلبہ کے آئیلٹس آف لنگرہانز کے الفاخلیوں میں پیدا ہونے ہارمون۔گلائیکوجن کوگلوکوس میں تبدیل کرتا ہے۔اس طرح کونی شکر کومزید ہونے سے روکتا ہے۔جانوروں کے لبلبوں سے حاصل کیاجاتا ہے۔چونکہ پولی پپٹائیڈہارمون ہے اس لئے انجکشن کے ذریعے دیاجاناچاہئے۔

Glucocorticoid *(gloo-ko-kor'-ti-koid)*. A steroid hormone which promote gluconeogenesis (i.e. the formation of gluco and glycogen from protein) and whic antagonizes the action of insulin. Occurin naturally in the adrenal cortex as cortiso and hydrocortisone, and produced synthe cally as, for example, prednisone and pred solone.

وکوکارٹی کائڈ: ایک سٹرائڈہارمون۔ایڈرینل کارٹیکس میں قدرتی طور رٹیسون اور ہائیڈروکارٹیسون پایاجاتا ہے۔

Glucogenesis *(gloo-ko-jen'-e-sis)*. Production glucose.

وکونیوجینس: گلائیکونیوجینس۔

Gluconeogenesis *(gloo-ko-ne-o-jen'-e-sis)*. T formation of sugar from protein or fat wh there is lack of available carbohydrate.

Glucophage *(gloo'-ko-fag)*. Metformin (q.v.).

وکوفیج: میٹفارمن۔

Glucose *(gloo'-kos)*. Dextrose or grape sugar. monosaccharide. The form in which carboh drates are absorbed through the intestinal tr and circulated the blood. It is stored as glyc gen in the liver.

وکوس۔قندانگور: ڈکٹروزیاانگوری شکر۔مونوسیکرائیڈ۔کاربوہائیڈریٹس

گلوکوس کی صورت میں آنت میں جذب ہوتے ہیں اور خون میں گردش کرتے ہیں۔ جگر میں بطور گلائیکو جن ذخیرہ ہوتا ہے اس کا ۲۵ فیصد ۲۵ سی سی کا ایک وریدی ٹیکہ صبح ایک شام برائے یرقان اس کا ۵ فیصد ۴۰ قطرے فی منٹ وریدی ڈراپ برائے یوریمیا یعنی سمیت بول۔

Glucoronic acid *(gloo-kur-on'-k)*. An acid which acts on bilirubin to form conjugated bilirubin.

Glutaminase *(gloo-tam'-in-az)*. An amino acid-degrading enzyme, being used in the treatment of cancer.

Gluteal *(gloo'-te-al)* [G. gloutos, but tock]. Pertaining to the buttocks.

الوی : چھوتڑوں سے متعلق چوتڑ کے تین عضلات کا سیٹ۔

Guten *(gloo'-ten)* [L.]. A protein constituent of wheat flour. Insoluble in water but an essential component of the elastic 'dough'. It is not tolerated in coeliac disease (q.v.).

Glutethimide *(gloo-teth'-i-mid)*. Hypnotice of medium action. Useful when an alternative to the barbiturates is required.

گلوٹیتھی مائیڈ: درمیانی درجے کا خواب آور۔

Glycerine (e) *(glis'-e-rin)*. A clear, syrupy liquid prepared synthetically or obtained as a by-product in soap manufacture. It has a hygroscopic action. **glycerine and borax,** useful for softening sordes (q.v.). **glycerine and honey,** useful as a softening agent for ora l toilet. **glycerine and ichthyol,** used to relieve inflammation. **glycerine and mangesium sulphate,** useful for boils, etc.

گلسرین : ایک صاف مائع۔ صابن بنانے کے دوران یا تالیفی طور پر حاصل کیا جاتا ہے۔ اس کا دوائی کے ساتھ محلول عموماً گلے میں لگانے کے کام آتا ہے۔ گلسرول نقطۂ جوش ۲۹۰ س۔ پانی میں حل پذیر، فارمیسی میں مستعمل۔

Glycerophosphates *(glis-er-o-fos'-fatz)*. Appetite stimulant.

Glyceryl trinitrate *(glis'-er-il-tri-nit'-rat)*. Vasodilator used in angina pectoris. Given mainly as tablets which should be chewed, or dissolved under the tongue.

گلسرائل ٹرائی نائٹریٹ : چبانے یا چوسنے والی گولیوں کی صورت میں دیا جاتا ہے۔ درد دل یا انجینہ پیکٹورس میں نصف تا ایک گولی حسب ضرورت زبان کے نیچے رکھی جائے۔ درد کی حالت میں رکھی جائے۔

Glycine *(gli'-sen)* . A non-essential amino acid (q.v.).

گلائی سین : ایک غیر ضروری سادہ ترین امینوایسڈ، نقطہ پگھلاؤ ۲۳۲ س، بے رنگ حل پذیر نامیاتی تالیف میں مستعمل۔

Glycinuria *(gli-sin-u'-ri-a)*. Excretion of glycine in the urine. Associated with mental subnormality.

گلائی سینوریا: پیشاب میں گلائی سین کا اخراج۔

Glycogen *(gli'-ko-jen)* [G. glykys, sweet]. Animal starch, the form to which glucose is linked in branched chains for storage in the body. **glycogen storage disease,** inborn error of carbohydrate metabolism. Associated with mental subnormality.

گلائیکوجن۔ نشاستہ حیوانی : حیوانی نشاستہ، گلوکوس اس میں تبدیل ہو کر جسم میں ذخیرہ ہو جاتا ہے۔

Glycogenase *(gli-ko-jen-az)* [g. glykys, sweet; genesis, descent]. An enzyme necessary for the conversion of glycogen into glucose.

شکر زائی: خامرہ جو گلائی کوجن کو گلوکوس میں تبدیل کرنے کے لئے ضروری ہے۔

Glycogenesis *(gli-ko-jen'-e-sis)*. Glycogen formation from blood glucose.

گلائی کوجینوسس : گلائی کوجن کے ذخیرہ میں زیادتی جس کی وجہ سے میٹابولزم میں گڑبڑ ہے۔

Glycolysis *(gli-kot'-i-sis)* [G. glykys, sweet; lysis, a loosening]. The hydrolysis of sugar in the body--glycolytic, adj.

گلائی کولیسز۔ شکر پاشیدگی: جسم مین شکر کی ہائیڈرولسس۔

Glycogenosis *(gli-ko-jen-o'-sis)* [G. glykys, sweet; genesis,descent; -osis, condition]. Metabolic disorder leading to increased storage of glycogen. Leads to glycogen myopathy.

Glyconeogenesis *(gli-ko-ne-o-jen'-e-sis)* [G. glykys, sweet; noes, new; genesis, descent]. Gluconeogenesis (q.v.).

گلائیکونیوجینیسز : جب مہیا شدہ کاربوہائیڈریٹ کی کمی ہو تو پروٹین یا چکنائی سے شکر کا بننا۔

Glycosides *(gli'-ko-sidz)*. Natural substances composed of a sugar with another compound. The non-sugar fragment is termed an 'aglycone,' and is sometimes of therapeutic value. Digoxin is a familiar example of a glycoside.

گلائیکوسائیڈز: قدرتی اشیاء جن میں شکر کے ساتھ کوئی دوسرا مرکب ہو۔ اگر انہیں تیزاب کے ساتھ ملایا جائے تو گلوکوس اور دوسرے مرکبات بنتے ہیں۔

Glycosuria *(gli-ko-su'-ri-a)*. [G. glykys, sweet; rhize, root]. Liquoric root, demulcent, slightly laxative, expectorant and used as a flavouring agent Results in an increase in extracellular fluid, retention of sodium and increased excretion of potassium.

جنس ملیٹھی: کھانسی کے شربت میں مستعمل مائع۔خوشبو دینے والا عامل۔

Glymidine *(gli'-mi-den)*. Oral antidiabetic agent.

گلائمیڈین : شکر کم کرنے والا عامل۔

Gnathalgia *(nath-al'-ji-a)* [G. gnathos, jaw; algos, pain]. Pain in the jaw.

الم الشدق۔وجع الفلک: جبڑے میں درد۔

Gnathoplasty *(nath'-o-plas-it)* [G. gnathos, jaw; plassein, to form]. Plastic surgery of the jaw.

ترقیع الشرق: جبڑے کی پلاسٹک سرجری۔

Goblet cells Special secreting cells, shaped like a goblet, found in the mucous membranes.

جام نما خلیے: میوکس جھلیوں میں پائے جانے والے مخصوص اخراجی خلیے۔

Goeckerman regime *(ga'-ker-man)*. A method of treatment for psoriasis; exposure to ultraviolet) light alternating with the application of a tar paste.

گوئیکرمین ریجیم: سوریاسس کے لئے علاج کا طریقہ۔

Goitre *(goi'-ter)*[L. guttur, throat]. An enlargement of the thyroid gland, **simple g.**, in which the patient does not show any signs of excessive thyroid activity. **toxic g.**, in which the enlarged gland secretes an excess of thyroid hormone. The patient is nervous, loses weight and often has palpitations and exophthalmos. See COLLOID.

گلہڑ: تھائیرائیڈ گلینڈ کا بڑھا ہوا حصہ۔گلسوؤں کا مرض جانا۔جسم میں آیوڈین کی کمی سے ہوتا ہے۔گردن خی سامنے ابھار دکھائی دیتا ہے۔

Goitrogens *(goi'-tro-jens)* [L. guttur, throat' G. genesis, descent]., Agents causing goitre. Some occur in plants, e.g turnip, cabbage, brussels sprouts and peanuts. Drugs, e.g. propylthiouracil, carbimazole, potasium perchlorate and thiocyanate, iodide.

گائٹروجنز: گلہڑ پیدا کرنے والا عوامل۔بعض پودوں میں پائے جاتے ہیں۔مثلاً شلجم، بند گوبھی، مٹر وغیرہ۔

Golden eye ointment Ung. hyd. ox. flav. Yellow oxide of mercury ointment.

زریں عینی مرہم: پارے کے زرد آکسائیڈ کا مرہم۔

Gold injections See AUROTHIOMALATE.

زریں ٹیکے : آروتھومیلیٹ۔

Goldthwait belt Wide belt with steel support for back injuries.

گولڈتھویٹ بیلٹ: کمر کے زخموں کو سہارا دینے کے لئے فولاد کا سہارا جو چوڑی پٹی پر ہوتا ہے۔

Goldthwait strap Strap to support foot injuries. [Joel Goldthwait, American orthopaedic surgeon, 1866-1961].

گولڈتھویٹ سٹرپ: پاؤں کے زخموں وک سہارا دینے کے لئے سٹرپ۔

Gonad *(gon'-ad)* [G. gone, generation]. A male or female sex gland. See OVARY, TESTIS--gonadal, adj.

غدہ تناسلی: زیادہ مادہ جنسی گلینڈ۔

Gonadotrophic *(gon-ad-o-tro'-fik)* [G. gone, generation; atrophe, nourishment]. Having an affinity for or influence on the gonads.

مولد الفی: غدہ تناسلی پر اثر انداز ہونا یا ان سے الف رکھنا۔

Gonadotrophin *(gon-a-do-tro'-fin)* [G. gone, generation; trophe, nourishment]. Any gonad-stimulating hormone. See FOLLICLE STIMULATING HORMONE.

گونیڈوٹرافن: کوئی غدہ یا تناسلی کو تحریک دینے والا ہارمون۔

Gonadylseric Serum gonadotrophin for oral administration for acne. An extended course of treatment is essential

گونا: کیل کے لئے سیرم گونیڈوٹرافن منہ کے ذریعے دیا جاتا ہے۔

Gonan Serum gonadotrophin.

گونین: سیرم گونیڈوٹرافن۔

Gonioscopy *(gon-i-os'-kop-i)* [G. gonia, angle;

skopein, to examine]. Measuring angle of anterior chamber of eye with a gonioscope.

زاویہ بینی: گونیوسکوپ کی مدد سے آنکھ کے امامی خانہ کے زاویہ کی پیائش۔

Goniotomy *(gon-i-ot'-o-mi)* [G. gonia, angle; tome, a cutting]. Operation for glaucoma. Incision through the anterior chamber angle to the canal of Schlemm.

گرینوٹومی: گلاکوما کے لئے اپریشن۔

Gonococcus *(gon-o-kok'-us)* (Neisseria gonorrhoeae). A Gram-negative diplococcus, the causative organism of gonorrhoea. It is a strict parasite. Occurs characteristically inside polymorph leucocytes in the tissues--gonococci, pl.; gonococcal, adj.

نبقۂ سوزاک: گونوکوکس۔ایک گرام منفی ڈپلوکاکسس۔سوزاک پیدا کرتا ہے۔طفیلی ہے۔نوزائیدہ بچے کی آنکھ میں سوزش اس جرثومہ کی وجہ سے ہوتی ہے۔اس تکلیف میں پنسلین استعمال کرتے ہیں۔

Gonorrhoea *(gon-or-re'-a)* [G. gone, generation; rheein, to flow]. An infectious disease of venereal origin in adults. In children infection is accidental, e.g. gonococcal ophthalmia of the newborn, gonococcal vulvovaginitis of girls, before puberty. Chief manifestations of the disease in the male are a purulent urethritis with dysuria. In the female, urethritis and endocervicitis which may be symptomless. Incubation period is usually 2 to 5 days--gonorrhoeal, adj.

سوزاک: بالغوں میں چھوت کی بیماری۔بچوں میں اتفاقیہ ہو جاتی ہے۔مجامعت کرنے کے بعد دوسرے تیسرے روز پیشاب کی نالیس رُخ اور متورم ہو جاتی ہے اور اس میں جلن اور خراش ہوتی ہے۔تین چار روز بعد جلن اور درد میں زیادتی ہو جاتی ہے اور سنہری مائل زرد رنگ کی گاڑھی پیپ زیادہ مقدار میں آنے لگتی ہے۔کولہوں اور کمر میں درد ہو جاتا ہے۔بھوک کم لگتی ہے اور قبض ہو جاتی ہے۔پیشاب رک رک کر آتا ہے اور بعض اوقات پیشاب میں خون لوتھڑے یا چھلکے ہوتے ہیں۔عضو تناسل متورم ہو جاتا ہے۔

Gonorrhoeal *(gon-or-re'-al)*. Resulting from gonorrhoea. **gonorrhoeal arthritis** is a metastatic manifestation of gonorrhoea.

gonorrhoeal ophthalmia is one form of ophthalmia neonatorum.

سوزاکی: سوزاک سے پیدا ہونے والا۔

Goodpasture's syndrome Association of haemorrhagic lung disorder with glomerulonephri- tis. [Ernest W. Goodpasture. American pathologist, 1886-1960].

گڈپاسچر سنڈروم: پھیپھڑوں کا ایک مرض۔

Gordh needle *(gort')*. An intravenous needle with a rubber diaphragm. Through it repeated injections can be given.

گارٹ سوئی: ربڑ ایا فرام کے ساتھ انٹراوینس سوئی اس سے ٹیکے بار بار لگائے جاسکتے ہیں۔

Gouge *(gowj)*. A chisel with a grooved blade for removing bone.

روکھانی: ہڈی ختم کرنے کے لئے بلیڈ کے ساتھ چھینی۔

Gout *(gowt)* [L. gutta, drop]. A form of metabolic disorder in which sodium biurate is deposited in the cartilages of the joints, the ears, and elsewhere. The big toe is characteristically involved and becomes acutely painful and swollen. See TOPHUS, PURINS, URIC ACID.

نقرس: میٹابولک گڑبڑ جس میں جوڑوں' کانوں وغیرہ کی چبنی ہڈیوں میں سوڈیم بائی یوریٹ جمع ہو جاتا ہے۔پاؤں کا انگوٹھا سوج جاتا ہے اور تکلیف دہ ہوتا ہے۔

Gout

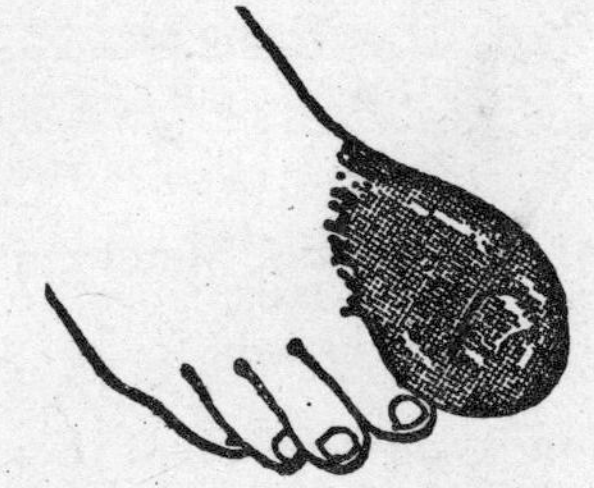

GPI, General paralysis of the insane (q.v.).

جی پی ائی: پاگل شخص کو پاگل پن کا دورہ۔

Graefe's knife *(gra'-fes)*. Finely pointed knife with narrow blade, used for making incisions across anterior chamber of eye prior to removal of cataract. [Albrecht von Graefe, German ophthalmologist, 1828-70].

گریفی کا چاقو: تنگ بلیڈ کے ساتھ باریک نوکدار والا چاقو۔

Graft [G. graphein, to write]. A tissue or organ which is transplanted to another part of the same animal (autograft), to another animal of the same species (homograft), or to another animal of a different species (heterograft). Only autograft and homorgrafts are used in man.

پیوند: نسیج یا عضو جو اسی جانور کے کسی اور حصے کے ساتھ یا اسی نوع کے کسی دوسرے جانور کے ساتھ یا مختلف نوع کے کسی جانور کے ساتھ پیوند کیا جاتا ہے۔

Gramicidin *(gram-is-i'-din)*. A mixture of antibiotic substances obtain from tyrothricin. Too toxic for systemic use, but valuable for topical application when local antibiotic therapy is required.

گریمی سائڈن: ٹائروتھریسن سے حاصل شدہ اینٹی بایوٹک اشیاء کا آمیزہ۔

Gram's stain A bacteriological stain for differentiation of germs. Those retaining the stain are Gram-positive (+), those unaffected by it are gram negative (-). [Hans Christian Joachim Gram, Danish physician, 1853-1938].

گرام سٹین: جراثیموں میں فرق معلوم کرنے کے لئے ایک جراثیمی رنگ جن پر رنگ چڑھ جائے گرام مثبت ہوں گے جو رنگ نہ پکڑیں گرام منفی ہوں گے۔ اس کا نام فزیشن کریسچین گرام پر ہے۔ بلغم میں گرام سٹین سے کوئی جراثیم دکھائی نہیں دیتے۔

Grand mal *(g-ong mal)*. Major epiepsy. See EPILEPSY.

صرع کبیر: بڑی مرگی۔

Granulation *(gran-u-la'-shun)* [L. granulum, small grain]. The outgrowth of new capillarieis and connective tissue cells from the surface of an open wound. **g. tissue,** the young, soft tissue so formed--granulate, v.t., v.i.

انگور زخم: ایک کھلے زخم کی سطح سے رابطی نسیج کے خلیوں اور نئی نسوں کا بڑھاؤ۔

Granulocyte *(gran'-u-lo-sit)* [L. granulum, small grain; G. kytos, cell]. A cell containing granules in its cytoplasm. Used as syn. for polymorphonuclear leucocytes which have neutrophil, eosinophil or basophil granules.

گرینولوسائیٹ۔ ذرہ خلیہ: ذرات۔ دانوں یا گرینولز پر مشتمل کوئی خلیہ۔

Granulocytopenia *(gran-u-lo-sit-o-pe'-ni-a)* [L. granulum, small grain; G. kytos, cell; penia want]. Decrease of granulocytes (polymorphs not sufficient to warrant the term agranulocytosis (q.v.).

غیر تقوینی نقص الام: گرینولوسائیٹس کی کمی۔

Granuloma *(gran-u-lo'-ma)* [L. granulum, smal grain; G. -oma, tumour]. A tumour formed of granulation tissue. **g., venereum,** see LYMPHOGRANULOMA--granulomata, pl.; granulomatous, adj.

دانہ دار سلعہ: گرینولیسن نسیج کا بنا ہوا ناسور۔

Gravel *(grav'l)* A sandy deposit which, if present in the bladder, may be passed with the urine.

پتھری: ایک ریتلا ذرہ جو بلیڈر میں ہونے کی صورت میں پیشاب کے ساتھ جاسکتا ہے۔

Graves' disease Thyrotoxicosis (q.v.), [Robert James Graves, Irish physician, 1797-1853].

غدۂ درقیہ کے فعل کی خرابی سے مرض: تھائروٹاکسیکوسس۔ اس کا نام آئرلینڈ کے فزیسن رابرٹ جیمز گریوز کے نام پر ہے۔

Gravid *(grav'-id)* [L. gravis, heavy or pregnant]. Pregnant.

حاملہ: جسے حمل ہو۔

Gravitational *(gra-vi-ta'-shun-al)*. Being attracted by force of gravity. **g. ulcer,** varicose ulcer (q.v.).

تجاذبی: کشش ثقل کی وجہ سے کھینچنا۔

Gravity *(gra'-vi-ti)* [L. gravis, heavy]. Weight. **specific g.,** the weight of the substance compared with that of an equal volume of water.

کشش ثقل: وزن۔ زمین یا دوسرے سیارے یا سیٹلائیٹ اور اس کی سطح پر یا اس کی ثقلی میدان میں موجود جسم کے درمیان ثقلی قوت۔

Grawitztmour Hypernephroma (q.v.). [Paul Albert Grawitz, German pathologist, 1850-1932].

گراوٹوز سلعہ: ہائپر نفروما۔

Green monkey disease See MARBURG DISEASE.

غول پسند: گروہ میں رہنے کو ترجیح دینا۔ میل ملاپ کرنے والا۔

Griffith's types Antigenic subdivisions of Lancefield group A streptococci by virtue of their characteristic M protein antigens.

اقسام گرفت: سٹرپٹوکاکسی کی تقسیم۔

Grinders *(grin'-derz)*. The molars or double teeth.

طواحن: مولرز یا ڈبل دانت۔

Grinder's asthma One of the many popular names for silicosis arising from inhalation of metallic dust.

ڈاڑھوں کا دمہ: دھاتی گرد سانس کے ذریعہ اندر جانے کی وجہ سے سلیکوس۔

Gripe *(grip)*. Colic.

قولنج: کولک۔

Griseofulvin *(gri-se-o-ful'-vin)*. An oral fungicide, useful in ringworm.

گریسیوفلوین: منہ کے ذریعے دیئے جانے والا سماروغ کش رنگ ورم میں مفید۔ فلسین۔ گریسوون۔

Grocer's itch Contact dermatitis, especially from flour or sugar.

جرب بقالین: خصوصاً آٹے یا چینی کی وجہ سے بیماری۔ ہاتھوں کی ترکھلی۔ متعدد ی قسم کی سوزش جلد۔

Groin The jucntion of the thigh with the abdomen.

چڈا۔ پیغول: ران کا بطن کے ساتھ جوڑ۔

Group psychotherapy See PSYCHOTHERAPY.

گروہی سائیکوتھراپی: سائیکوتھراپی۔

Growing pains Pain in the limbs during youth; differential diagnosis rheumatic fever.

شباب کے اعصابی درد: عالم شباب میں جوارح میں درد۔

Guanethidine *(gwan-eth'-i-den)*. A hypotensive, sympathetic blocking agent. Gives sustained reduction of intraocular pressure in glaucoma. Applied locally to block the sympathetic fibres to the eye in exophthalmos. Absorbed more regularly and permits a smoother control of hypertension than mecamylamine.

گوٹنے تھائی ڈین: سمپتھیٹک بلاک کرنے والا عامل راسے کین' ہائپرٹنشن یا بلڈ پریشر میں اس کی ایک گولی صبح ایک دوپہر ایک شام۔

Guanimycin *(gwan-i-mi'-sin)*. Streptomycin, sulphagaunidine and kaolin. Antidiarrhoeal.

گوٹنے مائی سین: اسہال روکنے والی دوا۔ بے سری پیچش اور بچوں کے دستوں کے لئے مفید۔

Guanoclor *(gwan'-o-klor)*. Antihypertensive.

گوانوگلور: دافع پیش طنابی۔

Guanoxan sulphate *(gwan-oks'-an-sul'-fat)*. Antihypertensive.

گوانوکسان سلفیٹ: دافع بیش طنابی۔

Guillotine *(gil'-o-ten)*. A surgical instrument for excision of the tonsils.

گلوٹین۔ گردن زن۔ لوزہ تراش: گلے کاٹنے کے لئے آپریشن کا ایک آلہ۔

Guinea worm *(gin'-i)* Dracunculus medinensis (q.v.).

نارو: ڈریکنکولس میڈینس۔ لمبے اور پتلے کیڑے۔ لمبائی تقریباً ایک فٹ۔ نر اور مادہ علیحدہ۔ جوہڑوں کا پانی پینے سے جسم کے اندر انڈے چلے جاتے ہیں۔ ڈیرہ غازی خان اور راجن پور کے اضلاع میں مرض پایا جاتا ہے۔

Gullet *(gul'-et)*. The oesophagus.

گلا۔ گلو۔ مری۔ غذا کی نالی: ایسوفیگس۔ زخرا۔

Gumma *(gum'-a)*. A localized area of vascular granulation tissue which develops in the later stages (tertiary) of syphilis. Obstruction to the blood supply results in necrosis, and gummata near a surface of the body tend to break down, forming chronic ulcers, e.g. on the nose, the lower leg, the palate, etc. Probably these ulcers are not infectious.

دل آتشک: اسکولر گرینولیشن نسیج کا ایک مقامی ایریا۔ بعد میں آتشک کی آخری سٹیج ظاہر ہوتی ہے۔

Gut The intestines.

آنت۔ معا۔ گٹ: انتڑیاں۔

Gynaecography *(gi-ne-kog'-ra-fi)* [G. gyne, woman; graphein, to write]. Radiological visualization of internal female genitalia after pneumoperitoneum--gynaecographical, adj.; gynaecographically, adv.

گائینیکوگرافی: نیوموپیری ٹونیم کے بعد اندرونی مادہ تولید اعضاء کو ریڈیالوجی کے ذریعے نوٹ کرنا۔

Gynaecologist *(gi-ne-kol'-oj-ist)*. A surgeon who specializes in gynaecology.

ماہر نسوانی امراض: نسوانی مرضیات کا ماہر۔

Gynaecology *(gi-ne-kol'-o-ji)* [G. syne, woman; logos, discourse]. The science dealing with the disease which are peculiar to women.

نسوانی مرضیات : ان امراض کی سائنس جو صرف عورتوں کے ساتھ مخصوص ہیں۔

Gynaecomastia *(gi-ne-ko-mas'-ti-a)* [G. gyne, woman; mastos, breast]. Enlargement of the male mammary gland.

گائینکو ماسٹیا : نر پستان کا بڑھاؤ۔

Gypsona *(jip-so'-na)*. Ready-made quick-setting plaster of Paris bandage made by impregnating fine plaster of Paris into specially woven (interlock) cotton cloth. For immobilization in fracture treatment and orthopaedic conditions generally.

جپسونا : پلاسٹر آف پیرس کی ریدی میڈ پٹی۔

Gypsum *(jip'-sum)*. Plaster of Paris (calcium sulphate).

پلاسٹر آف پیرس

Gyretomy *(ji-rek'-to-mi)* [G. gyros, circle; ektome, excision]. Surgical removal of a gyrus, a convoluted portion of cerebral cortex.

جائیکریکٹومی : سیر برل کارٹیکس کے ایک حصے کو سرجری کے ذریعے کاٹنا۔

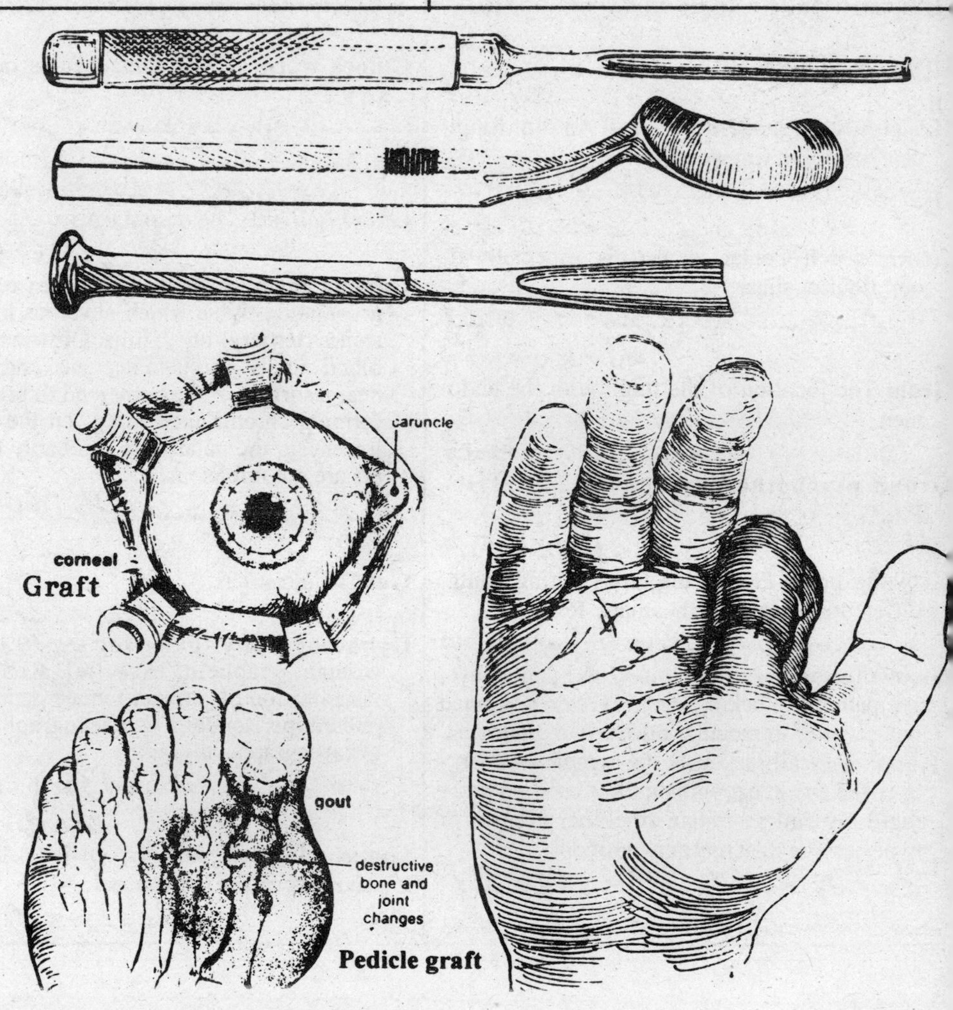

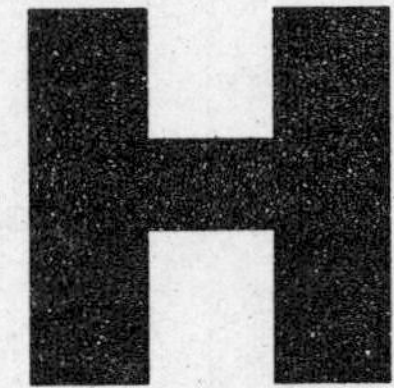

H Symbol for Hydrogen, enthelpy and magnetic field strength.

ایچ: علامت ہے ہائیڈروجن، حرارت اور مقناطیسی قوتِ میدان کی۔

h Symbol for hecto-d, hour, Plank't constant and height.

ایچ: علامت ہے ہیکٹو اور گھنٹہ کی، پلانک کے مستقل اور اونچائی کی۔

Habit *(hab'it)* [L. *habitus,* from habere to hold]. A fixed or constant practice established by frequent repetition. It is also a state of predisposition or bodily temperament.

خصلت، عادت: کسی صورت میں بار بار دہرانے سے حاصل کردہ ایک مستقل آٹومیٹک تاثر۔

Habituation *(ha-bich'-oo-a-shan)* The gradual adaptation to a stumulus or to the environment. A conditions resulting from the repeated consumption of a drug, with a desire to continue its use, but with little or no tendency to increase the dose, there may be psychic but no physical, dependence on the drug and delrimental effects, if any, are primarily on the individual.

عادت ڈالنا: کسی شے یا محرک یا ماحول کو آہستہ آہستہ اختیار کر لینا۔ کسی دوا یا نشہ کی چیز کو بار بار استعمال کر کے عادت ڈال لینا۔ یہ نفسیاتی مسئلہ بن جاتا ہے اور پھر اس کا مریض کے ذہن پر اتنا زیادہ اثر نہیں ہوتا۔

Haem *(him)* The pigments which carry the portion of haemoglobin.

خون: ہیموگلوبن کا پگمنٹ لے جانے والا حصہ۔

Haemangioma *(ha'm-an-jioma)* [G. *heme,* blood; *aggeon,* vessel; *ome,* mass]. A malformation of blood vessels. This may occur in any part of the body. When this thing occurs in the skin, it is sign since birth.

دموی عروقی سلعہ: خونی رگوں کی خلعت ناقص جو جسم کے کسی بھی حصے میں ہو سکتی ہے۔ جب جلد میں ہو تو یہ پیدائش کا نشان ہوتا ہے۔

Haemarthrosis *(hemar-thro-sis)* [G. *heme,* blood; *arthros,* joint; *osis,* condition]. This is a condition in which blood goes into joint cavity. The hemoglobin and plasinin with their irritant and chondrolytic effects destroy the joint.

نزف مفصلی: جوڑ کے کہفہ میں خون کی موجودگی۔

Haematemesis *(he-ma-te-mesis)* [G. *heme,* blood; *emesis,* vomiting]. The vomiting of blood.

خونی قے: خون کی قے۔

Haematinic *(he-ma-ti-nik)* [G. *heme,* blood; *tinik,* produce]. The substances which are required for the formation of hemoglobin and red blood cells.

مقوی خون: ایسی اشیاء جو سرخ خونی خلیے اور اس کے اجزاء کی پیداوار کے لئے لازم ہوں۔

Haematobia *(he-ma-to'be-a)* A genus of flies of the family Muscidae. **H. irritans,** a genus of small flies "hornflies" which are very troublesome to cattle.

مکھی: مکھی کی قسم جو کہ فیملی مسیڈی سے تعلق رکھتی ہے۔ اسکی قسم ارٹینس ہے جو کہ شور مچانے والی چھوٹی مکھیاں ہوتی ہیں اور مویشیوں کو بہت تنگ کرتی ہیں۔

Haematogenous *(he-mat-oj'-en-us)* [G. *haima,*

blood; kolpos, vagina]. See CRYPTOMENO-RRH- OEA.

مہبلی نزف الام : یونانی الفاظ ہیما بمعنی کون اور کولپوس بمعنی ویجائنا کا مجموعہ۔ کرپٹومنوریا۔

Haematogenous *(he-mat-oj'-en-us)* [g. haima, blood; genesis, descent]. 1. Concerned with the formation of blood. 2. Carried by the blood stream

خون سے حاصل کردہ : (۱) خون سے بننے سے متعلق۔ (۲) خون کے ذریعے جانا۔

Haematology *(he-mat-ol'-o-ji)* [G. haima, blood; logos, discourse]. The science dealing with the formation, composition, functions and diseases of the blood--haematological, adj.; haematologically, adv.

دمویات۔ علم عوارض خون : سائنس جو خون کی بناوٹ' کمپوزیشن' افعال اور بیماریوں سے متعلق ہے۔

Haematoma *(he-ma-to'-ma)* [G. haima, blood; -oma, tumour]. A swelling filled with blood--haematomata, pl.

خون کا گومڑ۔ دموی سلعہ : ابھار جو خون سے بھرا ہو۔

Haematometra *(he-ma-to-me-tra)* [G. haima blood; metra, womb]. An accumulation of blood (or menstrual fluid) in the uterus.

رحمی اجتماع۔ سیلان رحم رحمی : یورٹرس میں خون کا اجتماع۔

Haematopoiesis *(he-ma-to-poi-e'-sis)* See HAEMOPIESIS.

خون زائی : ہیموپائسس۔

Haematosalpinx *(he-ma-to-sal'-pinks)* [G. haima, blood; salpigx, trumpet]. Blood in the Fallopian tube.

انبوبی اجتماع الام۔ امتلاء قنات : فلوپ دموی۔ فلوپئین نالی میں خون۔

Haematozoa *(he-ma-to-zo'-a)* [G. haima, blood; zoion, living theing] Parasites, living in the blood-haematozoon, sing.

خونی طفیلی : طفیلی۔ خون میں رہتے ہیں۔

Haematuria *(he-ma-tu'-ri-a)* [G. haima, blood; ouron, urine]. Blood in the urine-haematuric, adj.

بول الام : پیشاب میں خون۔

Haemochromatosis *(he-mo-kro-ma-to'-sis)* [G. haima, blood; chroma, colour; -osis, condition]. A congenital error in iron metabolism with increased iron deposition in tissues, resulting in brown pigmentation of the skin and cirrhosis of the liver. Syn,. 'bronzed diabetes.'--haemochromatotic, adj.

خون لونیت : لوہے کے میٹابولزم میں غلطی جس سے جلد میں بھورا پگمنٹ بن جاتا ہے۔

Haemoconcentration *(he-mo-kon-se n-tra'-shun)*. [G. haima, blood; L. con, together; centrum, centre]. Relative increase of volume of red blood cells to volume of plasma, usually due to loss of the latter.

دموی ارتکاز : پلازما کی جسم کی نسبت سرخ خونی خلیوں کے جسم میں اضافہ جو عموماً پلازما کے ضیاع کی وجہ سے ہوتا ہے۔

Haemocytometer *(hem-o-si-tom'-et-er)* [G. haima, blood; kytos, cell; metron, a measure]. An instrument for measuring the number of blood corpuscles.

دانہ ہائے خون پیما : خونی خلیوں کی تعداد کی پیمائش کرنے کا ایک آلہ۔

Haemodialysis *(he-mo-di-al'-is-is)* [G. haima, blood; dialysis, a separating]. A process of removing waste products from an dreplacing essential constituents in blood by a process of dialysis (q.v.). Such a technique is used in the artificial kidney.

ہیموڈایالائی سس : ڈایالائسس کے طریقے سے خون سے فضول مادوں کو نکالنے اور خون میں لازمی اجزا شامل کرنی کا ایک طریقہ۔ یہ تکنیک مصنوعی گردے میں استعمال کی جاتی ہے۔

Haemoglobin *(he-mo-glo'-bin)* [G. haima, blood; L. globus, ball]. The respiratory pigment in the red blood corpuscles. it is composed of an iron containing substance called 'haem', combined with globin. It has the reversible function of combining with, and releasing oxygen. See OXYHAEMO- GLOBIN.

ہیموگلوبن : سرخ خون خلیوں میں تنفسی پگمنٹ۔ یہ لوہے پر مشتمل ہیم جو گلوبن کے ساتھ ملا ہوتا ہے سے بنا ہوتا ہے۔ یہ آکسیجن کے ساتھ ملتا ہی اور پھر آکسیجن کو علیحدہ کر دیتا ہے۔ خون میں ۹۰ فیصد اس میں پروٹین ہوتی ہے۔

Haemoglobinaemia *(he-mo-glo-bin-e'-mi-a)*. Haemoglobin in the blood plasma--haemoglobinaemic, adj.

ہیموگلوبن دمویت : خونی پلازما میں ہیموگلوبن۔

aemoglobinometer *(he-mo-glo-bin-om'-et-er)* [G. haima, blood; globus, ball; metron, a measure]. An instrument for estimating the percentage of haemoglobin in the blood.

ہیموگلوبن پیما : خون میں ہیموگلوبن کی فیصد مقدار کے تعین کرنے کا آلہ۔

aemoglobinopathy *(he-mo-glob-in-op'-ath-i)* [G. haima, blood; globus, ball; pathos, disease]. Abnormality of the haemoglobin--haemoglobinopathic. adj.

ہیموگلوبن پیتھی : ہیموگلوبن کا نارمل نہ ہونا۔

aemoglobinuria *(he-mo-glob-in-u'-ri-a)* [G. haima, blood; globus, ball; ouron, urine]. Haemoglobin in the urine--haemoglobinuric, adj.

ہیموگلوبن بولیت : پیشاب میں ہیموگلوبن۔

aemolysin *(he-mo-li-sin)* [G. haima, blood; lysis, a loosening]. An agent which causes disintegration of erythrocytes. See ANTIBODIES.

ہیمولائی سن : ارتھروسائیٹس کوختم کرنے والا عامل۔

emolysis *(he-mol'-is-is)* [G. haima, blood; lysis, a loosening]. Disintegration of red blood cells, with liberation of contained haemoglobin. Laking. See ANAEMIA, HAEMOGLOBINAEMIA--haemoly-tic, adj.

خون پاشیدگی : سرخ خونی خلیوں کا خاتمہ۔ جس سے ان میں موجود ہیموگلوبن خارج ہو جاتی ہے۔

emolytic disease of the newborn A pathological condition in the newborn child due to rhesus incompatibility between the child's blood and that of the mother. Red blood cell destruction occurs with anaemia, often jaundice and an excess of erythroblasts or primitive red blood cells in the circulating blood. Immunization of women at risk, using gammaglobulin containing a high titre of anti-D can prevent haemolytic disease of the newborn. Exchange transfusion of the infant may be essential.

emopericardium *(he-mo-per-ri-kar'-di-um)* G. haima, blood; peri, around; kardia, heart]. Blood in the pericardial sac.

تاموری اجتماع الام : پیریکارڈیئل تھیلی میں خون۔

Haemoperitoneum *(he-mo-per-it-on-e'-um)* [G. haima, blood; peri, around; teinein, to stretch]. Blood in the peritoneal cavity.

نزف باریطونی : پیریٹونیئل کہفہ میں خون۔

Haemophilia *(he-mo-fil'-i-a)* [G. haima, blood; philein, to love]. Deficiency of antithaemophilic globulin (AHG Factor VIII). An inherited bleeding disease found only in males and transmitted through carrier females, who are daughters of affected males. Under special genetic circumstances, females with haemophilia may be produced. patient is subject to prolonged bleeding following even minor injuries--haemophiliac, adj.

ہیموفلیا : صرف آدمی میں پائے جانے والی بیماری جس میں خون نہیں جمتا۔ اس لئے زخم سے خون بہتا رہتا ہے۔ مریض دانت وغیرہ نہ اکھڑوائے انتقال خون تازہ دیجئے۔

Haemophilus *(he-mof'-il-us)* [G. haima, blood; philein, to love]. A genus of bacteria. Small Gram-negative rods which show much variation in shape (pleomorphism). They are strict parasites, and accessory substances pre sent in blood, are usually necessary for growth. They are found in the respiratory tracts of vertebrates and are often associated with acute and chronic disease, e.g. Haemophilus influenzae. See DUCREY'S BACILLUS.

خون پسند جرثومہ : جراثیم کا ایک جنس۔ چھوٹے گرام منفی سلاخی جراثیم۔ طفیلی۔

Haemophthalmia *(he-mof-thal'-mi-a)* [G. thor'-aks) [G. haima, blood; pneumon, lung; thorax, thorax]. The presence of blood and air in the pleural cavity causing compression of lung tissue.

دموی استرواح الصدر : پلیورل کہفہ میں خون اور ہوا کی موجودگی جس سے پھیپھڑوں کے نسیج پر دباؤ پڑتا ہے۔

Haemopoiesis *(he-mo-poi-e-sis)*. [G. haima, blood; poiesis, production]. The formation of blood--hae- opoietic, adj.

تدمیہ۔ تکوین دم : خون کا بننا۔

Haemoptysis *(he-mop'-tis-is)* [G. haima, blood; ptysis, spitting]. The coughing up of blood-haemoptyses, pl.

سل۔خون تھوکنا : خون کی کھانسی میں تھوکنا۔فائیٹو میناڈی اون انجکشن روزانہ لگایئے یاایک گولی دن میں ۳مرتبہ۔کاربازوکروم ۵سی سی کا ٹیکہ صبح وشام کولہے میں لگایئے۔

Haemorrhage *(hem'-or-raj)* [G. haima, blood; rhegnynai, to burst]. The escape of blood from a vessel. Arterial, capillary, venous designates the type of vessel from which it escapes. **primary h.,** that which occurs at the time of injury or **operation. reactionary h.,** that which occurs within 24 hours of injury or operation. **secondary h.,** that which occurs within 7 to 10 days of injury or operation. **accidental antepartum h.,** bleeding from separation of a normally situated placenta, after the 28th week of pregnancy. the term placental abruption now preferred. **antepartum h.,** vaginal bleeding after the 28th week and before labour, **intrapartum h.,** that occurring during labour. **postpartum h.,** excessive bleeding after delivery of child. In Great Britain it must be at least 500 ml to qualify as haemorrhage. **secondary postpartum h.,** excessive uterine bleeding more than 24 hours after delivery--haemorrhagic, adj.

ہمیرتج۔جریان خون : رگ سے خون کا بہنا۔جسم کے کسی حصے سے خون بہنا۔اس کی مختلف حالتیں یہ ہیں۔(۱) بنیادی: زخم لگنے یا اپریشن سے خون کا فوری اجراء (۲) نیتجتاً۔ زخم لگنے یا اپریسن کے ۲۴ گھنٹوں کے اندر خون کا اجراء۔(۳) ثانوی زخم لگنے یا اپریشن کرنے سے ہفتہ عشرہ میں کون کا اجراء (۴) غیر متوقع بچے کی پیائش سے پہلے حادثاتی طور پر حمل ٹھہرنے کے بعد فرج سے خون جاری ہونا اور قبل ولادت ہونے والے دردوں سے پہلے۔(۶) بچے کی پیدائس کے دوران جریان خون۔ جب بچے کی پیدائش کے سلسلے میں درد ہونا شروع ہو چکے ہوں۔(۷) بچے کی پیدائش کے بعد جریان خون کثرت سے ہونا۔(۸) ثانوی بچے کی پیدائش کے بعد ۲۴ گھنٹوں سے زیادہ کثرت سے جریان خون ہونا۔

Haemorrhagic disease of newborn. Characterized by gastrointrestinal, pulmonary or intracranial haemorrhage occuring from th second to the fifth day of life. Due to physiological variation in clotting power d to change in prothrombin content which fal on second day, and returns to normal at end

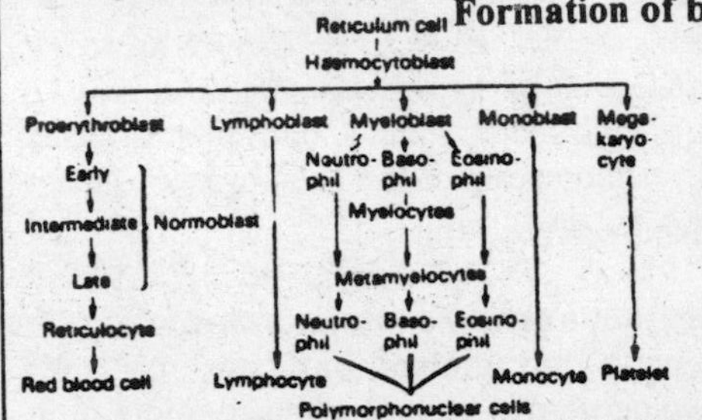

Formation of bloo

of first week when colonization of gut wi bacteria results in synthesis of vitamin K, th permitting formation of prothrombin by t liver. Responds to administration of vitan K.

ودکانزفی مرض : زندگی کے دوسرے سے پانچویں دن تک واقع ہونی ٹروانٹسٹائینل، ششی یا انٹراکرانیکیل ہیمرتج۔ اس کی دو اقسام ہیں۔ یکل اور ثانوی۔

Haemorrhoidal *(hem-or-roid'-al)* [G. hain blood; rheein, to flow]. 1. Pertaining to hae orrhoids. 2. Applied to blood vessels and n ves in the anal region.

یری۔مقعدی : (۱) ہیمرائڈز سے متعلق۔(۲) مقعد والے حصہ اقع خونی رگوں اور اعصاب پر اطلاق کیا جاتا ہے۔

Haemorrhoidectomy *(hem-or-roid-ek'-to-* [G. haima, blood; rheein, to flow; ektor excision]. Surgical removal of haemorrhoid

ربراری : ہیمرائڈز کو اپریشن کے ذریعے ختم کرنا۔

Haemorrhoids *(hem'-or-rodiz)* [G. hain blood rheein, to flow]. Varicosity of the ve around the anus; piles **external h.,** th outside the anal sphinceter covered with sk **internal h.,** those inside the anal sphin covered with mucous membrane.

ائڈز۔بواسیر (واحد: باسور : بواسیر ہو جانا۔مقعد کے گرم متورم یں بیرونی اگر صفرے سے باہر کھال سے ڈھکی ہوں اور اندرونی اگر

صفرے کے اندر میوکس جھلی سے ڈھکی ہوں۔

aemosalpinx *(he-mo-sal'-pinks)*. See HAEMATO- SALPINX.

انبوبی اجتماع الدم : ہیمٹیو سلپنکس۔

aemosiderosis *(he-mo-sid-er-os'-is)* [G. haima, blood; sideros, iron] Iron deposits in the tissues.

ہیموسائیڈرین کا جماؤ : بافتوں میں لوہے کا اجتماع۔

aemospermia *(he-mo-sper'-mi-a)* [G. haima, blood; sperma, seed]. The discharge of blood-stained semen.

منی الدم : خون آلود منی کا اخراج۔

aemostasis *(he-mo-sta'-sis)* [G. haima, blood; stasis, a standing]. 1. Arrest of bleeding. 2. Stagnation of blood within its vessel.

احتباس الدم : (۱) روانی خون کا رکنا۔ (۲) خون کا اپنی رگ میں کھڑا ہونا۔

aemostatic *(he-mo-stat'-ik)* [G. haima, blood; starikos, causing to stand]. Any agent which arrests bleeding. **haemostic forceps**, artery forceps.

حابس الدم : روانی خون کو روکنے والا عامل۔

aemothorax *(he-mo-thor'-aks)* [G. haima, blood; thorax, thorax]. Blood in the pleural cavity.

نزف صدری : بلیورل کہفہ میں خون۔

ir *(har)*. Thread-like appendage present on all parts of human skin except palms, soles, lips, glans penis and that surrounding the terminal phalanges. **exclamation-mark h.**, the broken-off stump found at the periphery of spreading bald patches in alopecia areata. Atrophic thining of the hair shaft gives this characteristic shape--hence its name.

بال : دھاگہ نما لوازمہ جو انسانی جلد کے تمام حصوں پر موجود ہوتا ہے۔ سوائے ہتھیلیوں، تلووں، لبوں، عضو تناسل کے سروں اور انگلیوں کے اگلے سروں کے۔

ldol *(hal'-dol)* Haloperidol (q.v.).

libut liver oil. A very rich source of vitamins A and D. The smaller dose required makes it more acceptable than cod liver oil.

قفندر (ماہی) کے جگر کا تیل : اس میں حیاتین اے اور ڈی کثرت سے ہوتے ہیں۔

Halitosis *(hal-i-to'-sis)* [L. halitus, breath; G. -osis, condition]. Bad breath.

بدبودار دم : خراب سانس۔

Hallucination *(hal-u-sin-a'-shun)* [L. alucinari, to wander in the mind]. A false perception occurring without any true sensory stimulus. A common symptom in severe psychoses (q.v.) including schizophrenia, paraphrenia, confu- sional states. Also common in delirium, duri- ng toxic states and following head injuries.

واہمہ۔ ہزیان : ایک غلط تصور جو پریشانی کی صورت میں پیدا ہوتا ہے۔

Hallucinogens *(hal-us-in-o'-jens)*. Chemicals, e.g. mescaline, LSD, capable of producing hallucina- tion. Psychotomimetics.

ہلوسینوجنز : کیمیائی مرکبات۔ مثلاً ایل ایس ڈی وغیرہ جن سے انسان تخیل میں پرواز کرتا ہے۔

Hallucinosis *(hal-u-sin-o'-sis)*. [L. alucinari, to wander in the mind; G. -osis, condition]. A psychosis in which the patient is grossly hallucinated. Usually a subacute delirious state; the predominant symptoms are auditory illusions (q.v.). and hallucinations.

واہمیت : ایسی حالت جس میں مریض تخیل پرواز کرتا ہے۔

Hallux *(hal'-uks)* [L. allex, big tow]. The great toe, **hallux valgus,** bunnion (q.v.). **hallux rigidus,** ankylosis of the metatarsophalangeal articulation caused by osteoarthritis.

انگوٹھا : پاؤں کا انگوٹھا۔

Halogen *(hal'-o-jen)* [G. hals, salt, sea]. Any one of the non-metallic elements--bromine, chlorine, fluorine, iodine.

ہیلوجن۔ برقی منفی عناصر : چار عناصر فلورین۔ کلورین۔ برومین اور آیوڈین مذکورہ چار ادھاتی عناصر میں سے ایک۔

Haloperidol *(hal-o-per'-i-dol)*. Tranquillizer. Useful in acute mania. Useful for premedication.

ہیلوپیری ڈال : سکون بخش دوا۔ شدید مانیا میں مفید۔

Halothane A clear colourless liquid used as an inhalation anaesthetic. Advantages; non-explosive and non-inflammable in all circumstances. Ordour is not unpleasant. It is non-irritant.

ہیلوتھین : ایک صاف بے رنگ مائع جو سانس کے ذریعے بے ہوش کرنے میں استعمال کیا جاتا ہے۔

Hamamelids *(ham-am-el'-ids)*. Witch **hazel, aqua h.,** 'extract of witch hazel', made from the bark. Astringent lotion.

ہیلمیلڈز : وچ بندوق۔ اس کی چھال سے عرق کشید کیا جاتا ہے۔

Hamamelids leaf incorporated in suppositories for non-inflammatory piles.

Hammer toe

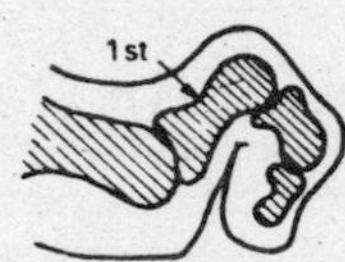

Hammer toe A permanent hyperextension of the first phalanx and flexion of second and third phalanges.

مطرقی انگوٹھا : پہلے فیلنکس کا مستقل بڑھاؤ اور دوسری و تیسری انگلیوں کا مستقل خم۔

Handicapped The term applied to a person with a defect tha t interferes with normal activity and achievement.

کوتاہ : ایسا شخص جس میں کوئی نقص یا کمی پائی جائے۔

Hand-Schuller Christian disease A rare condition usually manifesting in early child-hood with histiocytic granulomatous lesions affecting many tissues. Regarded as a form of histiocytosis X. Cause unknown and course relatively being [Alfred Hand, American paediatrician, 1868-1949. Artur Schuller, Austrian neurologist, 1876-1958. Henry Asbury Christian, Boston internist, 1876-1951].

ہینڈ شلر کرسچین مرض : ہیسٹو سائی ٹوسس۔ خواتین کی نسبت مردوں پر اثر ہوتا ہے۔

Hangnail *(hang'-nal)*. A narrow strip of skin, partly detached from the nail fold.

ردناخن : ناخن سے جزوی طور پر الگ ہونے والی کھال۔

Hansen's disease and bacillus See LEPROSY

ض ہنسن۔ جذام۔ کوڑھ : کوڑھ

Hare-lip A congenital defect in the lip; a fissur extending from the margin of the lip to th nostril; may be single or double, and is ofte associated with cleft palate.

ٔرمیت : ہونٹ میں نقص۔ ہونٹ کے کنارے سے نتھنے کی طرف شگاف۔ نگل یا ڈبل۔

Harris's operation. A transvesical, suprapub type of prostatectomy (q.v.). [S. Harvy Harri Australian surgeon, 1880-1936].

یشن۔ ہیرث : پروسٹاٹیکٹومی کی ایک قسم۔ اس کا نام آسٹریلوی سرجن ں ہاردی حارث کے نام پر ہے۔

Hartmann's solution. An electrolyte repla ement solution. Contains sodium lactate a chloride, potassium chloride and calciu chloride. [Alexis hartmann. American phy ician, 1898].

ن کا محلول : الیکٹرک ولائیٹ کی جگہ متبادل محلول۔ سوڈیم لیکٹیٹ و رائیڈ، پوٹاشیم کلورائیڈ اور کیلشیم کلورائیڈ پر مشتمل۔

Hartnup disease Inborn error of protein met bolism. Associated with mental subnormalit Can be treated with nicotinamide and ne mycin.

ٹنپ مرض : پروٹین میٹابولزم کی پیدائشی غلطی۔ اس میں ذہنی پسماندگی تی ہے۔

Hashimoto's disease Affliction of an enlarg thyroid gland occurring in middle-ag females, and producing mild hypothyroidis Result of sensitization of patient to her ov thyroid protein, thyroglobulin. See AUT IMMUNIZATION [H. Hashimoto, Japane surgeon, 1881-1934].

ں مونو کا مرض : درمیانہ عمر کی خواتین میں بڑھی ہوئی تھائیرائڈ گلینڈ۔

Hashish *(hash'-ish)*. Cannabis indica (q.v.).

یش : گنابس انڈیکا۔

Haustration *(haws-tra'shun)*. Sacculation, as

the colon--haustrum, sing; haustra, pl.

ہاسٹریشن : سیکولیشن۔ جیسے قولون کی۔

ay fever. A form of allergic rhinitis in which attacks of catarrh of conjunctiva, nose and throat are precipitated by exposure to pollen.

تپ کاہی : زردانوں سے ناک۔ گلے وغیرہ کی ترسیب۔

aygarth's nodes. Swelling of joints sometimes seen in the finger joints of patients suffering from arthritis. [John Haygarth, English psysician, 1740-1827].

نوڈز ہائی گارتھ : جوڑوں کا ورم۔

CG. Haman chorionic gonadotrophin; obtained from the placenta. Used for eryptorchism.

ایچ سی جی : پلیسنٹا سے حاصل شدہ انسانی کوریانی گوینڈوٹرافن۔

ealing *(he'-ling)* [A.S.]. The natural process of cure or repair of the tissues, **healing by first intention,** when the edges of a clean wound are accurately held together, healing occurs with the minimum of scarring and deformity. **healing by second intention,** when the edges of a wound are not held together, the gap is filled by granulation tissue before epithefium can grow over the wound-heal, v.t., v.i.

شفا۔ اندمال زخم : بافتوں کی مرمت یا علاج کا قدرتی طریقہ۔

ealth *(helth).* World Health Organization states, 'Health is a state of complete physical, mental and social well-being and not merely the absence of disease or infirmity, 'Office of Health Economics states, 'A person should be regarded as healthy provided he can remain socially and economically active, even though he may have to suffer, some health disability or discomfort.

صحت۔ تندرستی : ورلڈ ہیلتھ آرگنائزیشن کے مطابق مکمل طبیعی صحت۔ ذہنی اور سماجی بہتری ہے تاکہ صرف بیماری یا کمزوری کی غیر موجودگی۔ ہیلتھ اکنامکس کے آفس کے مطابق ایسے شخص کو صحت مند سمجھنا چاہئے جو سماجی و معاشی طور پر عامل ہو خواہ وہ معذور ہی کیوں نہ ہو۔

Heart

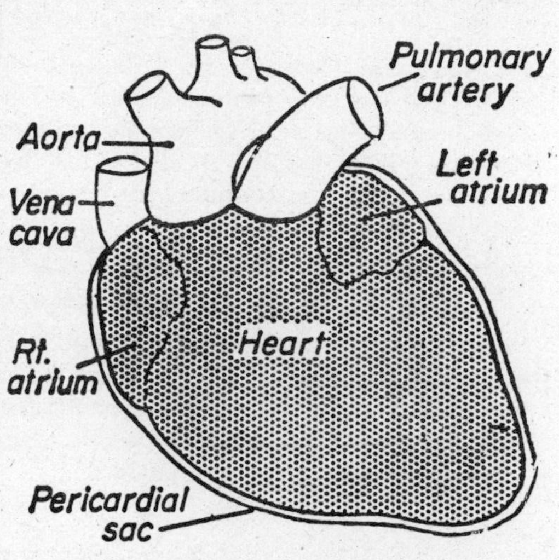

Heart *(hart)* [A.S. heorte]. The hollow muscular organ which pumps the blood through the body; situated behind the sternum, lying obliquely between the two lungs. It weighs 2.24 to 3.36 hg in the female and 2.80 to 3.36 hg in the male. **heart-lung,** apparatus for extra corporeal oxygenation of the blood. Used with heparin to prevent blood clotting.

دل۔ قلب : کھوکھلا عضلاتی عضو جو خون کو جسم میں پمپ کرتا ہے۔ دونوں پھیپھڑوں کے درمیان۔

Heartblock Partial or Complete inhibition of the speed of conduction of the electrical impulse from the atrium to the ventricle of the heart. The cause may be an organic lesion or a functional disturbance. In its mildest form, it can only be detected electrocardiographically, whilst in its complete form the ventricles beat at their own slow intrinsic rate uninfluenced by the atria.

سکوت قلب : دل کے ایٹریم سے وینٹریکل کی طرف برقی امپلس کی رفتار کی مکمل یا جزوی رکاوٹ اس کی تشخیص میں الیکٹرا کارڈیوگرام مدد ہے۔

Heartburn See PYROIS and HOT-FAT HEARTBURN SYNDROME.

وجع الفواد : سٹرنم کے پیچھے جلن کا احساس۔

Heat exhaustion. Heat syncope. Collapse, with or without loss of consciousness, suffered in conditions of heat and high humidity; largely resulting from loss of fluid and salt by sweating. If the surrounding air becomes saturated, heat-stroke will ensue.

حرارتی خستگی : حرارت اور زیادہ نمی کی حالتوں میں مبتلا ہوش میں ہوتے ہوئے یا ہوش کے بغیر موت پسینے سے سیال اور نمک کا ضیاع ہو جاتا ہے اگر آس پاس کی ہوا سیر شدہ ہو تو ہیٹ سٹروک ہوگا۔

Heat-stoke Final stage in heat exhausion. When the body is unable to !ose heat, hyperpyrexia occurs and death may ensue. A complica tion of electropyrexia (q.v.). See STROKE.

[ہیٹ سٹروک' لولگنا : جب جسم حرارت ضائع کرنے کے ناقابل ہو جائے تو موت واقع ہو جاتی ہے۔

Hebephrenia *(he-be-fre'-ni-a)* [G. hebe, puberty; phren, mind]. A type of schizophrenia (q.v.)--hebephrenic, adj.

جنون شباب۔شبابی دیوانگی : شائزوفرمیا کی ایک قسم۔

Helberden's disease Angina pectoris.

Heberden's nodes small osseous swellings at terminal phalangeal joints occurring in many types of arthritis.

وجع القلب۔درد دل: انجینا پکٹورس۔

Hedonism *(hed'-on-izm)* [G. hedone, pleasure]. Excessive devotion to pleasure, so that a person's conduct is determined by an unconscious drive to seek pleasure and avoid unpleasant things.

لذتیت : مسرت وشادمانی کی طرف زیادہ رجحان۔

Hegar's sign. Marked softening of the cervix in early pregnancy. [Alfred Hegar, German gynaecologist, 1830-1914].

علامت ہیگر : وضع حمل کے اولین دنوں میں سروکس کا نمایاں طور پر نرم ہونا۔

Heinz body. Refractile, irregularly shaped body present in red blood cells in some haemoglobino- pathies.

ہینز باڈی : درون خلوی ہیموگلوبن میں موجود انعطافی بے قاعدہ شکل کا

م۔

Helium *(he'-li-um)* [G. helios, the sun]. an ine gas of low density. Sometimes mixed wi oxygen for treatment of asthma, as it ai inspiration.

م : ایک عنصر۔جوہری وزن ۴٫۰۰۲۶۔جوہری عدد ۲۔ایک ہلکی' غیر
س اور غیر آتش گیر گیس۔کم کثافت والی گیس۔بعض دفعہ دمہ کے علاج کے
ے آکسیجن کے ساتھ ملائی جاتی ہے کیونکہ یہ اندر کی طرف سانس لینے میں مدد
ن ہے۔

Heller's operation Division of the muscle co at the junction between the oesophagus a the stomach; used to relieve the defficulty swallowing in cases of cardiospasm. [Ern Heller, Professor of Surgery and Surgeon St. Georg Hospital, Leipzig, 1877-1964].

رز اپریشن : ایسوفیگس اور معدہ کی درمیان جنکشن پر عضلی کوٹ کی
یم۔

Helminthagogue *(hel-minth'-a-gog)*. [helmins, worm; agogos, leading]. See ANT ELMINTIC.

م کش' دافع دیدان : انتھلمنٹک۔

Helminthiasis *(hel-minth'-a-sis)* [G. helmi worm; N.L. -iasis, condition]. The conditi resulting from infestation with worms.

انیت : کیڑوں سے بھرے ہونے کی حالت۔

Helminthology *(hel-min-thol'-o-ji)* [G. helmi worm; logos, discourse]. The study of pa sitic worms.

انیات : طفیلی کیڑوں کا مطالعہ۔

Heloma *(hel-o'-ma)* [G. helos, a nail]. Co callosity--helomata, pl.

ن۔ گٹا : پاؤں یا انگوٹھے کا سخت ہو جانا۔

Hemeralopia *(hem-er-al-o'-pi-a)* [G. heme day; alaos, blind; ops, eye]. Defective visi in a bright ıight. Term has been incorrec used for nyctalopia, nigh blindness(q.v.).

کوری : تیز روشنی میں ناقص نظر آنا۔

Hemianopia *(hem-i-an-o'-pi-a)* [G. hemi, h a-, not; opsis, visision]. Blindness in one h of the visual field of one or both eyes.

وری۔نیم بصری : دونوں آنکھوں یا آنکھ کے بصارت کا نصف

دائرہ نظر نہ آنا۔

emiatrophy *(hem-i-at'-ro-fi)* [G. hemi, half; atrophia, lack of food]: Atrophy of one half or one side. **hemiatrophy facialis,** a congenital condition, or a manifestation of seleroderma (q.v.)., in which the structures on one side of the face are shrunken.

ذبول نصفی : ایک طرف یا نصف کی اثرانی

emichorea *(hem-i-kor-e'-a)* [G. hemi, half; choreia , dance]. Choreiform movements limited to one side of the body. See CHOREA.

قطرب نصفی : جسم کے ایک طرف محدود کوریفارم حرکات۔

emicolectomy *(hem-i-ko-lek'-to-mi)* [G. hemi, half; kolon, colon; ektome, excision]. Removal of approximately half the colon.

جزوی قولون براری : قریبا نصف قولون ختم کرنا۔

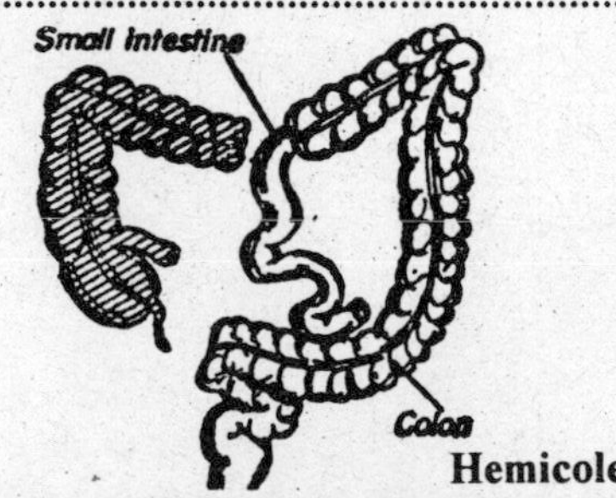

Hemicolectomy

emicrania *(hem-i-kran'-i-a)* [G. hemi, half; kranion, skull]. Unilateral headache as in migraine.

یک طرفہ سردرد

emidiaphoresis *(hem-i-di-a-for-e'-sis)* [G. hemi, half; diapkerein, carry through]. Unilateral sweating of the body.

تعرق نصفی : جسم کا یک طرفہ پسینہ۔

emiglossectomy *(hem-i-glos-ek'-to-mi)* [G. hemi, half; glossa, tongue; ektome, excision]. Removal of approximately half the tongue.

نیم زبان براری۔نصف لسان براری : قریبا نصف زبان کا خاتمہ۔

eminevrin *(hem-in-ev'-rin).* Chlorme thiazole (q.v.).

ہیمی نیوزین : کلورمیتھازول

Hemiparesis *(hem-i-pa-re'-sis).* [G. hemi, half; paresis, paralysis]. A slight paralysis or weakness of one half of face or body.

فالج نصفی خفیف : چہرے یا جسم کے نصف حصے کی کمزوری۔

Hamiplegia *(hem-i-ple'-ji-a)* [G. hemi, half; plege, stroke]. Paralysis of one side of the body, usually resulting from a cerebrovascular accident on the opposite side--**hemiplegic,** adj.

فالج نصفی : جسم کا ایک طرف کا دورہ۔

Henoch's purpura *(hen'-oks).* See PURRURA. [Edvard H. Henoch, German paediatrician, 1820-1910].

Hepar *(he'-par)* [G.]. The liver--hepatic, adj.

کبد : جگر جسم کی سب سے بڑی غدہ۔

Heparin *(hep'-ar-in).* an acid present in liver and lung tissue. When injected intravenously it inhibits coagulation of the blood, and it is widely used in the treatment of thrombosis, often in associated with orally active anticoagulants such as phenindone.

ہیپارین: جگر اور پھیپھڑے کے نسیج میں موجود ایک ترشہ کاروزی تھارامبوسز میں اس کا دس ہزار یونٹ کا ایک ٹیکہ صبح ایک شام ڈیڑھ لاکھ یونٹ دے کر بند کر دیجئے۔

Hepatectomy *(hep-at-ek'-to-mi)* [G. hepar, liver; ektome, excision]. Excision of part of the liver.

جگر براری : جگر کا ایک حصہ کاٹنا۔

Hepatic *(hep-at'-ik)* [G. hepar, liver]. Pertaining to the liver.

جگری : جگر سے متعلق۔

Hepaticocholedochostomy *(hep-at'-id-o-ko-l-e-dok- os'-to-mi)* [G. hepar, liver, chole, bile; docke, reception; stoma, mouth]. End-to-end union of the severed hepatic and common bile ducts.

ہیپیکو سٹول ڈاکوسٹومی : کٹی ہوئی جگری اور مشترک صفراوی نالیوں کے سرے کو سرے سے ملانا۔

Hepaticoenteric *(hep-at'-ik-o-en-ter'-rik).* [G. hepar, liver; enteron, intestine]. Pertaining to the liver and intestine.

کبدی معائی : جگر اور آنت سے متعلق۔

Hepaticojejunostomy *(hep-at'-ik-o-je-joon-os'-to-mi)* [G. hepar, liver; L, jejunus, empty; G. stoma, mouth]. Anastomosis of the hepatic duct to a loop of proximal jejunum.

ہیپیٹیکو نوسٹومی : جگری نالی کا امامی جیجونم کے لوپ کے ساتھ جال۔

Hepatitis *(hep-a-ti'-tis)* [G. hepar, liver; -itis, inflammation]. Inflammation of the liver; **infective h.,** Syn. 'catarrhal jaundice,' hepatitis-A virus infection of liver with an incubation period of two to six weeks, causing jaundic after a brief influenzalike illness. Notifiable in Britain since 1968. Spread by faecaloral route. Virus B or SH is spread only by contact or inoculation with human blood products and causes **serum h.** Incubation period six weeks to six months, but infection can be severe, even fatal. It is estimated that 2 to 3 per-cent of world adult population are carriers of hepatitis-B virus. **Australia antigen** *(an'-ti-jen),* associated with hepatitis virus B. Discovered by Dr. Blumberg in 1965 in the blood of an Aborigine. In the United Kingdom it is found in about 1/800 to 1/1000 of the population, mostly without manifestations of disease. Rates are higher in tropical areas. The majority of patients with serum hepatitis give a positive reaction to the Australia antigen during the acute phase of illness, but because of technical limita tions a negative reaction does not exclude serum hepatitis. Persons whose serum contains the antigen are, through their blood, infective to others. Their blood must never be used for transfusion because of this risk. See JAUNDICE.

ورم جگر : جگر کی سوزش۔

Hepatization *(hep-a-ti-za'-shun)* [G. hepar, loiver]. Pathologica l changes in the tissues, which cause them to resemble liver. Occurs in the lungs in pneumonia.

جگر سازی : بافتوں میں تبدیلیاں جن سے وہ جگر سے مشابہ ہوتی ہیں۔ نمونیہ میں پھیپھڑوں میں واقع ہوتی ہیں۔

Hepatocellular *(hep-at-o-sel'-u-lar)* [G., hepar, liver; L. cellula, small cell]. Pertaining to, affecting liver cells.

گری خلوی : جگری خلیوں یا ان سے متاثر کرنے کی متعلق۔

Hepatocirrhosis *(hep-at-o-si-ro'-sis)* [G. hepa liver; kirrhos, tawny; -osis, condition]. Cirrhosis (q.v.). of the liver.

ال الکبد : جگر کا سروس۔

Hepatoma *(hep-at-o'-ma).* [G. hepar, live -oma, condition]. Primary carcinoma of th liver hepatomata, pl.

گری سلعہ : جگر کا اولین کرسینوما۔

Hepatomergaly *(hep-at-o-meg'-al-i)* [G. hepa liver; megas, large]. Enlargement of the live It is palpable below the costal margin.

لانی جگر۔ کبر الکبد : جگر کا بڑھنا۔

Hepatosplenic *(hep'-at-o-splen'-ik)* [G. hepa liver; toxikon, poison]. Having an injurio effect on liver cells hepat.otoxicity, n.

بدی کمی : جگری خلیوں پر نقصان دہ اثرات۔

Heptalgin *(hep-tal'-jin).* Phenadoxone (q.v.).

ہیپلیجن : فیناڈوکسون۔

Hereditary *(he-red'-it-a-ri)* [L. heredita heirship]. Inherited ; capable of being inherited.

وروثی : وراثت میں جانے کا اہل۔ وراثت میں ملوا ہوا۔

Heredity *(he-red'-i-ti)* . That factor responsib for the persistence of characteristics in successive generations.

راث : وہ عامل جو تواتر سے نسل در نسل خصوصیات کے مستقل پن کا زمہ دار

-

Hermaphrodite *(her-maf'-ro-dit)* [L. hermaphroditus, from G. Hermes and Aphr- odite Individual possessing both ovarian and testicular tissue. Although they may approximat either to male or femal type, they are usuall sterile from imperfect development of the gonads.

جنسے : بیضہ دان اور خصیوں کی بافتوں کے حامل افراد۔

Hernia *(her'-ni-a)* [L.]. The abnormal protrusio of an organ, or part of an organ, through a aperture in the surrounding structure commonly the protrusion of an abdomin organ through a gap in the abdominal wall. **diaphragmatic h.,** protrusion through the diaphragm, the commonest one involv-

Types of hernia

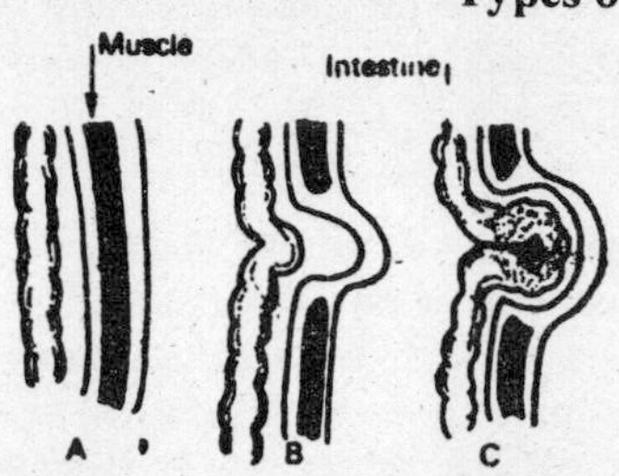

A Normal
B SB Simple hernia
C Strangulation of loop of intestine
Type of hernia

ing the stomach at the oesophageal opening (**hiatus h.**). **femoral h.,** protrusion through the femoral canal, alongside the femoral blood vessels as they pass into the thigh. **inguinal h.,** protrusion through the inguinal canal in the male. **strangulated h.,** hernia in which the blood supply to the organ involved is impaired, usually due to constriction by surrounding structures. **umbilical h.,** protrusion through the area of the umbilical scar. See IRREDUCIBLE.

ہرنیا۔فتق : اردگرد کی ساختوں میں سوراخ میں سے کسی عضو یا کسی عضو کے کسی حصے کا غیر معمولی طور پر باہر نکل آنا۔ زیریں پیٹ میں زیر جلد پیٹ کی دیوار میں راستہ ہوتا ہے جس میں سے سپر میٹک کارڈ نکل کر فولوں تک پہنچ جاتی ہے۔ یہ راستہ دونوں جانب ہوتا ہے۔ بعض اوقات راستہ زیادہ کھلا ہوتا ہے اور آنتوں کے کچھ حصے پیٹ میں سے اتر کر فوطوں تک آ جاتے ہیں۔

Hernioplasty *(her-ni-o-plas'-ti)* [L. hernia, rupture; G. plassein, to form]. An operation for hernia, in which an attempt is made to prevent recurrence, by refashioning the structures to give greater strength hernioplastic, adj.

ہرنیو پلاسٹی : ہرنیا کا اپریشن۔

Herniorrhaphy *(her-ne-or'-raf-i)* [L. hernia, rupture; G. rhaphe, a suture]. An operation for hernia, in which the weak area is reinforced by some of the patient's own tissues, or by some other material.

فتق دوزی : ہرنیا کا اپریشن جس میں کمزور حصے مریض کی اپنی بافتوں سے بھر دیئے جاتے ہیں یا کسی دوسرے میٹریل سے۔

Herniotome *(her'-ne-o-tom)* [L. hernia, rupture; G. tomos, a cutting]. A special knife with a blunt tip, used for hernia operations.

ہرنیوٹون : ہرنیا کے اپریشن کیلئے مستعمل ایک مخصوص چاقو جس کا راس کند ہوتا ہے۔

Herniotomy *(her'-ne-ot'-o-mi)* [L. hernia, rupture; G. tome, a cutting]. An operation to cure hernia, by the return of its contents to their normal position, and the removal of the hernial sac.

فتق شگافی : ہرنیا کے علاج کے لئے اپریشن۔

Heroin *(her'-o-in)*. Diamorphine (q.v.).

ہیروئن : ڈایامارفین۔

Herpangina *(her-pan-jin-a')* [G. herpein, to creep; L. angere, to strangle]. Minute vesicles and ulcers at the back of the mouth Short, febrile illness in children caused by Coxsackie viruses.

ہرپینجینا : منہ کی پشت پر چھوٹے آبلے اور السر۔

Herpes *(her'-pez)*. [G. herpein, to creep]. Vesicular eruption due to a virus infection, **herpes facialis, febrillis and labialis** are names used when blisters appear around the mouth (cold sores). Caused by the virus of herpes simplex type 1. Can a lso cause dendrritic corneal ulcer. Genital herpes caused by herpes simplex virus type. 2. **herpes zoster** (shingles) is caused by varicella-zoster virus; the virus attacks sensory nerves, with sever pain and appearance of vesicles along the distribution of the nerves involved (usually unilateral). herpes simplex virus and varicella-zoster virus often cause recurrent infection as they remain latent in nerve ganglia after the initial infection--herpetic, adj.

ہرپیز : حملہ وائرس کی وجہ سے آبلہ نما شگاف۔

Herpetiform *(her-pet'-i-form)* [G. herpein, to

creep; L. forma, form]. Resembling herpes.

نملہ نما۔ داد جیسا : ہرپیز سے مشابہ۔

Hesperidin *(hes-per'-i-din)*. Functions as vitamin P (q.v.). See CITRIN.

Hetacillin *(het-a-sil'-in)*. Synthetic antibilotic of the penicinate group. Destroyed by penicillianase, thus not active agaisnt Staphylococcus resistant to penicillin G.

ہیٹاسلین : پینی سینیٹ گروہ کا تالیفی اینٹی بایوٹک۔

Heterogenous *(het-er-oj'-en-us)* [G. heteros, other; genesis, descent]. Of unlike origin; not originating within the body; derived from a different species, e.g. the use of beef bone pegs in orthopaedic surgery. See AUTOGENOUS, HOMOGENOUS.

مختلف الاوضاع : مختلف ماخذ کا جسم کے اندر پیدا نہ ہونا۔ مختلف انواع سے حاصل شدہ۔

Heterologous *(het-er-ol'-o-gus)* [G. heteros, other; logos, relation]. Of different origin; from a different species.

دگرزاد : مختلف انواع سے۔

Heterophile *(het'-er-o-fil)* [g. heteros, other; philos, fond]. Activity of a product of one species agaisnt that of another, for example human antigen against sheep's red blood cells.

Heteroplasty *(het-e-ro-plas'-ti)* [G. heteros, other; plassein, to form]. Plastic operation using a graft from another individual--heteroplastic, adj.

دگر پیوندکاری: پلاسٹک اپریشن جس میں پیوند کسی دوسرے فرد سے استعمال کیا جائے۔

Heterosexual *(he-te-ro-seks'-u-al)* [G. heteros, other; L.sexuas, sex]. Attracted towards the opposite sex. Opp. homosexual.

دگرجنسیہ : جنس مخالف کی طرف کشش۔

Hetrazan *(het'-ra-zan)*. Diethyl carbamazine (q.v.).

ہیٹروزان : ڈائی ایتھائل کاربامیزین۔

Hexachlorophane *(heks-a-klor'-o-fan)*. An antiseptic used in skin sterilization, and in some bactericidal soaps. Any medicinal product containing, hexachlorophane (irrespective of the amount) must bear a warning on the container 'not to be used for babies', or 'not to be administered to a child under 2'. Under suspicion as being a possible cause of brain damage in babies.

ہیکساکلوروفین : دافع تعفن جو جلد کو صاف کرنے اور بعض جراثیم کش صابنوں میں مستعمل ہے۔

Hexamethonium bromide *(heks-a-meth-o'-ni-um bro'-mid)*. One of the earlier ganglionic blocking agents, used in the treatment of hypertension, given by subcutaneous or intramuscular injection. It is now being replaced by orally active drugs such as pentolinium or mecamylamine (q.v.).

ہیکسامیتھونیم۔ برومائیڈ : ہائپرٹنشن کے علاج میں استعمال کیا جاتا تھا۔ ٹیکے کے ذریعے لگاتے تھے اب اس کی جگہ دوسری ادویات دینے لگے ہیں۔

Hexamine *(heks'-a-men)*. A urinary antiseptic of low toxicity. Action is due to liberation of formaldehyde in the urine, and is increased by acidification. Often prescribed with sodium acid phosphate. **Hexamine hippurate**, especially useful before urinary tract surgery.

ہیکسامین : ایک بولی دافع تعفن جس میں زہریلا پن کم ہوتا ہے۔
ہیکسا۔تھائیلین ٹیٹرامین۔ یوروٹرومین۔

Hexobarbitone *(heks-o-bar'-bit-on)*. A short-acting barbiturate, useful when a prompt but relatively brief action is required.

ہیکسوباربی ٹون : ایک مختصر العمل باربیٹوریٹ۔

Hexoestrol *(heks-es'-trol)*. A synthetic compound related to stiboestrol, and used for similar purposes.

ہیکسوایسٹرول : سٹلبواسٹرول سے ملتا جلتا تالیفی مرکب اور انہی مقاصد کے لئے استعمال کیا جاتا ہے۔

Hexopal *(heks'-o-pal)*. Nicotynil alcohol. Vasodilator in peripheral vascular disease.

ہیکسوپال : نکوٹائنل الکوحل۔

Hexose *(heks'-os)* A class of simple sugars, monosaccharides, $C_0H_{12}O_6$. Examples are glucose, mannose, galactose.

ہیکسوز : سادہ شکروں کی ایک جماعت۔ مونوسیکرائیڈز۔ مثلاً گلوکوس، گلیکٹوز

وغیرہ۔ سالمہ چھ کاربن جوہروں پر مشتمل۔

Hexylresorcinol *(heks-il-re-sor'-sin-ol)*. An anthelminitic with a wide range of activity, being effective against threadworm, roundworm, hookworm and intestinal fluke. It is followed by a saline purge. Treatment may have to be repeated at 3 day intervals. Also used in cystitis and other infections of the urinary tract.

ہیکسائل ریسارسینول : چرنوں راؤنڈورم، ہک ورم اور آنتوں کی فلوک کے لئے موثر۔ ایک زرد قلمی ٹھوس۔

HGH. Human growth hormone secreted by pituitary gland. Has now been synthesized.

ایچ جی ایچ : پچوٹری گلینڈ کا ہارمون جو اب تالیف کیا جاتا ہے۔

Hiatus *(hi-a'-tus)* [L.]. A space or opening. See HERNIA--hiatal, adj.

وقفہ۔ گم حصہ : ایک سوراخ یا جگہ۔

Hibb's operation Operation for spinal fixation, following spinal tuberculosis. No bone graft is used (as in Albee's operation), but the split vertebral spines are pressed outwards, and laid in contact with the lamina e. Bony union occurs, and the spine is rigid. [Russell Aubra Hibbs, American orthopaedic surgeon, 1869-1932].

ہنبر اپریشن : سپائنل فکسیشن کے لئے اپریشن۔

Hibitane *(hi'-bi-tan)*. Chlorhexidine (q.v.).

ہبی ٹین : کلورہکسیڈین۔

Hiccough *(hi-kuf)*. An involuntary inspiratory spasm of the respiratory organs, ending in a sudden closure of the glottis, with the production of a characteristic sound. Hiccip.

ہائی کف۔ ہچکی : تنفّسی اعضا کا غیر ارادی اندر کی طرف سانس لینے کا عمل جس سے گلاٹس اچانک بند ہو جاتا ہے اور مخصوص آواز نکلتی ہے۔

Hiccup *(hi-kup)*. Hiccough (q.v.).

ہچکی : ہائی کف۔ فواق۔

Hidrosis *(hid-ro-sis)* [G. hidros, sweat; -osis, condition]. Sweat secretion.

کثرت پسینہ : پسینے کا اخراج۔

Higginson's syringe Compression of the rubber bulb forces fluid forward through the nozzle for irrigation of a body cavity. [Alfred Higginson,

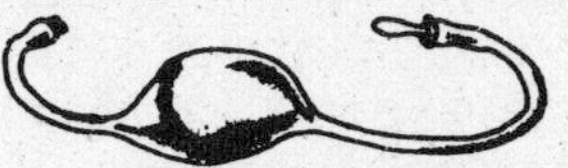

Higginson's syringe

Liverpool surgeon of the 19th century].

ہگنسنز سرنج : جسمانی کہفے کو سیراب کرنے کے لئے ربڑ کے بلب کا دباؤ سیال کو نوزل میں سے آگے دھکیلتا ہے۔

Hilum *(hi-lum)* [L. a trifle]. A depression on the surface of an organ where vessels, ducts, etc. enter and leave--hilar, adj.; hili, pl.

ناف : عضو کی سطح پر نشیب جہاں رگیں، نالیاں داخل و خارج ہوتی ہیں۔

Hippocrates *(hi-pok'-ra-tez)*. Famous Greek physician and philosopher (460 to 367 BC) who established a school of medicine at Cos, his birthplace. He is often termed the 'Father of Medicine'.

بقراط : مشہور یونانی طبیب و فلسفی۔ بابائے ادویات۔

Hippuran *(hip'-u-ran)*. One of the iodine-containing media used in X-ray Depts. **radioa ctive H.,** see RENOGRAM.

ہپوران : آیوڈین پر مشتمل میڈیا میں سے ایک جو شعبہ ہائے ایکسرے میں استعمال کیا جاتا ہے۔

Hiprex *(hip-reks)*. Hexamine hippurate (q.v.).

Hirschsprung's disease. Megacolon. Congenital intestinal aganglionosis. There is marked hypetrophy and dilation of the colon. Treated by Swenson's operation (q.v.), Duhamel's operation (q.v.).[Harold Hirschsprung, Danish physician, 1830-1916].

اتساع قولون ذاتی : میگا قولون۔ اس میں قولون پھیل جاتا ہے۔

Hirsute *(her'-sut)* [L. hirsutus]. Hairy or shaggy.

موئی : بالدار۔

Hirudiin *(hi-roo'-din)*. A substance secreted by the leech, which prevents the clotting of blood.

جونک۔ ہیروڈن : جونکوں سے خارج ہونے والا مادہ جو خون کو انجماد سے روکتا ہے۔

Hirudo *(hi-roo'-do)* [L.]. The leech.

علقہ : جونک

Hirudoid cream. *(hi-ru'-doid).* Non-greasy cream containing heparin lg in an absorbable base. Useful for acute and chronic inflammatory skin lesions, haemotoma, haemorrhoids and phlebothrombosis.

ہیرُوڈائڈ کریم : اس کریم میں گریس نہیں۔

Histalog *(his'-ta-log).* Betazole hydrochloride (q.v.).

ہسٹالاگ : بیٹاہائیڈروکلورائیڈ۔

Histamine *(his'-ta-men).* A naturally occurring chemical substance in body tissues wich, in small doses, has profound and diverse actions on muscle, blood capill, iries, and gastric secretion. Sudden excessive release from the tissues, into the blood, is believed to be the cause of the main symptoms and signs in anaphylaxis (q.v.)--histaminic, adj. Used in circulatory and gastric function tests. There are two types of **h. receptor** cells in the body, H_1 in the cells of bronchial muscle, and H_2 in the cells that secrete gastric juice.

ہسٹامین : جسمانی بافتوں میں قدرتی طور پر پایا جانے والا کیمیائی مادہ۔ نقطۂ پگھلاؤ ۸۶°س ایک سفید قلمی مرکب۔ معدہ میں نمک کے تیزاب کے اخراج کو تحریک دیتا ہے۔

Histidinaemia *(his-ti-din-em'-i-a).* Genetically determined increase in histidine in blood. Gives rise to speech defects without mental retardation.

ہسٹڈی رنیمیا : خون میں ہسٹڈین کی زیادتی۔ اس سے ذہنی پسماندگی کے بغیر تقریری نقائص پیدا ہوتے ہیں۔

Histidine *(his'-ti-den).* An essential amino acid which is widely distributed and is present in haemoglobin. It is a precursor of histamine.

ہسٹڈین : ایک لازمی امینو ایسڈ جو ہیموگلوبن میں موجود ہوتا ہے۔ حل پذیر۔

Histiocytes *(his'-ti-o-sits).* Derived from reticuloendothelial cells; act as scavengers.

Histiocytoma *(his-ti-o-si-to-ma).* Benign tumour of histiocytes.

Histiocytosis X *(his-ti-o-sit-o'-sis).* See HAND-SCHULLER-CHRISTIAN DISEASE.

سٹیوسائی ٹوسس : ہینڈشلر کرسچین کی بیماری۔

Histocompatibility *(his-to-kom-pat-ib-il'-it-i)* Cells ability to be accepted and to function in a new situation; important in organ transplantation.

Histology *(his-tol'-o-ji)* [G. histos, web; logos, a discourse]. Microscopic study of tissues histological, adj.; histologically, adv.

سیجیات : بافتوں کا خوردبینی مطالعہ۔

Histolysis *(his-tol'-is-is)* [G. histos, web; lysis, a loosening]. Disintegration of organic tissue--histolytic, adj.

سیج پاشی : نامیاتی نسیج کا خاتمہ۔

Histones *(his'-tons).* Recent research shows that h. are a system of proteins that may control genes.

سٹونز : لحمیات کا ایک نظام جو جینز کو کنٹرول کرتا ہے۔

Histoplasmosis *(his-to-plas-mo'-sis)* [G. hystos web; plasma, anything formed; -osis condition]. One of the infective reticuloses Disease involving the reticuloendothelial system, resulting from infection by the fungus Histoplasma capsulatum.

سٹو پلاسموسس : سماروغ سے ہونے والی بیماری جس سے ریٹیکولو اینڈو تھیلیل نظام متاثر ہوتا ہے۔

Hives *(hivs).* Nettle-rash; urticaria (q.v.).

چھپاکی : نبات ایلیل اڑٹیکیریا۔

Hobnail liver Firm nodular liver, may be found in cirrhosis.

سختی جگر : جگر کا سروسس۔

Hodgkin's disease. Lymphadenoma. A malignant lymphoma causing progressive enlargement of lymph nodes and involvement of reticuloendothelial tissues including bone marrow. Some causes show Pel-Ebstein fever (q.v.). [Thomas Hodgkin, English physician, 1798-1866].

مرض ہائی جیکن : لمفاڈنوما۔ ریٹیکولو اینڈو تھیلیل نظام کی ارتقاء پذیر بیماری۔ لمفٹک گلینڈز بڑھ جاتی ہے۔ بخار ہوتا ہے اور خون کی کمی واقع ہوتی ہے۔ علاج کے لئے ایکسرے پیوری نتھال اور لیوکیران۔

Homans' sign. Passive dorsiflexion of foot

causes pain in calf muscles. Indicative of incipient or established venous thrombosis of leg. [John Homans, American surgeon, 1877-1954].

ہومینز سائین : کاف عضلاتی میں درد ہوتا ہے کیونکہ پاؤں کا غیر معمول پشتی خم ہوتا ہے۔

Iomatropine *(hom-at'-ro-pen).* A mydriatic similar to atropine, but with a more rapid and less prolonged effect. Often used as a 2 percent solution with a similar amount of cocaine, which addition increases the mydriatic action and deadens pain.

ہوماٹروپین : ایٹروپین سے ملتا جلتا مڈریاٹک لیکن زیادہ موثر لیکن کم عرصہ کے لئے ۲ فیصد محلول کوکین کی مساوی مقدار کے ساتھ مستعمل ہے۔ درد کو ختم کرتا ہے۔

Iomeopathy *(hom-i-op'-ath-i)* [G. homoios, like; pathos, disease]. A method of treating disease by prescribing minute does of drugs which, in miximum dose, would produce symptoms of the disease. First adopted by Halnemann-- homeopathic, adj.

Iomicide *(hom'-i-sad)* [L. homo, man; coedere, to kill]. Killing of another person; manslaughter it accidental, murder if intentional.

علاج بالمثل، ہومیوپیتھی : دوائی کی تھوڑی سی مقدار سے بیماری کا علاج کرنے کا طریقہ۔ اس طریق علاج کا بانی ہنی من ہے۔

Iomocystinuria *(ho-mo-sis-tin-u'-ri-a)* [G. homos, same; kystis, bladder; ouron, urine]. Excretion of homocystine (a sulphur containing amino acid, homologue of cystine) in the urine. Gives rise to slow development of mental retardation of varying degree, lens and growth abnormalities and thrombotic episodes which are often fatal in childhood-homocystinuric, adj.

ہوموسسٹی نیوریا : ہوموسسٹین کا اخراج جو کہ پیشاب میں ہوتا ہے۔

Iomogeneous *(hom-o-jen'-e-us)* [G. homos, same; genos, race]. Of the same kind; of the same quality or consistency throughout.

ہم جنس : ایک ہی قسم کا یکساں ترکیب کے۔

Iomogenize *(ho-moj'-en-iz).* To make into the same consistency throughout.

ہوموجینائز : جو سارا ایک ہی طرح کا ہو۔

Homogenous *(hom-oj'-en-us)* [G. homos, same; genos, race]. Having a like nature, e.g. a bone graft from an-other human being.

ہم نسل : ایک جیسی خصلت۔

Homograft *(ho'-mo-graft)* [G. homos, same]. A tissue or organ which is transplanted from one individual to another of the same species. Syn. allograft.

ہم پیوند : ایک نسیج یا عضو جو ایک فرد سے اسی نوع کے دوسرے فرد کے ساتھ پیوند کیا جائے۔

Homolateral *(ho-mo-lat'-er-al)* [G. homos, same; L. lateralis, side]. On the same side--homolaterally, adv.

ہم جانب : اسی طرح۔ ایک ہی طرف۔

Homologous *(hom-ol'-o-gus)* [G. homos, same; logos, word]. Corresponding in origin and structure. **homologous chromosomes,** those that pair during reduction cell division and contain identical arrangement of genes in their DNA pattern.

مماثل : سب کی اصل اور ساخت ایک ہونا۔

Homonymous *(hom-on'-im-us)* [G. homos, same; enyma, name]. Corresponding halves.

ہم نام : متعلقہ نصف

Homosexual *(ho-mo-skes'-u-al)* [G. homos, same; L. sexus, sex]. Of the same sex. Often used to describe a person who indulges in homosexuality.

ہم جنسیہ : اسی جنس کو کشش کرنے کا رجحان۔

Homosexuality *(ho-mo-skes-u-al-it-i)* Attraction for, and desire to establish an emotional and sexual relationship with a member of the same sex.

Homotransplant *(ho-mo-trans'-plant)* [G. homos, same; L. transplantare, to transplant]. Tissues or organ transplanted from non-identical members of the same species. Syn. allotransplant; homograft.

ہوموٹرانس پلانٹ : بافتیں یا عضو جن میں اسی نوع کے غیر مشابہ اراکین سے پیوند کیا جائے۔

Homozygous *(hom-o-zi'-gus).* Having identical genes in the same locus on one of the chromosome pairs.

مشابہ زواجہ : کروموسوموں کے جوڑوں میں سے ایک پر ایک ہی مقام پر ایک جیسے جینز رکھنا۔

Hanvan *(hon'-van)*. Stilboestrol diphosphate, broken down by prostatic tissue to release stilboestrol in situ, thus reducing systemic side effects,

ہانوین : سٹلبوایسٹرول ڈائی فاسفیٹ۔

Hookworm See ANCYLOSTOMA.

ہک ورم : انسائیلوسٹورما۔ انسانی انتڑیوں میں رہ کر خون چوستے ہیں۔ ننگے پاؤں چلنے والوں کے پاؤں میں جلا کر اندر لاردے گھس جاتے ہیں۔ علاج کے لئے بیفی نیم گرینیولز کی بتی بنائی جاتی ہے۔ ایک خوراک شربت میں گھول کر صبح خالی پیٹ دیں اور چار گھنٹے بعد مریض کو سالٹ کا جواب دیں۔

Hordeolum *(hor-de'-o-lum)* [L. hordeum, grain of barley]. A stye; a furuncle on the eyelid.

انجن ہاری : آنکھ کے پپوٹے پر گلٹی۔

Hormone *(hor'-mon)* [G. hormaein, to excite]. Specific chemical substances secreted by an endocrine gland a nd conveyed in the blood to regula te the functions of tissues and organs elsewhere in the body.

ہارمون مہیجہ : بغیر نالی والی غدد سے اخراج ہونے والی رطوبت جو خون میں شامل ہو کر دوسری بافتوں میں عاملیت پیدا کرتی ہے۔

Hormonotherapy *(hor-mo-no-ther'-a-pi)*. Treatment by hormones.

ہارمونی علاج : ہارمونز کے ذریعے علاج۔

Horner's syndrome Clinical picture following paralysis of cervical sympathetic nerves, on one side. There is myosis, slight ptosis with enophthalmos, and anhidrosis. [Johann Friedrich Horner, Swiss ophthalmologist, 1831-86].

ہارنرز سنڈ ورم : کلینکل پکچر۔

Horton's syndrome. Severe headache due to the release of histamine in the body. To be differentiated from migraine. [Bayard Taylor Horton, American physican, 1895].

ہارٹونز سنڈ ورم : جسم میں ہسٹامین خارج ہونے کی وجہ سے سخت سردرد۔

Host *(host)* [L. hospes]. The organic structure upon which parasites thrive. **intermediate h.,** one in which the parasite passes its larval or cystic stage.

یزبان : نامیاتی ساخت جس پر طفیلی رہتے ہیں یا پرورش پاتے ہیں۔

Hot-dog-headache. Post-prandial; induced by sodium nitrite content of frank furters.

Hot-fat heartburn sysndrome. Due to excessive leak from stomach to oesophagus producing hypersensitivity in the oesophageal mucosa; tends to be worse after fatty or fried food or drinking coffee. May be associated with hiatus hernia.

Hour-glass contraction A circular constriction in the middle of a hollow organ (usually the stomach or uterus), dividing it into two portions.

یت گھڑی سکڑاؤ : کسی کھوکھلے عضو کے درمیان میں سے اتنا تنگ ہونا کہ اسے دو حصوں میں تقسیم کردے۔

Housemaid's knee See BURSITIS.

رم در جک : برسٹس۔

HPFSH. Human pituitary follicle (q.v.) stimulating hormone.

یچ پی ایف ایس ایچ : انسانی پیٹوایٹری فولیکل جو ہارمون کو تحریک کرتا ہے۔

HPV-77. High passage virus of the 77th passage level. Attenuated rubella virus used to produce active immunity.

یچ پی وی۔ ۷۷ : ۷۷ویں لیول کا ہائی پیسج وائرس

Humatin *(hu'-mat-in)*. Paromomycin (q.v.).

ومیٹن : پرومائی سین۔

Humerus *(hu'-mer-us)* [L.]. The bone of the upper arm, between the elbow and shoulder joint--humeral, adj.; humeri, pl.

ضہ۔ ہیومرس : کہنی اور شانے کے جوڑ کے درمیان بالائی بازو کی ہڈی لمبی ہوتی ہے۔ بالائی کنارہ گول اور چکنا۔ زیرین کنارہ چوڑا اور گراری نما س پر زیریں بازو کی ہڈیاں جڑ کر کہنی بناتی ہیں۔ بالائی کنارہ شانہ کی ہڈی سے ف یا گلینائیڈ کیویٹی میں رہتا ہے اور حرکت کرتا ہے۔

Humidity *(hu-mid'-it-i)* [L. humidus, moist]. The amount of moisture in the atmosphere as measured by a hygrometer. **relative h.,** the ratio of the amount of moisture present in the air to the amount which would saturate it (at the same temperature).

وبت نمی : فضا میں نمی کی مقدار جسے رطوبت پیما سے ناپا جائے

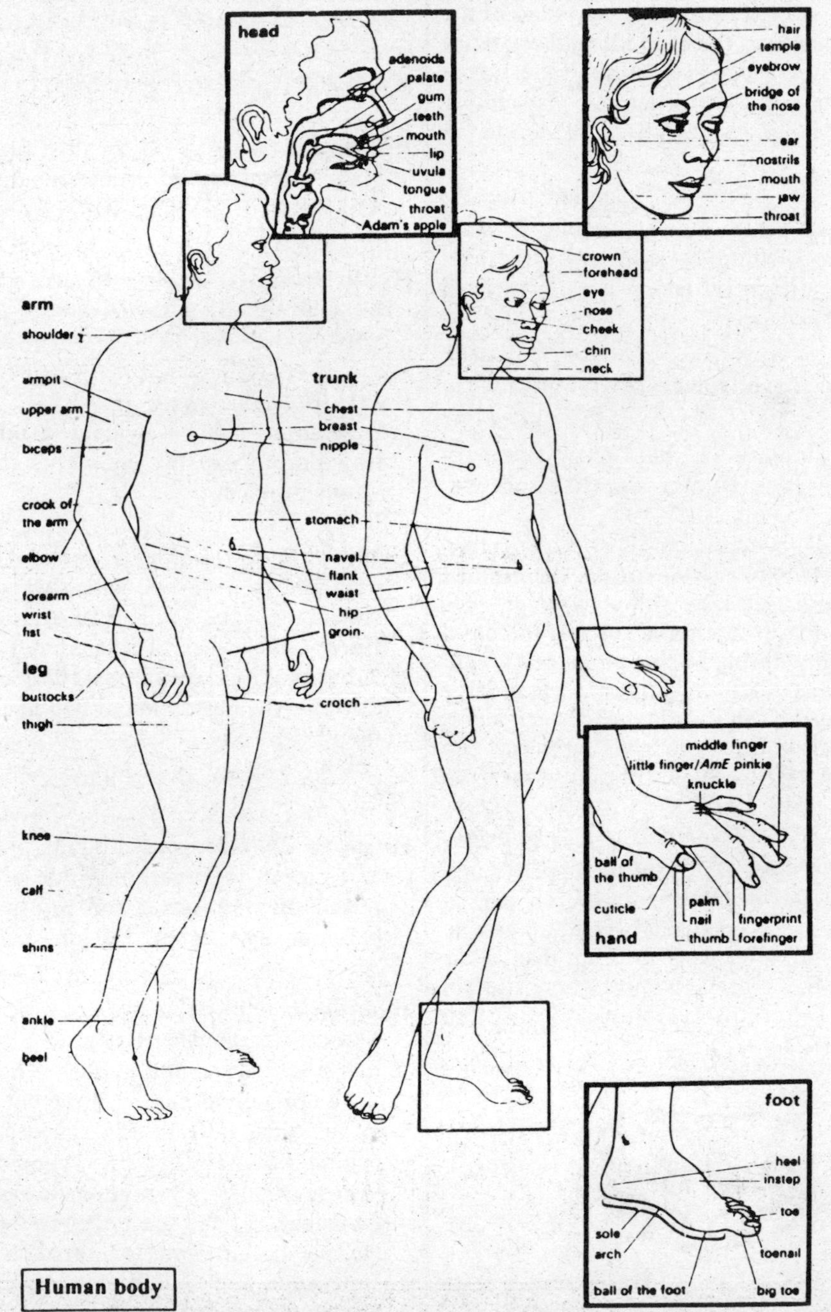
head
adenoids
palate
gum
teeth
mouth
lip
uvula
tongue
throat
Adam's apple
hair
temple
eyebrow
bridge of the nose
ear
nostrils
mouth
jaw
throat
crown
forehead
eye
nose
cheek
chin
neck
arm
shoulder
armpit
upper arm
biceps
crook of the arm
elbow
forearm
wrist
fist
leg
buttocks
thigh
knee
calf
shins
ankle
heel
trunk
chest
breast
nipple
stomach
navel
flank
waist
hip
groin
crotch
middle finger
little finger/AmE pinkie
knuckle
ball of the thumb
cuticle
palm
nail
thumb
fingerprint
forefinger
hand
foot
heel
instep
toe
sole
arch
toenail
ball of the foot
big toe

Human body

Humor *(hu'-mor)* [L. a liquid]. any fluid of the body, **aqueous h.,** the fluid filling the anterior and posterior chambers in front of the optical lens. **vitreous h.,** the gelatinous mass filling the interior of the eyeball from the lens to the retina.

رطوبت : جسم کا کوئی سیال۔

Hunger *(hung'-ger)* A longing, usually for food. **air h.,** see air. **hunger pain,** epigastric pain which is relieved by taking food; associated with doudenal ulcer.

بھوک : خواہش جو عموماً خوراک کے لئے ہوتی ہے۔

Hunter-Hurler syndrome. Gargoylism (q.v.).

ہنٹر ہرلر سنڈ ورم : گارگائلزم

Hunterian chancre The hard sore of primary syphillis. [John Hunter, Scottish surgeon, 1728-93].

ابتدائی آتشکی زخم : اولین آتشک کا سخت ناسور۔

Huntington's chorea Genetically determined heredofamilial disease with slow progressive degeneration of the nerve cells of the basal ganglia and cerebral cortex. Affects both sexes, and is due to a dominant gene of large effect. Develops in middle age, or later, and is associated with progressive demintia. See CHOREA [George Huntington, American physician, 1862-1927].

رعشۂ مزمن : توارثی کوریا۔

Hutchinson's teeth Defect of the upper central incisors (second dentition) which is part of the facies of the congenital syphilitic person. The teeth are broader at the gum than at the cutting edge, and each shows an elliptical notch. [Jonathan Hutchinson, English surgeon, 1828-1913].

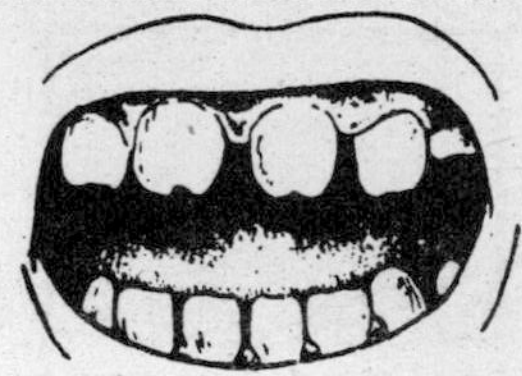

Hutchinson's teeth

[...]ندان ہچنسن : بالائی مرکزی دانتوں کا نقص مسوڑھوں کے پاس چوڑے [...]رنوک کی طرف پتلے یعنی کم چوڑے ہوجاتے ہیں۔

Hyalase *(hi'-a-laz).* Hyaluronidase (q.v.).

[...]یالیز : ہیالرونیڈز۔

Hyaline *(hi'-a-len)* [G. hyalos, glass]. Lik[e] glass; transparent. **h. membrane disease.** Se[e] RESPIRA- TORY DISTRESS SYNDROME

[...]یالین زوجاجی : سیشے کی طرح شفاف۔

Hyalitis *(hi-al-i'-tis)* [G. hyalos, glass; -iti[s] inflamm- ation]. Inflammation of the optic[al] vitreous humor or its enclosing membrane.

[...]رم زجاجیہ : بصری وٹریس ہیومر یا اس کو بند کرنیوالی جھلی کی سوزش۔

Hyaloid *(hi'-a-loid)* [G. hyalos, glass] Resembling hyaline, **hyaloid membrane,** th[e] transparent capsule enclosing the optica[l] vitreous humor.

[...]وجاجی۔شفاف : ہیالین سے مشابہ۔

Hyaluronidase *(hi-al-u-ron'-i-daz).* An enzym[e] obtained from testes, which when injecte[d] subcutaneously, promotes the absorption o[f] fluid. Given with or immediately before subcutaneous infusion; 1000 units wi[ll] facilitate the absorption of 500 to 1000 ml o[f] fluid.

[...]یالرونیڈیز : خصیوں سے حاصل کردہ ایک خامرہ۔ اسے جب انجکشن [...]کے ذریعے اندر پہنچایا جائے تو سیال کے انجذاب میں مدد دیتا ہے۔

Hycal *(hi-cal')* Flavoured liquid; protein-fre[e] low-electrolyte; carbohydrate preparatio[n] based on demineralized liquid glucose providing 240 kcal per 100 ml.

[...]ئیکل : ایک خوشبودار مائع۔لحمی اجزاء سے پاک۔

Hydatid *(hi'-dat-id)* [G. hydatis, watery vesicle] The cyst formed by larvae of a tapeworm Echinococcus, found in dogs. The encyste[d] stage normally occurs in sheep but can occu[r] in man after he eats with soiled hands fro[m] petting a dog. The cysts are commonest in th[e] liver and lungs. Cysts grow slowly and onl[y] do damage by the space they occupy. If the[y] leak, or become infected, urticaria and feve[r] supervene and 'daughter' cysts can resul[t] Treatment surgical. See Test (CASONI)

کیسآ بہ : کتوں میں پائے جانے والے کدو کیڑے اکینو کاکسس کے لاردوں سے بننے والا سسٹ۔ کتے پر ہاتھ پھیرنے سے انسان میں منتقل ہو جاتے ہیں جگر اور پھیپھڑوں میں پائے جاتے ہیں۔

datidiform *(hi-da-tid'-i-form)* [G. hydatis, watery vesicle; L. forma, shape]. Pertaining to or resembling a hydatid. **hydatidifrorm mole,** see MOLE.

ہائیڈاٹڈی فارم : کیسآ بہ سے مشابہ۔

draemia *(hi-dre'-mi-a)* [G. hydor, water; haima, blood]. A relative excess of plasma volume compared with cell volume of the blood; it is normally present in late pregnancy--hydraemic, adj.

خونابی : خون کے مقابلے میں پلازما کی زیادتی۔ ایسا عموماً حمل کے آخر ایام میں ہوتا ہے۔

dramnios *(hi-dram'-ni-os)* [G. hydor, water; amnion, membrane around fetus]. An excess of amniotic fluid.

افراط رحل : اینانک سیال کی زیادتی۔

dragyrum *(hid-rar'-ji-rum)* [L.]. Mercury or quicksilver.

سیماب : کوئک سلور کا پارہ۔

drathrosis *(hi-drar-thro'-sis)* [G. hydor, water; arthron, joint; -osis, condition]. A collection of fluid in a joint cavity. **intermittent h.,** afflicts young women; probably due to allergy. Synovitis develops spontaneously, lasts a few days, and disappears as mysteriously.

استسقاء مفاصل : جوڑ کے کہفہ میں سیال کا اجتماع۔

drate *(hi'-drat)*. Combine with water--hydration, n.

آبید : پانی کے ساتھ ملاپ۔ ہائیڈ ریشن ہائیڈ روفلومیتھازائیڈ۔

droa *(hi-dro'-a)* [G. hydreno, water; oion, egg]. Syn., dermatitis herpetiformis (q.v.). **hydroa aestivale,** or Hutchinson's summer prurigo, is a vesicular or bullous disease occurring in children. It affects exposed parts and probably results from photosensitivity. **hydroa vacciniforme** is a more severe from of this in which scarring ensues.

تقفع : ڈرمٹیٹس ہرپیٹفارمس

Hydrocele *(hi'-dro-sel)* [G. hydor, water; kele, tumour]. A swelling due to accumulation of serous fluid in the tunica vaginalis of the testis, or in the spermatic cord.

ہائیڈروسیل : منوی ڈوری یا خصیے کا ٹیونیکا ویجینیلس میں سیرس سیال کے اجتماع کی وجہ سے ورم خصیوں کی تھیلی یا بڑھ میں پانی آجانا۔

Hydrocephalus *(hi-dro'-kef'-a-lus)* [G. hydor, water; kephale, head]. 'Water on the brian'. An excess of cerebrospinal fluid inside the skull due to an obstruction to normal CSF circulation. **external h.,** the excess of fluid is mainly in the subarachnoid space. **internal h.,** the excess of fluid is mainly in the ventricles of the brian. Spitz-Holter valve (q.v.) used in drainage operations for this condition--hydrocephalic, adj.

استسقاء دماغ : کھوپڑی میں سروبروسپائینل سیال کی زیادتی۔

Hydrochloric acid *(hi-dro-klor'-ik-as'-id)*. Secreted by the gastric oxyntic cells and present in gastric juice (0.2 per-cent). The strong acid is caustic, but a 10 percent dilution is used orally in the treatment of achlorhydria.

نمک کا تیزاب : گیسٹرک آکسنٹک خلیوں سے خارج ہوتا ہے اور گیسٹرک جوس میں ۰٫۲ فیصد ہوتا ہے۔

Hydrochlorothiazide *(hi-dro-klor-o-thi'-a-zid)*. More powerful diuretic than chlorothiazide (q.v.).

ہائیڈروکلوروتھیازائیڈ : کلوروتھیازائیڈ سے زیادہ طاقتور پیشاب آور دوا۔ ہائپرٹنشن یا بلڈ پریشر میں اس کی ایک گولی صبح ایک دوپہر ایک شام۔ کنجیسٹو ہارٹ فیلیور اور دمہ قلبی میں پیٹ میں پانی۔ سوزش گردہ کے لئے ایک گولی روزانہ ناشتے کے بعد دن میں تین گولیاں برائے میینیئر۔

Hydrocortisone *(hi-dro-kor'-ti-zon)*. Cortisol an adrenal cortical steroid essential to life. It is more effective locally than cortisone, and is used extensively in inflamed conditions of the skin, eyes and ears, frequently in association with locally effective antibiotics. Also used by intrarticular injection for arthritis and bursitis; intravenously in

(A)Congenital hydrocele B) Infantile hydrocele

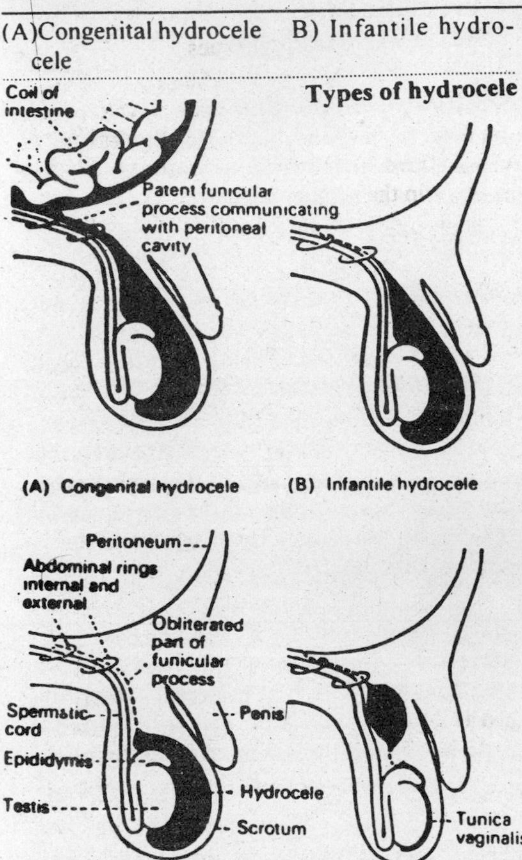

C) Vaginal hydrocele D) Hydrocele of the cord

Type of hydrocele

Addisonian crisis, by retention enema in ulcerative colitis, and as spray or snuff in hay fever.

ہائیڈروکارٹی سون : کورٹیسول۔ایک ایڈرینل کارٹیکل سٹیرائڈ جوزندگی کے لئے لازمی ہے۔مختلف امراض میں مفید۔پوٹوں کی سوزش میں مفید۔

Hydrocyanic acid *(hi-dro-si-an'-ikas'-id)*. Pressuic acid. The dilute acid (2 per-cent) has a sedative action on the stomach, and has been given with bismuth carbonate and other antacids in the treatment of vomiting. In large doses, pressic acid is rapidly fatal by causing respiratory and cardiac paralysis.

ہائیڈروسیانک ایسڈ : پرسک ایسڈ۔معدہ پر اثر کرتا ہے۔قے میں دوسروں کے ساتھ ملا کر دیا جاتا ہے۔اس کی زیادہ مقدار نقصان دہ ہے۔

Hydrofl.umethiazide *(hi-dro-flu-meth'-i-azid)*. Diuretic. Decreases reabsorption of sodium and chloride in kidney tubules.

ہائیڈروفلومیتھازائڈ : پیشاب آور۔گردے کی نالیوں میں سوڈیم اور کلورائیڈ کے انجذاب میں کمی پیدا کرتا ہے۔

Hydrogen *(hi'-dro-jen)*. A colourless, odourless combustile gas. **hydrogen ion oncentration** a measure of the acidity or alkalinity o solution, ranging from pH 1 to 14,7 being approximately neutral; the lower numbers denoting acidity; the higher ones denoting alkalinity. **hydrogen peroxide, H2 O2,** a powerful oxidizing and deodorizing agent used for cleaning wounds; diluted with 4 to 8 parts of water as a mouthwash, and with 50 percent alcohol as ear drops.

ہائیڈروجن : ایک بے رنگ، بے لوث، آتش گیر گیس۔ایک عنصر۔جوہڑی وزن ۱۰۰۷ء۱ جوہری عدد ۱۔سب سے ہلکی شے۔آکسیجن کیساتھ مل کر پانی بناتی ہے۔تمام جاندار اشیاء ساتھ مل کر پانی بناتی ہے۔تمام جاندار اشیاء اور کیمیاتی مرکبات میں پانی کے طور پر پائی جاتی ہے۔آکسی ہائیڈروجن برنر، تکلیفی امونیا کی تیاری میں اور بطور تخفیفی عامل استعمال ہوتی ہے۔ہائیڈروجن کے ساتھ ملنے کو ہائیڈروجنیت کہا جاتا ہے۔ہائیڈروجن کے عمل سے کوئلہ سے مصنوعی معدنی تیل تجارتی پیمانہ پر تیار کیا جاتا ہے۔ہائیڈروجن آئنز کے گراموں کی تعداد فی لٹر (محلول کا) کسی محلول کا تیزابیت جاننے کے لئے مفید ہے اور اسے پی ایچ کی اصطلاحات میں ظاہر کیا جاتا ہے۔ہائیڈروجن پر آکسائیڈ ایک گاڑھا مائع ہے جس کا نقطۂ جوش ۱۵۰٫۲°س ہے۔مارلیٹ میں فروخت ہونی والا اس مرکب کا آبی محلول ہوتا ہے۔یہ آکسیجن خارج کرتا ہے۔بطور دافع تعفن اور رنگ کاٹ استعمال ہوتا ہے۔

Hydrolysis *(hi-drol'-is-is)*. [G. hydor, water lysis, a lossening]. The splitting into more simple substances by the addition of water--hydrolytic, adj.; hydrolyse, v.

آب پاشیدگی: کسی شے کا پانی کے ذریعے تجزیہ پانی کا بھی کیمیائی تجزیہ ہے۔

ydrometer *(hi-drom'-et-er)* [G. hydor, water, metron, a measure]. An instrument for determining the specific gravity of fluids--hydrometry, n

آب پیما : مائعات کی کثافت یا کثافت اضافی ناپنے کے لئے ایک آلہ۔

ydrometria *(hi-dro-met'-ri-a)* [G. hydor, water; metra, uterus]. A collection of watery fluid within the uterus.

استسقاءالرحم : رحم یا یورٹرس میں آبی سیال کا اجتماع۔

ydronephrosis *(hi-dro-nef-ro'-sis)* [g. hydor, water; nephros, kidney; -osis, condition]. Distension of the kidney pelvis with urine, from obstructed outflow. If unrelieved, presure eventually causes atrophy of kidney tissue. Operations are pyeloplasty (q.v.). and Hamilton Stewart nephroplasty. See NEPHROPLASTY.

استسقاءگردہ : رکے ہوئے پیشاب کی وجہ سے گردے پیلوس کا پھیلاؤ۔

ydropericarditis *(hi-dro-pe-ri-kard-i'-tis)* [G. hydor, water; peri, around; kardia, the heart; -itis, inflammation]. Pericarditis with effusion.

تاموری آبی التہاب : پیریکارڈیٹس اخراج کے ساتھ۔

ydropericardium *(hi-dro-pe-ri-kard'-i-um)* [G. hydor, water; peri, around; kardia, the heart]. Fluid in the pericardial sac in the absence of inflammation. Can occur in heart and kidney failure.

استسقاءحجاب قلب : سوزش کی غیر موجودگی میں پیراکارڈیئل تھیلی میں سیال۔

ydroperitoneum *(hi-dro-pe-ri-to-ne'-um)* [G. hydor, water; peritonaion, peritoneum]. See ASCITES.

استسقائے زقی : اسائیٹس۔

ydrophobia *(hi-dro-fo'-bi-a)* [G. hydor, water; phobos, fear]. Rabies in man.

ہلکا۔آب ترسیدگی : آدمی کو پاگل کتے کا کاٹنا۔مریض شوروغل سے گھبراتا ہے۔غذا نگلنے میں دقت ہوتی ہے۔چیختا ہے۔نبض تیز ہو جاتی ہے۔درجہ حرارت بڑھ جاتا ہے۔تشنج کے دورے پڑتے ہیں مریض پانی کو دیکھ کر ڈرنے لگتا ہے۔

ydropneumothorax *(hi-dro-nu-mo-thor'-asks)* [G. hydor, water; pneuma, breath; thorax, chest]. Pneumothorax further complicated by effusion of fluid in the pleural cavity. Usually tubercular.

آبی استرواح الصدر : پلیورل کہفہ میں سیال کے اخراج کی ساتھ نیوموتھوریکس۔

Hydrops *(hi'-drops)* [G.]. Dropsy--hydropic, adj. **hydrops fetails,** severe form of erythroblastosis fetalis (q.v.).

استسقاءجلندھر : ڈراپسی

Hydrosaplinx *(hi-dro-sal'-pinks)* [g. hydor, water; salpigx, trumpet]. Distension of the Fallopian tube with watery fluid.

استسقائے انبوبی : آبی سیال کے ساتھ فلوپیئن نلی کا پھیلاؤ۔

Hydrosaluric. Hydrochlorothiazide (q.v.).

ہائیڈروسیلورک : ہائیڈروکلوروتھیازائیڈ۔

Hydrotherapy *(hi-dro-the'-ra-pi)* [G. hydor, water; therapeia, treatment]. The science of therapeutic bathing for diagnosed conditions.

آبی علاج : تشخیص شدہ حالت کے لئے آبی علاج کی سائنس۔

Hydrothorax *(hi-dro-thor'-asks)* [G. hydor, water; thorax, chest]. The presence of fluid in the pleural cavity.

استسقاءسینہ : پلیورل کہفہ میں سیال کی موجودگی۔

Hydroureter *(hi-dro-u-re'-ter)* [G. hydor, water; oureter, ureter]. Abnormal distension of the ureter with urine.

استسقاءصالبی : پیساب کے ساتھ مثانے کا غیر معمولی پھیلاؤ۔

Hydroxocobalamin *(hi-droks-o-ko-bal'-a-men).* A longer-acting form of vitamin B_{12}. See CYANOCOBALAMIN.

ہائیڈروکسوکوبالامین : حیاتین ب۱۲ کی ایک قسم۔

Hydroxychloroquine *(hi-droks-i-klor'-o-kwin).* Antimalarial. Can cause retinopathy.

ہائیڈروکسی کلوروکوئن : ملیریا کے خلاف استعمال ہونے والی دوا۔

Hydroxyl *(hi-droks'-il).* The monovalent group OH, consisting of a hydrogen atom linked to an oxygen atom.

ہائیڈروکسل : یک گرفتہ گردہ او ایچ۔آکسیجن ایٹم کے ہائیڈروجن ایٹم پر مشتمل۔

Hydroxyprogesterone caproate *(hi-droks-i-pro- jes'-ter-on kap-ro-at).* Given intramuscularly for recurrent and threatened abortion.

Hydroxystilbamidine *(hi-droks-i-stil-ba-m'-i-den)*. Useful in aspergillosis.

ہائیڈروکسی سٹل بیمیڈین :اس پرجلوسس میں مفید۔

Hydroxyurea *(hi-droks'-i-u-re'-a)*. Simple compound given orally. Mode of action uncertain, may be of value in patients with chronic myeloid leukaemia who no longer show a response to busulphan.

ہائیڈروکسی یوریا :سادہ مرکب جومنہ کے ذریعے دیا جاتا ہے۔

Hydroxyzine *(hid-roks'-i-zen)*. Atarax. Tranquillizer. See ATARACTIC.

ہائیڈروکسی زین :سکون بخش دوا۔

Hygiene *(hi'-jen)* [G. hygieinos, healthy]. The science dealing with the maintenance of health. **communal h.,** embraces all measures taken to supply the community with pure food and water, good sanitation, housing, etc. **industrial h.** (occupational health) includes all measures taken to preserve the individual's health whilst he is at work. **mental h.** deals with the establishment of healthy mental attidues and emotional reactions. **personal h.,** includes all those measures taken by the individual to preserve his own health--hygenic, adj.

اصول صحت :سائنس جوصحت قائم رکھنے سے متعلق ہے۔

Hygraphen *(hi'-gr-gen)*. Organic mercurial useful when trichomonal infections do not respond to metronidazole.

ہائیگرافین :نامیاتی کیوریل۔

Hygroma *(hi-gro'-ma)* [G. hygros, moist; -oma, tumour]. A cystic swelling containing watery fluid, usually situated in the neck and present at birth-- hygromata, pl.; hygromatous, adj.

سلعۂ مائی : آبی سیال پر مشتمل سسلک ورم جو گردن میں ہوتا ہے۔اور پیدائش کے وقت موجود ہوتا ہے۔

Hygrometer *(hi-grom'-et-er)* [G.hygros,moist; metron, a measure].An instrument for measuring the amount of moisture in the air. See HUMIDITY.

رطوبت پیما :ہوامیں نمی کی مقدار کی پیائش کے لئے ایک آلہ۔

Hygroscopic *(hi-gro-skop'-ik)* [G. hygros, moist; skopein, to examine]. Readily absorbing water, e.g. glycerine.

نم گیر :پانی کو جذب کرنے والا۔مثلاً گلیسرین

Hygroton *(hi-gro'-ton)*. Chlorthalidone (q.v.).

ہائیگروٹون : کلورتھیلیڈون

Hymen *(hi'-men)* [G. membrane]. A membranous perforated structure stretching across the vaginal entrance. **imperforate h., a** congenital condition leading to haematocolpos. See CRYPTOMENO- RRHOEA.

ہائمن۔ پردۂ بکارت :ایک جھلی دار سوراخوں والی ساخت جو دیجائنا کے دخول کے پار ہوتی ہے۔ بالغ عورت کی اندام نہانی کے گرد باریک سی جھلی۔ کنوار پن کا پردہ' وزنی کام کرنے' زیادہ جسمانی کام کرنے یا اچھلنے کودنے سے پردہ پھٹ سکتا ہے۔ بعض اوقات پردہ پھٹنے سے خون خارج نہیں ہوتا۔ انگلی

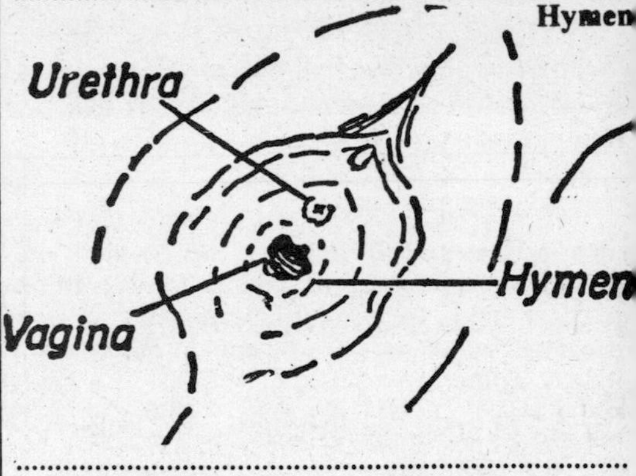

Hymen

Urethra

Hymen

Vagina

: اندر داخل کرنے سے بھی پردۂ بکارت پھٹ سکتا ہے۔ اندرونی چھوٹے لبوں کے درمیان باریک سی جھلی جس کے درمیان ایک سوراخ ہوتا ہے۔ اس میں شریانیں اور اعصاب ہوتے ہیں اس لئے پہلی مباشرت کے دوران اس کے پھٹنے سے درد ہوتا ہے اور اخراج خون بھی ہوتا ہے۔

Hymenectomy *(hi-men-ek'-to-mi)* [G. membrane; ektome, excision]. Surgical excision of the hymen.

بکاہ براری :پردۂ بکارت یا ہائمن کا سرجیکل انقطاع۔

Hymenotomy *(him-men-ot'-o-mi)* [G. membrane; tome, a cutting]. Surgical incision of the hymen.

غشاء تراشی :پردۂ بکارت یا ہایمن میں اپریشن کے ذریعے شگاف۔

Hyoid *(hi'-oid)* [G. y-eidos,; shaped like letter 'Y']. A U-shaped bone at the root of the tongue.

عظم لامی : زبان کی جڑ پر واقع ایک یو کی شکل والی ہڈی یہ چھوٹی ہڈی گردن میں لیرنکس کے ذرا اوپر پائی جاتی ہے۔اس پر زبان کے عضلات جڑتے ہیں۔

Hyoscine *(hi'-o-sen)*. A hypnotic alkaloid obtained from belladonna and hyoscyamus. Often used for pre-operative sedation in association with morphine, papaveretum or pethidine. Also **mydriatic** and cycloplegic. Syn. scopolamine.

ہائیوسین : ایک خواب آور الکلائڈ۔حمل میں صبح کے وقت متلی میں ہائیوسین بذریعہ دہن دی جاتی ہے۔۲۰۰/۱تا۱۰۰/۱ اگرین زیر جلد ٹیکہ کیجئے تسکین دہ اور نیند آور ہے۔

Hyoscyamus *(hi-o-si'-a-mus)*. Henbane leaves and flowers. Resembles belladonna in its properties. Sometimes given with potassium citrate for urinary trct spasm.

تخم بھنگ : بھنگ کے پتے اور پھول۔خصوصیات میں بیلاڈونا سے مشابہ۔

Hyperacidity *(hi'-per-as-id'-it-i)* [G. hyper, above; L. acidus, acid]. Excessive acidity. See HYPERCHL- ORHYDRIA.

بیش (ترشی معدہ): زائد تیزابیت

Hyperactivity *(hi'-per-ak-ti-vi-ti)* [G. hyper, above; L. activus, active]. Excessive activity.

تیز رفتاری : زائد عاملیت۔

Hyperaemia *(hi'-per-e'-mi-a)* [G. hyper, above; haima, blood]. Excess of blood in an area. **active h.** caused by an increased flow of blood to a part. **passive h.** occurs when there is restricted flow of blood from a part--hyperaemic, adj.

اجتماع خون : کسی ایریا میں خون کی زیادتی۔

Hyperaesthesia *(hi'-per-es-the'-zia-a)* [G. hyper, above; aisthesis, sensation]. Excessive sensitiveness of a pa rt--hyperaesthetic, adj. (Cf. anaesthesia).

تیز حسی : کسی حصے کی زائد حساسیت۔

Hyperaldosteronism *(hi-per-al-dos-ter'-on-izm)*. Production of excessive aldosterone **primary h.**, see ALDOSTERONE. **secondary h.**, the adrenal responds to an increased stimulus of extra adrenal origin.

Hyperalgesia *(hi-per-al-jez'-i-a)* [G. hyper, above; algesis, sense of pain]. Excessive sensibility to pain. Also HYPERALGIA--hyperalgesic, adj.

حساسیت درد : درد کو زیادہ محسوس کرنا۔

Hyperbaric *(hi-per-bar'-ik)* [G. hyper, above; baros, weight].At greater pressure, specific gravity or weight, than normal **hyperbaric oxygen chamber**, sealed cylinder containing oxygen under pressure. Accommodates patient, attendant and equipment. In some units surgery can be performed. Anaerobic organisms and their ability to produce toxins are adversely affected by oxygen. O_2 saturated tissues respond better to radiotherapy.

ہائیپر برک : نارمل سے زیادہ دباؤ، وزن مخصوص یا وزن۔

Hyperbilirubinaemia *(hi'-per-bi-li roo'-b-in-e'-mi-a)* [G. hyper, above; L. bilis, bile; ruber, red; G. haima, blood]. Excessive bilirubin in the blood. Present in physiological jaundice of the newborn. See PHOTOTHERAPY--hyperbilirubinaemic,adj

ہائیپر بلی روبی نیمیا : خون میں زائد بلیر دین۔نوزائیدہ بچے کے طبعیاتی یرقان میں موجود۔

Hypercalcaemia *(hi'-per-kal-se'-mi-a)*.[G. hyper, above; L. calx, lime; G. haima, blood]. Excessive calcium in the blood. **idiopathic h.**, disorder of calcium storage. Cause unknown. Hypersensitivity to vitamin D has been suggested. Some infants recover. Those who are severely affected show osteosclerosis, developmental retardation and hypertension. Fatal cases show nephrocalcinosis at autopsy. Survivors later present with a typical facies. mental subnormality and aortic stenosis. Treatment includes one of the calcium-free milks. In acute stages, steroids may be useful. Clinical picture may closely resemble renal acidosis (q.v.). Nephrocalcinosis may occur in both. Diagnosis rests on raised blood calcium and urea without a consistently alkaline urine--hypercalcaemic, adj.

بیش کلسیت :خون میں زائد کیلشیم۔

Hypercalciuria *(hi-per-kal-si-u'-ri-a)* [G. hyper, above; L. calx, lime; G. ouron, urine]. Greatly increased calcium excretion in urine, as seen in hyperparathy-roidism. **idiopathic h.,** used when there is no known metabolic cause, hypercalciuria of importance in pathogenesis of nephrolithiasis.

بیش کلس بولی :پیشاب میں کیلشیم کے اخراج کی بہت زیادہ مقدار۔

Hypercapnia *(hi'-per-kap'-ni-a)* [g. hyper, above; kapnos, smoke]. Excessive CO_2 in the blood-hypercapnic, adj.

ہیپر لپنیا۔بیش دخانی :خون میں زائد کاربن ڈائی آکسائیڈ۔

Hypercarbia *(bi-per-kar'-bi-a)*. Hypercapnia (q.v.).

ہائپر کاربیا :ہائپر کپنیا۔بیش دخانی۔

Hypercatabolic *(hi-per-kat-ab-ol'-ĭk)* [g. hyper, above; kata, down; ballein, to throw]. Excessive breakdown of complex substances into simpler ones within the body. Can occur in acute renal failure.

Hyperchloraemia *(hi'-per-klor-e'-mi-a)* [G. hyper, above; chloros, pale green; haima, blood]. Excessive chloride in the blood. One form of acidosis (q.v.)--hyperchloraemic, adj.

ہائپرکلوریمیا :خون میں زائد کلورائیڈ۔

Hyperchlorhydria *(hi'-per-klor-hi'dri-a)* [G. hyper, above; chloros, pale geen; hydor, water]. Excessive hydrochloric acid in the gastric juice--hyperchlor- hydric, adj.

ہائپر کلور ہائیڈریا :گیسٹرک جوس میں زائد نمک کا تیزاب۔

Hypercholesterolaemia *(hi-per-kol-es-te-r-ol-e'-mi-a)* [G. hyper, above; chole, bile; stereos, stiff; haima, blood]. Excessive cholesterol in the blood. Predisposes to atheroma and gall-stones. Also found in myxoedema--hypercholesterolaemic, adj.

ہائپر الیکٹرولائی ٹیمیا :زیادہ سیرم سوڈیم اور کلورائیڈ لیولز کے ساتھ ڈی ہائیڈریشن۔

Hyperemesis *(hi-per-em'-es-is)* [G. hyper, above; emesis, vomiting]. Excessive vomiting, **hyperemesis gravidarum,** a complication of pregnancy which may become serious.

رت قے :زائد قے۔

Hyperextension *(hi-per-eks-ten'-shun)* [G. hyper, above; L. extendere, to stretch]. Ove extension.

ں توسیع :زیادہ پھیلاؤ۔

Hyperflexion *(hi-per-flek'-shun)* [G. hype above; L. flexio, a bending]. Excessive fle ion.

ں خمیدگی عضو :زیادہ خمیدہ

Hyperglycaemia *(hi-per-gli-se'-mi-a)* [(hyper, above; glykys, sweet; haima, blood Excessive sugar in the blood--hypergly aemic, adj.

ں شکردمویت :خون میں زائد شکر۔

Hyperglycinaemia *(hi-per-gli-sin-e'-mi-a* Excess glycine in the serum. Can cau acidosis and mental retardation-hyperg ycinaemic, adj.

رگلائیسنیمیا :سیرم میں زائد گلائیسین ۔ذہنی پسماندگی پیدا کرسکتا ہے۔

Hyperhidrosis *(hi'-per-hi-dro'-sis)* [G. hyp above; hidros, sweat; -osis, condition]. Exce sive sweating--hyperhidrotic, adj.

ثرت پسینہ :زائد پسینہ۔

Hyperinsulinism *(hi-per-in'-sul-in-izm)* [hyper, above; L. insula, island]. Intermitte or continuous loss of consciousness, with without convulsions. Due to excessive insu from the pancreatic islets lowering the blo sugar.

ولینی صدمہ :ہوش کا ضیاع متواتر یا وقفوں کے ساتھ لبلہ کے خلیوں سے رانسولین کی وجہ سے خونی شکر کی مقدار کم ہو جاتی ہے۔

Hyperinvolution *(hi'-per-in-vo-loo'-shun)* [hyper, above; l. involutus, infolded]. Redu tion to below normal size, as of the uter after parturition.

ں انحطاط :نارمل سائز سے کم میں تخفیف۔

Hyperkalaemia *(hi'-per-kal-e'-mi-a)* [G. hyp above; N.L. kalium, potassium; G. haima, ood]. Excessive potassium in the bloo hyperkalaemic, adj.

رکیلیمیا :خون سے زائد پوٹاشیم۔

Hyperkeratosis *(hi'-perke-ra-to-sis)* [G. hyper, above; keras, horn; -osis, condition]. Hypertrophy of the cornea or the horny layer of the skin--hyperkeratotic, adj.

بیش قرنیت : جلد کی ہارنی تہہ یا کورنیا کی ہائپر ٹرافی۔

Hyperkinesis *(hi-per-kin-e'-sis)* [G. *hyper,* above; *kinesis*, motion]. Excessive movement-- hyperkinetic, adj.

اضطراب بیش حرکیت (عضلہ) : زائد حرکت۔

Hyperkinetic syndrom First described in 1962; usually appears between the ages of 2 and 4 years. The child is slow to develop intellectually. There is a marked degree of distractability and a tireless unrelenting exploration of the environment, together with agressivness, especially towards siblings, even if unprovoked. He is fearless and undeterred by threats of punishment. The parents complain of his cold unaffectionate character and destructive behaviour. Condition often responds to chlorpromazine, primidone óramphetamine and can tolerate large doses of these. Many also improve spontaneously between 7 and 10 years old. Some consider tha t genetic and environmental factors are important, because studies have shown that the child often reacts to changes in his social circumstances.

Hyperlipaemia *(hi-per-li-pem'-i-a)* [G. *hyper, above; lipos,* fat; haima, blood]. Excessive fat in the blood--hyperlipaemic. adj.

ہائپر لائی پیمیا : خون میں زائد چکنائی۔

Hypermagnesaemia *(hi-per-mag-nes-e'-mi-a)* [G. *hyper,* above; *Magnesie lithos* Magnesian stone; haima, blood]. Excessive magnesum in the blood-- hypermagnesaemic, adj.

ہائپر میگنیمیا : خون میں زائد میگنیشیم۔

Hypermetabolism *(hi-per-met-ab'-ol-izm)* [G. *hyper,* above; *metabole,* change]. Production of excessive body heat. Characteristic of thyrotoxicosis-- hypermetabolic, adj.

بیش تحویل یا میٹابولزم : زائد جسمانی حرارت پیدا ہونا۔

Hypermetropia *(hi'-per-me-tro'-pi-a)* [G. *hyper,* above; *metron,* a measure; ops, eye]. Longsightedness caused by faulty accommodation of the eye, with the result that the light rays are focused beyond, instead of on, the retina-- hypermetropic, adj.

بعیدی نظری : آنکھ کی غلط تطبیق کی وجہ سے نزدیک کی نگاہ کمزور ہونا۔ روشنی کی شعاعیں ریٹینا پر فوکس نہیں ہوتیں۔ بلکہ اس سے آگے جا کر ہوتی ہیں۔ اسے محدب عدسوں کے چشمے سے صحیح کیا جا سکتا ہے۔

Hypermobility *(hi-per-mo-bil'-i-ti)* [G. *hyper,* above; L. *mobilitas,* mobality]. Excessive mobility.

شدت حرکت : زائد متحرک ہونا۔

Hypermotility *(hi'-per-mo-til'-i-ti)* [G. *hyper,* above; L. *movere,* to move]. Increased movement, as peristalsis.

شدت حرکت : حرکت زیادہ ہو جانا مثلاً پیرا سٹالسس۔

Hypernatraemia *(hi'-per-na-re'-mi-a)* [G. *hyper,* above; *nephros,* kidney; -oma, tumour]. Grawitz tumour. A malignant neoplasm of the kidney--hypernephromata, pl.; hypernephromatous, adj.

ہائپر نیٹریمیا : خون میں زائد سوڈیم۔

Hypernephroma *(hi'-per-nef-ro'-ma)* [G. *hyper,* above; *nephros,* kidney; -oma tumour]. Grawitz tumour. A malignant neoplasm of the kidney--hypernephromata, pl.; hypernephromatous, adj.

برکلوی سلعہ : گردے میں خرابی۔

Hyperonychia *(hi'-per-on-ik'-i-a)* [G. *hyper,* above; *onyx,* nail]. Excessive growth of the nails.

کلاں ناخنی : ناخنوں کا زیادہ بڑھنا۔

Hyperosmolar diabetic coma *(hi-per-os-m-o'-lar).* Coma characterized by a very high blood sugar without accompanying ketosis.

ہائپر آسمولر شکری بے ہوشی : زیادہ ہائی بلڈ پریشر کے ساتھ بے ہوشی۔

Hyperosomalrity *(hi'-per-os-mo-lar'-i-ti)* [G. *hyper,* above; *osmos,* impulse]. Syn. hypertonicity. A solution exerting a higher osmotic pressure than another, is said to have a hyperosmolarity, with reference to it. In medicine, the comparision is usually made with nromal plasma.

ہائپر آسمولیریٹی : محلول جس کا نفوذی دباؤ دوسرے سے زیادہ ہو۔ ادویات میں عموماً نارمل پلازما سے موازنہ کیا جاتا ہے۔

Hyperostosis *(hi'-per-os-to'-sis)* [G. *hyper,* above; *osteon,* bone; -osis, condition]. See EXOSTOSIS.

بیش تعظم : ایکسوسٹوسس۔

Hyperoxaluria *(hi-per-oks-al-u'-ri-a)* [G. *hyper,* above; *oxalis,* garden sorrel; ouron, *urine*]. Excessive oxaluria (q.v.)--hyperoxaluric, adj.

ہائپر اوکسیلوریا : زائد کسیلوریا۔

Hyperparathyroidism *(hi'-per-pa-ra-t-hi'-roid-izm)* [G. *hyper,* above; para, near; *thureoeides,* sheild-shaped]., Overaction of the parathyroid glands with increase in serum calcium levels; may result in osteitis fibrosa cystica with decalcification and spontaneous fracture of bones. See TEST. INTRAVENOUS CALCIUM **tertiary h.,** development of parathyroid adenomata causing hypercalcaemia on top of reactive of secondary parathyroid hyperplasia due to malabsorption of chronic glomerular failure.

بیش درقیت : پیراتھائیرائڈ گلینڈز کا زائد ایکشن جس سے سیرم کیلشیم لیول زیادہ ہو جاتا ہے۔ ہڈیاں سیرم کیلشیم لیول زیادہ ہو جاتا ہے۔ ہڈیاں دکھتی ہیں۔ گردوں میں کنکریاں بننے لگتی ہیں۔ ہڈیاں نرم اور کمزور ہو جاتی ہیں۔

Hyperperistalsis *(hi'-per-pe-ri-stal'-sis)* [G. *hyper,* above; *peri,* around; *stellein,* to draw in]. Excessive peristalsis--hyperperistalic, adj.

افراط حرکت دودی : زائد پیراسٹالسس

Hyperphenylalaninaemia *(hi-per-fe-nil-al-anin-e'-mi-a).* Excess of phenylalamine in the blood.

ہائپر فینا مل ایلانینیمیا : خون میں فینائل الانین کی زیادتی۔

Hyperphagia *(hi'-per-fa'-ji-a)* G. *hyper,* above; *phagein,* to eat]. Overeating.

ہائپر فیجیا : زیادہ کھانا۔ خوش خوراکی۔

Hyperphosphataemia *(hi-per-fos-fat-e'-mia-a)* [G. *hyper,* above; *phosphoros,* light-bringer; *haima,* blood]. Excessive phosphates in the blood-- hyperphosphataemic, adj.

ہائپر فاسفاٹیمیا : خون میں زائد فاسفیٹس۔

Hyperpiesis *(hi-per-pi-es'-is)* [G. *hyper,* above *piesis,* pressure]. Hypertension (q.v.).

زیادتنش خون : ہائی بلڈ پریشر۔

Hyperpigmentation *(hi-per-pig-men-ta'-shun)* [G. *hyper,* above; *L. pigmentum,* pigment] Increased or excessive pigmentation.

بیش لونیت : زائد پگمنٹ ہونا۔

Hyperpituitarism *(hi-per-pit-u'-it-ar-izm).* Overactivity of the anterior lobe of the pituitary producing gigantism or acromegaly (q.v.).

بیش نخامیت : پیٹوایٹری کے امامی لوب کی زائد عاملیت جس سے گگانٹزم ہوتا ہے۔

Hyperplasia *(hi'-per-pla'-zi-a)* [G. *hyper,* above; *plasis,* a moulding]. Excessive formation of cells-- hyperplastic, adj.

زائد خلوی : خلیوں کا زائد بننا۔

Hyperpnoea *(hi'-perp-ne'-a)* [G. *hyper,* above *pnoe,* breath]. Rapid, deep breathing; panting gasping--hypernoeic, adj.

افراط تنفس : تیز گہرے سانس۔

Hyperpotassaemia *(hi'-per-pot-as-e'-mi-a).* Increased potassium in the blood. Hyperkalaemia. Theoretically can cause heart block cardiac arrest and muscle paralysis-hyperpotassaemic, adj.

ہائپرٹوپاسیمیا : خون میں کیلشیم کی بڑی ہوئی مقدار۔

Hyperpyrexia *(hi'-per-pi-reks'-i-a)* [G. *hyper* above; *pyressein,* to be feverish]. Body temperature above 40-41°C (105°F)--hyperpyrexial, adj.

تپ شدید : جسم کا درجہ حرارت ۴۰ تا ۴۱ س یا ۱۰۵ ف۔

Hypersecretion *(hi'-per-se-kre'-shun)* [G. *hyper,* above; L. *secretus,* separated]. Excessive secretion.

بیش افراز : رطوبت کا زائد اخراج۔

Hypersensitivity *(hi-per'-sen-si-ti'-vi-ti)* [G. *hyper,* above; L. *sentire,* to feel]. A state of being unduly sensitive to a stimulus or an allergen (q.v.)--hypersensitive, adj.

بیش حساسیت : زیادہ حساس ہونے کی حالت۔

Hypersplenism *(hi-per-splen'-izm)* [G. *hyper,* above; *splen,* spleen]. Term used to describe depression of erythrocyte, granulocyte and platelet counts by enlarged spleen in presence of active bone marrow.

ہائپر سپلنزم : بڑھی ہوئی تلی کی بڑھی ہوئی ہیمولائیٹنگ عاملیت۔

Hypertelorism *(hi-per-tel'-or-izm)* [G. *hyper,* above; *tele,* far off; *horos,* a boundary]. Genetically determined cranial anomaly (low forehead and pronounced vertex) associated with mental subnormality.

ہائپر تیلورزم : ذہنی پسماندگی۔ ماتھے نیچے دبا ہوا۔

Hypertensin *(hi-per-ten'-sin).* Angiotensin (q.v.).

ہائپر ٹنسن

Hypertension *(hi-per-ten'-shun)* [G. *hyper,* above; *tendere,* to stretch]: Abnormally high tension, by custom alluding to blood pressure and involving systolic and/or diastolic levels. There is no universal agreement of their upper limits of normal, especially in increasing age. Many cardiologists consider a resting systolic pressure of 160 mm of mercury (mmHg), and/or a resting diastolic pressure of 100 mm Hg, to be pathological. The cause may be renal, endocrine, mechanical or toxic (as in toxaemia of pregnancy) but in many cases it is unknown and this is then called 'essential h.' **primary pulmonary h.,** constriction of blood vessels in the lungs with consequent resistance to blood flow which increases pressure in the right cardiac ventricle and atrium. Cause unknown. Usually leads to death from congestive heart failure in 2 to 10 years-- hypertensive, adj.

بیش طنابی : غیر معمولی زیادہ دباؤ۔ ہائی بلڈ پریشر۔ عموماً زیادہ کھانے والوں کو ہوتا ہے۔ علاج کے لئے کم غذا۔ سبزی خوری۔ موٹاپے اور قبض خوری کا علاج ضروری ہیں اور ریزرپین۔ (سرپاسل) ایک گولی صبح ایک دوپہر ایک شام۔ میتھائل ڈونا (ایلڈومیٹ) ۱ تا ۳ گولیاں اور فروسے مائیڈ (لاریکس) ۱ تا ۲ گولیاں۔

Hyperthermia *(hi'-per-ther'-mi-a)* [G. *hyper,* above; *therme,* heat]. Very high body temperature-- hyperthermic, adj.

بیش تپشی : بہت زیادہ جسمانی درجہ حرارت۔

Hyperthyroidism *(hi'-per-thi'-roid-izm)* [G. *hyper,* above; *thureoeides,* sheild shaped]. Thyrotoxicosis (q.v.).

زہریلا گلھڑ : تھائیرو ٹوکسیکولسس۔ گوپوزڈیزیز۔ تھائرائیڈ گلینڈ معمولی سی بڑھ جاتی ہے اور ہارمون تھائیروکین کی مقدار بہت زیادہ ہو جاتی ہے۔ یہ مرض عورتوں میں زیادہ ہے۔ علاج کے لئے لیوگالز آیوڈین پروپائیل تھایو یورسیال نیومرکازول۔ پوٹاشیم پرکلوریٹ اور برومائیڈ مکسچر۔

Hypertonia *(hi'-er-to'-ni-a)* [G. *hyper,* above; *tonos,* tension]. Increased tone in a muscular structure-- hypertonic, adj,; hypertonicity, n.

بیش طنابی : کسی عضلاتی ساخت میں بڑھی ہوئی ٹون۔

Hypertonic *(hi'-perton'ik)* [G. *hyper,* above; *tonos,* tension]. 1. Pertaining to hypertonia. 2. Pertaining to saline. h. saline has a greater osmotic pressure than normal physiological (body) fluid.

بیش ولوجہ : (۱) ہائپر ٹونیا سے متعلق۔ (۲) سیلائن سے متعلق۔

Hypertoxic *(hi-per-toks'-ik)* [G. *hyper,* above; *toxikon,* poison]. Very poisonous.

سخت سمی : زیادہ زہریلا

Hypertrichiasis *(hi'-per-trik-i'-a-sis)* [G. *hiper,* above; *thrix,* hair; -osis, condition]. Excessive hairiness. Also HYPERTRICHOSIS.

گھنے بال : زیادہ بال ہونا۔

Hypertrophy *(hi'-per-trof-i)* [G. *hyper.* above; *trophe,* nourishment]. Increase in the size of tissues or structures, independent of natural growth. It may be congenital (see PYLORIC STENOSIS), compensatory, complementary or functional--hypertrophic, adj.

بیش نمو : قدرتی بڑھاؤ کے ساتھ ساختوں یا بافتوں کے سائز میں بڑھاؤ۔

Hyperuricaemia *(hi-per-u-ris-e'-mi-a).* Excessive uric acid in the blood Characteristic of gout. Occurs in untreated reticulosis, but is increased by radiotherapy, cytotoxins and corticosteroids-- hyperuricaemic, adj.

ہائپر یوریسیمیا : خون میں زائد یورک ایسڈ۔ جوڑوں کے درد کی خصوصیت۔

Hyperventilation *(hi'-per-ven-til-a'-shun)* [G. *hyper,* above; L. *ventilare,* below]. Syn., hypernoea (q.v.).

ہائپرونٹی لیشن : ہائپرینا۔

Hypervitaminosis *(hi'-per-vi-ta-min-o'-sis)* [G. *hyper,* above; L. *vita,* life; G. -osis, condition]. Any condition arising from an excess of vitamins, especially vitamin D.

بیش وٹامنیت : وٹامنز خصوصاً وٹامن ڈی کی زیادتی سے ہونے والی حالت۔

Hypervolaemia *(hi-per-vol-e'-mi-a)* [G. *hyper,* above; L. *volume,* volume; G. *haima,* blood]. Plethora (q.v.).

ہائپروولیمیا : پلیتھورا۔

Hypaema *(hi-fe'-ma)* [G. *hypo,* under; *haima,* blood]. Blood in the anterior chamber of the eye.

قلت الام۔ دردوں چشمی نزف : آنکھ کے امامی چیمبر میں خون۔

Hypnosis *(hip-no'-sis)* [G. *hypnos,* sleep; *-osis,* condition]. A state resembling sleep, brought about by the hynotist utilizing the mental mechanism of suggestion. Can be used to produce painless labour; dental extractions, and is occasionally utilized in minor surgery and in psychiatric practice--hypnotic, adj.

خواب مصنوعی۔ تنویم : نیند سے مشابہ حالت۔

Hypnotherapy *(hip-no-ther'-a-pi)* [G. *hypnos,* sleep; *therapeia,* treatment]. Treatment by prolonged sleep or hypenosis.

تنویمی علاج : طویل نیند یا ہپنوسس سے علاج۔

Hypnotic *(hip-not'-ik)* [G. *hypnos,* sleep]. 1. Pertaining to hypnotism. 2. A drug which produces a sleep resembling natural sleep.

تنویمی۔ خواب آور : (۱) ہپناٹزم سے متعلق۔ (۲) قدرتی نیند سے مشابہ نیند پیدا کرنے والی دوا۔ زیادہ کھا لینے کی صورت میں سانس فیل ہونے لگتا ہے۔ جسم ٹھنڈا، نبض کمزور سانس میں خراٹے کی آواز۔ فوراً معدہ دھونا چاہئے۔ مصنوعی سانس۔ کورامین۔ تیز چائے۔ ایمافیٹامین اور مالش مفید ہیں۔

Hypoaesthesia *(hi-po-es-the'-zi-a)* [G. *hypo,* below; *aisthesis,* sensation]. Diminished sensitiveness of a part--hypoaesthetic, adj.

ہائپوایستھیسیا : کسی حصے کی حساسیت میں کمی۔

Hypocalcaemia *(hi-po-kal-se'-mi-a)* [G. *hypo,* under L. *calx,* lime; G.l *haima,* blood]. Decreased calcuium in the blood. See TETANY hypocalcaemic, adj.

ص دموی کلسیت : خون میں کیلشیم کی مقدار میں کمی۔

Hypocapnia *(hi-po-kap'-ni-a)* [G. *hypo,* und *kapnos,* smoke]. Diminished CO_2 content the blood; can be produced by hyperventila on-- hypocapnial, adj.

Hypochloraemia *(hi-po-klor-e'-mi-a)* [G. *hyp* under; *chloros* pale; *haima,* blood]. Reduc chlorides in the circulating blood. A form alkalosis--hypochloraemic, adj.

کلوریمیا : گردشی خون میں تخفیف شدہ کلورائیڈز

Hypochlorhydria *(hi-po-klor-hi'-dri-a)* [*hypo,* under; *chloros,* pale green; *hyp* water]. Decreased hydrochloric acid in gastric juice--hypochlorhydric, adj.

نمک ترشگی : گیسٹرک جوس میں نمک کے تیزاب کی مقدار میں کمی۔

Hypochlorite *(hi-po-klor'-it)*. Salts of hy chlorous acid. They are easily decomposed yield active chlorine, and have been wid used on that account in the treatment wounds--Dakin's solution and eusol be examples. Miltion is a proprietary prod that contains a stabilizer of therefore ret its activity over a longer period.

لورائیٹ : ہائپوکلورس ایسڈ کے نمکیات۔ اس سے کلورین بنتی ہے اس خموں کے علاج میں مستعمل ہے۔

Hypochondria *(hi-po-kon'-dri-a)*. Excess anxiety about one's health. Commor depressive and anxiety states--hypochon ac,adj.; hypoch- ondriasis,

۔ سودا: صحت کے متعلق بلاوجہ پریشانی۔ پریشانی کی حالتوں میں عام

Hypochondrium *(hi-po-kon'-dri-um)*. upper lateral region (left and right) of abdomen, below the lower ribs--hypoch riac, adj.

بطن کا بالائی جانبی ریجن جو دائیں اور بائیں زیریں پسلیوں کے نیچے ۔

Hypochromic *(hi-po-kro'-mik)* [G. *hypo,* u *chroma,* colour]. Defficiency in colourin pigmentation. Decreased haemoglobin red blood cell.

ہائپوکرومک :رنگ یا پگمنٹ میں کمی۔سرخ خونی خلیے میں کم ہیموگلوبن۔

Hypodermic *(hi-po-der'-mik)* [G. *hypo,* below, *derma,* skin]. Below the skin Subcutaneous--hypodermically, adv.

زیریں جلد

Hypodermic

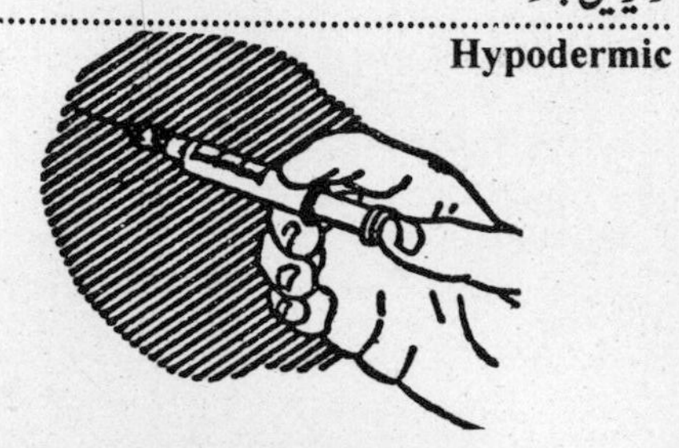

Hypofibrinogenaemia *(hi-po-fi-brin'-o-j-en-e'-mi-a).* See AFIBRINOGENAEMIA and ACUTE DEFIBRINATION SYN. DROME--ypofibrinogenacanic. adj.

ہائپوفجبر نیوجنیمیا :افیبر نیوجنیمیا۔رحم الٹ جانے سے اینا ٹک۔سیال ماں کے خون میں مل سکتا ہے۔جس میں تھرمبو پلاسٹین کی مقدار زیادہ ہوتی ہے جو ماں کے خون میں یہ مرض پیدا کرسکتا ہے۔یہ مرض بہت کم ہوتا ہے۔

Hypofunction *(hi-po-fungk'-shun)* [G. *hypo,* below; L. *functio,* performance]. Diminished performance.

قلت فعل۔کاہلی : گھٹی ہوئی ادائیگی۔

Hypogammaglobulinaemia *(hi-po-gam-m-a-glob'-u- lin-e'-mi-a).* Decreased gammaglobulin in the blood. Lessens resistance to infection.See DYSGAMMAGLOBULINA-EMIA-- hypogamma- globulinaemic, adj.

ہائپوگیما گلوبولینیمیا : خون میں گیما گلوبولن کی کمی۔بیماری سے مدافعت میں کمی ہوجاتی ہے۔

Hypogastrium *(hi-po-gas'-tri-um)* [G. *hypo,* below; *gaster,* belly]. That area of the anterior abdomen which lies immediately below the umbilical region. It is flanked on either side by the iliac fossae--hypogastric, adj.

زیرمعدہ :امامی بطن کا وہ ایریا جو امبلیکل ریجن کے فوراً نیچے واقع ہوتا ہے۔

Hypoglossal *(hi-po-glos'-al)* [G. *hypo,* below; *glossa,* togue]. Under the tongue, **hypoglossal nerve,** the twelfth pair of cranial nerves.

زیرزبانی : زبان کے نیچے۔زیرعصابی عصب یا نزد میڈلا آبلانگیٹا سے نکلتی ہے اور زبان کی عضلات کو سپلائی دیتی ہے۔

Hypoglycaemia *(hi-po-gli-se'-mi-a)* [G. *hypo,* below; *glykys,* sweet; *haima,* blood]. Decreased blood sugar, attended by anxiety, excitement, perspiration, delirium or coma, **insulin h.** can be produced intentionally (insulin treatment) in schizophrenia. **idiopathic h.,** associated with mental subnormality. ACTH useful. **leucine-induced h.,** a genetic metabolic disorder due to sensitivity to the amino acid leucine-- hypoglycaemic, adj.

کم شکر دمویت : کم خونی شکر سے جس سے پریشانی ہو۔جوش پسینہ اور بے ہوشی ہوتی ہے۔

Hypokalaemia *(hi-po-ka-le'-mi-a)* [G. *hypo,* below; L. *kalium,* potassium]. Abnormally low potassium level of the blood-- hypokalaemic, adj. See POTASSIUM DEFICIENCY.

ہائپوکیلیمیا :خون کا پوٹاشیم لیول جو غیر نارمل طور پر کم ہے۔

Hypomagnesaemia *(hi-po-mag-nes-e'-mi-a)* [G. *hypo,* below; *magnesie lithos,* Magnesian stone; *haima,* blood]. Decresed magnesium in the blood-- hypomagnesaemic, adj.

قلت مفنیس دمویت :خون میں کم میگنیشم۔

Hypomania *(hi-po-ma'-ni-a)* [G. *hypo,* below; *mania,* madness]. A less intense form of mania (q.v.)., in which the patient is easily distracted-- hypomanic, adj.

سادہ جنون :پاگل پن کی ایک ہلکی قسم۔

Hypometabolism *(hi-po-met-ab'-ol-izm)* [G. *hypo,* below; *metabole,* change]. Decreased production of body heat. Characteristic of myxoedema.

ہائپومیٹابولزم :جسمانی حرارت کی کمی یا کم پیداوار۔

Hypomotility *(hi-po-mo-ti'-li-ti)* [G. *hypo,* under; L. *movere,* to move]. Decreased movement as of the stomach or intestines.

خفیف حرکت : تخفیف شدہ حرکت مثلاً معدہ یا انتڑیوں۔

Hyponatraemia *(hi-po-nat-re'-mi-a)* [G. *hypo,* below; *natros,* sodium; *haima,* blood]. Decreased sodium in the blood--hyponatraemic, adj.

ہائپونیٹریمیا : خون میں سوڈیم کی کمی۔

Hypo-osmolarity *(hi-po-os-mo-lar'-it-i)* [G. *hypo,* below; *osmos,* impulse]. Syn., hypotonicity. A solution exerting a lower osmotic pressure than another, is said to have a h.-o. with reference to it. In medicine the comparison is usually made with normal plasma.

قلیل نفوذی دباؤ : محلول میں دوسرے کی نسبت کم نفوذی دباؤ ہونا۔

Hypoparathyroidism *(hi-po-pa-ra-th-i'-roid-izm)* [G. *hypo,* under; para, near; *thureoeides,* shield shaped]. Underaction of the parathyroid glands with decrease in serum calcium levels, producing tetany (q.v.).

ناقص نزدورقیت : سیرم کیلشیم لیولز میں پیراتھائیرائیڈ گلینڈز کے ایکشن میں کمی۔ پیراتھارمون کی کمی سے خون میں کیلشیم کی مقدار کم ہو جاتی ہے جس سے عضلات زیادہ حساس ہو جاتے ہیں اور تشنج کے دورے پڑنے لگتے ہیں۔ ہاتھ کی انگلیاں اکڑ کر ٹیڑھی ہو جاتی ہیں۔ پاؤں اکڑ جاتے ہیں چہرے کے عضلات پھڑکتے ہیں۔

Hypopharynx *(hi-po-far'-ingks).* That portion of the pharynx lying below and behind the larynx, correctly called the laryngopharynx.

زیربلعوم : فیرنکس کا وہ حصہ جو لیرنکس کے پیچھے اور نیچے ہوتا ہے۔

Hypophoria *(hi-po-fo'-ri-a).* [G. *hypo,* below; *phoros,* bearing]. A state in which the visual axis in one eye is lower than the other.

ہائپوفوریا : ایسی حالت جس میں ایک آنکھ میں بصری محور دوسری سے کم ہے۔

Hypophosphataemia *(hi-po-fos-fat-e'-mi-a).*[G. *hypo,* below; *phosphoros,* light-bringer; *haima,* blood]. Decreased phosphates in the blood-- hypophosphataemic,

ہائپوفاسفیٹیمیا : خون میں فاسفیٹس کی کمی۔

Hypophysectomy *(hi-pof-i-sek'-to-mi)* [G. *hypo,* below; *physis,* growth; ektome, excession]. Surgical removal of the pituitary gland.

نخامیہ براری : پیٹوایٹری گلینڈ کا سرجیکل خاتمہ۔

Hypophysis cerebri *(hi-pof'-i-sis).* The sm oval-shaped gland lying in the pituitary fos of the sphenoid bone and connected to t under surface of the brain by a stalk; t pituitary gland-- hypophyseal, adj.

ہ نخامیہ : پیٹوایٹری گلینڈ۔ چھوٹی بیضوی شکل کی غدجو دماغ کے نچلے پر ہوتی ہے۔

Hypopiesis *(hi-po-pi-es'-is)* [G. *hypo,* belo *piesis,* pressure]. Hypotension (q.v.).

تنش خون : کم بلڈ پریشر۔

Hypopigmentation *(hi-po-pig-men-ta'-shun)* [G. *hypo,* below; L. *pigmentum,* pigmen Decreased or poor pigmentation.

پگمنٹیشن : پگمنٹ کی کمی۔

Hypopituitarism *(hi-po-pit-u'-it-ar-izm)* [*hypo,* under; L. *pituita,* slime]. Pituitary gla insufficiency, especially of the anterior lo Absence of gonadotrophins leads to failure ovulation, uterine atrophy and amenorrho Loss of trophic hormones to other endocri produces mental inertia, laziness, weakne lack of sweating, sensitivity to cold (may hypothermia), hypoglycaemia, pale sk depigmentation of mammary alveolae a perineum. Can result from post-part infarction of the pituitary gland.

نخامیت : پیٹوایٹری گلینڈ کا ناکافی ہونا خصوصاً امامی لوب کا۔

Hypoplasia *(hi-po-pla'-zi-a)* [G. *hypo,* und *plassein,* to form]. Defective development any tissue--hypoplastic, adj.

س : کسی نسیج کی ناقص ترقی۔

Hypopotassaemia *(hi-po-pot-as-se'-mi-a).* HYPOKALAEMIA.

پوٹاشیم : خون کا پوٹاشیم لیول جو غیر معمولی کم ہو۔

Hypoproteinaemia *(hi-po-pro-ten-em'-i-a)* *hypo,* below: *proteios,* **primary;** *hai* blood]. Deficient protein in blood plas from dietary deficiency or excessive excret (albuminuria)-- hypoproteinaemic, adj.

لحمیات : خونی پلازما میں پروٹین کی کمی۔

Hypoprothrombinaemia *(hi-po-pro-thr bin-e'-mi-a)* [G. *hypo,* below;*pro,* bef *thrombos,* clot; *haima,* blood]. Deficiency prothrombin in the blood which retards its clotting ability. See VITAMIN K and JAUNDICE-- hypoprothrombinaemic. adj.

قلت پروتھرومبین : خون میں پروتھرومبین کی کمی جو اس کے جمنے کا خاصیت کو ختم کرتا ہے۔

ypopyon *(hi-po'-pi-on)* [G. *hypo*, below; *pyon*, pus]. A collection of pus in the anterior chamber of the eye.

قرنیائی پیپ۔کوشکی رحم : آنکھ کے امامی چیمبر میں پیپ کا اجتماع۔

'posecretion *(hi-po-sek-kre'-shun)* [G. *hypo*, below; L. *secretio*, secretion]. Deficient secretion.

قلت افراز : اخراج رطوبت میں کمی۔

'posmia *(hi-pos'-mi-a)* [G. *hypo*, below; *osme*, smell]. Decrease in the normal sensitivity to smell. Has been observed in patients following laryngectomy.

ضعف قوت شامہ : سونگھنے کی نارمل حس میں کمی۔

'pospadias *(hi-po-spa'-di-as)* [G. *hypo*, below; *spein*, to draw out]. A congenital malformation of the male urethra. Sub-divided into two types; (1) penile, when the terminal urethral orifice opens at any point along the posterior shaft of the penis; (2) perineal, when the orifice opens on the perineum and may give rise to problems of sexual differentiation. Cf. epispadias.

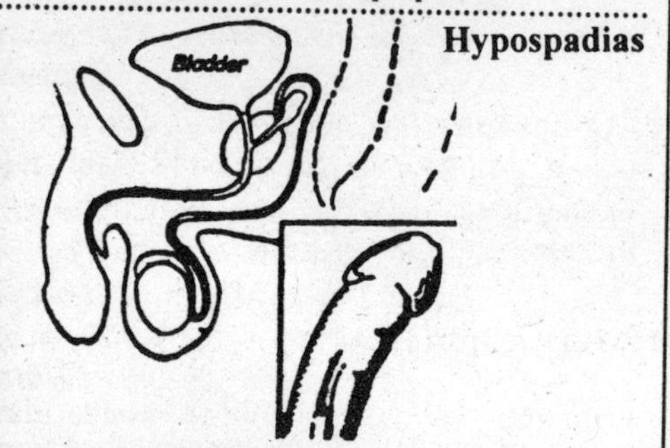

Hypospadias

تحت مبالی نقص : ایک ناقص ساخت جس میں زیریں تھر اعضو تناسل کی زیریں سطح پر کھلتا ہے۔

Hypostasis *(hi-po-sta'-sis)* [G. a standing under]. 1. A sediment. 2. Congestion of blood in a part due to impaired circulation--hypostatic, adj.

زیروکود : کسی حصے میں خون کا اجتماع۔

Hypotension *(hi-po-ten'-shun)* [G. *hypo*, below; L. *tensio*, a stretching]. Low blood pressure (systolic below 110 mm Hg, diastolic below 70 mmHg), may be primary, secondary (e.g. shock, Addison's disease) or postural. It can be produced by the administration of drugs to reduce bleeding in surgery--hypotensive, adj.

کم تنش خون : کم بلڈ پریشر۔

Hypothalamus *(hi-po-thal'-a-mus)* [G. *hypo*, below; *thalamos*, chamber]. Below the thalamus. Part of the midbrain closest to the pituitary. Under control of the emotions and even of the conscious brain.

زیرعرشہ : تھیلامس کے نیچے۔

Hypothenar eminence *(hi-po-the'-nar)* [G. *hypo*, below; *thenar*, palm]. The eminence on the ulnar side of the palm below the little finger.

ریزراحی فراز : چھوٹی انگلی کے نیچے ہتھیلی کی الز جانب ابھار۔

Hypothermia *(hi-po-ther'-mi-a)* [G. *hypo*, below; *therme*, heat]. Below normal body temperature, ascertained by the low-reding thermometer. Occurs in the very young and in old people. An artificially induced hypothermia (30° C or 86° F) can be used in the treatment of head injuries and in cardiac surgery. It reduces the oxygen consumption of the tissues and thereby allows greater and more prolonged interference of normal blood circulation. **hypothermia** of the **newborn,** failure of the newborn child to adjust to external cold; may be associated with infection. **local h.** has been tried in the treatment of peptic ulcer. See REFRIGERATION.

ہایپوتھرسیا : نارمل درجہ حرارت سے نیچے۔

Hypothyroidism *(hi-po-thi'-roid-izm)* [G. *hypo*, below; *thureoeides*, sheild-shaped]. Defines those clinical conditions which result from suboptimal circulating levels of one or both thyroid hormones. See THYROXINE, TRIIODOTHYRONINE. Hypothyroidism currently classified as; (1) overt (see MYXOEDEMA);(2)mild;(3)preclinical; (4)automimmune thyroid disease without thyroid failure. See CRETINISM and MYXOEDEMA

ناقص درقیت : کلینکل حالات جو تھائیرائڈ ہارمونز کی وجہ سے ہوتے ہیں۔

Hypotonic *(hi-po-ton'-ik)* [G. *hypo,* below; *tonos,* tension]. Having a low osmotic pressure; less than isotonic; lacking in tone, tension, strength-- hypotonia, hypotonicity, n.

کم دلوجہ : کم نفوذی دباؤ ہونا۔

Hypovase *(hi'-po-vas).* Prazosin (q.v.).

Hypoventilation *(hi-po-ven-til-a'-shun)* [G. *hypo*, below; L. *ventilare,* below]. Diminished breathing or underventilation.

کم تنفس : سانس میں کمی۔

Hypovitaminaemia *(hi-po-vi-ta-min-e'-mi-a)* [G. *hypo,* below; L. *via,* life; -amine; *haima,* blood]. Deficiency of vitamins in the blood-hypovitamin-- aemic adj.

قلت حیاتینیت۔ناقص حیاتینیت : ایسی حالت جو وٹامنز کی کمی کی وجہ سے ہو۔

Hypovolaemia *(hi-po-vol-e'-mi-a).* See OLIGAEMIA--hypovolaemic, adj.

ہائپوو ولیمیا : اولیگیمیا

Hypoxaemia *(hi-poks-e'-mi-a)* [G. *hypo,* under; *oxys,* sharp; *haima,* blood]. Diminished amount (reduced saturation) of oxygen in the arterial blood-- hypoxaemic, adj.

قلت آکسیجن : شریانی خون میں آکسیجن کی مقدار میں کمی۔

Hypoxia *(hi-pok'-si-a)* [G. *hypo,* under; *oxys,* sharp]. Diminished amount of oxygen in the tissues-- hypoxic, adj. **anaemic h.,** resulting from a deficiency of haemoglobin. **histotoxic h.,** interference with the cells in their utilization of O_2, e.g. in cyanide poisoning. **hypoxic h.,** interference with pulmonary oxygenation. **stagnant h.,** a reduction in blood flow, as seen in the finger nails in surgical shock or in cold weather.

ہائپوکسیا : بافتوں میں آکسیجن کی کم مقدار۔

Hysterectomy *(hi-ter-ek'-to-mi)* [G. *hystera,* womb; *ektome,* excision]. Surgical removal of the uterus. **abdominal h.,** effected via a lower abdominal incision. **subtotal h.,** removal of the uterine bodyt,leaving the cervix in the vaginal vault. Rarely performed because of the risk of a carcinoma developing in the cervical stump. **total h.,** complete removal of the uterine body and cervix. **viginal h.,** effected per vaginam. **Wertheim's h.,** total removal of the uterus, the adjacent lymphatic vessels and glands, with a cuff of the vagina.

رحم براری : رحم یا یورٹرس کا اپریشن سے خاتمہ۔

Hysteria *(his-te'-ri-a)* [G. *hystera,* womb]. A neurosis usually arising from mental conflict anb repression (q.v.), and characterized by the production of a diversity of symptoms, e.g tics, paralysis, anaesthesia, etc. The disorder is characterized by dissociation (q.v.)--hysterical, adj

شدید جذباتیت۔خلل اعصاب۔اختناق الرحم : نیوروسس جو عموماً ذہنی تکرار کی وجہ سے ہوتا ہے۔اس میں بے ہوشی بھی ہو جاتی ہے۔مریضہ کا دم گھٹتا ہے۔یہ مرض رحم کی خرابی سے ہوتا ہے۔باؤ گولہ۔آنکھوں سے پانی۔سر درد، سستی وضعف اور تاریکی دو پرچشم کی شکایات ہوتی ہیں۔پھر شکم میں ایک گولہ سا اٹھ کر اوپر جا کر گلے میں اٹک جاتا ہے۔دم گھٹنے لگتا ہے۔گردن سخت ہو جاتی ہے۔مریضہ روتی یا ہنستی ہے ہاتھ پاؤں میں تشنج ہو جاتا ہے۔پیشاب زیادہ آتا ہے۔

Hysterography *(his-te-rog'-ra-fi)* [G. *hystera,* womb; *graphein,* to write]. X-ray examination of the uterus--hysterograph, hysterogram, n hysterographical. adj. hysterographically, adv

رحم نگاری : رحم یا یورٹرس کا ایکسرے کے ذریعے ٹیسٹ۔

Hysterosalpingectomy *(his-te-ro-sal-pin-jek'-to-mi)* [G. *hystera,* womb; *salpigx,* trum,pet; *ektome,* excision]. Excision of the womb and usually both uterine tubes (oviducts).

رحم دانبوبہ براری : بطن اور عموماً دونوں نالیوں کا انقطاع۔

Hysterosalpingography *(his-te-ro-sal-ping-og'-ra-fi)* [G. *hystera,* womb; *salpigx,* trumpet; *graphein,* to write]. X-ray exami ation of the uterus and tubes after injection of a contrast medium--hysterosalpin- gograph.

ہسٹیر وسیلپنگو گرافی: کنٹراسٹ میڈیم کے انجکشن کے بعد یوٹرس اور نالیوں کی ایکس رے کے ذریعے جانچ پڑتال۔

ysterosalpingostomy *(his-te-ro-sal-pin-g-os'-to-mi)* [G. *hystera,* womb; *salpigx,* trumpet; *stoma,* mouth]. Anastomosis between an oviduct and the uterus.

رحمی انبوی تفویہ :یوٹرس اوراوویڈکٹ کے درمیان جال

ysterotomy *(his-te-rot'-o-mi)* [G. *hystera,* womb; *tome,* a cutting].

رحم شگافی۔ قیصری تراش : ۲۸ویں ہفتے سے قبل حمل کوختم کرنے کیلئے یورٹرس کا شگاف۔

Hysterotrachelorraphy *(his-te-ro-trak-el -or'a-fi)* [G. *hystera,* womb; *trachelos,* neck; *rhaphe,* suture].

ہسٹیر وٹریکلورافی :لیرٹیڈ سروکس یوٹری کی مرمت۔

Hystiocytosis X. *(his-ti-o-si-to'-sis)* See HISTIOCYTOSIS.

ناسور

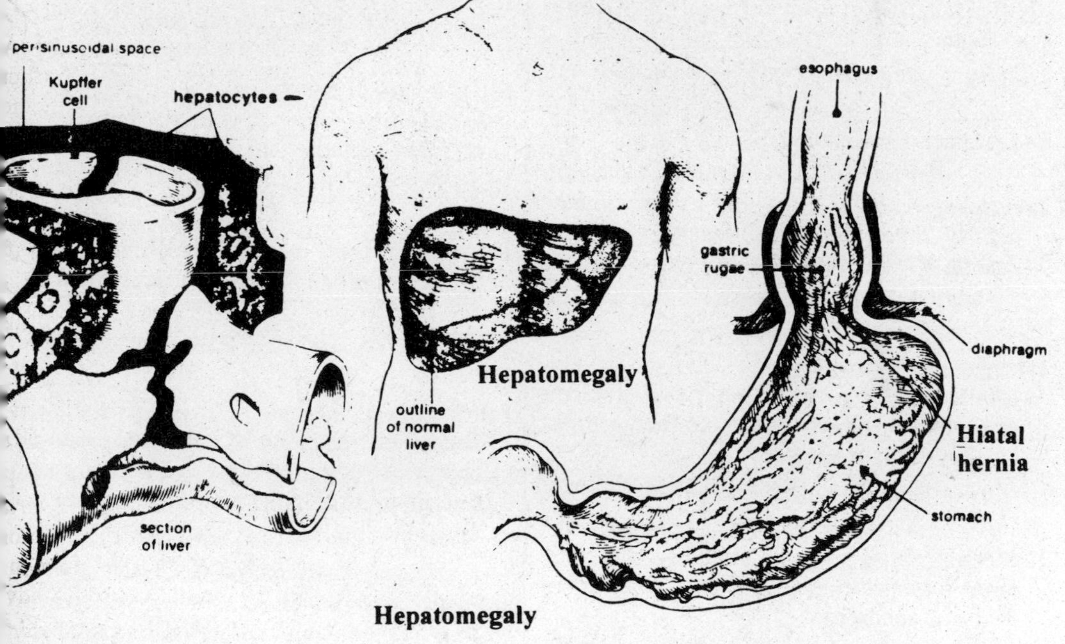

Hepatomegaly

I

I Symbol for Iodine, inosine, electric current, intensity (of radiant energy) and ionic strength.

آئی: علامت ہے آئیوڈین، آئنوسین، برقی رو، شعاعی توانائی کی شدت اور چارج کی طاقت کی۔

IAEA Internationl Atomic Energy Agency.

آئی اے ای اے: بین الاقوامی ادارہ برائے ایٹمی توانائی۔

Iamatology *(i-am-a-tol-o-je)* [G. *ioma,* iomate remedy; *logos,* discourse]. Branch of science dealing with the study of remedies.

تریاقی سائنس: سائنس کی وہ شاخ جس میں علاج وغیرہ کا مطالعہ کیا جائے۔

Iatrogenesis *(i'-atro-jen-a-sis)* [G. *genesis,* production]. The creation of additional problems or complications resulting from the treatment of a physician or surgeon.

ایاٹروجینسس: طبیب یا ماہر جراحت کے علاج سے پیدا ہونے والے اضافی مسائل یا نقصانات کیلئے یہ اصطلاح استعمال ہوتی ہے۔

Ibufenac *(i'bufa-nak)* An analgesic and anti-inflammatory formerly used inthe treatment of heumatic conditions.

آئیبوفینک: درد اور سوزش سے آرام کیلئے دوا ہے۔ پہلے یہ جوڑوں کے درد اور علاج وغیرہ کے لئے استعمال ہوتی تھی۔

Ibuprofen *(i'bu-pro-fen)* It is a nonsteroidal, analgesic, antipyretic and anti-inflammatory agent. It is a derivation of propionic acid. It is used for relief of pain, reduction of fever and in the treatment of osteoarthritis and rheumatoid arthritis.

آئبوپروفن: یہ ایک غیر سٹیرائیڈ درد، بخار اور سوزش کے لئے دوا ہے۔ یہ پورپیونک تیزاب سے اخذ کردہ ہے۔ یہ روماٹائیڈ آرتھرائٹس اور اوسٹیو آرتھرائٹس کے لئے بھی موثر ہے۔

Ice *(i's)* One of the six solid form of water, but usually the common low-density form melting at 0°C at 1 atmosphere.

برف: پانی کی چھ ٹھوس اقسام میں سے کوئی ایک قسم۔ یہ عموماً صفر درجہ سینٹی گریڈ اور ایک اسٹماسفیئر دباؤ پر پگھل جاتی ہے۔

Ichthyol *(ik-the-ol)* A trade mark for the preparation of ichkrammol. It is local skin anti-infective.

اکتھاٹیول: یہ اکتھمول کی تیاری کا تجارتی نام ہے۔ یہ جلدی امراض کے لئے موثر ہے۔

Ichthyosis *(ik'the-o-sis)* [G. *ichthy,* fish; *osis,* condition]. A group of cutaneous disorders characterized by increased or aberrant keratinization, resulting in non-inflammatory scaling of the skin. It is a congenital condition.

سمک جلدی: خشک اور سکیلی کھال۔ مچھلی والی جلد۔

Icterus *(ik-ter-us)* [L. G. *ikteros,* yellowness] Jaundice. **epidemic catarrhel i.**, a mild form of infection hepatitis. **i. gravis neonatorum** severe jaundice in newborn, usually a form of isoimmunization with Rh factor. **i. neonatorum,** the jaundice sometimes seen in newborn children.

زردی: یرقان۔ دورانِ زچگی یہ مرض نوزائیدہ بچوں کو ہو جاتا ہے۔

Idea *(i'-de-a)* A mental impression or conception

تصور۔ خیال: احساس۔ تاثر۔ ذہنی رو۔

Ideaction *(i-de-a'-shun)* [g. *idea,* form]. The process concerned with the highest function of awareness the formatin of ideas. It includes thought, intellect and memory.

تفکر : بیداری کے اعلیٰ ترین فعل۔نظریات بنانے والے متعلق طریق۔ اس میں خیال ذہانت اور یادداشت شامل ہیں۔

Identical twins *(i-den'-tik-al)*. Two off-spring of the same sex, derived from a single fertilized ovum. See BINOVULAR and UNIOVULAR.

مماثل جڑواں : ایک ہی جنس کے دو بچے جو ایک ہی بارور بیضے سے بنتے ہیں۔

Identification *(i-den-ti-fi-ka'-shun)* [L. *idem,* same]. Recognition. In psychology, the way in which we form our personality by modelling it on a chosen person, e.g. identification with the parent of same sex--helping to form one's sex role; identification with a person of own sex in the hero-workship of adolescence.

شناخت : پہچان۔نفسیات میں وہ طریقہ جس میں ہم کسی شخص پر اپنی شخصیات بناتے ہیں۔

Ideomotor *(i-de-o-mo'-tor)* [G. *idea,* form; L. *movere,* to move]. Mental energy, in the form of ideas, producing automatic movement of muscles, e.g. mental agitation producing agitated movements of limbs.

تصوری حرکی : نظریات کی صورت میں ذہنی توانائی جس سے عضلات کا خودکار حرکت ہوتی ہے۔

Idioventricular *(id-i-o-ven-trik'-u-lar)* [G. *idios,* one's own; L. *ventriculum,* ventricle]. Pertaining to the cardiac ventricles and not affecting the atria.

خالص بطینی : قلبی وینٹریکلز سے متعلق اور ایٹریا پر اثر نہ ہونا۔

Idiopathy *(id-io-pa'-thi)* [G. *idios,* one's own; *pathos,* disease]. A pathologic state of unknown or spontaneous origin--idiopathic, adj.

مخصوص عارضہ : بیماری کی حالت میں جس کے متعلق پتہ نہ ہو۔

Idiosyncrasy *(id-i-o-sing'-kra-si)* [G. *idios,* own; *synkrasis,* mingling together]. A peculiar variation of constitution or temperament. Unusual individual response to certain drugs, proteins, etc. whether by injection, ingestion, inhalation or contact.

خاص مزاج : طبیعت کی ایک مخصوص تبدیلی۔بعض اوقات ادویات وغیرہ کی طرف انفرادی ردعمل۔

Idoxuridine *(i-doks-u'-ri-din)* 5-Iodo-2-deoxyuridine, Antiviral chemotherapeutic agent for corneal herpetic uicers. It interferes with synthesis of DNA in herpes simplex virus and prevents it from multiplying. Active against vaccinia infection.

اڈوکسوریڈین : وائرس کے خلاف عامل۔

Ileal bladder *(il'-e-al blad'-er)*. See BLADDER.

Ileitis *(il-e-i'-tis)*. [L. *ilia,* flanks; G. *itis,* inflammation]. Inflammation of the ileum **regional i.,** non-specific chronic recurrent granulomatous disease affecting mainly young adults and characterized by a necrotizing, ulcerating inflammatory process, there usually being an abrupt demarcation between it and healthy bowel. There can be healthy bowel ('skip' area) intervening between two diseased segments.

ورم لفافی : معاءِ لفاف یا الیم کی سوزش۔

Ileocaecal *(i-le-o-se'-kal)* [L. *ilia,* flanks; caecus, blind]. Pertaining to the ileum and the caecum.

لفافی : اعوری الیم اور سیکم سے متعلق۔

Ileocolic *(i-le-o-kol-i'-tis)* [L. *ilia,* flanks; G. *kolon,* colon; -itis, inflammation] Inflammation of the ileum and the colon.

لفافی قولونی التہاب : الیم اور قولون کی سوزش۔

Ileocolostomy *(i-le-o-kol-os'-to-mi)* [L. *ilia,* flanks; G. *kolon,* colon; stoma, mouth]. A surgical made fistula between the ileum and the colon, usually the transverse colon. Most often used to bypass an obstruction or inflammation in the caecum or ascending colon.

لفافی قولونی ناسور : الیم اور قولون کے درمیان اپریشن کے ذریعے سٹولا بنانا۔

Ileocutaneous ureterostomy. See BLADDER and URETEROSTOMY.

الیوکوٹینیس یورٹروسٹومی : بلیڈر۔

Ileocystoplasty *(i-le-o-sis'-to-plas-it)* [L. *ilia,* flanks; G. *kystis,* bladder; *plassein,* to form]. Operation to increase the urinary bladder.See COLOCYSTOPLASTY for diagram-- ileocystoplastic, adj.

الیوسسٹو پلاسٹی :بولی بلیڈر کو بڑھانے کے لئے اپریشن۔

Ileoproctostomy *(i-le-o-prok-tos'-to-mi)* [L. *ilia,* flanks; G. *proktos,* anus; *stoma,* mouth]. An anastomosis between the ileum and rectum; used when disease extends to the sigmoid colon.

لفائفی مستقیمی لفویہ : ایلم اور ریکٹم کے درمیان جال۔

Ileorectal *(i-le-o-rek'-tal)* [L. *ilia,* flanks; *rectus,* straight]. Pertaining to the ileum and the rectum.

الیوریکٹل :ایلم اور ریکٹم سے متعلق۔

Ileosigmoidostomy *(i-le-o-sig-moid-os'-to-mi)* [L. *ilia,* flanks; G. *sigmoides,* E shaped; *stoma,* mouth]. An anastomosis between the ileum and sigmoid colon; used where most of the colon has to be removed.

لفائفی سینی تفویہ :سگمائڈ قولون اور ایلم کے درمیان اپریشن سے بنا ہوا۔
فسٹولا۔عموماً مصنوعی مقعد کی مستقل صورت۔

Ileostomy *(i-le-os'-to-mi)* [L. *ilia,* flanks; G. *stoma,* mouth]. A surgical made fistula between the ileum and the anterior abdominal wall; usually a permanent form of artificial anus when the whole of the large bowel has to be removed, e.g. in severe ulcerative colitis. **ileostomy bags,** rubber or plastic bags used to collect the liquid discharge from an ileostomy.

لفائفی تفویہ : امامی بطنی دیوار اور ایلم کے درمیان اپریشن سے بنا ہوا
فسٹولا۔عموماً مصنوعی مقعد کی مستقل صورت۔

Ileo-ureterostomy *(i-le-o-ur-et-er-os'-to-mi)* [L. *ilia,* flanks; G. *oureter,* ureter; *stoma,* mouth]. Treansplantation of the lower ends of the ureters from the bladder to an isolated loop of small bowel which in turn, is made to open on the abdominal wall. See BLADDER.

الیویوریٹروسٹومی :یوریٹرز کے ذریعہ سروں کی پیوندکاری۔

Ileum *(il'-e-um)* [L. *ilia,* flanks]. The lower three fifths of the small intestine, lying between the jejunum and the caecum--ileal, adj.

معالفائف۔پیچیدہ آنت : چھوٹی آنت کا نچلا ۳/۵ حصہ جو جیجونم اور
سیکم کی درمیان ہوتا ہے۔

Ileus *(il-e'-us)* [G. *eileos,* intestinal obstruction]. Intestineal obstruction. Usually restricted to paralytic as opposed to mechanical obstruction and characterized by abdominal distension. vomiting and the absence of pain. See MECONIUM.

معائی قولنج :آنت کی رکاوٹ۔

Ilococcygeal *(i-li-o-koks-ij'-e-al)* [L. *ilium,* flank; G. *kokkyx,* cuckoo]. Pertaining to the ilium and coccyx.

رقفی عصعصی :ایلم کا کاکس سے متعلق۔

Iliofemoral *(i-li-o-fem'-or-al)* [L. *ilium,* flank; *femur,* thigh].

رقفی خفذی :ایلم اور فیمر سے متعلق۔

Iliopectineal *(i-li-o-pek-tin'-e-al)* [L. *ilium,* flank; *pecton,* crest]. Pertaining to the ilium and the pubis.

رقفی اور مشطی :ایلم اور پیوبس سے متعلق۔

Iliopsoas *(i-il-o-so'-as)* [L. *ilium,* flank; G. *psoai,* loins]. Pertaining to the ilium and the loin.

ھلہ٬ حرقفی خصری :ایلم کمر سے متعلق۔

Ilium *(il'-i-um)* [L. flank]. The upper part of the innominate bone, a separate bone in the fetus. The flank--iliace, adj.

رقفہ۔نشتگاہ کی ہڈی۔پہلو :انامینیٹ ہڈی کا بالائی حصہ۔کولہے کی
ی یا ہپ بون کا بالائی چوڑا حصہ جو ایک طرف سیکرم سے جڑتا ہے۔

Illusion *(i-lu'-shun)* [L. *illusio-illudere,* to deceive]. A misidentification of a sensation e.g. of sight, a white sheet being mistaken for a ghost, the sheet being misrepresented in consciousness as a figure.

یب نظر۔التباس: کسی احساس کی غلط شناخت مثلاً سفید چادر کو بھوت
ھ لینا۔

Ilotycin *(i-lo-ti'-sin).* Erythromycin (q.v.).

ٹی سین : ارتھرومائی سین۔ارتھروسین۔ٹانسی لائی ٹس میں ایک گولی ہر
گھنٹے بعد۔

Image *(im'-aj)* [L. imago]. A revived experien

of a percept recalled from memory. (Small and taste).

خیال۔ذہنی تصویر :یادداشت سے کسی تجربے کو دیکھنا۔

magery *(im'-aj-er-i)* [L. imago, image] Imagination. The recall of mental images of various types depending upon the special sense organs involved when the images were found, e.g. **auditory i.,** motor i., visual i. (sight), tactile i. (touch), olfactory i.

متخیلہ۔سماں بندی : تخیل۔ذہنی تصورات۔

nbalance *(im-bal'-ans).* Want of balance. Term refers commonly to the upset of acid-base relationship and the elctrolytes in body fluids.

عدم توازن :توازن کی کمی۔

nferon *(im'-fer-on).* An iron-dextran complex for parental iron therapy. Used as a total dose infusion to obtain a rapid response in marked iron deficiency anaemia.

امفیرون :دروں عضلاتی ٹیکے کے لئے ڈیکسٹران اورلوہے کا کمپلکس۔

ipramine *(im-ip'-ra-men).* Antidepressant, anticholinergic, antihistaminic, anti-Parkinson and antiserotonin properties. Chemically related to chlorpromazine. Raises levels of serotonin and catecholamines in brain.

امپرامین :پریشانی ومایوسی کوختم کرنے والی دوا۔

mune *(i-mun')* [L. immunis, exempt from public burden]. Not susceptible to an infection. **immune body,** antibody. **immune reaction response,** that which causes a body o reject a transplanted organ, to respond to bacterial disease which develops slowly, and o act against malignant cells; cellular mmunity is the term used for these various eactions. This does not occur in hymectomized mice.

معنون :جسے کوئی بیماری نہ لگ سکے۔

nunity *(im-mun'-i-ti)* [L. *immunis,* exempt rom public burden]. A state of relative esistance to an infection. **cellular i.,** roduced by the T-lymphocytes (see IMMNE). **humoral i.,** from antibodies produced y B-lymphocytes. Immunity can be **innate** rom inherited qualities), or it can be acquired, actively or passively, naturally or artificially. **active i.** is acquired, naturally during an infectious disease or articficaclly by vaccination with dead or living organisms. **passive i.** is acquired, naturally when maternal antibody passes to the child via the placenta or in the milk, or artifically by administering imm- une sera containing antibody--obtained from animals or human beings.

قوتِ مدافعت۔مناعت :بیماری کے خلاف۔مدافعت کی حالت یہ توراثی یا اکتسابی ہوتا ہے۔جسم میں وائرس یا جراثیم کے خلاف قوتِ مدافعت پیدا ہوجاتی ہے۔ویکسین لگاکرقوت مدافعت پیدا کی جاتی ہے۔

Immunization *(im-mu-ni-za'-shun)* [L. *immunis,* exempt from public burden]. The process of increasing specific antibody in the tissues.

معنون سازی :بافتوں میں مخصوص اینٹی باڈی بڑھانے کے لئے۔

Immunogenesis *(im-mun-o-jen'-e-sis)* [L. *immunis,* exempt from public burden; G. genesis, descent]. The process of production of immunity--immunogenetic, adj.

امینوجینیسس :امیونٹی پیدا کرنے کا طریقہ۔

Immunogenicity *(im-mun-o-jen-is-i-ti).* The ability to produce immunity.

امینوجینی سٹی :امیونٹی پیدا کرنے کی صلاحیت۔

Immunoglobnlins *(im-mun-o-glob'-u-lins).* Syn., gamaglobulins (q.v.).

امینوگلوبولنز :گیماگلوبولنز۔

Immunology *(im-mun-ol'-oj-i).* The special study of immunity--immunological, adj.; immunologically, adv.

مناعیات :امیونٹی کامخصوص مطالعہ۔

Immunopathology *(im-mun-o-path-ol'-oj-i)* Abnormal immune reaction as when a person becomes sensitized.

امیونوپتھیالوجی :غیرنارمل امینوردعمل۔

Immunosensitivity *(im-mun-o-sen-sit-iv'-ti).* The state produced by immunopathology.

مزاحمتی حساسیت :امینوپتھیالوجی سے پیداشدہ صورت۔

Immunosuppressive *(im-mun-o-sup-res'-iv).* [L. *immunis,* exempt from public burden; *supprimere,* to press down]. That which prevents the occurence of an immune reaction (q.v.).

مزاحمتی روک : وہ جو کسی امیون ردعمل کے وقوع پذیر ہونے کو روکے۔

Immunotherapy *(im-mun-o-ther'-a-pi)*. Any treatment used to produce immunity.

مناعتی علاج : امیونٹی پیدا کرنے کے لئے استعمال ہونے والا کوئی طریقہ۔

Immunotransfusion *(im-mun-o-trans-fu'-zhun)* [L. *immunis,* exempt from public burden; *trransfundere,* to trasnfuse]. Transfusion of blood from a donor previously rendered immune by repeated inoculations with a given agent from the recipient.

اعفائی نقل الدم : امیون شخص سے خون کا انتقال۔

Impacted *(im-pak'-ted)* [L. *impactum,* from *impingere,* to strike against]. Firmly wedged, abnormal immobility, as of faeces in the rectum; fracture; a fetus in the pelvis; a tooth in its socket or a calculus in a duct.

متصادم : فریکچر۔ ساکٹ میں دانت۔ غیر معمولی طور پر غیر متحرک۔

Impalpable *(im-pal'-pa-bl)* [L. in, not; palpare, to feel]. Not palpable. Incapable of being felt by touch (palpation).

لمس ناپذیر : چھونے سے محسوس کرنے سے عاری۔

Imperforate *(im-per'-for-at)* [L. in, not; perforare, to bore through]. Lacking a normal opening. **imperforate anus,** absence of an opening into the rectum. **inperforate hymen,** a fold of mucous membrane at the vaginal entrance which has no natural outlet for the menstrual fluid.

بے سوراخ : نارمل سوراخ نہ ہونا۔

Impatigo *(im-pet-i'-go)* [L.]. An inflammatory, pustular, skin disease usually caused by staphylococcus, occasionally by Strept- ococcus. **impetigo contagiosa,** a highly contagious form of impetigo, commonest on the face and scalp, characterized by bullae which become pustules and then honey-coloured crusts. See ECTHYMA-- impetiginous, adj.

زرد زخم : ایک جلدی مرض۔ جراثیمی مرض۔ جلد سرخ و متورم ہو کر چھوٹے چھالے بنتے ہیں جن سے پانی بہتا ہے۔

Implantation *(im-plan; ta'-shun)* [L. in, into; plantare, to plant]. The insertion of livin[g] cells or solid materials into the tissues, e.g accidental implantation of tumour cells in wound; implanation or radium or solid drugs.

خال : بافتوں میں جاندار خلیے یا ٹھوس مادے لگانا۔

Implants *(im'-plantz)* [L. *in,* in; *planta,* sprout Tissues or drugs inserted surgically into th human body, e.g. implantation of pellets testosterone under the skin in treatment carcinoma of the breast, implantation deoxycortone acetate (DOÇAS) in Addison disease.

صبیہ : انسانی جسم میں بذریعہ اپریشن بافتیں یا ادویات رکھنا۔

Impotent *(im'-po-tent)* [L. impotentia, inability By custom referring to the male. Absence sexual power.

د : عام طور پر نر کے لئے مستعمل جنسی قوت کی غیر موجودگی، قوتِ مردی کی
ور، عضو تناسل یا خصیتین میں پیدائشی نقص، کثرت، مباشرت، حلق یا اغلام
عادت یا عرصہ تک جریان منی اور کثرتِ احتلام کی وجہ سے ہوتا ہے۔

Impregnate *(im'-preg-nat)* [L. *in,* in; *prae nans,* pregnant]. Fill. Saturate, Render p gnant.

ہ : بھرا ہوا۔ سیر شدہ۔ حاملہ کرنا۔

Impulse *(im'-puls)* [L. *impulsus,* striki against]. 1. The tendency to act without del eration. 2. A sudden push or communica force.

ن۔ ترنگ۔ ضرب : (۱) سوچے سمجھے بغیر کام کرنے کا رجحان۔
چانک دھکیلنا۔

Imuran. Azathioprine (q.v.).

ران : امیونٹی کم کرنے والی دوا۔

Inaccessibility *(in-ak-ses-ib-il'-i-ti)*. In ps hiatry denotes absence of patient response.

ل رسائی : مریض کے ردعمل کی غیر موجودگی۔

Inassimilable *(in-as-sim'-a-bl)* [L. *in, carcer,* prison]. The abnormal imprisonn of a part, as in a hernia which is irreduci and a pregnant uterus held between the sa promontory.

ل پذیر: انجذاب کے ناقابل۔

Incarcerated *(in-kar'-se-ra-ted)* [L. in carcer, prison]. The abnormal imprison of a part, as in a hernia which is irreducible, and a pregnant uterus held beneath the sacral promontory.

مقید : کسی حصے کا غیر معمولی طور پر مقید ہوجانا۔ مثلاً ہرنیا' حاملہ یورٹرس۔

Incest *(in'-sest)* [L. *incestus,* unchaste]. Sexual intercourse between near kindred, whose marriage is prohibited by law.

حرمت : قریبی رشتہ دار جن کی شادی قانوناً نہیں ہوسکتی ان کا جنسی ملاپ۔

Incipient *(in-sip'-i-ent)* [L. incipere, to begin]. Initial, beginning, in early stages.

ابتدائی : ابتدائی یا اولی مرحلوں میں۔

Incision *(in-sizh'-un)* [L. *incisio,* cut]. Cutting into body tissue, using a sharp instrument--incise, v.t.; incisional, adj.

قطع۔شگاف : تیز آلہ استعمال کرتے ہوئے جسمانی نسیج کو کاٹنا۔

Incisors *(in-si'-sorz)* [L. *incisus,* cut into]. The eight front cutting teeth, four in each jaw.

قاطع دانت : آٹھ آگے والے قاطع دانت۔ ہر جبڑے میں چار۔

Inclusion bodies *(in-klu'-zhun bod'-iz).* Minute particles found in the cells of affected tissues.

دخیل اجسام : متاثرہ بافتوں کی خلیوں میں پائے جانے والے باریک ذرات۔

Incompatibility *(in-kom-pat-ib-il'-it-i)* [L. *in,* not; *compatibilis,* compatible]. Usually refers to the bloods of donor and recipient in transfusion, when antigenic differences in the red cells result in reactions such as haemolysis or agglutination. When two or more medicaments are given concurrently or consecutively they can attenuate, counteract or even potentiate the desired result of one another.

تضاد۔تناقض : یہ اصطلاح عموماً انتقال خون میں خون دیتے اور خون لینے والے سے متعلق استعمال ہوتی ہے۔ اگر ان کے سرخ خلیوں کے اینٹی منی ایک جیسے نہ ہوں تو ردعمل ہوگا۔

Incompetence *(in-kom'-pe-tens)* [L. *incompetens,* insufficient]. Inadequacy to perform a natural function, e.g. mitral incompetence--incompetent, adj.

نااہلی : قدرتی عمل کی ادائیگی کے لئے غیر موزونیت۔

Incontinence *(in-kon'-tin-ens)* [L. *incontinentia,* inability to retain]. Inability to control the evacuation of urine or faeces. **overflow i.,** dribbing of urine from an overfull bladder. **stress i.,** occurs when the intra-abdominal pressure is raised as in coughing and sneezing; there is usually some weakness of the urethral sphincter muscle coupled with anatomical stretching and displacement of the bladder neck.

ضعف ضبط : فضلے یا پیشاب کے اخراج کو کنٹرول کرنے کی نااہلیت۔ حرقتہ البول۔ تقطیر البول پیشاب کا قطرہ قطرہ آنا۔ پیشاب سرخ یا زردی مائل بہ سرخی اور جلن کے ساتھ آتا ہے۔ پیشاب کے کرنے کے بعد قطرہ قطرہ دیر تک ٹپکتا ہے مریض کو ایسا معلوم ہوتا ہے گویا ابھی مثانہ میں پیشاب باقی ہے۔

Incoordination *(in-ko-or-din-a'-shun).* [L. *in,* not; *cum,* together; *ordinare,* to regulate]. Inability to produce smooth, harmonious muscular movements.

عدم ارتباط : یکساں عضلاتی حرکات پیدا کرنے کی نااہلیت۔

Incubation *(in-ku-ba'-shun)* [L. *incubare,* to hatch]. The period from entry of infection to the appearance of the first symptom.

اخفائے مرض : مرض کی ابتداء سے پہلی علامت کے ظہور تک کا عرصہ۔

Incubator *(in'-ku-ba-tor)* [L. *incubare,* to hatch]. A temperature-regulated apparatus in which premature or delicate babies can be reared, or bacteria cultured.

انکوبیٹر۔جراثیم زا مشین : ایک بکس جو اس طرح تیار کیا جاتا ہے کہ تھرموسٹیٹ کے ذریعے اندرونی درجہ حرارت مستقل رہے۔ اس میں جراثیم کو کلچر کیا جاتا ہے یا قبل از وقت پیدا ہونے والے بچوں کو رکھا جاتا ہے۔

Indema *(in'-de-ma).* Phenindione (q.v.).

Inderal *(in'der-al).* Propranolol (q.v.).

انڈرال : پروپرینول۔ آئی۔ سی۔ آئی کمپنی کی تیار کردہ گولیاں۔ وجع القلب اور قلبی بے قاعدگیوں میں مفید۔

Indian hemp Cannabis indica (q.v.). Hashish.

ہنڈی بھنگ۔گانجا : حشیش۔ بھنگ کا پودا۔

Indicanuria *(in-di-kan-u'-ri-a).* Excessive potassium salt (indican) in the urine. Traces in normal urine. See INDOLE.

نیلی بولی : پیشاب میں زائد پوٹاشیم نمک۔

Indicator *(in'-dik-a-tor)* A substance used to make visible the completion of a chemical reaction.

کاشفہ : ایک شے جو کیمیائی تعامل کی تکمیل کو مرئی بنانے کے لئے استعمال

کی جاتی ہے۔

Indigenous *(in-dij'-e-nus)* [L. *indigena,* a native]. Native to a certain locality or country, e.g. Derbyshire neck (simple colloidal goitre).

ملکی۔دیسی : کسی خاص جگہ یا ملک کا رہنے والا۔

Indigestion *(in-di-jes'-chun).* Dyspepsia.

بدہضمی : ڈسپیپسا۔

Indigestion *(in-dig-o-kar'-min).* A dye used as an 0.4 percent solution for testing renal function. Given by intravenous or intramuscular injection. The urine is coloured blue in about 10 min if kidney function is normal.

انڈیگوکارمین : ایک رنگ جو بولی فعل کی جانچ کے لئے بطور ۰٫۴ فیصد محلول استعمال کیا جاتا ہے۔ یہ ٹیکے کے ذریعے دیا جاتا ہے۔ اگر گردے صحیح کام کر رہے ہوں تو پیشاب کا رنگ قریباً دس منٹ میں نیلا ہو جاتا ہے۔

Indocid *(in'-do-sid).* Indomethacin (q.v.).

انڈوسڈ : انڈومتھاسن چائے والا چمچ دن میں ۳ مرتبہ نصف گلاس پانی میں گھول کر کھانے سے پہلے برائے اکیوٹ گوؤٹ یا نقرس۔ جوڑوں کے درد میں مفید اینٹی ریومیٹک۔

Indol *(e) (in'-dol).* A product of intestinal putrefaction: it is oxidized to indoxyl in the liver and excreted in urine as indican. See INDICANURIA.

انڈول ای : انتڑیوں میں گلنے سے حاصل ہوتا ہے۔

Indolent *(in'-do-lent)* [L. *in,* not; *dolere,* to feel pain]. A term applied to a sluggish ulcer which is generally painless and slow to heal.

بے حسی۔کاہلی : السر جس میں درد نہ ہو اور جلد ٹھیک۔

Indometha-cin *(in-do-meth'-a-sin).* An analgesic with anti-inflammatory properties. Useful in the rheumatic disorders. Can be given orally and by suppository.

انڈمیتھاسین : جوڑوں کے درد میں مفید۔ انڈوسنا۔ مفید برائے اکیوٹ گوؤٹ یا نقرس۔

Induction *(in-duk'-shun)* [L. *inducere,* to lead into]. The act of bringing on or causing to occur, as applied to anaesthesia and labour.

استقراء : واقع ہونے کا عمل جیسے دردزہ یا بے ہوش کرنا۔

Industrial disease A disease contracted by reason of occupational exposure to an industrial agent known to be hazardous, e.g. dust, fumes, chemicals, irradiation, etc., the notif ication of, safety precautions against and co mpensation for which are controlled by law Syn., occupational disease. See DERMATIT IS.

صنعتی مرض : گرد، دھواں، تابکاری وغیرہ سے مرض۔

Industrial therapy Current organization o outside industrial working conditions within a unit in a psychiatric hospital. The main purp ose is preparation of patients for their retur to the working community.

انڈسٹریل تھراپی : مریضوں کو صحت یابی کے بعد کام کرنے کے قابل بنانا۔

Induration *(in-du-ra'-shun)* [L. *indurare,* t harden]. The hardening of tissues as in hyp eraemia, infiltration by neoplasm, etc.--in durated, adj.

صلب : تشنج کا سخت ہونا۔

Inertia *(in-er'-shi-a)* [L. inactivity]. Inactivity **uterine i.,** lack of contraction of parturien uterus. It may be primary due to constitutiona weakness; secondary due to exhaustion fro frequent and forcible contractions.

جمود : غیر عاملیت۔

In extremis *(in-eks-tre'-mis)* [L.]. At the poi of death.

حالتِ نزع : موت کے کنارے پر۔قریب المرگ۔

Infant *(in'-fant)* [L. *infans,* without speech]. A baby or a child of less than 1 year old.

نابالغ۔ننھا شیر خوار : ایک سال سے کم عمر کا بچہ۔ قانون میں اکیس سال سے کم عمر شخص۔

Infantile paralysis See POLIOMYELITIS.

فالج الاطفال : پولیو۔

Infantilism *(in-fant'il-izm)* [L. *infantilis,* of in ants]. General retardation of developme with persistence of childish characteristi into adolescence and adult life.

طفلیت : سن بلوغت میں بچگانہ خصوصیات۔ تکمیل میں عام کمی۔

Infarct *(in'-far-kt)* [L. *infarcire,* to stuff into Area of tissue affected, when end artery su plying it is occluded, e.g. in kidney or hea Common complication of subacute end carditis.

مفصمہ : متاثر نسیج کا ایریا۔

Infarction *(in-fark'-shun)* [L. *infarcire,* to stuff into]. Death of a section of tissue because the blood supply has been cut off.

انسداد : خون کی سپلائی بند ہونے سے نسیج کے ایک حصے کی موت۔

Infection *(in-fek'-shun)* [L. *infectio,* infection]. The successful invasion, establishment and growth of micro-organisms in the tissues of the host.

چھوت ۔ بیماری کا حملہ ۔ سمیت : میزبان کی بافتوں میں خوردجسیموں کا کامیاب حملہ ۔ قیام اور نشوونما۔

Infectious disease *(in-fek'-shus diz-ez')* A disease caused by a specific, pathogenic organism and capable of being transmitted to another individual by direct or indirect contact. 'Fevers.'

چھوت کی بیماری ۔ متعدی مرض : بیماری جو مخصوص جسمے سے ہوتی ہے اور ایک دوسرے کو لگتی ہے۔

Infectious monoucleosis *(in-fek'-shus mon-o-nu- kle-o'-sis)* [L. *infectio,* infection; G *monos,* one; L. *nucleus,* kernel; G-osis, condition]. Most common cause of the glandular fever syndrome (q.v.). Infecting agent is the Epstein-Barr virus. Most primary infections occur in childhood and in early a dolescence and may be symptomless, but 60 per-cent manifest the glandular fever syndrome. As well as production of specific antibodies to EBV in infectious mononucleosis there is an abnormal antibody which has 'heterophile' activity directed against sheeps red blood cells--the basis of the Paul-Bunnell test (q.v.). which is positive in IM. One attack confers complete immunity and also lifelong harbouring of the virus in the body--as viral particles in saliva (hence the synonym 'kissing disease') and in the lymphocytes.

Infective *(in-fek'-tiv).* Infectious. Disease transmissible from one host to another. infective **hepa titis,** see HEPATITIS.

متعدی : چھوت کی بیماری جو ایک میزبان سے دوسرے میں منتقل ہوتی ہے۔

Inferior *(in-fer'-i-or)* [L.]. Lower, beneath.

اسفل : کمتر ۔ نیچے۔

Inferiority complex. Term first used by A dler to describe a complex (q.v.) arising from conflict between fear a nd wish for recognition which results often in compensatory or a aggresive behaviour.

احساس کمتری : کمپلکس جو خوف اور خواہش کے درمیان چپقلش سے ابھرتا ہے۔

Infertility *(in-fer-til'-i-ti)* [L. *infertilis,* unfruitful]. Lack of ability to reproduce. Psychological and physical causes play their part. The abnormality can be in the husband and/or wife.Special clinics exist to investigate this condition.

بانجھ پن : تولیدی اہلیت کی کمی۔

Infestation *(in-fes-ta'-shun)* [L. *infestare,* to infest]. The presence of animal parasites in or on the human body--infest, v.t.

ابتلاء : انسانی جسم میں یا پر حیوانی طفیلیوں کی موجودگی۔

Infiltration *(in-fil-tra'-shun).* Penetration of the surrounding tissues; the oozing or leaking of fluid into the tissues. **Infiltration anaesthesia,** analgesia produced by infiltrating the tissues with a local anaesthetic.

سرایت : گردوالی بافتوں کی دخل اندازی ۔ بافتوں میں سیال جانا۔

Inflammation *(in-flam-ma'-shun)* [L. *inflammare,* to set on fire]. The reaction of living tissues to injury, infection, orirrita tion; characterized by pain, swelling, redness and heat--inflammatory, adj.

سوزش : زندہ بافتوں کا زخم ۔ بیماری وغیرہ کی لئے ردعمل جو صحت کے لئے ضروری ہے ۔ اس جگہ ضروری ورم گرمی اور درد ہوسکتا ہے یا عضو کا فعل معطل ہو جاتا ہے۔

Influenza *(in-floo-en'-za)* [It. influence]. An acute viral infection of the nasopharynx and respiratory tract which occurs in epidemic or pandemic form--influenzal, adj.

انفلوئنزا ۔ وبائی زکام : وائرس کی بیماری جو نیزوفیرنکس اور تنفسی راہ کو متاثر کرتی ہے۔

Infrared rays, Long, invisible rays of the spectrum. Used therapeutically for the production of heat in the tissues.

زیرسرخ شعاعیں : طیف کی طویل۔ غیر مرئی اشیاء۔ بافتوں میں حرارت پیدا کرنے کے لئے استعمال کی جاتی ہے۔

Infundibulum *(in-fun-dib'-u-lum)* [L.]. Any funnel-shaped passage--infundibular, adj.; infundibula, pl.

قیفی ساخت۔قیف : کوئی قیف نما راستہ۔

Infusion *(in-fu'-zhun)* [L. *infundere,* to pour into]. 1. Fluid flowing by gravity into the body. 2. An aqueous solution containing the active principle of a drug, made by pouring boiling water on the crude drug. 3. **Amniotic fluid i.** (q.v.).

القاء۔نقاعت :(۱) سیال کا کشش ثقل سے جسم میں بہنا۔(۲) ایک آبی محلول۔(۳) امنیاٹک سیال۔

Ingestion *(in-jest'-chun)* [L. *ingestio,* from *ingerere,* to put into]. The act of taking food or medicine into the stomach.

ادخال : خوراک یادوا کو معدہ میں لے جانا کا عمل۔

Ingrowing toenail Spreading of the nail into the lateral tissue, causing inflammation.

لحمی
درجی ناخن : جانبی نسیج میں ناخن کا پھیلنا۔جس سے سوزش ہوتی ہے۔

Inguinal *(ing'-gwin-al)* [L. *inguen,* groin]. Pertaining to the groin. **inguinal cana l,** a tubular opening through the lower part of the anterior abdominal wall, parallel to and a little above the i. (Poupart's) liga ment. It measures 38.0 mm. In the male it contains the spermatic cord; in the fema le the uterine round ligaments. **inguinal hernia,** one occurring through the internal abdominal ring of the i. canal.

اربی۔جڈے کا : پیغول سے متعلق۔

Inhalation *(in-hal-a '-shun)* [L. *in,* in; *halare,* brea the]. 1. The breathing in of air, or other vapour, etc. 2. A medicinal substance which is inhaled.

بھپارہ۔لخلخہ : (۱) ہوا یا دوسرے بخارات کو سانس کے ذریعے اندر لے جانا۔(۲) ایک ادویاتی مادہ جسے سانس کے ذریعے اندر لے جاتے ہیں۔

Inherent *(in-he'-rent)* [L. *inhoerere,* to adhere to]. Innate; inborn.

جبلی : پیدائشی۔وراثت میں حاصل کردہ۔

Inhibition *(in-hib-i'-shun)* [L. *inhibere,* to restrain]. Loss or partial loss of function either mental or physical as a result of mental (psychic) influences.

امتناع۔رکاوٹ : عمل کا مکمل یا جزوی ضیاع جو ذہنی یا جسمانی ہو۔ یہ ذہنی یا نفسی اثرات کی وجہ سے ہوتا ہے۔

Injected *(in-jek'-ted)* Congested, with full vessels.

پر : بھری ہوئی رگوں کے ساتھ بہت زیادہ ہونا۔

Injection *(in-jek'-shun)* [L. *injectio*]. 1.The ac of introducing a fluid (under pressure) int the tissues, a vessel, cavity or hollow organ (Air can be injected into cavity. See PNEU MOTHORAX.) 2. The substance injected See HYPODERMIC. INTRA -ARTERIAL INTRACUTANEOUS, INTRADERMAL INTRAMUSCULAR, INTRATHECAL INTRAVASCULAR, INTRAVENOUS SUBCUTANEOUS.

کا۔انجکشن : (۱) سیال کو بافتوں۔رگ۔کہفہ یا کھوکھلے عضو میں داخل کرنے کا عمل۔زیر جلد، عضلاتی یا وریدی (۲) اندر داخل ہونے والا مادہ۔

Innate *(in-at)* [L. innatus, born]. Inborn dependent on genetic constitution.

طری : جینز پر منحصر۔پیدائشی۔

Innervation *(in-ner-va'-shun)* [L. *in,* in; ders Can be given orally and by suppository.

تقویت اعصاب : کسی حصے کو عصب کی سپلائی۔

Innocent *(in'-no-sent)* [L. *in,* not; *nocere,* t harm]. Benign; not malignant.

لیم : بداندیش نہ ہونا۔

Innocuous *(in-ok'-u-us)* [L. *innocuus,* harmless Harmless.

بے ضرر : بے ضرر۔جس سے نقصان نہ ہو۔

Innominate *(in-non'-in-at)* [L. *innominat*]. Ur named.

بے نام۔لااسمی : بغیر نام کے۔

Inoculation *(in-ok-u-la'-shun)* [L. *inocular* engraft]. Introduction of material (usuall vaccine). into the tissues. Introduction micro-organisms into culture medium fc propagation. Mode of entry of bacteria int body.

ٹا : بافتوں میں مادہ۔عموماً 'ویکسین' کا دخول۔پھیلاؤ کے لئے کلچر میڈیم میں خوردجسموں کا دخول۔

Inorganic *(in-or-gan'-ik)* Neither animal n vegetable in origin.

غیرعضوی۔غیرنامیاتی : جس کی اصل حیوانی یا نباتی نہ ہو۔

nosital *(in-os'-it-ol).* A member of the vitamin B_2 complex.

حیاتیہ : وٹامن بی۲ کمپلکس کا ایک رکن۔

notropic *(i-no-tro'-pik)* Having an effect on the contractility of muscles.

notropic agents Currently being used in a three-year study of left ventricular function during and after open- heart surgery.

quest *(in;qwest).* A legal enquiry, held by a coroner, into the cause of suddent or unexpected death.

تفتیش : اچانک موت کی وجہ معلوم کرنے کے لئے قانونی انکوائری۔

nsecticide *(in-sek'-ti-sid)* [L. *insectum,* cut into; *coedere,* to kill]. An agent which kills insects-- insecticidal. adj.

حشرات کش : حشرات کو مارنے والا عامل۔

nsemination *(in-sem-in-a'-shun)* [L. *inseminare,* to implant]. Introduction of semen into the vagina, normally by sexual intercourse. **artificial i.,** instrumental injection of semen into the vagina. See AID and AIH.

تخم ریزی : عموماً جنسی ملاپ کے ذریعے منوی مادے کا ویجائنا میں دخول۔

nsensible *(in-sens'-i-bl)* [L. *insensibilitis*]. Without sensation or consciousness. Too small or gradual to be perceived, as i. perspiration (q.v.).

بے ہوش۔ بے حس : ہوش کے بغیر۔

nsertion *(in-ser'-shun)* [L. *inserere,* to graft into]. The act of setting or placing in. The attachment of a muscle to the bone it moves.

اندغام: کسی شے کو اندر رکھنے کا عمل۔ عضلے کا اس ہڈی کے ساتھ الحاق جسے وہ حرکت دیتا ہے۔

nsidious *(in-sid'-i-us)* [L. *insidiosus,* cunning]. Having an imperceptible commencement, as of a disease with a late manifestation of definite symptoms.

غافل گیر : غیر محسوس طور پر واقع ہونا۔

nsight *(in'-sit).* Ability to accept one's limitations but at the same time to develop one's potentialities. In psychiatry means; (1) knowing that one is ill; (2) a developing knowledge of one's present attitudes and past experiences and the connection between them.

بصیرت : کسی کی مجبوری کو قبول کرنے کی اہلیت لیکن اس کی صلاحیتوں کو ترقی دینا۔

In situ *(in-sit'-u)* [L.]. In the correct position; undisturbed.

برمحل : صحیح حالت میں۔ ڈسٹرب کئے بغیر۔

Insomnia *(in-som'-ni-a)* [L.]. Sleeplessness.

بے خوابی : بے خوابی کی حالت۔

Inspiration *(in-spi-ra'-shun)* . The drawing of air into the lungs; inhalation--inspire, v.t.; inspiratory, adj.

دم درکشی : پھیپھڑوں میں ہوا کھینچنا۔ اندر کی طرف سانس لینا۔

Inspissated *(in'-spis-a'-ted)* [L. *in,* in; *spissare,* to thicken]. Thickened, as by evaporation or withdrawal of water applied to sputum and culture media used in the laboratory.

گاڑھا : گاڑھا کیا ہوا۔ پانی نکال کر یا بخارات سے پانی کو اڑا کر گاڑھا کیا ہوا۔

Instep *(in'-step).* The arch of the foot on the dorsal surface.

پشتِ پا : بطنی سطح پر پاؤں کی محراب۔

Instillation *(in-stil-a '-shun)* [L. *instillare,* to pour in drop by drop]. Insertion of drops into a cavity, e.g. conjunctival sae, external auditory meatus.

تلقین۔ اقطار: کسی کہفہ میں قطروں کا دخول۔

Instinct *(in'-stingkt)* [L. *instinctus,* incite]. An inborn tendency to act in a certain way in a given situation, e.g. **paternal i.,** to protect children-- instinctive, adj.; instinctively, adv.

وجدان۔ جبلت : کسی دی گئی صورت حال میں کسی طریقے سے عمل کرنے کا پیدائشی رجحان۔

Insufflation *(in-suf-fla'-shun)* [L. *insufflare,* to breathe out]. The blowing of air along a tube (Eustachian, Fallopian) to establish patency. The blowing of powder into a body cavity.

تنفس مصنوعی : جسمانی کہفہ میں سفوف کو پھونک کر داخل کرنا کسی نلی میں ہوا داخل کرنا۔

Insulin *(in'-su-lin).* A pancreatic hormone, made in the islet cells of Langer-hans, secreted into the blood, and having a profound influence on carbohydrate metabolism by stimulating the transport of glucose into cells. The hormone is prepared commercially in various forms a nd strengths which vary in their speed, length and potency of action and which a re used in the treatment of diabetes mellitus (q.v.).

انسولین: ایک ہارمون جو لبلبہ میں پیدا ہوتا ہے اور جسمانی شکر کو کنٹرول کرتا

ہے۔جسم میں داخل کرنے سے خون میں شکر کی مقدار کو کم کرتا ہے اور اس طرح ذیابیطس کو آرام پہنچاتا ہے۔ یہ ایک پروٹین ہے۔ یہ ہارمون لینگر ہارموز کے آئیلیٹ خلیوں میں بنتا ہے اور خارج خون ہوتا ہے۔

Insulinase *(in'-su-lin-az)*. An enzyme that inactivates insulin. **insulina se antagonists and inhibitors,** growth hormone, cortisol, glucagon, thyroxine and adrenaline.

انسولی نیز : ایک خامرہ جوانسولین کے اثر کو ختم کرتا ہے۔

Insulinoma *(in-su-lin-o'-ma)*. Adenoma of the islets of Langerhans in the pancreas. Also insuloma.

انسولی نوما : لبلبہ میں آئیلیٹس آف لینگر ہانز کا ایڈینوما اسے انسولوما بھی کہتے ہیں۔

Intal *(in'-tal)*. Disodium cromogycate (q.v.).

انٹیل ڈائی : سوڈیم کروموگلائیکیٹ۔

Integrin *(in-teg'-rin)*. Oxypertine (q.v.).

Integument *(in-teg'-u-ment)* [L.]. A covering, especially the skin.

غلاف جلد : باہر کا غلاف۔خصوصاً جلد۔

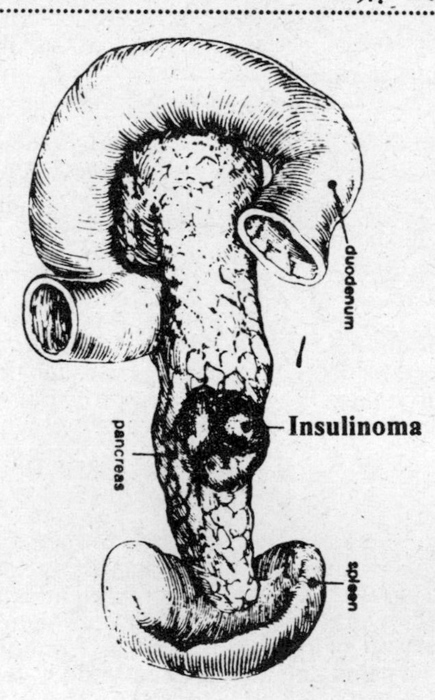

Intellect *(in-te-lekt)* [L. *intellectus,* understanding]. Reasoning power, thinking faculty.

فہم۔عقل : دلیل دینے کی طاقت۔

Intelligence *(in-tel'-i-jens)* [L. *intelligentia]* Inborn mental ability **intelligence tests,** designed to determine the level of intelligence. **intelligence quotient,**or **1Q**. the ratio of mental age to chronological (acute) age.

ذہانت : پیدائشی ذہنی قابلیت۔

Interarticular *(in-ter-ar-tik'-u-lar)* [L. *inter,* between; *articulus,* joint]. Between the articulating surfaces of a joint.

بین مفصلی : جوڑ کی گھومنے والی سطوح کے درمیان۔

Interatrial *(in-ter-a'-tri-al)* [L. *inter,* between *atrium,* ha!l]. Between the two atria of the heart. Previously interauricular.

بین الماتی : دل کے دوایٹریا کے درمیان سابقہ انٹرآریکولر۔

Interauricular *(in-ter-awr-ik'-u-lar)*. See INTERA-TRIAL.

بین اذینی : انٹرایٹریل۔دل کے دوا ایٹریا کے درمیان۔

Intercellular *(in-ter-sel'-u-lar)* [L. *inter,* between; *cellula,* little cell]. Between the cells of a structure.

بین خلوی : ساخت کے خلیوں کے درمیان۔

Intercostal *(in-ter-kos-tal)* [L. *inter,* between *costa,* rib]. Between the ribs.

بین الاضلاعی : پسلیوں کے درمیان۔

Intercourse *(in'-ter-kors)* [L. *inter,* between *currere,* to run]. A second disease arising in a person already suffering from one disease.

اختلاط۔میل جول : رابطہ۔ملاپ۔محبت۔

Intercurrent *(in-ter-kur-ent)* [L. *inter* between *currere,* torun]. A second disease arising in a person already suffering from one disease.

عارضہ : ایسے شخص میں دوسری بیماری پیدا ہونا جو پہلے ہی ایک مرض کا شکار ہو۔

Interferon *(in-ter-fe'-ron)* [L. *inter,* between *ferire,* to strike]. A protein effective against most viruses. When a virus infects a cell, it triggers off the cell's production of i. This then interacts with surrounding cells and renders them resistant to virus attack

Available only in very limited amounts for clinical use as bulk production in the laboratory is difficult and expensive.

انٹرفیران : خلیے میں وائرسوں کی موجودگی کے نتیجے میں کئی حیوانی خلیوں میں پیدا ہونے والی پروٹین یہ ان وائرسوں کے خلاف حفاظت کرتی ہے۔

Interlobar *(in-ter-lo'-bar)* [L. *inter*, between; *lobos*, lobe]. Between the lobes, e.g. interlobar pleurisy.

بین لختی : لوبوں کے درمیان۔

Interlobular *(in-ter-lob'-u-lar)* [L. *inter*, between; *lobulus*, small lobe]. Between the lobules.

بین لخیخی : لوبیلز کے درمیان۔ مثلاً پھیپھڑے یا جگر کے بیچ میں۔

Intermenstrual *(in-ter-men'-stru-al)* [L. *inter*, between; *menstrualis*, monthly]. Between the menstrual periods.

بین طمثین : حیضوں کے درمیان۔

Intermittent *(in-ter-mit'-ent)* [L. *inter-mettere*, to leave off]. Occuring at intervals.

وقفہ دار : وقفوں کے ساتھ واقع ہونا۔ باری کا بخار۔

Internal *(in-ter'-nal)* [L. *internus*]. Inside, **internal ear**, that part of the ear which comprises the vestibule, semicircular canals and the cochlea. **internal secretions,** those produced by the ductless of endocrine glands and passed directly into the blood stream; hormones.

اندرونی : اندر۔ اندر کی طرف۔

Interosseous *(in-ter-os'-e-us)* [L. *inter* between; *os*, bone]. Between bones.

بین عظمی : ہڈیوں کے درمیان۔

Interphalangeal *(in-ter-fal-an'-je-al)*. Between the phalanges.

بین سلامی : پوروں کی ہڈیوں کے درمیان۔

Interposition operation Vein graft to eardrum.

تداخلی اپریشن : کان کے پردے کے ساتھ ورید کا پیوند۔

Interserosal *(in-ter-se-ros'-al)* [L. *inter*, between; *serum*, whey]. Between serous membrane as in the pleural, peritoneal and pericardial cavities-- interserosally, adv.

انٹرسیروسیل : سیرس جھلی کے درمیان۔

Intersexuality *(in-ter-seks-u-al'-i-ti)* [L. *inter*, between; *sexus*, sex]. The possession of both male and femal characteristics. See TURNER'S and KLINEFELTER'S SYNDROME.

دوجنسی : نر اور مادہ دونوں خصوصیات ہونا۔

Interspinous *(in-ter-spi-nus)* [L. *inter*, between; *spina*, thorn]. Between spinous processes, especially those of the vertebrae.

بین شوکی : سپائن کے زائدوں کے درمیان، خصوصاً مہروں کے زائدوں کی درمیان۔

Interstices *(in-ter'-sti-sez)* [L. *interstitium*, a place between]. Spaces.

خلو: جگہیں۔

Interstitial *(in-ter-stish'-al)* Situated in the interstices of a part; distributed through the connective structures.

جگہیں شگافی : کسی حصے کی جگہوں میں واقع۔

Intertrigo *(in-ter-tri'-go)* [L. *inter*, between; *terere*, to rub]. Superficial inflammation occurring in moist skin folds--intertrigenous, adj.

تشمیط : نمدار جلدی تہوں میں واقع سطحی سوزش۔

Intertrochanteric *(in-ter-tro-kan'-ter-ik)* [L. *inter*, between; G. *trochanter*]. Between trochanters.

بین طرونی۔ بین الطروفاء : طروفا کے درمیان۔

Intervantricular *(in-ter-ven-trik'-u-lar)* [L. *inter*, between; *ventricula*, small cavity]. Between ventricles, as those of the brain or heart.

درمیانی دیوار : بطینوں کے درمیان جیسے دل اور دماغ کے۔

Intervertebral *(in-ter-ver'-ti-bral)* [L. *inter*, between; *vertebra*]. Between the vertebrae, as discs and formaina. See NUCLEUS. PROLAPSE.

بین فقراتی : مہروں کے درمیان۔

Intima *(in'-tim-a)* [L. *intimus*, innermost]. *The internal coat of a blood vessel--intimal, adj.*

استرجھلی : خونی رگ کا اندرونی کوٹ۔

Intocostrin. A curare muscle relaxant. See MUSCLE.

انٹوکاسٹرن : عضلے کو سکون پہنچانے والا۔

Intolerance *(in-tol'-e-rans)* [L. *intolerans*]. Inability to bear pain or discomfort. Idiosyncrasy (q.v.) to certain drugs, etc.

نارواداری : درد برداشت کرنے کی نااہلیت۔

Intra-abdominaol *(in-tra-ab-dom'-in-al)* [L. *intra,* within; *a bdomen,* belly]. Inside the abdomen.

درون شکمی بطن کے اندر۔

Intra-amniotic *(in-tra-am-ni-ot'-ik)* [L. *intra,* within ; G. *amnio,* fetal membrane]. Within , or into the amniotic fluid.

انٹراامنیاٹک: امیناٹک سیال میں۔

Intra-arterial *(in-tra-art-er-i-al)* [L. *intra,* within; G. *arteria,* artery]. Within an artery--intra- arterially,adv.

درون شریانی: شریان میں۔

Intra-articular *(in-tra-art-ik'-u-lar)* [L. *intra,* within; *articulus,* joint]. Within a joint.

دروں مفصلی :

Intrabronchial *(in-tra-brong'-ki-al)* [L. *intra,* within; G. *brogchos,* windpipe]. Within a bronchus.

دروں شعبی : ہوا کی نالی کے اندر۔

Intradural *(in-tra-du'-ral)* [L. *intra,* within; dura *mater,* hard mother]. Inside the dura mater.

Intracanalicular *(in-tra-kan-al'-ik'-u-lar)* [L. *intra,* within, *canaliculus,* a small channel]. Within a canaliculus.

دروں قنالچی: قنالچہ کے اندر۔

Intracpillary *(in-tra-kap'-il'-a-ri)* [L. *intra,* within; *capillus,* hair]. Within a capillary.

انٹراکیپلری : نس کے اندر۔

Intracapsular *(in-tra-kap'-su-lar)* [L. *intra,* within; *capsula,* small box]. Within a capsule, e.g. tha t of the lens or a joint. Opp. extracapsular.

درون کیسوری: کیپسول کے اندر۔

Intracardiac *(in-tra-kar'-di-ak)* [L. *intra,* within; *kardia,* heart]. Within the heart.

درون قلبی : دل کے اندر۔

Intracaval *(in-tra-ka'-val)*. Within the vena cava, by custom referring to the inferior one--intracavally, adv.

انٹراکیول : وینا کیوا کے اندر۔

Intracerebral *(intra-sel'-u-lar)* [L. *intra,* within *cellula,* small cell]. Within a cell. Opp. extr acellular.

رون خلوی :خلیے کے اندر۔

Intracellular *(intra-sel'-u-lar)* [L. *intra,* within *cerebrum,* brain]. Within the cerebrum.

رون دماغی : سربرم کے اندر۔

Intracorpuscular *(in-tra-kor-pus'-ku-lar)* [L *intra,* within; *corpusculum,* small body]. Wit hin a corpuscle.

رون جسیمی : خلیے کے اندر۔

Intracranial *(in-tra-kra-ni-al)* [L. *intra,* within G. *kranion,* skull]. Within the skull.

رون قحفی : کھوپڑی کے اندر۔

Intracutaneous *(in-tra-ku-ta'-ne-us)* [L. *intra* within; *cutis,* skin]. Within the skin--intra dermally, adv.

رون جلدی : جلدی بافتوں میں۔

Intradermal *(in-tra-der'-mal)* [L. *intra,* withir G. *derma,* skin]. Within the skin--intrad ermally, adv.

رون جلدی : کھال کے اندر۔

Intraflodex *(in-tra-flo'-deks)*. Low molecula weight dextran 10 per-cent in normal saline c in 5 per-cent dextrose solution. Given as i.v infusion for prevention and treatment of intr vascular sludging and to improve capillar circulation.

ٹرافلوڈیکس : کم سالمی وزن والا ڈیکسٹران نارمل سیلائن میں دس فیصد یا
نچ فیصد ڈیکسٹروز محلول میں۔ شعری گردش کو بہتر بنانے کے لئے مستعمل ہے۔

Intragastric *(in-tra-gas'-trik)* [L. *intra,* withi G. *gaster,* belly]. With the stomach.

رون معدی : معدی کے اندر۔

Intragluteal *(in-tra-glu-te'-al)* [L. *intra,* withi G. *gloutos,* buttock]. Within the glute muscle compressing the buttock--intraglu eally, adv.

راگلوٹیل : چتون بنانے والے عضلات کے اندر۔

Intrahepatic *(in-tra-hep-at'-ik)* [L. *intra,* wit in; G. *hepar,* liver]. Within the liver.

ون کبدی : جگر کے اندر۔

Intralipid *(in-tra-li-pid)*. Intravenous fluid 1.

litre, 20 per-cent contains 1000 kca l. Prepared from soya bean oil and egg yolk phosphatides.

انٹرالائیپڈ : آئی۔وی۔سیال۔سویابین کے تیل اور انڈے کی زردی کے فاسفیٹائڈز سے تیار کیا جاتا ہے۔

Intralobular *(in-tra-lob'-u-lar)* [L. *intra,* within; *lobulus,* small lobe]. Within the lobule, as the vein draining a hepatic lobule.

انٹرالوبیولر : چھوٹے لوب کے اندر۔

Intraluminal *(in-tra-lu'-min-al)* [L. *intra,* within; *lumen,* light]. Within the hellow of a tube-like structure--intraluminally, adv.

انٹرالیومینل : نلی نما ساخت کی کھوکھلی جگہ میں۔

Intralymphatic *(in-tra-lim-fat'-ik)* [L. *intra,* within; *lympha,* water]. Within a lymphatic gland or vessel.

دروں لمفی : لمفیٹک گلینڈ یا رگ کے اندر۔

Intreamedullary *(in-tra-med-ul'-a-ri)* [L. *intra,* within; *medulla,* marrow]. Within the bone marrow.

دروں لبی : ہڈی کے گودے میں۔

Intramural *(in-tra-mur'-al)* [L. *intra,* within; *murus,* wall]. Withing the layers of the wall of a hollow tube or organ--intramurally, adv.

دروں دیواری : کسی کھوکھلی نلی یا عضو کی دیوار کی تہوں میں۔

Intramuscular *(in-tra-mus'-ku-lar)* [L. *intra,* within; *musculus,* muscle]. Within a muscle--intramuscularly, adv.

عضلاتی : عضلہ کے اندر۔عضلاتی ٹیکہ۔عضلات میں گہرا کر کے لگایا جاتا ہے۔چھوٹے ٹیکے بازو میں عضلات میں اور زیادہ مقدار کے ٹیکے کولہے کے عضلات میں بہتر رہتے ہیں۔

Intranasal *(in-tra-na'-zal)* [L. *intra,* within; *nasus,* nose]. Within the nasal cavity--intranasally, adv.

درانفی : ناک کے کہفہ کے اندر۔

Intranatal *(in-tra-na'-tal)* [L. *intra,* within; *natus,* birth]. At the time of birth. Syn., intrapartum (q.v.)--intranatally, adv.

انٹرانیٹل : پیدائش کے وقت پر۔

Intraocular *(in-tra-ok'-u-lar)* [L. *intra,* within; *oculus,* eye]. Within the globe of the eye.

دروں چشمی : آنکھ کے گلوب کے اندر۔

Intraocular

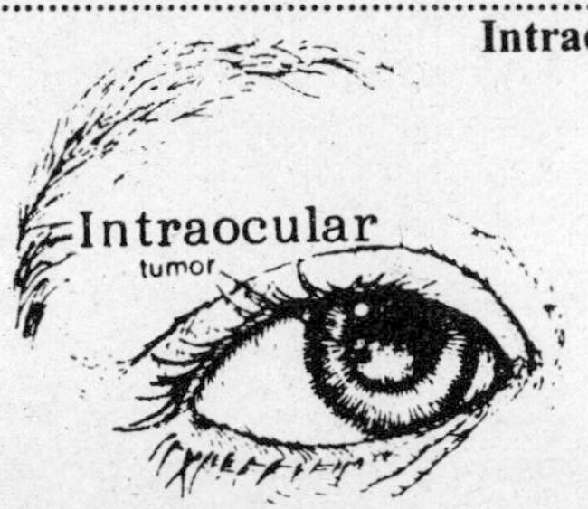

Intraoral *(in-tra-o'-ral)* [L. *intra* within; *os,* mouth]. Within with mouth as an i. appliance--intraorally, adv.

دروں دہنی : منہ کے اندر۔

Intraobital *(in-tra-orb'-it-al)* [L. *intra*, within; *orbita,* orbit]. Within the orbit.

دروں محجری : آربٹ کے اندر۔

Intraosseous *(in-tra-os'-e-us)* [L. *intra,* within; *osseus,* of bone]. Inside a bone.

دروں عظمی : ہڈی کے اندر۔

Intrapartum *(in-tra-par'-tum)* [L. *intra,* within; *partus,* a birth]. During labour, as asphyxia, haemorrihage or infection.

انٹراپارٹم : دردزہ کے دوران بیماری یا خون کی روانگی۔

Intraperitoneal *(in-tra-per-i-ton-e'-al)* [L. *intra,* within; G. *peri,* around; *teinein,* to stretch]. Within the peritoneal cavity--intraperitoneally, adv.

انٹراپیری ٹونیل : پیریٹونیل کہفہ کے اندر۔

Intrapharyngeal *(in-tra-far-in-je'-al)* [L. *intra,* within; G. *pharygx,* pharynx]. Within the pharynx--intrapharyngeally, adv.

دروں بلعومی : فیرنکس کے اندر۔

Intraplacental *(in-tra -pla-sen'-al)* [L. *intra,* within; *placenta,* cake]. Within pleural cavity--intrapleurally, adv.

دروں مشیمی : پلیسنٹا کے اندر۔

Intrapleural *(in-tra-ploo'-ral)* [L. *intra,* within; G. *pleural,* side]. Within the pleural cavity--intrapleurally, adv.

دروں پلورائی: پلیورل کہفہ کے اندر۔

Intrapulmonary *(in-tra-pul'-mon-a-ri)* [L. *intra*, within; *pulmo,* lung]. Within the lungs, as i. pressure.

درون ششی ۔ دروں ریوری : پھیپھڑوں کے اندر۔

Intrapunitive *(in-tra-pun'-it-iv)*. Tending to blame oneself.

انٹراپیونیٹو : اپنے آپ کو موردِ الزام ٹھہرانا۔

Intraretinal *(in-tra -ret'-i-nal)* [L. *intra,* within; *rete,* not]. Within the retina.

دروں شبکیتی : ریٹنا کے اندر۔

Intraserosal *(in-tra-ret'-i-nal)* [L. *intra,* within; *serum,* whey]. Within a serous membrane. See INTERSEROSAL--intraserosally, adv.

انٹراسیروسیل : سیرس جھلی کے اندر۔

Intraspinal *(in-tra-spi'-nal)* [L. *intra,* within; *spina,* thorn]. Within the spinal canal, as i. anaesthesia-- intraspinally, adv.

دروں شوکی : سپائنل قنال کے اندر۔

Intrasplenic *(in-tra-splen'-ik)* [L. *intra,* within; G. *splen,* spleen]. Within the spleen.

دروں طحالی : تلی کے اندر۔

Intrasynovial *(in-tra-si-no'-vi-al)* [L. *intra,* within; N.L. *synovia]*. Within a synovial membrane or cavity--intrasynovially, adv.

دروں زلالی : سائینویل جھلی یا کہفہ کے اندر۔

Intrathecal *(in-tra-the'-kal)* [L. *intra,* within; G. *theke,* a case]. Within the meninges; into the subarachnoid space--intrathecally, adv.

دروں صری : سب ارقنائڈ جگہ میں۔

Intrathoracic *(in-tra-thor-as'-ik)* [L. *Intra,* within; G. *thorax,* chest]. Within the cavity of the thorax.

دروں صدری : تھوریکس کے کہفہ میں۔

Intratracheal (in-tra-trak-e'-al) [L. *intra,* within; L.L. *trachia,* windpipe]. Within or through the trachea. **intratracheal anaesthesia,** the administra tion of an anaesthetic through a special tube passed down the trachea--intracheally, adv.

درون قصبی : ہوا کی نالی میں سے یا اس کی اندر۔

Intratumour *(in-tra -tu'-mor)* [L. *intra,* within; L. *tumor,* swelling]. Within a tumour.

درون سلعہ : ناسور کے اندر۔

Intrauterine *(in-tra-u'-te-rin)* [L. *intra,* within; *uterus,* womb]. Within the uterus. See IUCD.

درون رحمی : یورٹرس کے اندر۔

Intravaginal *(in-tra-va-ji'-nal)* [L. *intra,* within; *vagina,* sheath]. Within the vegina--intravaginally, adv.

درون مہبلی : ویجائنا کے اندر۔

Intraval *(in'-tra-val)* Thiopentone (q.v.).

انٹراوال : تھیوپنٹون۔

Intravascular *(in-tra-vas'-ku-lar)* [L. *intra,* within; *vasculum,* small vessel]. Within the blood vessels--intravascularly, adv.

انٹراواسکولر : خونی رگوں کے اندر۔

Intravenous *(in-tra-ve'-nus)* [L. *intra,* within; *vena,* vein]. Within or into a vein-intravenously. adv.

درون وریدی : ورید کے اندر۔ وریدی ٹیکا۔ جو زیریں بازو کے سامنے والی وریدوں میں لگاتے ہیں۔ یہ ٹیکہ آہستہ آہستہ لگانا چاہئے۔ پہلے خون کھینچ کر دیکھ لیتے ہیں کہ سوئی ٹھیک رگ میں ہے۔

Intraventricular *(in-tra-ven-trik-u-lar)* [L. *intra* , within *ventriculus,* cavity]. Within a ventricle, especially cerebral ventricle.

درون بطینی : بطین کے اندر، خصوصاً سر برل بطین۔

Intrinsic *(in-trin'-sik)* [L. *intrinsecus,* inward]. Inherent or inside; from within; real; natural.**intrinsic factor,** a protein released by gastric glands, essential for the satisfactory absorption of the extrinsic factor vitamin B_{12}.

درونی : پیدائشی ۔ اندر۔ اندر میں سے حقیقی ۔ قدرتی۔

Introitus *(in-tro'-it-us)* [L.]. Any opening in the body; an entrance to a cavity particularly the vegina .

Introitus

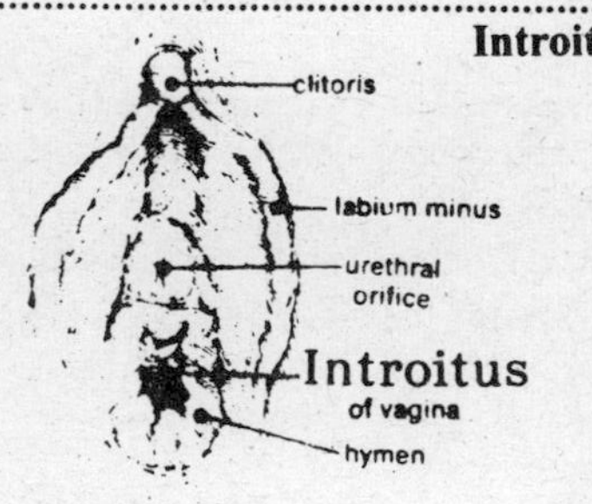

مدخل، مولج : جسم میں کوئی سوراخ۔ کسی کہفہ خصوصاً ویجائنا میں داخل ہونے کا راستہ۔

trojection *(in-tro-jek'-shun)* [L. *intro,* inward; *jacere,* to throw]. A mental process whereby a person identifies himself with another person or object.

بلع ذہنی : ایک ذہنی طریق جس سے کوئی شخص اپنے آپ کو دوسرے شخص یا شے کے ساتھ شناخت۔

trospection *(in-tro-spek'-shun)* [L. *intro,* within; *spicere,* look]. Study by a person of his own mental process. Seen in an exaggerated form in schizophrenia.

معائنہ نفس : کسی شخص کا اپنے ہی ذہنی طریقوں کا مطالعہ۔

troversion *(in-tro-ver'-shun)* [L. *intro-versus,* inward]. The direction of thoughts and interest inwa rds to the world of ideas, instead of outwards to the external world--introvert, n.

باطنیت ۔ خانہ نشینی : خیالات اور دلچسپی کی سمت اندرونی جانب نظریات کی دنیا کی طرف ہوتی ہے۔ بیرونی جانب باہر کی دنیا کی طرف نہیں ہوتی۔ باہر گھومنے پھرنے کی بجائے تصنیف وتالیف کا مشغلہ اختیار کرنا۔

tubation *(in-tu-ba'-shun)* [L. *in,* in; *tubus,* tube]. Insertion of a tube into a hollow organ, especially into (or via) the larynx. Used, prior to anaesthesia, to promote suction of the respiratory tract, to maintain an airway--See INTRATRA- CHEAL. **doudenal i.,** a double tube is passed as far as the pyloric antrum under flouroscopy. The inner tube is then passed along to the doudenojejunal flexure. Barium can then be passed to outline the bowel.

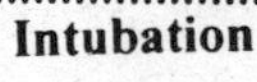

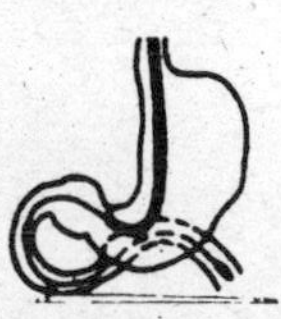

ادخال نلی : کھوکھلے عضو خصوصاً لیرنکس میں ایک نلی رکھنا تاکہ سانس جاری رہے۔

Intussusception *(in-tus-sus-sep'-shun)* [L. *intus,* within; *suscipere,* to receive]. A condition in which one part of the bowel slips into (invaginates) the lower part, causing intestinal obstruction. It occurs most commonly in infants.

انغماد : ایسی حالت میں جس میں معا کا ایک حصہ پھسل کر نچلے حصہ میں چلا جاتا ہے جس سے آنت بند ہو جاتی ہے۔ عموماً چھوٹے بچوں میں ایسا ہوتا ہے۔ انیما کیجیے اور گر افاقہ نہ ہو تو فوراً اپریشن۔

Intussusception

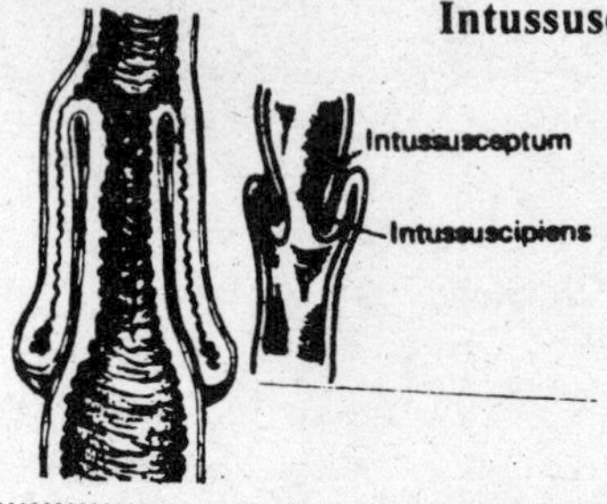

Intussusceptum *(in-tus-sus-sep'-tum)* The invaginated portion of an intussusception.

مغمود : انغماد کا حصہ جو اندرونی جانب دبا ہوتا ہے۔

Intussuscipiens *(in-tus-sus-sip'-i-ens)* The receiving portion of an intussusception.

غامد : انغماد کا وصول کرنے والا حصہ۔

Inunction (in-ungk'-shun) [L. *inunctio,* anointing]. The act of rubbing an oily or fatty substance into the skin.

مالش تیل: کھال میں کوئی تیلدار یا چکنا مادہ ملنے کا عمل۔

Invagination *(in-vaj-in-a'-shun)* [L. *in,* in; *vagina,* sheath]. The act or condition of being ensheathed; a pushing inward, forming a pouch--invaginate, v.t.

انغماد: شید ہونے کی حالت یا عمل۔ اندرونی جانب دبا ہوا جس سے ایک تھیلی بن جاتی ہے۔

Invasion *(in-va'-zhun)* [L. *invasio,* attack]. The entry of bacteria into the body.

حملہ : جسم میں جراثیم کا داخلہ۔

Inversine *(in'-ver-sen)* Mecamylamine (q.v.).

انورسین : میکامائلامین

Inversion *(in-ver'-shun)* [L. *inversio,* upside down]. Turning inside out, as i. of the uterus. See PROCIDENTIA.

تقلیب : الٹ جانا۔ جیسے یورٹرس کا الٹ جانا۔

Invertase *(in'-ver-tas)* [L. *invertere,* to turn into]. A sugar-splitting enzyme in intestinal juice.

شکر آبپاش : آنتوں کے جوس میں شکر پھاڑنے والا خامرہ سکریز۔ شکر کو گلوکوس اور فرکٹوز میں تبدیل کرتا ہے۔

In vitro *(vi'-tro)* [L.]. In glass, as in a test-tube.

درز جاج : حیاتیاتی یا حیاتی کیمیا کے اعمال سے متعلق ان تجربات کو کہا جاتا ہے جو تجربہ گاہ میں کئے جائیں تا کہ جاندار کی جسم کے اندر کئے جائیں۔

In vivo *(vi'-vo)* [L.]. In living tissue.

وراحیاء : جاندار نسیج میں۔

Involucrum *(in-vol-uk'-rum)* [L. covering]. A shea th of new bone, which forms around necrosed bone, in such conditions as osteomyelitis. See CLOACA.

ہڈی کا خول : نئی ہڈی کی شید۔

Involuntary *(in-vol'-un-ta-ri)* [L. *involuntarius*]. Independent of the will, as muscle of the chest and abdominal organs.

غیر ارادی : بلا ارادہ۔ جس میں مرضی کا داخل نہ ہو۔ مثلاً چھاتی کے عضلات اور بطنی اعضاء۔

Involution *(in-vol-u'-shun)* [L. *involutus,* rolled up]. The normal shrinkage of an organ after fulfilling its functional purpose, e.g. uterus after labour. In psychiatry, the period of decline after middle life-- involutional, adj.

انحطاط : فعلیاتی مقصد کے حصول کے بعد کسی عضو کا نارمل سکڑاؤ۔ مثلاً دردزہ کے بعد یوٹرس درمیانی عمر کے بعد زوال پذیر عرصہ۔

Iodatol *(i-od'-at-ol)*. Iodized Oil (q.v.).

آیوڈیٹال : خشخاش کی بیجوں کا تیل۔

Iodex *(i'-o-deks)*. A non-staining iodine ointment. Used as a counterirritant in sprains, chilblains, etc.

آیوڈیکس : آیوڈین کا مرہم۔ دافع تعفن۔ ورم دور کرتا ہے۔ درد کے لئے فائدہ مند ہے۔

Iodides *(i'-o-didz)*. Compounds of iodine and a base. Potassium and sodium iodide are the most common medicinal iodides.

یوڈائیڈز : آیوڈین کے مرکبات اور ایک اساس۔ پوٹاشیم اور سوڈیم وڈائڈ ادویات میں عام مستعمل ہے۔

Iodine *(i'-o-den)*. Powerful 'antiseptic used as tincture for skin prepara tion and emergen treatment of small wounds. Orally it antithyroid, e.e. it decreases release of th horm- ones from the thyroid gland **povido** **i.,** anti bacterial. See BETADINE. **prote** **bound i.,** (PBI), estimated in thyroid inves gations. **radioactive i.** (^{181}I) is used investiga tion and treatment of thyrotoxicosi

وڈین : طاقتور دافع تعفن۔ چھوٹے زخموں کے علاج کے لئے ٹنکچر۔

Iodism *(i'-o-dizm)*. Poisoning with iodides; t symptoms are those of a common cold a the appearance of a rash.

یت یود : آیوڈائڈز کے ساتھ زہریلا پن۔ عام زکام علامات میں شامل

Iodized oil *(i'-od-izd)* Poppy-seed oil containi 40 percent of organically combined iodi Should be colourless or pale yellow; dark solutions have decomposed. Used as contr agent in X-ray examination of bronchial tra sinuses and other cavities.

ڈین سے متاثر تیل: خشخاش کے بیجوں کا تیل جس میں چالیس فیصد تی طور پر ملی آیوڈین ہوتی ہے۔

Iodoform *(i-o'-do-form)*. Antiseptic iodi compound of yellow colour and characteris odour. Now used chiefly as BIPP (q.v.).

فارم : دافع تعفن پیلے رنگ اور مخصوص بو کا مرکز۔

Iodosin *(i-o-dop'-sin)*. A protein substar which with vitamin A, is a constituent of v ual purple present in the rods in the retina the eye.

ڈاپسن : ایک پروتینی مادہ جو وٹامن اے کے ساتھ آنکھ کے ریٹنا میں وں میں موجود بصری اودے کا ایک جزو ہے۔

Iodoxyl *(i-o-doks'-il)* . A contrast agent cor ining 50 per-cent of combined iodine. Gi by slow intravenous injection in pyelograp The solution is irrita nt, and extravenous ection must be avoided. For this reason d done (q.v.) is often preferred.

ایوڈالسل : ملی ہوئی آیوڈین کے پچاس فیصد پر مشتمل کنٹراسٹ عامل۔

n *(i'-on)*. A charged atom which, in electrolysis, passes to one or the other pole, or electrode--ionic, adj.

آئن۔ برق پارہ : ایک برق جوہر یا جواہر کا گروہ۔ایک چارج شدہ ایٹم جو برق پاشیدگی میں ایک سے دوسرے قطب یا برقیرے کی طرف جاتا ہے۔

nization *(i-on-i-za'-shun)*. Treatment whereby ions of various substances, e.g. zinc, chlorine, iodine, histamine, are introduced into the skin by means of a constant electrical current.

روانیت : آئنز کا بننا۔علاج جس میں مختلف اشیاء مثلاً جست۔کلورین۔ آیوڈین۔ ہسٹامین کے آئنز مستقل برقی کرنٹ کے ذریعے کھال میں داخل کئے جاتے ہیں۔

panoic acid *(i-o-pan-o'-ik-as'-id)*. A complex iodine derivative of butyric acid; used as a contrast agent in cholecystography. Side reactions are few, and it gives denser shadows than the earlier pheniodol.

آیوپینونک ایسڈ : بوٹائرک ایسڈ سے حاصل شدہ ایک پیچیدہ آیوڈین۔

ecacuanha *(ip-i-kak-u-an'-a)*. Dried roo0t from Brazil and other South American countries. Principal alkaloid is emetine (q.v.). Has expectorant properties, and is widely used in acute bronchitis and relief of dry cough. A safe emetic in la rger doses.

عرق آپیکا : برازیل اور دوسرے جنوبی امریکی ممالک سے خشک جڑ۔زیادہ تر الکلائڈ امیٹین ہے خشک کھانسی کو آرام پہنچاتا ہے۔

P. Intermittent positive pressure. Used to inflate the lungs (inspiration). Expiration is by recoil of elastic lung tissue.

آئی پی پی : وقفوں کے درمیان مثبت دباؤ۔پھیپھڑے پھلانے کے لئے مستعمل۔

rindol *(ip-rin'-dol)* Tricyclic antidepressant. Has few side effects; tolerated well by most people, slight risk of jaundice in allergic people.

اپرنڈال : ٹرائی سائیکلک پریشانی کم کرنے والا دوا جنہیں الرجی ہو۔انہیں یرقان کا خطرہ ہوتا ہے۔

roniazid *(ip-ro-ni'-az-id)*. Antidepressant. MAOI. (q.v.). Antituberculosis.

اپرونیازڈ : پریشانی کم کرنے والی دوا۔دافع تپ دق۔

Ipsilateral *(ip-si-lat'-er-al)* [L. *ipse,* self; *latus,* side]. On the same side--ipsilaterally, adv.

ہم جانب : اسی جانب۔ایک ہی طرف۔

IQ. Intelligence (q.v.). quotient.

اشاریہ ذہنی : ذہانت کا پیمانہ۔ذہانت کی اکائی۔

Iridectomy *(ir-i-dek'-to-mi)* [L. *iris,* rainbow; G. *ektome,* excision]. Excision of a pa rt of the iris, thus forming an artifical pupil.

قزحیہ براری : آئرس کے ایک حصے کو کاٹنا اس طرح ایک مصنوعی پتلی بن جاتی ہے۔

Iridencleisis *(ir-id-en-kli'-sis)*. A filtering operation. Scleral incision made at angle of anterior chamber; meridian cut in iris; either one or both pillars are left in scleral wound to contract as scar tissue. Decreases intraocular tension in glaucoma.

اریڈن کلائی سس : ایک فلٹرن اپریشن۔

Iridocele *(ir-id-o-sel')* [L. *iris,* rainbow; G. *kele,* hernia]. Protrusion of part of the iris through a corneal wound (prolapsed iris). Iridoptosis.

فتق قزحیہ : کورنیا کے زخم میں سے آئرس کے ایک حصے کا باہر نکلنا۔

Iridocyclitis *(ir-id-o-si-kli'-tis)* [L. *iris,* rainbow; G. *kyklos,* circle; -itis, inflammation]. Inflammation of the iris and ciliary body.

التہاب قزحیہ وجسم ہدبی : آئرس کی اپنے ہدبی جسم کی سوزش۔

Iridodialysis *(ir-id-o-di-al'-i-sis)* [L. *iris,* rainbow; G. *dialysis,* a separating]. A separation of the iris from its ciliary attachment.

تخلیص قزحیہ : آئرس کی اپنے ہدبی الحاق سے علیحدگی۔

Iridoplegia *(ir-id-o-ple'-ji-a)* [L. *iris,* rainbow; G. *plege,* stroke]. Paralysis of the iris.

شلل قزحیہ : آنکھ کی پتلی کی قوتِ حس کا زوال۔

Iridoptosis *(ir-id-op-to'-sis)* [L. *iris,* rainbow; G. *ptosis,* a failing]. Prolapse of the iris.

سقوط قزحیہ : آنکھ کی پتلی کا سقوط۔

Iridotomy *(ir-id-ot'-om-i)* [L. *iris,* rainbow; G. *tome,* a cutting]. An incision into the iris.

قزحیہ تراشی : آنکھ کی پتلی میں شگاف۔

Iris *(i'-ris)* [L. rainbow). The circular coloured membrane forming the anterior one-sixth of the middle coat of the eyeball It is perforated in the centre by an opening named 'the pupil.' Contraction of its muscle fibres regulates the amount of ligh entering the eye. **iris bombe,** bulging forward of iris due to pressure of aqueous behind, when posterior synechiae are present.

قزحیہ : گول رنگین جھلی جو آنکھ کے گولے کے درمیانی کوٹ کا اگلا چھٹا حصہ بناتی ہے اس کے مرکز میں سوراخ ہوتا ہے جسے پتلی کہتے ہیں اس کے عضلاتی ریشے آنکھ میں داخل ہونے والی روشنی کو کنٹرول کرتے ہیں۔

Iritis *(i-ri'-tis)* [L. *iris*, rainbow; G. *-itis*, inflammation]. Inflammation of the iris.

سوزش قزحیہ : قزحیہ یا آئرس کی سوزش۔

Iron and ammonium citrate A soluble non-irritant iron complex, now rarely used in the oral treatment of iron deficiency anaemia.

آئرن اور امونیم سٹریٹ : ایک حل پذیر آئرن کمپلکس۔ خون میں لوہے کی کمی کے علاج میں مستعمل۔

Iron gluconate *(gloo'-kon-at)*. An organic salt of iron, less irritant and better tolerated than ferrous sulphate.

آئرن گلوکونیٹ : لوہے کا ایک نامیاتی نمک۔

Irreducible *(ir-re-du'-si-bl)* [L. *irredux*, does not bring back]. Cannot be brought to desired condition **irreducible hernia,** when the contents of the sac cannot be returned to the appropriate cavity, without surgical intervention.

تحلیل ناپذیر : مطلوبہ حالت کی طرف نہیں لایا جاسکتا۔

Irritable *(ir'-it-abl)* [L. *irritare*, to irritate]. Capable of being excited to activity; responding easily to stimulirritability, n.

حساس : عاملیت کے لئے موثر بنانے کا اہل۔ تحریکوں کے لئے ردعمل رکھنے والا۔

Irritant *(ir'-it-ant)* [L. *irritare*, to irritate]. Any agent which causes irritation.

خراش آور : سوزش یا خراش پیدا کرنیوالا کوئی عامل جلد پر خراش پیدا ہونے سے دوران خون تیز ہو جاتا ہے۔ گرمی پیدا ہوتی ہے اور درد کو آرام آتا ہے۔ سب لازمی تیل ایسے ہیں مثلاً تارپین اور رنگ کا تیل۔

Ischaemia *(is-ke'-mi-a)* [G. *ischein*, to check; *haima*, blood]. Deficient blood supply. S ANGINA, VOLKMANN--ischaemic, adj.

ـ الدام : خون کی سپلائی کی کمی۔

Ischiorectal *(is-ki-o-rek'-tal)* [G. *ischion*, h *rectus*, stra ight]. Pertaining to the ischiu and the rectum, as an i. abscess which occu between these two structures.

مستقیمی : اسکیئم اور ریکٹم سے متعلق۔

Ischium *(is'-ki-um)* [G. *ischion*, hip]. The low part of the innominate bone of the pelvis; bone on which the body rests when sittin ischial, adj.

ـ سرین کی ہڈی : پیڑو کی لااسمی ہڈی کا زیریں حصہ۔ ہڈی جس ٹھے ہوئے جسم ٹکا ہوتا ہے۔ چوتڑ کی ہڈی جس سے کولہے کی ہڈی یا ہپ بون یریں حصہ بنتا ہے۔ یہ حصہ موٹا اور مضبوط ہوتا ہے۔ یہ ہڈی ایک طرف سے اور دوسری طرف پیوبس سے ملتی ہے۔

Islets of Langerhans *(i'-lez- lan'-ger-han* Collections of special cells scatered throu hout the pancreas. They secrete insulin wh is poured directly into the blood stream. [P Langerhans, German pathologist, 1847-88].

ر ہینز کے جزیرے : سارے لبلبہ میں منتشر خصوصی خلیوں کا اجتماع سولین پیدا کرتے ہیں جو خون میں براہ راست شامل ہوتی ہے اور گلوکوس کو سے نکالنے اور گلائیکوجن میں تبدیل کرنے میں مدد دیتی ہے اس کی کمی رض ذیابیطس ہو جاتا ہے۔

Ismelin *(is'-me-lin)*. Guanethidine (q.v.).

ے لین : گوانیتھیڈین۔ ہائپرٹنشن یا بلڈ پریشر میں اس کی ایک گولی صبح دوپہر ایک شام انتہائی زود اثر۔

Isocarboxazid *(i-zo-kar-boks'-a-zid)*. Antidepressant. MAOI.

ﺴوکاربوکسازڈ : پریشانی کم کرنے والی دوا۔

I-so-gel *(i'-so-jel)*. Granules prepared from husks of mucilaginous seeds, and used a bulk-forming laxative in chronic constipatio

ﺴوجیل : بیجوں کے چھلکوں سے تیار شدہ دانے۔

Isoimmunization *(i-so-im-mu-ni-za'-shun)*

isos, equal; L. *immunis,* exempt from public burden]. Development of anti-Rh agglutins in the blood of an Rh-negative person who has been given an Rh-positive transfusion, or who is carrying an Rh-positive fetus.

آئیسوامیونائزیشن :اینٹی آر ایچ کی تکمیل۔

Isolator *(i'-so-la-tor).* Apparatus ranging from what is virtually a large plastic bag in which a patient can be nursed to that in which an operation can be performed. It aims to prevent bacterial entry to or exit from the enclosed space.

حاجز : سامان جو ایک بڑا پلاسٹک کا تھیلا ہوتا ہے جس میں مریض کی تیمارداری کی جاتی ہے جس میں اپریشن بھی کیا جاسکتا ہے۔

Isoleucine *(i'-so-lu-sen).* One of the essential amino acids (q.v.).

آئیسولیوسین :لازمی امینوایسڈز میں سے ایک۔ بے رنگ قلمی مرکب۔ مالیکیولی وزن ۱۳۱ء۲۔

Isolevin *(i-so-lev'-in)* Isoprenaline sulphate (q.v.).

آئیسولیون :آئیسوپرینالین سلفیٹ۔

Isometric *(i-so-met'-rik).* Of equal proportions. **isometric exercises,** carried out without movement; maintain muscle tone.

Isoniazid *(i-so-ni-az-id)* A derivative of isonicotinic acid. It has a specific action against the tubercle bacllus, and is widely employed in the treatment of tuberculosis. Combined treatment with other tuberculostatic drugs such as streptomycin and PAS is not only more effective than any drug alone, but the risk of bacterial resistance is also reduced. Can be neurotoxic.

آئیسونایازڈ : آئیسونکوٹینک ایسڈ کا حاصل۔ اس کا تپ دق کے جرثومے کے خلاف مخصوص ایکشن ہے۔ اس لئے تپ دق کے علاج کے لئے مستعمل ہے۔ آئیسوفیکس۔ تپ دق اور پیری کارڈائی ٹس میں روزانہ ایک گولی صبح ایک دوپہر ایک شام دو سال تک۔ پلیوریسی میں ایک گولی صبح ایک دوپہر ایک شام۔

Isoprenaline sulphate *(i-so-ren'-a-len).* An adrenaline derivative with similar broncho-dilator properties. Given in asthma, etc., as sublingual tablets of 20 mg; also by spray inhalation. Speeds up the heart in heart block (Stokes-Adams syndromne).

آئیسوپرینالین سلفیٹ :ایڈرینا کا حاصل۔ دمہ میں دیا جاتا ہے۔

Isotonic *(i-so-ton'-ik)* [G. *isos,* equal; *tonos,*tension]. Equal tension; applied to any solution which has the same osmotic pressure as blood. isotonic saline (syn., normal saline), 0.9 per-cent solution of salt in water.

ہم طناب: مساوی ٹنشن۔ اس اصطلاح کا اطلاق ایسے محلول پر ہوتا ہے جس کا نفوذی دباؤ خون کے برابر ہو۔

Isotopes *(i'-so-topz)* [G. *iso,* equal; *topos,* place]. Two or more forms of the same element having identical chemical, but differing physical properties. Those isotopes with radioactive properties are used in medicine for research, diagnosis and treatment of disease.

ہم جا : ایک ہی عنصر کی دو یا زیادہ اقسام جن کے ایک جیسی کیمیائی لیکن مختلف طبعی خصوصیات ہوں۔ امراض کی تشخیص، تحقیق اور علاج میں مستعمل۔

Isoxazole penicillins *(i-soks'-a-zol).* Can be taken orally. Given high blood levels of penicillin in a freely available form to act against staphylococci, afterabsorption. Particularly effective for boils and carbuncles.

آئیسوکسازول پینسلینز : منہ کے ذریعے یہ دوا لی جاسکتی ہے ابلوں کے لئے مفید۔

Isoxuprine *(is-oks'-u-pren).* Peripheral vasodilator, and spasmolytic. Acts on myometrium preventing contractions, thus useful in premature labour.

آئیسوکسوپرین :وقت سے پہلے دروزہ میں مفید۔

Isoxyl *(is-oks'-il).* New drug used for tuberculosis, in conjunction with other antituberculous drugs.

آئی سا کسل : تپ دق کے لئے مستعمل نئی دوا۔ جو دوسری ادویات کے ساتھ دی جاتی ہے۔ تھایوکارلائیڈ۔ ایک گولی صبح ایک دوپہر ایک شام۔

Itch See SCABIES. **itch mite,** Sarcoptes scabiei (q.v.).

خارش۔ لت۔ چداس : ایک طفیلی جلدی مرض۔ چھوت کی بیماری۔

IUCD. Intrauterine contraceptive device. See IUD.

آئی یوسی ڈی : دروں یوٹرس مانع حمل طریق۔ اس کی ساتھ سے زیادہ مختلف اقسام ہیں۔

IUD. Intrauterine divice. Over 60 different forms known by the International Planning Perenthood Federation.

آئی یوڈی: دروں یوٹرس طریق۔ پلاسٹک کے سپرنگ یوٹرس یا رحم کے اندر رکھا جاتا ہے۔

Types of IUD

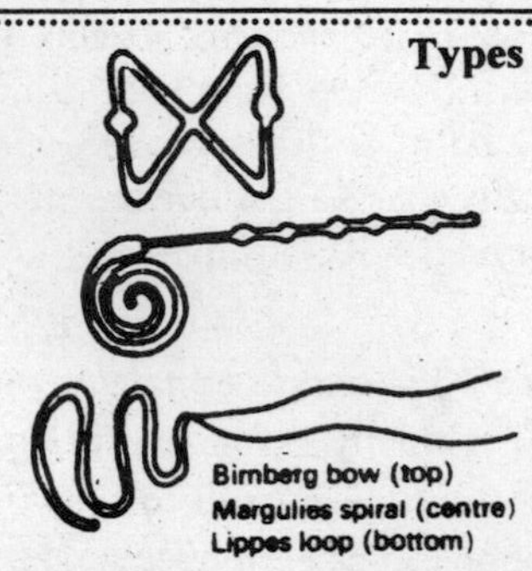

Izal *(i'-zal).* An emulsion of tar oils, widely used as a general disinfectant and deodorant for drains, skins, floors, etc. 'White fluid'.

آئیزیل : کولتار کے تیلوں کا ایملشن۔ دافع تعفن۔ فرش نالیوں وغیرہ میں ڈالا جاتا ہے۔ سفید سیال۔

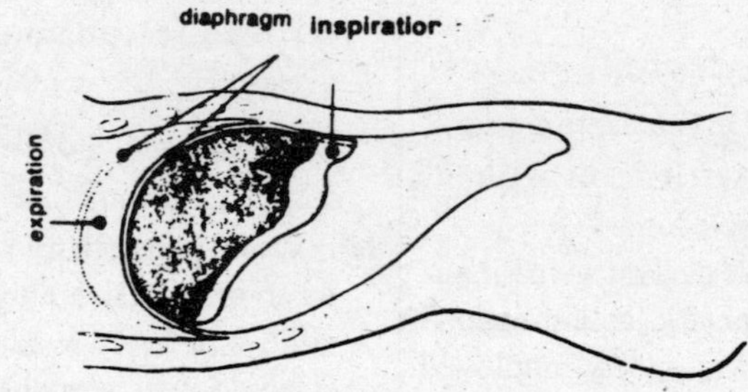

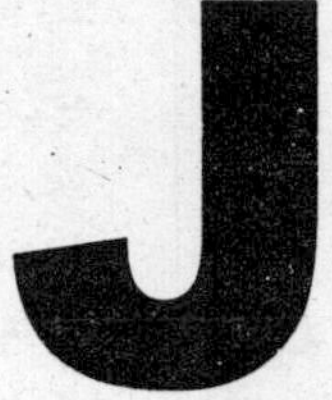

J. Symbol for Joule.

جے: کام کی اکائی ''جول'' کی علامت ہے۔

Jacket *(jak'et)* An enveloping structure or garment especially a covering for the trunk or for the upper part of the body.

جیکٹ: ڈھانپنے والی چیز یا لباس جو کہ زیادہ تر جسم کے اوپر والے حصے کو ڈھانپنے کے کام آتا ہے۔

Jacksonian epilepsy march [John Hughlings Jackson, English neurologist 1835-1911]. Epilepsy characterized by local motor seizures with unilateral clonic movements that starts in one group of the muscles and spread systematically to the adjacent groups, reflecting the march of epileptic activity through the motor cortex. The seizures are due to discharging focus in the contralateral motor cortex.

مرگی: صرع قشری۔ مرگی کا مرض۔ یہ قسم عضلات کے ایک خاص حصے میں حرکت سے شروع ہو کر ساتھ والے موٹر نیوران کے گروہ میں بھی منتقل ہو جاتے ہیں۔

Jactitation *(jak-ti-ta'-shan)* [L. *jactitatio, jactilare,* to toss]. The tossing to and fro of a patient in acute disease.

اچھلنا: شدید بیماری کی حالت میں مریض کا اِدھر اُدھر یا آگے پیچھے اچھلنا۔ لاطینی زبان جیکٹیشیو، جیکٹیشیئر بمعنی اچھالنا سے ماخوذ ہے۔

Janiceps *(jan-i-seps)* [L. *janus,* a two faced god; *caput,* head]. Conjoined twins with one head and two opposite faces.

دو چہروں والے جڑواں: ایسے جڑواں بچے جن کا سر ایک ہی ہو اور ان کے دونوں طرف چہرے ہوں۔ لاطینی لفظ جینس بمعنی دو چہروں والا دیوتا اور کیپٹ بمعنی سر سے ماخوذ ہے۔

Jaundice *(jawn'dis)* [F. *jaunisse from jaune,* yellow]. A syndrome characterized by hyperbilirubinemic and deposition of bile pigment in the skin, mucous membrane and sclera with resulting yellow appearance of the patient called also icterus. **acholuric j.,** jaundice without bilirubin in urine. It is associated with elevated unconjugated bilirubin. **hemolytic j.,** jaundice caused by increased production of bilirubin from hemoglobin under conditions causing accelerated degradation of crythrocytes **infectious j.,** infectious hepatitis, Weil's syndrome. **latent j.,** hyperbilirubimemia without yellow staining of the tissues. **physiologic j.,** mild icterus neonatorum lasting the first few days after birth. **obstructure j.,** that which is due to an impediment to the flow of the bile from the liver cells to the duodenum.

یرقان: ایک حالت جس میں بلیروبن کا لیول خون میں زیادہ ہوتا ہے۔ زیادہ ہونے کی صورت میں جلد پیلی ہو جاتی ہے۔

Jejunum *(je-joo'-num)* [L. *jejunus,* empty]. That part of the small intestine between the duodenum and the ileum. It is about 2.483 m in length--jejunal, adj.

صائم۔خالی آنت: ڈیُ ینم اور ایلیم کے درمیان چھوٹی آنت کا حصہ۔

Jelonet *(jel-on-et')*. Paraffi . gauze dressing consisting of specially woven (interlock) gauze impregnated with a soft paraffin mass for burns and wounds, etc.

جیولٹیٹ : پیرافین گاز ڈریسنگ۔

Jigger *(ji'-ger)* (Tunga penetrans). A flea, prevalent in the tropics. It burrows under the skin to la y its eggs, causing intense irritatin. Secondary infection is usual.

چچڑی : ٹنگاپینیٹریز۔ پسو۔ جلد کے نیچے سوراخ کر کے انڈے دیتا ہے۔ جس کی وجہ سے سخت سوزش ہوتی ہے۔

Joint. The articulation of two or more bones (arthrosis). There are three main classes: (1) fibrous (synarthrosis), e.g. the sutures of the skull; (2) cartilaginous (synchondrosis), e.g. between the manubrium and the body of the sternum; and (3) synovial, e.g. elbow or hip charcot's j., syphilitic degeneration of joint surfaces and surrounding structures. See CHARCOT.

Types of Joints

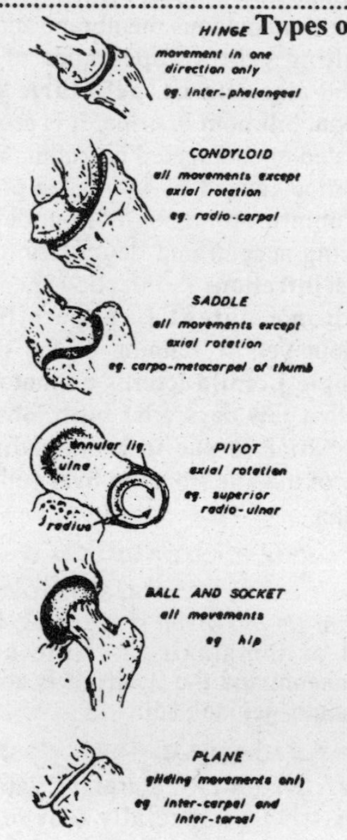

جوڑ : دو یا زیادہ ہڈیوں کا گھومنا۔ دو یا زیادہ ہڈیاں جہاں ملتی ہیں۔ اسے جوڑ کہتے ہیں جوڑ کی ہڈیوں کے سرے ریشے دار کیپسول میں بند ہوتے ہیں۔ جوڑ کے غلاف کے اندر جھلی میں لعاب پیدا ہوتا ہے جو چکناہٹ کا کام دیتا ہے۔ جوڑوں کی اقسام یہ ہیں۔ (۱) گولی اور پیالہ والا جوڑ یعنی بال وسباکٹ والا جوڑ جیسا کہ کولہے کا جوڑ اور شانہ کا جوڑ۔ (۲) قبضہ والا جوڑ جیسے کہنی اور ٹخنے کے جوڑ (۳) پھسلنے والا جوڑ جیسا کہ گھٹنے اور جبڑے کے جوڑ۔ (۴) گدی نما جوڑ جیسا کہ انگوٹھے کا جوڑ اور ہنسلی وسینے کی ہڈی کا جوڑ۔

Juole. The SI (International System of Units) unit for measuring energy, work and quantity of heat. The unit (J) is the energy expended when 1 kg (kilogram) is moved 1 m (metre) by a force of 1 N (newton). The kilojoule (kJ=10^3 J) and the megajoule (MJ = 10^6 J) is used by physiologists and nutritionists for large amounts of energy.

Joint-breaker fever Syn., o'nyong-nyong fever (q.v.).

جوڑ توڑ بخار : وائرس سے ہونے والا بخار، وائرس مچھر کے ذریعے جسم میں پہنچتا ہے۔ مشرقی افریقہ میں یہ مرض بہت زیادہ ہوتا ہے۔

Jugular *(jug'-u-lar)* [L. *jugulum,* collarbone]. Pertaining to the throat. j. veins, two veins passing down either side of the neck.

وداجی : گلے سے متعلق۔

Junket *(jun'-ket).* Milk predigested by the addition of rennet. Curds and whey.

پھٹا دودھ : دودھ جو رینٹ کے اضافہ کی وجہ سے پہلے ہی ہضم ہو جائے۔

Juxtaposition *(juks'-ta- po-zish-un)* [L. near; *position,* a placing]. The act of placing side by side.

پیوستگی : ساتھ ساتھ ملحقہ۔ بالکل نزدیک۔

Giiding Joint

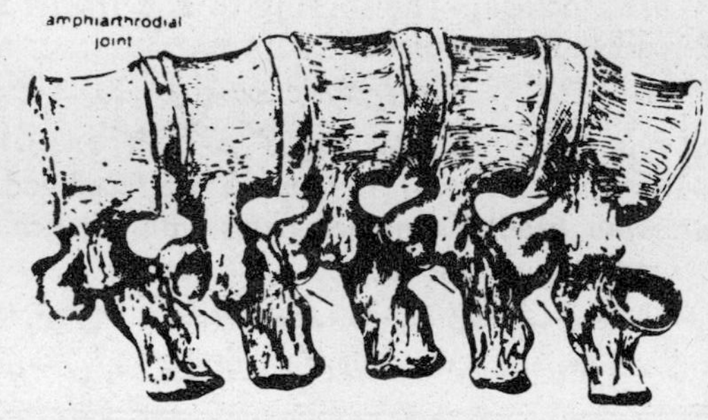

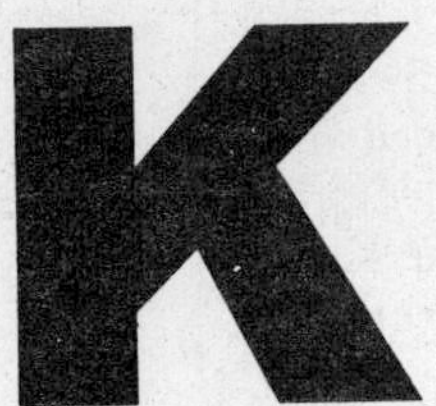

K Symbol for **potassium** [L. *kalium*]. Kelvin, equilibrium constant, kilo, Boltzman's constant & rate constant.

کے: علامت ہے پوٹاشیم (کیلیم)، کیلون، توازن کے مستقل، کلو، بالٹز مین کے مستقل اور شرح کے مستقل کی۔

(*keppa*) The tenth letter of Greek alphabet symbol for one of the two types of immunoglobulin light chains.

کے۔ کاپا: علامت جو کہ یونانی حروف تہجی کا دسواں حرف ہے اور امینوگلوبولن کی ہلکی زنجیروں میں سے ایک کی علامت۔

K_{285} Starch powder used in place of talc in rubber gloves. Its advantage is that granulome is not resulted in its use.

کے ۲۸۵: نشاستہ کا سفوف جو ربڑ کے دستانوں کے لئے ٹالک کے متبادل کے طور پر استعمال ہوتا ہے۔

Kaledana *(kal'-a-daina)* The dried seed of Ipomoeanill. It is used in India & China for its purgative and authemintic properties.

کالا دانہ: یہ اپومیائل کا خشک بیج ہے۔ انڈیا اور چین میں استعمال ہوتا ہے۔ یہ جلاب آور اور کیڑے مار دوا ہے۔

Kalagua *(ka-lah-gwa)* It is a drug used in South America for the treatment of tuberculosis.

کالاگوآ: ٹی بی کی دوا ہے۔ تپ دق کے لئے یہ جنوبی امریکا میں استعمال کی جاتی ہے۔

Kaliuresis *(ka-le-u-re-sis)* [L. *kalium*, potassium; G. *ouresis*, a making water]. The excretion of potassium in the urine.

کالیوریسس: پیشاب میں پوٹاشیم کا خارج ہونا۔ یہ لاطینی لفظ کیلیم بمعنی پوٹاشیم اور یونانی لفظ اوریسیس بمعنی پیشاب کرنا سے ماخوذ ہے۔

Kanamycin *(kan-a-mi'-sin)* An aminuglycoside antibiotic complex derived from streptomyces kanamyseticus, consisting of three components designated A, B, & C. Common available form is a mixture of A & B. It is effective against aerobic gram negative bacilli and gram positive bacteria. It is also effective in T.B.

کینامائی سین: نیومائیسین جیسا۔ تپ دق کے لئے استعمال کیا جاسکتا ہے۔ جدید اینٹی بائیوٹک ہے۔

Kaolin *(ka-o-lin)* A hydrated aluminiam silicate, powdered and freed from gritty particles by elutriation. A soft white or yellowish white powder with a clay like taste, used as an adsorbent and in kaolin mixture.

گل چینی: قدرتی ایلومینیم سلیکیٹ۔ منہ کے ذریعہ دیا جائے تو زہریلے مادے کو جذب کرلیتا ہے۔ اس لئے خوراک کے زہریلے پن میں مفید ہے۔

Karyogenesis *(kar-e-o-jen-a-sis)* [G. *karyo-nal*, kernal; *genesis*, production]. The development of the nucleus of a cell.

نیوکلیس کا بننا: یونانی لفظ کیریو بمعنی مرکزہ اور جینیسز بمعنی بننا سے ماخوذ ہے۔ نیوکلیس یا مرکزے کا بننا۔

Karyolysis *(kar-e-ol-asis)* [G. *lysis*, dissolution] A form of necrobiosis in which the nucleus of a cell swells and gradually loses its chromatin.

نیوکلیس کا ٹوٹنا: یونانی لائیسز بمعنی ختم ہونا سے ماخوذ ہے۔ مرکزہ ٹوٹنے کا عمل جس میں خلیے کا مرکزہ پھول جاتا ہے اور آہستہ آہستہ کروماٹن ضائع کر دیتا ہے۔

Keller's operation For hallux valgus or rigidus.

Excision of the proximal half of the proximal. phalanx, plus any osteophytes and oxostoses on the metatarsal head. The toe is fixed in the corrected position; after healing a fibrous arthroplasty results.[William Lordan Keller, US Army surgeon (retired) of Washington, 1874-1959].

کیسلرز اپریشن : ایک اپریشن۔

Kelly-Paterson syndrome. Also called 'Plummer- Vinson syndrome' (q.v.).

کیلی پیٹرسن سنڈورم : سنڈورم کی ایک قسم۔

Kellin *(kel'-lin)*. Has properties similar to glyceryl trinitrate, and is given in angina pectoris.

کیسلن : خصوصیات کے لحاظ سے گلسرائل ٹرائی نائٹریٹ سے مشابہ۔

Kelocyanor *(kel-o-si'-an-or)* See COBALTEDETATE.

Keloid *(ke'-loid)* [G. *kelis,* spot; *eidos,* form]. An overgrowth of scar tissue, which may produce a contraction deformity.

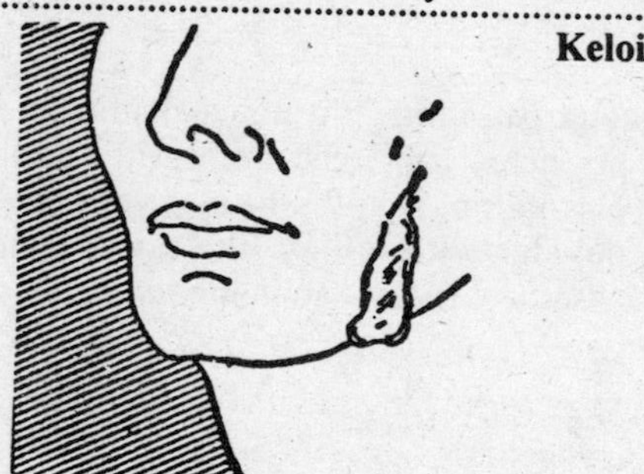

انگور : نشان زدہ نسیج کا زیادہ بڑھاؤ۔

Kemardrin *(ke'-ma-drin)*. Procyclidine (q.v.).

کیماڈرن : پروسائیکلیڈین۔ اس کی ایک گولی صبح ایک دوپہر ایک شام برائے پارکن سوزم یعنی رعشہ۔

Kemithal *(ke'-mi-thal)*. Thialbarbitone (q.v.).

کیمی تھیل : تھیل باربیٹون۔

Keratectomy *(ke-ra-tek'-to-mi)* [G. *keras,* horn; *ektome* excision]. Removal of a portion of the cornea.

قرنیہ براری : قرنیہ کے ایک حصے کا خاتمہ۔

Keratitic precipitates (KP) *(ker-a-ti'-tik pre-ip'-i-taz)*. Large cells adherent to posteri surface of cornea; present in inflammation iris, ciliary body and choroid.

کے پی : بڑے خلیے جو قرنیہ کی خلفی سطح کے ساتھ ہوتے ہیں۔ آئرس۔
بی۔ جسم اور کورائڈ کی سوزش میں موجود۔

Keratin *(ker'-a-tin)* [G. *keras,* horn]. A protei found in all horny tissue. Used to coat pil given for their intestinal effect, since k. ca withstand gastric juice.

راتین : تمام ہارنی نسیج میں پائی جانے والی پروٹین۔

Keratinization *(ker-a t-in-iz-a'-shun)* [G. kera horn]. Conversion into horny tissue .Occu as a pathological process in vitamin deficiency.

رنیت : ہارنی نسیج میں تبدیلی۔

Keratitis *(ke-ra-ti'-tis)* [G. *keras,* horn; -itis, in lammation]. Inflammation of the cornea.

رم قرنیہ : قرنیہ کی سوزش۔

Keratoconjunctivitis *(ker-a-to-kon-jung k-tiv-i'-tis)* [G. *keras,* horn; L. *conjunctivus* serving to connect; G. -itis, inflammation] Inflammation of the cornea and conjunctiva **epidemic k.,** due to an adenovirus (q.v.) Presents as an acute follicular conjunctiviti with pre-auricular and submaxillary adenitis **keratoconjunctivitis siccas,** see SJOGREN'S SYNDROME.

کیریٹوکنجیکٹیوٹیس : قرنیہ اور کنجیکٹیوا کی سوزش۔

Keratoconus *(ke-ra-to-ko'-nus)* [G. *keras,* horn *konos,* cone]. A cone-like protrusion of the cornea, usually due to a non-inflammatory thinning

مخروطی قرنیہ : قرنیہ کا مخروط نما ابھار۔

Keratoiritis *(ke-ra-to-i-ri'-tis)* [G. *keras,* horn, L. *iris,* rainbow; G. -itis, inflammation]. Inflamation of the cornea and iris.

قرنیتی قزحیتی التہاب : قرنیہ اور آئرس کی سوزش۔

Keratolytic *(ke-ra -tol'-i-tic)*. Having the property of breaking down keratinized epidermis.

کیریٹولائی سس : اپی ڈرمس کا جھڑنا۔

Keratoma *(ke-ra-to'-ma)* [G. *keras,* horn; *-oma,* tumour]. An overgrowth of horny tissue. Callosity--keratomata, pl.

قرنی سلعہ :ہارنی نسیج کا ایک زائد بڑھاؤ۔

Keratomalacia *(ke-ra -to-mal-a'-se-a)* [G. *keras,* horn; *malakia,* softness]. Softening of the cornea; ulceration may occur; frequently caused by lack of vitamin A.

لینت قرنیہ : قرنیہ کا نرم ہونا۔ السر ہوسکتا ہے۔ عموماً وٹامن اے کی کمی سے ہوتا ہے۔

Keratome *(ker'-a-tom)* [G. *keras,* horn; *tomos,* cutting]. A special knife with a trowel-like blade for incising the cornea.

قرنیہ تراش : قرنیہ کے اپریشن کے لئے ایک مخصوص چاقو۔

Keratomileusis *(ker-a-to-mil-u'-sis)* [G. *keras,* born; *mileusis,* to carve]. Surgical treatment for correction of myopia.

کیریٹومیلوسس :دوری نگاہ کی کمزوری کے لئے سرجیکل علاج۔

Keratopathy *(ke-ra-top'-a-thi)* [G. *keras,* horn; *pathos,* disease]. Any disease of the cornea --keratopathic, a dj.

مرض قرنیہ :قرنیہ کی کوئی بیماری۔

Keratophakia *(ker-a-to-fak'-i-a)* [G. *keras,* horn; *phakos,* lentil (lens)]. Surgical treatment for correction of hypermetropia.

کیریٹوفیکیا :ہائپر میٹروپیا کی تصحیح کے لئے سرجیکل علاج۔

Keratoplasty *(ke-ra-to-plas'-ti)* [G. *keras,* horn; *plassein,* to form]. Corneal grafting. Replacing of unhealthy tissue with healthy tissue obtained from a donor--keratoplastic, adj.

قرنیہ پیوندی : قرنیہ کی پیوندکاری۔ غیر صحت مند نسیج کی جگہ صحت مند نسیج لگانا جو کسی دوسرے شخص سے حاصل کیا جاتا ہے۔

Keratosis *(ke-ra-to'-sis)* [G. *keras,* horn; *-osis,* condition]. Theickening of the horny layer of the skin. Also referred to as 'hyperkeratosis.' Has appearance of warty excrescences. **keratosis palmaris et plantaris** (or tylosis) is a congenital thickening of the horny layer of the palms and soles. **splar k.** (Peasant's neck) is a form of chronic dermatitis on exposed areas and is a reaction to excessive sunlight.

قرنیت : جلد کی ہارنی تہہ کا دبیز ہونا۔

Kerecid *(ker'-e-sid).* Idoxuridine (q.v.).

کیریسڈ :اڈوکسورڈین۔

Kerion *(ke'-ri-on)* [G. *kerion,* honey-comb]. A boggy suppurative mass of the scalp associated with ringworm of the hair.

چھتے داردانے :بالوں کے رنگ ورم کے ساتھ جلد سر۔

Kernicterus *(ker-nik'-ter-us).* Bile staining of the basal ganglia in the brain which may result in mental deficiency, and occurring in icterus gravis neona torum (q.v.).

کرنکٹیرس : دماغ میں اساسی ابھاروں کی بائیل سٹیننگ۔

Kerning's sign *(ker'-nigs).* Inability to straighten the leg at the knee joint when the thigh is flexed at right angles to the trunk. Occurs in meningitis. [Vladimir Kerning, Russian physicina, 1840-1917].

علامت کرنگ : گھٹنے کے جوڑ پر ٹانگ سیدھی کرنے کی نااہلیت۔

Ketalar *(ket'-al-ar).* Ketamine hydrochloride (q.v.).

کٹیلیر : کیٹلامین ہائیڈروکلورائیڈ۔

Ketamine Hydrochloride *(ket'-a-men-hi-dro-klor'-id).* Intravenous or intramuscular ana esthetic agent. Initial dose determined by patient's weight. Does not have muscurla relaxation properties and is therefore unsuitable for intra-abdominal procedures.

کیٹامین ہائیڈروکلورائیڈ : ٹیکے کے ذریعے سن کرنے والا عامل۔

Ketogenic diet *(ke-to-jen'-ik).* A high fat content producing ketosis (acidosis).

کیتون زاغذا : چربی کی زیادہ مقدار ہونا۔

Ketonaemia *(ke-ton-e'-mi-a)* [Ger' *keton;* G. *haima,* blood]. Ketone bodies in the blood--ketona emic, adj.

کیتون الدم :خون میں کیتون اجسام۔

Ketone *(ke-ton).* K. bodies in ketosis (q.v.). Also used of the CO group (carbonyl) in the structural formulae of organic compounds, e.g. ketosteroids (q.v.).

کیتون : کیٹوسس میں کیتون اجسام۔ نامیاتی مرکبات کا سلسلہ۔

Ketouria *(ke-ton-u-ri-a)* [Ger,keton; G. ouron, urine]. Ketone bodies in the urine--ketonuric, adj.

کیتون بولی: پیشاب میں کیتون۔

Ketonuria *(ke-ton-u'-ri-a)* [Ger. *keton*; G. *-osis*, condition]. Clinical picture arises from accumulation in blood stream of ketone bodies, *B*hydroxybutyric acid, acetoacetic acid and acetone. Syndrome includes drowsiness, headache and deep respiration--ketotic, a dj.

کیتونیت : خون میں کیتون اجسام' ایسٹیو ایسٹیک ایسڈ اور ایسیٹون کے جمع ہونے سے ابھرنے والی کلینکل پکچر۔

Ketosteroids *(ke-to-ste'-roids)*. Steroid hormones which contain a keto group, formed by the addition of an oxygen molecule to the basic ringstructure. The 17-ketosteroids (which have this oxygen at carbon 17) are excreted in normal urine, and are present in excess in overa ctivity of the adrenal glands and the gonads.

کیٹوسٹیرائڈز : سٹیرائڈز ہارمونز جن میں ایک کیٹو گروہ ہوتا ہے اور بنیادی رنگ ساخت میں آکسیجن کے ایک سالمے کے اضافہ سے بنتے ہیں۔

Ketovite *(ket'-ȯ-vit)*. Tablets and liquid. Contains vitamins A, D, C, B12, B6, B2, B1, folic acid, nicotinamide, calcium pantothenate, inositol, boitin, acetomenaphthone, tocopheryl acetate and choline chloride.

کیٹووائیٹ : مائع اور گولیوں کی صورت میں دستیاب بہت سے وٹامنز پر مشتمل۔

Kidneys *(kid-niz)*. Two glands situated in the upper, posterior abdominal cavity, one on either side of the vertebral column. Their function is to secrete urine.

Urinary organs

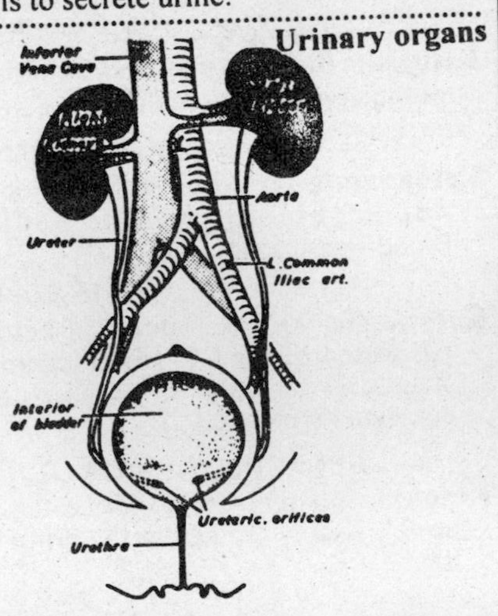

گردے : بالائی، خلفی، بطنی، کہفہ میں واقع دو گلینڈز ریڑھ کی ہڈی کے دونوں طرف۔ ان کا کام پیشاب خارج کرنا ہے۔ دایاں گردہ بائیں گردے کی نسبت ذرا نیچے ہوتا ہے۔ ان کی لمبائی اوپر سے نیچے کی طرف ۱۲ سنٹی میٹر یا ۴½ انچ چوڑائی، ۷ سنٹی میٹر یا ۲½ انچ اور موٹائی ۴ سے یا ۱½ انچ ہوتی ہے گردوں کے گرد کچھ مقدار چربی کی ہوتی ہے۔ دائیں گردے کے اوپر گلینڈ رینل گلینڈ ہوتی ہے۔ گردوں کے گرد ایک کیپسول ہوتا ہے۔

Killian's operation. Curetting of the fronta sinus, leaving the supraorbital ridge intact t reduce deformity. [Gustav Killian, Germa laryngologist and rhinologist, 1860-1921].

پریشن کلیان : ایک اپریشن۔

Kimmelstiel-Wilson syndrome Intercapillar glomerulosclerosis present in diabetics, wit hypertension, albuminuria and oedema. [Pa Kimmelstiel, German pathologist, 1900. Cli ford Wilson, English physician. 1906].

ل سٹائل ولسن سنڈورم : ذیابیطس کے مریضوں میں موجود بین شعری میرولوسکلیروسس۔

Kenaesthesis *(ki-nes-the'-sis)* [G. *kinein*, move; *aisthesis*, sensation]. Muscle sens perception of movement--kinaesthetic, adj.

س حرکت عضلہ : عضلاتی حس۔

Kinase *(ki'-nas)*. An enzyme-activator. Sy co-enzyme. See ENTEROKINASE, TH OMBOKINASE.

ں کارخمیر : خامرہ کو عامل بنانے والا۔

Kineplastic surgery *(ki-ne-plas'-tik sur'-jer-* Operative measures, whereby certain mus groups are isolated, and utilized to work ce ain modified prostheses.

ین پلاسٹک سرجری : اپریشن کے ایسے اقدامات جن سے بعض اتی گروہ علیحدہ ہوجاتے ہیں۔

Kinetic *(kin'-et-it)* Pertaining to, or produci motion.

ں : حرکت یا حرکت پیدا کرنے سے متعلق۔

Kirschner wire *(kirsch'-ner)*. A wire drilled i a bone to apply skeletal traction. A hand electric drill is used, a stiurup attached the wire rendered tuat by means of a spe wire- tightener. [Martin Kirschner, Ger surge- on, 1879-1942].

کرشنز تار : استخوانی ٹریکشن کے لئے ہڈی میں کھینچی گئی تار۔

ss of life Method of artificial respiration. Exhaled breath of operator inflates the patient's lungs. Routes: (1) mouth to mouth; (2) mouth to nose; (3) mouth to nose and mouth.

بوسۂ تار۔ مصنوعی عمل تنفس : مصنوعی تنفس کا طریقہ۔ اپریٹر کا بیرونی جانب سانس مریض کے پھیپھڑوں کو پھلا دیتا ہے۔ (۱) منہ سے منہ (۲) منہ سے ناک (۳) منہ سے ناک اور منہ۔

bsiella Genus of bacteria . *Klebsiella pneumoniae* is the cause of a rare form of pneumonia. See FRIEDLANDER'S BACILLUS.

ebs-Loeffler bacillus (syn., *Corynebacterium diphtheriae)*. A clinicolaboratory term for the diphtheria bacillus named after the discoverers of the organism. [Theodor Klebs, German bacteriologist, 1834-1913. Friedrich A. J. Loeffler, German bacteriologist. 1852-1915].

جرثومۂ خناق : ایک جرثومہ۔

ptomania *(klep-to-ma'-ni-a)* [G. *kleptein,* to steal; *mania,* madness]. Compulsive stealing due to mental disturbance, usually of the obsessional neurosis type.

چوری کا جنون : دماغی خرابی کے سبب چوری کرنا۔

nefelter's syndrome A person with 44 autosomes and XXY sex chromosomes, making a total complement of 47. Individual appears to be male, but he has large breasts, small genitalia , atrophied testes and is sterile. Genetic female, pragmatic male. Increased height apparent before puberty. It is possible that the violence and aggression have an organic basis which may be reflected in the EEG. Commonly recognized only in adult life sterility clinic.

کلائین فیلٹر سنڈورم : ایسا شخص جس میں چوالیس آٹوسوم اور تین کروموسوم یعنی ایک ایکس وائی ہوں اس طرح کل سنتالیس کروموسوم ہوں ایک زائد کروموسوم۔ ایکس کروموسوم کی زیادتی فرد زکھائی دیتا ہے چھاتیاں بڑی ہوتی ہیں۔ نامرد ہوتا ہے۔

mpke's paralysis Paralysis and atrophy of muscles of forearm and hand, with sensory and pupillary disturbances due to injury to cervical sympathetic nerves. Clawhand results [Madame Klumpke, French neurologist, 1859-1927].

فالج کلمپکے : ہاتھ اور اس کے ساتھ والے بازو کے حصے کے عضلات کا فالج اور اثرانی۔

Knee. The hinge joint formed by the lower end of the femur and the head of the tibia. **knee cap,** the patella . **knee jerk,** a reflex contraction of the relaxed quadriceps muscle elicited by a tap on the patellar tendon; usually performed with the lower femur supported behind. the knee bent and the leg limp. Persistent varia tion from normal usually signifies organic nervous disorder.

Knee joint

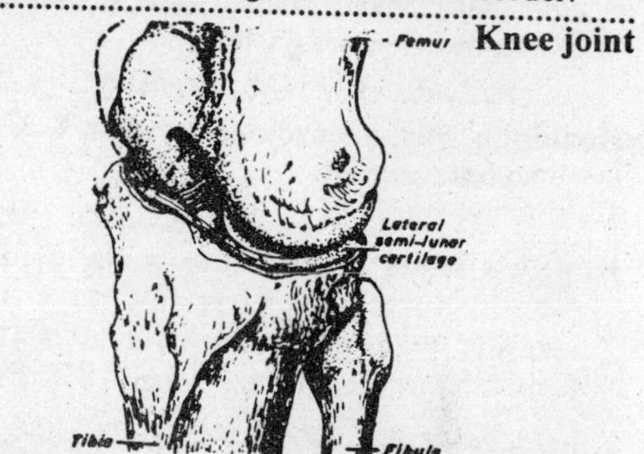

زانو۔ گھٹنا: ٹیبیا کے سر اور فیمر کے زیریں سرے سے بننے والا جوڑ۔ اس جوڑ پر گھٹنے کے موڑنے یا گھولنے کی حرکت ہوتی ہے۔

Knuckles *(nuk'-ls)*. The doresal aspect of any of the joints between the phalanges and the metacarpal bones, or between the phalanges.

بند انگشت: پوروں کے درمیان یا پوروں اور میٹا کارپل ہڈیوں کے درمیان جوڑوں میں سے کسی ایک کی ڈارسل صورت۔

Koch's bacillus (Syn., *Mycobacterium tuberculosis)*. A term used for the tubercle bacillus in clinicolaboratory parlance and named after Koch, who first described the bacillus. [Robert Koch, German bacteriologist, 1843-1910].

کاکس بیسلس : مائیکو بیکٹریم ٹیوبرکولوسس۔ تپ دق کا جرثومہ۔ اس کا نام جرمن ماہر جراثیم رابرٹ کاک کے نام پر رکھا گیا ہے۔

Koch-Weeks bacillus (Syn., *haemophilus*

aegyptius). A small Gram-negative rod, characteristically intracellular in polymorphs in exudate. The cause of a form of acute infectious conjunctivitis. [Robert Koch, German bacteriologist, 1843-1910. John E. Weeks, American ophthalmologist, 1853-1949].

کاک ویکس بیسلس : ایک چھوٹا گرام منفی سلاخی جرثومہ۔

Kohler's disease *(ke'-lers).* Osteochondritis of the navicular bone. Confined to children of 3 to 5 years. [Alban Kohler, German physician, 1874-1947].

مرض کوہلر۔ورم عظم کعب: ہڈیوں کا ایک مرض۔

Koilonychia *(koil-o-nik'-i-a)* [G. *koilos,* hollow; *onyx,* nail]. Spoon-shaped nails, characteristic of iron deficiency a naemia.

قعری ناخن : چمچ نما ناخن جو خون میں لوہے کی کمی سے ہو جاتے ہیں۔

Konakion. Phytomenadione. Vitamin K. Can be given intravenously.

کون کیون : وٹامن 'کے' بذریعہ ٹیکہ دیا جا سکتا ہے۔

Koplik's spots Small white spots inside the mouth, during the first few days of the invasion (prodromal) stage of measles. [Henry Kopik, New York paediatrician, 1858-1927].

کوپلکس سٹاپ: خسرہ والے حملہ کے مرحلہ کے پہلے چند ایام کے دوران منہ کے اندر چھوٹے سفید نشان۔

Korsakoff's psychosis or-syndrome. A condition which follows delirium and toxic states. Often due to alcoholism. The consciousness is clear and alert, but the patient is disorientated for time and place. His memory is grossly impared, especially for recent events. Often he confabulates to fill the gaps in his memory. Alcoholic dementia. Polyneuritic psychosis. Afflicts more men than women in the 45-55 age group. [Sergei S. Korsak off, Russian neurologist, 1854-1900].

ہذیانی کیفیت : الکحل کی وجہ سے زہریلے پن کی حالت۔

Krabbe's disease. Genetically determined degenerative disease associated with mental subnormality. [Knud H. Krabbe, Danish neurologist.

کربیز مرض: ذہنی پسماندگی کا ایک مرض۔

Kraurosis vulvae *(kraw-ro'-sis-vul-ve)* degenerative condition of the vaginal introi associted with postmenopausal lack oestrogen.

دگی (فروج) : ویجائینل انٹرائٹس کی تباہ کن حالت۔

Krukenberg tumour *(kroo'-ken-kerg).* secondary malignant tumour of the ovary. primary growth is usually in the stoma [Friedrich Ernst Krukenberg, German pa ologist, 1871 , 1946].

بز مرض : ذہنی پسماندگی کا ایک مرض۔

Kraurosis vulvae *(kraw-ro'-sis vul'-ve)* secondary malignant tumour of the ovary. primary growth is usually in the stom [Friedrich Ernst Krukenberg, German pat ogist, 1871-1946].

ن برگ سلعہ : بیضہ دان کا ثانوی ناسور۔اولی بڑھاؤ عموماً معدہ تا ہے۔

Kuntscher nail Used for intramedul fixation of fractures of long bones, espec the femur. The nail has a 'clover-leaf' c section. [Gerhard Kuntscher, orthopa surgeon of Kiel, 1902].

نیل : طویل ہڈیوں خصوصاً فیمر کے فریکچر کو ٹھیک کرنے کے لئے

Kuru *(koo'-roo).* Slow virus disease of ce nervous system. Probably transmitte cannibalism. Rare and declining in incid Occurred exclusively among New Gu highlanders.

: وائرس کی بیماری خصوصاً نیو گنی میں ہوتی ہے۔عموماً مہلک۔

Kwashiokor *(kwash-e-or'-kor).* A nutrit disorder of infants and young children the diet is persistently deficient in esse protein; commonest in primitive tropical where maize is the staple diet. Cha racte features are anaemia, wasting, deper oedema and a fatty liver. Untreate progresses to death.

رکور : چھوٹے اور نوعمر بچوں میں خوراک کی گڑبڑ جب غذا میں مستقل ی پروٹین کم ہو۔

KY jelly. A mucilaginous lubrica ting jelly

کے وائی جیلی : جیلی کی ایک قسم۔

mograph *(ki'-mo-graf)* [G. *kyma* wave; *graphein,* to write]. An apparatus for recording movements, e.g. of muscles, columns of blood. Used in physiological experiments--kymogra phic, adj.; kymographically, adv.

نبض شمار : حرکات ریکارڈ کرنے کیلئے سامان۔

pholordosis *(ki-fo-lor-do'-sis)* Co-existence of kyphosis and lordosis (q.v.).

کائیفو لارڈوسس : کفوسس اور لورڈوسس کا اکٹھے ہونا۔

Kyphoscoliosis *(ki-fo-skol'-i-o-sis).* Coexistence of kyphosis and scoliosis (q.v.).

کوزالتوا : کفوسس اور سکولیوسس کا اکٹھے ہونا۔

Kyphosis *(ki-fo'-sis)* [G. hunch-backed]. As in Pott's disease, an excessive backward curvature of the dorsal spine.

کوزپشتی ۔ کبڑاپن : ڈارسل سپائن کا پیچھے کی طرف زیادہ خم۔

L

L Symbol for lambert, liter, length.

ایل: علامت ہے لیمبرٹ، لٹر اور لمبائی کی۔

λ *(lambda)* The eleventh letter of the Greek alphabet. Symbol for wavelength, decay constant and one of the two types of immunoglobulin light chains, former symbol for microliter.

لیمبڈا: یونانی حروف تہجی کا گیارہواں حرف۔ ویولینتھ، تابکاری کے مستقل کی علامت ہے۔ امینوگلوبولن کی ہلکی زنجیر کی علامت بھی ہے۔

Labetalol *(la-bet-a-lol)* A beta advenergic & alpha adrenergic blocking agent. It is a good anti-hypertensive drug.

لابیٹالول: بیٹا اور الفا بلاکنگ عامل ہے۔ دونوں گروہ ہونے کی وجہ سے بلند فشار خون کے لئے بہترین دوا ہے۔

Labia *(la-be-a)* [L.]. A fleshy border or edge, used in anatomical nomenclature as a general term to designate such a structure. In the plural often used alone to designate the labia majora and minora pudencli.

شفتین فرج: ہونٹ۔ مثلاً ویجائنا کے گرد پائے جانے والے دو بڑے لب یا ان کے اندر پائی جانے والی دو چھوٹی تہیں۔ بیرونی لب بڑے اور واضح ہوتے ہیں۔ بلوغت کے وقت ان پر بال اگتے ہیں۔ یہ زیادہ حساس نہیں ہوتے۔ ان کے اندر اندرونی لب، پردۂ بکارت، بظر، سوراخ، فرج اور بولی سوراخ ہوتے ہیں۔ کنواری لڑکیوں میں یہ لب ایک دوسرے سے کافی ملے ہوتے ہیں لیکن مباشرت کے بعد یہ لب ایک دوسرے سے جدا ہو جاتے ہیں۔

Labialism *(la-be-al-izm)* Defective speech, with use of labial sounds.

نقص آواز: بولنے میں نقص ہونا۔ صرف ہونٹوں سے آواز نکال کر بولنے کی

ش کرنا۔

Labile *(la-bi'l)* [L. *lobilis,* unstable]. Glidi moving from point to point over the surf unstable, fluctuating, chemically unstable.

پذیر، ناپائیدار: ناپائدار۔ بدلی ہوئی جیسا کہ ادویات محلول میں اکثر جاتی ہیں۔

Lability *(la-bil-e-te)* The quality of being stable in psychiatry emotional instabili rapidly changing emotions.

ن مزاجی: ناپائداری۔ مزاج میں اچانک تبدیلی آجانا۔ ایسا عموماً پے میں ہوتا ہے۔ اس کا سبب ذہنی خلفشار بھی ہوسکتا ہے۔

Labioglossolaryngeal *(la-be-o-glos-o-lar- je-al)* [L. *labium,* lip; *glossa,* tongue]. Pert ing to the lips, tongue and larynx. **l. par sis,** a nervous disease characterized progressive paralysis of the lips, tongue larynx.

ں کا فالج: ہونٹوں کے پٹھوں کی مرضی سے حرکت میں رکاوٹ۔

Labioglossopharyngeal *(la-be-o-glos-o-fa- je-al)* Pertaining to the lips, tongue and p ynx.

، لسانی، حلقومی: لبوں، زبان اور فیرنکس کے متعلق۔

Labiomycosis *(la-be-o-mi'-ko-sis)* [L. *lab* lip]. Any disease of lip due to fungus, suc thrush.

کی بیماری: فنجائی کی وجہ سے ہونٹوں کی بیماری۔ جیسے تعرش۔

Labyrinthitis *(lab-ir-in-thi'-tis)* [G. *labyrin* labyrinth; *-itis,* inflammation]. Inflamma of the internal ear, Syn., otitis interna.

ورم تیر۔سوزش تیہ :اندرونی کان کی سوزش۔

Laceration *(las-er-a'-shun)* [L. *lacerare,* to tear]. A wound with torn and ragged edges- lacerate, v.t.

جراحت۔چیر پھاڑ:پھٹے ہوئے کناروں والا زخم۔

Lachesine *(lash'-es-en).* E3. An alternative mydriatic in atropine sensitivity.

لیشن ایسائین :ایٹروپین حسیت میں ایک متبادل۔ای ۳۔

Lachrymal *(lak'-ri-mal).* Also spelt lacrymal. See LACRIMAL.

اشکی : آنسوؤں سے متعلق۔کوئے کی ہڈی۔یہ چہرے کی سب سے چھوٹی ہڈیاں ہوتی ہیں۔ہر آنکھ کی اندرونی دیوار کے سامنے کے حصے میں ایک نالی ہوتی ہے۔اس کے ذریعہ آنسو آنکھوں سے ناک میں پہنچ جاتے ہیں۔

Lacrimal *(lak'-ri-mal)* [L. *lacrima,* a tear]. Pertaining to tears. **lacrimal bone,** a tiny bone at the inner side of the orbital cavity. **lacrimal duct,** connects I. gland to upper conjunctival sae. **lacrimal gland,** situated above the upper. outer canthus of the eye.

اشکی :آنسوں سے متعلق۔

Lacrimation *(lak-ri-ma'-shun).* An outflow of tears; weeping.

کثرت اشک :آنسوؤں کا بہہ نکلنا۔رونا۔

Lacrimonasal *(lak-ri-mo-na'-zal)* [L. *lacrima,* tear; *nasus,* nose]. Pertaining to the lacrimal and nasal bones and ducts.

لیکریمونیزل :لیکریمل،نیزل ہڈیوں اور نالیوں سے متعلق۔

Lactagogue *(lak'-ta-gog)* [L. *lac,* milk; G. *agogos,* leading]. Any substance to stimulate lactation; none are very effective as yet.

مدرلبن۔شیر افزاء: دودھ کو تحریک دینے والی شے۔دودھ اتارنے والی دوائی۔

Lactalbumin *(lakt-al-bu'-min)* [L.*lac,* milk; *albumen,* egg-white]. The more easily digested of the two milk proteins. See CASEINOGEN.

شیری البومین۔زلال لبن: زیادہ آسانی سے ہضم ہونے والی دودھ کی دو پروٹینز۔

Lactase *(lak'-tas).* A saccharolytic enzyme of intestinal juice; it splits lactose into glucose (dextrose) and galactose.

شیر پاش۔لکتاز :ایک خامرہ جو لکٹوز کو گلوکوس میں تبدیل کرنے کیلئے عمل انگیزی کرتا ہے۔ممالیہ کے ہضمی رسوں میں موجود ہوتا ہے۔آنت کے جوس کا سیکرولائیٹک خامرہ۔لیکٹوز شیر پاش گلوکوس (ڈیکسٹروز)+ گلیکٹوز۔

Lactase deficiency Clinical syndrome of milk intolerance. In severe intolerance the infant may pass a litre or more of fluid stool per day. Temporary intolerance can follow neonatal alimentary tract obstructions, but rarely gives long term problems.

Lactate dehydrogenase *(lak'-tat de-hid-r-oj'-en-as).* An enzyme of which there are five versions (isozymes) in the body. LDH-I is the one in the heart; its blood level rises rapidly when heart tissue dies. After heart transplant, rejection is imminent wh3en the LDH-1 activity is greater than that of its isozyme LDH-2 during the first 4 post-operative weeks. After 6 months this diagnostic indication disappears.

لکتات ڈیہائیڈروجینز :خامرہ جس کی جسم میں پانچ اقسام ہیں۔

Lactation *(lak-ta'-shun)* [L. *lactare,* to suckle]. Secretion of milk Suckling; the period during which the child is nourished from the breast.

شیر آوری : دودھ کا اخراج۔دودھ پلانا۔وہ عرصہ جس کے دوران بچے کو چھاتی سے دودھ پلایا جاتا ہے۔

Lacteals *(lak'-te-als)* [L. *lac,* milk]. The commencing lymphatic ducts in the intestinal villi; they absorb split fats and convey them to the receptaculum chyli.

عروق لبنیہ : آنت کی ولائی میں واقع لمفیٹک نالیاں جو لمف کو جمع کرتی ہیں جس میں ہضم شدہ چکنائی کے اجزاء زیادہ پائے جاتے ہیں۔اس لئے اس کی رنگت سفید ہوتی ہے۔

Lactic acid *(lak'-tik as'-id).* The acid that causes the souring of milk. It is obtained by the fermentation of lactose; used as a vaginal douche, 1 per-cent. Sometimes added to milk (1 drachm to 1 pint) to produce fine curds for the treatment of gastroenteritis in infants.

دودھ کا تیزاب :ایک بے رنگ قلمی نامیاتی تیزاب،نقطۂ پگھلاؤ ۱۸°س۔یہ لیکٹوز کی تخمیر سے حاصل ایک ہے۔ویجائنل ڈوش کے طور پر ایک فیصد استعمال کیا جاتا ہے۔بچوں میں انتڑیوں کی بیماری کے علاج کے لئے دودھ میں ڈالا جاتا ہے۔

Lactiferous *(lak-tif'-er-us)* [L. *lac,* milk; *ferre,* to carry]. Conveying or secreting milk.

شیرآور : دودھ پیدا کرنا۔

Lactifuge *(lak'-te-fuj)* [L. *lac,* milk; *fugare,* to put to flight]. Any agent which suppresses milk secretion.

مانع افروزلین : اخراج شیر کو کم کرنے والا عامل۔ دودھ خشک کرنے والی دوا۔

Lactobacillus *(lak-to-bas-il'-us).* A genus of bacteria. A large Gram-positive rod which is active in fermenting carbohydrates, producing acid. No members are pathogenic.

لیکٹوبےسلس : جراثیم کا ایک جنس۔ ایک بڑا گرام مثبت سلاخی جرثومہ جو کاربوہائیڈریٹس کی تخمیر کر کے ایسڈ بناتا ہے۔ اس کے اراکین مرض پیدا نہیں کرتے۔ یہ آنتوں میں پائے جاتے ہیں۔ حرکت نہیں کرتے۔ سپورز نہیں بناتے۔ دودھ سے دہی بناتے ہیں۔ دہی معدے اور آنتوں کے دوسرے جراثیم مارنے میں مدد دیتا ہے اس لئے آنتوں کے امراض میں مفید ہے۔

Lactoflavin *(lakL-to-fla-vin).* Riboflavin (q.v.).

لکٹوفلیون : ریبوفلیون

Lactogenic *(lak'-to-jen-ik)* [L. *lac,* milk; G. *genesthai* to be produced]. Stimulating milk production. See LUTEOTROPHIN.

لکٹوجینک۔ شیراز : دودھ کی پیداوار کو تحریک دینا۔

Lactometer *(lak-tom'-et-er)* [L. *lac,* milk; G. *metron,* a measure]. An instrument for measuring the specific gravity of milk.

شیرپیا۔ مقیاس۔ اللبن : دودھ کے وزن مخصوص کی پیمائش کے لئے آلہ۔

Lactose *(lak'-tos).* Milk sugar. Less soluble and less sweet than ordinary sugar. Used in infant feeding to increase the carbohydrate content of diluted cow's milk. In some infants the gut is intolerant to lactose. See LACTASE. In severe intolerance the infant may pass a litre or more of fluid stool per day. Temporary intolerance can follow neonatal alimentary tract obstructions, but rarely gives long-term problems.

قندشیر۔ شکرشیر۔ لیکٹوز : ملک شوگر۔ ایک سخت قلمی حل پزیر ڈائی سیکرائڈ نقطۂ پگھلاؤ ۲۰۳ س گنے کی شکر سے کم شیریں۔ یہ سکر دودھ میں پائی جاتی ہے۔ لیکٹوز یا قند شیر دودھ پر بعض جراثیم کے عمل میں لیکٹک ایسڈ میں تبدیل ہو جاتا ہے۔ کھانڈ جو ماں اور گائے کے دودھ میں قدرتی طور پر پائی جاتی ہے عام کھانڈ سے ڈیڑھ گنا زیادہ استعمال کرنا پڑتی ہے۔

Lactosuria *(lak-to-su'-ri-a)* [L. *lac,* milk; G *ouron,* urine]. Lactose in the urine--lactosuric adj.

شیرقندبولی : پیشاب میں لیکٹوز۔

Lacuna *(la-ku'-na)* [L. cavity]. A space between cells; sinus--lacunae, pl.; lacunar, adj.

[...]وف : خلیوں کی درمیان جگہ۔

Laevulose *(lev'-u-los).* Fructose or fruit sugar sweeter and more easily digested tha[n] ordinary sugar, and is useful for diabetics also used as a test for hepatic function, as does not normally increase the blood suga[r] level, except in hepatic damage.

[...]پ گرداں شکر۔ قندمیوہ : فرکٹوز، فروٹ شوگر، عام شکر کی نسبت زیادہ [...]ریں اور آسانی سے ہضم ہونے والی شکر۔ ذیابیطس کے مریضوں کے لئے [...]ید۔ جگر کی خرابی کی صورت میں اس کی مقدار خون میں بڑھ جاتی ہے۔

Lambliasis *(lam-bli' a-sis).* Giardiasis (q.v.).

[...]بلیاسس : جیاڈیاسس۔

Lamella *(la-mel'-a)* [L. small plate]. A thi[n] plate-like scale or partition. A gelatine-coate[d] disc contanning a drug; it is inserted under t[he] eyelid--lamellae, pl.; lamellar, adj.

[...]قہ : ایک پتلا پلیٹ نما سکیل یا منقسم کرنے والا دوائی پر مشتمل ڈسک۔

Lamina *(lam'-in-a)* [L.]. A thin plate or lay[er] usually of bone--laminae, pl.

[...]قہ : ایک پتلی پلیٹ یا تہہ، عموماً ہڈی کی۔

Laminectomy *(lam-in-ek'-to-mi)* [L. *lamina,* thin plate; G. *ektome,* excision]. Removal [of] laminae of vertebrae-- to expose the spinal c[o]rd and menninges. Most often performed [in] lumbar region, for removal of degenerat[ed] invertebral disc.

[...]ہ براری : مہروں کے لیمنا کا خاتمہ۔

Lamprene *(lam'-pren).* Clofazimine (q.v.).

[...]رین : کلوفازمین

Lanatoside C. *(lan-at'-o-sid).* A glycoside [of] the Austrian foxglove, usually employed ntravenous injection when rapid digitaliz-ation is required. Oral therapy is less reliable.

لینٹوسائیڈسی : عموماً دروں وریدی ٹیکہ کے ذریعہ دیا جاتا ہے۔

ncefield's groups Subdivision of the genus Streptococcus on the basis of antigenic struc-ure. The members of each group have a characteristic capsular polysaccharide. The majority of streptococci of epidemiological mportance to man belong to Group A. [Rebe-cca Lancefield, New York bacteriologist, 1895].

لانس فیلڈ کے گروہ : اینٹی جینک ساخت کی بنیاد پر جنس سٹرپٹوکاکسز کی مزید تقسیم۔

nolin(e) *lan'-o-len).* wool fat containing 30 percent water. **anhydrosl,** is the fat obtained from sheep's wool. They are used in ointment bases, as such bases can form water-in-oil emulsions with aqueous constituents, and are readily absorbed by the skin. Adeps lanae hydrosus.

روغن پشم۔لانولین : موم ایسا مادہ۔اس میں کولسٹرول ہوتا ہے دوسر۔ مخلوط نامیاتی مادے بھی پائے جاتے ہیں۔جلد اسے فوراً جذب کر لیتی ہے مرہم اور کاسمیٹکس میں مستعمل ہے۔تیس فیصد پانی پر مشتمل ادن کی چکنائی۔

noxin *(lan-oks'-in).* Digoxin (q.v.).

ugo *(lan-u'-go)* [L. down]. The soft, downy hair often present on newborn infants, especially when they are premature.

پشم جنین : نرم رواں جو اکثر نوزائیدہ بچوں پر موجود ہوتا ہے۔یہ بال عمو بچے کے کندھوں اور کانوں پر ہوتے ہیں لیکن بچے کی ابتدائی زندگی کے چ ہفتوں ہی میں جھڑ جاتے ہیں۔

aroscopy *(lap-ar-os'-ko-pi)* [G. *lapara,* soft part of flank; skopein, to examine]. Endo-scopic examination of the pelvic organs by the transperitoneal coute. Laparoscope intr-oduced through the abdominal wall after ind-uction of a premoperitoneum. For biopsy, aspiration of cysts and division of adhesions. Tubal ligation for sterilization and even ven-osuspension can be performed via the lapa-roscope--laparoscopic, adj.; laparoscopic-ally, adv.

معدہ بینی : پلوک اعضاء کی انڈوسکوپک جانچ۔

Laparotomy *(lap-ar-ot'-o-mi)* [G. *lapara,* soft part of flank; *tome,* a cutting]. Incision of abdominal wall. (Usually reserved for exploratory operationo.

(دیوار) معدہ شگافی : بطنی دیوار کو کاٹنا۔پیٹ کے درمیان میں لمبا عمودی چیرا دے کر پیٹ کا اندرونی معائنہ کیا جاتا ہے اور نقص دور کیا جاتا ہے۔

Largactil *(lar-gak'-til).* Chlorpromazine (q.v.).

لارجیکٹل : کلورپرومازین قے روکنے کے لئے ایک گولی صبح ایک دوپہر ایک شام ہچکی روکنے کے لئے بھی مذکورہ خوراکیں یا ۲۵ ملی گرام کا عضلاتی ٹیکہ کولہے پر لگایئے۔

Laroxyl. Amitriptyline (q.v.). See ANTIDEPR-ESSANT.

بے روکسل : ایمی ٹرائی ٹائیلین۔

Larva *(lar'-va)* [L. *larva,* ghost]. An embryo which is independent before it has assumed the characteristic features of its parents. **larva migrans,** itching tracks in the skin with formation of blisters caused by the burrowing of larvae of some species of fly and normally animal-infesting Ancylostoma--larvae, pl.; larval, adj.

لاروا : ایک جنین جو آزاد ہو اس سے پہلے کہ اپنے والدین کی نمایاں خصوصیات حاصل کرے۔

Larvicide *(lar'-vi-sid)* [L. *larva,* ghost; L. *caedere,* to kill]. Any agent which destroys larvae--larvicidal, adj.

لارواکش دوا : لاروؤں کو تباہ کرنے والا عامل۔

Laryngeal *(lar'-in-jel)* [G. *largx.*] Pertaining to the larynx.

حنجری : لیرنکس سے متعلق۔

Larngectomy *(lar-in-jek'-to-mi)* [G. *larygx,* larynx; *ektome* excision]. Excision of the larynx.

حنجرہ براری : لیرنکس کا خاتمہ۔

Laryngismus stridulus *(lar-in-jis'-mus strid'-u-lus).* Momentary attack of laryngeal spasm as in infantile tetany associated with rickets.

خناق کاذب : لیرنجیل سپازم کا عارضی حملہ۔

Laryngitis *(lar-in-ji'-tis)* [G. *larygx,* larynx;

-*itis,* inflammation]. Inflammation of the larynx.

ورم حنجرہ : لیرنکس کی سوزش۔

Laryngofissure *(lar-in-go-fish'-ur)* [g. *larygx,* larynx; L. *fissura,* fissure]. The operation of opening the larynx in midline.

حنجرہ آشکاری : میانی لکیر میں لیرنکس کھولنے کا اپریشن۔

Laryngopharynx *(lar-in'-go-far'-ingks)* [G. *larygx,* larynx; *pharygx,* pharynx].The lower portion of the pharynx--laryngopharyngeal, adj.

حنجری بلعوم : فیرنکس کا زیریں حصہ۔

Laryngoscope *(lar-in'-go-skop)* [g. *larygx,* larynx; *skopein,* to examine]. Instrument for exposure and visualization of larynx--laryngoscopy, n.; laryngoscopic, adj.

حنجرہ بین : زخرے یا لیرنکس کو ظاہر کرنے والا آلہ۔

Laryngospasm *(lar'-in-go-spazm)*. Convulsive involuntary muscular contraction of the larynx, usually accompanied by spasmodic closure of the glottis.

حنجرہ کی اینٹھن۔ تشنج المزمار : زخرے یا لیرنکس کا بے ارادہ عضلاتی سکڑاؤ۔

Laryngologist *(lar-in-gol'-oj-ist)* [g. *larygx,* larynx; *logos,* discourse]. A specialist in laryngeal diseases.

ماہر حنجریات : لیرنجیل امراض کا ماہر۔

Laryngoparalysis *(lar-in'-go-par-al'-is-is)* [G. *larygx,* larynx; G. *paralysis*]. Paralysis of the larynx.

زخرے کا لقوہ : زکرے یا لیرنکس کا فالج زخرے کا لقوہ جو عصبی نوعیت کا ہو۔

Laryngopharyngetomy *(lar-in-go-far-in-je-k'-to-mi)*. [G. *larygx; pharygx; ektome,* excision]. Excision of the larynx and lower part of pharynx.

قطع حنجرہ و بلعوم : زخرے یا لیرنکس اور فیرنکس کے زیریں حصے کا انقطاع۔

Laryngostenosis *(lar-in-go-sta-no'-sis)* [G. *larygx,* larynx; *stenosis,* straitened]. Narrowing of the glottic aperture.

یق حنجرہ : گلاٹک سوراخ کا تنگ ہونا۔

Laryngotomy *(lar-in'-go-tra-ke'-al)* [G. *laryg* larynx; *trachus,* rough]. Pertaining to th larynx and trachea.

جرہ شگافی : زخرہ یا لیرنکس کھولنے کا اپریشن۔

Laryngotracheal *(lar-in'-go-tra-ke'-al)* [C *larygx,* larynx; *trachus,* rough]. Pertaining the larynx and trachea.

ری قصبی : زخرہ یا لیرنکس اور ٹریکیا سے متعلق۔

Laryngotracheitis *(lar-in-go-tra-e-i'-tis)* [C *larygx, trachus,* rought; -itis, inflammation Inflammation of the larynx and trachea.

م حنجرہ و قصبۃ الریہ : زخرہ یا لیرنکس اور ٹریکیا کی سوزش۔

Laryngotracheobronchitis *(lar-in-go-trak'-o-brong-ki-tis)* [g. *larygx,* larynx; *trachus,* rough; brogchos, windpipe; *-itis,* inflan mation]. Inflammation of the larynx, trach and bronchi.

لوٹریکیو برونکائی ٹس : زخرہ یا لیرنکس، ٹریکیا اور برونکائی کی سوزش۔

Larynx *(lar'-ingks)* [G. *larygx*]. The organ voice situated below and in front of th pharynx and at the upper end of the trachea laryngeal, adj.

رہ۔ زخرہ۔ آلۂ صوت : آواز کا عضو۔ سانس کی نالی کا ابتدائی حصہ کی دیواریں کرکری ہڈی کی ہوتی ہیں جو ایک دوسرے کے ساتھ عضلات رباط سے جڑی ہوتی ہیں۔ اندرونی سطح پر میوکس جھلی ہوتی ہے۔

Laser beam *(la-ser)*. Light Amplification Stimulated Emission of Radiation. Ener transmitted as heat that can coagulate tiss Has been used for detached retina and cance

ربیم : روشنی کی ایمپلیفیکیشن۔ علیحدہ ریٹنا اور سرطان کے لئے مستعمل۔

Lassa fever Previously an African mala diagnosed first in 1969; human beings ing food or water contaminated by rat excreme containing the arenavirus which can then transmitted from person to person. Strong suspected that primary cases are more high contagious than secondary ones, Incubati period 3 to 16 days, early symptoms resem typhoid and septicaemia. By the sixth d ulcers develop in the mouth and throat; fe is variable, sometimes being very hig

Fatality rate in some areas is as high as 67 percent. Infected people must be nursed in strict isolation.

ssar's paste *(las'-sars)*. Contains zinc oxide, starch and salicylic acid in soft paraffin. Used n eczema and similar conditions as an antiseptic protective.

لیسرس پیسٹ : نرم پیرافین میں زنک آ کسائیڈ نشاستہ اور سیلیسائیلک ایسڈ، خارش میں اور دافع تعفن کے لئے مستعمل۔

tent heal *(la'-tent)* [L. *latens* lying hidden]. That heat which is used to bring about a change in state, not in temperature.

مخفی حرارت : وہ حرارت جو حالت میں تبدیلی لانے کے لئے استعمال ہوتی ہے۔ تا کہ درجہ حرارت میں۔ حرارت کی وہ مقدار جو فیز کی آئیسوتھرمل تبدیلی میں جذب یا خارج ہو۔ پگھلاؤ اور پگھولاؤ کے نقطوں پر حرارت میں اضافہ کرنے سے درجہ حرارت بلند نہیں ہوتا جب تک حالت کی تبدیلی مکمل نہ ہو۔

teral *(iat'-e-ral)* [L. latus, side]. At or belonging to the side; away from the median the--laterally, adv.

جانبی : جو ایک طرف ہو۔

udanum *(lawd'-num)*. Old name for tincture of opium.

لودانم : افیون کی ٹنکچر کا پرانا نام۔

ghing gas Nitrous oxide.

خندہ آور گیس : نائٹرس آکسائیڈ ہنسانے والی گیس۔ ایک بے رنگ گیس۔ دندان سازی میں ہلکا پن سن کرنے کے لئے استعمال ہوتی ہے۔

vage *(lav-azh'-* [F.]. Irrigation of or washing out a body cavity.

غسل معدہ : جسمانی کہفہ کا غسل۔

xative *(laks'-a-tiv)*. A mild aperient.

ملین دوا : ہلکا جلاب لانے کے لئے دوا۔ قبض دور کرتی اور پاخانہ لاتی ہے لیکن زیادہ دست نہیں لگتے مثلاً فینا فتھے لین۔

H. Lactate dehydrogenase (q.v.).

ایل ڈی ایچ : لیکٹیٹ ڈیہائیڈروجینز۔

opa *(el-do'-pa)*. Levodopa (q.v.).

ایل ڈوپا : لیووڈوپا۔

d *(led)*. A metal, the salts of which are astringent when applied externally.

سیسہ : ایک عنصر جوہری وزن ۲۰۷،۱۹ء جوہری عدد ۸۲ کثافت اضافی ۳۴،۱۱ نقطۂ پگھلاؤ ۳۲۷،۴ء°س۔ ایک نرم نیلگوں سفید دھات یہ عموماً سلفائیڈ کی صورت میں قدرتی حالت میں پایا جاتا ہے۔ اس کے مرکبات زہریلے ہوتے ہیں۔ مرکبات رنگ و روغن کی تیاری میں کام آتے ہیں۔ ایک سفید قلمی مرکب لیڈ آرسینیٹ کرم کش کے طور پر استعمال کیا جاتا ہے۔

Leadbetter-Politano operation. An anti-reflux measure by tunne] reimplantation of ureter into urinary bladder.

لیڈ بیٹر پولیٹانو اپریشن : بولی مثانہ میں یورٹیر کی پیوندکاری سے ایک اینٹی ریفلکس اقدام۔

Lead lotion *(led-lo'-shun)* . A weak solution of lead subacetate used as a soothing astringent lotion for sprains and bruises.

لیڈ لوشن : لیڈ سب ایسیٹیٹ کا ہلکا محلول۔

Lead poisoning *(led)*. Acute poisoning is unusual, but chronic poisoning due to absorption of small amounts over a period, is less uncommon. This can occur in young children by sucking articles made of lead alloys, or painted with lead paint. In spite of legislation and safety precautions, industrial poisoning is still the commonest cause. Anaemia, loss of appetite, and the formation of a blue line round the gums are characteristic.

سیسے کا زہر : سیسے کی بنی ہوئی اشیاء چوسنے سے بچوں کو ہو جاتی ہے۔ خون کی کمی۔ بھوک کی کمی یا مسوڑھوں کے گرد نیلی لکیر کی بناوٹ اس کی علامات ہیں۔

LE cells Characteristic cells found in patients with lupus erythematosus.

ایل۔ ای خلیے : مخصوص مریضوں کی ہڈیوں کے گودے میں پائے جانے والے مخصوص خلیے۔

Lecithin *(les'-i-thin)* [G. *lekithos*, egg yolk]. A nitrogenous, fatty substance in cell protoplasm.

زردین : خلوی پروٹوپلازم میں نائٹروجنی چکنا مادہ۔ لپڈز کی قسم۔ کیمیائی طور پر چکنائیوں جیسی ہے لیکن اس میں نائٹروجن اور فاسفورس زائد ہوتے ہیں۔

Ledermycin *(led-er-mi'-sin)* . Demethylchlortetracycline. One of the tetracyclines (q.v.).

Leech *(lech)*. *Hirudo medicinalis.* An acquatic worm which can be applied to the human body to suck blood. Its saliva contains hirudin, an anticoagulant.

جونک۔ خون کش : ایک آبی کیڑا جو خون چوسنے کے لئے انسان کو لگایا

جاتا ہے۔اس کالعاب دہن خون کو جمنے نہیں دیتا۔

Legumen *(leg-u'-men)*. The protein present in pulses--peas, beans and lentils.

لگومن : پروٹین جو دالوں میں ہوتی ہے۔ دالوں میں ماش' لوبیا' مٹر وغیرہ شامل ہیں۔

Leishman-Donovan bodies *(lesh'-man don'-ov-an)*. The rounded forms of the protozoa Leishmania found in the endothelial cells and macrophages of patients suffering from leishmaniasis (q.v.).

لشمان ڈونووان اجسام : پروٹوزوا لشمانیہ کی کروی اقسام۔ یہ کالا زار بخار کے مریض کی تلی و جگر میں پائے جاتے ہیں۔

Leishmania *(lesh-ma'-ni-a)* Genus of flagellated protozoon. *Leishmania donovant* is responsible for disease of kalaazar, or leishmaniasis (q.v.).

لشمانیا : ایک پروٹوزون جو بیماری پیدا کرتا ہے۔ انسانی جسم میں ناقابل حرکت۔ عموماً پس سیلز میں ہوتا ہے۔ انسان میں لاہوری پھوڑے یا اوورینٹل سورز کا سبب ہے مچھر کی انت میں حرکت کرسکتا ہے۔

Leishamaniasis *(lesh-man-i'-a-sis)*. Infestation by Leishmania, spread by sandflies. Generalized manifestation is kala-azar (q.v.). Cutaneous manifestation is such as Aleppo or Delhi boil (oriental sore) (q.v.). Nasopharyngeal manifestation is espundia (q.v.).

کالا آزار۔ لاہوری پھوڑا : پشمانیا پروٹوزون سے ہونی والی بیماری' ریٹ مکھی یا مچھر کے کاٹنے سے یہ مرض ہوتا ہے۔ تشخیص کے لئے پھوڑے کا پانی گلاس سلائیڈ پر رکھ کر سٹین کرکے خوردبین میں دیکھیئے۔

Lens *(lenz)*. 1. The small biconwex crystalline body which is supported in the suspensory ligament immediately behind the iris of the eye. On account of its elasticity, the lens can alter in shape, enabling light rays to focus exactly on the retina. 2. A piece of transparent material, usually glass, with a regular curvature of one or both surfaces, used for conveying or diffusing light rays.

عدسہ : (۱) کوئی ایسی شے جس سے گزر کر کرنوں کی بیم مرکوز یا منتشر ہو جائے۔ چھوٹا دوہرا محدب قلمی جسم جو آنکھ کی آئرس کے پیچھے ہوتا ہے۔ اس سے روشنی کی شعاعین یا کرنیں ریٹنا پر مرکوز ہوتی ہیں۔ (۲) عدسہ شفاف شیشے کا ٹکڑا ہوتا ہے۔ عدسے شفاف واسطوں سے بنائے جاتے ہیں ان کی ایک یا

نوں سطحوی کروی ہوتی ہیں۔ عدسے محدب یا مقعر ہوتے ہیں۔ محدب سے درمیان سے موٹے ہوتے ہیں جبکہ مقعر عدسوں کے کنارے موٹے تے ہیں۔ محدب عدسے شعاعوں کو مرکوز اور مقعر عدسے شعاعوں کو منتشر رتے ہیں۔ محدب عدسہ دوہرا' مستوی یا مقعر محدب عدسہ ہوتا ہے۔ مقعر سہ بھی دوہرا مستوی یا محدب مقعر عدسہ ہوتا ہے۔

Lenticular *(len-tik'-u-lar)* [L. *lenticula,* lentil Pertaining to or resembling a lens.

رسی : عدسہ سے مشابہ یا عدسہ سے متعلق۔

Lentigo *(len-ti'-go)* [L.]. A freckle--lent-igne pl.

ھائیں : جلد کا داغ۔

Lentil *(len'-til)*. A cheap and nutritious legume containing a large amount of protein.

سور : مسور کی دال۔ پروٹین کی کافی مقدار پر مشتمل ایک سستا اور غذادار لومن۔

Lentizol *(len'-tiz-ol)* A tricyclic antidepressan Useful for depression when accompanied b agita tion. Amitripty-line hydrochloride (q.v.)

Leontiasis *(le-on-ti'-a-sis)* [G. *leon,* lion; N. *-iasis,* condition]. Enlargement of face an head giving a lion-like appearance; most ofte caused by fibrous dysplasia of bone.

ءالاسد : چہرے اور سر کا بڑھاؤ جو بعض امراض میں شیر کی طرح دکھائی تا ہے۔

Leprologist *(lep-rol'-oj-ist)* [G. lepros, scal logos, discourse]. One who specializes in t study and treatment of leprosy--leprology, n.

ہر جزام : کوڑھ کے مطالعہ اور علاج میں ماہر۔

Lepromata *(lep-rp'-ma-ta)* [G. *lepros,* scal *-oma,* tumour]. The granulomatous cutaneo eruption of leprosy--leproma, sing., lepron atous, adj.

رومیٹ : کوڑھ کی جلدی آبلے۔

Leprosy *(lep'-ro-si)* [G. *lepros,* scaly]. progressive and contagious disease, endem in warmer climates, and characterized b granulomatous formation in the nerves or the skin. Caused by *Mycobacterium leprae* (Hansen's bacillus). BCG vaccination confe red 87 percent protection in one large-sca trial. leprous. adj.

جذام کوڑھ : ایک مرض جو گرم ممالک میں ہوتا ہے۔ بی' سی۔ جی کی ویکسین مفید ہے۔ اس کے جراثیم گرام مثبت اور ایسڈ فاسٹ ہوتے ہیں اور ۵ء۱ سے ۸ مائیکرون تک طویل ہوتے ہیں۔

.eptazol *(lep'-ta-zol)*. Powerful central stimulant.

لیپٹازول : طاقتور مرکزی محرک باربیٹوریٹ کے زہریلا پن میں مستعمل۔

.eptocytosis *(lep-to-si-to'-sis)* [G. *leptos,* thin; *-osis,* condition]. Thin, flattened, circulating red blood cells (lepotocytes). Characteristic of Cooley's anaemia (q.v.). Also seen in jaundice, hepatic disease and sometimes after splenectomy.

لیپٹوسائی ٹوسس : پتلے' چپٹے' گردشی سرخ خونی خلیے۔ یرقان وغیرہ کے امراض میں نظر آتے ہیں۔

.eptomeningitis *(lep-to-men-in-ji'-tis)* [G. *leptos*, thin; *menigx*, membrane; *-itis*, inflammation]. Inflàmmation of the inner covering membranes (meninges) of brain or spinal cord.

ورم سحایائے رفیعہ : شوکی ڈور سے یا دماغ کی اندرونی غلافی جھلیوں کی سوزش۔

.eptospira *(lep-to-spi'-ra)* [G. *leptos,* thin; *speisa,* coil]. A genus of bacteria. Very thin, finely coiled bacteria which require dark ground microscopy for visualization. Common in water as saprophytes; pathogenic species are numerous in many animals and may infect man. *Leptospira icterohaemorrhagiae* causes Weil's disease in man; *Leptospira canicola,* 'yellows' in dogs and pigs, transmissible to man. See CANICOLA FEVER.

حمی زرد : جراثیم کا ایک جنس۔ بہت تاریک۔ پانی میں بطور گندخور عام ہوتے ہین۔ مرض پیدا کہنے والی انواع بہت سے جانوروں میں ہوتی ہے۔

.eptospirosis *(lep-to-spri-ro'-sis)* [G. *leptos,* thin; *speira,* coil; *-osis,* condition]. Spirochaetal disease. Leptospirosis haemorrhagica, Weil's disease (q.v.).

لیپٹوسپائروسس : ایک مرض۔

.eptothrix *(lep'-to-thriks)* [G. *leptos,* fine; *thrix,* hair]. A genus of bacteria. Gram-negative; found in water; non-pathogenic. A term also used in medical bacteriology to describe filamentous bacteria resembling actinomycetes.

لیپٹوتھرکس : جراثیم کا ایک جنس۔ گرام منفی' پانی میں پایا جاتا ہے۔ مرض پیدا نہیں ہوتا۔

Lesbianism *(les'-bi-an-izm)* . Sexual attraction of one woman to another.

Lesch-Nyhan disease *(lesh-ni'-an)*. Described in 1965; transmitted via mother to only male children. Overproduction of uric acide, associated with brain damage resulting in cerebral palsy and mental retardation. Victims are complelled, by a self-destructive urge, to bite away the sides of their mouth, lips and fingers.

Lesion *(le'-zhun)* [L. laesio, a hurting]. Pathological change in a bodily tissue.

خلل اعضاء۔ زخم : جسمانی نسیج میں مرض والی تبدیلی۔

Lethane *(le-than)*. A mixture of thiocyanate derivatives with insecticidal properties; used for pediculosis capitis.

لیتھین : ایک آمیزہ جس میں تھیوسانیٹ کے حاصلات شامل ہیں۔

Lethidrone *(leth'-i-dron)*. Nalorphine (q.v.).

لیتھڈرون : فلورفین۔

Leucarsone *(lu'-kar-son)*. Carbarsome (q.v.).

لیوکارسون : کاربرسوم۔

Leucine *(lu'-sen)*. One of the essential amino acids (q.v.).

لیوسین : لازمی امینوایسڈز میں سے ایک سفید حل پذیر امینوایسڈ۔ نقطۂ پگھلاؤ ۲۹۳ تا ۲۹۵°س۔ ممالیہ جانوروں کے لئے لازمی۔

Leucocytes *(lu'-ko-sits)* [G. *leukos,* white; *kytos,* cell]. The white corpuscles of the blood. In the blood stream they are colourless, nucleated masses, and some are motile and phagocytic. See BASOPHIL, EO: INOPHIL, LYMPHOCYTE, MONONUCLE R, POLY MORPHONUCLEAR--leucocytic, dj.

خلیہ ابیض۔ سفید خلیے : سفید خون خلیے۔ خون کی وہ خلیے جن میں ہیموگلوبن نہیں ہوتا۔ یہ بیماری کے خلاف مدافعت پیدا کرتے ہیں۔ وہ گول اور بے رنگ ہوتے ہیں۔ ان میں مرکزہ ہوتا ہے۔ ان میں سے بعض متحرک ہیں۔

Leucocytolysis *(lu-ko-si-tol'-is-is)* [G. ***leukos,***

white; *kytos*, cell; *lysis*, a loosening]. Destruction and disintegration of white blood cells--leucocytolytic, adj.

خلیات ابیض پاشی : سفید خونی خلیوں کی تباہی یا خاتمہ۔

Leucocytosis *(lu-ko-si-to'-sis)* [G. *leukos*, white; *kytos*, cell; *-osis*, condition]. Increased number of leucocytes in the blood. Often a response to infection--leucocytotic, adj.

لیوکوسائی ٹوسس۔ کثرت خلیا ابیض : خون میں لیوکوسائیٹس کی بڑھی ہوئی تعداد۔

Leucoderma *(lu-ko-der'-ma)* [G. *leukos*, white; *derma*, skin]. Defective skin pigmentation, especially when it occurs in patches or bands.

پھلبہری۔ برص : ناقص جلدی پگمنٹیشن۔ جلد کا رنگ اڑ جاتا ہے اور سفید داغ پڑ جاتے ہیں۔ اس میں میتھا کسالین مفید ہے۔

Leucoma *(lu-ko'-ma)* [G. white spot on the eye]. White opaque spot on the cornea--leucomata, pl.; leucomatous, adj.

پھولا : قوزیہ پر سفید غیر شفاف داغ۔

Leuconychia *(lu-kon-ik'-i-a)* [G. *leukos*, white; *onyx*, nail]. White spots on the nails.

لیوکونکیا : ناخنوں پر سفید داغ۔

Leucopenia *(lu-ko-pe'-ni-a)* [G. *leukos*, white; *penia*, want]. Decreased number of leucocytes in the blood--leucopenic, adj.

قلت خلیات ابیض : خون میں لیوکوسائیٹس کی تخفیف شدہ تعداد۔

Leucopoiesis *(lu-ko-poi-e'-sis)* [G. *leukos*, white; *poiesis*, making]. The formation of white blood cells--leucopoietic, adj.

تولید خلیات ابیض : سفید خون خلیوں کا بننا۔

Leucorrhoea *(lu-ko-re'-a)* [G. *leukos*, white; *rheein*, to flow]. A sticky, whitish vaginal discharge-- leucorrhoeal, adj.

سیلان رحم۔ لیکوریا : اندام نہانی یا ویجائنا کا چمٹنے والا سفید ڈسچارج۔ نئی شادی شدہ عورتوں میں کثرت جماع سے لیکوریا ہو جاتا ہے اور اس کی وجہ جراثیمی سرایت ہے۔

Leucotomy *(lu-kot'-o-mi)* [G. *leukos*, white; *tome*, cutting]. **perfrontal l.**, an operation devised by Moniz (1936) for the treatment of certain forms of chronic insanity by cutting the frontothalamic connection fibres in the brain. Moniz's original method was to inje alcohol into the prefrontal white matt Freeman, Wattas and others (194 introduced surgical cutting of the fibres a other modifications.

ف ابیض تراشی : پاگل پن کے لئے اپریشن

Laryn

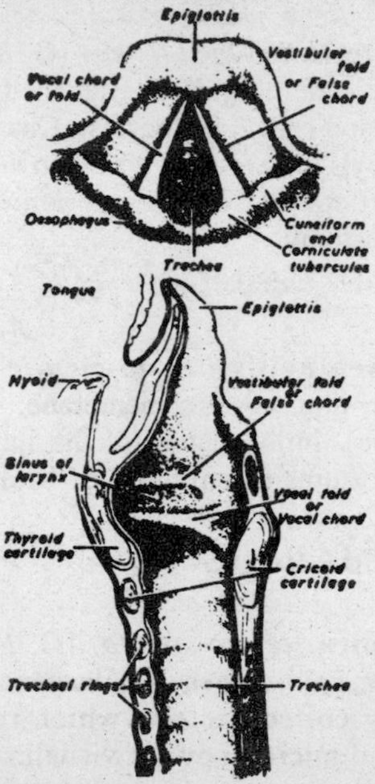

upper figure = laryngoscopic view
lower figure =
sagital section

Leucovorin *(lu-kov'-or-in)*. Folinic acid Citrorovam Factor given by mouth i.m. or i as an antidote to methotrexate. Used 'rescue' patients from high dose methotrex therapy for malignant disease.

دورن : فولینک ایسڈ۔

Leukaemia *(lu-ke'-mi-a)* [G. *leukos*, white; *haima*, blood]. A malignant proliferation the leucopoietic tissues usually producing abnormal increase in leucocytes in the blo with immature cells among them. T varieties are **acute lymphatic, myeloid monocytic l.** and **chronic lymphatic**

myeloid l. Acute leukaemia rapidly results in infection, haemorrhage and anaemia. The process in slower in the chronic types, with splenomegaly and lymjph node enlargement in the lymphatic variety. The term **aleukaemic l.** is used when the leucocyte count remains normal or below.

کثرت خلیات ابیض : خون کی بیماری جس میں سفید خلیے قسم یا تعداد میں غیر معمولی ہوتے ہیں۔ کنسر یا سرطان کی قسم علاج کے لئے ٦ مرکیپ ٹوپیورین۔ پریڈنی سولوں اور انتقال خون۔

eukeran *(lu'-ker-an)*. Chlorambucil (q.v.).

لیکوران : کلورمبوسل۔ مفید برائے مرض ہاجکین۔ سرطان یا کینسر۔

eukoplakia *(lu-ko-pla'-ki-a)* [G. *leukos*, white; *plax*, flat and broad]. White, thickened patch occurring on mucous membranes. Occurs on lips, inside mouth or on genitalia. sometimes denotes precancerous change. sometimes due to syphilis. See KRAUROSIS VALVAE.

تقشر اللسان : میوکس جھلیوں پر واقع سفید۔ دبیز پٹی ہونٹوں پر، منہ کے اندر یا جنسی اعضاء پر ہوتی ہے۔

evallorphan tartrate Narcotic antagonist.

لیویلیورفین ٹارٹریٹ : خواب آور دوا۔

evamisol *(lev-a-mi'-sol)*. Synthetic anthelmintic. Better tolerated than piperazine citrate and virtually free of toxic effects. Currently being used for treatment of reheumatoid arthritis as an immunostimulant.

لیویمیسول : زہریلے اثرات سے آزاد۔

evator *(le-va'-tor)* [L. *levare*, to lift up]. A muscle which acts by raising a part. An instr ument for lifting a depressed part.

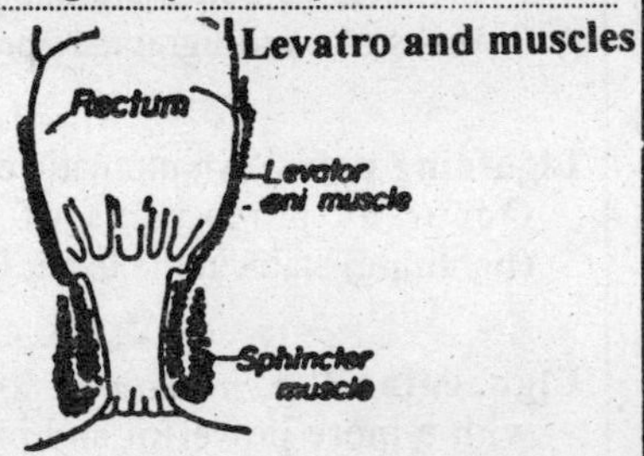

Levatro and muscles

رافع۔ رافعہ : عضلہ جو ایک حصہ اٹھانے سے کام کرتا ہے۔ دبے ہوئی حصے کو اٹھانے کے لئے ایک آلہ۔

Levin's tube Used in gastric acid tests.

لیون کی ٹیوب : گیسٹرک ایسڈ ٹیسٹوں میں مستعمل۔

Levodopa *(lev-o-do'-pa)* L-dopa, Synthetic anti-Parkinson drug. In Parkinson's disease there is inadequate dopamine (a transmitter substance), in the basal ganglia. In these ganglia l. is converted into dopamine and replenishes the stores. Unlike dopamine levodopa can cross the blood-brain barrier. See CARBIDOPA.

لیووڈوپا : تالیفی اینٹی پارکنسن ڈرگ۔

Levophed *(lev'-o-fed)*. Noradrenaline (q.v.).

لیووفیڈ : نارایڈرینالین۔

Levorphanol *(lev-or'-fan-ol)* A synthetic substitute for morphine. It is less hypnotic than morphine buyt has a more extended action. Almost as effective by mouth as by injection.

لیوورفینول : متبادل کا متبادل۔ مارفین سے کم خواب آور۔

Levulose *(lev'-u-los)*. Fruit sugar; fructose. Also LAEVULOSE (q.v.).

چپ گرداں شکر۔ قند میوہ : فروٹ شوگر۔ فرکٹوز۔ عام شکر کی نسبت زیادہ شیریں اور آسانی سے ہضم ہونے والی شکر۔ ذیابیطس کے مریضوں کے لئے مفید۔

L-form. A bacterium whose cell wall has been destroyed. In this condition it can survive harmlessly for months. Under certain conditions it can quickly change into a pathogenic bacterium.

ایل فارم : جرثومہ جس کی دیوار خلیہ تباہ ہوگئی ہو۔

LGVCFT. Lymphogranuloma venereum complement fixation test.

ایل جی وی سی ایف ٹی : لمفوگرینولوما وینیریم کمپلیمنٹ فکسیشن ٹیسٹ۔

Libido *(li-bi'-do)* [L. longing]. Freud's name for the urge to obtain sensual satisfaction which he believed to be the mainspring of human behaviour. Sometimes more loosely used with the meaning of sexual urge. Freud's meaning was satisfaction through all the senses.

شہوت : جنسی مسرت حاصل کرنے کے لئے خواہش کے لئے فرائڈ کا نام، انسانی رویہ کی تشریح، جنسی تسکین کی بنیاد پر کی گئی ہے۔

Librium *(lib'-ri-um)*. Chlordiazepoxide (q.v.).

لبریم : کلورڈائزپ آکسائیڈ۔ نامردی اور جریان یا پروٹیسٹوریا کے علاج کے لئے ایک گولی صبح ایک شام ایک دوپہر طبعیت میں سکون ذہنی پریشانی کو ختم اور بے خوابی کو رفع کرتی ہے۔

Lice *(lis')* See PEDICULUS.

جوئیں : پیڈیکولس

Lichen *(li-ken)* [G. *leichen* lichen]. Aggregations of papular skin lesions. **Lichen nitidus,** characterized by minute, shiny, flat-topped, pink papules of pinhead size. **lichen planus,** aggregaters of small papules, polygonal in shape, flat-topped, and of violaceous hue. **lichen scrofulosorum,** a form of tuberculide, **lichen simplex,** a psychosomatic condition which produces areas of irritating, leathery, shiny papules (lichenification). Syn., neurodermatitis. **lichen spinulosus,** a disease of children characterized by very small spines protruding from the follicular openings of the skin and resulting from vitamin A deficiency. **lichen urticatus,** papular urticaria (q.v.)--lichenoid, adj.

لائیکن : جلدی زخموں کا اجتماع۔

Lichenification *(li-ken-i-fik-a'-shun)* [G. leichen, lichen; L. *facere,* to make]. Thickening of the skin, usually secondary to scratching. Striae become more prominent and the area affected appears to be composed of small, shiny rhomboids.

لائیکینی فیکیشن : جلد کی دبازت۔

Lidocaine *(lid'-o-kan)*. Lignocaine (q.v.).

لیڈوکین : لگنوکین۔

Lidothesin. Lignocaine (q.v.).

لیڈوتھیسین : لگنوکین۔

Lien *(li-en)* [L.]. The spleen.

طحال : تلی۔

Lienculus *(li-en-i'-tis)* [L. *lien,* spleen; G. *itis,* inflammation]. Inflammation of the spleen.

...ندتلی : تلی کی سوزش۔

Lienitis *(li-en-i'-tis)* [L. *lien,* spleen; G. *it*... inflammation]. Inflammation of the spleen.

...م تلی : تلی کی سوزش۔

Lienorenal *(li-en-o-re'-nal)* [L. *lien,* spleen; *re*... kidney. In 1. shunt, the splenic vein ... anastomosed to the left renal vein to relie... portal hypertension.

...رینل : تلی اور گردے سے متعلق۔

Ligament *(lig'-a-ment)* [L. *ligamentum,* ban... A strong band of fibrous tissue serving ... bind bones or other parts together, or ... support an organ--ligamentous, adj.

...ط : عضو کو سہارا دینے کے لئے یا ہڈیوں یا دوسرے حصوں کو اکٹھے باندھنے ... لئے ریشہ دار نسیج کی ایک مضبوط پٹی۔

Ligate*(li-gat')* [L. *ligare,* to bind]. To tie ... blood vessels, etc. at operation--ligation, n.

...ش۔ پٹی۔ ربط شریان : اپریشن کے وقت خونی رگوں وغیرہ کو ...ھنا۔

Ligature *(lig'-a-tur)* [L. *ligatura,* a band]. T... material used for tying vessels or sewing ... tissues. Silk, horse-hair, catgut, kangaroo te... don, silver wire, nylon, linen and fascia ... be used.

...یان بندی۔ پٹی : بافتوں وک سینے یا رگوں کو باندھنے کے لئے ...عال ہونے والا میٹریل۔

Lightening *(li;'-ten-ing)*. Term used to den... the relief of pressure on the diaphragm by ... abdominal viscera, when the presenting p... of the fetus descends into the pelvis in the ... 3 weeks of a primigravida's pregnancy.

...گ : ڈایافرام پر دباؤ کی کمی۔

Lightning pains Symptomatic of tabes dorsal... Occur as paroxysms of swift cutti... (lightning) stabs in the lower limbs.

...م صاعقہ : زیریں جوارح میں شدید درد۔

Lignocaine *(lig'-no-kan)* A local anaesthe... with a more powerful and prolonged acti... than procaine. The strength of solution var... from 0.5 per-cent for nerve block. Adrenali...

is usually added to delay absorption. Also effective for surface anaesthesia as ointment (2 per-cent) and for urethral anaesthesia as a 2 percent gel. Now widely accepted as a antiarhythmic agent, especially in the management of ventricular tachycardia and ventricular ectopic beats occurring as complica tions for acute myocardial infarction.

لگنوکین : مقامی طور پر سن کرنے والی دوائی۔ پروکین سے زیادہ طاقتور اور لگاتار ایکشن۔

Lime water Solution of calcium hydroxide (about 0.15 percent). It is used in a number of skin lotions, and with an equal volume of linseed or olive oil it forms a soothing application. It is also used in infant feeding as it hinders the formation of large curds.

چونے کا پانی : کیلشیم ہائیڈروآکسائیڈ کا آبی محلول۔ یہ کاربن ڈائی آکسائیڈ کے تحمل سے دودھیا ہو جاتا ہے کیونکہ اس میں ناحل پزیر کیلشیم کاربونیٹ بن جاتا ہے۔ جلدی لوشن میں مستعمل بچے کو دودھ پلانے میں بھی مستعمل۔

Liminal *(lim'-in-al)* [L. *limen,* threshold]. The lowest intensity of a stimulus which can be perceived by the human senses. See SUBLIMINAL.

اقل شعوری : محرک کی کم ترین شدت۔ اسے انسانی خواس محسوس کر سکتے ہیں۔

Lincocin *(lin'-ko-sin).* Lincomycin (q.v.)

Lincomycin *(lin-ko-mi'-sin).* Antibiotic for infections caused by Gram-positive pathogens.

لکنو مائی سین : گرام مثبت جراثیم سے ہونے والے امراض کے لئے اینٹی بیاٹک ۔لکنوسین۔ اس کا ایک کیپسول صبح دوپہر شام برائے پراپرا۔

Linctus *(ling'-tus)* [L. *Iinctus* , a licking]. A sweet, syrupy liquid; it should be slowly sipped. See GEES L.

لعوق : ایک شیریں شربتی مائع۔ اسے ایک ایک گھونٹ کر کے پینا چاہیئے۔

Linea:*(lin-i-a)* A line. **Linea alba,**the whitle line visible after removal of the skin in the centre of the abdomen, stretching from the ensiform cartilage to the pubis, its position on the surface being indicated by a slight depression. **linea nigra,** pigmented line from umbilicus to pubis which appears in pregnance. **lineae albicantes,** white lines which appear on the abdomen after reduction of tension as after childbirth, tapping of the abdomen, etc.

خط : لکیر

Lingua *(ling-gwa)*[L.] The tongue -lingual, adj

لسان : زبان

Liniment *(lin-i-ment)* [L. *linire,* to smear] A liquid to be applied to the skin gentle friction.

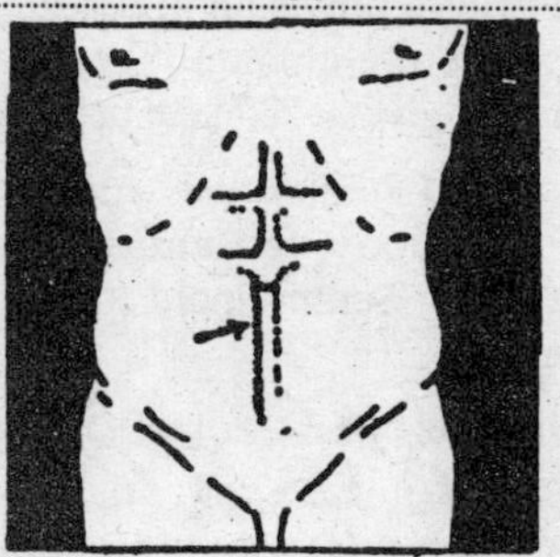

Linea alba

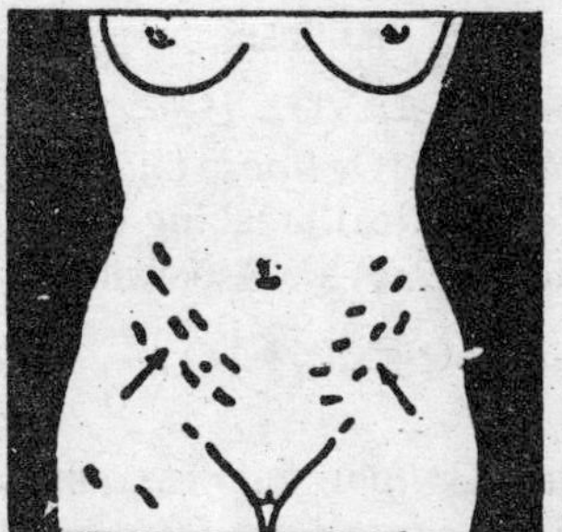

Lineae albicantes

مالشی تیل : لنی منٹ تھوڑی رگڑ سے جلد پر مائع کا اطلاق

Linolenic acid *(lin-o-le-nik)* An unsaturated, essential fatty acid. Found in vegetablats.

لنولنیک ایسڈ : ایک سیر شدہ لازمی فیٹی ایسڈ۔ نباتی چکنائیوں میں پایا جاتا ہے۔

Lioreal *(li-o-re-sal)* Baclofen (q.v.)

Liothyronine *(li-o-thi-ron-in)* Secretion of thyroid gland. Together with thyroxline stimulates metabolism in body tissues.

لیوتھائیرونین : تھائیرائیڈ گلینڈ کی رطوبت۔

Lipaemia *(li-pe-mi-a)* [G. *lipos,* fat; haima, blood] Increased lipoids (especialy cholesterol) in the blood lipaemic, adj.

شحمیت الدم : خون میں بڑے ہوئے لیائڈز خصوصاً کولیسٹرول

Lipase *(li-paz)* Any fat-splitting enzyme. **pancreatic** l. , steapsin. (q.v.)

شحم پاشمیر : ایک خامرہ جو چکنائیوں پر عمل کرتا ہے۔

Lipiodol *(lip-i-o-dol)* lodized oil (q.v.)

لیپوڈول : خشخاش کے بیجوں کا تیل جس میں ۴۰ فیصد آیوڈین ہوتی ہے۔

Lipiphysan, Lilocarlorie provision in parenteral feeding. Ten per cent emulsion gives 1240 kcal and 15 per cent gives 1780 kcal per litre.

لپی فائیسین : خوراک میں کلوکلوری کا اہتمام

Lipoid *(li-poid)* [G. lipos, fat; *eidos,* form] Resembling fat or oil. Serum lipoids raised in thynotd deficiency.

شحم ۔ چربی: نامیاتی مرکبات کا ایک گروہ جو فیٹی ایسڈز کے ایسٹرن ہوتے ہیں۔ پانی میں ناحل پذیر بہت سے نامیاتی محللوں میں حل پذیر۔

Lipoidosis *(li-poid-o-sis)* [G. *lipos, fat; eidos,* form; *osis,* condeition] Disease due to disorder of fat metabolism. lipoidoses, pl.

لپائڈوسس: چربی کے میٹابولزم میں گڑبڑ کی وجہ سے مرض۔

Lipolysis *(li-pol'-i-sis)* [G. *lipos,* fat; *lysis,* a lossening]. The chemical breaking down of fat. The lipolytic enzymes are responsible.

لیپو[illegible] : چربی کا کیمیائی طور پر ٹوٹنا جس کے لئے خامرات ذمہ دار ہیں۔

Lipoma *(li-po-ma)* [G. *lipos,* fat; *oma,* tumour] A benign tumour containing fatty tissue. lipomata, pl: lipomatous,adj.

شحمی سلعہ : فیٹی نسیج پر مشتمل ناسور۔ زیر جلد چربیلے۔ گوشت کی رسولی۔ آپریشن سے نکل سکتی ہے۔

Lipotrophic substances *(li-po-tro-fik)* Factors which cause the removal of fat from the liver by transmethylation.

لیپوٹرافک اشیاء : وہ عوامل جو چربی ختم کرتے ہیں۔

Lipuria *(li-pu-ri-a)* [G. *lipos,* fat; *ouron* urine]. Fat in the urine. Adiposuria lipuric, adj.

[illegible]بی دار پیشاب : پیشاب میں چکنائی

Liquemin *(lik-we-min)* Heparin (q.v.)

[illegible]یکوائمن :ہیپرن

Liquor *(lik-er)* [L. liquid] A soloution 1. **amni[illegible]** the fluid surrounding the fetus. **liquor episp[illegible] asticus,** a blistering fluid. **liquor folliculi,** th[illegible] fluid surrounging? a developing ovum in [illegible] Graafian follicle. **liquor picis carb** an alcoh[illegible] olic extract of coal tar. Used in eczema an[illegible] other conditions requiring mild tar treatmen[illegible] **liquor sanguinis,** the fluid part of bloo[illegible] (plasma).

[illegible]وشاندہ: محلول ۔ دوائی اور پانی یا الکحل کا محلول عموماً کچھ عرصہ تک رکھا جا [illegible]کتا ہے۔

Liquorice *(li-sid-on-il)* Has a relaxing effec[illegible] onthe neurogenic bladder.

[illegible]لیٹھی : گلرائزا۔

Lisidonil *(li-sid-on-il).* Has a relaxing effect o[illegible] the neurogenic bladder.

[illegible]سڈونل : نیوروجینک بلیڈر اچھا اثر کرتا ہے۔

Lithiasis *(lith-i'-a-sis)* [G. *lithos,* stone; N.I[illegible] *lasis,* condition]. Formation of calculi.

[illegible]یدائش سنگ مثانہ: پتھریوں کا بننا۔

Lithium carhbonate *(li-thi-um kar-bon-a[illegible]* Used inj manic depressive illness. Possib[illegible] side effects include diarrhoea, vomiting[illegible] drowsiness, ataxia, coarse tremor. Contra[illegible] ndicated in cardiac or renal disease. Regul[illegible] blood serum levels necessary and thyroid fu[illegible] ction should be assessed before and at regul[illegible] intervals during treatment.

[illegible]تھم : مرض میں مستعمل

Litholapaxy *(lith-ol-a-pak-si)* [G. *lithos, ston[illegible]* *lapaxis,*evacuation] Crushing a stone withi[illegible] the urinary bladder and removing the fragm[illegible] ents by irrigation. Syn. lithopaxy.

[illegible]لیل حصات : بولی مثانے میں پتھری کو توڑنا اور ٹکڑوں کو وہاں سے [illegible]

Lithopaedion *(lith-o-pe-di-on)* A dead fetu[illegible] retained in the uterus, e.g. in the case of o[illegible] dead twin, which becomes mummified an[illegible] sometimes impregnated with lime salts.

متحجر جنیں : یوٹرس میں رہ جانے والا مردہ بچہ

Lithotrite *(lith-o-trit)* [G. *lithos,* stone; 1. *terere,* to wear] An instrument for crushing a stone in the urinary bladder.

حصاہ شکن یا سنگ شکن آلہ ۔ پتھری توڑ آلہ : بولی مثانے میں پتھری توڑنے کے لئے آلہ

Lithuresis *(lith-u-re-sis)* [G. *lithos,* stone; *ouron,* urine] Voiding of gravel in the urine.

بول رملی : پیشاب میں پتھریلے ذرات آنا۔

Litmus *(lit-mus)* A vegetable pigment used as an indicator of acidity or alkalinity. Blue 1. papér turns red when in contact with an acid. Red 1. paper turns blue when in contact with an alkali.

لٹمس: ایک حل پذیر مادہ۔ تیزاب سے لال اور الکلی سے نیلا ہو جاتا ہے۔ انڈیکیٹر کے طور پر استعمال کیا جاتا ہے۔ ایک نباتی پگمنٹ۔

Little's disease Diplegia of spastic type causing scissor leg deformity. Congenital disease in which there is cerebral atrophy or agenesis [Willian John Little, English surgeon, [18-0-94]

صلابت عضلات ۔ مولودی : مرض جس میں سر برل اٹرافی ہو جاتی ہے۔

Liver *(liv-er)* The largest organ in the body, varying in weight in the adult from 13.59 to 18. 12 hg or about one-thirtieth of body weight. It is relatively much larger in the fetus. It is situated in the right upper section of the abdominal cavity. It secretes bile, forms and stores glycogen and plays an important part in the metabolism of proteins and fats.

جگر : جسم میں سب سے بڑی گلینڈ۔ بطنی کہفہ کے دائیں بالائی حصے میں واقع ہے۔ یہ بائل خارج کرتا ہے۔ گلائیکوجن بناتا اور ذخیرہ کرتا ہے۔ وزن میں جسم کے وزن کا تیسواں حصہ لیکن بطن میں بچے کا جگر نسبتاً بڑا ہوتا ہے۔ ہضم شدہ خوراک جگر میں جاتی ہے۔ جہاں وہ جمع رہتی ہے یا جسم کے دوسرے حصوں میں بھیجی جاتی ہے۔ نشاستہ والی اغذیہ گلوکوس اور لیوولز بن کر جگر میں جاتی ہے۔ جگر ان دونوں کو گلائیکوجن میں تبدیل کر دیتا ہے یہ علمی اجزاء کو کنٹرول کرتا ہے۔

Livid *(liv-id)* [L. *lividus,* of a leaden, bluish colour] Blue discolouration due to bruising. congestion or insufficient oxygenation.

سرمئی : نیلی رنگت ہو جانا

L-lytic compound *(el-lit-ik)* Isoxuprine (q.v.)

ایل لائیٹک مرکب : آئیسوکسوپرین

LOA. Midwifery. Left occipitoanterior presentation.

ایل او اے : مڈوائفری۔ بائیں اکسیپو امامی ساحت جنین کا طبعی رخ۔ اس میں جنین لمبے رخ پر ہوتا ہے۔ اس کا سر نیچے ہوتا ہے۔ اس رخ میں ولادت سہل ہوتی ہے۔

Lobe *(lob)* [G. *lobos,* lobe] A rounded section of an organ, separated from neighbouring sections by a fissure or septum etc. -lobar, adj.

لوب ۔ لختہ ۔ فص: کسی عضو کا گول حصہ جو نزدیکی حصوں سے کسی پردے وغیرہ کے ذریعے الگ ہو۔

Lobectomy *(lob-ek'-to-mi)* [G. *lobos,* lobe; *ektome,* excision] Excision of **lobe** , as the lung

فص براری : لوب کا کوٹنا۔ مثلاً پھیپھڑے کا

Lobeline *(lob-el'-en)* Occasionally used for resuscitation of the newborn by **injection** into the umbilical cord.

لوب لائن : نوائیدہ بچے کو ہوش میں لانا

Lobotomy *(lob-o'-to-mi)* [G. *lobos,* lobe; tome, a cutting] Section of brain tissue. Used in surgical treatment of emotional disease.

فص شگافی : دماغی بافت کا حصہ۔ جذباتی مرض کے سرجیکل علاج میں مستعمل

Lobule *(lob'-ul)* [G. *lobos,* lobe] A small lobe or a subdivision of a lobe-lobular, lobulated, adj.

فصیص : چھوٹا لوب۔ لوب کا حصہ

Localize *(lo'-kal-iz)* [L. *localis,* place] To limit the spread; to determine the site of a lesion localization.

محدود کرنا: پھیلاؤ محدود کرنا۔ زخم کی جگہ کا تعین کرنا

Lochia *(lo-ki-a)* [G. Discharge after childbirth]. The vaginal discharge which occurs during the puerperium. Af first pure blood. it later becomes paler, diminishes in quantity and finally ceaseslochial, adj.

نفاس : ویجائنل ڈسچارج بچے کی پیدائش کے تقریباً ایک ماہ بعد تک عورت کے رحم سے رطوبت خارج ہوتی ہے اور رحم خود بھی سکڑ کر پھولی ہوئی رگوں کو سکیڑتا ہے۔ جس کی وجہ سے خون باہر کی طرف نکلتا ہے اس خون اور رطوبت کے اخراج کو نفاس کہا جاتا ہے۔ نفاس کی رنگت تبدیلی ہوتی رہتی ہے۔ شروع میں لال رنگ۔ بعد میں سبزی مائل اور آخر میں گدلے پانی کے رنگ کا ہو جاتا ہے۔

Lockjaw Tetanus (q.v.)

چاندنی : تشنج

Locomotor *(lo-ko-mo'-tor)* Can be applied to any tissue or system used in human movement. Most usually refers to nerves and muscles. Sometimes includes the bones and joints. **locomotor ataxia,** the discordered gait and loss of sense of position in the lower limbs, which occurs in tabes dorsalis (q.v.) Tabes dorsalis is sometimes referred to, still, as 'locomotor ataxia.'

متحرک : انسانی حرکت میں مستعمل کوئی نسیج یا نظام

Loculated *(lok'-u-la-ted)* [L. *loculus,* little place]. Divided into numerous cavities.

لاکولیٹڈ : مختلف کھوں میں تقسیم۔

Loiasis *(loi-as-is)* Special form of filariasis (Filaria *Loa loa)* which occurs in West Africa, Nigeria and the Cameroons. The vector, a large horse-fly, Chrysops, bites in the daytime. Larvae take 3 years to develop and may live in a man for 17. They creep about and cause intense itching. Accompanied by nophilia.

لوئیسس : فلیریاسس کی مخصوص قسم

Loin [*L. lumbus*]. That part of the back. between the lower ribs and the iliac crest; the area immediately above the buttocks.

کمر : پیٹھ کا حصہ۔ الیائیک کرلیٹ اور نچلی پسلیوں کے درمیان۔

Loin *(lo-mo-till)* Diphenoxylate hydrochloride and atropine sulphate. Useful for loose colostomy and postvagotomy diarrhoea. Reduces molitity of gut and allows time for absorption of water from faeces. Single dose lessens desire to defeacate after one hour and is effective for 6 hours.

موٹل : ڈائی فناکسی لیٹ ہائیڈروکلورائیڈ اور ایٹروپین سلفیٹ۔ اس کی دو ولیاں ہر تین گھنٹے بعد برائے دست یا اسہال۔

Lomulizder *(lom'-ul-i-zer)* Device whic disperses fine powder (contained in a tin plastic cartridge) through a mouth piece.

سولائزر : آلہ جو باریک سفوف کو ماؤتھ پیس میں سے منتشر کرتا ہے۔

Long-sighted Hypermetropic See HYPERMET ROPIA.

ید بین، دراز نظر : ہائپر میٹروپک۔

Lorazepam *(lor-az-e-pam)* Tranquillizer (q.v.).

Lordosis *(lor-do-sis)* [G. a spinal curvature]. A exaggerated formward, convex curve of th lumbar spine.

مار : لبر سپائن کا زائد آگے کی طرف محدب خم۔ کبڑا پن۔

Lorexane *(lor-eks-an)* Gamma benzen hydrochloride (q.v.).

Lorfan. Levallorphan tartrate (q.v.).

رفین : لیویلورفن ٹارٹریٹ۔

Lotio rubra. See RED LOTION.

شیور برا : سرخ لوشن۔

Loupe *(loop)* [F.]. A magnifying lensused i opthalmology.

ئینہ مکبر : ایک عدسہ آفتھلمولوجی میں مستعمل۔

Louping ill. Tick-borne virus meningoenc ephalitis in sheep. Antibodies have been fo und in human serum.

پنگ اِل : بھیڑوں میں پایا جانے والا وائرس۔ انسانی سیریم میں اینٹی یز پائی گئی ہیں۔

Louse *(lows)* A small parasitic insect, there ar three varieties affecting man lice. *pl.* Se PEDICULUS.

ں : ایک چھوٹا طفیلی حشرہ۔ اس کی تین اقسام انسان کو متاثر کرتی ہیں۔

Low birth-weigh. Term used to indicate weight of 2.5 kg or less at birth, whether o not gestation was below 37 weeks.

LSD. Lysergic acid diethylamide (q.v.).

ں ایس ڈی : لائیزجک ایسڈ ڈائی میتھائل ایمائیڈ۔

L-tryptophan *(l-trip-to-fan)* See TRYPTOPH ANE.

Lubb-dubb. Words descriptive of the hea sounds as appreciated in auscultation.

ب ڈپ : دل کی آوازوں کو ظاہر کرنے والے الفاظ۔

ucanthone *(lu-kan-thon)* Synthetic oral drug for the treatment of schistosomiasis.

لیوکینتھون: منہ کے ذریعے کھائی جانے والی تالیف دوا۔

ucid *(loo-sid)* [L. *lucisus*, clear]. Clear; mental clarity.

واضح۔صاف: ذہنی صفائی۔

ues *(lu-ez)* [L. pestilence]. Syphilis leuetic, *adj*.

وبا: آتشک۔

ugol's solution *(loo-gols)* An aqueous solution of iodine and potassium iodide. Used in the preoperative stabilization of thyrotoxic patients. It has been given by slow intravenous injection in thyro- toxic crisis. [Antoine Lugol, physician in Paris, 1786-1851].

لیوگول کامحلول: پوٹاشیم آیوڈائیڈاور آیوڈین کا آبی محلول۔

umbago *(lum-ba-go)* [L.]. Incapacitating pain low down in the back. A symptom of fibrositis of lumbar muscles, spondylitis, prolapsed interverteb- ral disc, etc.

کمری: پیٹھ سے متعلق۔لمبر درٹبری یا کمر کے مہرے تعداد میں پانچ ہوتے ہیں۔لمبر پنکچر یعنی حرام مغز سے پانی نکالنے کے لئے سوئی چبھوتے اور پانچویں لمبر مہرے کے درمیان چبھوتے ہیں۔

umbocostal *(lum-bo-kos-tal)* [L. *lumbus*, loin; *costa*, rib]. Pertaining to the loin and ribs.

قطنی ضلعی: پیٹھ اور پسلیوں سے متعلق۔

umbosacral *(lum-bo-sa-kral)* [L. *lumbus*, loin; *sacrum*, sacred]. Pertaining to the loin or lumbar vertebrae and the sacrum.

قطنی عجزی: سیکرم اور لمبر مہروں سے متعلق۔

umbricus *(lum-brik-us)* [L.]. A genus of earthworms. See ASCARIDES.

کیچوا: کیچوؤں کا ایک جنس۔نیماٹوڈ ورم یا کیڑا۔کیچوے کے اگلے سرے پر منہ اور خلفی سرے پر مبرز ہوتی ہے۔اس کی غذائی قنال یک سیدھی ٹیوب ہوتی ہے۔یہ دوز وجیہ ہے۔اس میں دونوں نر اور مادہ تولیدی اعضاء موجود ہوتے ہیں۔اس میں خود باروری نہیں ہوتی۔

umen *(loo-men)* [L. light]. the space inside a tubular structure—lumina *pl.*; luminal, *adj*.

نوریہ: (ا) نلی نما ساحت کے اندر جگہ۔(۲) نوری فلکس کی ماخوذ ایس آئی اکائی۔نوری فلکس یا نوری نفاذ سے مراد ہے کسی علاقہ میں سے گزرنے والی روشنی جو ایک سیکنڈ یا ثانیہ میں گزرتی ہے۔

uminal *(loo-min-al)* Phenobarbitone (q.v.).

لیومی نیل: فینا باربیٹون۔

Lungs. The two main organs of respiration which occupy the greater part of the thoracic cavity; they are separated from each other by the heart and other contents of the mediastinum. Together they weigh about 11.88 hg and they are concerned with the oxygenation of the blood.

Lungs

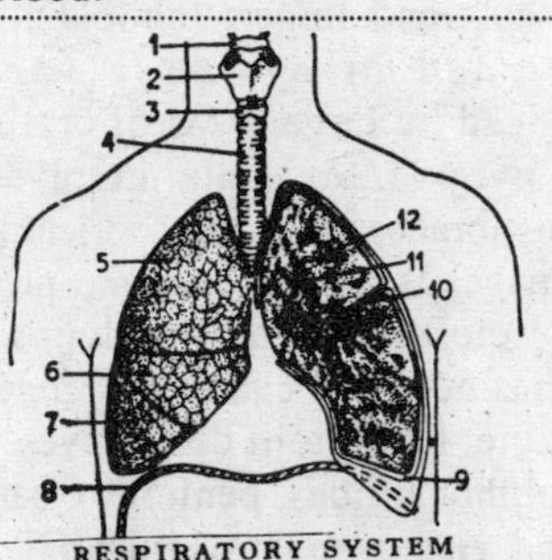

DIAGRAM OF LUNGS WITH LEFT SIDE IN SECTION

1. Hyoid bone. 2. Thyroid cartilage. 3. Cricoid cartilage. 4. Trachea. 5. Upper lobe of lung. 6. Middle lobe of lung. 7. Lower lobe of lung. 8. Diaphragm. 9. Pleura. 10. Pulmonary veins. 11. Bronchus. 12. Pulmonary artery

پھیپھڑے: تنفس کے دو بڑے اعضاء جو تھوراسک کہفہ کے زیادہ حصے میں موجود ہوتے ہیں۔وہ خون کو آکسیجن مہیا کرتے ہیں۔ان کے بیچ میں دل اور اس کی مخصوص بڑی نالیوں کے جو کچھ حصے ہوتے ہیں۔پھیپھڑے کسی قدر مخروطی شکل کے ہوتے ہیں۔ان کی نوک گردن کی جڑ تک پہنچتی ہے۔نیچے کا چوڑا حصہ ڈایافرام پر رکا ہوتا ہے۔دایاں کسی قدر بڑا اور تین حصوں میں منقسم ہوتا ہے۔بایاں کسی قدر چھوٹا اور دو حصوں میں منقسم ہوتا ہے۔

Lunula *(loo-nu-la)* [L. little moon]. The semilunar pale area at the root of the nail.

Lunula

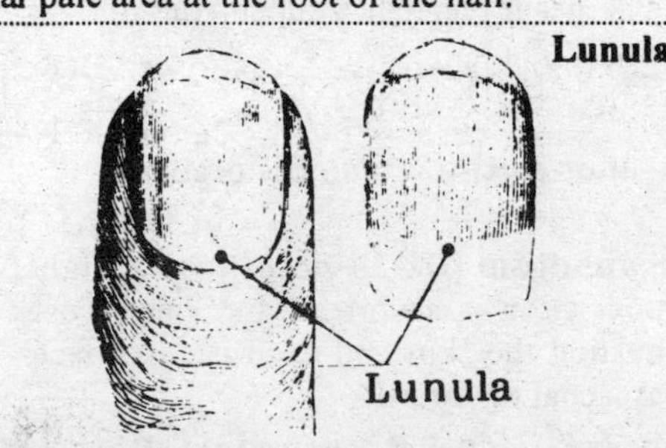

ہلال الظفر : ناخن کی جڑ پر نظر آنے والا نصف قمری پیلا ایریا۔

Lupus *(loo'-pus)* [L. wolf]. A nodular skin condition with many manifestations. **lupus erythematosus,** see COLLAGEN, I.E. CEI I.S. The discoid variety is charaterized by patulous follicles, adherent scales, telangiectasis and atrophy; commonest on nose, malar regions, scalp and fingers (chilblain 1.). The disseminated or systemic variety is characterized by large areas of erythema on the skin, pyrexia, toxaemia, involvement of serous membranes (pleurisy, pericardits) and renal damage. Is an autoimmune process. A syndrome closely resembling lupus erythematosus has been associated with ingestion of hydrallazine, hydantoin derivatives, griseofulvin, sulphonamides, penicillin, carabamazepine and guanoxan. **lupuspernio,** a form of sarcoidosis (q.v.) **lupus vulgaris,** the commonest variety of skin tuberculosus; ulceration occurs over cartilage (nose or ear) with necrosis and ficial disfigurement.

آکلہ (مرض): جلد کی مخصوص حالت۔

Luteotrophin *(loo'-te-o-tro-fin)* Secreted by the anterior pituitary gland; it assists the formation of the corpus luteum in the ovary.

لیوٹیوٹرافین: امامی اپٹوایٹری گلینڈ کی رطوبت۔ یہ بیضہ دان میں کارپس لوٹیم بنانے میں مدد دیتی ہے۔

Luteum *(loo'-te-um)* [L. *luteus,* yellow] yellow. **corpus 1.** a yellow mass which forms in the ovary after rupture of a Graafian follicle. It secretes progester one and persists and enlarges if pregnancy supervenes.

لیوٹیم: پیلا یا زرد۔ کارپس لیوٹیم ایک زرد مادہ جو بیضہ دان میں گرافی فولیک کے پھٹنے کے بعد بنتا ہے۔ یہ پروجیسٹرون خارج کرتا ہے۔

Luxation *(luks-a'-shun).* Dislocation.

موچ: اپنی جگہ سے ہل جانا۔

Lycopodium *(lik-ko-po-di-um)* A light, dry powder; it is adsorbent and can be used for dusting the skin and excoriated surfaces and as a coating for pills.

لائکوپوڈیم: ایک ہلکا خشک سفوف۔ یہ جاذب ہے اور جلد پر چھڑکنے کے لئے استعمال کیا جاسکتا ہے۔

Lying-in-period Early postnatal period, not less than 10 days after the end of labour during which the continued attendace of a midwife on the mother and/or infant is requisite.

عرصہ زچگی: بچے کی پیدائش کے بعد کم از کم دس ایام جس میں زچہ و بچہ کا خیال رکھا جاتا ہے۔

Lymeccline *(lim-s'i-klin)* A complex of tetracycline, formaldehyde and lysine that provides a higher blood level than given by tetracycline alone.

Lymph *(limf)* [L. *lympha,* water]. The fluid contained in the lymphatic vessels. It is transparent, colourless or slightly yellow. Unlike blood,lymph contains only one type of cell, the lymphocyte.

لمف: لمفی رگوں میں موجود سیال۔ یہ شفاف۔ بے رنگ یا ہلکا زرد ہوتا ہے۔ اس میں خلیے کی صرف ایک قسم لمفوسائیٹ ہوتی ہے۔

Lymphadenectomy *(limf-ad-en-ek-to-mi)* [L. *lympha,* water; G, *aden,* gland; *ektome,* excision]. Excision of on or more lymph nodes.

لمفاڈین ایکٹومی: ایک یا زیادہ لمف نوڈز کا قطع

Lymphadenitis *(limf-ad-en-i-tis)* [L. *lympha,* water; G. *aden,* gland; *itis,* inflammation] Inflammation of a lymph node.

ورم غدود لمفی: لمف نوڈ کی سوزش۔

Lymphadenoma *(limf-ad-en-o'-ma).* Hodgkin's disease (q.v.)

سلعہ غدود لمفی: ایک مرض۔

Lymphadenopathy *(limf-ad-en-op'-ath-i)* [L. *lympha,* water; G. *aden,* gland; *pathos,* disease]. Any disease of the lymph nodes--lymphadenopathic, adj.

ورم و تہیج غدد لمفادیہ: لمف نوڈز کی کوئی بیماری

Lymphangiectasis *(limf-an-ji-ek-ta-sis)* [L.*lympha,* water, G. *aggeion,* vessel; *ektasis,* extension] Dilation of the lymph vessels--lymphangietatic, adj.

تمدد اوعیہ لمفادیہ: لمفی رگوں کا پھیلاؤ۔

Lymphangiogram *(limf-an'-ji-o-gram)* [L.*lympha,* water; G.*aggeion,* vessel;

gramma, letter]. Radiograph demonstrating the lymphatic system after injection of an opaque medium-- lymphangiography, n; lymphangiographical, adj; lymphangiographically, adv.

لمف انجیکٹو گرام: ریڈیوگراف جوغیر شفاف میڈیم کے انجکشن کے بعد لمفی نظام کوظاہر کرتا ہے۔

ymphangioma *(limf-an-ji-o'-ma)* [L. *lympha,* water; G. *aggeion,* vessel; *-oma,* tumour;]. A simple tumour of lymph vessels frequently associated with similar formations of blood vessels-- lymphangiomata, pl; lymphangiomatous, adj.

سلعہ عروق لمفی: لمفی رگوں کا مصنوعی راہوں سے تبادلہ

ymjphangioplasty *(limf-an'-ji-o-plas-ti)* [L.*lympha,* water, G. *aggeion* vessel; *plassein,* to form]. Replacement of lymphatics by artificial channels (buried silk threads) to drain the tissues. Relieves the brawny arm after radical mastectomy-- lymphangioplastic, adj.

لمفی رگوں کا مصنوعی راہوں سے تبادلہ

ymphagitis (limf-an-ji'-tis) [L. lympha, water; G. aggeion, vessel; -itis, inflammation]. Inflammation of a lymph vessel.

ورم عروق لمفی: لمفی رگ کی سوزش۔

ymphangits *(limf-at-ik)* [L.*lympha,* water] Pertaininhg to, conveying or containinhg lymph.

بلغمی مزاج لمفی: لمف پر مشتمل یا اس سے متعلق

ymphaticovenous *(limf'-at-ik-o-ven-us)* [L. *lympha,* water; *vena,* vein]. Implies the presence of both lymphatic vessels and veins to increase drainage from the area.

لمفیٹیکو وینس: ایریا سے نکاس کو بڑھانے کے لئے لمفی رگوں اور وریدوں دونوں کی موجودگی

ymphoblastoma *(limf-o-blass-to-ma)* [L.*lympha,* water; G. *blastos,* germ; *oma,* tumour]. Malignant lymphoma in which single or multiple tumours arise from lymphoblasts in lymph nodes. Sometimes associated with acute lymphatic leukaemia. **lymphoblastoma malignum,** Hodgkin's disease. (q.v.).

لمفو بلاسٹو ما: لمفو ما جس میں ایک یا زیادہ ناسور لمف نوڈز میں لمفو بلاسٹس سے بنتے ہیں۔

Lymphocyte *(limf-o-sit)* [L. *lympha* water; G. *kytos,* cell.]. One variety of white blood cell. The lymphocytic stem cells under go transformation to Y-lymphoeytes (in the thymus) which provide cellular immunity; and B-lymphocytes (in a site as yet unkown) with form anitbodies and provide humoral immunity. The transformation is humoral immunity. The transformation is usually complete a few months after birth.--- lymphocytic. adj.

لمفی خلیہ: لمف نوڈز میں بننے والے لیوکوسائیٹ کی ایک ورائٹی۔ خون میں ۲۵ فیصد۔

Lymphocytosis *(limf-o-si-to'-sis)* An increase in lymphocytes in the blood.

کثرت خلایا لمف: خون میں لمفوسائیٹس کی زیادتی۔

lymphoedema *(limf-e-de-ma)* [. *lympha,* water; G. *oidema,* swelling]. Excess of fluid in the tissues from obstruction of lymph vessels. See ELEPHANTIASIS and FILARIASIS.

اویمائے سیرمی: لمفی رگوں میں رکاوٹ کی وجہ سے بافتوں میں سیال کی زیادتی۔

Lymphoepithelioma *(limf-o-ep-i-thel-i-o'-ma)* [L. *lympha,* water; G. *epi,* on; *thele,* nipple; *oma,* tumour]. Rapidly growing malignant pharyngeal tumour .May involve the tosil. Often has metastases in cervical lymph nodes -- lymphoepitheliomata, pl.

لمفو اپی پھیلوما: تیزی سے بڑھنے والا فیرنجیل ناسور

Lymphogranuloma inguinale *(lim-fo-gran-u-lo'-ma in-gwin-a-le)* [L.*lympha,* water; *granulum,* grain; G. *oma,* tumour; L. *inguinalis,* of the grooin]. Called 1.Venereum in USA. Tropical venereal disease caused by a virus. Primary lesion on the genitalia may be an ulcer or herpetiform eruption and is usually evanescent. Soon buboes (q.v) appear in regional lymph nodes. They form a painful mass called proadenitis and commonly produce sinuses. Further spread by lymphatics may cause severe periproctisis or rectal stricture in women. Patch skin test (lygranum) and a complement-flixation test of patient's serum are used in diagnosis.

لمفو گرینو ما انگوا ینلی :وائرس سے پیدا ہونے والی بیماری

Lymphograophy *(limf-og-ra-fi)* [L. *lympha,* water; G. *graphein,* to write]. X-ray examination of the lymphatic system after it has been rendered radio opaque. **therapeutic 1.** endolymphatic radiontheraphy. See RADIO THERAPY-- lymphographical, adj; lymphographically, adv.

لمفو گرافی :لمفی نظام کی ایکس رے کے ذریعے جانچ پڑتال۔

Lymphoid *(limf-oid)* [L. *lympha,* water; G. *eidos,* form]. Pertaining to lymph.

لمف نما: لمف سے متعلق۔

Lymphoma *(limf-o'-ma)* [L. *lympha,* water; G. *oma,* tumour] A benign tumour of lymphatic tissue. malignant 1., term now applied to include malignant tumours arising from reticuloendothelial tissues. Previously called malignant reticulosis---lymjphomata, pl; lymphom atous, adj.

لمفو ما :لمفادی رسولی۔لمفی نسیج کا ناسور۔

lymphorrhagia *(limf-or-aj-e-a)* [L.l *lympha,* water; G. *rhegnynai,* to burst forth] An outpouring of lymph from a severed lymphatic vessel.

لمفو ریجا سیلان رطوبت طلمیہ :کٹی ہوئی لمفی رگ سے لمف کا بھاؤ۔

Lymphosarcoma *(limf-o-sar-ko-ma)* [. *lympha,* water; G., *sarkoma,* fleshly overgrowth]. A malignant tumour arising from lymphatic tissue--lymphosarcomats, pl; lymophosarcomatous, adj.

لمفی نسیج سے بننے والا ناسور۔

Lypressin *(li-of-rin)* Adrenaline preparation. Should be used only in open angle glaucoma.

ایڈرینالین سے تیار شدہ

Lyophilization *(li-of-il-iz-a-shun)* A special method of preserving such biological substances as plasma, sera, bacteria and tissue.

Lyphilized skin *(li-of-li-izd).* Skin which has been subjected to lyophilization. It is reconstituted and used for temporary skin replacement.

Lypressin *(li-press-in)* Antidiuretic. See VASOPR-ESSIN.

Lysergic acid diethylamide *(lik-ser-gikas-id-dei-eth-ii-a-mid).* Potent hallucinogenic agent. An amino oxidase inhibitor. See MAOI

لائیسر جک ایسڈ :ارگٹ سے حاصل شدہ قلمی مرکب۔ایل ایس ڈی کی تیاری میں مستعمل۔

Lysin *(li-sen)* A cell dissloving substance in blood. See BACTERIOLYSIN. HAEMOLYSIN.

خون سے خلیے کو حل کرنے والا مادہ۔

lysin *(li-sen)* An essential amino acid necessary for growth. Deficiency may cause nausea, dizziness and anaemia. It is destroved by heating.

ایک لازمی قلمی حل پذیر امینو ایسڈ جو نشو نما کے لئے ضروری ہے اس کی کمی سے متلی اونگھ اور خون کی کمی ہو سکتی ہے۔نقطہ پگھلاؤ ۲۲۴س مالیکیولی وزن ۲" ۱۴۶ امینو ایسڈز میں امینو گروہ اور کاربوکسل گردہ دونوں موجود ہوتے ہیں۔اور ان سے پروٹین بنتی ہے۔

Lysis *(li-sis)* [G.] 1.A gradual return to normal, used especially in relation to pyrexia. Opp, crisis. 2. Dissolution and disintegration of bacteria and cells the action of a lysin.

خلیہ پاشی :اینٹی باڈیز۔لائی سنز کے ذریعہ ملیات خصوصاً خون اور جراثیم کے خلیات کی تباہی یا خاتمہ۔

lysol *(li'-sol)* Well known disinfectant containing 50 per cent cresol in soap solution. It has a wide range of activity.

لائسول: نرم صابن کے محلول کے ساتھ کریسولز کا آمیزہ۔ یہ دافع تعفن کے طور پر استعمال کیا جاتا ہے۔

sozyme *(li'-so-zim)* [G. *lysis,* dissolution; *zyme,* leaven] A bacteriolytic enzyme. See TEARS.

:ایک جراثیم پاش خامرہ۔

Lytic cocktail Consists of promethazine (Phenergan), meperidine (pethidine) and chlorpromazine (Largactil) diluted in normal saline solution. Used during the induction and maintenance of hypothermia. Ablishes shivering and convulsions.

: پرومیتھازین پیتھیڈین اور لارجیکٹل پر مشتمل نارمل سیلائن محلول میں ہلکا کیا ہوا کپکپاہٹ کو ختم کرتا ہے۔

M

M *(em)* Symbol for mega, molar, median, meter, milli and mass etc.

ایم: علامت ہے میگا، مولر، میڈین، میٹر، ملی اور حجم وغیرہ کی۔

μ *(mu)* The twelfth letter of the Greek alphabet. Symbol for linear attenuation co-efficient, population, mean, micro, micron, electrophoritic, mobility and the heavy chain of IGM.

میو: یونانی حروف ابجد کا بارہواں حرف۔ لینئر اٹینوئیشن کوئیفیشینٹ، آبادی کی اوسط، مائیکرو، مائیکرو، الیکٹروفوریٹک، موبلیٹی اور آئی جی ایم کی بھاری زنجیر کی علامت ہے۔

MacConkey's agar *(ma-kong-kez)* [Alfred Theodore MacConkey, English bacteriologist 1861-1931]. An agar medium containing peptone, lectose, bile salts, sodium chloride, neutral red and crystal violet, used to differentiate fermenters coliforms from non-lactose fermenters among the enteric bacilli.

میکانگی ایگر: یہ میڈیم پیپٹون، لیکٹوز، بائیل، نمکیات، عام نمک، نیوٹرل ریڈ اور کرسٹل وائیلٹ پر مشتمل ہوتا ہے۔ یہ میڈیم لیکٹوز میں خمیر پیدا کرنے اور نہ کرنے والے بیکٹیریا میں فرق کرنے کے لئے استعمال کیا جاتا ہے۔

Maceration *(ma's-ar-a'-shan)* [L. *maceratio,* to soften]. Softening of the solid by soaking in histology. The softening of tissues by soaking in acid, until the connective tissue fibres are so dissolved that the tissue components can be teased apart.

Machine *(ma-she'n)* [L. *machina,* machine]. A conttrivance or appatus for the production, conversion or transmission of some form of energy or force.

ن: ایک ایسا آلہ یا اوزار جو کہ پیداوار، تبدیلی یا توانائی کی ایک قسم کو قسم میں تبدیل کرنے میں مدد دے یا کرے۔

Macroanalysis *(mak-ro-a-nal-a-sis)* Chem analysis using 0.1 to 0.2 g of the substa under study.

و تجزیہ: ایسا کیمیائی تجزیہ جس میں سو یا دو سو ملی گرام مرکب استعمال کیا ۔

Macroblast *(mak-ro-blast)* [G. *blastos,* cells large young normoblast with megalobla features.

ے جرثومے: بہت بڑے مرکزے والے خون کے سرخ جرثومے۔ اس گالوبلاسٹک خوبیوں والے نئے نارموبلاسٹ بھی شامل ہوتے ہیں۔

Macroblepharia *(mak'ro-bla-far-e-a)* [G. *b haron,* eyelid]. Abnormal largeness of eyelid.

ے پپوٹے: آنکھ کے بہت ہی بڑے پپوٹے ہونا۔

Macrocephalous *(makro-sef-a-les)* [G. *keph* head]. Having an excessively large head.

Macrocheiria *(mak-ro-ki-le-a)* [G. *cheir,* h *macro,* large]. Excessive size of the hand.

ہاتھ: ہاتھوں کا بہت زیادہ بڑا ہونا۔

Macrocrania *(mak'ro-kra-ne-a)* Abnorm increase in the size of skull, the facial being disproportionately small in comparis

و کرینک: کھوپڑی کا حد سے زیادہ بڑا ہو جانا۔ اس میں چہرہ کھوپڑی ابلے میں بہت چھوٹا رہ جاتا ہے۔

Macromastia *(mak-ro-mas-ti-a)* G. *makr*

large; *mastos,* breast] Abnormally large breast.

بڑے پستان: چھاتی جو غیر معمولی طور پر بڑی ہوئی ہو۔

acrophage *(mak-ro-faj)* [G. *makros,* large; *phagein,* to eat]. A phagocytic cell, which plays an important part in organization and repair of tissue.

میکروفیج: ایک فیگو سائیٹ خلیہ جو نسیج کی تنظیم اور مرمت میں اہم کردار ادا کرتا ہے۔

acroscopic *(mak-ro-skop'-ik)* [G.*makros,* large; *skopein,* to examine0 Visible to the naked eye; gross . Opp microscopic.

کلاں: جو چیز آنکھ سے دیکھی جا سکے۔

acula *(mak'-u-la)* [L.] A spot -- macular, adj. **macula lutea,** the yellow spot on the retina, the area of clearest vision. **macula solaris,** a sunspot, a freckle.

داغ جلد: ایک داغ۔ دھبہ۔ دانہ۔ میکولا لوٹیا آنکھ میں عدسہ کی سیدھ میں زرد نشان جو ریٹینا کا حساس حصہ ہے۔

acule *(mak'-ul)* [. *macula,* spot] A discoloured spot, not raised above the skin's surface -- macular, adj.

داغ: ایک بدنما دھبہ جو جلدی سطح سے اوپر ابھرا ہوا نہ ہو یا جس کا رنگ اڑ چکا ہو۔

aculaopapular *(mak'-u-lo-pap-u-lar)* [L. *icula,* spot; *papula,* pustule]. The presence of acules and raised palpable spots (papules) on : skin.

میکولوپیپولر: ایسے دھبوں کی موجودگی جو جلد پر ابھرے ہوئے ہوں۔

adecassol *(mad-ek'-as-ol)* Ointment with 1 per cent plant extract from *centela asiatica.* promotes healing due, to sitmulation of collagen formation and fibroblastin proliferation.

adribon *(mad-rib-on)* A sulphonamide, useful as a prophylactic of urinary infection as resistance does not occur.

میڈری باں: ایک سلفونامائیڈ۔

adua foot *(ma-du-ra)* Mycetoma. Fungus disease of the foot found by India and the tropics. Characterized by swelling and the development of nodules and sinuses. May terminate in death from sepsis.

فطر پا: مستوما۔ پاؤں کا سمارذغی مرض۔

Magnesuim carbonate *(mag-ne-zi-um)* A powder widely used as an antacid in peptic ulcer and as a laxative.

میگنیشیم کاربونیٹ: ایک سفوف السر میں اور ہلکے جلاب کے طور پر مستعمل۔

Magnesium hydroxide A valuable antacid and taxative, usually given as an aguenous suspension referred to as cream of magnesia or mist. maghydrox. It is sometimes preferred to magn- esium and other carbonates, as it does not liberate carbon dioxide in the stomach. Also used as an antidote in noisoning by mineral acids.

میگنیشیم ہائیڈرو آکسائیڈ: ایک سفید قلمی مرکب۔ اسے میگنیشیم اور دوسرے کاربونیٹس پر ترجیح دی جاتی ہے کیونکہ یہ معدہ میں کاربن ڈائی آکسائیڈ پیدا نہیں کرتا۔ معدنی ترشوں سے زہریلا پن میں بطور تریاق مستعمل۔

Magnesium sulphate. Epson salts; an effective rapid- acting laxative, especially when given in dilute solution on an empty stomach. It is used as a 25 per-cent sulution as a wet dressing for inflamed conditions of the skin and as a paste with glycerin for the treatment of boils and carbuncles.

میگنیشیم سلفیٹ: میگنیشیم سلفیٹ ایک سلفیٹ قلمی حل پذیر نمک ہے جو دوائیوں اور چمڑے کی صنعت میں کام آتا ہے۔ اپسی نمک۔ ہلکے جلاب کے طور پر استعمال ہوتا ہے۔ کھال جل جانے کی صورت میں اس کا پچیس فیصد محلول تر ڈریسنگ کے طور پر استعال کیا جاتا ہے۔ آبلوں کے علاج کے لئے گلسرین کے ساتھ ملا کر پیسٹ کے طور پر استعال کیا جاتا ہے۔

Magnesium trisilicate Tasteless white powder with a mild but prolonged antacid action. It is therefore used extensively in peptic ulcer, often combined with more rapidly acting antacids. It does not cause alkalosis, and large doses not cause alkalosis, and large doses can be given withcut side effects.

میگنیشیم ٹرائی سیلیکیٹ: ڈائی میگنیشیم ٹرائی سیلیٹ۔ ایک سفید بے ذائقہ

سفوف۔ السر میں مستعمل اسے زیادہ مقدار میں بھی دیا جاسکتا ہے۔

Magnum *(mag-num)* [L. *magnus,* large]. Large or great of great, as foramen m. in occipital bone.

میگنم: بڑا۔ جیسے آکسیپٹل میں بڑا سوراخ۔

Majeptil *(ma-jap-til)* Closely resembles chlorpromazine. (q.v.)

میجپٹل: کلور پرومازین سے مشابہ۔

Mal [F] . Disease **mal de mer,** seasickness **grand m,** major epilepsy. **petit m.** minor epilepsy.

عارضہ: مرض۔ بیماری۔

Malabsorption *(mal-ab-sorb-shun)* Poor or disordered absorption. **malabsorption syndrome,** losws of weight and steatorrhoea, varying from mild to severe. Caused by (1) lesions of the small intestine; (2) lack of digestive enzymes or bile salts; (3) surgical operations.

کم جذب: کم انجذاب۔

Malacia *(mal-a-si-a)* [G. *malakia,* softness]. Softening of a part.See KERATOMALACIA, OSTEOMALACIA.

لینت عضو: کسی حصے کی نرمی۔

Maladjustment *(mal-ad-just-ment)* [L. *malus,* bad; a,to; *justus,* right].Bad or poor adaptation to enviro ment. socially, mentally or physically.

عدم مطابقت: ماحول کے مطابق صحیح طور پر نہ ڈھلنا۔

malaise *(mal-az)* [F]. A feeling of illness and discomfort.

بے قراری: بیماری اور بے سکونی کا احساس۔

malalignment *(mal-al-in-ment)* [L] *malus,* bad; *linea,* line] Faulty alignment -- as of the teeth, or fracture.

میل ایلائنمنٹ: ناقص صف بندی جیسے دانتوں یا فریکچر کی۔

Malar *(mal-ar)* [L. *mala*-cheek] Relating to the cheek.

خدی: رخسار سے متعلق۔ رخساروں کی ہڈیاں جن سے رخساروں کے ابھار بنتے ہیں۔ نیز یہ آنکھ کے حلقوں کی زیریں سطح اور ناک کی اطراف بنانے میں مدد دیتی ہے۔

Malaria *(mal-ar-i-a)* [It. *malaria,* badair]. tropical disease caused by one of the gu Plasmodium carried by infected mosquit of the genus Anopheles, *plasmodi flaciparum* causes malignant tertian *plasmodium vivax* causes benign tertian and *Plasmodium malariae* causes quartan Signs and symptoms are caused by t presence in the red blood cells of t erythrocytic (E) stages of the parasite. In falciparum malaria *only* the blood-forms the parasite exist. There is an additio persistent infection in the liver (t extraerythrocytic or EE form) in all ot forms of malaria and it is the fact responsible for relapses. Clinical picture one of recurring rigors, anaemia, toxaen and splenomegaly -- mnalarial , adj.

یا: ملیریا کی وجہ پلازموڈی ہے جو ۱۸۸۰ء میں دریافت ہوا۔ اس کی فت کا سہرا فرانسیسی طبیب لیوران کے سر ہے۔ ملیریا بخار میں سخت سردی ں ہوتی ہے۔ رونگٹے کھڑے ہو جاتے ہیں اور دانت بجتے ہیں۔ اس کے ریض کو گرمی لگتی ہے۔ اس کے بعد مریض کو گرمی لگتی ہے۔ اس کا جسمانی حرارت ۱۰۵ تک جا پہنچتا ہے۔ اسے سر درد اور متلی ہوتی ہے پھر پسینہ آتا اور بخار اتر جاتا ہے۔ چونکہ بخار وقفوں کے ساتھ ہوتا ہے اس لئے اسے ں کا بخار کہتے ہیں۔

ہ بیماری کی حالت میں دل کی دھڑکن اور تنفس کی شرح بڑھ جاتی ہے مریض و یہ بدل جاتا ہے اور چڑچڑا ہو جاتا ہے۔ اس کی سوچ بچار کی صلاحیت کار ہو جاتی ہے یہ مرض پاکستان میں عام ہے۔ مچھروں سے پھیلتا ہے۔ ن میں مچھروں کی بھرمار ہے۔ مچھروں سے بچاؤ ضروری ہے۔ ملیریا کی ت میں میٹا کیلفن کی دو گولیاں یا کلوروکوئن کی چار گولیاں دی جاتی ہیں۔

Malarial therapy Induction of hyperpyrexia inoculation with benign form of malar Used in the treatment of neurosyphilis.

یائی تھراپی: نیوروسائفلس کے علاج میں مستعمل۔

Malariologist *(mal-ar-i-ol-o-jist)* [It *malar* bad air; G. *logos,* discourse]. An expert in study of malaria.

لیریا: ملیریا کے مطالعہ میں ماہر۔

Malassimilation *(mal-a-sim-il-a-shun)* Poor disordered assimilation.

ں انجذاب: استحالہ کی کمی۔

Malathion *(mal-ath-i-on)* Organophosphorus compound, used as insecticide in agriculture. Powerful and irreversible anticholinesterase action following excessive inhalation. Potentially dangerous to man for this reson. Currently being used for treatment of head lice.

میلیتھون: آرگینو فاسفورس میں مرکب۔ زراعت میں بطور حشرات کش مستعمل۔

ale fern. Filix mas (q.v.)

نرفون: کدو کیڑے کو نکالنے کے لئے مستعمل نرفون کا عرق۔

lformation *(mal-for-ma-shun)* [L. *malus,* bad; *formare,* to form] Abnormal shape or structure; deformity.

خلقت ناقص: غیر معمولی شکل یا ساخت۔ بدشکلی۔

lignant *(mal-ig-nant)* [L. *malignus,* wicked]. Virulent and dangerous; that which is likely to have a fatal termination. malignant growth or tumour, cancer or sarcoma. malignant pustule, anthrax malignancy, n.

مہلک شدید: خطرناک جو مہلک بھی ہوسکتا ہے۔

lingering *(mal-ing-er-ing)* Deliberate (volitional) production of symptoms to evade an unpleasant situation.

تمارض: ناخوشگوار صورتحال سے بچنے کیلئے علامات کی سوچی سمجھی پیداوار۔

lleolus *(mal-le-o-lus)* [L. hammer] A part or process of a bone shaped like a hammer, **external m,** at the lower end of the fibula. **internal m,** situated at the lower end of the tibia melleoli, pl; malleolar, adj.

Malleolus

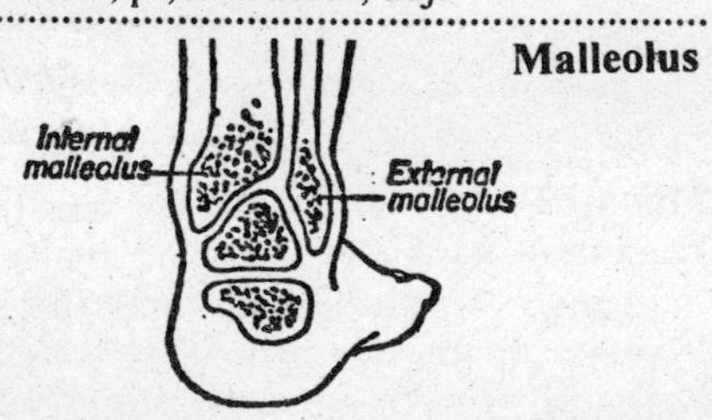

(عظم) کعبیہ: ہڈی کا حصہ یا زائدہ جس کی ہتھوڑی۔

Malleus *(mal-i-us)* [L] The hammer shapped lateral bone of the middle ear.

مطرقی ہڈی: درمیانی کان کی ہتھوڑی نما جانبی ہڈی۔

Malnutrition *(mal-nu-trish)* [L. *malus,* bad; *nature,* to nourish] . The state of being poorly nourished. May be caused by inadequate intake of one or more of the essential nutrients or by malassimil- ation.

سوتغذیہ۔ ناقص غذا: کم تغذیہ کی حالت۔

Malocclusion *(mal-ok-klu-shun)* [L. *malus,* bad; *occludere,* to close] Failure of the upper and lower teeth to meet properly when the jaws are closed.

دندان بے نظم: جب جبڑے بند ہوں تو بالائی و زیریں دانتوں کے مناسب طور پر ملنے میں ناکامی۔

Malposition *(mal-po-zi-shun)* [L. *malus,* bad; *positio,* palce]. Any abnormal position of a part.

غلط جگہ: کسی حصے کی غیر معمولی پوزیشن۔

Malpractice *(mal-prak-tis)* [L. *malus,* bad; G. *praktikos,* fit for doing] Malpraxia. Unethical, improper or injurious treatment.

غفلت مجرمانہ: غیر اخلاقی۔ نامناسب یا تکلیف دہ رویہ۔

Malpresentation *(mal-prez-en-ta-shun)* [L. *malus,* bad; *proesentere,* to present]. Any unusual presentation of the fetus in the pelvis.

سوءوضع (جنین): پیلوس یا پیڑو میں بچے کی غیر معمولی پیش کش۔

Malta fever See BRUCELLA, BRUCELLOSIS, The condition is also called abrotus f. Mediterranean f, and undulant f.

مالٹا بخارا: اسے انڈولینٹ بھی کہتے ہیں۔

Maltase *(mawl-tas)* A sugar splitting (saccharolytic) enzyme found in the body, especially in intestinal juice.

خمیر شعر مالٹیز: ایک خامرہ جو خمیر میں پایا جاتا ہے۔ یہ مالٹوز کو گلوکوز میں تبدیل کردیتا ہے۔ مالٹوز پانی مالٹیز دو گلاس۔ آنت کے جوس میں پایا جاتا ہے۔

Maltose *(mawl'-tos)* Malt sugar a disacharide; produced by the hydrolysis of strach during digestion.

شکر شعیر: مالٹ شکر۔ ایک سخت قلمی حل پذیر ڈائی سیکرائڈ۔ گنے کی شکر

سے کم شیریں ۔ یہ مالٹ میں نشاستہ پر خامرہ ۔ ڈایاسینٹر کے عمل سے بنتا ہے۔ ہضم کے دوران نشاستہ کی آب پاشیدگی سے بنتا ہے۔

Malunion *(mal-un'-yon)* [L. *malus,* bad; *unite,*] Union of a fracture in bad position.

ناقص ملاپ: فریکچر کا خراب حالت میں ملنا۔

Mamma *(ma'-ma)* [L. breast] The breast; milk -secreting gland mammae, pl;mammary. addkj.

ممہ ۔ پستان ۔ ثدی: چھاتی ۔ دودھ خارج کرنے والی گلینڈ۔

Mammaplasty *(ma'-ma-plas-ti)* [L. *mamma,* breast; G. *plassein,* to from.] Any plastic operation on the breast mammaplastic, adj.

ممہ پلاسٹی: چھاتی پر کوئی پلاسٹک اپریشن۔

Mammilla *(mam-li'-a)* [L. nipple] The nipple; a small papilla -- mammilae, pl.

حلمہ: ایک چھوٹا ابھار ۔ چوچی ۔ نپل۔

Mammography *(mam-og-ra-fi)* [L. *mamma,* breast, G. *graphein,* to write]. X-ray examination of the breast after injection of an opaque agent. Syn. mastography - mamographic, adj; mammograp- hically, adv.

مموگرافی: کسی غیر شفاف عامل کے انجکشن کے بعد چھاتی کی ایکس رے جانچ۔

Mammotrophic *(mam-o-tro'-fik)* [L. *mamma,* breast; G. *trephein,* to noursih] Having an effect upon the breast.

مموٹرافک: چھاتی پر اثر ہونا۔

Manchester operation See FORTHERGILL'S OPERATION.

مانچسٹر اپریشن: اپریشن فودرگل۔

Mandelamine *(man-del'-a-men)* See MAN-DELIC ACID.

میڈلامین: مینڈلک ایسڈ ۔ دافع تعفن کے طور پر مستعمل۔

Mandelic acid *(man-del'-ik- as'-id)* A urinary antiseptic used mainly as the calcium or ammonium salts. A high degree of uninary acidity is essectial for activity, and supplementary administration of ammonium chloride may be required. Limitation of fluids is also desirable.

مینڈیلک ایسڈ: ایک سفید قلمی مرکب ۔ دافع تعفن کے طور پر استعمال کیا

ا ہے۔

mandible The lower jawbone.

نہ: زیریں جبڑے کی ہڈی ۔ گھوڑے کی نعل کی شکل کی کھوپڑی کی واحد ں جو حرکت کر سکتی ہے اس میں ایک درمیانی حصہ اور دو شاخیں ہوتی ہیں ۔ ہر خ کے آخری کنارے پر ایک چکنا نوکیلا حصہ ہوتا ہے ۔ جو کنپٹی کی ہڈی سے طرح جڑا ہوتا ہے کہ جبڑے کی ہڈی حرکت کر سکتی ہے ۔ اس ہڈی کی نوں کے ساتھ عضلات جڑے ہوتے ہیں ۔ جن میں چبانے کے لئے مال کیا جاتا ہے۔ اس ہڈی میں سولہ خانے ہوتے ہیں۔

Mandrax *(man'-draks)* Methaqualone (q.v.) a diphenhydramine (q.v.)

ڈریکس: یہ دوائی الکوحل کے ساتھ نہیں دینی چاہیئے۔

Mania *(ma'-ni-a)* [G. madness] One phase manic depressive psychoses in which t prevailing mood is one of undue elation. a there is pronounced psychomotor overactiv and often pathological excitement-- mani adj.

: نفسیاتی مرض کا ایک مرحلہ ۔ مریض بے چین رہتا ہے ۔ ہنستا ہے ۔ قہقے ہے ۔ اپنی تعریف کرتا رہتا ہے ۔ ناراض ہونے پر مارنے کو دوڑتا ہے۔

Manic depressive psychosis *(man-i de-pres-iv- si-ko-siz)* A type of ment disorder which alternates between phases excitement and phases of depression. Oft between these phases there are periods complete normality.

ی اختلال دماغی: ذہنی مرض کی ایک قسم ۔ دماغی فتور ۔ جنونی یا جذباتی بت ۔ صرف تھوڑی دیر کیلئے حالت معمول پر ہوتی ہے۔

Manipulation *(man-ip-u-la'-shin)* Using t hands skilfully as in reducing a fracture hernia, or changing the fetal position.

ج بالید ۔ علاج دستکاری: ہاتھوں کو مہارت سے استعمال کرنا ۔ جیسے ر یا ہرنیا کی تخفیف میں یا بچے کی پوزیشن بدلنے میں۔

Mannitol *(man'-i-tol)* A natural sugar that is metabolized in the body and acts as osmotic diuretic. When the renal blood fl is low, mannitol probably exerts a dir action on the renal vessels and restores flow with a rapid improvement in rea function. Mannitol-induced diuresis used tranquillizer and barbiturate poisoning, and head injuries to shrink brain.

مینی ٹول: ایک سفید قلمی الکحل۔ایک قدرتی شکر پیشاب آور۔

nnityl hexanitrate *(man'-i-til-heks-a-it'-rat)* A long acting vasodilator, used nainly for the prophylactic treatment of ngina pectoris. Prolonged administration nay cause methaemoglo- binaemia.

مینٹی ٹول ہیکسا نائٹریٹ: ایک بے رنگ ناحل پذیر مرکب۔نقط پگھلاؤ112س۔دھماکہ خیز اشیاء اور دوائیوں میں مستعمل ہے۔

nnomustine *(man-o-mus-ten)* Antimitotic gent useful in cancer.

مینومسٹین: مائی ٹوسس کو روکنے والا عامل۔سرطان میں مفید۔

annose *(man'-os)* A fermentable nonosaccharide.

مینوز: مانوسیکرائیڈ۔

nometer *(man-om-et-er)* [G. *manos,* rare; *netron,* a measure]. An instrument for neasuring the pressure exerted by liquids or ;ases. See SPHYGMOMANOMETER.

دباؤ پیما: مائعات یا گیسی دباؤ کی پیمائش کا ایک آلہ کسی جگہ پر ہوائی دباؤ ک پیمائش بیرومیٹر اور کسی برتن میں سطح کے دباؤ کے پیمائش دباؤ پیما سے کی جاتی ہے۔

ntoux reaction *(man'-too)* An intradermal nethod of determining the degree of ensitivity of a patient to old tuberculin by ısing serial dilutions 1:10 000, 1:1000 and :100. Purified protein derivative (PPD) is a urified type of tuberculin.[Charles Mantoux, rench physician, 1877-1947.1

مینٹو تعامل: کسی مریض کا ٹوبر کولن سے حساسیت معلوم کرنے کا معلوم

nubrium *(man-u-bri-um)* [L. handle]. A andle-shaped structure; the upper part of the reast bone or sternum.

دستہ: ہینڈل کی شکل ایسی ساخت۔چھاتی کی ہڈی یا سٹرنم کا بالائی حصہ۔

OI. Monoamine oxidase inhibitor (q.v.)

ایم اے او آئی: مانوامین آکسیڈ۔

ıple syrup urine disease. Genetic disorder o recessive familial type. Leucine, isoleucine nd valine are excreted in excess in urine iving the smell of maple syrup. Sypptoms nclude spasticity, feeding and respiratory ifficulties; severe damage to the CNS mayu occur. A diet low in the three amino acids may be effective started early enough. otherwise the disorder is fatal. Genetic counselling may be indicated. In the pregnant woman, examination may reveal evidence of the disorder and in such cases it may be wise to advise termination of pregnancy.

میپل شربت بولی مرض: پیشاب سے میپل سیرپ کی بو لیوسین۔آئیسو لیوسین اور ویلین کی وجہ سے آنا۔اس سے غذائی اور تنفسی مشکلات ہوتی ہیں۔

Marasmus *(mar-az-mus)* [G. a withering]. Wasting away of the body, especially that of a baby, without apparent cause. The currently preferred term is failure to thrive (q.v.) -- marasmic, adj.

لاغری۔سوکڑا: جسم کا ضائع ہونا۔خصوصاً بچے کا بغیر کسی ظاہری سبب کے۔چھوٹے بچے غذا کی کمی کی وجہ سے سوکھ جاتے ہیں۔دودھ اور خوراک ہضم نہیں کر سکتے۔دست لگے رہتے ہیں۔علاج کیلئے سٹینوز دلول شربت ایک چھوٹی چمچی دن میں ایک دو دفعہ دو ماہ تک ملٹی وٹامن ڈراپس ۵ قطرے روزانہ ایک دفعہ اور اینزائم وٹامن کمپاؤنڈ سیرپ ایک چمچ دن میں تین مرتبہ۔

Marboran *(mar-bor-an)* Methisazone (q.v.)

مربورین: تھیسازون۔

Marburg disease Syn green monkey disease. Highly infectious viral disease characterized by a sudden onset of fever, malaise, headache and myalgia especially in the lumbar region. Between day five and seven, a rash appears on the buttocks, trunk, outer aspects of arms and around the hair roots. Treatment is symptomatic. Virus can persist in the body for two to three months after the initial attack. Cross infection probably occurs by the aerosol route. Incubation period believed to be four to nine days and mortality rate in previous outbreaks has been approximately thirty per cent

Marcain *(mar-kan)* Bupivacaine (q.v.)

مارکین: بوپیوکین۔

Marevan *(mar-e-van)* Slow-acting anticoagulant. Warfarin (q.v.)

میریوین: آہستہ عمل کرنیوالا خون نہ جمنے دینے والا۔

Marfan's syndrom. Hereditary genetic disorder of unknown cause. There is dislocation of the lens, congenitl heart disease and arachnodactyly with hypotonic musculature and lax ligaments, occasionally excessive height and abnormalities of the iris. [B.J.A.] Marfan, Paris physician, [1858-1942]

مرفینس سنڈورم: نامعلوم سبب کی توارثی جینی خرابی۔

Marihuana. Indian hemp (q.v.) Hashish.

میری ہوانا: حشیش۔

Marion's disease. Hypertrophic stenosis of the internal urinary meatus.

میریونس: مرض۔اندرونی بولی می ایٹس کی ہائپرٹرافک سٹینوسس۔

Marmite. A proprietary concentrated extract obtained from yeast by autolysis with salt and flavoured wirth vegetables and spices.It contains vitamins of the B_2 complex (riboflavin 1.5 mg per g; niacin (nicotinic acid), 16.5 mag per g).

مرمائیٹ: خمیر سے حاصل شدہ عرق۔

Marplan. Isocarboxozid(q.v.).

مرپلین: آئیسوکاربوکسازڈ۔

Marrow *(mar-o)* [A.S *mearg,* pith] The soft, pulpy substance present in bones, and is concerned with blood formation. **yellow m.** is a fatty substance, present in the shafts of long bones.

گودا: نرم گودا جو ہڈیوں میں موجود ہوتا ہے۔لال گودے کا تعلق خون بنانے سے ہے۔زرد گودا چکنا مادہ ہوتا ہے۔

Marshal-Marchetti- Krantz operation. For stress incontinence. Usually undertaken in patients who have not been controlled by a colporrphaphy. 85 per cent success rate.

مارشل مارکیٹی کرانٹز اپریشن: یہ اپریشن ۸۵ فیصد کامیاب ہے۔

Marsilid. A monoamine exidase inhibitor. (q.v.)

مرسیلڈ: ایم۔اے۔او۔وائی۔

Marsupialization *(mar-sup-i-al-iz-a-shun)* [G. *marsippion,* bag]: An operation for cystic abdominal swellings, which entails stitching the margins of an opening made into the cyst, to the edges of the abdominal wound, thus forming a pouch.

تھیلی بننا: سسٹک بطنی ابھاروں کے لئے ایک اپریشن۔اس میں تھیلی سی بن جاتی ہے۔

Marzine *(mar-zen)* Cyclizine. Action quick a short. Sould not be given in pregnancy. S ANTIHISTAMINES.

ین: سائیکلیزین۔ایکشن تیز اور مختصر۔حمل کے دوران نہ دی جائے۔

Masochism *(mas-o-kizm)* Punishing the self may be a conscious or unconscious prec Opp, sadism. [Leopold von Sacher Mashoch, Austrain historian, 1836-95].

کیت: اپنے آپ کو سزا دینا۔

Mastalgia *(mas-tal-ji-a)* [G. *masios,* brea *algos,* pain]. Pain in the breast.

ن کا درد: الم الثدی۔چھاتی میں درد۔

Mastectomy *(mas-tek-to-mi)* [G.*mastos,* brea *ektome,* excision] Surgical removal of t breast. **Simple m,** removal of the breast w the overlying skin. Combined wi radiotherapy this operation is the usu treatment for carcinoma of the breast. **radi m.**removal of the breast with the skin a underlying pectoral muscle together with the lymphatic tissue of the axilla.

ن براری: چھاتی کا سرجیکل خاتمہ۔

Masteril *(mas-ter-il)* Drostanolone (q.v).

ٹریل: ڈروسٹینولون۔

Mastication *(mas-tik-a-shun)* [L.*msticare,* chew]. The act of chewing.

نا: چبانے کا عمل۔

Mastitis *(mas-ti-tis)* [G. *mastos,* breast; it inflammation] Inflammatiopn of the brea Chronic m. the name for the merly applied the nodular changes in the breasts no usually called fibrocystic disease.

پستان: چھاتی کی سوزش۔

Masti

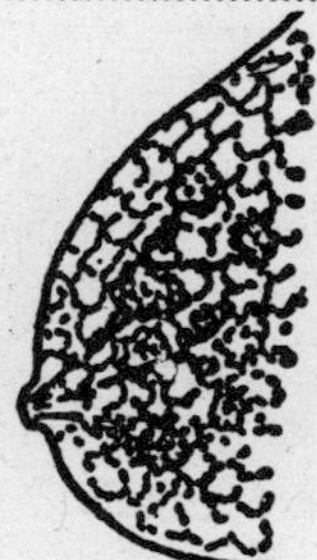

Mastography *(mas-tog-ra-fi)* See mammography mastographic, adj., mastographically, adv.

ماسٹوگرافی: مموگرافی۔

Mastoid *(mas-toid)*[G. *mastos, breast;eidos,* form]. Nipple shaped. **mastoid air cells** extended in a backward and downward direction from the antrum. **mastoid antrum** the air space within the mastoid process, lined by mucous membrane continuous with that of the tympanum and mastoid cells. **mastold process,** the prominence of the mastoid portion of the temporal bone just behind the ear.

حلمہ نما: پستان نما۔ نپل نما۔

Mastoidectomy *(mas-toid-ek-to-mi)* [G. *mastos,* breast; *eidos,* form; *edtome,* excision] Drainage of the mastoid air cells and exision of diseased tissue. **cortical m,.** all the mastoid cells are removed making one cavity which drains through an opening (aditus) into the middle near. The external meatus and middle ear are untouched. **radical m.,** the mastoid antrum, and middle ear are made into one continuous cavity for drainage of infection. Loss of hearing is inevitable.

عظم حلمیہ براری: مسٹائیڈ ہوا خلیوں کی صفائی۔

Mastoiditis *(mas-toid-i-tis)* [G. *mastos,* breast; *eidos,* form; *itis,* inflamation]. Inflammation of the mastoid air-cells.

ورم عظم حلمیہ: مسٹائڈ ہوا۔ خلیوں میں سوزش۔

Mastoidotomy *(mas-toid-o-to-mi)* [G. *mastos,* breast; *eidos,* form; *stoma,* mouth]. Incision into the mastoid process of temporal bone.

مسٹائڈوٹومی: ٹیمپورل ہڈی کے مسٹائڈ زائد سے شگاف۔

Masturbation *(mas-tur-ba-shun)* [L. *masturbari,* to defile oneselt]. The production of sexual excitement by friction of the genitals.

مشت زنی: تولیدی اعضاء کو رگڑ کر جنسی خواہش پیدا کرنا۔

Masteria medica *(mat-e-ri-a med-i-ka)* [L.] The science dealing the origin, action of drugs.

علم الادویہ: ادویات کے عمل۔ خوراک وغیرہ سے بحث کرنے والی سائنس۔

Matrix *(ma-triks)* [L.] The foundation substance in which the tissue cells are embedded.

بچہ دانی۔ بستی بین خلویہ۔ غلاف لونیہ: (1) بنیادی مادہ جس میں نسیجی خلیے ہوتے ہیں۔ (2) کاسٹ کو شکل دینے کیلئے سانچہ۔ (3) طولی مساواتوں کے سیٹ کو حل کرنے کے لئے ریاضی کے عناصر کو قطاروں اور کالموں میں ترتیب دینا۔ (4) کمپیوٹر میں ایک کوڈ سے دوسرے میں ترجمہ کرنے کے لئے اجزاء۔ (5) بھرت میں قلمی فیز جس میں دوسری فیزیں بھی شامل ہیں۔

Mastromycin *(mat-ro-mi-sin)* Oleandomycin (q.v).

میٹرومائی سین: اولینڈ مائی سین۔

Maturation *(mast-u-ra-shun)* [L. *maturare,* to make ripe]. The process of attaining full development.

پھوڑے کا پکنا: پوری تکمیل حاصل کرنے کا طریقہ۔ مکمل نشونما۔ کامل بالیدگی۔

Maurice Lee tube Combine nasogastric aspiration and jejunal feeding.

مارس لی ٹیوب: نیزوگیسٹرک اسپرین اور جیجونل فیڈنگ کو ملاتی ہے۔

Maxilla *(maks-il-a)* [L. jaw]. The jawbone; in particular the upper jawmaxillary, adj.

Maurice lee tube

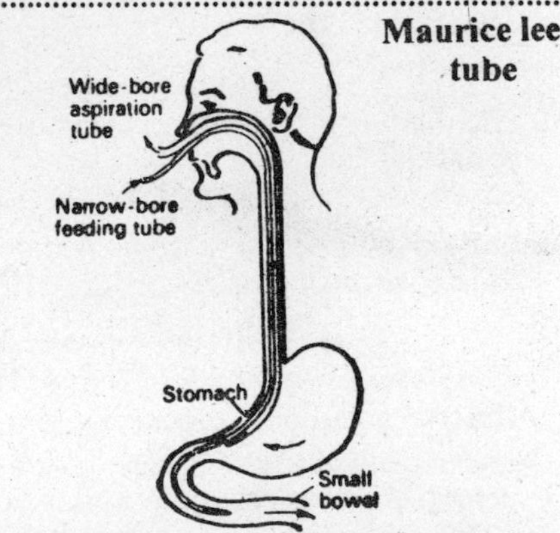

فک اعلیٰ: جبڑے کی ہڈی۔ خصوصاً بالائی جبڑے اوپر کی ہڈیاں جو تعداد میں دو ہوتی ہیں اور مل کر بالائی جبڑا بنتا ہے۔ تالو کا اگلا حصہ سخت حصہ اپنی سے بنتا ہے۔ ناک کی اطراف اور آنکھوں کے آر بٹ کا کچھ زیریں حصہ

Maxillafocial *(maks-il-o-fa-shal* [L. *maxilla,*

jaw; *facies,* face] Pertaining to the maxilla and face, A subdivisioin in plastic surgery.

فکی وجہی: میکسلا اور چہرے سے متعلق۔

Maxolon *(maks-o-lon)* Metoclipramide (q.v.)

میکسولون: میٹوکلوپرامائیڈ۔

Meatotomy *(me-at-ot-o-mi)* [L; G. *tome,* a cutting]. Surgery to uninary meatus for meatal uncer and stricture in men.

منفذ البول شگافی: بولی میس سرجری۔

M and B 7714 (3 -methyl -4-bromo-5-for mylisoth- aiazole thio semicarbazone). Samallpox prophylactic agent.

میڈلی ۷۷۱۴: چیچک کی دوائی۔

McBurney's point A point one-third of the way between the anterior superior iliac spine and the umbilicus, the site of maximum tenderness in cases of acute appendicitis [Charles McBurney, New York surgeon, 1845, 1913].

نقطہ مکبرنی: ایک نقطہ۔

Measles *(mez-lz)* Morbilli. An acute infectious disease caused by a virus. Characterized by fever, a blotcyhy rash and catarrh of mucous membranes. Endemic and worldwide in distribution.

سونڈی: وائرس سے پھیلنے والی چھوت کی بیماری۔

Meatus *(me-a-tus)* [L.] An opening or channel-meatal, adj.

منفذ: ایک سوراخ یا راستہ۔

Mebanazine *(meb-an'-a-zen).* A monoamine oxidase inhibitor (q.v.)

میبنازین: ایم۔اے۔او۔آئی مانوامین آکسیڈیز۔

Mecamylamine *(me-ka-mi-la-min)* An orally effective ganglionic blocking agent used in the treatment of hypertension. It is much more potent that hexamethonium, and the response is smoother and more predictable. Like similar drugs,it may cause severe constipation, but this does not interfere significantly with absorption. The action lasts over six to twelve hours,and three doeses daily afford adequate control.

میکامائل امین: ہائپرٹنشن کے علاج میں مستعمل۔

Mechanism of labour The forces which extrude the fetus through the birth canal together with the opposing, resisting forces which affect its positions. [See diagram on opposite page.]

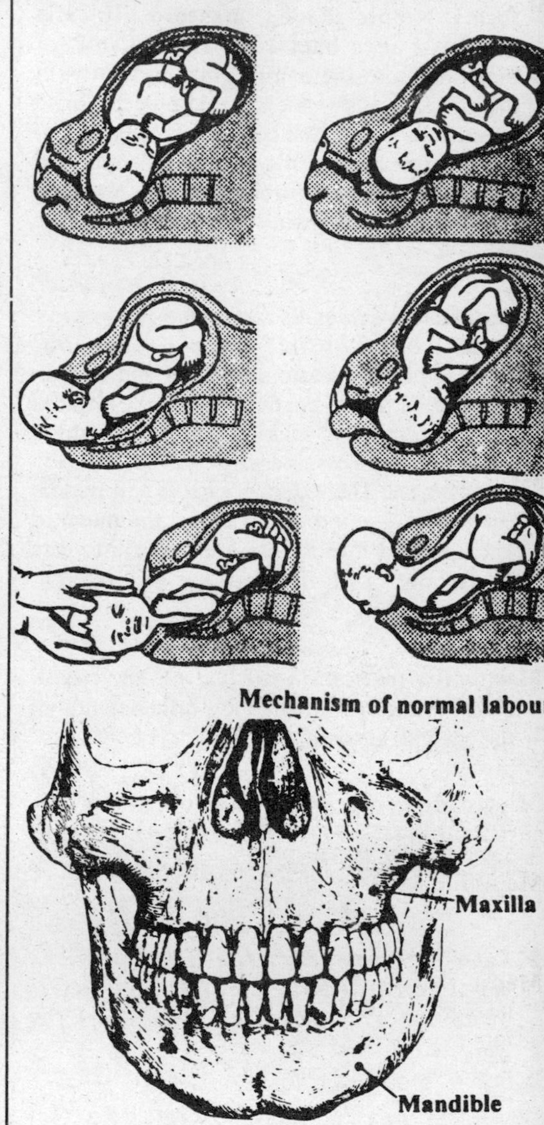

Mechanism of normal labour

میکانیت وضع حمل: قوتیں جو بچے کو پیدائشی قنال سے باہر دھکیلتی ہیں۔

Mechlorethamine hydrochloride *(me-klor-eth -a-men)* Cytotoxic agent.

میکلورتھیمین ہائیڈروکلورائڈ: سائیٹوٹاکسک عامل۔

Mecholyl. Cholinergic agent.

میکولل: کولینرجک عامل۔

Meckel's diverticulum *(mek-els- di-ver-tik-ū-lum)* A blind pouch like sac sometimes arising from the free border of the ileum. Occurs in two per-cent of population. usually symptomless. May cause Gl bleeding may intussuscept or obstruct. [John Freidrich meckel, German anatomist and gynaecologist, 1714-74]

ڈائی ورٹی کولم میکل: ایک بند تھیلی جو بعض دفعہ ایلم کے آزاد باڈر سے ابھرتی ہے۔

Meclozine *(mek-lo-zen)* Antihistamine (q.v.)

میکلوزین: اینٹی ہسٹامین۔ حمل میں متلی کے لئے مفید ہے۔ میکلوزین بی چھ گولیاں ایک صبح ایک شام۔

Medetron *(me-kon-i-um)* [G. *mekonion*]. The discharge form the bowel of newly born baby. It is a greenish-black, viscid substance. It is a greenish black, impaction of m. in bwel. Associated with smelly, fatty stools and chest infection. Earliest sign of mucoviscidosis.

کیٹی میگونیم: نوزائیدہ بچے کا اخراج فضلہ۔ بچہ اپنی پیدائش کے ابتدائی چند ایام کے دوران کولتار کی طرح کالا ایک مادہ میکونیم خارج کرتا ہے۔ حمل کے دوران اس نے رحم میں جو کچھ کھایا ہوتا ہے یہ اس کا فضلہ ہوتا ہے۔ باقی ماندہ ایسے فضلات ناڑ و اور آنول کے راستے ہو چکے ہوتے ہیں۔ صرف میکونیم ہی ایسا مادہ ہوتا ہے جو جنین کی بڑی آنت میں رہ گیا ہوتا ہے جسے بچہ منہ یا مقعد کے راستے خارج کرتا ہے۔

Meconium *(med-e-tron)* Stethoscopr (q.v.) that can be used over clothing.

میڈیٹرون: سٹیتھو سکوپ جو کپڑوں کے اوپر بھی استعمال ہو سکتی ہے۔

Media *(me-di-a)* [L. *medius,* middle,]. The middle coat of a vessel. Nutritive jelly used for culturing bacteria.

شامہ میان: رگ کا درمیانی کوٹ۔ جراثیم کے کلچر کے لئے استعمال ہونے والی غذادار جیلی۔

Medial *(me-di-al)* [L. medius, middle]. Pertaining to or near the middle--medially, adv.

وسطی: درمیان کے نزدیک یا متعلق۔

Median *(med'-i-an)* [L. *medius,* middle].The middle. **median line,** an imaginary line passing through the centre of the body from a point between the eyes between the closed feet.

میانی خط وسطی: درمیان۔ ایک فرضی خط جو جسم کے مرکز میں سے ہوتا ہوا آنکھوں کے درمیان ایک نقطہ سے بند پیروں کے درمیان تک گزرتا ہے۔

Mediastinum *(med-i-as-ti-num)* [L. *mediusm,* middle]. The space between the lungs-- mediastinal adj.

غشائے وسطی: پھیپھڑوں کے درمیان جگہ۔

Mediastinoscopy *(med-i-as-tin-os-ko-pi)* [L.*medius,* middle; G. *skopein,* to examine]. Minor surgical procedure for visual inspection of the mediastinom. May be combined with biopsy of lymph nodes for historical examination.

Medical jurisprudence *(med-ik-al-joo- ris -proo -dens)* syn., forensic medicine.

طبی قانون: فورینسک میڈیسن۔

Medicament *(med-ik-a-ment)* [L. *medicamentum,* remedy]. A remedy or medicine.

مرہم۔ دوا۔ علاج: علاج یا میڈیسن۔

Medicated *(med-i-ka-ted)* [L. *medicare,* to heal]. Impregnated with a drug or medicine.

دواملا: دوا سے بھرا ہوا۔

Medicinal *(med-is-in-al)* pertaining to a medicine.

ادویاتی: میڈیسن سے متعلق۔

Medicine *(med-sin)* 1.Science or art of healing, especially as distinguished form surgery and obstetrics. 2. A therapeutic substance.

طب۔ دوا: (1) صحت مند بنانے کا آرٹ یا سائنس۔ (2) علاج کیلئے مادہ۔

Medicohirurgical *(med-i-ko-ki-rur-ji-kal)* Pertaining to both medicine and surgery.

طبی جراحی: میڈیسن اور سرجری دونوں سے متعلق۔

Medicosocial *(med-i-ko-so-shall)* Pertaining to medicine and sociology.

طبی سماجی: میڈیسن اور سوشیالوجی سے متعلق۔

Medinal *(med-in-al)* Barbitone sodium (q.v).

میڈینل: باربیٹون سوڈیم۔

Mediolateral *(me-di-o-lat-er-al)* [L. *medius,* middle; *latus,* side]. Term used in midwife.

متوسط جانبی: مڈوائفری میں مستعمل اصطلاح۔

Mediterranean fever See BRUCELLA, BRUCE- LLOSIS, Also called 'abrotus f, 'Malta f. and 'undulant f.'.

مالٹا بخار: مالٹا بخار۔

Medium *(med-di-um)* A substance used in bacteriology for the growth of organisms - media, pl.

بدرقہ: جسیموں کی نشونما کے لئے جرثومیات میں مستعمل مادہ۔

Medomin *(med-o-min)* One of the barditones. Hypno/sedative cabsules.

میڈومن: باربیٹونز میں سے ایک۔

Medresco *(med-res-ko)* National Health issue hearing aid, So named after the Medical Research Council.

میڈریکسو: آلہ سماعت۔

Medrogestone *(med-ro-jes-ton)* A female hormone, given orally or by injection. Shrinks diseased prostate gland.

میڈروجیسٹون: ایک مادہ ہارمون۔ غیر صحتمند پروسٹیٹ گلینڈ کو سکیڑتا ہے۔

Medrone *(med-ron)* Methylprednisolone (q.v.)

میڈرون: میتھائل پریڈنیسولون۔

Medroxyprogesterone acetate*(m- ed -ok s-i-pro -jes -ter-on as-e-tat)* Long act-ing (90) days contracep tive given by injection.

Medulla *(me-dul-a)* [L.] 1. The marrow in the centre of a long bone. 2. The soft internal portion of glands, e.g. kidneys, adrenals, lymph nodes, edc. **meddulla oblongats,** the upper part of the spinal cord between the foarmen magnum of the occipital bone and the pons cerebri -- medullary, adj.

گودا۔ نخاع: (1) طویل ہڈی کے مرکز میں گودا۔ (2) گلینڈز کا نرم اندرونی حصہ مثلاً گردے۔ میڈلا آبلانگیٹا سپائنل کارڈ کا بالائی حصہ ہے اور کھوپڑی کے اندر ہوتا ہے۔

Medullated *(med-ul-a-ted)* Containing or surrounded by a medulla or marrow, partucularly referring to nerve fibres.

مغزی غلاف دار: میڈلا یا گودے پر مشتمل یا اس سے گھرا ہوا۔ خصوصاً عصبی ریشوں سے متعلق۔

Medulloblastoma *(med-ul-o-blas-to-ma)* [L. *medullab* marrow; G. *blastos,* germ; *-oma,* tumour]. Malignant, repidly growing tumour of children; appears in the midline of the cerebellum.

میڈلو بلاسٹوما: بچوں کا تیزی سے بڑھنے والا ناسور۔

Mefenamic acid *(mef-en-am-ik)* Analgesic that does not interfere with uricosuric action of sulphnpy- razone, therefore useful in gout. Also has antiinflammatory and antipyretic actions.

میفینمک ایسڈ: جوڑوں کے درد میں مفید۔

Mefenide acetate *(mef-en-id as-e-tat)* Antiseptic dermatotogical cream.

Mefruside *(mef-ru-sid)* Diuretic, Smooth prolonged action, maximal in first 12 hours, produces salt and water loss with little potassium depletion. In hypertensive patients m. has a useful hypotensive action.

میفروسائیڈ: پیشاب آور۔

Megacephalic *(me-ga-kef-al-ik)* [G. *megas,* large; *kephale,* head]. Large headed.Syn., macrocephalic, megalocephalic.

کلان سر: بڑے سر والا۔

Megacolor *(meg-a-klor)* Clomocycline (q.v.)

میگا کلور: کلوموسائیکلین۔

Megacolon *(meg-a-klon)* [G. *megas* large; *kolon,* colon]. Condition of dilated and elongated colon. in an adult the cause is unknown. in a child the parasympathetic ganglion cells are absent in the distal part of the colong (Hirschsprung's disease. (q.v.)

قلا قولون: قلون کی بڑی اور پھیلائی حالت۔

Megakaryocyte *(mega-kar-i-o-sit)* [G. *megas,* large; *karyon,* kernal; *kytos,*cell]. Large multinucleated of the marrow which produce the blood platelets.

میگا کیریوسائیٹ: گودے کے بڑے مرکزائی خلیے جو خونی پلٹیلٹ بناتے

ہیں۔

Megaloblast *(meg-a-lo-blast)* [G. *megas,* large; *blastos,* germ]. A large , nucleated, primitive red blood cell formed where there is a deficiency of vitamin B_{12} or folic acid-megaloblastic, adj.

ایک بڑامرکزائی: اوّلی سرخ خونی خلیہ۔

Megalomania *(meg-a-lo-man-i-a)* [G. *megas,* large; *mania,* madness]. delusion of grandeur, characteristic of general paralysis of the insane (q.v.)

کبیرالراس: جس کاسر بڑاہو۔

Megalomaina *(meg-a-lo-man'-i-a)* [G. *megas,* large; *mania,* madness]. Delusion of grandeur , chara- cteristic of general paralysis of the insane (q.v.)

خطب عظمت: پاگلوں کی تشنج والی خصوصیات۔

Megimide , Bemegride *(q.v)*

میجیمائیڈ: بمیگرائڈ۔

Meibmian cyst *(mi-bom-i-an)* See CHALAZION.

پپوٹوں کی گرہ دار گلٹی: گلازیون۔

Meibomian glands *(mi-bom-i-an)*. Sebaceous glands lying in grooves on the inner surface of the eyelids, their ducts opening on the free margins of the lids. [Heinrich Meibom, German anatomist. 1638 -- 1700-].

غدد مقعدہ: سیبشس گلینڈز جوآنکھ کے پپوٹوں کی اندرونی سطح پرواقع ہوتی ہے۔

Meig's syndrome (megz). Benign solid ovarian tumour associated with bydroperitoneum and hydrothorax. [Joe V. Meigs, American surgeon, 1892.]

میگزسنڈورم: بیضدان کاٹھوس ناسور۔

Meiosis *(me-I-o-sis)* Miosis (q.v.) Also myosis.

Melaena *(mel-e-na)* [G. *melas,* black]. Black, tar-like stoods . Evidence of intestinal bleeding.

خونی پاخانہ: کالافضلہ۔انتڑیوں میں روانی خون کاثبوت۔

Melancholia *(mel-an-ko-li-a)* [G.*melagcholia*]. Term reserved in psychiatry to mean severe forms of depression -melancholic, adj.

مالیخولیا: پریشانی ومایوسی کی انتہائی اقسام۔

Melanin *(mel-an-in)* [G. *melas,* black]. A black pigment found in hair, skin and the choroid of the eye.

سیاہی ۔جلدی سیاہی: آنکھ کے کورائڈ۔جلداور بالوں میں پایاجانے والا ایک سیاہ پگمنٹ ۔ایک گہرے بھورے رنگ کا پگمنٹ جو جلدی خلیوں میلینوسائیٹس میں بنتاہے۔

Melanoma *(mel-an-o-ma)* [G. *melas,* black; *-oma,* tumour]. A tumour arising from the pigment-producing cells of the deeper layers in the skin, or of the eye melanomata. pl; melanomatous. adj.

سیاہ سلعہ: آنکھ کے یاجلدمیں گہری تہوں کے پگمنٹ پیداکرنے والاخلیوں سے بننے والاناسور۔

Melanosarcoma *(mel-an-o-sar-ko-ma)* [G. *melas,* black; *sarkoma,* fleshy overgrowth]. One form of malignant melamelanosar-comatous, adj.

میلانوسرکوما: میلانوماکی ایک قسم۔

Melanosis *(mel-an-o-sis)* [G. *melas,* black; *-osis,* Condition]. Dark pigmentation of surfaces as in sunburn addison's disease, etc. melanotic, adj.

سیاہ سرطان: سطوح کی ڈارک پگمنٹیشن۔

Melanuria *(mel-an-ur-i-a)* [G. *melas,* black; *ouron,* urine]. elanin in the urine.melanuric, adj.

بول سیاہ: پیشاب میں سیاہی۔

Melarsoprol *(mel-ar-so-prol)* Organicarsenical given i.v. in trypanosomilasis.

میلرسوپرول: نامیاتی آرسینک۔

Melarsonyl potassium *(mel-ar-son-il)* Organic arsenical given i.v. intrypanosomiasis. Less toxic than melarsoprol.

میلرسونل پوٹاشیم: نامیاتی آرسینک مگرکم زہریلا۔

Melitensis. See BRUCELLOSIS.

میلی ٹینس: بروسیلوس۔

Melleril Thioridazine (q.v.)

ملیرل: تھیوڑازین۔

Melphalan *(mel-fa-lan)* Alky lating cytotoxic agent

میلفیلین: سائیٹوٹاکسک عامل۔

Membrane *(mem-bran)* A thin lining or covening sustance. **basement m.** a thin layer beneath the epithelium of mucous surfaces. **hyloid m.,** that surrounding the vitreous humor of the eye. **mucous m.,** contains glands which secrete mucus, It lines the cavities and passages that communicate with the exterior of the body. **serous m,** a lubricating membrance lining the closed cavities, and reflected over their enclosed organs.**synovial m.** that lining the intra-articular parts of bones and ligaments **tympanic m.** the eardrum -- membranous adj.

جھلی: ایک غلافی مادہ۔

Menadione *(men-a-di'-on)* Chemical name of vitamin K. (q.v.)

میناڈی اون: وٹامن کے کا کیمیکل نام۔

Menaphthone *(men-af'-thon)* Vitamin K is an essential factor in blood coagulation. and menaphthaone is a synthetic oil-soluble. Compound with similar activity. Used in haemorrhage and obstructive jaundice. Given intramusculary.

مینفتھون: ایک تالیفی مرکب۔ تیل میں حل پذیر۔ خون کو منجمد کرتا ہے۔

Menarche *(men-ar-ke)* [G. *men,* month, *arche,* beginning]. When the menstrual periods commence and other bodily changes occur.

مینر کی: جب حیض کے ایام شروع ہوتے ہیں اور دوسری جسمانی تبدیلیاں واقع ہوتی ہیں۔

Mendel's law. A thoery of heredity evolved by an Austrian monk which deals with the interaction of dominant and recessive characters in cross- breeding [Gregor Johann Mendel, 1822-84]

قانون منڈل: گریگر جان مینڈل کا باپ ایک کسان اور پھل اگانے والا تھا۔ شروع میں وہ پادری بن گیا بعد میں اس کا تقرر ہائی سکول میں ہوگیا جہاں وہ یونانی اور ریاضی پڑھاتا تھا۔ مینڈل نے خوردنی مٹر پر تجربات کیئے۔ قانون علیحدگی یا گیمٹوں کے خالص پن کے قانون کی رو سے اگر دو گیمٹوں کے ملاپ کے ذریعہ دو متضاد خصوصیات کے حامل جین یکجا کر دیئے جائیں تو وہ اولاد کے خلیوں میں قائم رہتے ہیں لیکن پھر گیمٹ بننے پر علیحدہ ہو جاتے ہیں۔ اس طرح ہر گیمٹ میں صرف ایک جین ہوتا ہے اس کا تناسب ایک تین ہوگا۔ قانون خودمختار آرائشگی کی رو سے کسی مخلوط میں متضاد خواص کے ایک جوڑے کا عمل دوسرے جوڑوں کے عمل سے بالکل آزاد و خودمختار ہوتا ہے اور وہ اتفاقا جدا ہوتے ہیں۔ اس میں تناسب 3:9 1:3 ہوگا۔

Mendelson's syndrome. Inhalation of regurgitated stomach contents,which can cause immediate death from anoxia, or it may produce extensive lung damage or pulmonary oedema with severe brounchsopasm.

مینڈلسن سنڈروم: معدے کے اجزاء کا سانس کی نالی میں جانا۔ اس سے موت واقع ہوسکتی ہے۔ یا پھیپھڑوں کو نقصان پہنچ سکتا ہے۔

Meniere's disease *(Man-yers)* Distension of membranous labyrinth of middle ear from excess fluid. Pressure cause ischaemia and failure of function of nerve of hearing and balance, thus there is fluctuating deafness. tinnitus and repeated attacks of vertigo,[Prosper Memere, French otologist 1799-1862]

مرض مینیئر: زائد سیال کی وجہ سے درمیانی کان میں خرابی کا کلیا کی خرابی سے جسمانی توازن برقرار رکھنے میں دشواری۔ چکر آتے ہیں۔ علاج کے لئے وٹامن بی کمپاؤنڈ۔ اینزائم وٹامن کمپاؤنڈ۔ ہائیڈروکلورتھایازائیڈ۔ سٹے مٹل ورنکوٹینک استعمال کیجئے۔

Meninges *(men-in-jes)* [G. *menigx,* membrane] The surrounding membranes of the brain and spinal cord. They are three in number (1) the dura mater (outer); (2) arachnoid membrane (middle); (3) pia mater (inner)-- meninx (me-ningks), sing; meningeal, adj.

سحایا۔ دماغی پردے: شوکی ڈوراا ور پرندے کے گرد جھلیاں۔ بیرونی موٹا پردہ۔ دیوار میٹر۔ اس کے نیچے ارکنائڈ میٹر اور تیسرا پردہ پایا میٹر ہے۔

Meningioma *(men-in-ji-o-ma)* [G. *menigx,* membrance; *oma,* tumour]. A slowly growing fibrous tumour arising in the meninges meningiomata, pl; mening- iomatous, adj.

سلعہ سحایا: رفتہ رفتہ بڑھنے والا ریشہ دار ناسور۔

Meningism meningismus *(men-in-jism or men-in-jis-mus)* Condition presenting with signs and symptoms of meningitils (e.g. neck stiffness): meningitis does not develop.

سحایت: مینجیٹس کی علامت ظاہر کرنے والی حالت مثلاً گردن کا اکڑاؤ۔

Meningitis *(men-in-ji-tis)* [G. *menigx,* membrance; *-titis,* inflammation]. Inflammation of the meninges. An epidemic form is known as cerebrospinal fever, the infecting organism is *Neisseria meningitidis* (meningococcus). The term meningococcal Meningitis is now preferred. See LEPTOMENINGITIS. PACHYMENINGITIS- meningitides, pl.

گردن توڑ بخار: سحایا (مینجز) ایک جراثیمی مرض۔

Meningocele *(men-ing-go-sel)* [G. *menigx,* membrance, *kele,* hernia]. Protrusion of the meninges through a bony defect. It forms a cyst filled with cerebrospinal fluid See SPINA BIFIDA.

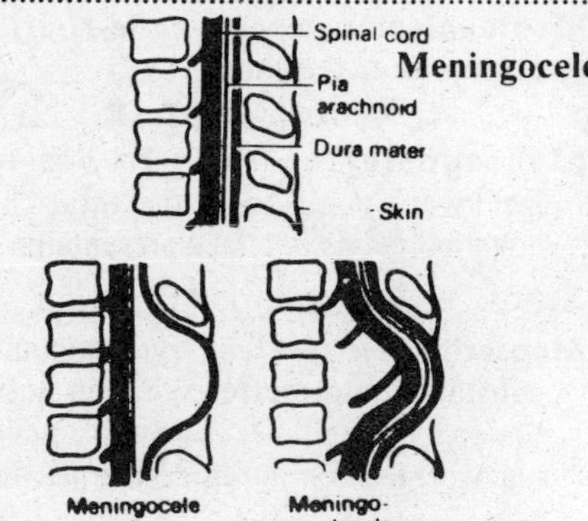

Meningocele

قلیہ سحایہ: استخوانی نقص میں سے سحایا کا ابھار۔ یہ ایک سسٹ بناتا ہے جس پر سربروسپائنل سیال بھرا ہوتا ہے۔

Meningococcus *(men-ing-go-ko-kus)* Syn. *neisseria meningitidis* meningococcal, adj.

مینگو کاکس: نسریا مینجینڈس۔

Meningoencephalitis *(mening-go-en-kef-al-i-tis)* Inflammation of the brain and the meninges -- meningoencephalitic, adj.

التہاب المخ والسحایا۔ التہاب۔ سحائی و دماغی: دماغی اور سحایا کی سوزش۔

Meningomyelocele *(men-ing-go-mi-el-o-el)* [G.*menigx,* membrance, *myelos,* marrow, *kele,* hernial].l Protrusion of a portion of the spinal cord and its enclosing membranes through a bony defect Syn. myelomeninggocele.

فتق سحائی غشائی: استخوانی نقص میں سے نخاع اور اس کے گرد جھلیوں کے ایک حصے کا نکل آنا۔

Meniscectomy *(men-i-sek-to-mi)* [G. *meniskos,* crescent-shaped; *edtome,* excision]. The removal of a semilunar cartilage of the knee joint, following injury and displacement. The medial injury and desplace ment. The medical cartilage is damaged most commonly.

مینی سیکٹومی: گھٹنے کے جوڑ کو ایک چسنی ہڈی کا قطع۔

Menicus *(men-is-kus)* [G. *meniskos,* crescent]. 1. semilunar cartilage, particularly in the knee joint. 2. The curved upper surface of a column of liquid menisci, pl.

ہلالیہ: (1) کسی برتن میں کسی مائع کی خمیدہ سطح (2) ایک مقعر محدب عدسہ۔ (3) ایک ہلالی کرکری ہڈی۔ خصوصاً گھٹنے کے جوڑ میں۔

Menopause *(men-o-pawz)* [G. *men,* montn; *pausis,* stopping] The cessation of menstruation: occurring normally between the ages of 45 and 50. The change of life. Climacteric. **artificial m.,** an earlier menopause induced by radiotherapy or surgery for some pathological condition menopausal, adj.

سن یاس: حیض کی بندش۔ عموماً ۴۵ تا ۵۰ سال کے درمیان ایسا ہوتا ہے۔

Menorrhagia *(men-or-a-ji-a)* [G. *men,* month; *rhegnynai,* to burst forth]. And excessive regular menstrual flow.

جریان حیض۔ کثرت حیض: زائد باقاعدہ حیض۔ اس کی وجوبات رحم کی سوزش رحم کی سولی۔ پروجسٹرون ہارمون کی کمی کیلشیم کی کمی اور رحم کی سرطان ہیں۔ علاج کے لئے پروجیسٹرون انجکشن دن میں دو دفعہ یا کیلشیم سینڈوز ۱۰ سی سی کا وریدی ٹیکہ روزانہ دس دن تک لگائیں یا ارگونامین کی گولیاں ایک صبح ایک دوپہر ایک شام۔

Menses *men-sez)* [L.months.]. The sanguineous fluid discharged from the uterus during menstruation; menstrual flow.

حیض: حیض کے دوران یوٹرس سے سیال کا بہاؤ۔ ماہواری آنا۔

Menstrual *(men-stroo-al)* Relating to the menses. **menstrual cycle,** the cyclical chain of events that occurs in the uterus in which a flow of blood occurs for four to five days every twenty days. The cycle is governed by hormones form the anterior pituitary gland and the ovaries.

ماہواری ۔ حیضی: حیض سے متعلق ۔ حیضی دور ۲۸ ایام کے بعد ۴ یا ۵ ایام کے لئے ہوتا ہے جس میں خون کا بہاؤ جاری رہتا ہے۔

Menstruation *(men-stroo-a-shun)* [L. *menstruare*, to menstruate]. The flow of blood from the uterus once a month in the female. It commences about the age of 13 and ceases about 45.

حیض ۔ طمث: مادہ میں ماہ میں ایک بار یوٹر سے خون کا بہاؤ ۔ یہ عمل قریباً ۱۳ سال کی عمر سے شروع ہوتا ہے اور قریباً ۴۵ سال کی عمر میں بند ہو جاتا ہے ۔ اگر بیضہ زرخیز نہ ہو تو ہارمونز رحم یا یوٹرس کی دیواروں کو سکڑ دیتے ہیں ۔ اور ان میں بھرا ہوا خون اندرونی دیواروں کے شکستہ حصے لے کر اندام نہانی کے راستے باہر نکل آتا ہے ۔ اس خون کے اخراج کو حیض کہا جاتا ہے ۔ چونکہ یہ عمل عورت کے جسم سے ہر ماہ بعد ہوتا ہے اس لئے اسے ماہواری بھی کہتے ہیں۔

Mental *(men-tal)* [L. *mentum,* chin]. Pertaining to the chin.

ذقنی ۔ دماغی: ٹھوڑی سے متعلق ۔ ذہنی فتور سے مراد ذہنی مرض ہے۔

Mental disorder: Mental illness, arrested or incomplete development of mind, psychopathic disorder and any other disorder of disability of mind, and mentally disordered shall be construed accordingly. **mental subnormality,** see SUBNORMALITY.

Mental Health Review Tribunal. A body set up in each Regional Health Administration area to deal with patients applications for discharge on alternation of their conditions of detention in hospital.

مینٹل ہیلتھ ریویو ٹریبونل: ایک باڈی جو ہسپتال سے ڈسچارج ہونے کے لئے مریضوں کی درخواستوں کا جائزہ لیتی ہے۔

Mental Welfae Officer . Appointed by the Local Health Authority to deal with; (1) applications for compulsory or emergency admission to hospital, or for conveyance of patients there; (2) applications concerning guardianship, the functions of the nearest relative if so appointed; (3) returning patients absent without leave, or apprehending patients escaped from legal custody. In addition, the MWO may have a wide range of functions in the care and aftercare of the mentally disordered in the community. This includes home visiting training centres, clubs and general supervision of the discharged patient.

افسر ذہنی بہبود: مقامی ہیلتھ اتھارٹی کا مقرر کردہ افسر۔

Menthol *(men-thol)* Mild analgesic obtained from oil of peppermint. Used in liniments and ointments for rheumatism, and as an inhalation or drops for nasal catarrh.

جوہر پودینہ: کافور گروہ کے نامیاتی مرکبات کے سلسلہ میں سے ایک ۔ ایک سفید قلمی مرکب جو قدرتی تیلوں میں پایا جاتا ہے ۔ نقطہ پگھلاؤ ۔ ۴۲س سالمی وزن ۔ ۱۵۴٫۲۷ مخصوص بو ۔ دوائی میں مستعمل ہے۔

Mentoanterior *(men-to-an-te-ri-or)* Forward positio- ns to the chin.

ذقنی امامی: ماں کے پیڑو میں بچے کی ٹھوڑی کی فارورڈ پوزیشن۔

Mentoposterior *(men-to-pos-te-ri-or)* Backward position of the fetal chin in the maternal pelvis in a face presentaion.

ذقنی خلفی: ماں کے پیڑو میں بچے کی ٹھوڑی کی بیک ورڈ پوزیشن۔

Mepacrine *(me-pa-kren)* Synthetic antimalarial substance, more effective than quinine, and better tolerated. Occasionally used against tapeworm, and in lupus erythematosus.

میپاکرین: تالیفی ضد ملیریائی مادہ ۔ کونین سے زیادہ موثر اور بہتر طور پر برداشت کیا جاسکتا ہے ۔ بعض دفعہ کدو کیڑے کے خلاف بھی استعمال کیا جاتا ہے اس کی گولی صبح ایک شام برائے لیوپس اریتھیمے ٹوسس۔

Mepazine *(mep-a-zen)* Similar to chlorpr- omazine (q.v) Useful in midwifery.

میپازین: کلوپرومازین سے مشابہ ۔ مڈوائفری میں مفید۔

Mephenesin elixir. Mild muscle relaxant. Can be given through stomach tube.

میفنسین اکسیر: عضلے کو سکون پہنچانے والا ۔ معدے کی نلی میں دیا جاسکتا ہے۔

Mephine *(mef-en)* A sympathomimetic hypertensive agent.

میفین: مفنٹر مین سلفیٹ۔

ephyton *(me-fi-ton)* Phytomenadione. An emulsion of vitamin K for oral administration.

مفی ٹان: وٹامن کے کا ایملشن۔منہ کے ذریعے دیا جاتا ہے۔

lepilin *(mep-il-in)* Androgen-oes- trogen mixture, Useful at the menopause. Theoretically the oestrogens give relief and prevent masculinization by the androgens, while the latter prevent undue stimulation of the breasts and of the endometruim, and also by their anobolic effects promote a feeling of well-being.

میپی لن: اینڈروجن ایکسٹروجن مکسچر۔مینوپاز کے وقت مفید۔

eprobamate *(mep-ro-bam-at)* One of the carbamates, A tranquillizer which, by central nervous action, produces mental relaxation. For poisoning, see p. 337.

میپروبیمیٹ: کاربامیٹس میں سے ایک۔ذہن کے لئے سکون بخش۔

epyramine *(me-pir-a-men)* An effective antihista- mine, useful inallergic skin conditionsl. The sedative side effects may cause drowsiness in some patients.

میپرامین: ایک موثر اینٹی ہسٹامین۔الرجک جلدی حالتوں میں مفید۔

erbentyl *(mer-ben-til)* Dicyclomine (q.v.)

مربینٹل: ڈائی سائیکلومین۔

ercaptopurine *(mer-kap-to-pur-in)* Used in the treatment of acute leukaemia in children. Prevents synthesis of nucleic acid.

مرکیپٹوپیورین: بچوں میں لیوکیمیا کے علاج میں مستعمل۔نکلیک ایسڈ کی تالیف روکتا ہے۔مفید برائے علاج کینسر یا سرطان۔

ercurialism *(mer-ku-ri-al-izm)* Toxic effects on human body of mercury -- the ancient cure for syphilis. May result from use of teething powdcers (cf. pink disease) or calome (as an abortifacient). Symptomatology includes stomatitis, loosening of teeth, gastroenteritis and skin eruptions.

سیمابی مرض: انسانی جسم پر پارے کے زہریلے اثرات آتشک کا پرا: علاج۔

ercuric oxide *(mer-ku-rik oks-id)* A bright yellow powder, used mainly as oculent hydrarg. ox. flav. (golden eye ointment). It is antiseptic and is used in conjuctivitis and other eye conditions

مرکیورک آکسائیڈ: ایک حل پذیر زہریلا سفوف جو زرد یا لال قلموں کی صورت میں پایا جاتا ہے۔پگمنٹ اور دافع تعفن کے طور پر استعمال کیا جاتا ہے۔آنکھ کے لئے مستعمل ہے۔

Mercurochrome *(mer-ku-ro-krom)* Red dye containing mercury in combination. Has antiseptic properties, and is sometimes used for skin sterilizatiopn as a 2 per cent solution in a mixture of acetone, alcohol and water.

مرکیوروکروم: سرخ رنگ جس میں پارہ شامل ہے۔دافع تعفن اور بعض جگہ جلد کو صاف کرنے کیلئے ایسیٹون الکحل اور پانی کے مکسچر میں دو فیصد محلول کے طور پر استعمال کیا جاتا ہے۔

Merthiolate *(mer-thi-o-lat)* Thiomersalate (q.v.) Used in bone bank (1 in 1000 to 1 in 3000) Organic iodine solution. Useful for preparation of skin prior to surgery.

مرتھیولیٹ: تھیومرسلیٹ۔استخوانی بنک میں مفید نامیاتی آیوڈین محلول۔اپریشن سے پہلے جلدی تیاری میں مفید۔

Mesateritis *(mes-art-er-i-tis)* [G. *mesos,* middle; *arteria,* artery; *-itis,* inflammation]. Inflammation of the middle coat of an artery.

التہاب طبقہ وسطی شریانی: شریان کے درمیانی کوٹ کی سوزش۔

Mescaline *(mes-kal-en)* A hallucinogenic agent. Can be used to produce abreaction.

میسکیلین: واہمہ والا عامل۔

Mesencephalon *(mes-en-te-ri)* [G. *mesos,* middle; *egkephalos,* brain]. The midbrain.

میان دماغ: درمیانی دماغ۔

Mesentery *(mes'-en-te-ri)* [G. *mesos,* middle; *enteron,* intestine]. A large fold of peritoneum passing between a portion of intestine and the posterior abdominal wall - mesenteric, adj.

رودہ بند: بڑی پیری ٹونیم کی تہہ جو خلفی بطنی دیوار اور آنت کے ایک حصے کے درمیان سے گزرتی ہے۔

Mesontion *(mes-on-tion)* Methoin (q.v.)

میسنٹائن: میتھوئن۔

Mesothelioma *(mes-o-the-li-ma)* A rapidly fatal tumour that spreads over the pleural covering of the lung. Of current interest because of its association with the asbestos industry.

میسوتھی لیوما: ایک ہلاکت آفرین ناسور جو پھیپھڑے کے پلیورل غلاف پر پھیلتا ہے۔

Mestinon *(mes-tin-on)* Pyridostigmine (q.v.)

میسٹینون: پائیریڈوسٹگمین۔

Metabolic *(met-àb-ol-ik)* [G. *metabloe,* change]. Pertaining to metabolism. **basal m. rate (BMR)** , The expression of basal metabolism in terms of kcal per sz.m of body surface per hour -metabolic- ally, adv.

تحویلی: میٹابولزم سے متعلق۔

Metabolism *(met-ab-ol-zim)* [G. *metabole,* change]. The series of chemical changes in the living body by which life is maintained. The tissues are broken down by wear and tear (catabolism) and rebuilt (ababolism) continuously, **basal m.** the energy used by a body at complete rest, being the minimum necessary to maintain life. Se ADENOSINE DIPHOSTHATE and TRIPHOSPATE metabolic. adj.

تحول: ایسے کیمیائی اعمال جن کا تعلق جاندار اشیاء سے ہے۔ تعمیری یا تخریبی عمل ہوتے ہیں۔ دونوں اقسام کے کیمیائی اعمال کو مجموعی طور تحول کہا جاتا ہے۔

Metabolite *(mct-ab-ol-it)* [G. *metabole,* change]. Any product of metabolism, **essential m,.** a substance necessary for proper metabolism. e.g. vitamins.

متحول مادہ: ایسی کوئی بھی شے جو تحول یا میٹابولزم میں حصہ لے۔

Metaca pophalangeal *(met-a-kar'-po- fal-an -je-al)* [G. *meta,* after; *karpos,* wrist; *phalagx,* series]. Pertaining to the metacarpus and the phalages.

مشطی سلامی: میٹا کارپس اور سلامیات سے متعلق۔

Metacarpus *(met-ak-ar'-pus)* [G. *mela,* atter; *karpos,* wrist]. The five bones which from that part of the hand between the wrist and fingures metacarpal, adj.

Metacarp

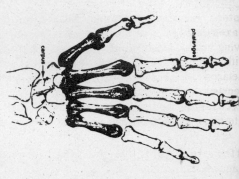

ت دست: پانچ ہڈیاں جو کلائی اور انگلیوں کے درمیانی ہاتھ کا حصہ بناتی

Metaraminol *(met-ar-a-min'-ol)* Vasopress agent used in hypotensive shock.

ریمینول: کم تنش خون، میں مستعمل۔

Metastab *(met'-a-stab)* Methylprednisolon (q.v.)

سٹیب: میتھائل پریڈنیسولون۔

Metastasis *(me-tas-ta-sis)* [G. removal]. T trans- ference of disease from one part of body to another, usually by blood or lymp Asecondary growth metastases, pl; metastat adj: metastasize. v.

ال مرض: جسم کے ایک حصے سے دوسرے حصے میں انتقال مرض۔ عموما یا لمف سے۔ ثانوی نشونما۔

Metatarsalgia *(met-a-tar-sal-ji-a)* [G. *me after;*L. *tarsus,* ankle; G. *algos.*Pain]. Pa under the metatarsal heads.

مشط پا: میٹا ٹارسل سروں کے نیچے درد۔

Metatarsophalangeal *(met-a-tar-so- -an-je-al)* [G. *meta,* after; L. *tarsus,* ank *phalagx,* series] Pertaining to the metatars and the phalanges.

ی سلامی: میٹا ٹارس اور سلامیات سے متعلق۔

Metatarsus *(met-a-tar-sus)* [G. *meta,* after; *tarsus,* ankle]. The five bones of the fo between the ankle and the toes -- metatars dj.

عظم پشت پا: ٹخنے اور پیروں کی انگلیوں کے درمیان پاؤں کی پانچ ہڈیاں

atone *(met-aton)* Glycerophosphates (q.v.)

:azoa *(met-a-zo-a)* [G. *mta,* after ; *zoion,* ving being]. Multicellular animal organisms ith differentation of cells to form tissues -- ietazoal, adj.

eorism *(me-te-or-izm)* [G. *meteoros,* lofty]. xcessive accumulation of gas in the itestines. Tympanites.

بادشکم: آنتوں میں گیس کا جمع ہونا۔

tformin, *(met-form-in)* One of the iaguanides. Antidiabetic agent.

میٹفورمن: ضد ذیابیطس عامل۔ڈایا گوانا نائیڈز میں سے ایک۔

thacycline *(meth-a-si-klin)* Antibiotic articularly useful in exacerbations of chronic ronchitis.

میتھا کولین: ایک مرکب جو عمل میں ایسٹائل کولین سے مشابہ ہے۔لیک زیادہ عامل اور پائیدار۔

thadone *(me-tha-don)* A synthentic iorphine -like analgesic, but with a reduced :dative action. Can be given orally or by ijection. Particullary valuable in visceral ain, and useful in the treatment of useless ough. May cause addiction if treatment is rolonged. Can be used in withdrawal rogrammes for heroin addicts.

میتھاڈون: ایک تالیفی مارفین کی طرح مسکن دوا۔بیکار کھانسی کے علاج مفید ہے۔ہیروئن چھڑانے کے لئے استعمال کیا جاتا ہے۔

haemalbumin *(met-hem-al-bu-min)* bnormnal compound in blood from ombination of haem with plasma albumen.

haemoglobin *(met-hem-o-glob-in)* A form haemoglobin consisting of a combination globin with an oxidized haem, containing rric iron. This pigment is unable to transport xygen. May be formed following the lministration of a wide variety of drugs, cluding the sulphonamide. May be present the blood as a result of a congenital normality.

میٹ ہیموگلوبن: فیرک لوہے پر مشتمل تکسید شدہ ہیم کے ساتھ گلوبن کے ملاپ پر مشتمل ہیموگلوبن کی ایک قسم۔یہ پگمنٹ آکسیجن لے جانے کے ناقابل ہے۔

Methaemoglobinaemia *(met-hem-o-glob-in-e'-mi-a)* Methaemoglobin in the blood. If large quantities are present, individuals may show cyanosis, but otherwise no abnormality except, in severe cases, breathlessness on exertion, because the methaemoglobing cannot transport oxygen -- methaemoglobinaemic, adj.

میتھا ایموگلوبی نیمیا: خون میں میتھیموگلوبن۔اگر زیادہ مقدار موجود ہو تو نیلا یرقان ہو جاتا ہے۔لیکن اس کے علاوہ کوئی غیر معمولی بات نہیں ہوتی سوائے اس کے کہ سخت کام کرنے کی صورت میں سانس پھول جاتا ہے کیونکہ میتھیموگلوبن آکسیجن نہیں لے جاتا۔

Methaemoglobinuria *(met-hem-o-glob-in-ur'-i-a)* Methaemoglobin in the urine -- methaemoglob- inuric, adj.

پیشاب میں میتھیموگلوبن۔

Methandienone *(meth'-an-di-en-on)* Anticatabolic agent, useful in muscle wasting occurring as a result of the body's attempt to restore nitrogen balance, as when protein nitrogen is lost in serum from a large wound or pressure sore, and in senile debility.

:اینٹی کیٹابولک عامل۔عضلے کے لئے مفید۔ڈائی اینابال۔قلبی بے قاعدگی یا کارڈیک ارتھیمیا اور سربرل ہیموریج یا فالج میں اس کی ایک گولی صبح ایک شام۔یہی خوراک برائے مسکولر ڈس بڑائی۔

Methane *(meth-an)* Most important component of natural gas. See BENZTROPINE and THAM.

Methaqualone *(meth-a-qwal-on)* Oral hypnotic; useful alternative to the barbiturates. Has been used i.v. to produce loss of consiousness as an alternative to thiopentone. For poisining.

میتھا کوالون: خواب آور۔

Methedrine *(meth-i-drin-)* See METHYLA-MPHETAMINE.

میتھیڈرین: میتھائل امینٹامین۔

Methenolone enanthate *(meth-en-o-lon-en-an-that)* Anabolic steroid.

Methicillin *(meth-i-sil-lin)* A semisynthetic

penicillin active against pernicillin-resistant staphylococci. Destroyed by gastric juice. Given by injection.

میتھیکلین: ایک نیم تالیفی پنسلین جو ایسے سٹیفائلو کاکسی کے خلاف عمل کرتی ہے جن پر پنسلین اثر نہیں کرتی۔ گیسٹرک جوس سے تباہ ہوتی ہے۔ ٹیکے کے ذریعے دی جاتی ہے۔

Methionine *(meth-i-o-nen)* One of the essential sulphur-containing amino acids. Occasionally used in hepatitis and other conditions associated with liver damage.

میتھولین: گندھک پر مشتمل لازمی امینوایسڈز میں سے ایک۔ بعض اوقات جگر کے امراض میں استعمال کیا جاتا ہے۔ اون گیسین اور لحمیات میں پایا جاتا ہے۔

Methohexitone (Methohexital) Sodium*(meth-o-heks-i-ton)* Ultrashort-acting barbiturate given i.v. pre-operatively.

ایک باربیٹوریٹ۔

Methoin *(meth-oin)* Anticonvulsant used for major, focal and psychomotor epilepsy.

میتھوئن: دافع تشنج۔

Methotrexate *(meth-o-treks-at)* Amthopterin (q.v.)

ضد فولک ایسڈ: اس خامرہ کو روک دیتا ہے۔ جو فولک ایسڈ کو تبدیل کر کے عامل بناتا ہے۔ اس لئے تقسیم کے دوران خلیوں کے خلاف عمل کرتا ہے۔

Methotrimeprazine *(meth-oks-a-men)* A pressor drug used to restore blood pressure. It has few side effects on the heart or central nervous system. Given intravenously or intramuscularly.

دوا جو خونی دباؤ کو برقرار رکھنے کے لئے استعمال کی جاتی ہے۔ ناک بند ہونے کی صورت میں اس کے نیزل ڈراپس ہر تین گھنٹے کے بعد ناک میں ڈالئے۔

Methoxyflurane *(mth-oks-i-flur'-an)* Obstetric inhalational analgesic.

میتھوکسی فلیورین: آبسٹرڈک سانس کے ذریعے اندر لی جانے والی مسکن دوا۔

Methsuximide *(meth-suks'-i-mid)* For control of temporal lobe epilepsy and petit mal.

میتھ سیکسیمائڈ: ٹیمپورل لوب مرگی کے کنٹرول کے لئے مستعمل۔

Methyclothizide *(meth-i-klo-thi-az-id)* See CHLOROTHIAZIDE

ئل کلوتھیازائیڈ: کلورتھیازائیڈ۔

Methylamphetamine hydrochloride *(m*
-il - am-fet'-a-men hid-dro-klor'-id) A cen
nervous system stimulant similar
amphetamine (q.v.) Produces a marked
prolonged rise in blood pressure if injec
Can be given orally, intramuscularly
intravenously. Dependence on drug i
danger.

ئل امفیٹامین ہائیڈروکلورائیڈ: امفیٹامین کی طرح مرکزی عصبی
تحریک دینے والا۔ اگر ٹیکے کے ذریعہ دیا جائے تو خونی دباؤ کو زیادہ کرتا
صدمہ۔ بیٹوریٹ کے زہریلا پن اور ہلکی پریشانی میں دیا جاتا ہے۔ اس
پر انحصار خطرناک ہے۔

Methylated spirit Alcohol containing 5 per c
of wood naphtha to make it non-potable.
methylated spirit used for spirit stoves, et
less pure, and is coloured to distinguis
from the above.

ل سپرٹ: میتھی سپرٹ ۵ فیصد چوبی نفتھا پر مشتمل الکحل ہے۔ یہ ایک
یندھن ہے جس میں حجم کے لحاظ سے ۹۰ فیصد ایتھانول ۹،۵ فیصد
ل۔ ۰،۶۵ فیصد پائرڈین شامل ہیں۔ اس میں پیٹرولیم اور میتھائل بنفشی
بھی قلیل مقدار رہتی ہے۔

Methyldopa *(meth-il-do'-pa)* Cau
decarboxylase inhibition. Hypotensive ag
Action increased with thiazide diuretics.

ئیل ڈوپا: کم تنش خون والی دوا۔ ایلڈومیٹ۔ ہائی بلڈ پریشر کے لئے
تین گولیاں روزانہ حسب ضرورت۔

Methylene blue *(meth'-i-len)* Antiseptic
sometimes used in urinary infections, o
with hexamine (q.v.). The intramusc
injection of a 2.5 per cent solution has b
used a a renal function test.

نلین نیلا: دافع تعفن رنگ۔ بعض اوقات بولی امراض میں
ں۔ اکثر ہکسامین کے ساتھ۔ ایک حل پذیر مرکب انتہائی نیلا رنگ۔
ت میں رنگ کے طور پر استعمال کیا جاتا ہے۔

Methylpentynol *(meth-il-pen'-tin-ol*
short-acting mild sedative. One of
carbamates. It reduces apprehesion in s
cases, and is useful in conditions of emoti
stress.

میتھا ئیل پینٹی: مختصر عمل والی ہلکی مُسکن دوا۔ کار بامیٹس میں سے ایک جذباتی دباؤ کی حالتوں میں مفید۔

thyl phenidate *(meth-il-fen-i-dat)* ntidepressant. Acts by stimulation of central ervous system.

میتھا ئیل فنٹی ڈیٹ: مایوسی ختم کرنے والی دوا۔ مرکزی عصبی نظام کو تحریک دینے سے عمل کرتی ہے۔

hylphenobarbitone *(meth-il-fe-no-ar'-bit-on)* Greater anticonvulsant action an phenobarbitone. Useful in epilepsy, xiety states and or senile tremor.

میتھا ئیل فینو باربیٹون: فینو باربیٹون کی نسبت زیادہ دافع تشنج۔ مرگی پریشانی کی حالتوں میں مفید۔

hylprednisolone *(meth-il-pred-nis'-o-lon)* teroid suitable for rheumatoid arthritis, flammtory and allergic conditions. ometimes injected locally for exophthalmos.

میتھا ئیل پریڈنی سولون: سٹیرائڈ جو الرجی وغیرہ کی حالتوں میں مناسب ہے۔

hylsalicylate *(meth-il-sal-is'-il-at)*. intergreen. Used externally as a mild unterirritant and analgesic in rheumatic and milar conditions. Supplied as ointment or iment.

میتھا ئیل سلسیا ئیلیٹ: ایک بے رنگ تیل۔ نقطہ جوش ۲۲۳ء۳° خوشبوؤں اور ادویات میں استعمال کیا جاتا ہے۔

hlscopolamine *(meth-il-sko-pol-a-min)* ntisp- asmodic, especially useful for laxing gastric and intestinal muscle.

ltestosterone *(meth-il-tes-tos-ter-on)* An ally active form of testosterone (q.v.) Given sublingual tablets.

میتھائل ٹیسٹوسیٹرون: ٹیسٹوسیٹرون کی ایک قسم۔ ٹیسٹوویرون سن یاس مرض یا مینو پازل سنڈروم میں ایک گولی صبح ایک شام نامردی کے علاج لئے ایک گولی صبح ایک دوپہر ایک شام تین ماہ تک۔

ylthiouracil *(meth-il-thi'-o-u'-ra-sil)* An tithyroid compound used in thyrotoxicosis. inhibits the formation of thyroxine. eactions have followed its use, and rbimazole (q.v.) is often prferred.

متھائیل تھایوریسل: اینٹی تھائیرائڈ مرکب۔ تھائیروکسن کے بننے کو روکتا ہے۔

Methyprylone *(meth-ip-ril-on)*. Non-barbiturate hypno-sedative.

میتھائیل پرائی لون: باربیٹوریٹ سے آزاد۔ خواب آور مُسکن آور۔

Methysergide *(meth-i-ser-jid)* Used for migraine. Can cause retroperitoneal fibrosis.

میتھی سرجائیڈ: مائیگرین کے لئے مستعمل۔

Metiamide *(met'-i-a-mid)* Gastric secretory inhibitor thus encouraging healing of peptic ulcers.

Metoclopramide *(met-o-klo'-pra-mid)* Gastric sedative. Antiemetic that can be given orally or by injection. Not so effective in vomiting of labyrinthine origin.

میٹوکلوپریمائیڈ: گیسٹرک مسکن دوا۔ دافع قے۔

Metritis *(me-tri-tis)* [G. *metra*, womb; *-itis*, inflamm -ation]. Inflammation of the uterus.

ورم رحم: رحم یا یوٹرس کی سوزش۔

Metronidazole *(met-ro-ni-da-zol)* Antimicrobial agent especially useful for treating severe anaerobic sepsis. Can be given intravenously and orally. Drug of choice of amoebiasis, Tricho- monas, bacteroides and Vincent's infection.

میٹرو نائیڈازول: ملجیل۔ اینٹی امیبک۔ منہ اور مسوڑھوں کی بیماری میں مفید۔ سردکس یا رحم کے منہ کی سوزش میں ایک گولی صبح ایک دوپہر ایک شام سات دنوں تک۔ امیبائی پیچش میں دو گولیاں صبح دو دو پہر دو شام دس ایام تک۔

Metropathia haemorrhagica *(met-ro-path-i-a hem-or-aj'-ik-a)*. Irregualr episodes of uterine bleeding due to excessive and unopposed oestrin in the blood stream. Usually associated witha follicular cyst in the ovary.

مرض رحم: یوٹرس میں روانی خون کے بے قاعدہ سلسلے۔

Metrorrhagia *(met-ro-ra-[illegible]-a)* [G. *metra*, womb; *rhegnynai*, to burs[illegible] forth] Uterine bleeding between the menstr[illegible]al periods.

نزف الدم رحم: حیضی وقفوں کے درمیان یوٹرس کی روانی خون۔

Metrulen *(met-ru-len)* Ethynodiol diacetate (q.v.)

Metycaine *(me-ti-kan)* A local anaesthetic of the cocaine type, used for infiltration, spinal anaes- thesia,and as eye drops.

میٹی کین: کوکین قسم کا مقامی طور پرسن کرنے دوا۔

Mexiteline hydrochloride Antiarrhythmic agent. Controls existing ventricular arrhythmia and can be used as a prophylactic.

Mexiti. Mexiteline bydrochloride (q.v.)

Michel's clips *(mi-shels)* Small metal clips used instead of sutures for the closure of a wound. [Gaston Michel, French surgeon in Nancy, 1875-1937]

مشیں کلپس: زخم کو بند کرنے کے لئے مستعمل چھوٹے دھاتی کلپ۔

Microangiopathy *(mi-kro-an-ji-op'-ath-i)* Thickening and reduplication of basement membrance in blood vessels. Occurs in diabetes mellitus.

مائیکرو اینجیو پیتھی: خونی رگوں میں بیسمنٹ جھلی کا دبیز ہونا۔ ذیابیطس میں ایسا ہوتا ہے۔

Microbe *(mi-krob)* [G. *mikros,* small; *bios,* life]. A microscopic organism (syn. micro-organis) microbial microbic, adj.

خردبینی: ایک خوردبینی جسیمہ۔

Microbiology *(mi-kro-bi-lo-ji)* [G. *milkros,* small; *bios,* life; *logos,* discourse] The science of micro-organisms.

میکروبیات: خودجسیموں کی سائنس۔ خوردبینی اجسام کا مطالعہ۔

Microcephalic *(mi-kro-kef-al-ik)* [G. *milkros,* small; kephale, head]. Pertaining to an abnormally small head.

مائیکروکیفیلک: غیر معمولی چھوٹے سرے متعلق۔

micrococcus *(mi-kro-kok'-us)* [G. *milkros,* small; *coccus,* a berry] A genus of bactria. Gram-positive spherical bacteria occurring in irregular masses. They comprise saprophytes, parasites and pathogens.

کروی نبقہ: جراثیم کا جنس۔ بے قاعدہ مادوں میں واقع گرام مثبت گول جراثیم۔ وہ گند خود۔ طفیلی اور بیماری پیدا کرنے والے ہوتے ہیں۔

Microcyte *(mi-kro-sit)* [G. *milkros,* small; *kytos,* cell] An undersized red blood cell found especially in iron deficiency anaemia. **microcytosis,** an increased number of microcytes microcytic, adj.

...یہ خون: انیمی خون میں پایا جانے والا سائز سے کم سرخ خونی کلیہ۔

Mecrofilaria. Tiny worms, Cause filari... (q.v.)

...فلیر: چھوٹے کیڑے۔

Micrognathia *(mi-kro-nath'-ia-a)* ... *milkros*-small; *gnathos,* jaw]. Small ... especially the lower one.

...ی: چھوٹا جبڑا۔ خصوصاً زیریں (شکل دیکھیے) جبڑوں کا چھوٹا پن۔

Microgynon *(mi'-kro-gi-nin)* Low oestr... oral contraceptive.

Micron *(mi-kron)* [G. *milkros,* smal... millionth part of a metre, represented b... Greek letter mu (*u*)

...ن: میٹر کا دس ہزاروں حصہ۔ اس کا سابقہ نام مائیکرو میٹر ہے۔ اسے ...ف میور۔ (u) سے ظاہر کیا جاتا ہے۔

Micro- organism *(mi'-kro-or-gan-izm...* micros- copic cell. (Often synonymous ... bacterium but includes virus, protoz... rickettsia, fungus alga and lichen.)

...ی جسیمہ: یک خلوی جاندار جو صرف خوردبین کی مدد سے دیکھا جا... ...اندار شے جو سائز میں بہت چھوٹی ہو۔ اس میں اکثر جرثومہ پروٹوزون ...اروغ الگا اور لائیکن کو شامل کیا جاتا ہے۔

Microscopic *(mi-kro-skop-ik)* [G. *mil...* small; *skopein,* to examine] Extremely s... visible only with the aid of microscope.

...: انتہائی چھوٹا جو صرف خوردبین کے ذریعے دیکھا جاسکے۔

Microsporum *(mi-kro-spo-rum)* [G. *mil...* small; *sporos,* seed] A genus of f... Parasitic, living in keratin-containing ti... of man and aminals. Cause of ringw... *Microsporum audouini* is the comm... cause of scalp ringworm.

...سپورم: سماروغ کا ایک جنس۔ طفیلی۔ آدمی اور حیوانات کی کیراٹین ...ں میں رہتا ہے۔ رنگ کا ورم سبب۔

Microsurgery *(mi-kro-sur-je-ri)* Use o... binocular operating microscope durin... performance of operation, usually au... microsurgical, adj.

...ی: اپریشنوں کی ادائیگی کے دوران دو چشمی خوردبین کا استعمال۔ ...سرجری کے دوران اعضاء بڑے نظر آتے ہیں۔

icturition *(mik-tu-rish-un)* L. *micturire* , to make water] The act of passing urine,

سلس البول: پیشاب کرنے کا عمل۔

idbrain *(mid-bray-n)* Amiloride (q.v.)

میڈ برین: امیلورائیڈ۔

idamro The mesencephalon (q.v.)

میان دماغ۔ وسطی دماغ: میز نسفالان۔ دماغ کا وسطی حصہ۔ یہ سر برم اور پانز ویرولاتی کے درمیان ہوتا ہے۔

idriff. The diaphragm. (q.v.)

پردہ۔ ءول: ڈایافرام۔

igraine *(mē'-gren)* Hemicrania. Periodic. throbbing headache, unilateral initially, with at least three of the following features; (a) sensory prodromata; (b) photophobia (c) nausea or vomiting (d) family history of m., and (e) fluid retention before or diuresis during the attack. Tyramine in food has been investigated as a cause migrainous, adj.

شقیقہ: سر درد کی قسم۔ اس کا سبب خوراک میں ٹائرامین کی موجودگی ہے۔ عموماً نصف سر کا درد اس میں ارگوڑامین کیفین۔ سٹے مےٹل اور پینٹ ایزوسین دیجئے۔

ikulicz's disease. Chronic hypertrophic enlargement of the lacrimal and salivary glands. Now thought to be an autoimmune process. [Johannes von Mikulcz-Radecki, Rumanian surgeon. 1850-1905].

مرض مکولکز: لکریمل اور سلوری گلینڈز کا بڑھاؤ۔

iliaria *(mil-e-er-i-a)* [L. *miliarius,* millet]. Prickly heat. Common in the tropics, and affects waistline , cubital fossae and the chest. Vesicular and erythematous eruption, caused by blocking o sweat ducts. ducts, and their subsequent rupture, or their infection by fungi or bacteria.

مبارکی: پرکلی ہیٹ۔ گرمی دانے۔

iliary *(mil-i-ri)* [L. *miliarius,* millet] Resembling a millet seed. **milliary tuberculosis,** a form in which tuberculous nodules are widely disseminated throughout the organs and tissues of the body.

باجرا برابر: چینا کے بیج سے مشابہ۔

Milium *(MIL-e-um)* [L. millet] Condition in which tiny, white cystic excrescences appear on the face, especially about the eyelids; associated with seborrhoea.

سلعہ بشریہ۔ موتی جھرا: ایسی حالت جس میں چھوٹے سفید سسٹک دانے چہرے پر ظاہر ہوتے ہیں خصوصاً آنکھ کے پپوٹوں۔

Milk sugar. Lactose.

شکر شیر: لیکٹوز۔

Miller-abbot tube A double lumen rubber tube used for intestinal suction. The second channel leads to a balloon near the tip of the tube. This balloon is inflated when the tube reaches the doudenum and it is then carried down the intestine by peristaltic activity.[Thomas Gier Miller, Emeritus Professor of Medicine, 1886 ; William Osler Abbot, Assistant Professor of Medicine and Lecturer in Pharmocology in the Univesity of Pennsylvania, 1902-43(he died of leukaemia)].

ملرابیٹ ٹیوب: ربڑ کی ایک ٹیوب۔

Milontin *(mil'-on-tin)* Phensuximide (q.v.)

ملان ٹن: فنیسکی مائیڈ۔

Miltherex *(mel-ther-eks)* Chlorine preparatioin, for safe disposal of tuberculous sputum.

ملتھریکس: کلورین کی تیاری۔

Milton A stabilized solution of sodium hypochlorite. Used as 2.5 to 5 per cent solution for wounds and other antiseptic purposes, as 1 per cent solution for sterilizing babies feeding bottles.

ملٹن: سوڈیم ہائپو کلورائٹ کا ایک پائدار محلول۔ زخموں کے لئے ۲.۵ تا ۵ فیصد محلو مستعمل اور دافع تعفن کے لئے بھی مستعمل۔ ایک فیصد محلول بچوں کے فیڈر کو پاک صاف کرنے کے لئے مستعمل ہے۔

Miltown . Meprobamate (q.v.)

ملٹاؤن: میپروبامیٹ

Minadex *(min-a-deks)* Ger.:ral tonic in covnvalescene.

میناڈیکس: آغاز صحت میں عام ٹانک فیرس سلفیٹ سیرپ۔ اس میں فولاد اور حیاتین الف ہیں۔ ایک چمچہ دن میں تین مرتبہ کھانے کے بعد خون کی کمی اور کمزوری کے لئے مفید ہے۔

Mineralocorticoid *(min-er-al-o-kor-ti-koid)* See AL- DSTERONE.

منر ملوکور ٹیکائڈ: اولڈسٹیرون۔

Miner's anaemia. Hookworm disease. See ANKYLOSTOMIASIS.

کان کن کا انیمیا: ہک ورم کی بیماری۔

Miner's elbow. Inflammation of the bursa over the point of the elbow. Syn. student's elbow.

کان کن کی کہنی: کہنی کے بوائنٹ پر برسا کی سوزش۔

Minovlar *(min-ov-lar)* Oral contraceptive.

Mintezol *(min-ov-lar)* Thiabendazole (q.v.)

مینٹزول: تھیابنڈزول۔

Miosis *(mi-os'-is)* [G.*meiosis,* diminution]. Excessive contraction of the pupil of the eye. Also MYSIS.

انقباض حدقہ: آنکھ کی پتلی کا سکڑاؤ۔

Miotic *(mi-ot-ik)* Pertaining to or producing miosis Also MYOTIC

قابض حدقہ: انقباض حدقہ سے متعلق یا اسے پیدا کرنا۔

Miraci D. Lucanthone (q.v.)

مریسل ڈی: لوکنتھون۔

Miscarriage *(Mis-kar-ij)* The lay term for an abortion.

اسقاط (حمل): اسقاط کے لئے عام اصطلاح۔ حمل ۲۸ ہفتوں سے پہلے گرتا ہے اور بچہ زندہ نہیں رہ سکتا۔ اسقاط کی پہلی علامت یہ ہے کہ تھوڑا بہت خون اندام نہانی سے نکلتا ہے۔ اور جنین خارج ہو جاتا ہے۔ اسقاط حمل کے اسباب یہ ہیں ورم گردہ مزمن یا رحم کا اپنی جگہ سے ٹل جانا۔ رحم کے غشاء مخاطی والے پرت میں خرابی۔ آتشک۔ تسمیم الدم۔ یعنی خون میں زہر پھیلنا۔ گردے گے پیٹرو کا ورم آرا بچ عنصر وغیرہ۔ اس کے علاج کے لئے حاملہ کو ہوادار کمرے میں آرام سے چارپائی پر لٹا دیں۔ اٹھنے بیٹھنے اور چلنے پھرنے سے روک دیں۔ خون کو روکنے والی دوائیں دیں۔ جب خون زیادہ خارج ہونے لگے تو حمل محفوظ نہیں رہ سکتا اس لئے انگلی فم رحم میں داخل کر کے بچے کو ہلا دینا چاہئے تاکہ بچہ جلد باہر آ جائے۔

Mistura *(mis-tu-ra)* A mixture.

چورن: ایک آمیزہ۔

Misuse of Drugs Act 1971. Combines and extends the Dangerous Drugs Acts 1965 and 1967 and the Drugs (Prevention of Misuse) Act 1964 which have been repealed. The Act is designed to control the manufacture, sale, prescribing and dispensing of certa habitforming drugs, to which an addicti may arise; these are now called controll drugs and are available to the public medical by medical prescription only, a heavy penalties may follow any illegal sale supply. The principal drugs concerned a opium, morphine, cocaine, diamorphi cannabis indica, and the many synthe morphin substtitutes as exemplified pethidine.

Mithramycin. *(mith-ra-mi'-sin)* Antitumo comp- ound. Derived from a micro-organi of the Streptomyces genus. Has been used Paget's disease. It probably acts directly osteoclasts.

ر امائی سین: دافع ناسور مرکب۔

Mitosis *(mito-sis)* [G. *mitos,* thread; *-os* condition]. A complicated method of c division occuring in specialized cells.

Mitral stenos

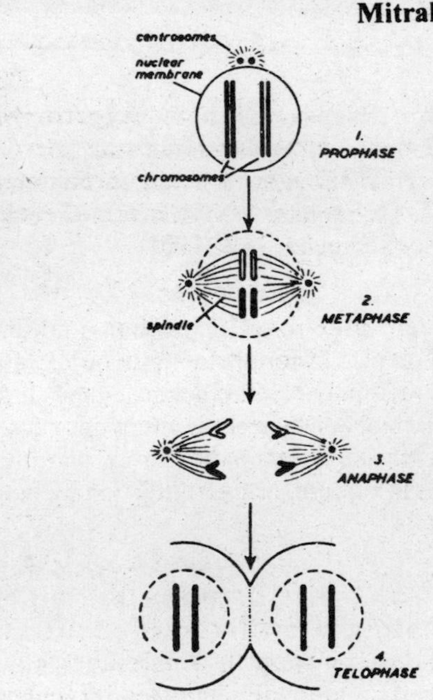

بلاراست تقسیم ۔ بالواسطہ تقسیم: تقسیم خلیہ کا طریقہ جو غیر تولیدی حصوں میں ہوتا ہے۔ اس میں کروموسوموں کی تعداد اتنی ہی رہتی ہے جتنی پہلی تھی۔ ایک سے دو خلیے بنتے ہیں۔ کروموسوم دوسروں یا قطبوں کے درمیان آجاتے ہیں۔ ہر ایک کروموسوم میں نصف ایک قطب کی طرف اور ف بقایا نصف دوسرے قطب کی طرف کھنچنے لگتا ہے۔ آخر کروموسوم قطب پر پہنچ جاتے ہیں۔ اس طرح ایک خلکیہ سے دو خلیے بن جاتے ہیں۔ اس تقسیم کے طریقہ میں ہر شے برابر دونوں نئے بننے والے خلیوں میں تقسیم ہو جاتی ہے۔ ہر نوع میں کروموسوموں کی تعداد مقرر رہوتی ہے۔ یہ تعداد اسی طرح رہتی ہے۔

Mitral *(mi-tral)* [G. *mitra,* turban]. Mitre-shaped, as the valve between the left atruim and ventricle of the heart (bicuspid valve) **mitral imcompetence,** a defect in the closure of the m.valve whereby blood tends to flow backwards into the left atrium from the left ventricle. **mitral stenosis, narrowing** of the m. orifice, usually due to rheumatic fever.

Mitral valvulotomy *(valvotomy)* an operation for splitting the cusps of a stenosed m. valve.

کلانما۔ کواڑی: پگڑی کی شکل کا۔ جیسے دل کے بطین اور بائیں ایٹریم کے درمیان ویلو۔

Mitral stenosis

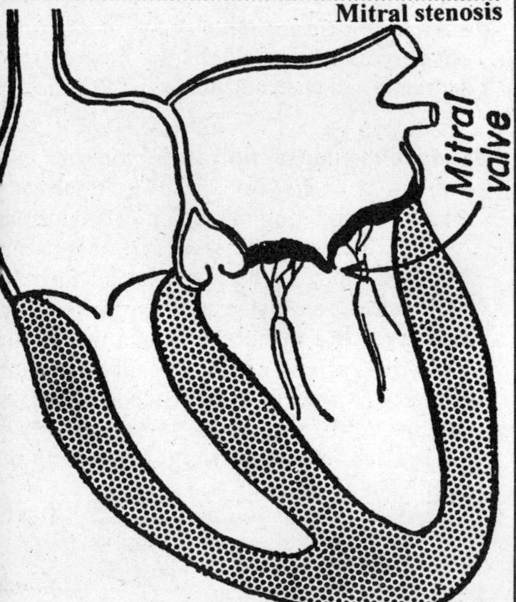

Mexogen *(miks-o-jen)* Androgenoestrogen mixture. See MEPLIN.

مکسوجن: اینڈروجن ایسٹروجن آمیزہ۔ میتھا ئیل ٹسٹو۔ سٹیرون کمپاؤنڈ۔ سن یاس کے مرض میں مفید ایک گولی دن میں تین دفعہ۔

MK-870 A potassium-sparing diuretic.

ایم کے ۸۷۰: پیشاب آور دوا۔

MLNS Mucocutaneous lymph node syndrome.

Modecate *(mod-e-kat)* Fluphenazine.(q.v.)

موڈ یکیٹ: فلوفینازین۔

Moditen. Fluphenazine. (q.v.)

موڈیٹن: فلوفینازین۔ طب دماغی میں مستعمل۔ ڈپو انجکشن کے طور پر دیا جا سکتا ہے۔

Moduretic *(mod-ur-et-ik)* Amiloride (q.v.) and hydrochlorothiazide (q.v.)

Mogadon *(mog-a-don)* Nitrazepam (q.v.)

موگیڈان: باربیٹو سے آزاد تنویمی مسکن دوا مرگی میں مفید۔

Molar tech *(mol-lar)* The double teeth or grinders, three on either side of each jaw.

ڈاڑھیں: ڈبل دانت یا پیسنے والے دانت۔ ہر جبڑے کے ایک طرف تین دانت۔

Mole *(mol)* [A.S., *mal,* spot]. See NAEVUS. **carneous m,.**the result of a missed abnortion, i.e. the uterus retains the dead and organized products of conception. **hydatidiform m.,** a condition in which the chorionic villi of the placenta undergo cystic degeneration and the fetus is absrbed. A proportion of the moled are active and if remnants are left in the uterus after abortion of the mole, malignant changes may ensue, giving rise to a chorionepithelioma. (q.v.)

مول ۔ خال: (۱) ایک جلدی ابھار جو پگمنٹ پیدا کرنے والے خلیوں یا خونی رگوں کی غیر معمولی تکمیل کی وجہ سے بنتا ہے۔ (۲) کسی شے کی مقدار کی بنیادی ایس۔ آئی اکائی۔

Molecule *(miks-o-jen)* The smallest particle into which matter can be divided and still retain its identity-- molecular, adj.

سالمہ: کسی شے کا سب سے چھوٹا حصہ جو آزادانہ طور پر وجود رکھتا ہے اور اصل مادے کی خصوصیات کا حامل ہوتا ہے۔

Mollities *(mol-ish-i-ez)* [L.]. Softness . **mollities ossium,** osteomalacia. (q.v.)

ملاسب عظام: نرمی۔ کسی عضو مثلاً ہڈی وغیرہ کا نرم پڑ جانا۔

Molluscum *(mol-us-lum)* [L. *molluscus,* soft]. A soft tumour. **molluscum contagiousum,** an infectious type of wart which appears on the skin as a waxy papule, often umbilicated; spread is by autoinoculation **mollusum fibrosum,** the superficial tumours of Rechlinghausen's disease.(q.v)

نرم پھوڑا: نرم یا ناسور جس کا منہ کھلا رہتا ہے۔

Monarticular *(mon-ar-tik'-u-lar)* [G. *monus,* single; L. *articulus,* joint] Relating to one joint.

متعلقہ جوڑ: جوڑ سے متعلق۔ جس کا تعلق جوڑ سے ہو۔

Monckeberg's sclerosis Senile degenerative change resulting in calcification of the media in arteries, especially of the limbs; leads to intermittent claudication or gangrene. [Johann Georg Monckeberg, German pathologist, 1877-1925]

سکلیر وسس منکیبرگ: تخریبی تبدیلی جو خصوصاً جوارح کی شریانوں مین میڈیا کیلسی فیکیشن کرتی ہے۔

Mongol *(mong-gol)* Preferred term is Down's syndrome. Refers to a type of congenital mentally subnormal child, with facial characteristics resembling the Mongolian races. Stigmata include oval tilted eyes, squint and a flattened occiput. Increased susceptibility to leukaemia. Abnormality of chromosome 21.Two types; 1 Failure of division of chromosome 21 results in an extra chromosome instead of the normal pair. The infant has 47 chromosomes. Usually born of elderly 21, total number of 46 being normal. Usually born of young mothers. Higher risk of recurrence in subsequent pregnancies.

منگول: اس سے بہتر اصطلاح ڈاؤن کا سنڈ دم ہے۔ ایسا بچہ جو ذہنی طور پر پسماندہ ہو اور چہرے کے خدوخال قوم منگول سے مشابہ ہوں۔ آنکھیں بیضوی اور جھکی ہوتی ہیں۔ اس میں کروموسوموں کی تعداد ۴۷ ہوتی ہے۔ جبکہ نارمل ۴۶ انسان میں ہوتی ہے۔ عموماً ایسی ماؤں کے ہاں ہوتے ہیں جن کی عمر زیادہ ہو ہوتی ہے۔ دوسری صورت میں کروموسوم ۲۱ غیر معمولی ہوتا ہے حالانکہ کروموسوم ۴۶ ہوتے ہیں۔

Monilia. Syn,. Candida (q.v.)

مونیلیا: کینڈا ایڈا

Moniliasis *(mon-il-i-a-sis)* Disease caused by infection with species of Monilia (Candida) Candidiasis (q.v.)

مونی لیاسس: کینڈا ایڈا کی نوع کے ساتھ چھوت سے ہونے والا مرض۔

Moniliform *(mon-nil-i-form)* [L. *monile* necklace; *forma,* form] Like a string of beads. Used to describe the arrangement of micro-organisms, or clinical features such as skin rash.

تسبیحی: تسبیح کے دانوں کیطرف خوبصورت۔ خورد جسیموں کی تنظیم بیان کرنے کے لئے مستعمل۔

Monitoring *(mon-it-or-ing)* Seouential recording. Term usually reserved for autim- atic visual display of such measur- ements as temperature, pulse, respir- ation and blood pressure.

Monitron *(mon-i-tron)* An apparatus for the autom- atic recording of temperature, pulse, respiration, and systolic and diastolic blood pressures.

Monoamine exidase *(mon-o-a-men-oks-i-dase)* An enzyme which inhibits the breakdown of serotonin and catecholamines in the brain.

مونوامین آکسیڈیز: ایک خامرہ۔

Monoamineoxidase inhibitor *(mon -o-a -men -oks -i-das in-hib-it-or)* MOAI. A substance which by inhibiting the action of monoamine oxidase, increases the level of serotonin and catecholamines in the brain; useful for relief of exogenous or reactive depression. Increases the effects of barbiturates and alcohol. Patient advised to abstain from cheese, Marmite, Bovril, broadbeans (because of episodic hypertension and possibility of subarachnoid haemorrhage) and drug not ordered by the doctor.

Monocular *(mon-ok'-u-lar)* [G. *monos,* single; L. *oculus,* eye] Pertaining to one eye.

یک چشم: ایک آنکھ سے متعلق۔

Monocyte *(mon'-o-sit)* [G. *monis,* single; *kytos,* cell] A mononuclear cell -- monocytic, adj.

یک نواتی خلیہ: ایک مرکزہ والا خلیہ۔ خون میں سات فیصد۔

Monomania *(mon-o-ma-ni-a)* [G. *monos,* one; *mania,* madness] Obsesseed with a single idea.

یک مانیا: ایک ہی نظریہ کا خبط۔

Mononuclear *(mon-o-nu-kle-ar)* [G. *monos,* one; L. *nucleus,* kerne]. With a single nucleus. Usually refers to a type of blood cell (monocyte), the largest of the cells in the normnal blood with a round, oval or indented nucleus.

یک نوائی: ایک مرکزہ کے ساتھ عموماً خونی خلیے کی قسم۔ نارمل خون میں گول یا بیضوی مرکزے کے ساتھ سب سے بڑا خلیہ۔

Mononucleosis *(mon-o-nu-kle-o-sis)* [G. *monos,* one; L. *nucleus,* kernal; G. *osis,* condition]. An increase in the number of circulating monocytes (monon- uclear cells) in the blood. **infection m.,** syn. glandular fever (q.v.)

تپ غدی: خون میں گردشی یک نواتی خلیوں کی تعداد میں اضافہ۔

Monoplegia *(mon-o-ple'-ji-a)* [G. *monos,* single; *pleg,* a stroke]. Paralysis of only one limb monoplegic, adj.

فالج یک عضو: صرف ایک جارح کی ایک اینٹھن۔ صرف ایک عضو کا فالج۔

Monosaccharide *(mon-o-sak'-a-rid)* A simple sugar ($C_6 H_{12} O_6$) Examples are glucose, fructose and galactose.

سادہ شکر: کاربوہائیڈریٹس کا ایک گروہ۔ مثلاً گلوکوس فرکٹوز اور گلیکٹوز۔

Monosomy *(mon'-o-so-mi)* Nondisjunction autoso- mal anomaly when one cell is left without one particular chromosome.

مانوسومی: ایک خلیہ ایک مخصوص کروموسوم کے بغیر رہ جاتا ہے۔

Monosulfiram *(mon-o-sul-fir-am)* Lotion for topical application inscabies. 25 per cent alchoholic solution which is diluted with 3 parts of water immediately before use. Chemically similar to disulfiram. Systemic toxic effects if alcohol is taken.

مانوسلفیریم: خارش تر کے لئے لوشن ۲۵۰ فیصد الکحل کا محلول جسے استعمال سے ذرا پہلے تین حصے پانی ڈال کر ہلکا کیا جاتا ہے۔ اسے بیرونی طور پر لگایا جاتا ہے۔

Monovular *(mon-ov-u-lar)* Uniovular (q.v.)

واحد بیضوی: ایک بیضے سے متعلق۔

Mons veneris *(mons-ven-er-is)* [L. *mons,* mountain]. The eminence formed by the pad of fat which lies over the pubic bone in the female.

ابھار زہرہ: چربی کے پیڈ سے بننے والا ابھار جو خواتین میں پیوبک ہڈی پر ہوتا ہے۔ زنانہ جنسی اعضا میں بیرونی لبوں کے اوپر کی طرف ہوتا ہے۔ یہ ابھار بہت نرم ہوتا ہے۔ بلوغت کے وقت اس پر بال اگ آتے ہیں۔ اس کی شکل مثلث کی طرح ہوتی ہے۔

Mooren's ulcer. Corneal rodent ulcer (q.v.) [Albert Mooren, German ophthalmologist, 1828-99]

قرحہ مورین۔ قرحہ قرینہ منزمن: کارنیل روڈنٹ السر۔

Morbili *(mor-bil-li)* Measles (q.v.)

خسرہ: خسرہ۔

Morbilliform *(mor-bil-i-form)* Describes a rash res - embling that of measles.

خسرہ نما: خسرہ سے مشابہ ریش۔

Moribund *(mor-i-bund)* [L. *moribundus,* dying]. In a dying state.

جان بلب: مرنے کی حالت میں۔

Moron *(mor'-on)* [G. *moros,* stupid]. American term. Syn. ESN (q.v.)

Moro reflex *(mor-o)* Contraction of an infant's limb and nech when he is allowed to drop a short distance through the air or is started by a sudden noise. [Ernst Moro, German physician, 1874-1951]

Morphine *(mor-fen)* The active principle of opium and a most valuable analgesic. Widely used in pain due to spasm, in haemorrhage, shock, and in useless cough. May cause some respiratory depression, especially in full doses.

مارفین۔ جوہر افیون: ایک سفید قلمی الکلائڈ جو افیم میں پایا جاتا ہے۔ نقطہ پگھلاؤ ۲۵۳س۔ یہ طاقتور نشہ ہے۔ طب میں درد دور کرنے کے لئے اس کی سلفیٹ یا ہائیڈروکلورائیڈ کی صورت میں دیا جاتا ہے۔ اس کا استعمال خطرناک ہے۔ پاکستان میں اس کا استعمال غیر قانونی ہے۔ صدمہ اور کھانسی میں مفید۔

Morphology *(mor-fol-oj-i)* [G. *morphe,* form; *logos,* discourse]. The science which deals with the form and structure of living things -- morphological, adj. morphologically, adv.

شکلیات: حیاتیات کی ایک اہم شاخ۔ علم کی یہ شاخ جانداروں کی دو شاخیں ہیں۔ بیرونی اور اندرونی شکلیات۔

Mortality *(mor-tal-i-ti)* [L. *mors,* death]l. The death-rate; the ratio of the total number of deaths to the total population.

شرح اموات: موت کی شرح۔ کل آبادی سے اموات کی کل تعداد کا تناسب۔

Mortha *(mor-tha)* Analgesic with morphine as a base. Is not a respiratory depressant. Can be given orally and by injection.

مورتھا: بطور اساس مافین کے ساتھ دافع دردوا۔

Mortification *(mor-ti-fik-a-shun)* [L. *mors,* death] Death of tissue. See GANGRENE.

فساد عضو: نسیج کی موت۔

Moryl *(mor-il)* Carbachol *(q.v.)*

مورل: پیرا سمپیتھٹک۔ عصبی نظام کے لئے متحرک۔ ایثائل کولین سے مشابہ۔ منہ سے کھانے پر عامل۔

Mortile *(mo-til)* [L. *mover,* to move]. Capable of spontaneous movement -- motility, n.

حرکیہ: اچانک حرکت کے قابل جو حرکت کر سکے۔

Motion *(mo-shun)* An evacuation of the bowel.

اجابت: فضلے کا اخراج۔ پاخانہ۔

Motor *(mo-ter)* [L. *mover,* to move]. Pertaining to action. See NEURONE.

موٹر: (۱) ایکشن سے متعلق۔ (۲) دوسری اقسام کی توانائی کی میکانکی توانائی میں تبدیل کرنے کا آلہ۔ موٹر اعصاب پیغام دماغ سے باہر کی طرف لے جاتے ہیں۔ انہیں افرنٹ نروبھی کہا جاتا ہے۔

Mould *(mold)* Multicellular fungus. Often used synonymously with fungus. Member of the plant kingdom with no differentation into root, stem or leaf, and without chlorophyll. Structurally consists of filaments or hyphae, which aggregate into a mycelium. Propagation is by means of spores. Occurs in infinite variety, as common saprophytes contaminating floodstuffs, and more rarely as pathogens.

پھپھوندی: کئی خلوی سماروغ۔ یہ اصطلاح سماروغ کے مترادف کے طور پر استعمال کی جاتی ہے۔ مملکت نباتات کا ایک رکن جس میں جڑ تنا اور پتے نہیں ہوتے۔ ان میں سبز مایہ یا کلوروفل نہیں ہوتا اس لئے اپنی خوراک خود نہیں بنا سکتے یہی وجہ ہے کہ یہ گندخور یا طفیلی ہیں۔ ساختی طور پر ریشوں پر مشتمل جو مل کر قطرومہ بناتے ہیں۔ ان کا پھیلاؤ بذروں کے ذریعہ ہوتا ہے۔ گند خود کھانے پینے کی اشیاء کو خراب کرتے ہیں۔ بہت کم سماروغ امراض پیدا کرتے ہیں۔

Moulding *(mold-ing)* The compression of the fetal head during its passage through the genital tract in labour.

ڈھلائی: بچے کی پیدائش کے دوران باہر آتے ہوئے بچے کے سر کا دباؤ۔

Mountain sickness Symptoms of sickness, tachycar- dia and dyspnoea, due to low oxygen content of rarefied air at a high altitude.

حمی کوہی: زیادہ بلندی پر لطیف ہوا کی وجہ سے کم آکسیجن ہونے کی بناء پر مرض کی علامات۔

Mucilage *(mu-sil-aj)* The solution of gum in water--mucilaginous, adj.

لعاب: پانی میں گوند کا محلول۔

Mucin *(mu'-sin)* [L. *mucus]* A mixture of glycoprot- eins found in or secreted by many cells and glands mucinous, adj.

میوسین: گلائیکو پروٹینز کا آمیزہ جسے بہت سے خلیے یا گلینڈز پیدا کرتے ہیں یا ان میں موجود ہوتا ہے۔

Mucinase *(mu-sin-as)* A specific mucindi- ssolving su- bstance contained in some aerosols. Useful in fibrocystic disease.

میوسی نیز: بعض ایروسائز میں موجود مخصوص مادہ جو میوسین کو حل کر لیتا ہے۔ فائبرو سسٹک بیماری میں مفید ہوتا ہے۔

Mucinolysis *(mu-sin-ol-i-sis)* [L. *mucus;* G. *lysis,* a loosening]. Dissolution of mucinmuc- inolytic, adj.

میوسینولائی سس: میوسین کی تحلیل۔

Mucocele *(mu'-ko-sel)* [L. mucus; G.*kele,* tumour] Distension of a cavity with mucus.

مخاطی قیلہ: کہفے کا میوکس کی وجہ سے پھیلاؤ۔

Mucocutaneous *(mu-ko-ku-tan-e-us)* Pertaining to mucous membrance and skin.

میوکوجلدی: میوکس جھلی اور کھال سے متعلق۔

Mucocutaneous lymphnode syndrome. MLNS. A dis ease affecting mainly babies and children; first noticed in Japan in the late 1960s. Characterized by fever, dry lips, red mouth and strawberry like tongue. A rash is in a glove-and-stocking distri- bution. There is cervical adenitis, polymorph- onuclear leucocytosis and raised ESR.

Mucoid *(mu-koiod)* Resembling mucus.

میوکس نما: میوکس سے مشابہ۔

Mucolytics *(mu-ko-lit'-iks)* [L. *mucus;* G. *lysis,* a loosening] Drugs which soften mucus and so reduce viscosity of secretion from the respiratory tract.

Mucopurulent *(muk-ko-pu'-ru-len)* [L. mucus; *pus,* pus] Containing mucus and pus.

ریمی: میوکس و پیپ پر مشتمل۔

Mucopus *(mu-ko-pus')* [L. *mucus,* mucus; *pus,* pus] Mucus containing. pus.

میوکوپس: پیپ پر مشتمل میوکس۔

Mucosa *(mu-ko-pus)* [L. mucus] A mucous membrance (q.v.) mucosal, adj; mucoae, pl.

غشاء مخاطی: میوکس جھلی۔

Mucous *(mu'-kus)* Pertaining to or containing mucus. **mucus colitis** mucomerbranous colitis. Possibly a functional disorder, manifested by passage of mucus in the stool, obstinate constipation and occasional colic mucus polypus, a growth (adenoma) of m. membrance which becomes pedunculated. See MEMBRANCE.

لعابی: میوکس پر مشتمل یا اس سے متعلق۔

Mucoviscidosis *(mu-ko-vis-kid-o'-sis)* [L. mucus; *viscidus,* sticky; G. *osis,* Condition]. A congenital hereditry disease with failure of development of normal mucus-secreting glands, sweat glands and pancreas. May present in a baby as meconium ilesus; in infancy with septic bronchitis and steatorrhoea. Stools contain excess fat; trypsin is absent from stool and duodenal juice. See CYSTIC.

میوکو وی ڈوسس: وراثت میں چلنے والی بیماری جس میں لبلبہ پسینہ گلینڈز اور نارمل میوکس خارج کرنے والی گلینڈز کی تکمیل میں ناکامی ہوتی ہے۔

Mucus *(mu-kus)* [L.] The viscid fluid secreted by mucous glands-- mucous mucoid, adj.

میوکس۔ بلغم۔ آؤں: میوکس گلینڈز سے خارج ہونے والا گاڑھا سیال۔ فضلے میں آؤں نہیں ہوتی۔

Multicellular *(mul-ti-sel-u-lar)* [L. *multus,* many; *cellula,* small cell] Constructed of many cells.

کثیر الخلایا: جو کئی خلیوں سے بنا ہو۔

Multigravida *(mul-ti-gra-ia-a)* [L. *multus,* many; *gravidus,* pregnant] A woman who has borne many children -- multigravidae, pl.

چند بار حاملہ: خاتون جو کہ کئی بچوں کو جنم دے چکی ہے۔

Multilobular *(mul-ti-lob-u-lar)* [L. *multus,* many; G. *lobos,* lobe]. Possessing many lobes.

کثیر الفصیص: کئی بولوں والا۔

Multilocular *(mul-ti-lik-u-lar)* [L. *multus,* many; *loculus,* Compartment] Possessing many small cysts, loculi or pockers.

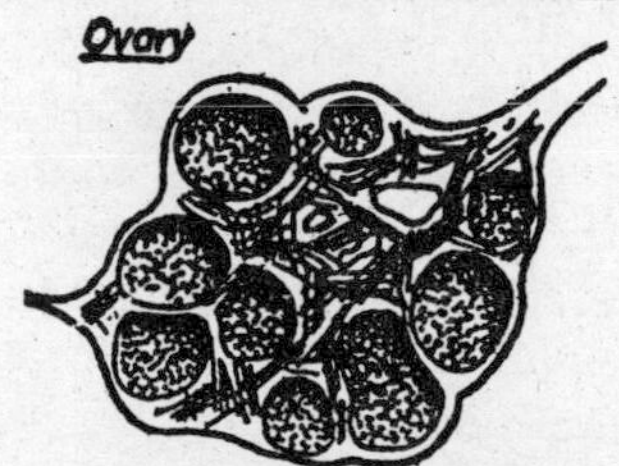

Multilocular cyst

Multilcular cyst

کثیر خانہ: بہت سے خانوں سسٹ یا جیبوں والا۔

Multinuclear *(mul-tin-nu-kle-ar)* [L. *multus,* many; *nucleus,* nut]. Possessing many nuclei multi- nucleate, adj.

بہت سے مرکزوں والا: جس میں کئی مرکزے ہوں۔

Multipara *(mul-tip-a-ra)* See MULTIGR-AVIDA. multiparae.pl.

کثیر زا عورت: کئی بچوں کو جنم دینے والی خاتون۔

Multiple sclerosis See SCLEROSIS.

Multivite *(mul-ti-vit)* tablets containing vitamin A 2500 units, aneurine hydrochloride 0.5 mg, ascorbic acid 12.5 mg and claciferol 6.25 g.

ملٹی وائٹ: وٹامن الف۔ انیورین ہائیڈروکلورائیڈ اسکاربک ایسڈ اور کیلسفیرول پر مشتمل گولیاں۔

Mumps An acute, specific inflammation of the parotid glands. caused by a virus. Syn. infectious parotitis.

کن پھیڑ: پیروٹڈ گلینڈز کی مخصوص سوزش۔ وائرس سے ہونے والا مرض۔

Mural *(mur-al)* [L. *murus* wall] pertaining to the wall of a cavity. organ or vessel.

دیواری: رگ عضو یا کہفہ کی دیوار سے متعلق۔

Mumur. Abnormal sound heard on auscultation of heart or great vessels. **Presystolic m.** characteristic of mitral stenosis in regular rhythm.

سرسراہٹ: دل سے غیر معمولی آواز سنائی دینا۔

Musca. *(mus-ka)* Genus of the common house-fly. capable of transmitting many enteric infections.

گھر کی مکھی: عام گھریلو مکھی جس سے کئی بیماریاں پھیلتی ہیں۔

Muscle *(mus-l)* [L. *musculus,* muscle]. Strong. contracile tissue which produces movement in the body. **cardiac m.** makes up the middle wall of the heart; it in involuntary. striated and innervated by autonomic nerves. **skeletal m.** surrounds the skeleton; it is voluntary, striated and innvervatedby the peripheral verves of the centrel nervous system. **visceral (internal) m.** is non-striated and involuntary and is innervated by the autonomic nerves. **muscle relaxants,** widely used in surgery. in tetanus to prevent spasm, in mechanically aided respiration and in the convulsive shock therapy for mental disorder muscular, adj.

عضلہ۔ پٹھا: مضبوط انقباضی نسیج جو جسم میں حرکت پیدا کرتا ہے۔ سکڑنے والے مضبوط ریشے۔ انکی اقسام قلبی ۔ڈھانچہ نما۔ اندرونی ریشے دار اور پھیلنے وسکڑنے والے عضلے ہیں۔ یہ عضلات میں بے شمار ریشے ایک بنڈل کی صورت میں بندھے ہوتے ہیں۔ ہر بنڈل ایک باریک جھلی میں لپٹا ہوتا ہے۔ ان پر دھاریاں دکھائی دیتی ہیں۔ ان کے کناروں پر رباط یا ٹنڈانز لگے ہوتے ہیں جن کے ذریعے وہ ہڈیوں سے جڑے ہوتے ہیں۔ غیر ارادی عضلات پر نہ تو دھاریاں ہوتی ہیں اور نہ ان کے کناروں پر رباط ہوتے ہیں۔ ان کا ریشہ تکلہ نما ہوتا ہے جن کے درمیان بیضوی شکل کی مرکز ہوتا ہے۔

Muscular dystrophies *(mus-ku-lar dis-tro-fez)* [. *musclus,* muscle; G. dysfaulty; *trophe,*nourishme- nt] Pseudohypertrophic or Duchenne, type is the most severe. Presents in early childhood. Runs a malignant course....there is a saying. Off his feet by ten dead by twenty. A clue to future treatment lies in recent advances in biochemical knowledge of the condition.

عضلی ڈس ٹرافی: سوڈوہائیپرٹرافک قسم سے زیادہ سخت ہے۔ بچپن کے شروع میں یہ مرض موجود ہوتا ہے۔

Musculature *(mus-ku-lat-ur)* [L. *musculus,* muscle] The muscular system or any part of it.

نظام عضلات: عضلاتی نظام یا اس کا کوئی حصہ۔

Musculocutaneous *(mus-ku-lo-ku-ta-ne-us)* [L. *mus- culus,* muscle; *cutis,* skin]. Pertaining to muscle and skin.

عضلی جلدی: جلد اور عضلے سے متعلق۔ عضلی جلدی عصب یا نرو بازو کی سائیڈ کو جاتی ہے۔ بالائی بازو کے عضلات اور زیریں بازو کی جلد کو سپلائی دیتی ہے۔

Musculoskeletal *(mus-ku-lo-skel-et-al)* [L. *musculus,* muscle; G. *skeletos,* dried]. Pertaining to the muscular and skeletal systems. Diseases of the musculoskeletal system is now a preferred term to rheumatism.

عضلی استخوانی: عضلاتی اور استخوانی نظاموں سے متعلق۔

Mustagen *(mus-ta-jen)* Mechlorethamine hydrochlo- ride (q.v.)

مسٹیجن: میکلورتھامین ہائیڈروکلورائیڈ۔

Mustard Crushed seeds of the m. plant which can be used orally as an emetic, or externally as a counter- irritant.

سرسوں۔ رائی: سرسوں کے کٹے ہوئے بیج جو قے آور کے طور پر استعمال کئے جاتے ہیں۔

Mustine *(mus-ten).* Nitrogen mustard, a cytotoxic alkylating agent (q.v.).

مستین: نائٹروجن مسٹرڈ۔ انٹراوینس انجکشن کے ذریعے دی جانے والی دوا۔

Mustagenesis *(mu-ta-jen-e-sis)* [L. *mutare,* to change; G. *genesis,* decent]. The production of mutatios mutagenic. mutagenetic. adj.;

mutagene- tically, *adv.*

میوٹاجینیس : تبدلات کی پیداوار۔

lutagenicity *(mu-ta-jen-is-i-ti)* [L. *mutare,* to chan- ge; G. *genes,* producing]. The capacity to produce gene mutations chromosome aberrations.

میوٹاجینی سٹی: غیر معمولی کروموسوم یا جینی تبدلات پیدا کرنے کی اہلیت۔

lutant *(mu-tan).* A cell which is the result of a gen- etic change.

متقلب : خلیہ جو جینی تبدیلی کا نتیجہ ہو۔

lutation *(mu-ta-shun)* [L. *mutare,* to change]. A change. An alteration in the genes of a living cell gives rise to genetic mutation, as a result of which the characters of the cell change. This change is heritable, remaining until a further mutation occurs. induced m., a gene mutation produced by a known agent outside the cell, e.g. ultraviolet radiation. **spontaneous m.,** a gene mutation taking place without apparent influence from outside the cell.

تبدل : توارثی مادہ میں معمولی تبدیلی ۔ کسی جیسے کے کروموں سوموں میں ڈی ۔ این اے کی کیمیائی ترکیب میں تبدیلی ۔ تبدیلیاں عموماً جینوں میں ہوتی ہیں ۔ لیکن بعض اوقات پورے کروموسوم بھی تبدیل ہو سکتے ہیں ۔ اگر گیمیٹوں میں تبدیلی آجائے تو بننے والے افراد متاثر ہوتے ہیں۔

lyalgia *(mi-al-ji-a)* [G. *mys.,* muscle; *algos,* pain]. Pain in the musclesmyalgic, *adj.*

دردعضلہ: عضلات میں درد۔

lyambutol *(mi-am-bu-tol).* Ethambutol (q.v.)

مائی ایمبوٹال : ایتھمبوٹول ۔ تپ دق میں صبح ناشتے کے روزانہ اکٹھی ۵ گولیاں۔

lyanesin *(mi-an-es-in).* Mephenesin (q.v.)

مایانیلسن: مفلیسن

lyasthenia *(mi-as-the-ni-a)* [G. *mys,* muscle; *astheneia,* weakness]. Muscular weakness myast- henia gravis, a disorder characterized by marked fatiguability of voluntary muscles, especially those of the eye. Due to a biochemical defect associated with abnormal behaviour of acetylcholine at neuromuscular junctions. There is considerable evidence for an autoimmune process. Patient forms antibody (to his own striated muscle fibres) which competes with acetylcholine and prevents if from carrying out its transmission duties especialy when only small quantities are available. Heredity, infections, environmental influences or a combination of these factors are all possible causes. Research on twins suggests that a rare recessive trait may be instrumental in causing the disease. See CRISIS.--myasthenic, *adj.*

عضلی ضعف: عضلاتی کمزوری۔

Myatonia *(mi-a-to'-ni-a)* [G. *mys,* muscle; a not; *tonos,* tone]. Absence of tone in muscle, myatonia congenita, a form of congenital muscular dyst- rophy in infancy. Child is unable to bear the we- ight of the head on the shoulders--myatonic, adj.

فقدان طن عضلی : عضلے میں ٹون کی غیر موجودگی ۔ عضلات میں ربط وہم آہنگی کا فقدان جس سے بچہ شانوں پر سر کا بوجھ برداشت نہیں کر سکتا۔

Mycardol *(mi-kar-dol).* Pentaerythrityl tetranitrate (q.v.)

مائی کارڈال: پینٹاارتھریٹائل ٹیٹرانائیٹریٹ۔

Mycelium *(mi-se-li-um)* [G. *mykes,* fungus]. A mass of branching filaments of moulds of fungi (hyphae) --mycelial, *adj.*

فطرومہ: سماروغ کے شاخ دار ریشوں کا گچھا۔

Mycetoma *(mi-se-to-ma)* [G. *mykes,* fungus; *-omas,* tumour] A fungus infection usually of the feet, occuring in tropical and subtropical regions . Similar to actinomycosis (q.v.) and aspergillosis. Syn, Madura foot.

سماروغی چھوت کی بیماری عموماً پاؤں میں ہوتی ہے۔

Mycifradin *(mi-si-fra-din)* Neomycin (q.v.)

مائیسی فریڈن: نیومائیسین۔

Mycobacterium *(mi-ko-bak-te-ri-um)* [G. *mykes,* fungus; *bacterium.* small rod]. Small slender rod bacteria. Grampositive and acid fast, both to a varying degree. Saprophytic, commensal and pathogenic species. *Mycobacterium tuberculosis* causes tuberculosis. *M. leprare,* leprosy. Anonymous mycobacteria are acid-fast bacilli with bacteriological differences from M.tuberculosis and have been subclassified. The pathogenic varieties. M. Kansassi and the Battery bacillus are elective human pathogens causing pulmonary and cervical tuberculosis.

مائیکو بیکٹیریم: چھوٹے سلاخی جراثیم۔ گرام مثبت گند خور اور مرض پیدا کرنے والی انواع۔ تپ دق اور جذام کے جراثیم۔

Mycology *(mi-kol-o-ji)* [G. *mykes,* fungus; *logos,* discourse]. The study of fungi--mycologist. n: mycological, adj; mycologically , adv.

فطریات ۔علم فطرات: نباتیات کی ایک شاخ جس کا تعلق سماروغ سے ہے۔

Mycoplasma *(mi-ko-plaz-ma)* [G. *mykes,* fungus; *plasma,* form] A small organism intermediate in size between viruses and bacteria. *Mycoplasma pneumoniae* proposed as syn. for Eaton agent (q.v.) One type of Mycoplasma associated with acute leukaemia. Now believed to play a signif- icant role in reproductive failure. Published evidence now associating m. with various and even NSU.

مائیکو پلازما: ایک چھوٹا جسیمہ جو سائز میں وائرس اور جراثیم کے درمیان ہے۔اس کا تعلق کئی چھوت کی بیماریوں کے ساتھ ہے۔

Mycosis *(mi-ko-sis)* [G. *mykes,* fungus; *-osis,* condition]. Disease caused by any fungus --mycotic, adj **mycosis fungoides** is a chronic and usually fatal disease, not fungal in origin. It is manifested by generalized pruritis, followed by skin eruptions of diverse character which become infiltrated and finally develop into granulomatous ulcerating tumours. A form of reticuloendothelial disease.

فطریت: کسی سماروغ سے ہونے والا مرض۔

Mydriacyl *(mid-ri-a-sil)* Mydriatic and cycloplegic.

مڈریاسل: اتساعی دوا۔آنکھ کی پتلی کے پھیلانے کے لئے دوا۔

Mydriatics *(mid-ri-a-sis)* [G. *dilatioin* of the pupil]. Abnormal dilation of the pupil of the eye.

اتساع حدقہ : آنکھ کی پتلی کا غیر معمولی پھیلاؤ۔

mydriatics *(mid-ri-at'-iks)* Drugs which cause mydri- asis.

تساعی ادویہ: ادویات جن سے اتساع حدقہ ہوتا ہے۔

Mydricaine *(mid-ri-kan)* Atropine, cocaine and adrenaline for ophthalmic work.

ڈریکین: آفتھلمک کام کے لئے ایٹروپین کوکین اور ایڈرینالین۔

Mydrilate *(mid-ril-at)* Cyclopentolate Mydriatic. Useful prior to examining the opti fundus.

ڈریلیٹ: سائیکلوپنٹولیٹ۔اتساعی دوا۔اوپٹک فنڈس کی جانچ سے پہلے فید۔

Myelin *(mi-e-lin)* [G. *myelos,* marrow] Th white, fatty substance constituting th medullary sheath of a verve.

حم اعصاب: سفید۔چربیلا مادہ جو عصب کی میڈلری شید بناتا ہے۔

Myelitis *(mi-e-li- tis)* [G. *myelos,* marrow, *-itis* infla- mmation of the spinal cord.

رم نخاع: ریڑھ کی ہڈی یا نخا کی سوزش۔

Myelocele *(mi-el-o-sel)* [G. *myelos,* marrow *kele,* hernbia] An accompaniment of spin bifida (q.v.) wherein development of th spinal cord itself has been arrested, and th central canal of the cord opens on the ski surface discharging cerebrospinal fluid Incompatible with life.

ق نخاع: نخاع کی تکمیل کا رک جانا۔

Myelocytes *(mi-el-o-sits)* [G. *myelos,* marrow *kytos,* cell] Precusor cells of granulocyti white blood cells normally present only i bone marrow--myelocytic, adj.

غز خلیہ: ہڈی کے مغز کے خلیے سے لیوکوسائیٹس بنتے ہیں۔

Myelofibrosis *(mi-el-o-fi-bro-sis)* Formation c fibrous tissue within the bone marrow cavity Interferes with the formation of blood cells.

ئیلو فائبروسس: استخوانی گودے کے کہفہ کے اندر ریشہ دار نسیج کا بننا۔ نی خلیوں کی بناوٹ میں دخل انداز ہوتا ہے۔

Myelogenous *(mi-el-oj-en-us)* [G. *myetos* marrow; *genesthai,* to be produced] Produce in or by the bone marrow.

اعی معززا: ہڈی کے گودے میں یا سے پیدا ہوتا ہے۔

yelogram *(mi-el-o-gram)* [G. *myelos,* marrow; *grmma,* letter]. Radiograph of spinal canal.

مائیلوگرام: سپائنل قنال کی ریڈیوگراف۔

yelography *(mi-el-og'-ra-fi)* [G. *myelos,* marrow; *graphein,* to write] Radiographic examination of the spinal canal by injection of a contrast medium into the subarachnoid space -- myelographic, adj; myelographcally, adv.

نخاعی تصویر کشی: سپائنل قنال کی ریڈیوگرافی جانچ۔

'eloid *(mi-e-loid)* [G. *myelos,* marrow; *eidos,* form]. Relating to the granulocuyte precursor cells in the bone marrow See LEUKAEMIA.

مغزی۔نخاع نما: گودے سے مشابہ سے متعلق۔

'eloma *(mi-el-o-ma)* [G. *myelos,* marrow; *oma,* tumour] A malignant condition arising from plasma cells, usually in the bone marrow. **multiple m.,**the formation of a number of myeloma tumours in bones -- nnyelomatous, adj.

مغزی سلعہ: ہڈی کے گودے کا ایک اولی ناسور یا رسولی۔

elomatosis *(mi-el-o-ma-to-sis)* Plasma cells neoplasia which can manifest as myeloma tumours in bones, diffuse change throughout the marrow or as extramedullary lesions. May produce changes in serum globulins (q.v.) and moist, Syn, meningomyelocele (q.v.)

شقاق نخاع۔شوکہ مشقوقہ: پتلی شفاف۔شفاف جھلی میں ملفوف۔

elopathy *(mi-el-op-ath-i)* [G. *myelos,* marrow; *pathos,* disease] . Disease of the spinal cord. Can be a serious complication of cervical spondyosis-- myelopathic, adj.

مرض نخاعی: نخاع کا مرض۔

'eran *(mi-ler-an)* Busulphan (q.v.)

مائیلیرین: بسلفان۔

carditis *(mi-o-kar-di-tis)* [G.*mysmuscle; ardia,* heart; *-itis* , inflammation]. Inflammation of the myocardiu.

ورم عضلات قلب: دل کی درمیانی تہہ کی سوزش یا سوج۔

ocardium *(mi-o-kar-di-um)* [G. *mysmuscle; ardia,* heart] The middle layer of the heart wall. See MUSCLE -- myocardia, adj.

Myocardium

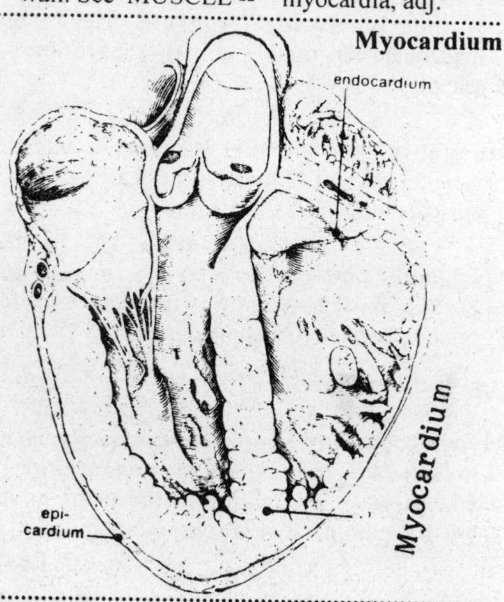

عضلیہ قلب: قلبی دیوار کی درمیانی پرت یا تہ۔

Myocele *(mi-o-sel)* [G. *mys,* muscle; *kele,* tumour]. Protrusion of a muscle through its ruptured sheath.

فتق عضلہ: پھٹے ہوئے غلاف میں سے عضلے کا ابھار۔

Myoclonus *(mi-o-klo-nus)* [G.*mysmuscle; konos,* confused movement] Clonic contractions of individual or groups of muscles.

رجفہ عضلہ: عضلاتی گروہوں یا فرد کے سکڑاؤ۔

Myocrisin *(mi-o-kri-sin)* Aurothiomalate (q.v)

مایوکرائی سین: آروتھیومیلیٹ۔یہ ٹیکہ ہفتے میں ایک بار برائے اکیوٹ ریو مائیڈ آرتھرائی ٹس۔

Myodil *(mi-o-dil)* An oily liquid used as a contrast agent in myelography. Given by intrathecal injec- tion.

مایوڈل: ایک تیلیا مائع۔

Myoelectric: *(mi-o-e-lek-trik)* Pertaining to the electrical properties of muscle.

عضلی برقی: عضلے کی برقی خصوصیات سے متعلق۔

Myofibrosis *(mi-o-fi-bro-sis)* Excessive connective tissue inmuscle. Leads to inadequate functioning of part -- mayofibroses, pl.

مایوفائبروسس: عضلے میں زائد رابطی نسیج۔

Myogenic *(mi-o-jen-ik)* [G. *mys,* muscle; *genesis,* decent] Orginating in, starting from, muscle.

عضلہ زاد۔ انقباض: عضلے سے ابتداء۔

Myolglobin *(m-o-glo-bin)* [G.*mys,* muscle; L. *glubus,* ball] Oxygen transporting muscle protein. Syn., myohaemoglobin.

حمرت العضلہ: آکسیجن لے جانے والی عضلاتی پروٹین۔ ہیموگلوبن کی قسم جو عضلاتی ریشوں میں پائی جاتی ہے۔

Myoglobinuria *(mi-o-glo-bin-u-ri-a)* [G. *mys,* muscle; L. *globus,* ball; G. *ouron,* urine]. Excretion of myoglobin in the urine as in crush syndrome. Syn. myohaemoglobinuria.

مایوگلوبی نیورا: پیشاب میں حمرت العضلہ کا اخراج۔

Myohaemoglobin *(mi-o-hem-o-globing)* A haem- oglobin present in muscle of much lower molecular weight than blood haemoglobing. It is liberated form muscle and appears in the urine in the crush syndrome.

عضلی ہیموگلوبن: عضلے میں موجود ہیموگلوبن جس کا سالمی وزن خونی ہیموگلوبن کے سالمی وزن سے کم ہوتا ہے۔ یہ عضلے سے خارج ہوتی ہے۔ کرش سنڈروم میں پیشاب میں ظاہر ہوتی ہے۔

Myohaemoglobinuria *(mi-o-hem-o-glob-in-ur-i-a)* Myohaemoglobin in the urine. CUSH SYNDRO- ME.

عضلی ہیموگلوبن بولی: پیشاب میں مایوہیموگلوبن۔

Myokymia *(mi-o-ki-mi-a)* [G. *mys,*muscies; *kyma,* wave] Muscle twitching. In the lower eyelid it is benign. **facial m.,** my result from long use of phenothiazine drugs; has aslo been observed in patients with disseminated sclerosis.

مایوکائیمیا: عضلاتی پھڑک یا تشنجی حرکت۔

Myoma *(mi-o-ma)* [G. mys, *muscle,* muscle; *-oma,* tumour]. A tumour of muscle tissue--myomata, pl; myomatous, adj.

سلعہ عضلہ۔ رسولی: عضلاتی نسیج کی رسولی۔

Myomalacia *(mi-o-mal-a-si-a)* [G. *mys,* muscle *malakia,* softness]. Softerning of muscle, a occurs in the myocardium after coronar occlusion.

نت عضلہ قلب: عضلے کی نرمی۔

Myomectomy *(mi-om-ek-to-mi)* [G.*mys* muscle; *-oma,* tumour; *ektome,* excision Enucleation of uterine fibroid(s).

لعہ رحم برادی: یوٹرن فائبرائڈ کا انقاف۔

Myometrium *(mi-o-me-tri-um)* [G. *mys* muscle; *metra,* womb]. The thick muscul wall of the uter- us

Myometriu

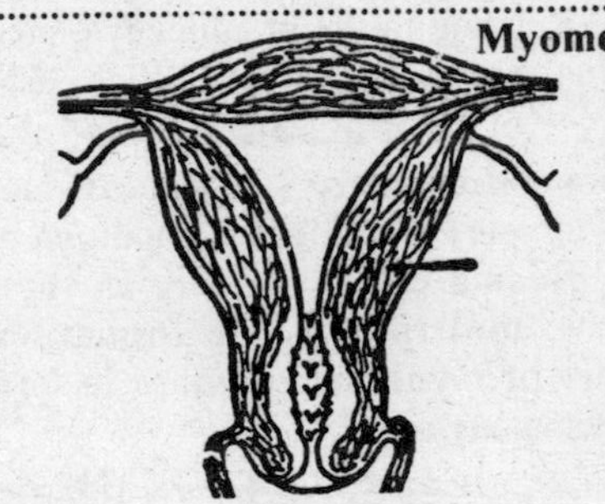

مدہ کا عضلاتی مواد: یوٹرس کی دبیز عضلاتی دیوار۔

Myoneural *(mi-o-nur-al)* [G. *mys,* musc *neuron,* verve]. Pertaining to muscle a nerve.

لی عصبی: عصب اور عضلے سے متعلق۔

Myopathy *(mi-op'-ath-i)* [G. *mys,* musc *pathos,* disease]. Any disease of t muscles--myopathic, adj. See GLYC GENOSIS.

س عضلہ: عضلات کا کوئی مرض۔

Myope *(mi-op)* [G.*myein,* to close; *ops,* eye] shortsighted person -- miopic, adj.

ب بین: نزدیک سے دیکھنے والا شخص۔

Myopia *(mi-o-pi-a)* [G.*myein,* to close; *o* eye]. Shortsightedness. The light rays come a focus in front instead of on, t retina--myopic, adj.

ب بینی۔ قریب نظری: دور کی نگاہ کا کمزور ہونا۔ نگاہ یا نظر کا ایک

نقص۔ اس میں ناظر دور کی اشیاء واضح طور پر نہیں دیکھ سکتا۔ اس نقص کو مقعر عدسوں سے درست کیا جاتا ہے۔

ıyoplasty *(mi-o-plas-ti)* [G. *mys,* muscle; *plassein,* to form]. Plasitc surgery of muscles--myoplastic , adj.

عضلات کا پلاسٹک عملیہ : عضلات کی پلاسٹک سرجری۔

yosarcoam *(mi-o-sar-ko-ma)* [G. *mys,* muscle; *sarkoma,* fleshy, overgrowth]. A malignant tumour derived from muscle--myosarcomata, pl; myosarcomatous, adj.

عضلی لحمی سلعہ : عضلے سے ماخوذ رسولی۔

yosin *(mi-o-sin)* [G. *mys,* muscle]. the main protein of muscle.

عضلین : عضلہ کی عام روٹین۔

yosis *(mi-o-sis)* Excessive contraction of the pupil of the eye. Also **miosis**--myotic, adj.

انقباض حدقہ : آنکھ کی پتلی کا زائد سکڑاؤ۔

yositis *(mi-o-si-tis)* [G. *mys,* muscle; *-itis,* inflammation of a muscle. **myositis ossificans,** deposition of active bone cells in muscle, resulting in hard swellings.

ورم عضلہ: عضلے کی سوزش۔ ایسے افراد جو کھانا زیادہ، بورزش کم، بیٹھنے، پیدل نہ چلنے ٹھنڈے مشروبات کے عادی ہوں یہ مرض انہیں زیادہ ہوتا ہے۔

yotics *(mi-ot-iks)* Drugs which cause myosis (q.v.) Also miotics.

انقباضی ادویات : ادویات جو آنکھ کی پتلی کے زائد سکڑاؤ کا سبب بنتی ہیں۔

yotomy *(mi-ot-om-i)* [G. *mys,* muscle; *tome,* a cutting]. Cutting or dessection of muscle tissue.

عضلہ تراشی : عضلاتی نسیج کی چیر پھاڑ یا اسے کاٹنا۔

yringa *(mi-ring-ga)* [L. *miringa;* G. *menigx,* membrance]. The eardrum or tympanic memb- rance.

طبل گوش : ٹمپینک جھلی یا کان کا پردہ۔

yringitis *(mir-in-ji-tis)* [G. *menigx,* membrance; *-itis,* inflammation]. Inflamm- ation of the eardrum (tympanic membrance).

ورم طبل گوش : کان کے پردے کی سوزش یا سوج

Myringoplasty *(mir-ing-o-plas-ti)* [G.*menigx,* membrance; *plassein,* to form]. This operation is designed to close a defect in the tympanic membrance. Grafts from a suitable vein, perichondrium of the tragus or temporalis fascia, have been used --- myring oplastic, adj.

ترقیع غشائے طبلی : کان کے پردے کے نقص کو ختم کرنے کے لئے اپریشن۔

Myingotome *(mir-ing-ot-om)* [G. *menigx,* mem- brance; *tomos,* a cutting]. A delicate instrument for incising the eardrum (tympanic memebrance)

طبلہ شگاف : کان کے پردے میں شگاف کے لئے ایک نازک آلہ۔

Myringotomy *(mir-ing-ot-o-mi)* [G. *menigx,* membrance; *tome,* a cutting]. Incision into the eardrum (tympanic membrance). Done previously to drain pus from the middle ear. Now donw for aspiration of non-suppurative exudates or transudates of the middle ear cleft. Middle ear ventilation maintained by insertion of teflon tube so that the fluid can drain down narrowed or malfunctioning pharyngotympanic tube; teflon tube removed when pharyngotympanic tube functioning normally.

صماخ شگافی : کان کے پردے میں شگاف۔

Mysoline *(mi-so-len)* Primidone (q.v.)

مائیسولین۔ پریمیڈون۔

Mysteclin F. Tetracycline, a broad spectrum antibiotic combined with an antitungal powder.

مسٹیکلن : ٹیٹراسائیکلین۔ ایک چوڑے طیف والا اینٹی بائیوٹک جو ضد ساروغ سفوف کے ساتھ ملا ہوتا ہے

Myxoedema *(miks-e-de-ma)* [G. *myxa,* mucus; *oidema,* swelling]. Clinical syndrome of hypothyr- oidism. (q.v.). Patient becomes slow in movement and dull mentally; there is bradycardia, low temperature,dry skin and swelling of limbs and face. the BMR (q.v.) is low, and the blood cholesterol is raised. No enlargement of gland as in Hashimoto's disease. preteibial m, unsightly thickening of skin over shins and feet which occurs rarely in patients with hyperthyroidism. Cause unknown; condition presists in spite of antithyroid treatment. **myxoedema coma,** impaired level of consciousness in severe m. Mortality rate of high from hypothermia, heart failure, cardiac arrhythmias or bronchopneumonia --myxoedemtous, adj.

مخاطی چبنل: ہائیپو تھائیرائڈزم کا کلینکل سنڈروم۔ مریض حرکت میں ست ہو جاتا ہے۔ عقل کم ہو جاتی ہے۔ بات چیت آہستگی تھکاوٹ زیادہ' حرکات آہستہ' جلد خشک موٹی و بھدی سی' سردی زیادہ لگنا اور جسم کی حرارت میں کمی ہو جاتی ہے۔ علاج کے لئے تھائی راکین مفید ہے۔

Myxoma *(miks-o-ma)* [G. *myxa,* mucus; *oma,* tumour]. A connective tissue tumour composed largely of mucoid material - myxomata, pl; myxomatous. adj.

سلعہ مخاطی: واصل نسیج کی رسولی جو عموماً میوکائڈ مادہ پر مشتمل ہوتی ہے۔

Myxosarcoma *(miks-o-sar-ko-ma)* [G. *myxa* mucus; *sarkoma,* fleshy overgrowth]. A malignant tumour of connectiv tissue with a soft, mucoid consistence - myxosarcomatous, adj.

سرطان مخاطی: واصل نسیج کی رسولی۔

Myxoviruses *(miks-o-vi-rus)* Name for the influenza group of viruses.

مکسووائرس: ۱۹۵۳ء میں انٹرنیشنل کانگریس آف مائیکروبیالوجی نے یہ نام تجویز کیا۔ وائرس کا انفلوئنزا گروہ۔ یہ میوکیہ خارج کرنے والے نسیج کو متاثر کرتے ہیں۔ اس میں پیراانفلوئنزا وائرس اور عقسی وائرس ہیں۔

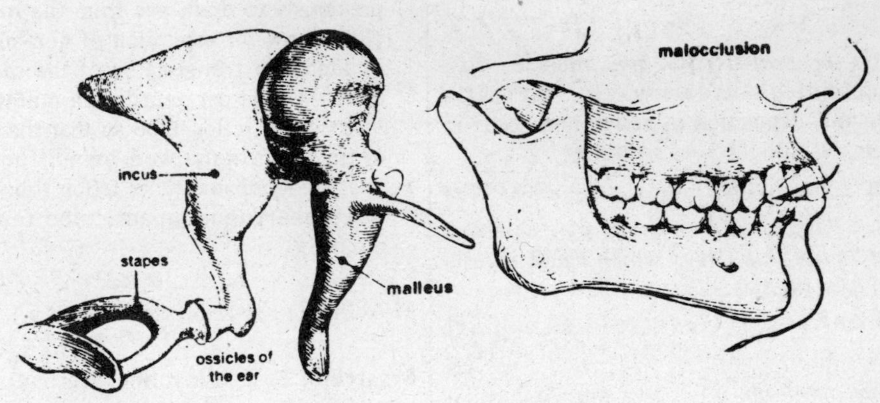

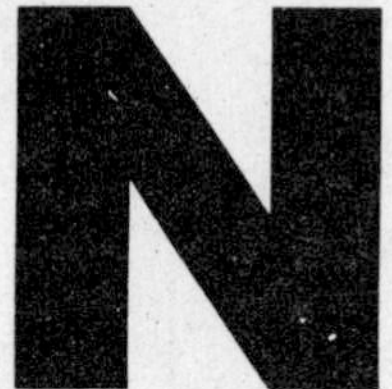

N *(en)* Symbol for neutron, nitrogen, normal, Avogadro's number and population size.

این: علامت ہے نیوٹران کی، نائٹروجن کی، نارمل محلول کی، آیوگاڈرو نمبر اور آبادی کے حجم کی۔

n *(en)* Symbol for nano, refractive index and nerve.

این: علامت ہے نینو، انعطافی معیار اور نرو کا۔

ν *(nu)* The thirteenth letter of the Greek alphabet and symbol for degrees of freedom and frequency.

نیو: یونانی حروف ابجد کا تیرہواں حرف۔ ڈگری آف فریڈم اور فریکوئنسی کی علامت ہے۔

Na Symbol for sodium [L. natrium].

این اے: سوڈیم کی علامت لاطینی لفظ نیٹریم کا مخفف۔

Nabothian follicles (systs galnds) Cystic enlargement of inflamed cervical glands of uterus. Here the duct is blocked by epithelium and normal flow of mucus is distubed.

Nafenopin *(na-fen-o-pin)* An anti-hyperlipidemic drug.

نیفنو پن: چکنائیوں کو کم کرنے والی دوا۔

Nalgele's obliquity In this case the fetal's head slids to one or other side to decrease the transverse diameter, presented to the pelvic brim.

Naevus *(na-vus)* [L. *mole*]. A mole, a lesion of the skin which is well circumscribed. This arises from the pigment producing cells (melanome) or due to developmental abnormality of blood vessels (angiome).

Nail *(na'l)* The horny cutaneous plate onthe dorsal surface of the distal and of a finger or toe. A rod of metal, bone or other natural used for fixation of the ends or the fragments or fractured bone.

ناخن: انگلی یا پاؤں کی انگلی کے اگلے اور اوپر والے سرے پر ایک سخت قسم کی پلیٹ کو کہتے ہیں۔ یا لوہے کی چھوٹی سلاخ جو کہ ٹوٹی ہوئی ہڈی کے سروں کو جوڑنے کیلئے استعمال کی جائے۔

Nailing *(na'l-ing)* The operation of fixing or fastening of a fractured long bone by insertion of a steel rod into the marrow cavity of the bone.

کیل سے جوڑنا: عمل جراحت کے ذریعے ٹوٹی ہوئی ہڈی کے لمبے سروں کے درمیان گودے والی جگہ پر سٹیل کی سلاخ لگا کر ہڈی کو جوڑنا۔

Nalidixic Acid *(nal-i-dik-sik a'sid)* A synthetic antibacterial agent used orally in the treatment of uriinary infections caused by gram-negative like proteus species.

Nalorphime *(na'l-or-fen)* A drug structurally related to morphine which acts as an antagonist to morphine and related narcotics. It counteracts respiratory depression due to nacotic overdosage, administered intravenously.

Name *(na'm)* A word or words used to designate a unique entity and distinguish it from other.

نام: ایک لفظ یا الفاظ جو کسی خاص چیز کو دیا جائے اور اس چیز کو دوسری چیزوں سے علیحدہ کرے۔

Napkin rash An erythema of the napkin area. Usual cause is ammoniacal of urine.

پیش گر چکتے: چھوٹے بچوں میں پیشاب کرنے کی وجہ سے نیپکن ایریا پر

نشان پڑ جاتا ہے جوعموماً پیشاب کی امونیاتی بوسیدگی کی وجہ سے ہوتا ہے۔

Naproxyn *(nap-ro-sin)*. Naproxen (q.v.)

Naproxen *(nap-roks-en)* Relieves pain, reduces infl- ammation and eases joint stiffness without causing gastric bleeding.

Narcissism *(nar-sis-izm)* [G. *narkissos*, a beautiful youth who fell in love with his own reflection]. Self-love. In psychiatry the narcissistic type of personality is one where the sexual love-object is the self.

نرگسیت: اپنے آپ سے محبت۔ ایک نفسیاتی بیماری جس میں انسان اپنی ہی خوبصورت شخصیت سے محبت کرتا ہے۔

Narcoanalysis *(nar-ko-an-al-i-sis)* [.G. *narco*, stupor; *analysis*, a loosening]. Analysis of mental content under light anaethesia, usually an intravenous barbiturate -- narcoanalytic, ajd; narcoanalytically, adv.

تحلیل خدری: خواب کی حالت طاری کر کے مریض کے ذہنی اجزاء کا معائنہ۔

Narcolepsy *(nar-ko-lep-si)* [G. *narco*, stupor; *lepsis*, a seizing]. An irresistible tendency to go to sleep. It is more usual to speak of the narcolepsies rather than of narcolepsy, for sudden, repetitive attacks of sleep occurring inthe day time arise in diverse clinical conditions -- narcoleptic, adj.

نومیت: نیند کا زبردست رجحان۔

Narcosis *(nar-ko-sis)* [G. *narco*, stupor]. Unconsciousness produced by a drug. **basal n,.** a state of unconsciousness produced by drugs prior to an anaesthetic or operation.l The drugs most commonly used for this purpose were avertin, paraldehyde or a barbiturate. Not so widely used as formerly. **carbon dioxide n,.** full bounding pusle, muscular twitchings. mental confusion and eventuatl coma due to increased CO_2 in the blood. **continuous n.,** treatment by prolonged sleep by spaced administration of narcotics. Introdued by Woolf in 1901. Used occasionally in mental illness to cut short attack of excitement or for severe emotional upset.

بے ہوشی: دوائی سے پیدا ہونے والی بے ہوشی جو کسی دوائی کے اثر سے ہو سکتی ہے۔ بنیادی بے ہوشی کے لئے کسی اپریشن سے پہلے بے ہوش کیا جاتا ہے۔ خون میں کاربن ڈائی آکسائیڈ کی زیادتی کی وجہ سے بے ہوشی طاری ہو جاتی ہے۔ یا مسلسل بے ہوش رکھا جاتا ہے جیسا کہ دماغی امراض کے علاج میں کیا جا سکتا ہے۔

Narcosynthesis *(nar-ko-sin-the-sis)* [G.*narc* stupor; *synthesis*, putting together]. Th building up of a clearer mental picture of a incident involving the patient by revivir memories of it. under light anaesthesia, s that both he and the therapist can examine t incident clearer perspective.

...لیف خدری: مریض کو ہلکا نشا دے کر گذشتہ واقعات یاد دلائے جاتے ... تا کہ اس کے ذہن میں صاف تصویر آ جائے۔ اس طرح مریض اور معالج ...علاج کے لئے کافی مدد ملتی ہے۔

Narcotherapy *(nar-ko-ther-a-pi)* See NAR OSIS.

...کوتھراپی: دوائی سے پیدا شدہ بے ہوشی۔

Narcotic *(nar-kot-ik)* [G.*narkotikos*, narcotic]. drug which produces abnormally deep sleep.

...اب آور: ایسی دوائی جو غیر معمولی طور پر گہری نیند پیدا کرے۔

Nardil Penelzine. (q.v.)

...ڈل فینلزین:

Nares *(nar-ez-)* [L.] The nostrils **anterior n.,** t pair of epenings from the exterior into t nasal cavities. **posterior n,.** cavities into t nasopharynx Syn. choanae -- naris, sing.

...نے: ناک کے سوراخ۔

Narphen *(nar-fen)* Phenazocine (q.v.)

...ین: فنازوسین۔

Nasal *(na-zal)* [L. *nasus*, nose] Pertaining to t nose.

...: ناک سے متعلق۔ ناک کی ہڈیاں دو ہوتی ہیں اور ناک کا بالائی حصہ بناتی ...۔ باقی ناک کرکری ہڈی کی بنی ہوتی ہے۔ ان ہڈیوں سے ناک کا ابھار بنتا ...

Naseptin *(na-sep-tin)* Cream containi

chlorhexidine hydrochloride 0.1 per cent and neomycin sulphate 0.5 per cent for nasal carries of staphylococci.

نیسیپٹن: ۱ء فیصد کلورا ہکسیڈین ہائیڈروکلورائڈ اور ۵ء فیصد۔ نیو مائیسین سلفیٹ پر مشتمل کریم۔

Nasogastric *(na-so-gas-trik)* [L. *nasus.* nose; G. *gast er,* belly] Pertaining to the nose and stomach, as passing a n. **tube** via this route usually for suction, lavage or feeding.

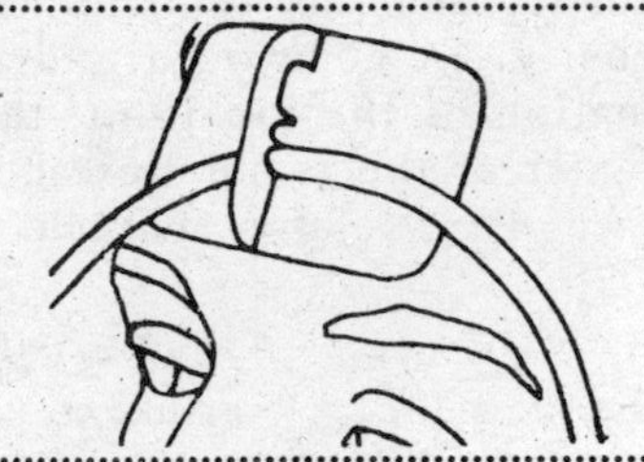

Disposable nasogastric tube holding device

نیزوگیسٹرک: ناک اور معدہ سے متعلق۔

Nasolacrimal *(na-zo-lak-ri-ma)* [L. *nasus,* nose; *lacrime,* tear] Pertaining to the nose an lacrimal apparatus.

انفی دمعی: ناک اور لیکریمل اپریٹس کے متعلق۔

Naso-oesopageal *(na-zo-es-of-a-je-al)* [L. *nasus,* nose; G. *oisophagos,* gullet].

انفی مریوی: ناک اور ایسوفیگس سے متعلق۔

Nasopharyngitis *(na-zo-far-in-ji-tis)* [L. *nasus,* nose; G. *pharygx,* pahrynx; *itis,* inflammation]. Inflammation of the nasopharynx.

ورم خلق انفی: نیزوفیرنکس کی سوزش۔

Nasopharyngoscope *(na-zo-far-in-go-skop)* [L. *nasus,* nose; G. *pharygx,* pharyns; *skopein,* to examine]. An endoscope for viewing the nasal pasendoscope for viewing the nasal passages and postnasal space nasopharygoscopic, adj.

نیزوفیرنگوسکوپ: نتھنے اور پچھلی جگہیں دیکھنے کے لئے اینڈوسکوپ۔

Nasopharynx *(na-zor-far-inks)* [L. *nasus,* nose; G. *pharygx,* pharynx]. The portion of the pharynx above the soft palate nasopharyngeal, adj.

خلق انفی: نرم پیلیٹ کے اوپر فلیرنکس کا حصہ۔

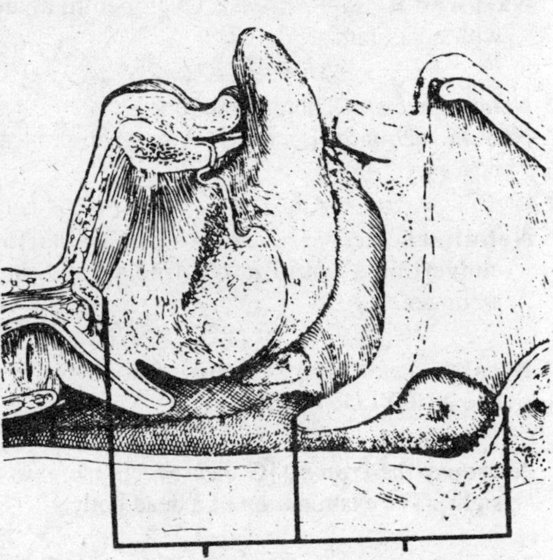

Oropharynx Nasopharynx

Oropharynx Nasopharynx

Nasosinusitis *(na-zo-si-nus-i-tis)* [L. *nasus,* nose; *sinus,* curve; G. *-itis* , inflammation]. Inflammation of the nose and adjacent sinuses.

التہاب حضرۃ الانف: ناک اور ملحقہ خانوں کی سوزش۔

Natulan *(nat-u-lan)* Procarbazine (q.v.)

نیٹولان: پروکاربازین۔

Nausea *(naw-se-a)* [G. *nausia,* sea-sickness]. A feeling of sickness without actual vomiting - neauseate, v.t. , v.i.

متلی: اصل قے کئے بغیر بیماری کا احساس۔ جی متلانا۔

Navane *(na-van)* Thiothixine (q.v.)

نیوین: تھیوتھکسین۔

Navel *(na-vl)* The umbilicus.

ناف: امبیلیکس۔

Navicular *(nav-ik-u-lar)* [L. *navicula,* smal boat]. Shaped like a canoe. The scaphoid bone of the tarsus and carpus.

عظم زوتی: کشتی نما۔ کارپس اور ٹارسس کی سکیفائڈ ہڈی۔ ٹخنے اور کلائی میں کشتی نما ہڈی۔

Navidrex *(nav-i-dreks)* Cyclopenthiazide.

نیویڈریکس : سائیکلوپنتھیازائڈ۔

Navidrex-K *(nav'-i-dreks).* Cyclopenthi azide with potassium.

نیویڈریکس ک: پوٹاشیم کے ساتھ سائیکلوپنتھیازائڈ۔

Nebcin *(neb-sin)* Tobramycin (q.v.)

Nebula *(neb-u-la)* [L. *mist)* A greyish, corneal opac- ity.

پھورا: کورنیا کی غیر شفافی۔آنکھ پر بھورے رنگ کا جالا آ جانا۔

Nebulizer *(neb-ul-iz-er)* An apparatus for converting a liquid into a fine spray.Syn,. atomizer.

عرق باش: مائع کو عمدہ سپرے میں تبدیل کرنے کا آلہ۔

Necator *(nek-at-or)* A genus of hook worms. See ANCYLOSTOMA.

نکیٹر: ہک ورمز کا ایک جنس۔

Necropsy *(ne-krop-si)* [G. *nekros,* corpse; *opsis,* sight]. The examination of a dead body.

لاش بینی۔معائنہ لاش: لاش کا معائنہ۔

Necrosis *(ne-kro-sis)* [G. mortification]. Localized death of tissue -- necrotic,adj.

نخیرہ: نسیج کی مقامی موت۔نسیج کا مردہ ہوجانا یا ناکارہ ہوجانا۔

Needling *(ned-ling)* Puncturing with a needle, especially of lens capsule to allow entry of quenous humor which wil absorb the lens or remnants thereof. Discission.

گودنا۔تابیر: سوئی ساتھ پنکچر کرنا۔سوتی سے سوراخ کرنے کا عمل۔

Nefrolan *(nef-ro-lan)* Clorexolone (q.v.)

نفرولان: کلطوریکسولون۔

Negativism *(neg-at-iv-izm)* [L. *negativus,* negative]. Active refusal to cooperate, ususally shown by the patient consistently doing the exact opposite of what he is asked. Common in schizophrenia.

منکریت: تعاون سے انکار مریض کو جو کچھ کرنے کو کہا جائے اس کو الٹ کرتا ہے۔شائزوفرینیا میں ایسا کثرت سے ہوتا ہے۔عدم تعاون علاج کے بارے میں مریض کا منفی رویہ۔

Negram *(na-gram)* Nalidixic-cid.

نیگریم: نالیڈکسک ایڈ۔

Neisseria. A genus of bacteria, Gramnegative diplicocci which are found as commensals man and animals, e.g. *Neisseria catarrha.* some are pathogenic to man. *Neisser genorrhoeae* causes gonorrhoea and *meninggitidis* causes men- ingitis.

ئے سیریا: جراثیم کا ایک جنس گرام منفی ڈپلوما کاکسی۔انسانی جسم میں ش پاتے ہیں نائے سیریا گانوریا جراثیم سوزک کا سبب ہیں اور چھوت ع کرنے لگتی ہے۔

Nelaton's line. An imaginary line joining anterior superior illac spine to the isch tuberosity. In coxa vara and upwa dislocation of the hip joint, the gre trochanter of the femur lies above t line.[Auguste Nelaton. French surge 1807-73]

۔نیلاٹون: ایک فرضی خط۔

Nematodes *(ne-ma-todz)* Wormlike creatures t have two sexes and an intesinal canal. Vari species are parasitic tc man and can be divi into two groups; (1) those that mainly live in intestine, e.g. hookworms and whipworms; those that are mainly tissue para- sites, e.g. gui worms, filarial worms.

ے: ورم ایسی مخلوق۔ان کی کئی انواع انسان پر طفیلی ہیں۔ان کی دو اقسام ۔(۱) جو آنت میں رہتے ہیں۔مثلاً ہک ورم اور وہپ ورم۔(۲) جو نسیج فیلی ہیں۔مثلاً گنی ورم۔فلیریل ورم۔

Nembutal *(nem-bu-tal)* Pentobarbitone (q.v.)

بیوٹل: پینٹوباربیٹون۔باربیچوریٹ خواب آور دوا۔

Neoarsphenamine *(ne-o-ars-fen-a-men)* organic arsenic compound, and one of t first chemotherapeutic drugs. Once wid used in the treatment of syphilis intravenous injection. Occasionally used Vincent's angina as a five per cent paint.

رسیفامین: ایک نامیاتی آرسینک مرکب۔

Neoathrosis *(ne-o-ar-thro-sis)* [G. *neos,* ne *arth- rosis* articulation]. Abnorm articulation; a false joint as at the site o fracture.

مل جدید۔نیا جوڑ: غیر معمولی آرٹیکولیشن۔

Neo-Cytamen *(ne-o-sit-a-men)* Hydroxc

obalamin (q.v.)

نیوسیٹامین: ہائیڈروکسوکوبلامن۔

Neo-epinine *(ne-o-ep-in-nen)* Tablets and spray solutions containing isopernaline (q.v.)

نیو اپی نین: آئیسو پرنیالین پر مشتمل گولیاں اور سپرے محلول۔ دمہ میں حسب ضرورت ایک گولی زبان کے نیچے رکھئے۔

Neologism *(ne-lo-oj-izm)* [G. *neos,* new; *logos,* discourse] A specially coined word, often nonsensical, may express a thought disorder.

الفاظ سازی: خیالی گڑبڑ۔

Neo-Mercazole Carbimazole (q.v.)

نیومرکازول: کاربیمزول۔ مفید برائے مرض ہائپر تھائیڈ ازم یعنی زہریلا گلہڑ۔

Neomin *(ne-o-min)* Streptomycin and neomycin.

نیومن: سٹریٹومائی سین اور نیومائی سین۔

Neomycin *(ne-o-mi-sin)* An antibiotic frequently used with corticosteoids in the treatment of inflamed andx infected skin conditions. Sometimes given orally for intestinal infections. See FRAMYCETIN SULPHATE.

نیومائی سن: اینٹی بایوٹک جو متاثرہ جلد کے لئے مستعمل ہے۔ بعض دفعہ آنت کی بیماریوں کے لئے منہ کے ذریعہ کھائی جاتی ہے۔ کیوٹسن دست روکنے کے لئے نیومائی سین سسپنشن چھوٹے بچوں کو ایک چمچہ دن میں چار مرتبہ پلائیے۔

Neo Naclex *(ne-o-na-kleks)* Bendroflyazide (q.v.)

نیونکلیکس: بنڈرو' فلوایزائڈ' ہائپر ٹنشن یا بلڈ پریشر میں اس کی ایک گولی روزانہ ناشتے کے بعد۔

Neonatal period *(ne-o-na-tal)* The first month of life in a baby. **neonatal mortality,** the death-rate of babies in th first month of life.

عرصہ نوخیز: بچے میں زندگی کا پہلا ماہ۔

Neonate *(ne-o-nat)* [L. *natus,* birth]. A newborn baby up to one month old.

نومولود: نوزائیدہ بچہ جس کی عمر ایک ماہ تک ہو۔

Neonatology *(ne-o-nati-ol-o-ji)* [G. *neos,* new; L. *natus,* birth; G. *logos,* discourse]. The scientific study of the new born.

Neonatorum *(ne-o-nat-or-um)* [G. *neos,* new; L. *natus,* birth]. Pertaining to the newborn.

نیونیٹوریم: نوزائیدہ بچے سے متعلق۔

Neoplasia *(ne-o-pla-zi-a)* [G. *neos,* new; *plassein,* to form]. Literally the formation of new tissue. By custom refers to the pathological process in tumour formation -- neoplastic, adj.

ورم۔ تسکون نسیج جدید: نئے نسیج کا بننا۔ رسولی بننا۔

Neoplasm *(ne-o-plazm)* [G. *neos,* new; *plasma,* form] A new growth; a tumour -- neoplastic, adj.

نو مایہ: نیا اگاؤ۔ رسولی۔ غیر معمولی بافت کا نیا اگاؤ یا نمو۔

Neoporin *(ne-o-spor-in)* Ophthalimic drops cont- aining polymixin, neomycin and grqamicidin.

Neostigmine *(ne-os-tig-men)* Synthetic compund used in myasthenia gravis; as a curarine antagonist, and in postoperative intestinal aotny. Given orally and by injection. Can cause excess bronchial sec- retion.

نیوسٹگمین: ایک تالیفی مرکب۔ پروسٹگمین۔ اختلاج القلب نوبتی میں اس کی ایک ایک گولی صبح' دوپہر' شام۔ یہی خوراک برائے انلار جڈ پراسٹی یعنی پیشاب رکنا' شدید عضلاتی کمزوری یا میاس تھنیا گریوس۔

Teothyt (ne-o-thil). An inhalation anaesthetic similar to ether.

نیوتھل: ایتھر سے مشابہ سانس کے ذریعے اندر جا کر سن کرنے والی دوا

Nepenthe (ne-pen-thel) an opium preparation resembling tincture of opium.

غم غلط دوا: افیم کی ٹنکچر سے مشابہ افیم

Nephralgia (nef-ral-ji-a) [G nephros, kidney. aigos, pain] Pain in the kidney. See Dietle's crists.

درد گردہ: گردے میں درد

Nephrectomy (nef-red-to-mi) [G. nephros, kidney, ektome, excision]. Removal of kidney.

گرد براری: گردے کا ہٹاؤ۔ گردہ نکالنا کا اپریشن۔

Nephril *(nef-ril)* Polythiazide. See CHLORO-THIAZIDE.

نفرل: پولی تھیازائیڈ۔

Nephritis *(nef-ri-tis)* [G. *nephros,* kidney; *-itis,* inflammation]. A term embracing a group of conditions in or an inflammatory-like reactioin,m focal or diffuse, in the kidneys. **acute glomerulo n,.**Syn. acute n. Bright's disease, Type 1 n. A diffuse inflammatory reaction of both kidneys, usually following a streptococcal infection, and classically manifest by puffiness of the face and scanty blood-stained urine. **chronic n.** syn,. Type III n. A chronic condition, sometimes the sequel to Type 1 or Type II n. in which there is a widespread fibrous replacement of functioning kidney tissue, resulting in progressive renal failure and an arterial hypertension and terminating ultimately in death. **nephrotic n.** syn,. Type II n. A chronic condition of unknown cause characterized by massive oedema and heavy proteinuria. See NEPHROTIC SYNDROME -- nephritic, adj.

ورم گردہ: گردے میں سوزش کی علامت۔

Nephrocalcinosis *(nef-ro-kal-sin-o-sis)* [G. *nephros,* kidney; L. *calx,* lime; *G. -osis,* condition] Multiple areas of calcification within the kidney substance.

نفروکیلسی نوسس: گردے کے مادے کے اندر بہت سے کلسی علاقے۔

Nephrocapsulectomy *(nef-ro-kap-sul-ek-to-mi)* [G. *nephros,* kidney; L. *capsula,* small box; G. *edtome,*excision] Surgical removal of the kidney capsule. Usually done for chronic nephritis.

کلاہ گردہ کا اخراج: گردے کے کیپول کا سرجیکل ہٹاؤ۔ عموماً گردے کی پرانی سوزش میں ایسا کیا جاتا ہے۔

Nephrogenic *(nef-ro-jen-ik)* [G. *nephros,* kidney; *gignesthai,* to be produced]. Arising in or produced by the kidney.

کلوی الاصل: گردے میں یا گردے سے پیدا ہونا۔

Nephrogram *(nef-ro-gram)* [G. *nephros,* kidney; *gramma,* letter]. Renogram (q.v.)

نیفروگرام: رینوگرام۔

Nephrolithiasis *(nef-ro-lith-i-a-sis)* [G.*nephros,*kid- ney; *lithos,* stone; N.L. *-iasis,* condition]. The pres- ence of stones in the kidney.

پتھری: گردے میں پتھریوں کی موجودگی۔

Nephrolithotomy *(nef-ro-lith-ot-o-mi)* [G. *nep-hros,* kidney; *lithos,* stone; *tome,* a cutting]. Removal of a stone from the kidney by a incision through the kidney substance.

یہ شگافی: گردے کے مادے میں سے شگاف کے ذریعے گردے سے
ری نکالنا۔

Nephrology *(nef-rol-o-ji)* [G. *nephros,* kidne *logos,* discourse]. Special study of th kidney's and the disease which afflict them.

گروہ: گردوں اوران کی بیماریوں کامخصوص مطالعہ۔

Nephron *(nef-ron)* [G. *nephros,* kidney]. Th basic unit of the kidney, comprising glomerulus, Bow- man's capsule, proxim and distal convoluted tubules, with loop Henle connecting them; a straight collecti tubule follows via which urine is conveyed the renal pelvis.

رجہ گروہ: گردے کی بنیادی اکائی۔ یہ پیشاب کو اکٹھا کرتے ہیں اوراسے
نے کی طرف بھیجتے ہیں۔

Nephropathy *(nef-ro-path-i)* [G. *nephro* kidney; *pathos,* disease]. Kidney disease nephropathic, adj.

ض گردہ: گردے کامرض۔

Nephropexy *(nef'-ro-path-i)* [G. *nephro* kidney; *pexis,* a fixing]. Surgical fixation of floating kidney.

بیت گردہ: تیرتے گردے کی سرجیکل فیکشن۔

Nephropexy *(nef-ro-peks-i)* [G. *nephro* kidney; plassein, to form]. Any plast operation on the kidney, especially for larg aberrant renal vessels that are dissected o the urinary tract and the kidney flode laterally upon itself. See HYDRONE PHROSIS.

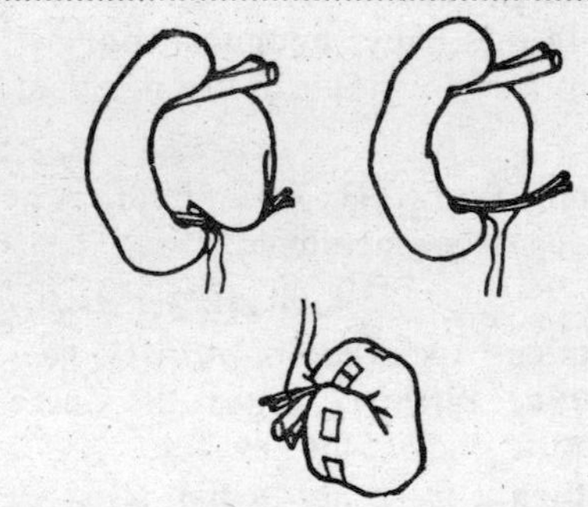

Hamilton-Stewart nephroplasty

نیفرو پلاسٹی: گردے پر کوئی پلاسٹک اپریشن۔

Nephroptosis *(nef-rop-to-sis)* [G. *nephros,* kidney, *ptosis,* a falling]. Downward displacement of the kidney.

سقوط گردہ: گردے کا نچلی طرف جھکاؤ۔

Nephropyosis *(nef-ro-skler-o-sis)* [G. *nephros,* kid- ney; *pyon,* pus; *-osis,* condition]. Pus formation in the kidney.

تقیح کلیہ: گردے میں پیپ کا بننا۔

Nephrosclerosis *(nef-ro-skler-o-sis)* [G. *nephros,* kidney; *slkerosis,* a hardening]. Renal insufficiency from hypertensive vascular disease, developing into picture identical with that of chronic nephritis -- nephrosclerotic adj.

صلابت گردہ: گردوں کی سوزش سے مشابہ مرض۔

Nephrosis *(nef-ro-sis)* [G. *nephros,* kidney, *-osis,* condition.].Any degenerative, non-inflammatory change in the kidney -- nephrotic, adj.

انحطاط گردہ: گردے میں کوئی تخریبی، غیر سوزشی تبدیلی۔

Nephrostomy *(nef-ros-to-mi)* [G.*nephros,* kidney; *stoma,* mouth]. A surgically established fistula from the pelvis of the kidney to the body surface.

کلوی تفویہ: گردے کے پیڈو سے جسمانی سطح کی طرف اپریشن سے فسٹولا بنانا۔

Nephrotic syndrome Used as synonym for type II nephritis (q.v.) Characteristics reduction in blood plasma albumen. albuminuria and oedema, usually with hyperlipaemia. May occur in other condition such as amyloid disease and glomerulosclerosis. (q.v.) of duabetes.

کلوی سنڈروم: گردے کی سوزش سے متعلق۔ خونی پلازما البومن میں تخفیف ہو جاتی ہے۔

Nephrotomy *(nef-rot-o-mi)* [G. *nephros,* kidney; *tomos,* a cutting]. An incision into the kidney sub- stance.

گردہ شگافی: گردے کے مادے میں شگاف۔

Nephrotoxic *(nef-ro-toks-ik)* [G. *nephros,* kidney; *toxikon,* poison]. Any susbtance which inhibits or prevents the functions of kidney cells, or causes their destruction -- nephrotoxin, n.

Nephroureterectomy *(nef-ro-ur-et-er-ek-to-mi)* [G.*nephros,* kidney; *oureter* ureter; *edtome,* exci- ssion].Removal of the kidney along with a part or the whole of the ureter.

قطع کلیہ وحالب: مکمل مثانے یا اس کے ایک حصے کے ساتھ عمل جراحت کے ذریعے گردے کا اخراج۔

Nerve an elongated bundle of fibres which serves for the transmission of impulses between the periphery and the verve centres. **afferent n.** one conveying impulses from the tissues to the n. centres; also known as receptor and sensory nerves. **efferent n.,** one which conveys inpulses outwards fron the n. centres; also known as 'effector' 'motor' 'secretory' 'trophci' ' vasoconstrictor' vasodilator' etc. accoding to function and location. See GANGLION NEURONE, PLEXUS.

عصب: ریشوں کا ایک طویل بنڈل جو عصبی مراکز اور اطراف کے درمیان پیغامات کی ترسیل کرتا ہے۔ نروفاسیرز یا عصبی ریشے ایک تنہا عصب میں تقریباً بارہ لاکھ ہوتے ہیں۔

Nervous *(ner-vus)* 1. Relating to nerves or nerve tissue. 2. Referring to a state of restlessness or timidity. **nervous system,** the structures controlling the actions and functions of the body; it comprises the brain and spinal cord and their nerv- es, and the ganglia fibres forming the autonomic system.

عصبی۔ اعصابی: (۱) اعصاب یا عصبی نسیج سے متعلق۔ (۲) بزدلی یا بے آرامی کی حالت۔

Nethaprin Dospan *(neth-a-prin-dos-pan)* Bronchial relaxant useful in asthma. Available as syrup, which is particullary useful for elderly patients.

نیتھپرن ڈوسپین: سانس کی نالی کے لئے آرام دہ۔ دمہ میں مفید۔ شربت کی صورت میں دستیاب جو عمر رسیدہ مریضوں کے لئے بالخصوص مفید ہے۔

Nettlerash *(net-tl)* Popular term to describe urticaria; weals of the skin.

پتی۔ شری: پتی اچھلنا۔ چھپا کی۔ جلدی امراض۔

Neulactil *(nu-lak-til)* Pericyazine (q.v.)

نیولیکٹل: پیری سیازین۔

Neural *(nur-al)* [G. *neuron* nerve] Pertaining to ner- ves.

عصبی ۔اعصابی: اعصاب سے متعلق۔ نیورل آرچ مہروں کے درمیان سوراخ بناتی ہے۔

Neuralgia *(nu-ral-ji-a)* [G. *neuron* nerve; *algos,* pain] Pain in the distribution of a nerve---neuralgic , adj.

درداعصاب: عصب کی شاخ میں درد۔

Neurapraxia *(nu-ra-praks-i-a)* [G.*neuron,* nerve; *apraxia,* nonaction]. Temporary loss of function in peripheral nerve fibres. Most commonly due to crushing or prolonged pressure. See AXONO- TMESIS.

نیوریپریکسا: جانبی عصبی ریشوں میں عمل کا عارضی ضیاع۔

Neurasthenia *(nu-ras-the-ni-a)* [G. *neuron* nerve; *asthenia,* weakness]. frequently misused term, the precise meaning of which is an uncommon nervous condition consisting of lassitude, interia, fatigue and loss of initiative. Restless fidgeting, over-sensitivity, undue irritability and often an asthenic physiaque are also present -- neurashenic, adj.

ضعف اعصاب: اصلاح جسے غلط طور پر استعمال کیا جاتا ہے۔ جموٗد' بھوک ہونا اور کارکردگی کا ضیاع۔ حساسیت میں اضافہ۔

Neurectomy *(nu-rek-to-mi)* [G. *neuron,* nerve; *ektome,* excision] Excision of part of a nerve.

عصب براری: عصب کے حصے کا اخراج۔

Neurilemma *(nur-i-lem-a)* [G.*neuron,* nerve; *lemma,* sheath]. The thin membranous outer covering of a nerve fibre surrounding the myelin sheath.

عصبی خلاف: مائیلن شید کے گرد عصبی ریشے کا پتلا جھلی دار بیرونی غلاف۔

Neuritis *(nu-ri-tis)* [G.*neuron,* nerve; *-itis.* inflammation]. Inflammation of a nerve -- neuritic, adj.

ورم عصب: عصب کی سوزش یا سوج۔ عموماً وٹامن ب کی کمی کی وجہ سے ہوتا ہے۔ کثرت تمباکونوشی یا شراب سے بھی یہ مرض ہوسکتا ہے۔ عصبی تار میں درد اور جلن، بعض اوقات بعض حصے سن ہوجاتے ہیں۔

Neuroblast *(nur-o-blast)* [G.*neuron,* nerve; *blastos,* germ]. A primitive nerve cell.

[...]بی نہوض: اولی عصبی خلیہ۔

Neuroblastoma *(nu-ro-blas-to-mia)* [G. *neuro[...]* nerve; *blastos,* germ; *-oma,* tumou[...] Malignant tunour arising in adrenal medu[...] from tissue of sympathetic origin. Most cas[...] show a raised urinary catecholamine excreti[...] -- neuroblastomata pl; neuroblastomatous, a[...]

[...]بی سلعہ: ایڈرینل میڈلا میں بننے والی رسولی۔

Neurodermatitis *(nu-ro-der-ma-ti-tis)* [G.*ne[...] ron,* nerve; *derma,* skin; *-itis,* infla- mmatio[...] Lichen simplex (q.v.) Leathy, thicken[...] patches of skin secondary to pruritus a[...] scraching. As the skin thickness, irritati[...] increases, scratching causes furth[...] thickening and so a vicious circle as set u[...] The appearance of the patch develo[...] characteristically as a thickened she[...] dissected into small, shiny, flattopp[...] papules.

[...]روڈرمیٹی ٹس: لائیکن سمپلکن ۔کھال کے چمڑے دار' دبیز ٹکڑے۔ کھال [...]دبازت سے سوزش بڑھتی ہے۔

Neurofibroma *(nu-ro-fi-bro-ma)* [G.*neuro[...]* nerve; L. *fibra,* fibre; G. *oma,* tumour] tumour arising from the connective tissue nerves. A generalized form of neurofib[...] omatosis (Recklinghausen's disease) recognized: multiple tumours occur in t[...] skin but may also be associated with visce[...] branches of the sympathetic nervous syetem neuroribromata, pl; neurofibromatous, adj.

[...]م عصبی لیفی: اعصاب کے واصل نسیج سے بننے والی رسولی۔

Neurogenic *(nu-ro-jen-ik)* [G. *neuron,* nerv[...] *gisnesthai,* to be formed]. Originating with[...] or forming nervous tissue. **neurogen[...] bladder,** See BLADDER.

[...]وجینک: عصبی نسیج بنانا۔

Neuroglia *(nu-rog-li-a)* [G. *neuron,* nerve; *gl[...]* glue]. The supporting tissue of the brain a[...] cord - neuroglial,.adj.

[...]ی سریش: دماغ اور نخاع کو سہارا دینے والا نسیج۔

Neuroleptanalgesia *(nur-ro-lept-an-al-je-zi-*

[G. *neuron,* nerve; *lepsis,* sezing; *a,* not; *algos,* pain]. Anaesthetic technique in which the major agents are neuroleptic and an analgesic drug, allowing patient to retain ability to co-operate.

نیورو پیسٹنل جیسیا: سن کرنے کے طریقہ۔

uroleptics *(nu-ro-lep-tiks)* [G. *neuron,* nerve; *lepsis,* seizing]. Drugs acting on the nervouos system. Includes the major antipshychotic tranquillizers.

نیورو لیپ ٹکس: اعصابی نظام کو متاثر کرنے والی ادویات۔

urologist *(nu-rol-o-jist)* [G.*neuron.* nerve; *logos,* word]. 'A specialist in neurology.

عصبیات دان: نیورولوجی میں ماہر۔

urology *(nu-rol-o-ji)* The sceince and study of nerves their structure, function and pathology; the branch of medicine dealing with diseases of the nervous system-neurological, adj.

عصبیات: اعصاب کا مطالعہ یا اعصاب کی سائنس عصبی نظام کے امراض کی ادویات کی شاخ۔

uromuscular *(nu-ro-mus-kul-er)* [G.*neuron,* nerve; L. *musculus,* muscle]. Pertaining to nerves and muscles.

عصبی عضلی: اعصاب وعضلات سے متعلق۔

uron (e) *(nu-ron)* [G. *nureon,* nerve]. The struct- ural unit of the nervous system comprising fibres (dendrites) which convey impulses to the nerve cell; the nerve cell itself, and the fibres (axons) which convey impulses from the cell. **lower motor n.** the cell is in the spinal cord and the axon passes to skeletal muscle. **upper motor n.,** the cell is in the cerebral cortex and the axon passes down the spinal cord to arborize with a lower motor n. -- neuroanl , neural, adj.

عصبانیہ: حیاتیاتی خلیہ کی ایک مخصوص قسم جو اعصابی نظام کی اکائی ہے۔ یہ ایک مرکزہ پر مشتمل ہوتا ہے۔ جس کے گرد سائیٹو پلازم ہوتا ہے جہاں سے دھاگے کے ایسے ریشے نکلتے ہیں۔ اکثر عصبانیوں میں تحریکوں کو کئی چھوٹے ریشے وصول کرتے ہیں۔ جنہیں ڈینڈرائیٹس کہتے ہیں اور خلیے سے ایک طویل ریشہ ایکسون واپس لے جاتا ہے۔

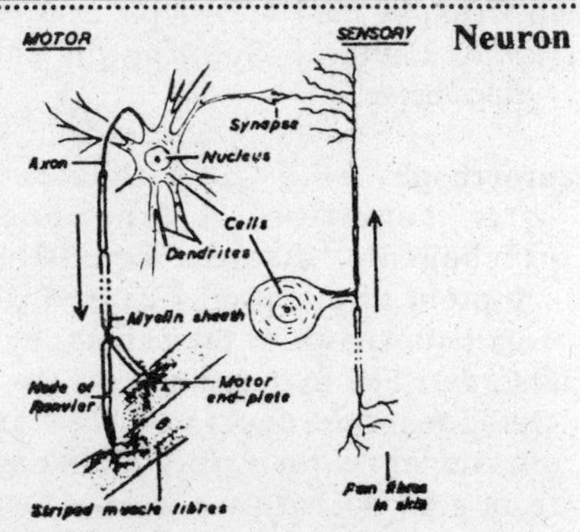

Neuropathic *(nur-ro-path)* [G.*neuron,* nerve; *pathos,* disease]. Relating to disease of the nervous system -- pathy, n.

عصبی مرضی: عصبی نظام کے مرض کے متعلق۔

Neuropathology *(nu-ro-path-ol-oj-i)* [G. *neuron,* nerve; *pathos,* disease; *logos,* discourage]. A bra- nch of medicine dealing with disease of the nervous system.

تشخیص امراض عصبی: علم ادویات کی ایک شاخ جو عصبی نظام کے امراض سے بحث کرتی ہے۔

Neuropharmacology *(mu-ro-far-ma-kol-o-ji)* [G. *neuron;* never; *pharmakon,* drug; *logus,* disc- ourage]. The branch of pharmacology dealing with drugs that affect the rervous system.

نیورو فارمیکالوجی: فارمیکالوجی کی شاخ جو عصبی نظام کو متاثر کرنے والی ادویات سے متعلق ہے۔

Neuroplasty *(nu-ro-plas-ti)* [G. *neuron,* nerve; *plassein,* to form]. Surgical repair of nerves -- neuroplastic, adj.

نیورو پلاسٹی: اعصاب کی عمل جراحی کے ذریعے مرمت۔

Neuropsychiatry *(nu-ro-sik-i-a-tri)* The combination of neurology and psychiatry. Specially dealing with organic and functional disease -- neuropsychiatric, adj.

عصبی نفسیات: نیورولوجی اور طبی نفسیات کو ملا کر نامیاتی اور فعلیاتی مرض اور اس کے علاج کا مطالعہ۔

Neurorrhaphy *(nu-ror'-a-fi)* [G. *neuron,* nerve; *raphe,* a suture]. Suturing the ends of a divided nerve.

طب عصبی دماغ: منقسم عصب کے سروں کو سینا۔

Neurorrhaphy *(nu-ror-a-fit)* [G. *neuron,* nerve; *-osis,* condition] A functional (i-e. psychogenic) disorder consisting of a symptom or symptoms caused, through usually unknown to the patient, by mental disorder. The four commonest are anxiety state. reactive deprssion, hysteria and obessional neurosis. (q.v.). Distinguished from a pschosis (q.v.). by the fact that a neurosis arises as a result of stresses and anxieties in the patient's environments. **institutional** n., apathy, withdrawal and non-participation occuring in long-stay patie-nt's enviroment. May be indistinguishable from the sings and symptoms for which the patient wa admitted to the institution --neurotic, adj.

خلل اعصاب: ذہنی عدم تسکین کا مرض جس سے مریض واقف نہیں ہوتا۔ یہ ذہنی نقص کی وجہ سے ہوتا ہے۔ یہ عام طور پر چار طرح اثر انداز ہوتا ہے۔ پریشانی کی حالت' اضطراب' ہسٹریا اور جنون۔ یہ مریض کے ماحول میں پریشانیوں اور دباؤ کی وجہ سے ہوتا ہے۔

Neurosurgery *(nu-ro-sur-jer-i)* [G. *neuron,* nerve; *cheirourgos,* working by hand]. Surgery of the nervous system -- NMR. Nuclear magnetic resonanc.

عصبی جراحی: عصبی نظام کی سرجری۔

Neurosyphilis *(nu-ro-si-fi-lis)* [G. *neuron,* nerve; N.L. *syphilus*]. Infection of brain or spinal cord, or both, by *Treponema pallidum.* The variety of clinical pictures produced is large,but the two common syndromes encountered are tabes dorsalis and general paralysis of the insane (GPI). The basic pathology is disease of the blood vessels, with later development of pathological changes in the meninges and the underlying nervous tissue. Very often symptoms of the disease do not arise until twenty years or more after the date of primary infection. See ARGLL. ROBERTSON PUPI -neurosyhphilitic, adj.

صبی آتشک: دماغ یا نخاع یا دونوں کا مرض جو ٹریپو۔نما پلیڈم سے ہوتا ہے۔

Neurotomy *(nu-rot-o-mi)* [G. *neruon* nerv *tome;* cutting]. Surgical cutting of a verve.

طع اعصاب: عصب کو عمل جراحت کے ذریعے کاٹنا۔

Neurotomy *(nu-ro-toks'-ik)* [G. *neuron,* nerv *toxiko,* poison]. Poisonous or destructive t nervous tissue--neurotoxin., n.

روٹاکسک: عصبی نسیج کے لیے زہریلا یا تباہ کن۔

Neurotoxic *(nu-ro-tiks)* [G. *neuron,* nerv *trepein,* to turn]. With predilection for th nervous system, used especially o *Treponema pullidum,* some forms of whic seem always to produce neurosyphiliti complications. n. viruses (rabies poliomyelitis, etc). make their major attack o the cells of nervous system.

صبانیہ الفی: وائرس جو عصبی نظام پر حملہ آور ہوتا ہے۔

neutron capture therapy, A new concept o treatment for carcinoma.

وٹران گروت علاج: کارسینوما کے علاج کے لئے نیا نظریہ۔

Neutropenia *(nu-tro-pe-ni-a)* [L. *neuter* neither; G. *penia,* want]. Shortage of the ter agranulocytosis neutropenic, adj.

لت خلیات ابیض: نیوٹروفلس کی کمی۔

Neutrophil *(nu-tro-fil)* [L. *neuter,* neither; G *philein,* to love]. The most common form o granulocyte (q.v.) in the blood, in which th granules are neither strongly basophilic o eosinophilic.

وٹروفل: کئی شکلی مرکزائی لیوکوسائیٹ کی ایک قسم۔

Neutrophlline *(nu-tro-fil-in)* Diprophyllin (q.v.)

وٹروفلین: ڈائی پروفلین۔

NGU. Non-gonococcal urethritis. See NSU.

ین جی یو: این ایس یو۔ نان گونوکوسل یریتھرین ٹیس۔

Niaiamide *(ni-al-a-mid)* A monoamine oxidas inhib- itor.

بلامائیڈ: ایم اے او آئی۔ مانو آمیجن آکسڈیز۔ یہ مسکن گولیاں اعصاب پر

مقوی اثر رکھتی ہیں۔ ہسٹیریا مین مفید۔ مقدار خوراک ایک گولی دن میں تین دفعہ۔

iamid. A monoamine oxidase inhibitor.

نیالمڈ: ایم اے او آئی۔ مانوامین آکسیڈیز۔ نائیلا مائیڈ۔ یہ مسکن گولیاں ہیں اور اعصاب پر مقوی اثر رکھتی ہیں۔ ہسٹریا میں مفید۔ خوراک ایک گولی دن میں تین دفعہ۔

icetal *(nik-e-tal)* See ISONIAZIDE.

iclosamide *(ni-klo-sa-mid)* Causes expulsion of adult tapeworm. Given in a single dose of 2 g. No starvation or purgation necessary.

نکلوسامائیڈ: بالغ کدو کیڑے کے اخراج کا سبب۔ بھوکا رہنا یا جلاب ضروری نہیں۔ صرف ایک ہی دوا کی خوراک دی جاتی ہے۔

icotinamide *(ni-ko-tin-a-mid)* A derivative of nicotinic acid and useful when the vasodilator action of that drug is not desired as in treatment of pellagra.

نکوٹینک ایسڈ: نکوٹینک ایسڈ سے حاصل شدہ۔

icotinic acid *(ni-ko-tin-ik as-id)* One of the essential food factor of the vitamin B complex. The vasodilator action of the compound is useful in chilblains, migraine, etc.

نکوٹینک ایسڈ: وٹامن بی کمپلکس میں لازمی غذائی عوامل میں سے ایک۔ بے رنگ قلمی ٹھوس۔ نقطہ پگھلاؤ ۲۳۵ ڈگری سینٹی گریڈ، گوشت اور خمیر میں پایا جاتا ہے۔ پیلاگرا کے مرض میں پچاس ملی گرام دو گولیاں دن میں تین دفعہ دو ماہ تک۔ شرائین کی سختی میں اس کی دو گولیاں صبح دو، دوپہر دو، شام یہی خوراک برائے مرض۔ فالج، لقوہ، وجع القلب ہائی بلڈ پریشر وغیرہ۔

ictitation *(nik-ti-ta-shun)* [L. *nictare,* to wink]. Rapik and involuntary blinking of the eyelids.

چشمک زنی: آنکھ کا تیزی سے بلا ارادہ جھپکنا۔

idation *(ni-da-shun)* [L. *nidus,* nest]. Implantation of the early embryo in the uterine mucosa.

مادہ گیری: رحمی میوکوسا میں اولی جنین کی پیوندکاری۔

idus *(ni-dus)* [L. nest] the focus of an infection. Septic focus.

بیضہ گاہ: سیپٹک فوکس۔ مرض کا فوکس۔

iemann-Pick disease. A lipoid metbolic disturba- nce, chiefly in female Jewish infants. Now thought to be due to absence or inadequacy of enzyme sphingomyelinase. There is enlargement of the liver, spleen and lymph nodes with mental subnormality. Now classified a lipid reticulosis. [Albert Niemann. German paediatrician, 1880-1921. Ludwin Pick, German paediatrician, 1868-1935.]

نیمپن پک مرض: ایک لپائڈ میٹالولک دخل اندازی زیادہ تر چھوٹی یہودی بچیوں میں ہوتی ہے۔ خیال ہے کہ یہ مرض خامرہ کی غیر موجودگی کی وجہ سے ہوتا ہے۔ ذہنی پسماندگی کے ساتھ جگر، لمف نوڈز اور تلی بڑھ جاتے ہیں۔

Nifenazone *(ni-fen-a-zon)* Antiarthritic drug.

نائیفینازون: اینٹی آرتھرٹک دوا۔

Night blindness Nyctalopia. Sometimes occurs in vitamin A deficiency and is maladaptation of vision to darkness.

شبکوری: اس بیماری میں اندھیرے میں نظر نہیں آتا۔ بعض دفعہ حیاتین الف کی کمی سے یہ مرض لاحق ہو جاتا ہے۔ نکٹا لوپیا رتوندھی۔ مریض تارے نہیں دیکھ سکتا۔ علاج کے لئے وٹامن اے ڈی کیپسول دن میں تین دفعہ تین ہفتے تک۔ کاڈلیور آئل تین کیپسول روزانہ کھانے کے بعد یعنی ایک کیپسول دن مین تین دفعہ۔

Night cry A shrill noise, uttered during sleep. May be of significance in hip disease when pain occurs in the relaxed joint.

چیخ شب: نیند کے دوران شور۔ کولہے کی تکلیف میں اہم۔

Night sweat Profuse sweating, usually during sleep; typical of tuberculosis.

پسینہ شب: عموماً نیند کے دوران پسینے آنا۔ تپ دق میں ایسا ہوتا ہے۔

Nihilistic *(ni-hil-is-tik)* [L. *nihil,* nothing]. Delusions and ideas of unreality; of not existing.

نائیفی لسٹک: غیر حقیقی نظریا جن کا وجود نہ ہو۔

Nikethamide *(ni-keth-a-mid)* Central nervous system (CNS) stimulant used in respiratory depression and collapse. Given intravenously or intramuscularly.

نکیتھے مائیڈ: مرکزی عصبی نظام کو تحریک دینے والا۔ تنفسی دباؤ میں مستعمل۔ کوارمین۔ ہیماپٹی۔ سیز ماخون تھوکنے، برتی برن اور پلومنری الیپولزم میں دل گھٹنے پر دوسی سی کا ٹیکہ لگایئے۔ مفید برائے ہٹ سٹروک، الرجی، سٹوپر یا مدہوشی، دوران خون گھبراہٹ، سانس رکنا، بے ہوشی، بلڈ پریشر کی کمی اور شاک یعنی صدمہ۔

Nikolsky's sign Slight pressure on skin causes

'slipping' of apparently normal epidermis, in the way that a rubber glove can be moved on a wet hand. Characteristic of pemphigus. [Pyotr V. Nickolsky, Russian dermatologist, 1858-1940]

علامات نکولسکائی: جلد پر معمولی دباؤ سے پھسلن ہوتی ہے۔ گیلے ہاتھ پر ربڑ کا دستانہ بھی پھسلتا ہے۔

Nilodin *(nil'-o-din)* Lucanthone (q.v.)

Nipple *(nip'-l)*. The conical eminence in the centre of each breast, containing the outlets of the milk ducts.

نپل۔ سر پستان۔ چوچی: ہر پستان کے مرکز میں مخروطی ابھار جو دودھ کی نالیوں کے سوراخوں پر مشتمل ہوتا ہے۔ یہ سوراخ ہر نپل میں سولہ یا پچیس ہوتے ہیں۔ چوچیوں کا مساج کرنے سے چوچیاں تن کر پوری طرح باہر نکل آتی ہیں۔ دودھ پلانے والی ماؤں کو چھاتیوں کا خاص خیال رکھنا چاہیئے۔

Niridazole *(ni-ri-daz-ol)* The drug of choice for *Schistosoma haematobius* infestation. Given orally in two divided doses, preferably at 12 hourly intervals; can be used as outpatient treatment if patient wanted that urine will be dark brown. Can also be used for *S. mansoni* and *S. japonicu,* infestations, but patient should be in hospital and outpatient treatment is no recommended. Toxic symptoms may be severe especially in patients with hepatosplenic disease.

نریڈیزوم: سات تا دس ایام کے لئے شسٹوسومیاسس اور امیباسس کے لئے منہ کے ذریعے کھائی جانے والی دعا۔

Nit The egg of the head louse (*Pediculus capitis*). It is firmly cemented to the hair.

لیکھ: سر کی جوں کا بیضہ۔ یہ بال کے ساتھ مضبوطی کے ساتھ چمٹا ہوتا ہے۔

Nitoman, Tetrabenazine (q.v.)

Nitrazepam *(ni-traz-e-pam)* A benzodiazepine hypnotic and as such drug of first choice. Is known to cause vivid dreams of a gradiose, futuristic nature in some people.

نائیٹرپسیم: نان باربیٹوریٹ خواب اور مسکن دوا۔

Nitric acid *(ni-trik as-id)* Dangerous caustic. Occasionally used in testing urine for albumen.

شورے کا تیزاب: شورے کا تیزاب ایک بے رنگ تیزاب مائع۔ نقطہ جوش ۸۶ ڈگری سینٹی گریڈ۔ ایک طاقتور تکسیدی عامل۔ یہ بہت سی دھاتوں اور کئی دوسری اشیاء پر عمل کر کے نائیٹروجن ڈائی آکسائیڈ کے بھورے بخارات بناتا ہے۔ یہ سوڈیم یا پوٹاشیم نائیٹریٹ پر مرتکز گندھک کے تیزاب کے عمل سے تیار کیا جاتا ہے۔ گرم پلاٹینم پر ہوا اور امونیا کا آمیزہ گزارنے سے بھی تیار ہوتا ہے۔ جس میں پلاٹینم عمل انگیز کے طور پر بھی استعمال ہوتا ہے۔ یہ تیزاب کیمیائی صنعت میں کافی زیادہ استعمال کیا جاتا ہے۔ خطرناک کاسٹک بعض دفعہ پیشاب میں البومن ٹیسٹ کرنے کے لئے استعمال کیا جاتا ہے۔

Nitrofurantion *(ni-tro-fur-an-tion)* Urinary antiseptic, of great value in Gram-positive and Gram-negative infections. Unrelated to sulphonamides or antibiotics.

نائیٹرو فیورین ٹائن: بولی دافع تعفن۔ فیوراڈین ٹن۔ دو دو گولیاں صبح دوپہر شام برائے پائی لائی ٹس یعنی سوزش حوض گردہ، سس ٹائی ٹس یعنی ورم مثانہ، انلارجڈ پراسٹیٹ گلینڈ یعنی پیشاب رکنا۔

Nitrofurazone *(ni-tro-fu-ra-zon)* Not for systemic administration by any route. Available as ointment and solution for topical application.

نائیٹرو فیورازن: مرہم اور محلول کے طور پر دستیاب۔ اسے جلی ہوئی جگہ پر لگا کر پٹی باندھیے۔ خواہ آگ سے جلے یا بجلی سے۔ فیوراسین مفید برائے سائی کوسس، لمفین جائی ٹس۔

Nitrogen *(nit-ro-jen)* A gaseous element; chief constituent of the atmosphere; essential connstituent of protein foods nitrogen balance is when a person's daily protein n. intake equals the daily excertion of n. exceeds the daily intake. Nitrogen is excrerted mainly as urea in the urine; ammonia, creatininie and uric acid account for a further small amount. Less than ten per cent total n. excreted in faeces. non-protein n. (NPN), nitrogen derived from all nitrogenous substances other than protein, i.e. urea, uric acid, ammonia nitrogen mustards, a group of cytotoxic drugs derivatives of mustard gasnitrogenous, adj.

نائیٹروجن: ایک گیسی عنصر جوہری وزن ۱۴٫۵۵۶۷، جوہری عدد ۷، ایک بے بو غیر مرئی کیمیائی طور پر غیر عامل گیس۔ زرخیز زمینوں میں نائیٹروجنی مرکبات پائے جاتے ہیں۔ یہ پروٹین، امینوایسڈز اور مادہ حیات کا اہم جزو ہے۔ نائیٹروجن کی کمی سے پتے پیلے پڑ جاتے ہیں۔ نائٹروجن کی وافر مقدار پھولداری کو بڑھاتی ہے۔ پیشاب میں نائیٹروجن کا اخراج یوریا کی صورت

میں ہوتا ہے۔

trous oxide, Widely used inhalation anaesthetic, especially for induction. Supplied in blue cylin- ders.

خندہ آور گیس: ہنسانے والی گیس۔ایک بے رنگ گیس۔دندان سازی میں ہلکا سا سُن کرنے کے لئے استعمال کی جاتی ہے۔

vaquine *(niv-a-kwin)* Chloroquine (q.v.)

نواکین: کلوروکوئین۔ملیریا کے علاج کے لئے مفید۔دن میں مفید تین گولیاں۔

becutane *(nob-e-ku-tan)* A soluble acrylic resin, which is sprayed over a wound and forms a transparent, non-inflammable elastic film. This permits the passage of air and water vapour but is impervious to bacteria. Nobecutane marking ink, a blue surgical marking ink. Nobecutane remover, a solvent for removal of n. plastic dressing and marking ink.

نوبیکیوٹین: ایک حل پذیر رال۔یہ زخم پر چھڑکی جاتی ہے شفاف الاسٹک فلم بناتی ہے۔اس میں سے ہوا اور آبی بخارات گذر سکتے ہیں لیکن جراثیم نہیں گذر سکتے۔

IR. Nuclear magnetic resonance (q.v.)

cturnal *(nok-tur-nal)* [L. *nocturnalis*]. Nightly; during the night; nocturnal enuresis, bed wetting during sleep.

شبانہ شمی: رات کے دوران۔ناکٹرنل اینوریسس یعنی بستر پر پیشاب نکل جا، تین سال سے زیادہ عمر کا بچہ سوتے میں پیشاب کرے تو یہ مرض ہے۔

cturia *(nok-tu-ri-a)* [L. *nox,* night; *G.* oiron, urine]. Passing urine at night.

de *(nod)* [L. *nodus,* knot]. A protuberance or swelling. A constriction. **atrioventricular n,.** the commencement of the bundle of His in the right at- rium of the heart.[. Wilhelm His, jun., German physician, 1863-1934]. **node of Ranvier,** the constriction in the neurilemma of a nerve fibre. [Louis Antoine Ranvier, French pathologis, 1835-1922] **sinoatrial n,.** situated at the opening of the superior vena cava into the right atrium; the wave of contraction begins here, then spreads over the heart.

نوڈ۔گلٹی۔عقدہ: (۱) ایک ابھار یا ورم۔(۲) جامد امواج کے نظام میں صفر ہٹاؤ کے نقاط۔(۳) دو نکات جن پر فلکی جسم کا مدار طریق الشمس کو قطع کرتا ہے۔(۴) خم یا سطح پر نقاط جو ایک ٹنجنٹ سے زیادہ رکھ سکتے ہیں۔(۵) پودے کے تنے کے وہ نقاط جن پر پتے لگے ہوتے ہیں۔

Nodule *(nod-ul)* [L. *nodulus,* knot]. A small node -- nodular, adj.

گلٹی: ایک چھوٹا نوڈ۔

Noludar *(nol-u-da)* Methyprylone (q.v.)

نلوڈیر: میتھاسپرائیلون۔

Non compos mentis *(non kom-pos men-tis)* [L.] Of unsound mind.

غیر صحیح دماغ: غیر صحت مند دماغ کا۔

Noradrenaline *(nor-ad-ren-a-len)* Endogenous nor- adrenaline is a neurohumoral transmitter which is released from adrenergic nerve endings. Although small amounts are associated with adrenalin in the adrenal medulla, its role as a hormone is a seco- ndary one. It has an intense vasoconstrictor action, and is given by slow intravenous injection in shock and peripheral failure.

نارایڈرینالین: ایک ہارمون جو ایڈرینل گلینڈ ایڈرینالین کے ساتھ موجود ہوتا ہے۔

Norethisterone *(nor-eth-is-ter-on)* Progestogen, said to suppress the gonadotrophin production by the pituitary. Given by tablet for irregular bleeding, dysmenorrhoea and premenstrual tension.

نارایتھسٹرون: پروجسٹوجن جو پیٹوایٹری سے گنیڈوٹروفن کی پیداوار کم کرتا ہے۔نوری جیسٹ۔ہر تین ماہ بعد ٹیکہ برائے کنٹراسیپشن۔

Norflex *(nor-fleks)* Orphenadrine (q.v.)

نارفلیکس: آرفنڈرین۔عضلات کے تشنج کے لئے مفید۔ایک گولی دن میں تین مرتبہ۔

Normoblast *(nor-mo-blast)* [L. *norma,* rule; G. *bla- stos,* germ]. A normal sized nucleated red blood cell, the precursor of the eryth- rocyte-normoblastic, adj.

طبعی حجم کا خون: نارمل سائز کا مرکزے والا سرخ خونی خلیہ۔

Normocyte *(nor-mo-sit)* [L. *norma,* rule; G. *kytos,* cell] A red blood cell of normal size --

normocytic, adj.

نرموسٹ: نارمل سائز کا سرخ خلیہ۔

Normoglycaemic *(nor-mo-gli-se-mik)* A normal amount of glucose in the blood normoglycaemia. n.

نرموگلائی سیمک: خون میں گلوکوز کی نارمل مقدار۔

Normotension *(nor-mo-ten-shun)* [G. *norma*, rule; *tender*, to strech]. Normal tension by current custom alluding to blood pressure -normotensive, adj.

نرموٹنشن: نارمل ٹنشن۔

Normothermia *(nor-mo-ther-mi-a)* [G. *norma*, rule; *therme*, heat]. Normal body temperature as opp- osed to hyperthermia and hyupothermia-- nor- mothermic, adj

نرموتھرمیا: نارمل جسمانی درجہ حرارت۔

Normotonic *(nor-mo-ton-ik)* [G.*norma*, rule; *tonos*, tension] Normal strength, tension tone, by current custom referring to muscle tissue. Spasmolytic drugs induce normotonicity in muscle, and can be used before radiography-normotonicity, n.

نرموٹونک: نارمل طاقت۔ٹنشن۔ٹون عموماً عضلاتی نسیج سے متعلق۔

Nortriptyline *(nor-trip-til-en)* Similar to amitriptyline. (q.v.).

نارٹرپٹائیلین: امیٹرٹائیلین۔

Nosocomial *(no-so-kom-i-al)* [G.*nosos*, disease; *komeo*, to take care of]. A n. patient is one which occurs in a patient who has been in hospital for at least 72 hours and did not have signs and symptoms of such infection on admission.

Nostagia *(nos-tal-ji-a)* [G. *nostos*, return home; *algos*, pain]. Homesickness-- nostalgic, adj.

دردوطن۔عارضہ وطن: گھر کی تنگی۔

Nostrils *(nos-trils)* The anterior opening in the nose; the anterior nares; choanae.

نتھنے: ناک میں امامی سوراخ۔

Novobiocin *(no-vo-bi-o-sin)* An orally active antibiotic. It should be reserved for use in infec- tions resistant to other drugs.

نووبایوسن: منہ سے کھایا جانے والا انٹی بایوٹک۔ایلباوائی سین۔اس کے دو

سول صبح تین شام برائے ریت مکھی' بخار' پین آفتھل مائی ٹس۔آسٹیو مائی
ٹس۔ایکوٹ اپنڈے خلیے کے مرکزوں میں پائے جانے والے نیوکلیک
ڈز اور لحمیات کے مرکبات جو زیادہ تر کروموسومز میں ہوتے ہیں۔وائرس
ل طور پر نکلیو پروٹین پر مشتمل ہوتا ہے۔زیست کا دارومدار نکلیو پروٹینز کی
یدی خصوصیات پر ہے۔

Nucleotoxic *(nu-kle-o-toks-ik)* [L. *nucleu* kernal; G. *toxikon*, poison]. Poisonous to c nuclei as some drugs toxins and viruses nucleotoxin, n.

وٹاسک: خلوی مرکزاؤں کے لئے زہریلا جیسے بعض ادویات' ٹاکس اور
س۔

Nucleus *(nuk-li-us)* [L.] 1.The inner essect part of a tissue cell, being necessary for t growth, nourishment and reproduction of t cell. 2. A circumscribed accummulation nerve cells in the certral nervous syste associated with a particular function. **nucle pulposus,** the soft core of an interverteb disc which can prolapse (q.v.) into the spi cord and cause sciatica -- nuclei, pl; nucle adj.

زہ: (۱) ایک اہم مرکزی نقطہ خصوصی طور پر کسی مادہ کا ذرہ جو قلموں کو بنانے
لئے بطور مرکزہ یا کہر آبی بخارات کی تکثیف کے لئے بطور مرکز فرض انجام
۔(۲) ایک سالمے میں جواہر کا ایک خالص حلقہ جو کیمیائی تبدیلیوں میں
شناخت قائم رکھتا ہے مثلاً بنزینی حلقہ میں چھ کاربن جواہر کا بنزین
ہ۔(۳) نسیجی خلیے کے اندرونی لازمی حصہ جو نشونما' تغذیہ اور خلیہ کی تولید
لئے ضروری ہے۔(۴) مرکزی عصبی نظام میں عصبی خلیوں کا ہجوم جن کا
ں فعل ہو۔

Nullipara *(nul-lip-a-ra)* [L. *nullus*, no *parere*, to bring froth]. A woman who has born a child-- nulliparous, adj; nulliparity, n

د عورت: ایسی خاتون جس نے کسی بچے کو جنم نہ دیا ہو۔

Nummular *(num-u-lar)* [L. *nummularis*, money]. Coin shaped; resembling rolls co as the sputum in phthisis.

ا: سکہ کی شکل کا۔سکوں کے رول سے مشابہ۔

Nupercaine *(nu-per-kan)* See CINCHOCAIN

ین: سنکوکین۔اس کا سطحی استعمال جلد کو سن کرتا ہے۔مرہم اور لوشن
ب ہیں۔خارش بند کرتے ہیں۔

Nutation *(nu-ta-shun)* [L. *nutare*, to no

Nodding; applied to uncontrolable head shaking.

چکرخوری: سر ہلانا۔

utrient *(nu-tri-ent)* [L. *nutrire,* to nourish]. Serving as or providing nourishment, **nutrient artery,** one which enters a long bone. **nutrient foramen,** hole in a long bone which admits the n. artery.

مقوی۔ مغذی: غذا مہیا کرنے یا غذا کے طور پر ہونا۔

utrition *(nu-tri-shun)* The sun total of the processes by which the living organism receives and utilizes the materials necessary for survival, growth and repair of worn-out tissue.

تغذیہ: ان تمام اعمال کا مجموعہ جن پر جاندار ایسی اشیاء وصول اور استعمال کرت ہے جو کہ زندہ رہنے' نشو نما اور بے کار بافتوں کی مرمت کر لئے ضروری ہے۔

x vomica *(nuks vom -ik-a)* The nuts from which strychnine is obtained. Occasionally used with other as a gastric stimulant.

کچلا: ایسے نٹ جن سے سٹرکنین حاصل ہوتا ہے۔ بعض اوقات گیسٹرک محرک کے طور پر استعمال کیا جاتا ہے۔ ذائقہ میں کڑوا زہریلا۔ اس کے کھانے سے سانس میں رکاوٹ ہوتی ہے۔ اس کے لئے گارڈینال سوڈیم کا تین گرین ٹیکہ اور ساتھ کورامین کا ٹیکہ لگایئے۔

ctalgia *(nik-tal-ji-a)* [G.*nyx,* night; *algos,* pain]. Pain occuring during the night.

الم اللیلی: رات کے دوران درد ہونا۔

ctalopia *(nik-tal-o-pi-a)* [G. *nyx,* night; *laosk,* blind; *ops,* eye]. Night blindness. (q.v.)

شب کوری: اندھیرے میں کچھ بھی دکھائی نہ دینا۔

ctophobia *(nik-to-fo-bi-a)* [G. *nyx,* night; *phobos,* fear]. Abnormal fear of the night and darkness.

شب ترسی: رات اور اندھیرے کا غیر معمولی خوف' شب خوفی کا مرض۔

Nycturia *(nik-tu-ri-a)* [G. *nyx,* night; *ouron,* urine]. Incontinence of urine at night.

نکٹوریا: رات کے وقت پیشاب کی بے اعتدالی۔

Nymphae *(nim-fe)* [G.]. The labia minora.

شفتین صغری: لیبیا مائنورا۔ لب صغیر۔

Nymphomania *(nim-fo-ma-ni-a)* [G. *nymphe,* a bride, nymph; *mania,* madness]. Excessive sexual desire in a female --nymphomaniac, adj.

شبق النساء۔ چداس: مادہ میں زائد جنسی خواہش۔ خواتین میں خواہش جماع کا غیر معمولی غلبہ۔

Nysrtaform *(nis-ta-form)* Fungicidal cream or nystatin with cortisone, in a water miscible base. Cortisone relieves the fungal irritation.

نسٹافارم: دافع سماروغ کریم۔

Nystagmus *(nis-tag-mus)* [G. *nystagmus,* nodding]. Involuntary and jerky repetitive movement of the eyeballs.

ڈیلہ کا پھڑکنا: آنکھ کے گولوں کی بلا ارادہ اور جھٹکے دار حرکت۔

Nystan betnovate *(nis-tan-bet-no-vat)* Nystain (q.v.) and betamethasone (q.v.).

Nystatin Antifungal antibiotic effective in the treat- ment of candidiasis (moniliasis). Prevents intestinal fungal overgrowth during broad spec- trum antibiotic treatment.

دافع سماروغ اینٹی بائیوٹک جو کینڈی ڈیاسس کے علاج میں موثر ہے۔ نوزائیدہ بچے کے منہ میں سفید چھالا سا نظر آتا ہے۔ تالو اور زبان پر بھی چھالے ہوتے ہیں۔ سفید دھبوں کی درمیانی جگہ سرخ ہوتی ہے اس کی وجہ ماں کی اندام نہانی میں موجود ایک پھپھوندی ایلبی کین ہے۔ بچے میں علامات چوتھے روز ظاہر ہوتی ہیں۔ سفید دھبوں کو صاف کرنے سے نیچے زخم ظاہر ہوتا ہے اس پر نسٹیٹین محلول لگاتے ہیں یہ ایک براڈ سپیکٹرم اینٹی فنگل دوا ہے۔ مقامی اندرونی طور پر استعمال کی جاتی ہے۔ بعض اوقات اسے آکسی ٹیٹرا سائیکلین کے ساتھ بھی ملا دیا جاتا ہے۔ یہ نیل سٹیٹ یا مائی کوسٹے ٹین کے برانڈ ناموں سے ملتی ہے۔

O

O Symbol for oxygen and ohne Hauch.

او: علامت ہے آکسیجن اور اوہنی ہاش کی۔

o *(o-mi'kron)* Omicron. The fifteenth letter of the Greek alphabet.

اومائیکرون: یونانی حروف ابجد کا پندرہواں حرف

OB Obstetrics.

زچگی: زچگی سے متعلق۔

Obcecation *(ob'-se-ka-shan)* Incomplete blindness.

نامکمل اندھاپن: جس میں آنکھیں مکمل طور پرناکارہ نہ ہوئی ہوں۔

Obese *(o-bes)* [L. *obesus*]. Excessively fat.

موٹاپا: بہت ہی موٹا ہونا۔

Obesity *(o-bes-ite)* [L. *obesus,* fat]. An increase in body weight beyond the limitation of skeletal and physical requirement as the result of an excessive accumulation of fat in the body.

موٹاپن: جسم کے وزن میں بہت زیادہ اضافہ ہو جانا۔ اتنا زیادہ کہ ڈھانچہ اور جسمانی ضروریات کو بھی پیچھے چھوڑ جائے۔ اس کی وجہ جسم میں بہت زیادہ چکنائی کا جمع ہو جانا ہے۔

Objective *(ob-jek'tiv)* [L. *objectivis)* Perceptible to the external senses. A result for whose achievement an effort is made. The lens or system of lenses in a microscope that is nearest to the object under examination.

مقصد: بیرونی حسوں سے سمجھنا۔ وہ مقصد جس کے حصول کے لئے کوشش کی جائے۔ عدسے یا عدسوں کا نظام جو کہ خوردبین میں لگے ہوتے ہیں اور زیر معائنہ شے کے قریب ہوتے ہیں۔

Obliteration *(ob-lit-ara-shan)* [L. *obliteratio,* to end]. Complete removal whether by disease, degeneration,surgical procedure, irradiatic or otherwise.

ع کرنا، ختم کرنا: کسی چیز کا مکمل خاتمہ چاہے کسی طرح سے بھی ہو۔ جیسے ی سے، ٹوٹ پھوٹ سے، عمل جراحت سے، شعاعوں سے یا کسی اور یقے سے مکمل ختم کیا جانا۔

Obsession *(ob-se-shan)* [L. *obsessio*]. A recı rent persistant thought, image or impulse tl is unwanted and distressing (egodystonic) a comes involuntarily to mind despite attem to ignore or suppress it. Common obsessic involve thoughts of violence, contaminati and self-doubt.

Obstetrician *(ob'-sta-tri-shan)* [L. *obstetrix,* m wife]. One who practices obstetrics.

Obstetrics *(ob-stet-riks)* [L. *obstetricia,* m wifery]. The branch of medical science esp ially surgery which deals with the mana ment of pregnancy, labor and puerperium.

Obstipation *(ob-sti-pa'-shan)* [L. *obstipatio,* c stipation]. Intractible constipation.

ی قبض: وہ قبض جسے قابو نہ کیا جاسکتا ہو۔

Obtundent *(ob-tun-dent)* [L. *obtundens,* soothe]. Having the power to soothe pain soothing or partially anesthetic medicines.

ن بخش دوا: وہ دوا جو درد سے آرام پہنچائے۔ درد سے آرام پہنچانے نیم بے ہوش کرنے والی دوا۔

Obturator *(obta-ra'tor)* [L. *obturare,* to clc Any structure natural or artificial that cl an opening.

Occipitofrontal *(ok-sip'-it-o-fron'-tal)* [L. *occiput*, back of head; *frons*, forehead]. Pertaining to the occiput and forehead.

(عضلہٴ) موخریہ جبہیہ : سر کے اگلے اور پچھلے حصہ سے متعلق۔

Occipitoposterior *(ok-sip'-it-o-pos-te'-ri-or)* [L. *occiput*, back of head; *posterior*, posterior]. When the fetal occiput is in the posterior half of the maternal pelvis.

موخری خلفی : جب بچے کے سر کا پچھلا حصہ مادری پیڈو کے پچھلے نصف میں ہو۔

Occiput *(ok'-si-put)* [L.]. The posterior region of the skull.

پشت سر : کھوپڑی کا پچھلا حصہ۔

Occlusion *(ok-kloo'-zhun)* [L. *occludere*, to close up]. The closure of an opening, especially of ducts or blood vessels. In dentistry, the fit of the teeth as the two jaws meet.

بستگی دندا : کسی سوراخ کی بندش۔ خصوصاً نالیوں یا خونی رگوں کی۔

Occult blood *(ok'-ul-t)*. Blood which is not visible to the naked eye but the presence of which can be detected by chemical means.

مخفی خون : خون جو آنکھ سے نظر نہ آئے بلکہ اس کی موجودگی کیمیائی وسائل سے معلوم کی جاسکے۔

Occupational delirium A psychiatric term for a condition which occurs in many cases of dementia .consisting of purposeless overactivity relating to pa tient's occupation.

مرض کسبی : مریض کے پیشے سے متعلق بلا مقصد زیادہ سرگرمی کا مظاہرہ۔

Occupational disease See INDUSTRIAL DISEASE.

کاروباری مرض : صنعتی مرض۔

Occupational therapy The use of occupations, usually manual, for therapeutic or remedial purposes in mental and physical disorders.

شغلی علاج : علاج کے لئے پیشوں کا استعمال۔

Ochsner-Sherran treatment Conservative measures sometimes used for patients with acute appendicitis. [Albert John Ochsner, American surgeon, 1858-1925].

اپنڈکس کے درد کے لئے بعض دفعہ پرانے طریقے استعمال میں لائے جاتے ہیں۔

Octapressin *(ok-ta-pres'-sin)*. Prilocaine with felypressin.

فیلیپریسن کے ساتھ پریلوکین۔

Octyl nitrite *(ok'-til-nit-rit)*. Vasodilator similar to amyl nitrate (q.v.). Given by inhalation.

ایمائیل نائٹریٹ سے مشابہ باسط شرائین۔

Ocular *(ok'-u-lar)* [L. *ocularis*, of the eyes]. Pertaining to the eye.

چشمی۔ عینی : آنکھ سے متعلق۔

Oculentum *(ok'-u-len-tum)*. Eye ointm-ent-oculenta, pl.

آکولینٹم : آنکھ کا مرہم۔

Oculist *(ok'-u-list)*. Medically qualified person who refracts and treats eye disease.

طبیب چشم : آنکھ کے امراض کا ماہر۔

Oculogenital *(ok-u-lo-jen'-it-al)* [L. *oculus*, eye; G. *genesis*, decent]. Pertaining to the eye and genital region, as the virus TRIC. It is found in the male and female genital canals and in the conjunctival sacs of the newborn.

آکولوجنیٹل۔ عینی تولیدی : آنکھ اور تولیدی حصے سے متعلق۔

Oculomotor *(ok-u-lo-ji'-rik)* [L. *oculus*, eye; G. *gyros*, circle]. Referring to movements of the eyeball. **oculogyric crises,** occur in Parkinsonism.

حرکات چشم سے متعلق : آنکھ کے گولے کی حرکات سے متعلق۔

Oculogyric *(ok-u-lo-mot'-or)* [L. *oculus*, eye; *movere*, to move]. The third cranial nerve which moves the eye and supplies the upper eye lid.

عصب محرک چشمی۔ عینی حرکی : تیسری کرینیل عصب جو آنکھ کو حرکت دیتی ہے اور بالائی پپوٹے میں جاتی ہے یہ عصب مذ برین یا وسطی دماغ سے شروع ہوتی ہے۔

Odontalgia *(o-don-tal'-ji-a)* [G.]. Tooth-ache.

دانت درد : د ت کا درد۔

Odontic *(o-don-tal'-tik)* [G. *od‹ ‹s*, tooth]. Pertaining to the teeth.

سنی۔ دندانی : دانتوں سے متعلق۔

Odontitis *(o-don-ti'-tis)* [G. *odous*, tooth; *-itis*, *inflammation*]. *Inflammation of the teeth.*

ورم دندان : دانتوں کی سوزش۔

Odontoid *(o-don'-toid)* [G. *odous,* tooth; *eidos,* form]. Resembling a tooth, **odontoid peg or process,** the toothlike projection of the body of the second cervical vertebra or axis.

دندان نما۔دندانی : دانت سے مشابہ۔

Odontolith *(o-don'-to-lith)* [G. *odous,* tooth; *lithos,* stone]. Tartar; the concretions which are deposited around teeth.

حضر۔قلح اسنان : دانت کے گرد جمع شدہ مواد۔

Odontology *(o-don-tol'-o-ji)* [G. *odous,* tooth; *logos,* discourse]. Dentistry.

علم دندان : دندان سازی۔

Odontoma *(o-don-to-ma)* [G. *odous,* tooth; *-oma,* tumour]. A tumour developing from or containing tooth structures--odontomata, pl.; odontomatous, adj.

دندانی سلعہ۔ورم دندان : دانتوں کی ساختوں پر مشتمل یا ان سے بننے والی رسولی۔

Odontoprisis *(o-don-to-pri'-sis)* [G. *odous,* tooth; *prisis,* sawing]. Grinding of the teeth.

دانت پیسنا : دانتوں کا پیسنا۔

Odontotherapy *(o-don-to-ther'-a-pi)* [G. *odous,* tooth; *therapeia,* treatment]. The treatment given for diseases of the teeth.

علاج دندان : دانتوں کی بیماریوں کے علاج۔

Odema *(e-de'-ma)* [G. *oidema,* swelling]. Dropsy. Abnormal infiltration of tissues with fluid. **cardiac o.,** a dependent oedema of subcutaneous tissues in cardiac failure. **hepatic o.** is caused by osmotic pressure changes in the blood. **hunger (famine) o.** results from reduced osmotic pressure of blood, secondary to protein starvation. **pulmonary o.** is a form of waterlogging of the lungs because of left ventricular failure or mitral stenosis. **renal o.** results from disturbed kidney filtration in nephritis. **subcutaneous o.** is demonstrable by the 'pitting' produced by pressure of the finger. See ANGIONEUROTIC O--oedematous, adj.

استسقاءِ لحمی : بافتوں کی سیال کے ساتھ غیر معمولی مداخلت مرض استقاء۔ جلندر۔

Oedipus complex *(ed'-i-pus kom'-pleks)* (Oedipus, King of Thebes, who unwitting killed his father and married his mother]. A unconscious attachment of a son to his moth resulting in a feeling of jealousy towards t father and then guilt, producing emotion conflict. This process was described by Fre as part of his theory of infantile sexuality a considered to be normal in male infants.

ری خلط : بیٹے کا اپنی ماں کی طرف جھکاؤ جس سے وہ باپ کے ساتھ د کرنے لگتا ہے۔اوڈیپس بادشاہ نے اپنے باپ کو قتل کر کے اپنی ماں سے ی کر لی تھی۔

Oesophageal *(e-sof-a-je'-al)* [G. *oisophago* gullet]. Pertaining to the oesophagus (q.v.).

Oesophagectasis *(e-sof-a-jek'-ta-sis)* [*oisophagos,* gullet; *ektasis,* extension]. dilated gullet (oesophagus).

باط مری : کشادہ ایسوفیکس۔حلق یا گلے کا پھیلاؤ۔

Oesophagectomy *(e-sof-a-jek'-to-mi)* [*oisophagos,* gullet; *ektome* excision Excision of part or the whole of t oesophagus.

ی براری : ایسوفیکس مکمل یا اس کا کوئی حصہ کاٹنا۔

Oesophagitis *(e-sof-a-ji'-tis)* [G. *oisophagos,* gullet; *-itis,* inflammation]. Inflammation the oesophagus.

Oesophagoscope *(e-sof'-a-gos-kop)* [*oisophagos,* gullet; *skopein,* to examine]. S ENDOSCOPE-- oesophagoscopy, n.; oesop agoscopic, adj

ی بین : اینڈوسکوپ۔ایسوفیکسن کو دیکھنے کا آلہ۔

Oesophagostomy *(e-sof-a-gos'-to-mi)* [*oisophagos,* gullet; *stoma,* mouth]. surgically established fistula between t oesophagus and the skin in the root of t neck. Used temporarily for feeding aft excision of the pharynx for malignant diseas

دیہ مری : گردن کی جڑ میں کھال اور ایسوفیکس کے درمیان اپریشن ذریعے سوراخ بنانا۔

Oesophagotomy *(e-sof-a-got'-o-mi)* [G. *oiso hagos,* gullet; *tome,* a cutting]. An incisi into the oesophagus.

تفویہ مری : ایسوفیگس میں شگاف۔

)esophagus *(e-sof'-a-gus)* [G. *iosophagos,* gullet]. The musculomembranous canal, 22.86 cm in length, extending from the pharynx to the stomach--oesophageal, adj.

مری۔غذا کی نالی : فیرنکس اور معدہ کے درمیان آنت کا حصہ۔

)estradiol *(es-trad'-i-ol).* Synthetic oestrogen. Given in amenorrhoea, kraurosis, menopause and other conditions of oestrogen deficiency. Given orally and by injection.

ایسٹراڈائی اول : تالیفی اسٹروجن۔زچہ میں دودھ کی زیادتی کے علاج کے لئے ایک انجکشن روزانہ تین۔

estriol *(es'-tri-ol)* . An oestrogen metabolite present in the urine of pregnant women. Fetus and placenta concerned in production. Oestriol excretion is an indicator of fetal well-being.

آسٹریلول : حاملہ خواتین کے پیشاب میں موجود اسٹروجن میٹابولائیٹ۔

estroform *(es'-tro-form).* Oestradiol (q.v.).

ایسٹروفارم : اوسٹراڈیول۔

estrogen *(es'-tro-jen)* A generic term referring to ovarian hormones. Three 'classical' ones; oestriol, oestrone and oestradiol. Urinary excretion of these substances increases throughout normal pregnancy--oestrogenic, adj.

شبق زاہارمون : ہارمون اوسٹراڈیول۔دماغی غدود ایف ایس ایچ ہارمون بناتے ہیں جو رحم کے خصیوں پر اثر انداز ہوتا ہے اور اس کے کچھ خلیے ایسٹروجن ہارمون بناتے ہیں جس کا کام رحم کی اندرونی تہہ کو دبیز کرنا اور پھیلانا ہے۔اس سے چھاتیاں بھی بڑھتی ہیں۔اس ہارمون کا ایک جفرہ اوسٹراڈیول ہے۔

estrone *(es'-tron).* A hormone similar to oestradiol, used mainly in local applications.

سبق زاہارمون: اوسٹراڈیول سے مشابہ ایک ہارمون۔ہارمون ایسٹروجن کا ایک جزو۔

dium *(o-id'-i-um)* Syn., Candida (q.v.).

اوئیڈیم : کینڈائیڈ

leandomycin *(ol-e-an-do-mi'-sin).* An antibiotic with a range of activity similar to that of penicillin. Should be reserved for infections resistant to other antibiotics.

اورلنڈومائیسین : پنسلین سے مشابہ اینٹی بایوٹک۔

Olecranon *(o-lek'-ra-non)* [G. *olekranon,* point of elbow]. The large process at the upper end of the ulna; it forms the tip of the elbow when the arm is flexed.

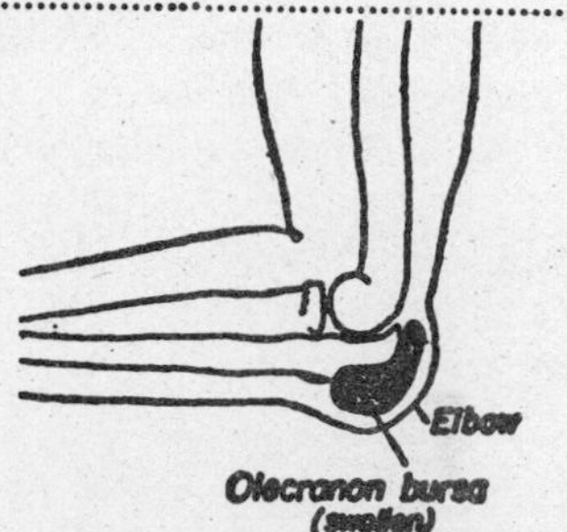

Olecranon bursitis

زج : کہنی کی ہڈی کے جوڑ کے آگے کی ہڈی۔النا کے بالائی سرے پر بڑا زائدہ۔جب بازو سیدھا کیا جائے تو کہنی کا اوپر والا سرا ہوتا ہے۔

Oleum olivae Olive oil (q.v.).

روغن زیتون : زیتون کا تیل۔

Oleum ricini *(ol'-e-um ri-si'-ni).* Castor oil (q.v.).

تیل ارنڈ : ارنڈ کا تیل۔کیسٹرائل۔

Olfactory *(ol-fak'-to-ri)* [L. *olfacere,* to smell]. Pertaining to the sense of smell. olfactory nerve, the nerve supplying the nose; the first cranial nerve. **Olfactory organ,** the nose--olfaction, n.

شمی : سونگھنے کی حس سے متعلق شمی عصب یا آلفیکٹری نروناک کی میوکس جھلی سے شروع ہوتی ہے اس کے ناک کی چھت میں اسفنجی ہڈی کی کربری فارم پلیٹ سے گزر کر آلفیکٹری بلب میں پہنچ جاتے ہیں۔

Oligaen *(ol-i-ge'-mi-a)* [G. *oligos,* little; *haima,* blood]. Diminshed total quantity of blood--oligaemic, adj

کمی خون : خون کی کل مقدار کی کمی۔

Oligohydramnios *(ol-i-go-hid-ram'-ni-os)* [G. *oligos,* little; *hydor,* water; *amnion,* fetal membrane]. Deficient amniotic fluid.

اولیگوہائیڈریم نیوس : ایمنا نک سیال کی کمی۔

Oligomenorrhoea *(ol-ig-o-men-or-re'-a)* [G.

oligos, little; *men,* month; *rheein,* to flow]. Infrequent menstruation, normal cycle is prolonged beyond 35 days.

قلت حیض : حیض میں بے قاعدگی۔ نارمل سائیکل ۳۵ ایام سے بھی بڑھ جاتا ہے۔

Oligophrenia *(ol-ig-o-fre'-ni-a)* Mental deficiency. 'Subnormality' and 'severe subnormality' are now the official terms-oligophrenic, adj.

اولیگوفرینیا : ذہنی کمی۔

Oligospermia *(ol-i-go-sper'-mi-a)* [G. *oligos,* little; *sperma,* seed]. Deficiency of spermatozoa in the semen.

قلت منی : منی میں سپر میٹازوآ کی کمی۔

Oliguria *(ol-ig-u'-ri-a)* [G. *oligos,* little; *ouron,* urine]. Deficient urine secretion--oliguric, adj.

قلت بول۔ کم بولی : پیشاب کا کم اخراج۔

Olive oil Used in gastric ulcer and as a laxative. Useful externally as emollient.

روغن زیتون : معدے کا السر میں اور بطور قبض کشا استعمال کیا جاتا ہے۔ زیتون کا تیل۔

Omentum *(o-men'-tum)* [L. apron]. A fold of peritoneum. **gastrosplenic o.** connects the stomach and spleen. The functions of the o. are protection, repair and fat storage. **greater o.,** the fold which hangs from the lower border of the stomach and covers the front of the intestines. **lesser o.,** a smaller fold, passing between the transverse fissure of the liver and the lesser curvature of the stomach--omental, adj.

ثرب : پرو ٹیونیئم کی تہہ۔

Omnopon *(om'-no-pon)* A preparation of opium alkaloids.

امنوپون : افیم کے الکلائیڈ سے تیار شدہ۔

Omphalitis *(om-fal-i'-tis)* [G. *omphalos,* navel; *-itis* inflammation]. Inflammation of the umbilicus.

ورم ناف : ناف کی سوزش۔

Omphalocele *(om'-fal-o-sel)* [G. *omphalos,* navel; *kele,* hernia]. Umbilical hernia.

امفیلوسیل : ناف کا ہرنیا۔

Onchoceriasis *(on-ko-ser'-ka).* Genus of filarial worms.

...کوسرکا : فلیریا کیڑے۔

Onchocerca *(on-ko-ser-ki-a'-sis)* Infestation o[f] man with Onchocerca. Adult worm[s] encapsulated in subcutaneous connectiv[e] tissue. Can cause 'river blindness'.

...وسرکیاسس : فلیریا کیڑے کا انسان پر حملہ۔ دریائی اندھا پن کا سبب۔

Oncogenic *(on-ko-jen'-ik)* [G. *onkos,* bul[k]; *genesis,* decent]. 1. Capable of tumo[ur] production. 2. The process of tumo[ur] formation. Currently used to describe th[e] carcinogenic viruses.

...وجینک : (۱) رسولی پیدا کرنے کا اہل۔ (۲) رسولی بننے کا طریقہ۔

Oncology *(on-kol'-o-ji)* [G. *onkos,* bulk; *logo[s]* discourse]. The scientific study [of] neoplasms--oncological, adj.; oncologicall[y] adv.

...عیات : نیوپلازمز کا سائنسی مطالعہ۔

Oncolysis *(on-kol'-i-sis)* [G. *onkos,* bulk; *lysis,* lossening]. Destruction of aneoplas[m] Sometimes used to describe reduction in si[ze] of tumour--oncolytic, adj.

...لائی سس : نیوپلازما کی تباہی۔ بعض دفعہ رسولی کے سائز میں تخفیف ...نے کو بیان کرنے کے لئے یہ اصطلاح استعمال کی جاتی ہے۔

Oncovin *(onk'-o-vin).* Vincristine (q.v.).

...ون : ونکرسٹین۔

Onychia *(o-nik'-i-a)* [G. *onyx,* nail]. Acu[te] inflammation of the nail matrix; suppurati[on] may spread beneath the nail, causing it [to] become detached and fall off.

...ناخن : ناخن کے میٹرکس کی انتہائی سوزش۔

Onychocryptosis *(on-ik-o-krip-to'-sis)* [G. *on[yx]* nail; *kryptos,* hidden; *-osis,* conditio[n]. Ingrowing of the nail.

...لظفر : ناخن کا اندر کی طرف بڑھنا۔

Onychogryphosis *(on-ik-o-gri-to'-sis)* [G. *on[yx]* nail; *griphos,* fishing net]. A ridge[d] thickened deformity of the nails. A[lso] ONYCHOGRYPOSIS.

...وتعقف والاظفار : ناخنوں کی دبیز بدصورتی۔

Onycholysis *(on-ik-ol'-i-sis).* [G. *onyx,* na[il]; *lysis,* a loosening]. Loosening of toe or fin[ger] nail--onycholytic, adj.

لخلتہ الاظافر : پاؤں یا ہاتھ کی انگلی کے ناخن کا ڈھیلا پن۔

Onychomycosis *(on-ik-o-mi-ko-sis)* [G. *onyx,* nail; *mykes,* fungus; *-osis* condition]. A fungal infection of the nails.

جذام الاظفار : ناخنوں کی سماروغی مرض۔

O'nyong nyong fever *(on-i'-ong-ni'-ong fe-ver).* Syn, joint-breaker fever. Caused by virus transmitted by mosquitoes in East Africa. First in north-west Uganda.

اونیا نگ نیا نگ بخار : مشرقی افریقہ میں مچھر کے ذریعے وائرس بخار پھیلتا ہے۔

Oocyte *(o-o-sit)* [G. *oion,* egg; *kytos,* cell]. An immature ovum.

بیضہ خلیہ : ایک کچا بیضہ۔

Oogenesis *(o-o-jen'-e-sis)* [g. *oion,* egg; *genesis,* production]. The production and formation of ova in the ovary--oogenetic, adj.

تولید بیضہ : بیضہ دان میں بیضوں کا بننا اور ان کی پیداوار۔

Oophorectomy *(o-o-for-ek'-to-mi)* [G. *oion,* egg; *ektome,* excision]. Excision of an ovary.

مبیض براری : بیضہ دانی کو کاٹ کر نکال دینا۔

Oophoritis *(o-o-for-i'-tis)* [G. *oion,* egg; *-itis,* inflammation]. Inflammation of an ovary.

ورم مبیض : بیضہ دان کی سوزش۔

Oophoron *(o-of'-er-on)* [g. *oion,* egg; *pherein,* to bear]. The ovary.

مبیض : بیضہ دان

Oophorosalpingectomy *(o-o-for-o-sal-pin-jek'-to-mi)* [g. *oion,* egg; *pherein,* to bear; *salpigx,* tube; *ektome*, excision]. Excision of an ovary and its associated Fallobian tube.

قطع خصیتہ الرحم وقناۃ المبیض : بیضہ دان اور اس سے متعلق فلوپین ٹیوب کاٹ کر نکال دینا۔

Oosperm *(o'-o-sperm)* [G. *oion,* egg; *sperma,* seed]. A fertilized ovum.

بارور بیضہ : ایک بارور بیضہ۔

Opacity *(o-pas'-i-ti)* [L. *opacus,* shaded]. Non-transparency; cloudiness; an opaque spot, as on the cornea or lens.

ناشفافی : غیر شفاف ہونا۔ دھندلا پن۔

Operidine *(o-per'-i-den).* A mixture of cuare and phenoperidine. Useful prior to use of ventilator for gravely ill asthmatic patients.

اوپیریڈین : ایک آمیزہ۔

Ophthalmia *(of-thal'-mi-a)* [G.]. Inflammation of the eye. **ophthalmia neonatorum,** defined by law in 1914 as a 'purulent discharge from the eyes of an infant commencing within 21 days of birth'. Only 6 percent of total cases are gonorrhoeal, but all are notifiable. **sympathetic o.,** iridocyclitis of one eye secondary to injury or disease of the other.

آشوب چشم : آنکھ کی سوزش۔

Ophthalmic *(of-thal'-mik)* [G. *ophthalmos,* eye]. Pertaining to the eye.

چشمی۔عینی : آنکھ سے متعلق۔

Ophthalmitis *(of-thal-mi'-tis)* [G. *ophthalmos,* eye; *-itis,* inflammation]. Syn., ophthalmia (q.v.).

ورم چشم : آفتھلمیا

Ophthalmologist *(of-thal-mol'-o-jist)* One who studies ophthalmology

ماہر عینیات : آفتھلمولوجی کا ماہر۔

Ophthalmology *(of-thal-mol'-o-ji)* [G. *opthalmos,* eye; *logos,* discourse]. The science which deals with the structure, function and disaeses of the eye--ophthalmological, adj.; ophthalmologically, adv.

عینیات : سائنس جو آنکھ کی ساخت، فعل اور بیماریوں کے متعلق بحث کرتی ہے۔

Ophthalmoplegia *(of-thal-mo-ple-ji-a)* [G. *ophthalmos,* eye; *plege,* stroke]. Paralysis of the eye muscles--op- hthalmoplegic, adj.

فالج چشم : آنکھ کے عضلات کی اینٹھن۔

Opthalmoscope *(of-thal-mo-skop)* [G. *ophthalmos,* eye; *skopein,* to examine]. An instrument fitted with a lens and illumination for examining the interior of the eye--ophthalmoscopic, *adj.*

شبکیہ بین : آنکھ کے اندرونی حصے کے معائنہ کے لئے عدسہ اور روشنی

کے ساتھ ایک آلہ۔

Ophthalmotonometer *(of-thal-mo- ton-om-eter).* Instrument for determining the intraocular press- ure.

قیاس تو ترالعین: انترا آ کولر دباؤ کی تعین کے لئے ایک آلہ۔

Opisthotonos *(op-is-thot-on-os)* [G. *opisthen,* behind; *tonos,* tension]. Extreme extension of the body occurring in tetanic spasm. Patient may be supported on his heels and his head alone--opisthotonic, *adj.*

کزاز عضلات ظہر: جسم کا انتہائی بڑھاؤ۔

Opium *(o'-pi-um).* Dried juice of o. poppy capsules. Contains morphine, codeine and other alkaloids. Valuable analgesic, but more constipating than morphine (q.v.). Also used as tincture of o. and as paregoric (camphorated tincture of o.).

افیم۔افیون: خشخاش کے غیر پختہ پھلوں سے خشک کیا ہوا دودھیا رس۔اس میں کئی الکائڈز ہوتے ہیں جن میں مارفین، فارسین اور کوڈین شامل ہیں۔

Opoidine *(op-oy-din).* Papaveretum (q.v.)

اوپائیڈین: پاپاورٹیم۔

Opportunistik infection A serious infection with a micro-organism which normally has little or no pathogenic activity but which has been activated by a serious disease or by a modern method of treatment.

موقعہ پرست چھوت: خورد جسیے کے ساتھ ایک تشویشناک بیماری۔

Opsonic index *(op-son-ik-in-deks)* [G. *opsonion,* provi- sions; L.*index,* a pointer]. A figure obtained by experiment which indicates the ability of ph agocytes to ingest foreign bodies such as bacteria.

نمائندہ اپسونین: تجربہ سے حاصل کردہ خاکہ جو بیرونی اجسام مثلاً جراثیم کو نگلنے کی فیگو سائٹس کی قابلیت ظاہر کرتا ہے۔

Opsonin *(op-son-in)* [G. *opsonion,* provisions]. An antibody which unites with antigen, usually part of intact cells, and renders the cells more susceptible to phagocytosis. See ANTIODIES opsonic, *adj.*

اپسونین: اینٹی باڈی جو اینٹی جن کے ساتھ ملتی ہے۔

Optic *(op-tik)* [G. *optikos,* of sight]. Pertaining to sight. **optic chiasma,** the X-shaped crossing of the fibres of the o. neve. **optic disc,** the point where the o. nerve ent- ers the eyeball.

نظری۔بصری: بینائی سے متعلق۔بصری عصب یا آپٹک نرو کی لمبائی قریبا چار سنٹی میٹر ہے۔ایسا شخص جو انعطافی غلطیوں کو ٹھیک کرنے کے لئے شیشے تجویز کرتا ہے۔

Optician *(op-ti'-shun)* [G.*optikos,* of sight]. One who pres- cribes glasses to correct refractive errors.

عینک ساز: ایسا شخص جو انعطافی غلطیوں کو ٹھیک کرنے کے لئے شیشے تجویز کرتا ہے۔

Optics *(op'-tiks)* [G. *opitkos,* of sight]. The branch of physics which deals with light rays and their relation to vision.

مناظریات: طبعیات کی وہ شاخ جو نوری شعاعوں اور ان کے نگاہ سے تعلق کے ساتھ بحث کرتی ہے۔

Optimax *(op'-ti-maks).* L-tryptophan with pryridoxine and ascorbic acid. Amino acid and vitamin preparation.

Optimum *(op'-tim-um)* [L.*optmus,* best]. Most favourable. optimum position, that which will be least awkward and most useful should a limb remain permanently para- lysed.

صحیح: سب سے زیادہ مناسب

Optometry *(op-tom'-et-ri)* [G. *optikos,* of sight; *metron,* a measure]. Measurement of visual acuity.

بصارت پیمائی: بصری اکوئٹی کی پیمائش۔

Orabase *(or'-a-bas).* Ointment; protects lesions on mucous membranes. **adeortyl in o.** (triamcinalone emolient), useful for mouth ulcers.

Oral *(o-ral)* [L. *os,* mouth]. Pertaining to the mouth orally, *adv.*

دہنی: منہ کے متعلق۔

Oratrol *(or-a-trol).* Dichlorphenamide (q.v.)

اوراٹرول: ڈائی کلورفینامائیڈ۔

Orbenin Cloxacillin (q.v.)

اوربلنیں: کلوکساسلین۔سپٹی سیمیا میں اس کا ٹیکہ مفید ہے۔ٹیکے۔کیپسول اور شربت دستیاب عام پنسلین سے زیادہ موثر۔نمونیا وغیرہ اور پھنسی پھوڑے

میں مفید۔

)rbicular *(or-bik'-u-lar)* [L. *orbicularis,* circular]. Rese- mbling the eyeball and its appendages--orbital, *adj.*

مستدیر: گلوب میں مشابہ۔کروی یا گول۔

)rbit *(or-bit)* [L. *orbita,* circuit]. The bony socket cont- aining the eyeball and its appendages--orbital, *adj.*

کاسہ چشم: آنکھ کا گولا اور اس کے زوائد پر مشتمل استخوانی ساکٹ۔

)rchidectomy *(or-ki-dek-to-mi)* [G. *orchis,* testis; *ektome,* excision]. Excision of a testicle.

خصیہ براری: خصیے کا کاٹ کر علیحدہ کرنا۔

)rchidopexy *(or-ki-do-pek-si)* [G. *orchis,* testicle; *pexis,* a fixing]. The operation of bringing an undescended testicle into the scrotum, and fixing it in this position.

خصیہ دوزی: ایسا خصیہ جو نیچے نہ اترا ہوا سے سکروٹم میں لانے کا اپریشن اور اسے اسی پوزیشن میں قائم رکھنا۔

)rchis *(or-kis)* [G.]. The testicle.

جنس سلحب: خصیہ۔فوطہ

)rchitis *(or-ki-tis)* [G. *orchis,* testicle; *-itis,* inflamma- tion]. Inflammation of the testicle.

)rciprenaline sulphate *(or-si-pren-a-lin-sul-tate).* Relax- ant for relief of bronchospasm. A derivative of adre- naline. Available as tablets or aerosol.

اورسی پرینالین سلفیٹ: برانکو سپازم کے آرام کے لئے دوا۔ایڈز ینالین سے حاصل شدہ۔

)rf. Skin lesions caused by a virus of sheep.

اورف: بھیڑوں سے انسان میں منتقل ہونے والا امراض بخار اور جوڑوں کا درد۔خون کی کمی اور جلد کا ٹھنا۔

)rganic *(or-gan'-ik).* Pertaining to an organ. Associated with life. **organic disease.** one in which there is struc- tural change.

عضوی: عضو سے متعلق۔حیات کے ساتھ تعلق۔

)rganism *(or'-gan-izm)* [G. *organon,* tool]. A living cell or group of cells differentiated into functionally distinct parts which are interdependent.

جسمیہ: جاندار شے۔جاندار یا پودہ۔

Orgasm *(or-gazm)* [G. orgasmos]. The crisis of sexual excitement.

انزال: جنسی جوش کا نقطہ عروج۔

Oriental sore *(o-ri-en'-tal sor).* Delhi boil. A form of cut- aneous leishmaniasis producing papular, crusted, gran- ulomatous eruptions of the skin. A disease of the tropics ad subtropics.

مغلی پھوڑا: جلد کا پھٹ کر آبلے بنانا۔

Orientation *(or-i-en-ta'-shun).* Clear awareness of one's position relative to the environment. In mental condi- toins o. 'in space and time' means that the patient knows where he is and recognizes the passage of time, i.e. can give the correct date. Disorientation means the reverse.

سمت بندی: ماحول کی نسبت سے اپنی پوزیشن کی واضح آگہی۔

Orifice *(or'-i-fis)* [L. *orificium,* opening]. A mouth or ope- ning.

روزن: منہ یا سوراخ۔شگاف۔گزرگاہ

Origin *(or-i-jin)* [L. *origo*]. The commencement or source of anything. **origin of a muscle,** the end that remains relatively fixed during contraction of the muscle.

مبدا۔آغاز۔ماخوذ: کسی چیز کا وقوع پذیر ہونا یا اس کی اصل یا مخرج۔ جائے اجزاء۔

Orinasee *(o'-rin-az).* Tolbutamide (q.v.)

اوری نیز: ٹولبوٹامائیڈ۔

Ornithine *(or'-ni-then).* An amino acid, obtained from ar- ginine, by splitting off urea.

آرنی تھین: یوریا کے پھٹنے سے آرجینین سے حاصل شدہ ایک امینوایسڈ۔

Ornithosis *(or-ni-thos'-sis)* [G. *ornis,* bird; *-osis,* cond- ition]. Human illness resulting from disease of birds.

اورنی تھوسس: پرندوں کی بیماری کے نتیجہ میں انسانی زندگی۔

Orogenital *(or-o-jen'-it-al)* [L. *os,* mouth; G. *genesis,* descent]. Pertaining to the mouth and the external gen- ital area.

دہنی تولیدی: منہ اور بیرونی تولیدی ایریا سے متعلق۔

Oropharynx *(or-o-far-inks)* [L. *os,* mouth; G. *pharygx,* pharynx]. 1. That portion of the pharynx which is below the level of the soft palate and above the level of the hyoid bone. 2. Pertaining to the mouth and pharynx--oroharyngeal, *adj*.

حلق۔گلا: فیرنکس کا وہ حصہ جو نرم پلیٹ کے لیول سے نیچے اور ہائی آئڈ ہڈی کے لیول سے اوپر ہے۔ ۲۔منہ اور فیرنکس سے متعلق۔

Oroya fever See BARTONELLA-FEVER.

اوریا بخار: برٹونیلا بخار۔

Orphenadrine *(or-fen'-a-dren)*. Tablets which counteract any tendency to Parkinsonism produced by tranquillizers. Sometimes useful in incontinence of urine.

آرفینڈرین: گولیاں جو سکون بخش ادویات سے پیدا شدہ پارکنسونزم کے رجحان کو زائل کرتی ہیں۔بعض اوقات پیشاب کے اعتدالی میں مفید۔

Orthocaine *(or'-tho-kan)*. Local anaesthetic similar to benzocaine (q.v.)

آرتھوکین: بنزوکین سے مشابہ مقامی طور پر سن کرنے والی دوا۔

Orthodontic *(or-tho-don'-tik)* [G. *orthos*, straight; *odous*, tooth]. A branch of dentistry dealing with prevention and correction of irregularities of the teeth.

آرتھوڈونٹک: دندان سازی کی ایک شاخ جو کولوموٹر نظام کو متاثر کرنے والی تمام حالتوں کے ساتھ بحث کرتی ہے۔

Orthopaedics *(or-tho-pe-diks)* [G. *orthos*, straight; *pais*, child]. Formerly devoted to the correction of defromities in children. It is now a branch of surgery dealing with all conditions affecting the locomotor system, whether by apparatus, maniplation or operation.

تقویم الاعضائیات: سانس پھولنا۔

Orthopnoea *(or-thop-ne'-a)* [G. *orhtos*, straight; *pnoe*, breath]. Breathlessness necessitating an upright, sitting position for its relief--orthopnoeic, *adj*.

وضعی ضیق النفس: آنکھ کے غیر عضلاتی غیر متوازن ہونے کا علاج و مطالعہ۔

Orthoptics *(or-thop-tiks)* [G. *orthos*, straight; *optikos*, optic]. Study and treatment of muscle imbalances of eye (squint).

علم التقویم البصر: آنکھ کے عضلاتی غیر متوازن ہونے کا علاج ومطالعہ۔

Orthostatic *(or-tho-stat-ik)* [G. *orthos*, straigh *statikos*, causing to stand]. Caused by th uprihgt stance . **ortho- static albuminuri** occurs in some healthy subjects ony when th take the upright position. When lying in be the urine is normal.

تادہ وضعی: یہ مرض بالکل سیدھا کھڑا رہنے سے ہوتا ہے۔

Orthotic *(or-thot-ik)* [G. *orthos*, straight]. Ar device app- lied to or around the body in th care of physical impairment or disability.

Ortolani's sign *(or-to-lan'-iz)*. Test performe shortly after birth to discern dislocation of th hip.

Os [L.]. A mouth. external o., the opening of th cervix into the vagina. internal o., the openi of the cervix into the uterine cavity--ora, pl.

Osicalcis calcaneu

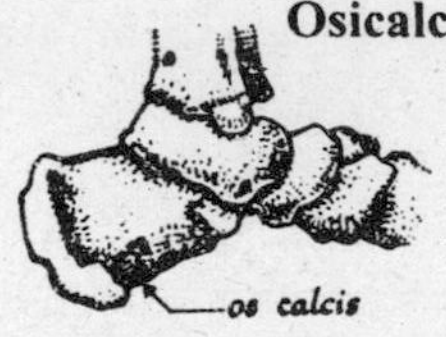

لم۔ہڈی: منہ۔

Oscillation *(os-il-a-shun)* [L. *oscillare*, swing]. A swinging or moving to and fro; vibration.

زاز: ادھر ادھر حرکت کرنا یا جھولنا۔ارتعاش۔دائیں بائیں جھولنے کی ت۔

Oscillometry *(os-il-om-et-ri)* [L. *oscillare*, swing; G. *metron*, a measure]. Measureme of vibration, using special apparat (oscillometer, osciloscope). Measures t magnitude of the pulse wave more precise than palpation.

عاشی پیمائش: مخصوص سامان کے ارتعاش کی پیمائش استعمال۔

Osler's nodes Small painful areas (due emboli) in pulp of fringers or toes, or pal and soles, occurring in sub- acute bacteri endocarditis. [William Osler, Engli physician (Candian birth), 1849-1919.].

آسلری گرہیں : ہتھیلیوں اور ایڑھیوں یا پاؤں اور ہاتھوں کی انگلیوں کے گوشت میں چھوٹے درد والے حصے۔

Osmolarity *(os-mo-lar-i-ti)* [G. *osmos,* impulse]. The osmotic pressure exerted by a substance in aqueous solution, defined in terms of the number of active parti- cles per unit volume.

نفوذیت : اکائی حجم میں عامل ذرات کی تعداد۔ آبی محلول میں کسی شے کا نفوذی دباؤ۔

Osmosis *(os-mo-sis)* [G. *osmos,* impulse]. The passage of water across a membrane under the influence of osmotic pressure.

عمل نفوذ۔ دلوج : نیم مسامدار جھلی میں سے محلل کی پراگندگی کا عمل۔ دراصل پراگندگی عمل نفوذ ہے لیکن خیال رہے کہ عمل نفوذ میں محلل کی پراگندگی ہوتی ہے۔ نہ کہ مخل کی اگر محلل پانی ہو تو پانی کی پراگندگی عمل نفوذ ہے۔ اندرونی پراگندگی کو داخلی نفوذ اور بیرونی پراگندگی کو خارجی نفوذ کہتے ہیں۔

Osmotic pressure *(os-mot-ik).* The pressure with which sodium chloride, sugars, urea and many other substances in solution draw water across a membrane, which allows the molecules of water to pass through, but which is relatively impermeable or semipermeable to other molecules.

نفوذی دباؤ : نفوذی دباؤ وہ دباؤ ہوتا ہے جو کسی محلول میں محلل کو نیم مسامدار جھلی کے ذریعے علیحدہ کرنے سے پیدا ہوتا ہے۔ پانی کی سطح بلند ہوتی ہے۔ پانی کی سطح بلند ہوتی ہے۔ نفوذی دباؤ کہلاتی ہے کسی محلول کے ارتکاز میں زیادتی سے نفوذی دباؤ میں بھی زیادہ ہو جاتا ہے۔ یہ محل کے ذرات کی تعداد پر منحصر ہوتا ہے۔ درجہ حرارت کے بڑھنے کے ساتھ ساتھ نفوذی دباؤ بھی بڑھتا ہے۔

Ospolot *(os'-pol-ot).* Sulthiame (q.v.)

اسپولاٹ : سلتھی ایم۔

Osset us *(os'-e-us)* [L. *osseus,* of bone]. bones, particularly those contained in the middle ear; the malleus, incus and stapes.

عظمی۔ استخوانی : ہڈی سے مشابہ یا متعلق۔

Ossicles *(os-ik-ls)* [L. *os.* bone]. Sma'' bones, particularly those contained in the middle ear; the mallus, incus and stapes.

کان کی چھوٹی ہڈی : چھوٹی ہڈیاں۔ خصوصاً درمیانی کان کی یعنی میلیس انکس اور سٹیپز۔

Ossification *(os-if-i-ka'-shun)* [L. *os,* bone; *facere,* to make]. The converstion of cartilage, etc. into bone-- os- sify, v.t., v.i.

ہڈی سازی : کارٹیلیج وغیرہ کی ہڈی میں تبدیلی۔

Osteitis *(os-te-i'-tis)* [L. *osteon,* bone *-itis,* inflammation]. Inflammation of bone. **osteitis deformans,** Paget's disease (q.v.) **osteitis fibrosa.** cavities form in the interior of bone. Cysts may be solitary or the disease generalized. Ths second condition is the result of exc- essive parathroid secretion and absorption of calcium from bone.

ورم عظم : ہڈی کی سوزش۔

Osteoarthritis *(os-te-o-arth-ri'-tis)* [G. *osteon,* bone; *arthron,* joint; *-itis,* inflammation]. Degenerative arth- ritis; may be primary, or may follow injury or disease involving the articular surfaces os synovial joints. The articular cartilage becomes worn, osteophytes form at the periphery of the joint surface and loose bodies may result--osteoarthritic, *adj.*

ورم مفصل و عظم : معدوس آرتھرٹیس۔

Osteoarthritis

ورم مفصل و عظم : جوڑوں کا مرض جو ۴۰ سال کی عمر کے بعد ہوتا ہے۔ عموماً موٹوں کو ہوتا ہے۔ ہڈیوں کے سرے گھس کر رگڑ کھاتے ہیں۔ فینائل بیوٹازون اور پریڈنی سولون مفید ہیں۔

Osteoblast *(os'-te-o-blast)* [G. *osteon,* bone;

blastos, ge- rm]. A bone-forming cellost-eoblastic, *adj.*

عظم ساز خلیہ : ہڈی بنانے والا خلیہ۔

Osteochondritis *(os-te-o-kon-dri'-tis)* [G. *osteon,* bone; *chondros,* cartilage; *-itis,* inflammation]. Originally an inflammation of one cartilage. Usually applied to non-- septic conditoins, especially avascular necrosis involv- ing joint surfaces, e.g. osteochondritis dissecans in whi- ch a portion of joint surface may separate to form a loo- se body in the joint. See SCHEUERMANS'S DISEA- SE.

التہاب عظمی وغضروفی: ہڈی اور کارٹیلج کی سوزش۔ دافع تعفن حالتیں۔

Osteochondroma *(os-te-o-kon-dro'-ma)* [G. *osteon,* bone; *chondros,* cartilage; *-oma,* tumour]. A benign bony and cartilaginous tumour.

ہڈی یا کارٹیلج کی رسولی:

Osteoclasis *(os-te-o-kla'-sis)* [G. *osteon,* bone; *klasis,* a breaking]. The therapeutic fracutre of a bone.

قطع عظم : ہڈی کا تھراپیوٹک فریکچر۔ ہڈیوں میں ٹوٹ پھوٹ کا عمل۔

Osteoclast *(os'-te-o-klast)* [G. *osteon,* bone; *klastos,* broken]. Bone destroyer; the cell which dissolves or removes unwanted bone.

قاطع عظم آلہ۔ مخرب عظم خلیہ : ہڈی کو تباہ کرنے والا۔ خلیہ جو غیر ضروری ہڈی کو ختم یا حل کرتا ہے۔

Osteoclastoma *(os-te-o-klas-to'-ma)* [G. *osteon,* bone; *klastos,* broken; *-oma,* tumour]. A tumour of the osteoclasts. May be benign, locally recurrent, or frankly malignant. The usual site is near the end of a long bone. See MYELOMA.

سلعہ عظمی: اوسٹیوکلاسٹس کی رسولی۔

Osteocyte *(os-te-o-sit)* [G. *osteon,* bone; *kytos,* cell]. A bo- ne cell.

آسٹیوسائیٹ : استخوانی خلیہ۔

Osteodystrophy *(os-te-o-dis-fro-fi)* [G. *osteon,* bone; *dys,* bad; *trophe,* nourishment]. Faulty growth of bone.

آسٹیوڈس ٹرافی: ہڈی کی ناقص نشو ونما۔

Osteogenic *(os-te-o-jen-ik)* [G. *osteon,* bone; *genesis,* descent]. Bone-producing. osteogenic sarcoma, malignant tumour originating in cells which normally produce bone.

آسٹیوجینک : ہڈی بنانے والی۔

Osteolytic *(os-te-o-lit'-ik)* [G. *osteon,* bone; *lysts,* a loosening]. Destructive of bone, e.g. osteolytic malign- ant deposits in bone.

آسٹیولائیٹ : ہڈی کو تباہ کرنے والا۔

Osteoma *(os-te-o'-ma)* [G. *osteon,* bone; *-oma,* tumour]. A tumour. (1) compact (ivory o.) (2) cancellous. May be single or multiple.

عظمی سلعہ : استخوانی رسولی۔

Osteomalacia *(os-te-o-mal-a'-se-a)* [G. *osteon,* bone; *malakia,* softness]. Infectious mineralization of the mature skeleton, with softening and bone pain. It is commonly caused by insufficient dietary intake of vitamin D.

ملاست عظام: کیلشیم اور فاسفیٹ کے زائد انجذاب کی وجہ سے نرم ہڈی۔

Osteomyelitis *(os-te-o-mi-el-i'-tis)* [G. *esteon,* bone; *myelos,* marrow; *-itis,* inflammation]. Inflammation commencing in the marrow of bone--osteomyelitic, *adj.*

ورم نخاع العظم : ہڈی کے مغز میں سوزش۔ یہ ایکوٹ یا کرانک ہوتی ہے۔

Osteopath *(os'-te-o-path)* [G. *osteon,* bone; *pathos,* dise- ase]. One who practises osteopathy.

عظم بند۔ مالشی جراح: ہڈیوں کی بیماریوں کا ماہر۔

Osteopathy *(os-te-op'-a-thi)* [G. *osteon,* bone; *pathos,* disease]. 1. Any disease of bone. 2. A theory which attributes a wide range of disorders to mechanical derangements of the skeletal system, which it is claimed can be rectified by suitable manipulations. Usually practised by medically unqualified persons--osteop- athic, *adj.*

مالشی علاج۔ دستی جراحی: ہڈی کی کوئی بیماری اور اس کا علاج۔

Osteopetrosis *(os-te-o-pet-ro'-sis)* [G. *osteon,* bone; *petros,* stone; *-osis,* condition]. See ALBERS SCHONBERG DISEASE.

مرمری ہڈیاں: مرض البرزشونبرک۔

Osteophony *(os-te-of-on-i)* [G. *osteon,* bone; *phone,* sound]. The conduction of sound waves to the inner ear by bone.

انتقال الصوت عظامی: صوتی لہروں کی اندرونی کان کی طرف ہڈی سے ترسیل۔

Osteophyte *(os'-te-o-fit)* [G. *osteon,* bone; *phyton,* plant]. A bony outgrowth or spur, usually at the margins of joint surfacs, e.g. in osteoarthritis--osteophytic, *adj.*

ہڈی کا ابھار: استخوانی بڑھاؤ۔عموماً جوڑ کی طرح کے کناروں پر ہوتا ہے۔

Osteoplasty *(os'-te-o-plas-ti)* [G. *osteon,* bone; *plassein,* to form]. Any plastic operation on bone--osteoplastic, *adj.*

عظم پیوندی: ہڈی پر کوئی پلاسٹک اپریشن۔

Osteosclerosis *(os-te-o-por-o'-sis)* [G. *osteon,* bone; *poron,* passage; *-osis,* condition]. Loss of bone density due to excessive absorption of calcium and phosphorus from the bone, due to progressive loss of the protein matrix of bone which normally carries the calcium deposits--osteoporotic, *adj.*

آسٹیوپوروسس: ہڈی سے فاسفورس اور کیلشیم کے زائد انجذاب کی وجہ سے استخوانی کثافت کا ضیاع۔

Osteosarcoma *(os-te-o-sar-ko'-ma)* [G. *osteon,* bone; *sarkoma,* fleshly overgrowth]. A sarcomatous tumour growing from bone--osteosarcomata, pl.; osteosarcomatous, *adj.*

ہڈی کا ورم: ہڈی سے اگنے والی گودے دار رسولی۔

Osteoporosis *(os-te-o-skle-ro'-sis)* [G. *osteon,* bone; *skle- rosis,* hardening]. Increased density or hardness of bone --osteosclerotic, *adj.*

تصلب العظام: ہڈی کی بڑھتی ہوئی سختی۔

Osteotome *(os'-te-ot-om)* [G. *osteon,* bone; *tomos,* cutting]. An instrument for cutting bone; it is similar to a chisel, ut it is bevelled on both sides of its cutting edge.

Osteotome

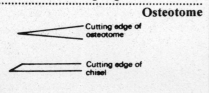

عظم تراش: ہڈی کا کاٹنے کا آلہ۔

Osteotomy *(os'-te-ot-om-i)* [G. *osteon,* bone; *tome,* a cutting]. Division of bone. **McMurray's o.,** division of femur between lesser and greater trochanter. Shaft displaced inwards beneath the head and abducted. This position maintained by a nail plate. Restores painless weight bearing. In congenital dislocation of hip, deliberate peivic o. reners the outer part of the socket (acetabulum) more horizontal. Pelvic o. now preferred to the shelf operation to provide a better roof at the acetabulum.

عظم تراشی: ہڈی کی تقسیم۔

Osteotomy

Ostium *(os'-ti-um)* [L.] The opening or mouth of any tub- ular passage--ostial, *adj.;* ostia, *pl.*

دہانچہ اسفج: کسی نلی نما راستے کا سوراخ یا منہ۔

Otalgia *(o-tal'-ji-a)* [G. *ous,* ear; *algos,* pain]. Earache.

کان کا درد: کان میں درد ہونا۔

Otitis *(o-ti'-tis)* [G. *ous,* ear; *-itis,* inflammation]. Inflam- mation of the ear. otitis externa, inflammation of the skin of the external auditory canal. **otitis intena,** see LABYR-

INTHITIS. otitis media, inflam- mation of the middle ear cavity. The effusion tends to be of a serious neture in adults; and of a mucous nature in children, giveing rise to the label 'glue ear'--otitic, *adj*.

ورم اذن: کان کی سوزش یا سوجن۔

Otolaryngology *(o-to-lar-in-gol'-o-ji)* [G. *ous,* ear; *tarygx,* larynx; *logos,* discourse]. The scince which deals with the structure, function and diseases of the ear and lary- nx.

اوٹولیرنگولوجی: سائنس جو کان اور لیرنکس کی ساخت، فعل اور امراض سے بحث کرتی ہے۔

Otoliths *(o'-to-liths)* [G. *ous,* ear; *lithos,* stone]. Tiny calcareous deposits within the membranous labyrinth of the internal ear.

حصاۃ الاذن: اندرونی کان کے جھلی دار لیبرنتھ کے اندر مواد۔

Otologist *(o-tol'-oj-ist)* [G. *ous,* ear; *logos,* discourse]. One specializing in the functions and diseases of the ear.

اذنیات دان: کان کے امراض و افعال میں ماہر کان کی امراض کا معالج۔

Otology *(o-tol'-o-ji)* [G. *ous,* ear; *logos,* discourse]. The science which deals with the structure, function and dis- eases of the ear.

اذنیات: سائنس جو کان کی ساخت، فعل اور امراض سے بحث کرتی ہے۔

Otomycosis *(o-to-mi-ko-sis)* [G. *ous,* ear; *mykes,* fungus; *-osis,* condition]. A fungal (Aspergillus, Candida) infectin of the external auditory meatus--otomycotic, *adj*.

اوٹومائی کوسس: بیرونی سمعی میٹس کا سماروغی مرض۔

Otorhinolaryngology *(o-to-ri-no-lar-in-gol'-o-ji)* [G. *ous,* ear; *rhis,* nose; *larygx,* larynx; *logos,* discourse]. The science which deals with the structure, function and diseases of the ear, nose and throat.

اذنخبریات: سائنس جو کان، ناک اور گلے کی ساخت فعل اور امراض کے متعلق بحث کرتی ہے علم امراض کان۔ ناک و گلو۔

Otorrhoea *(o-to-re'-a)* [G. *out,* ear; *rheein,* to flow]. A discharge from the external auditory meatus.

کان بہنا: بیرونی سمعی میٹیس سے ڈسچارج۔

Otosclerosis *(o-to'-skler-o-sis)* [G. *out,* ear; *sklerosis,* hardening]. New bone formatio affecting primarily the labyrinth of the inne ear and a common cause of progressiv deafness--otosclerotic, *adj*.

ملابت کان: نئی استخوانی بناوٹ جو اندرونی کان کی لیبرنتھ کو متاثر کرتی ہے اور بڑھے ہوئے بہرہ پن کی وجہ بنتی ہے۔

Ototoxic *(o-to-tok'-sik)* [G. *ous,* ear; *toxikon,* posion]. Having a toxic action on the ear.

وٹوٹیکسک: کان پر زہریلا ایکشن رکھنا۔

Ouabaine *(oo'-a-ban)* A cardiac glycoside. Like digoxin, it has a steadying effect on the heart.

Ova *(o'-va)* [L.]. The female reproductive cells--ovum, sing.

بیض (واحد بیضہ) بیضے: مادہ تولیدی خلیے۔ اودم حمل کے پہلے تین ہفتوں کے بیضہ کو کہتے ہیں رحم کے خصیے ایک ماہ میں صرف ایک بیضہ پیدا کرتے ہیں۔ جب یہ خارج ہوتا ہے تو فلوپین میں چلا جاتا ہے جہاں اسے باریک سلوٹیں (رحم کی) طرف دھکیلتی ہیں۔ اور یہ رحم کے منہ تک پہنچ جاتا ہے۔

Ovabain *(o'-va-ban).* Glycoside of digitalis.

ووابین: ڈجیٹیلس کا گلائیکوسائیڈ۔

Ovarian *(o-va'-ri-an)* [N.L. *ovarium,* egg] Pertaining to the ovaries, **ovarian cyst,** a ovarian tumour containing fluid--may b benign or malignant.

مبیضی: بیضہ دانوں سے متعلق۔

Ovariectomy *(o-ve-ri-ek'-to-mi)* [N.L. *ovarium* egg; *ektome,* excision]. Excision of an ovary Oopherectomy.

قطع المبیض: بیضہ دان کو کاٹ کر علیحدہ کر دینا۔

Ovariotomy *(o-ve-ri-ot'-om-i)* [N.L. *ovarium* egg; G. *tome,* cutting]. Literally mean incision of an ovary, but is the term usuall upplied to the removal of an ovary. Als OOPHORECTOMY.

مبیض شگافی: بیضہ دان نکالنا۔

Ovaritis *(o-ve-ri'-tis).* Oophoritis (q.v.)

ورم مبیض: اووفورئیٹس۔

Ovary *(o'-ver-i)* [N.L. *ovarium,* egg]. One o two small oval bodies situated on either sid of the uterus on the posterior surface of th broad ligament. The structures in which th ova re developed--ovarian, adj. **systic o.** rarely larger than a plum. Cysts contair oestrogenrich fluid. Causes menorrhagia.

بیضہ دانی۔خصیۃ الرحم : بیضہ دانیاں رحم کی دونوں جانب واقع ہوتی ہیں۔اس میں اللہ کی طرف بچہ یا جنین پیدا کرنے والا مادہ یا تخم پیدا ہوتا ہے جسے بیضہ کہتے ہیں۔ بیضوی شکل کی۔ بیضہ انثی عورت کے خصیۃ الرحم میں مہینے میں صرف ایک بار پیدا ہوتا ہے۔ جو قاذف نالی میں سفر کرتا ہوا رحم کی طرف اترتا ہے تاکہ مرد کے تولیدی مادہ مل کر حمل کا سبب بنے۔

'ercompensation *(o-ver-kom-pen-sa'-shun).* Name given to any type of behviour which a person adopts in order to cover up a deficiency in his personality, of which he is a ware. Thus a person who is afraid may react by becomng arrogant or boastful or quarrelsome.

اوور کمپنسیشن : اپنی شخصیت میں کمی کو پورا کرنے کے لئے کسی شخص کا رویہ۔ وہ ناراض، شیخی خور یا جھگڑالو ہوتا ہے۔

iduct *(o'-vi-dukt).* Syn., Fallopian tube (q.v.).

بیض نالی۔بیض قنات : نالی جس کے ذریعے بیضے، بیضہ دانیاں سے بیرونی جانب آتے ہیں۔فلوپین ٹیوب۔

ulation *(ov-u-la'-shun)* [L. *ovum,* egg]. The maturation and rupture of a Graafian follicle (q.v.) with the discharge of an ovum.

انڈے دینا۔بیض ریزی : بیضہ دانی کی جھلی سے تختہ بیضہ کا پھٹ کر نکلنا۔

acillin *(oks'-a-sil-in).* See FLUCLOX- ACILLIN.

آکساسلین : فلوکلوکساسلین۔

alate *(oks'-al-at).* Any salt of oxalicacid.

نمک ترش : ترشک کے تیزاب کا ایسڈ یا نمک۔

aluria *(oks-al-u'-ri-a)* [G. *oxalis,* garden *orrel;* ouron, urine]. Excretion of urine ontaining calcium oxalate crystals; ssociated often with dyspepsia.

ترشک بولی : کیلشیم اکسلیٹ کی قلموں پر مشتمل پیشاب کا اخراج۔

azepam *(oks-az'-e-pam).* Mild tranquillizer.

آکسازیپام : ہلکی سکون بخش دوائی فیل بوونیم۔

bile Fel bovinum (q.v.)

فیل بوونیم۔

ford inflator. A hand-operated bellows ttached to a face mask for emergency rtifical respiration.

آکسفورڈ دھونکنی : فوری مصنوعی تنفس کے لئے چہرے کے ماسک کے ساتھ ملحق ہاتھ سے کام کرنے والی دھونکنی۔

Oxidase *(oks-ے-i-das).* Any enzyme which promotes oxidation.

تکسیدیہ۔آکسی ڈیز : خامرہ جس سے تکسید ہوتی ہے۔

Oxidation *(oks-i-da-ے-shun).* The process of converting a substance into an oxide by the addition of oxygen. The carbon in organic compounds undergoes oxidation with the formation of carbon dioxide when they are combusted in air, or when they are metabolized in living material in the presence of oxygen. Also used in biochemistry for the process of the removal of hydrogen from a molecule (e.g. in the presence of air ascorbic acid undegoes o. with the formation of dehydroascorbic acid). The loss of an electron with an increase in valency (e.g. the conversion of ferrous to ferric iron) is also an oxidation. The greater part of the energy present in foods is made available to the body by the processes of o. in the tissues.

عمل تکسید : عمل تکسید میں آکسیجن کیمیائی طور پر مل کر نامیاتی مرکبات کی بوسیدگی کرتی ہے۔اس عمل میں توانائی کی کافی مقدار حاصل ہوتی ہے۔مثلاً تنفس کسی شے کو آکسیجن کی زیادتی سے آکسائیڈ میں تبدیل کرنے کا عمل۔

Oxycel *(oks-ے-i-sel).* This is oxidized cellulose, and is a useful haemostatic for plugging wounds when suturing is difficult. The material is subsequently is at a high pressure. See HYPERBARIC.

آکسیجن۔نسیم : ایک بے رنگ۔بے بو عنصر گیس۔حیات اور احتراق کے لئے لازمی۔علاج کے لئے سانس کے ذریعے آکسیجن اندر بھیجی جاتی ہے۔یہ گیس سلنڈروں میں مہیا کی جاتی ہے۔جن میں یہ زیادہ دباؤ پر ہوتی ہے۔

Oxygenation *(oks-i-jen-a-ے-shun).* The saturation of a substance (particularly blood) with oxygen--oxygenated, *adj.*

تکسید۔ترویج : کسی شے (خصوصاً خون) کا آکسیجن سے سیری۔

Oxygenator *(oks-ij'-jen-a-tor).* Artificial 'lung' as used in heart surgery.

آکسیجنیٹر : دل کی سرجری میں مستعمل پھیپھڑوں۔

Oxyhaemoglobin *(oks-i-he-mo-gl'-bin).* Oxygenated hae- moglobin, an unstable compound.

آکسیجنی حمرۃ الدم: ایک غیر پائیدار مرکب جو تنفس میں ہیموگلوبن پر آکسیجن کے عمل سے بنتا ہے۔

Oxyntic *(oks-in'-tik)* [G. *oxynein,* to make acid]. Producing acid. **oxyntic cells,** the cells in the gastric mucosa which produce hydrochloric acid.

مفرز تیزاب: ایسڈ پیدا کرنا۔

Oxypertine *(oks-i-per'-ten).* Tranquillizer, useful in anxiety neuroses.

Oxyphenbutazone *(oks-i-fen-bu'-ta-zon).* Anti-inflammat- ory, analgesic, anti-arthritic drug. Available as supposit- ories.

آکسی فین بیوٹازون: ضد آتش گیر، دافع درد دوا۔

Oxytetracycline *(oks-i-tet-ra-si'-klin).* An orally effective antibiotic with a wide range of activity. May be given by slow intravenous injection in severe infecions. Prolo- nged use may cause mo
nilial overgrowth in the intest- inal tract.

آکسی ٹیڑا سائیکلین: موثر اینٹی بایوٹک ٹیڑا ساء سن۔ نفخ شکم یا فبلیولینس کے علاج کے لئے ایک کیپسول دن میں ۴ مرتبہ۔ نمونیا میں ایک ٹیکہ روزانہ صبح دوشام۔ ہر چھ گھنٹے بعد ایک کیپسول برائے غذائی سمیت اس کا آئی آئنمنٹ برائے سٹائی۔

Oxytocic *(oks-i-to'-sik)* [G. *oxys,* sharp; *tokos,* childbirth]. Hastening parturition; an agent promoting uterine contr- actions.

منقبض الرحم: ایک ایجنٹ جو رحم کو سکیڑتا ہے۔

Oxytocin *(oks-i-to'-sin).* One of the poster pituitary hormones. Contracts muscle in m ducts and hence causes milk enjection preparation of pituitary extract that can ca uterine contrations, and so is useful postpartum heaemorrhage. Given intra uscularly, subcutaneously, orally, nasally intravenously in titration method wit positive pressure peristaltic pump.

بض ہارمون: ظلفی پچوایٹری ہارمونوں میں کو سکڑتا ہے۔ اس طرح کا اخراج ہوتا ہے۔ رحم کو سیکڑتا ہے۔ اور اس طرح خون کی بندش میں مفید ھاتیوں میں دودھ کی کمی کے مرض میں اس کا ٹیکہ روزانہ تین یام تک ۔

Oxyuris *(ok-si-ur'-is).* Nematoded, commo called threadworms (q.v.)

ک: نیماٹوڈن جنہیں عموماً چرنے کہا جاتا ہے۔

Ozeana *(o-ze-na)* [G. *ozein,* to smell]. Atro condition of the nasal mucous membrane associated crusting and foetor.

زلہ: ناک کی میوکس جھلی کی اٹرافک حالت۔

Ozone *(o'-zon).* An allotropic form of oxyg O_2. Has powerful oxidizing properties an therefore a disinfe- ctant.

ن: آکسیجن کی ایک بہروپی قسم جس کے سالمے میں تین جواہر ہوتے ہیں یہ نگوں گیس ہے۔ کیمیائی طور پر بہت عامل، ایک طاقتور تکسیدی عامل، یہ عام امیں قلیل مقدار میں ہوتی ہے۔ ہوا اور پانی کو صاف کرنے کے لئے اور رنگ ٹنے کے لئے استعمال کی جاتی ہے۔

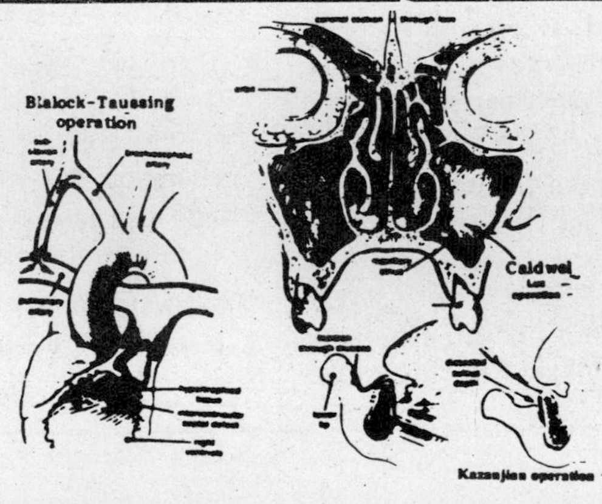

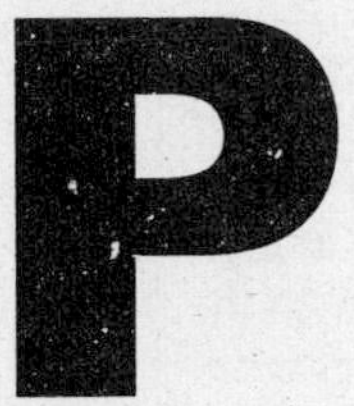

Symbol for phosphorous, para, posterior, pupil, power, pressure and probability.

پی: علامت ہے فاسفورس، پیرا، پچھلا، آنکھ کی پتلی، طاقت، دباؤ اور امکان کی۔

(pi') The sixteenth letter of Greek alphabet symbol for osmotic pressure.

پائی: یونانی حروف ابجد کا سولھواں حرف۔ اوسموٹک دباؤ کی علامت ہے۔

(fi') Phi. The twenty first letter of Greek alphabet.

فائی: یونانی حروف تہجی کا اکیسواں حرف۔

(si') Psi. The twenty third letter of Greek alphabet.

سائی: یونانی حروف ابجد کا تئیسواں حرف۔

ace-maker *(pa's ma'kar)* An object or substance that influences the rate at which a certain phenomenon occurs. The natural or artificial cardiac pace makers. A device that uses electrical impulses to reproduce or regulate the rhythons of hearrt.

achyblephron *(pak-e-blef-a-ron)* [G. *pachys,* thick; *blepharon,* eyelid]. A thickening of the eyelids chiefly near the border.

achycephaly *(pak-e-sef-a-le)* [G. *kephale,* head]. Abnormal thickness of the bones of skull, as in acromegaly.

achycheilia *(pak-e-kil-lea)* Thickening of the lips.

achydactyly *(pak-e-dak-til-ea)* [G. *daktylos,* fingers]. Abnormal thickening or enlargement of the fingers and toes.

دبیز انگشتی: ہاتھ اور پاؤں کی انگلیوں کا موٹا ہونا

Pachyglossia *(pak'-e-glose-a)* [G. *glossa,* tongue]. Abnormal thickness of the tongue.

دبیز زبان: زبان کا بہت زیادہ موٹا ہونا۔

Pachyonchia *(pak-e-o-nik-ea)* [G. *ony,* nail]. thickening of the nails.

دبیز ناخن: ناخن کا موٹا ہو جانا۔

Pack *(pa'k)* Treatment by wrapping a patient in blankets or sheets orr a limb in towels, wet or dry and either hot or cold, also the blankets, sheets or towels used for this purpose.

لپیٹنا: کسی مریض کو کمبل، چادر میں لپیٹ کر علاج کرنا۔ کسی ٹانگ کو تولیے، گیلے یا خشک گرم یا ٹھنڈے میں لپیٹ کر علاج کرنا۔ وہ چیزیں جو اس مقصد کے لئے استعمال کی جاتی ہیں۔

Pad *(pa'd)* A cushion like mass of soft material.

پیڈ: کسی نرم چیز کا، کشن کی طرح کی چیز۔

Paediatrics *(pe-de-at-riks)* The branch of medical science dealing with the disease of children.

Paget Schroethr syndrome *(pij-et-shra-tar-sin-drom)* [Sir James Paget, English surgeon 1814-1877]. Axillary or subclavian vein thrombosis, often associated with effort in fit young persons.

Paget's disease In this disease, alkaline phosphatase is in excess which causes a rapid bone formation and bone is thin.

Painter's colic Lead colic (q.v.).

رنگ ساز کا درد قولنج: لیڈ کولک۔ سیسے کا زہریلا پن۔ رنگ ساز کا درد

قولنج ۔ رنگ سازی کی صنعت کے ساتھ وابستہ افراد کے معدہ میں سیسے کا سفوف سانس کے ذریعے جا کر سمیت پیدا کرتا ہے. جس سے درد ہوتا ہے۔

Palate *(pal'-lat)* [L. *palatum*]. The roof of the mouth. artificial p., prosthesis for use in cleft palate. cleft p., a congenital cleft between the palatal bones, which leaves a gap in the roof of the mouth, opening directly into the nose. **hard p.,** the front part of the roof of the mouth formed by the two palatal bones. **soft p.,** situated at the posterior end of the p. and consisting of muscle covered by mucous membrane--palatal, palatine, *adj*.

Pharynx

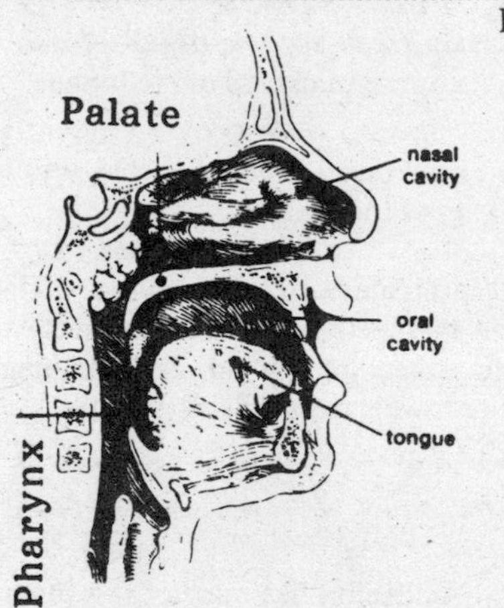

تالو ۔ منہ کی چھت ۔ تالو: منہ کا اوپری حصہ یعنی منہ کے اندر زبان کا بالائی گنبد نما ڈھانچہ۔ تالو کی ہڈیاں تعداد میں دو او. بالائی جبڑے کی ہڈیوں اور سیفنا ئڈ کے درمیان جڑی ہوئی ہیں۔ ان سے سخت تالو بنتا ہے۔

Palatoplegia *(pal-at-o-ple'-ji-a)* [L. *palatum,* palate, *plege,* stroke]. Parralysis of the soft palate--palat- oplegic, afj.

شلل حنگ: تالو سے متعلق۔

Palliative *(pal-i-a-tiv)* [L. *palliatus*, cloaked]. Any- thing which serves to alleviate but cannot cure a disease.

مسکن: درد کے آرام پہنچانے والی دوا لیکن بیماری کا علاج نہیں کرتی۔

Pallidectomy *(pal-id-ek-to-mi)* Destruction of a predetermined section of gloubs pallidus. See CHEMOPALLIDECTOMY and STER OTAXIS.

ں ڈیکٹومی: گلوس پلیڈس کے پہلے سے معین شدہ حصے کی تباہی۔

Pallidotomy *(pal-id-ot-o-mil)* [L. *pallidus,* pal G. *tome,* a cutting]. Srugical severance of t fibres the cerebral cortex to the corp striatum. Done to relieve the tremor in Parki son's disease. Less common now.

ڈوٹومی: سربرل کارٹیکس سے کاوپس سٹری ایٹم کو جانے والوں ریشوں کا یکل انقطاع۔

Palm *(pam)* [L. *palma*]. The anterior or flex surface of the hand.

یلی: ہاتھ کی اگلی یا فلیکسر سطح۔

Palmar *(pal-mar)* [L. *palmaris*]. Pertaining the palm of the hand. **palmar arche** superficial and deep, are formed by t anastomosis of the radial and ulnar arteries.

ی: ہاتھ کی ہتھیلی سے متعلق۔

Palpable *(pal-pa-bl)* [L..*palpare,* to tou softly]. Capable of being palpated.

پ ایبل: چھو کر محسوس کیے جانے کے قابل مثلاً نبض۔

Palpation *(pal-pa-shun)* [L. *palpare,* to tou sottly]. The act of manual examin tion-palpate, v.t.

ی معائنہ ۔ دستی معائنہ: جسمانی جانچ کا عمل ۔ اس میں مریض کی ٹٹولنا، دبا کر دیکھنا وغیرہ شامل ہیں۔

Palpebra *(pe-bra)* [L.]. The eyelidpalpebr adj.; palperbrae, pl.

ٹا: آنکھ کا پپوٹا۔

Palpitation *(pal-pit-a-shun)* [L. *palpitare,* pal- pitate]. Rapid forceful beating of t heart of which the patient is conscious.

ڑکن ۔ خفقان: دل کی تیز طاقتور دھڑکن جس سے مریض بھی باخبر ہوتا ۔ دل کی عام دھڑکن ۷۰ تا ۸۰ مرتبہ فی منٹ سے زیادہ۔

Palsy *(pawl-zi)*. See PARALYSIS. **Bell's** facial hemiparesis from oedema of t seventh (facial) cranial nerve. Cau unknown. [Charles Bell, Scottish physicia 1774-1842.] **Erb's p.,** involves the should and arm muscles from a lesion of the fifth a sixth cervical nerve roots. The arm han loosely at the side, with the forearm pronated ('waiter's tip position'). Most commonly a birth injury. [Wilhelm Heinrich Erb, German neur- ologist, 1840-1921.]

رعشہ تشنج۔ اینٹھن

ıludrine *(pal-u-drin)*. Proguanil (q.v.)

پیلوڈرین: پروگوائل۔

ımaquin *(pa-ma-kwin)*. Synthetic antimalarial, used mainly in association with quinine or chloroquine.

پاماکوئن: تالیفی طور پر تیارہ کردہ ضد ملیریائی۔کونین یا کلوروکوئن کے ساتھ مستعمل۔

ımergan. Pathidine and promethazine, with or without atropine. Used mainly as premedication.

پیمرگین: ایزوپین کے بغیر یا اس کے ہمراہ پتھیڈین اور پرومیتھازین۔

ınadol *(pan-a-dol)*. Paracetamol (q.v.)

پیناڈول: پیراسٹامول۔

ınarthritis *(pan-arth-ri-tis)* [G. *pas*, whole; *arthron*, joint; *-itis*, inflammation]. Inflammation of all the stru- ctures of a joint.

ورم ہمہ مفاصل: جوڑ کی تمام ساختوں کی سوزش۔

ıncarditis *(pan-kar-di-tis)* [G. *pas*, whole; *arthron*, joint; *-itis*, inflammation]. Inflammation of all the structures of the heart.

ورم ہمہ قلب: تمام قلبی ساختوں کی سوزش۔

ıncreas *(pan-kri-as)* [G. *pagkreas*]. A tongue-sh- aped glandular organ lying below and behind the stomatch. Its head is encircled by the duodenum and its tail touches the spleen. It is about 17.78 cm long and weighs about 98 g. It secretes the hormone insulin, and also pancreatic juice which contains enzymes involved in the digestion of fats and proteins in the small intestine.

لبلبہ: زبان کی شکل کی غدودوالی ساخت جو معدہ کے نیچے عقب میں واقع ہوتی ہے اس سے رطوبت خارج ہوتی ہے۔اس سے رطوبت خارج ہوتی ہے۔اور انسولین ہارمون بھی۔اس کے رس میں ہضمی خامرے ہوتے ہیں۔ اس کی لمبائی ۷۸ء۱۷ سم کے قریب ہوتی ہے اس میں چند مخصوص خلیوں کے گروہ ہوتے ہیں جو لینگر ہینز کے جزیرے کہلاتے ہیں۔

Pancreatectomy *(pan-kre-at-ek-to-mi)* [G. *pagkraes*, pancreas; *ektome*, excision]. Excision of part or the whole of the pancreas.

لبلبہ براری: پورا لبلبہ یا اس کا کوئی حصہ کاٹنا۔

Pancreatin *(pan-kre-atin)*. A mixture of enzymes obtained from the pancreas. Used in pancreatic diseases and deficiency. Standard and tirple- strength products are available.

بانقراسین: لبلبہ سے حاصل شدہ خامرات کا آمیزہ لبلبہ کی بیماریوں اور کمی میں مستعمل۔

Pancreatitis *(pan-kre-a-ti-tis)* [G. *pagkreas*, pancr- eas; *-itis*, inflammation]. Inflammation of the pancreas. Lipase level of blood and urine used as indicator of p. See DIASTASE.

ورم لبلبہ: لبلبہ کی سوزش۔

Pancreatrophic *(pan-kre-a-trof-ik)*. Stimulating the pancreas. Some of the anterior pituitary hormones have a p. actoin.

پین کریاٹرافک: لبلبہ کو تحریک دینا۔

Pancreozymin *(pan-kre-o-zi-min)*. A hormone secreted in the small intestine; stimulated flow of pancreatic enzymes.

Pancrex *(pan-kreks)*. Supplements deficient digestive enzymes in fibrocystic disease.

Pancuronium bromide *(pan-ku-ro'-ni-um)*. Muscle relaxant (q.v.)

Pancytopenia *(pan-si-to-pen'-i-a)*. Describes peripheral blood picture when red cells, granular white cells and platelets are reduced as occurs in suppression of bone marrow function.

Pandemic *(pan-dem'-ik)* [G. *pandemia*, the whole people]. An infection spreading over a whole country or the world.

عالمگیر وبا: پورے ملک میں اچھاں پر پھیلا ہوا چھوت کا مرض۔

Panhysterectomy *(pan-his- er-ek'-to-mi)*. An old term for the removal of the uterus and adnexa; more accurately d scribed as a total hysterectomy (q.v.) with bilateral salpingo-oophorectomy (q.v.)

کامل رحم براری: رحم اور ایڈنکسا کو کاٹ کر نکال دینا۔

Pannus *(pan'-us)* [L. cloth]. Corneal vascularization, often caused by conjunctival irritation.

غباری پردہ: پردہ قرنیہ کی سرخی۔

Panophthalmitis *(pan-of-thal-mi-tis)* [G. *pas,* whole; *ophthalmos,* eye; *-itis,* inflammation]. Inflam- mation of all the tissues of the eyeball.

ورم ہمہ چشم: آنکھ کے گولے کی تمام بافتوں کی سوزش۔ تقریباً پوری آنکھ میں ورم ہو جاتا ہے۔ آنکھ سرخ ہو جاتی ہے۔ آنکھ اور سر میں شدید درد، بخار اس کی علامات ہیں۔ نوووبائیوسین اور ٹیٹرامائی سین مفید ہیں۔

Panosteitis *(pan-os-ti'-i-tis)* [G. *pas,* whole; *osteon,* bone; *-itis,* inflammtion]. Inflammation of all constituents of a bone--medulla, bonv tissue and periosteum.

الم العظام: ہڈی کے تمام اجزاء کی سوزش۔

Pantie-girdle syndrome. The ankles of women of sedentary occupation, wearing a pantie-type of foundation garment, become swollen by night.

پینٹی گرڈل سنڈروم: مسلسل بیٹھ کر کام کرنے والی خواتین جو چست زیر جامہ پہنتی ہیں۔ ان کے ٹخنے رات کے وقت متورم ہو جاتے ہیں۔

Pantocaine. Amethocaine (q.v.)

پینٹوکین: امیتھوکین۔

Pantothenic acid *(pan-to-the-nik as-id).* A constituent of the vitamin B complex. Therapeutic value is uncertain.

پینٹوتھنک ایسڈ: وٹامن بی کمپلکس کا ایک جزو۔

PAO Peak acid output. See PENTAGASTRIN TEST.

Papaveretum *(pa-pa-ver-e-tum).* [L. *papaver,* pop- py]. A mixture of opium alkaloids containing 50 per cent of morphine.

پاپاوریٹم: ۵۰ فیصد مارفین پر مشتمل افیمی الکلائڈز کا آمیزہ۔

Papaverine *(pa-pav-er-en).* One of the less important alkaloids of opium, used mainly as a relaxant in spasm, asthma and peripheral vascular disorders.

پپاورین: ایک سفید غیر حل پذیر الکلائڈ۔ نقطہ پگھلاؤ ۱۴۷° س۔ افیم سے حاصل کیا جاتا ہے۔ دوائیوں میں اس کے ہائیڈروجن کلورائیڈ کی صورت میں

نعال کیا جاتا ہے۔

Papilla *(pa-pil'-a).* A minute nippleshape eminence, i.e. eminence. **anal p.,** epitheli projections on the edges of the anal valve **circumvallate p.,** the large papillae found the base of the tongue. **filiform p,** the fi hair-like papillae at the tip of the fongu **fungiform p.,** papillae shaped like a gungu found chiefly on the dorsocentral area of t tongue. **renal p.,** the summit of one of t renal pyramids papillae, *pl.*; papillary, *adj.*

پستان: چھوٹا نپل نما ابھار۔

Papillitis *(pap-il-i-tis)* [L. *papilla,* nipple; *-itis,* inflammtion]. Most usual inflammation of the optic disc. Otherwi inflammtion of a papilla. Can arise in t kidney after excessive phenacetin in- take.

حمی: زیادہ تر بصری قرص کی سوزش۔

Papilloedema *(pap-il-e-de'-ma)* [L. *papill* nipple; *oidema,* swelling]. Oedema of t optic disc; indicative of increased intracran pressure. Choked disc (q.v.)

ج لحمی: بصری قرص کا ورم۔

Papilloma *(pap-i-lo-ma)* [L. *papilla,* nipple, *-oma,* tumour]. A simple tumour arising fr a non-glan- dular epithelial surfacepapi omatous, adj.; papillomata, *pl.*

ی۔ پھوڑا: غیر غدودی بالائی سطح سے ابھرنے والی رسولی۔

Papule *(pa'-pul)* [L. *papula,* pimple]. A sm circumscribed elevation of the skin--papul *adj.*

ہ۔ مہاسا: ایک چھوٹا جلدی ابھار۔

Papulopustular *(pa-pu-lo-pus'-tul-ar)* [*papula,* pimple; *pustula,* blister]. Pertaining both papules and pustules (q.v.)

لوپسٹولر: پھنسیوں اور آبلوں دونوں سے متعلق۔

Para-aminobenzoic acid *(par-a a-mi'-no-ben o-ik-as- id).* An acid which acts as essential metabolite for many bactetr Sulphonamide drugs prevent some bacte from using PA and so stop their growth.

ıracentesis

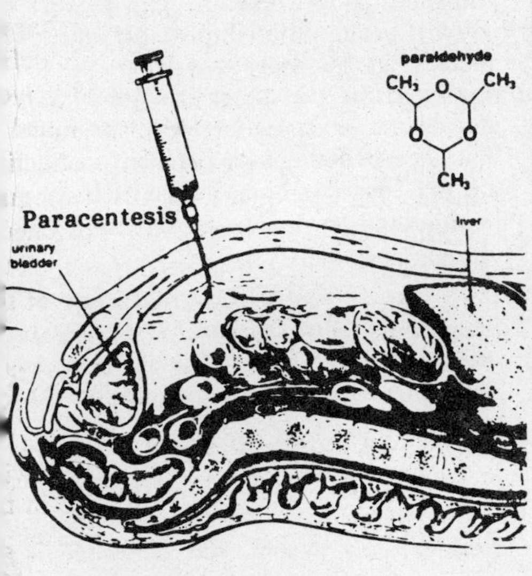

پیراامینونبزووئک ایسڈ: ایک تیزاب جو بہت سے جراثیموں کے لئے ایک لازمی میٹابولائیٹ کے طور پر عمل کرتا ہے۔

ra-aminosalicylic acid *(par-a a -min-o-sal-is-il-ik- as -id)*. Widely used antitubercular drug, usually in association with isoniazid or streptomycin. Has nauseous taste, so is usually given as cachets or granules.

پیراامینوسیلی سائیلک ایسڈ: ضد تپ دق کے طور پر مستعمل دوا۔

ra-aortic *(par-a a-or-tik)* [G. *para,* baside; *aorte,* aorta]. Near the aorta.

پیراایورٹک: ایورٹا کے قریب۔

ıracentesis *(par-a-sen-te'-sis)* [G. *parak-entesis,* a tapping]. The withdrawal of fluid from its containing , closed cavity by insertion of a hollow needle or cannula. Aspiration--paracenteses, *pl.*

بزل ثقب: ایک کھوکھلی سوئی گھسا کر بند کہفہ سے سیال باہر نکالنا۔ پیٹ سے پانی نکالنا۔

ıracetamol *(par-a-se'-ta-mol)*. An analgesic rese- mbling phenacetin in effect, but less liable to cause side effects in those patients sensitive to phena- cetin.

پیراسیٹامول: ایک دافع درد دوا۔ اثر میں فیناسٹین سے مشابہ۔ وہائیٹ لیک کے مرض میں ایک گولی صبح ایک دوپہر ایک شام ۲ ہفتے تک۔

Paracodol *(par-a-ko-dol)*. Soluble tablets of paraceta- mol with codeine.

Paradione *(par-a-di on)*. An anticonvulsant compo- und, useful in petit mal resistant ot trioxidone therapy.

پیراڈیون: ایک مرکب۔

Paraesthesia *(par-es-th-zi-q)* [G. *para,* beside; *aisth- esis,* perception]. Any abnormality of sensation.

لمس کاذب: محسوس کرنے کا غیر معمولی پن۔

Paraffin *(par-af-in)*. Medicinal paraffins are; liquid paraffin, used as a.laxative; soft paraffin, the familiar ointment base; and hard paraffin, used in wax baths for rheumatic conditions.

پیرافین: ادویات میں مستعمل پیرافین یہ ہیں۔ مائع پیرافین۔ بطور قبض کشا نرم پیرافین بطور مرہم بیس اور سخت پیرافین جوڑوں کے درد کے لئے ویکس باتھ میں مستعمل ہے۔

Paraformaldehyde *(par-a-form-al-de-hi-d)*. A solid modification of formaldehyde (q.v.), used for sterilizing catheters and disinfecting rooms.

پیرافارملڈ یہائیڈ: کیتھیٹر ز اور کمروں کو پاک صاف کرنے کے لئے فارملڈ یہائیڈ کی ٹھوس ترمیم استعمال کی جاتی ہے۔ گرم کرنے پر فارملڈ یہائیڈ میں تبدیل ہو جاتا ہے۔

Paraganglioma See PHAEOCHROMOC-YTOMA.

برعقود۔ زائد عقود: فیوکروموسائیٹوما۔

Paragesic *(par-a-gez-ik)*. Analgesic relaxant, useful for painful upper respiratory infection and migraie.

پیراجیسک: دافع درد دوا۔ پردرد بالائی تنفسی مرض اور مائیگرین کے لئے مفید۔

Parainfluenza virus. Causes acute upper respiratory infection.

پیراانفلوئنزا وائرس: یہ بالائی تنفسی مرض پیدا کرتا ہے۔

Paraldehyde *(par-al-de-hid)*. Liquid with

characteristic odour. Has sedative properties similar to chloral. Given orally or by intramuscular injection, or rectally as a solution in olive oil. Now rerely uses.

پیرلڈ یہائیڈ: ایسٹلڈ یہائیڈ کا ایک مائع پولیمر مخصوص بو کے ساتھ۔ نقطہ جوش ۱۲۴°س، دوائیوں میں نیند آور کے طور پر استعمال کیا جاتا ہے۔

Paralysis *(par-al-i-sis)* [G.] Complete or incomplete of nervous function to a part of the body. This may be sensory or motor or both. **paralysis agitans,** Parkinson's disease (q.v.) **bulbar p.,** involves the l abioglossopharyngeal region and results from degeneration of motor nuclei in the medulla oblongata. diver's p., see CAISSON DISEA-SE.**infantile p.,**see POLIOMYELITIS. flaccid p. results mainly from lower motor-neurone lesions. There are diminished or absent tendon reflexes. **Landry's** (acute ascending) p. is accompanied by fever and may terminate in respiratory stasis and death. pseudo p. of parrot, there is inability to move upper lilmb because of sysyphilitic osteochondritis; found in neonatal congenital syphilis. **pseudoblbar p,** there is gross disturbance in control of tongue, bilateral hemiplegia and mental changes following on a succession of 'strokes' **spas- tic p.** results mainly from upper motor neuroe lesions. There are exaggerated tendon reflexes. See PALSY.

فالج: جسم کے کسی حصے میں عصبی عمل کا مکمل یا نامکمل ضیاع۔ یہ سنسری، موٹر یا دونوں ہو سکتے ہیں۔

Paralytic *(par-al-it-ik)* [G. *paralytikos*]. Pertaining to paralysis. **paralytic ileus,** paralysis of the intestinal muscle so that the bowel content cannot pass onwards even though there is no mechanical obstruction. See APERISTALSIS.

مفلوج: فالج سے متعلق۔

Paramedian *(par-a-me-di-an)* [G. *para,* beside; L. *medianus,* middle]. Near the middle.

پیرامیڈین: درمیان کے نزدیک۔

Paramedical *(par-a-med-ik-al)* Associated w the medical profession. The p. servic include occup- ational, physical and spee therapy, and medical social work.

Paramenstrum *(par-a-men-stroo-um)* [G. *pa* beside; L. *menstruare,* to menstruate]. T four days before the start of menstruation a the first four days of the period itself.

Paramethasone *(para-a-meth-a-zon).* One the corticosteroids.

میتھاسون: کارٹیکاسٹیرائڈز میں سے ایک۔

Parametritis *(par-a-met-met-ri-tis)* [G. *par* beside; *metra,* womb; *-itis,* inflammatio Inflammation of the pelvic connective tissue

اب حول الرحم: پیڑو کے رابطی نسیج کی سوزش۔ بچہ دانی کے آس پاس سوزش۔

Parametrium *(par-a-met-ri-um)* [G. *par* beside; *metra,* womb]. The connective tissu immediately surrounding th uterus--parametrial, *adj.*

ط الرحم: رحم کے گرد رابطی نسیج۔

Paranasal *(par-a-na-zal)* [G. *para,* beside; *nasus,* nose]. Near the nasal cavities, as t various sinuses.

انیزل: ناک کے کھفوں کے قریب۔

Paraneoplastic *(par-a-ne-o-plas-tik)* [G. *par* beside; *neos,* new; *plasma,* form Paraneoplastic disease describes syndrom associated with mal- ignancy but not caus by the primary growth or its metastases.

رانیو پلاسٹک: سنڈروم کی ایک قسم۔

Paranoia *(par-a-noi-a)* [G. *para,* beyond; *noc* mi- nd]. Delusions of persecution--paranoi *adj.*

ت: ایک قسم کا جنون۔

Paranoit behaviour. Acts denoting suspici of others.

واسی رویہ: دوسروں کے شک کو ظاہر کرنے والے افعال۔

Paraoesophageal *(par-a-e-sof-a-jel)* [G. *par* bes- ide; *oisophagos.* gullet]. Near t oesophagus.

راالیسوفیجل۔ نزمریوی: ایسوفیگس کے نزدیک۔

Paraphimosis *(par-a-fi-mo-sis)* [G. *para,* beside; *phimosis,* a stopping up]. Retraction of the prepuce behind the glans penis so that the tight ring of skin interferes with the flood flow in the glans.

اختناق حشفہ: سرذکر کی جلد پیچھے ہٹ جانے اور آگے نہ آنے سے سرذکر تنگ رہ جانے کی حالت اس میں خونی بہاؤ میں رکاوٹ ہوتی ہے۔

Paraphrenia *(par-a-fre-ni-a)* [G. *para,* beyond; *phren,* mind]. A psychiatric illness in the elderly characterized by well-circumscribed delusions, usually of a persecutory nature--paraphrenic. *adj.*

بکواس: ڈیمنشیا کے بجائے کوئی ذہنی خرابی۔

Paraplegia *(par-a-ple-ji-a)* [G. *para,* beyond; *plege,* stroke]. Paralysis of the lower limbs, usually including the bladder and rectum--paraplegic. *adj.*

عناہت ذہنی: زیریں جوارح عموماً بشمول بلیڈر اور ریکٹم کا فالج۔

Pararectal *(par-a-rek-tal)* [G. *para,* beside; 1. *rectus,* straight]. Near the rectum.

پیراریکٹل: ریکٹم کے قریب۔

Parasitaemia *(par-a-sit-e-mi-a)* [G. *parasitos,* parasite; *haima,* blood]. Parasites in the blood-- parasitaemic, *adj.*

پیراسائی ٹیمیا: خون میں طفیلی۔

Parasigte *(par-a-sit)* [G. *parasitos*]. An organism which contains food shelter from another host organism--parasitic, *adj.*

طفیلی: ایسے جسیے دیگر جسیموں میں یا ان کے اوپر پرورش پاتے ہیں۔ اور ان سے ہی اپنی خوراک حاصل کرتے ہیں۔ جس جسیمہ پر وہ پرورش پاتے ہیں۔ اس کو میزبان جسیمہ کہتے ہیں۔ مثلاً پلازموڈیم مچھر اور انسان پر طفیلی ہے۔

Parasiticide *(par-a-sit-i-sid)* [G. *parasitos,* parasite; L. *caedere,* to kill]. An agent which will kill para- sites.

طفیلی کش: طفیلیوں کو مارنے والا ایجنٹ۔

Parasympathetic *(par-a-sim-path-et-ik)* [G. *para,* beside; *sympathes,* sympathetic]. A portion of the autonomic nervous system, derived from some of the cranial and sacral nerves belonging to the central nervous system.

نزمشاری عصبی: حرکی یا آٹونومک عصبی نظام کا ایک حصہ۔

Parasympatholytic *(par-a-sim-path-o-lit-ik).* Capable of neutralizing the effect of parasympathetic stimulation, e.g. atropine hyoscine.

پیراسمپتھو لائیٹک: نزمشاری عصبی تحریک کے اثر کی تعدیل کا اہل۔ مثلاً ایٹروپین۔

Parathion *(par-a-thi-on).* Organophosphorus compound uses as insecticide in agriculture. Powe- rful and irreversible anticholinesterase action. Potentially dangerous to man for this reason.

نامیاتی فاسفورس مرکب: جو زراعت میں حرارت کش کے طور پر استعمال کیا جاتا ہے۔

Parathormone *(par-a-thor-mon).* A hormone secreted by the parathyroid glands, which controls the calcium content of bone. Excess hormone cau- ses mobilization of calcium from the bones, which become rarefied.

جوہر غدہ جارالارقیہ: پیراتھائیڈ گلینڈز سے خارج شدہ ہارمون جو ہڈی کے کیلشیم جزو کو کنٹرول کرتا ہے۔

Parathyroid *(pra-a-thi-roid)* [G. *para,* beside; *thur- eieudes.* shield-shaped]. Four small endcrine glands lying close to or embedded in the posterior surface of the thyroid gland. They secrete a hor- mone. parathormone.

پیراتھائی رائڈ: چار چھوٹی اینڈوکرائن گلینڈز جو تھائیرائڈ گلینڈ کی خلفی سطح میں دھنسی ہوئیں یا قریب ہی واقع ہوتی ہیں۔ وہ ایک ہارمون پیراتھارمون خارج کرتی ہے۔ لمبائی قریباً چھ ملی میٹر اور چوڑائی اس سے ذرا کم۔

Parathyroidectomy *(par-a-thi-roid-ek-to-mi)* [G. *para,* beside; *thureoeides,* shield-shaped; *ektome,* excision]. Excision of one or more parathyroid glands.

شق جارالدرقیہ: ایک یا زیادہ پیراتھائیرائڈ گلینڈز کو کاٹ کر الگ کرنا۔

Paratracheal *(par-a-trak-e-al)* [G. *para,* beside; *trac- hus,* rough]. Near the trachea.

نزہوائی نالی: ٹریکیا کے نزدیک۔

Paratyphoid fever *(par-a-ti-foid-fe-ver)* [G. *para,* near; *typhodes,* delirious]. A variety of enteric fever, but less severe and prolonged than typhoid fever. Caused by *Salmonella paratyphi A* and *B.* and more rarely *C.* See TAB.

خفیف محرقہ تپ: بخار کی ایک قسم لیکن ٹائفائیڈ بخار سے شدت اور طوالت میں کم۔

Paraurethral *(par-a-u-reth-ral)* [G. *para,* beside; *ourethra,* urethra]. Near the urethra.

نزرحمی: یورتھرا کے قریب۔

Paravaginal *(par-a-va-ji-nal)* [G. *para,* beside; L. vagina]. Near the vagina.

نزصبلی: ویجائنا کے قریب۔

Paravertebral *(par-a-ver-te-bral)* [G. *para,* beside; L. *vertebra,* joint]. Near the spinal colum. **paravertebral block anaesthesia** (more correctly 'analgesia') is induced by infiltration of local anaesthetic around the spinal nerve roots as they emerge from the intervertebral foramina. **parav- ertebral injection** of local anaesthetic into sympathetic chain. Can be used as a test in ischaemic limbs of see if sympathectomy will be of value.

Injection points

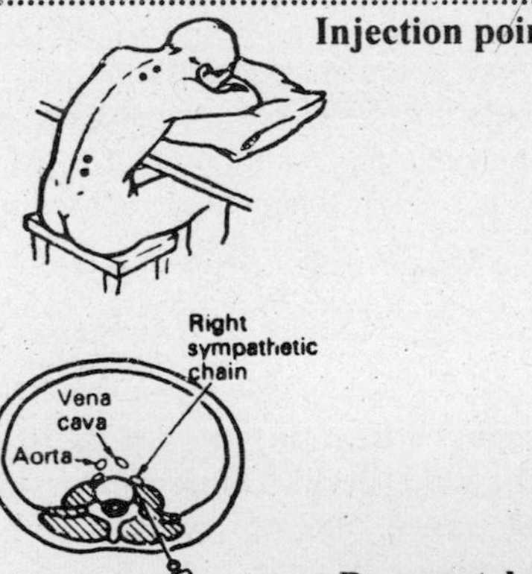

Paravertebral

نزمہروی: ریڑھ کی ہڈی کے قریب۔

Parenchyma *(par-eng-ki-ma)* [G. *para,* beside; *engchyma,* infusion]. The parts of an organ which in contradistinction to its interstitial tissue, are concerned with its function parencymal, parenchymatous, *adj.*

مسکن دوا: افیم کا فورزدہ ٹنکچر جو عموماً کھانسی کی سربتوں اور آمیزوں میں استعمال کیا جاتا ہے۔

Parenteral *(per-en-ter-al)* [G. *para,* beyond; *enteron,* intestine]. Not via the alimentary tract.

غیرامعائی: ہضمی قنال کے راستے نہیں یعنی جو ہضمی قنال کے راستے نہ ہو۔

Paresis *(par-e-sis)* [G. a letting go]. Partial or slight paralysis; weakness of a limb--paretic, *adj.*

فالج ناقص: جزوی یا ہلکا فالج۔ جارح کی کمی۔

Pareunia *(par-un-i-a)* [G. *pareunos,* lying beside]. Coitus, See DYSPAREUNIA.

مباشرت: ہم بستری۔

Pargyline. A monoamine oxidase inhibitor.

پیراگائی لین: مانوامین آکسیڈیز۔

Parietal *(par-i-et-al)* [L.*paries,* an enveloping structure]. Pertaining to a wall. **parietal bones,** the two bones which form the sides and vault of the skull.

جداری: جلد سے متعلق۔ کھوپڑی کی بالائی ہڈیاں جو دو ہوتی ہیں۔ ایک سر کے دائیں طرف اور دوسری بائیں طرف۔

Parity *(par-i-ti)* [L. *parere,* to bring forth]. Condition of a woman with regard to the number of children she has born.

مولدیت : جنم دیئے جانیوالے بچوں کی تعداد کی نسبت سے عورت کی حالت۔

Pakinsonism. A syndrome of mask-like expression, shuffing gait, tremor of the limbs and pill-rolling movements of the fingers. Can be drug-induced. The postencephalitic type comes on in the 30 to 40 age group and there may or may not be a clear history of encephalitis (sporadic type). Degenerative type of p. (paralysis agitans) comes on during middle life; arteriosclerotic type comes on in the elderly. Characterized by a distinctive clinical of termor and rigidity.

پارکن سن کا مرض ۔ رعشہ: اس بیماری میں مریض میں چال کی لڑکھڑاہٹ اور بدن میں رعشہ ہوتا ہے۔ انگلیاں اور ہاتھ کانپتے ہیں منشیات کے عادی لوگ اکثر اس کا شکار ہوتے ہیں۔ تنزلی جسم کا مرض ادھیڑ عمر میں ہی

اورمشریانی قسم کا مرض بڑھاپے میں ہوتا ہے۔ یہ مرض عام طور پر ۳۰ تا ۴۰ سال کی عمر میں ہوتا ہے۔ اس میں بینز ہکسیول۔ پروسائیکلی ڈین اور ہائیوسین ہائیڈرو برومائیڈ دیجئے۔

'arnate. Tranylcypromine. A monoamine oxidase inhibitor.

پرنیٹ: ٹرینائل سپرومین۔

'aromomycin *(par-om-o-mi-sin)*. Only administered orally. Useful for temporary or long-term suppr- ession of bowel flora; treatment of various forms of acute enteritis.

پیرومومائی سین: آنتوں کی بیماری کے لئے دوا۔

'aronychia *(par-on-ik-i-a)* [G. *para,* beside; *onyx,* nail]. A withlow. Suppurative inflammtion around a fingernail. The virus of herpes simplex can cause multiple vesicles over inflamed skin--**herpetic p.**

نختا: انگلی کے ناخن کے گرد سوزش۔

Paronychia

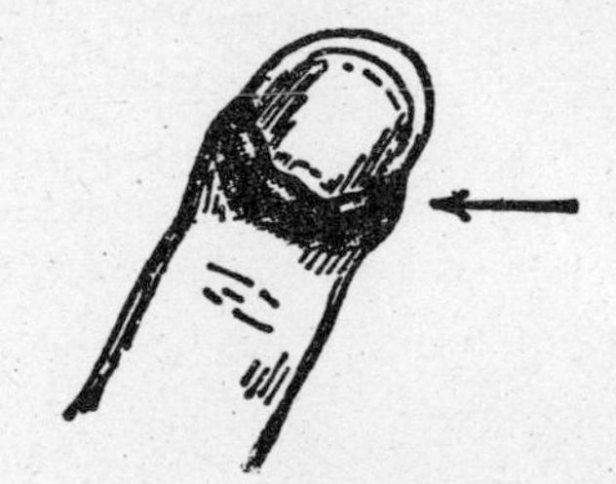

Parosmia *(par-os-mi-a)* [G. *para,* beside; *osme,* smell]. Perverted sense of smell, usually of an hallucinatory nature.

فتور شامہ: سونگنے کی حس میں خرابی۔

Parotidectomy *(par-ot-id-ek-to-mi)* [G. *para,* beside; *ous,* ektome, excision]. Excision of the parotid salivary gland.

اخراج غدہ نکفیہ: پیروٹڈ صلوری گلینڈ کو کاٹ کر الگ کرنا۔

Parotid gland *(par-o-tid)* [G. *para,* beside; *ous,* ear]. The salivary gland situated in front of and below the ear.-

نکفہ۔غدہ بنا گوشی: کان کے سامنے اور نیچے واقع سلوری گلینڈ۔

Parotid gland

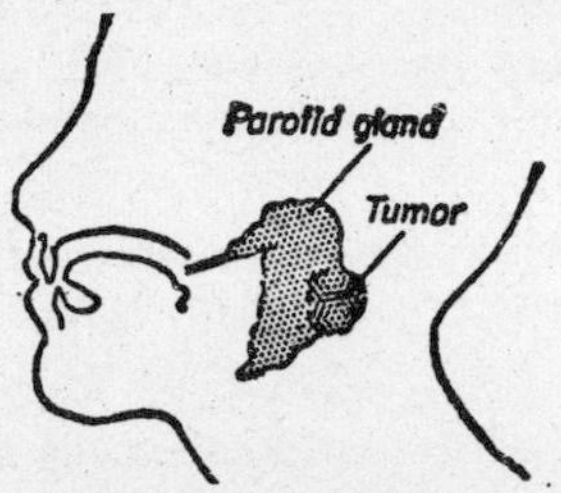

Parotitis *(par-o-ti-tis)* [G. *para,* beside; *ous,* ear; *-itis,* inflammtion]. Inflammation of parotid gland. **infectious (specific) p.,** mumps (q.v.) **septic p.** refers to ascending infection from the mouth via the parotid duct, when a parotid abscess may result.

کن پیڑ۔ ورم نکفہ۔: پیروٹڈ گلینڈ کی سوزش۔

Parous *(par-us)* [L. *parere,* to bring forth]. Having born a child or children.

حامل۔ پیدا کرنے والا: بچے یا بچوں کو جنم دینا۔

Paroxysm *(par-osk-izm)* [G. *paroxysmos,* irritation]. A sudden, temporary attack.

دورۂ مرض، شدت مرض: اچانک عارضی حملہ۔

Paroxysmal *(par-oks-iz-mal)* Coming on in attacks or paroxysms. **paroxysmal dyspnoea,** occurs mostly at night in patients with cardiac disease. **paroxys- mal fibrillation** occurs in the atrium of the heart and is associated with a ventricular tachycardia and total irregularity of the pulse rhythm. **paroxysmal tachycardia** may result from ectopic impulses arising in the atrium or in the ventricle itself.

دورے کا حملہ ہونا۔

Parrot disease. Psittacosis (q.v.).

طوطا روگ، مرض طوطی: سٹا کوسس۔

Parrot's nodes. Bossing of frontal bones in the congenital syphilitic. [Joseph Parrot, French phy- sician, 1829-83].

طوطی گرہیں: فرنٹل ہڈیوں کی خرابی۔ فرانسیسی طبیب جوزف پیرٹ کے نام پر۔

Parstelin *(pars-tel-in)* Tranylcypromine (q.v.)

and tri- fluoperazine (q.v.).

پارسٹیلین: پریشانی اور مایوسی میں مفید۔

Parturient *(par-tur-i-ent)* [L. *parturure,* to bring forth]. Pertaining to childbirth.

بچہ زا: بچے کی پیدائش سے متعلق۔

PAS. Para-aminosalicyclic acid. See AMINOSALI- CYCLIC ACID.

پی۔اے۔ایس: پیرا امینو سالیسائیکلک ایسڈ۔

Pasinah *(pas-in-a)* Antitubercular drug.

پیسینا: تپ دق کے خلاف دوا۔

Passive *(pas-iv)* Inactive. Opp. active. **passive hyper- aemia,** see HYPERAEMIA. **passive immunity,** see IMMUNITY. **passive move- ment,** performed by the physiotherapist, the patient being relaxed.

سست: غیر حاصل۔

Pasteurella *(pas-tur-el-la)* A genus of bacteria. Short Gram-negative rods, staining more deeply at the poles (bipolar staining). Pathogenic in man and animals. *Pasteurella pestis* is the causative organismm of classical plague. Currently preferred name is Yersinia. [Louis Pasteur, French scientist and bacteriologist, 1822-95].

پاسچورے لا: جراثیم کا ایک جنس۔ چھوٹے گرام منفی سلاخی جراثیم۔ اس کی نوع پیسٹیس طاعون کی ذمہ دار ہے۔

Pasteurization *(pas-tur-iz-a-shun)* A process where- by pathogenic organisms in fluid (especially milk) are killed by heat. **flash method of p. (H.T., S.T** —high temperature, short time), the fluid is heated to 72°C maintained at this temperature for 15 s, then rapidly cooled. **holder method of p.,** the fluid is heated to 63 to 65.5°C maintained at this temperature for 30 min then rapidly cooled. (Louis Pasteur, French scientist and bacteriologist, 1822- 95].

تطہیر پاسطوری، تطہیر حرارتی: جزوی طور پر پاک کرنا خصوصاً دودھ کو اس میں اتنے درجہ حرارت تک گرم کیا جاتا ہے کہ جراثیم مر جائیں لیکن جراثیم کے بذرے ختم نہیں ہوتے۔ یہ طریقہ فرانسیسی ماہر حیاتیات پاسٹیر کے نام پر رکھا گیا ہے۔

Patau's (13-15) syndrome. Autosomal trisomy Closely associated with mental subnormality Cells have 47 chromosomes.

سنڈروم پٹاؤ (۱۳ تا ۱۵): خلیوں میں ۴۷ کروموسومز ہوتے ہیں اس میں ذہن متاثر ہوتا ہے۔

Patella *(pat-el-a)* [L. small pan]. The knee-cap; a tri- angular, sesamoid bone—patellar, *adj.*; patellae, *pl.*

Patella

چپنی کی ہڈی: گھٹنے کی چپنی۔ ایک تکونی ہڈی۔ گھٹنے کے جوڑ کی حفاظت کرتی ہے۔ یہ ہڈی ۴ ارباط سے بندھی ہوتی ہے۔ اس ہڈی کی وجہ سے گھٹنا سامنے کی طرف ختم نہیں ہوسکتا۔

Patellectomy *(pat-el-ek-to-mi)* [L. *patella,* small pan G. *ektome,* excision]. Excision of the patella.

پٹیلیکٹومی: پٹیلا علیحدہ کرنا۔

Patent *(pa-tent)* [L. *patens,* open]. Open; not closed or occluded. **patent ductus anteriosus,** failure of ductus **arteriosus** to close soon after birth, so that the abnormal shunt between the pulmonary artery and the aorta is preserved. **patent interventricular septum,** a congenital defect in the dividing wall between the right and left ventricle of the heart— patency, *n.*

وسیع، کشادہ: کھلا، جو بند نہ ہو۔

Pathogen *(path-o-jen)* [G. *pathos,* disease; *genes,* producing]. A disease-producing agent, usually restricted to a living agent—pathogenic, *adj.*; pa- thogenicity, *n.*

مرض زا: مرض پیدا کرنے والا ایجنٹ۔ عموماً جاندار ایجنٹ تک محدود۔

Pathogenesis *(path-o-jen-e-sis)* [G. *pathos,*

disease; *genes,* producing]. The origin and development of disease—pathogenetic, *adj.*

تولید مرض: مرض کا اصل و تکمیل۔

Pathogenicity *(path-o-jen-is-i-ti)* The capacity to produce disease.

پیتھوجینی سٹی: مرض پیدا کرنے کی اہلیت۔

Pathognomonic *(path-og-no-mon-ik)* [G. *pathos,* disease; *gnomonikos,* skilled in one thing]. Charac- teristic of or peculiar to a disease.

(علامت) تشخیصیہ: کسی مرض سے مخصوص یا اسکی خصوصیت۔

Pathology *(path-ol-o-ji)* [G. *pathos,* disease; *logos,* discourse]. The science which deals with the cause and nature of diseasepath- ological, *adj.*; patholo- gically, *adv.*

مرضیات: سائنس جو مرض کی وجہ اور نیچر کے متعلق بحث کرتی ہے۔

Pathophobia *(path-o-fo-bi-a)* [G. *pathos,* disease; *phobos,* fear]. A morbid dread of disease.

خوف مرض: مرض کا خوف۔

Patterson-Kelly syndrome. See PLUMMERVI -N SON SYNDROME.

پیٹرسن کیلی سنڈروم: پلمر ونسن سنڈروم۔

Patulous *(pat-u-lus)* [L. *patulus,* standing open]. Opened out; expanded.

کشادہ: کھلا ہوا۔ پھیلا ہوا۔

Paul-Mikulicz operation *(pawl milk-u-litsh)* A meth- od for excision of a portion of the colon whereby the two cut ends of the bowel are kept out on the surface of the abdomen, and are joined at a later date without entering the peritoneal cavity. The method was designed to lessen the risk of periton- itis from leakage at the suture line. [Frank Thomas Paul, English surgeon, 1851-1941. Johann von Mikulicz-Radecki, Rumanian surgeon (in Polan), 1850-1905].

پال میکولکز اپریشن: قولون کے حصے کو کاٹنے کا طریقہ۔

Paul's tube. A flanged glass tube used to collect the contents after the bowel has been opened on the surface of the abdomen. [Frank Thomas Paul, Eng- lish surgeon, 1851-1941].

پال کی نلی: شیشے کی مخصوص نلی۔

Pavulon *(pav-u-lon)* Pancuronium bromide (q.v.).

Pawlik's grip. A method of determining the engage- ment or otherwise of the fetal head in the maternal pelvic brim. [Karel Pawlik, Czechoslovakian sur- geon, 1849-1914].

گرفت پالک: ماں کے پیڑو کے کنارے میں بچے کے سر کا تعین کرنے کا طریقہ۔

PBI (protein bound iodine). Iodine combined with protein as part of the thyroid hormone. Low in thy- roid deficiency.

پی بی آئی: تھائیرائیڈ ہارمون کے حصے میں پروٹین کے ساتھ آیوڈین۔

Pearson bed. A special type of hospital bed used for fractures. It is higher and narrower than the usual type. Instead of springs there are tight strips of webbing. The matters is in three or four sections. A Balkan beam is attached to the bed frame.

پیئرسن بیڈ: فریکچرز کے لئے مستعمل قسم کا ہسپتال کا بستر۔

Peauc d'orange *(po-dor-ongzh')* [F.]. Term applied to the appearance of the skin over the breast in acute inflammation or in advanced carcinoma, when lymphoedema causes the orifices of the hair follicles to appear as dimples, resembling the pits in the skin of an orange.

پیوڈی اورنج: چھاتی پر جلد کا ظہور۔

Pecazine *(pek-a-zen)* A phenothiazine derivative very similar to chloropromazine, and with similar therapeutic applications.

پیکازین: فینوتھیازین سے ماخوذ۔ کلورپرومازین سے مشابہ۔

Pectoral *(pek-tor-al)* [L. *pectoralis,* of the breast]. Pertaining to the breast.

صدری، قلبی: چھاتی سے متعلق۔

Pectus *(pek-tus)* [L.]. The chest. **pectus carinatum,** pigeon chest. **pectus excavatum,** funnel chest.

صدر: سینہ۔ چھاتی۔

Pedal *(ped-al)* [L. *pes,* foot]. Pertaining to the foot.

پیڈل، پائی: پاؤں سے متعلق۔ پاؤں کا۔

Pedascope *(ped-a-skop)* Allows shoe fitting under fluoroscopy.

پیڈ اسکوپ: فلوروسکوپی کے تحت پاؤں فٹ کرتا ہے۔

Pediatrician. See PAEDIATRICIAN.

ماہر طب اطفال: بچوں کے امراض میں ماہر۔

Pediatrics. See PAEDIATRICS.

پیڈیاٹرکس: بچوں سے بحث کرنے والی ادویات کی شاخ۔

Pedicle *(ped-ik-l)* [L. *pediculus,* little foot]. A stalk, e.g. the narrow part by which a tumour is attached to th **surounding** structures.

ساقچہ: ڈنڈی۔

Pediculosis *(ped-ik-u-lo-sis)* [L. *pediculus,* little foot; G. *-osis,* condition]. Infestation with lice (ped- iculi).

جوئیں پڑنا۔ قمل: جوؤں کے ساتھ تکلیف کی حالت۔

Pediculus *(ped-ik-u-lus)* [L.]. A genus of parasitic insectys (lice) important as vectors of disease. *Pediculus campitis,* the head louse. *Pediculus corporis,* the body louse. *Pediculus* (more correctly, *Phthiruius)pubis,* the public louse.

جنس جوں: طفیلی حشرات یعنی جوؤں کا ایک جنس۔

Ped-o-jet Apparatus of introduction of vaccines under pressure into the skin. Avoids the use of a needle with consequent danger of spreading serum hepatitis.

پیڈوجیٹ: کھال میں دباؤ کے تحت ویکسین داخل کرنے کا آلہ۔

Pedopompholyx *(pe-do-pom-fo-liks)* See CHEIROPOMPHOLYX.

پیڈوپومفولکس: کیروپوم فولکس۔

Peduncle *(ped-ungk-l)* [L. *pedunculus,* little foot.]. A stalk like structure, often acting as a support -- preduncular, pedunculated, adj.

مساق: ڈنڈی نما ساخت جو اکثر سہارے کے طور پر کام کرتی ہے۔

Peeling . Desquamation (q.v.)

چھیلنا: چھلنے کا عمل۔

Peganone *(peg-a-non)* Ethotion (q.v.)

پیگاں نون: ایتھوٹائن۔

Pel-Ebstein fever. Recurring bouts of pyrexia in reg- ular subsequnce found in lymphadenoma (Hodg- kin's desease). Less frequent man- ifestation with improving treatment. [Pieter Klazes Pel, Dutch physician, 1852-1919 Wilhelm Ebstein, German phys- ician 1836-1912].

بخار پیل ایب سٹائن: لمف اڈینو ماہوڈ گکنز بیماری میں پائے جانے والے باقاعدہ سلسلہ میں پائیریکسیا کے بار بار بوٹس۔

Pelizaeus-Merzbacher disease Geneticall deter- mined degenerative disease associate with mental subnormality. [Friedric Pelizaeus, German neurologist 1850----Ludwing Merzbacher, Germa physician in Argentina, 1875---].

پیلی زئیس مرز بیکر مرض: ذہنی تنزلی کے ساتھ تنزلی بیماری۔

Pellagra *(pel-a-gra)* A deficiency diseas caused by lack of vitamin B complex an protein. Syndrome includes glossitis dermatitis, peripheral neuritis and spinal cor changes (even producing ataxia), anaemia an mental confusion.

درشت جلدی: وٹامن بی کمپلکس کی کمی سے ہونے والا مرض۔ چہرے کی جلد متورم ہو جاتی ہے اور کالے نشان پڑ جاتے ہیں۔ آزاد کشمیر میں یہ مرض عام ہے۔ علاج کے لئے نیکوٹینک ایسڈ پچاس ملی گرام دو گولیاں دن میں تین دفعہ دو ہفتے تک اور وٹامن بی کمپلکس اور وٹامن سی ایک گولی روزانہ ایک ماہ۔

Pellet *(pel-et)* [L. *pila,* ball]. A little pill. Se IMPLA- NT.

قرص صغیر: ایک چھوٹی گولی۔

Pelvic floor repair . See FOTHERGILL'S OPER- ATION.

پیڑو کی فرش کی مرمت: اپریشن فودرگل۔

Pelvimeter *(pel-vim-et-er)* [L. *pelvis,* basin; G *metron,* a measure]. An instrument especiall devised to measure the pelvic diameters.

حوض پیما: پیڑوؤں کے اقطار کی پیمائش کے لئے خصوصی طور پر تیار کردہ آلہ۔

Pelvimete

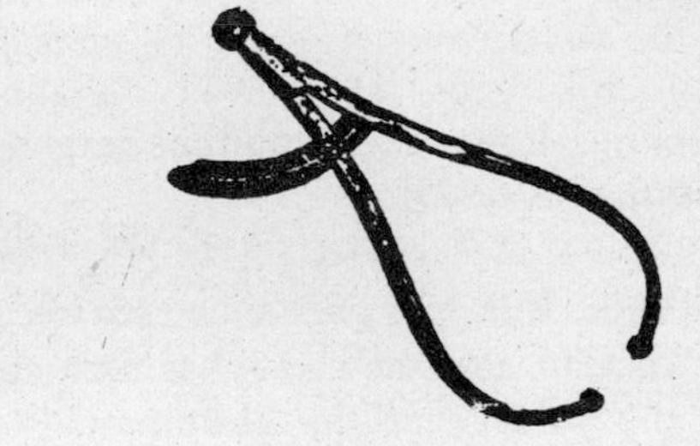

Pelvimetry *(pel-vim-et-ri)* [L. *pelvis,* basin; G. *metro- n,* a measure]. The measurement of the dime- nsions of the pelvis.

حوض پیمائی: پیڑن کے ابعاد کی پیمائش۔

Pelvis *(pel-vis)* [L.]. 1. A basin-shaped cavity. e.g. pelvis of the kidney. 2. The large bony basin-shaped cavity formed by the innominate bones and sacrum, containing and protecting the bladder, rectum and organs of generation. **contracted p,.**one in which one or more diameters are smaller than normal and this may result in difficulties in childbirth false p., the wide expanded part of the pelvis above the brim. **true p.,** that part of the pelvis below the brim--pelvic, adj.; pelves, pl.

حوض۔ پیٹرو کا حلقہ۔ ہکل عانی: (۱) بیسن نما کہفہ۔ (۲) بڑا استخوانی بیسن نما کہفہ جو لاامی ہڈیوں اور سیکرم سے بنتا ہے۔ اس میں بلیڈر یکٹم اور تولیدی اعضاء شامل ہیں اور یہ ان کی حفاظت بھی کرتا ہے۔

Human Pelvis And Perineum

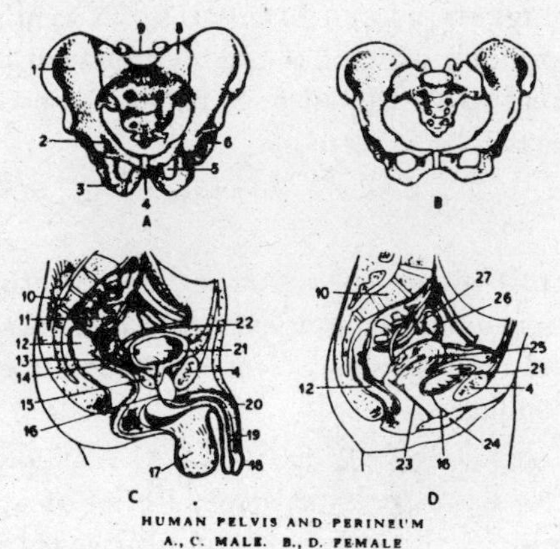

HUMAN PELVIS AND PERINEUM
A., C. MALE. B., D. FEMALE

Pemphigoid *(pem'-fi-goid)* [G. *pemphix* ,pustule]. Allied to pemphigus. A bullous eruption in the latter half of life. Of unknown cause. Histological exmamination of the base of a blister differenitates if from pemphigus.

فقاعی: چھالہ۔ آبلہ۔

Pemphigus *(pem-fig-us)* [G. *pemphix,* pustule]. Skin conditions with bullous (blister) eruptions, but more correctly used of a group of dangerous diseases called up 'p. vulgaris, 'p. vegetans and p. erythematosus'. neonatorum; (1) a dangerous form of impetigo occuring as an epidemic in the hospital nursery; (2) bullous eruption in congenital syphilis of the newborn. **pemphigus vulgris** is a bullous disease of middle age and later, of unknown aetiology. Oedema of the skin results in bister formation in the epidermis, with resulting secondary infection and rupture, so that large raw areas develop. Bullae develop also on mucous membrances Death is from malnutrition or intercurrent disease.

آبلہ۔ چھالہ: جلد پر چھالوں کی موجودگی کی حالت۔ علاج کے لئے پریڈنی سولون۔ سیپٹران۔ اے کی ٹی ایچ۔ ملٹی وٹامن پلس اور ڈائی اینا بال مفید ہیں۔

Pempidine *(pem-pi-den)* A blocking agent used for treatement of hypertension. It is active orally and the response is reliable and consistent in effect. Side effects are fewer than those experienced with other drugs of this type.

پمپیڈین: بیش طبانی کے علاج کیلئے مستعمل ایک بلاک کرنے والا ایجنٹ۔

Penbritin, Ampicillin (q.v.)

پین بریٹن: امپی سلین۔ گردے کی چھوت میں جراثیم اندام نہانی سے گردے میں پہنچ جاتے ہیں۔ گردہ دکھنے لگتا ہے۔ پیشاب کم آتا ہے۔ شدید بخار ہو جاتا ہے۔ اس میں یہ دوائی مفید ہے۔

Pendulous *(pen-du-lus)* [L. *pendere,* to hang]. Hanging down

معلق آویزاں: نیچے لٹکانا۔

Penethamate hydriodide *(pen-ne-tham-at hid-ri-o-did)* An iodine-containing form of pencillin. Said to be absorbed by lung tissue, and is therefore used respiratory infections.

پینتھیمیٹ ہائیڈرو آیوڈائیڈ: آیوڈین پر مشتمل پینسلین کی قسم۔ کہا جاتا ہے کہ اسے پھیپھڑے کی بافتیں جذب کر لیتی ہیں۔

Penicillamine *(pen-i-sil-a-men)* A degradation product of penicillin used in the treatment of heavy mental intoxication, Wilson's disease, lead pois- oning, cystinuria and rheumatoid arthritis.

پینی سلامین: پنسلین کا ایک پروڈکٹ۔ بھاری دھاتوں کے زہریلا پن میں مفید۔

Penicillin *(pen-i-sil-in)* . The first antibiotic, also known as 'p.G'. or 'benzyl p.' Widely used by injections due to Gram-positive bacteria, some cocci, and spirochaetes. High blood levels are obtained rapidly, and can by supplemented by injections of the slower acting procaine-p. **fortified pl.** is a mixture of p.G. and procaine p.p.V is an orally active form, as ordinary p. is rapidly destroyed by th gastric juice. The dose of penicillin varies widely according to the severity of infection, the largest being given in bacterial endocarditis (2 000 000 units).

پنسلین: سماروغ پنسلیم سے پیداشدہ پہلی ضدحیات یا جراثیم کش۔ یہ جراثیم کی بہت سی بیماریاں پیدا کرنے والی اقسام کی نشونمارو کنے کے لئے ایک بہت طاقتور ایجنٹ ہے۔ آتشک یا سفلس کے علاج کے لئے پنسلین کرسٹلان پانچ لاکھ یونٹ ایک ٹیکہ صبح ایک شام دس ایام تک۔ سوزاک میں پانچ ایام تک ایکٹینونائی کوسز میں ایک ماہ تک۔ مفید برائے اریی سپیلاز۔

Penicillinase *(pen-i-sil-in-az)* An enzyme which dest- royed penicillin.

پینی سلی نیز: پنسلین کو تباہ کرنے والا خامر۔

Penicillium *(pe-ni-sil-i-um)* [L. *penicillus,* brush] A genus of moulds. The hyphae bear spores characteristically arranged like a brush. Common contaminant of food. *Penicillium chrysogenum* is now used for the commercial production of the antibiotic. *P. noiatum* is a species shown by Fleming (1928) produce penicillin.

پینسلیم: سماروغ کا ایک جنس۔ ریشوں سے بذرے ہوتے ہیں اس لئے وہ برش کی طرح دکھائی دیتے ہیں۔ فلیمنگ نے اس سے پینسلین تیار کی۔

Penidural *(pen-i-du-ral)* Benzathine penicillin.

بنزاتھین: پینسلین۔

Penis *(pne-nis)* [L.]. The male organ of copulation-penile, adj.

آلہ تناسل۔ ذکر: مباشرت کا نرعضو۔ اس کا ایک حصہ اسفنجی اور دوسرا حشفیہ ہے۔ اسفنجی کے درمیان پیشاب کی نالی ہوتی ہے۔ جنسی ہیجان کے وقت اس میں خون بھر جاتا ہے اور تین کردو یا تین گنا بڑا ہو جاتا ہے۔ قضیب کا سرا یا حشفہ عضو کا حساس ترین حصہ ہے۔ اس میں سے بوقت حاجت پیشاب خارج ہوتا ہے اور یہی انزال کے وقت مادہ منویہ کو عورت کی اندام نہانی میں پہنچاتا ہے جو حمل کا باعث ہوتا ہے۔

Penofome *(pen-o-fom)* Mild detergent for therapeutic application to the skin and vagina.

Penotrane *(pen-o-tran)* Effective against Candida and pyogenic organisms.

Pentaerythrityl tetranitrate . Coronary vasodilator in tablet form.

پینٹااتھریٹائل ٹیٹرانائیٹریٹ: گولی کی صورت میں دستیاب۔

Pentacynium *(pen-ta-sin-i-um)* Ganglion blocking agent. Anti-hypertensive.

پینٹاسائی نیئن: بیش تابی کے علاج کے لئے مفید۔ گینگلیان بلاک کرنے والا ایجنٹ۔

Pentagastrin *(pen-ta-gas-trin)* A synthetic hormone which has largely replaced older drugs as the stimulant of choice foe evoking maximal acid secretion.

پینٹاگیسٹرین: زیادہ سے زیادہ ایسڈ پیدا کرنے کے لئے تحریک کرنے والا۔

Pentamidine *(pen-tam-i-din)*. Synthetic compound used in trypanosomiasis, kala-azar and leishmaniasis. Has also been used in moniliasis.

پنٹامیڈین: ایک تالیفی مرکب۔ کالا آزاداور کئی دوسری بیماریوں میں مفید۔

Pentazocine *(pen-taz-o-sen)* Relief of severe pain in the presence of bradycardia or hypertension pentazocine is better than morphine. Can be given orally, intramu- scularly, intravenously.

پینٹازوسین: سخت درد کو آرام دینے والا۔ ٹالون۔ پلیوریسی یا جرسام میں ایک گولی صبح ایک دوپہر ایک شام یہی خوراک برائے سر درد، درد شقیقہ۔

Penthrane *(pen-trhran)* Methoxyflurance (q.v.)

Pentobarbitone *(pen-to-bar-bit-on)* One of the

short-acting barbiturates. Often used for premed- ication in children.

پینٹو بار بی ٹون: مختصر العمل بار بیٹوریٹس میں سے ایک۔ اکثر بچوں کو احتیاط کے طور پر دیا جاتا ہے۔

ntolinium *(pen-to-lin-i-um)* A ganglionic blocking agent used in hypertension; active orally. Can be given by injection.

پینٹو لینیم: پیشاب میں پنج کاربنی شکر۔ میٹو بولک خرابی کی وجہ سے ایسا ہو سکتا ہے۔

ntose *(pen-tose)* A class of monosaccharides with five carbon atoms in their molecule.

مونو سیکرائڈز کی ایک جماعت جن کے سالمے میں پانچ کاربن ایٹم ہوتے ہیں۔ اہم ترین پنج کاربنی شکر ریبز ہے جو نکلیک ایسڈ کا لازمی جزو ہے۔

ntosuria *(pen-tos-u-ri-a)* [G. *pente,* five; *ouron,* urine]. Pentose in the urine. Can be due to a metabolic disorder pentosuric adj.

پیشاب میں پنج کاربنی شکر۔ میٹابولک خرابی کی وجہ سے ایسا ہو سکتا ہے۔

ntothal *(pen-to-thal)* Thiopentone (q.v.).

پینٹو تھال: تھیو پینٹون۔

ppermint *(pep-er-mint)* An aromatic carminative and stimulant. Also used as a flavouring agent.

پیپر منٹ۔ ست پودینہ: خوشبودار ہاضمہ دار اور محرک۔ فلیورنگ ایجنٹ کے طور پر بھی مستعمل۔

psin *(pep-sin)* A proteolytic enzyme of the gastric juice.

جوہر ہاضم: ایک ہاضمی خامرہ جو معدہ میں ہوتا ہے اور لحمیات کو پیپٹونز میں تبدیل کرتا ہے۔ یہ صرف تیزابی واسطہ ہے۔ یہ لحمیات پاش ہے اور لحمیات پر عمل کرتا ہے۔

psinogen *(pep-sin-o-jen)* Secreted by the peptic cells in the gastric mucoss and converted into pepsin by contact with hydrochloric acid.

پیپسینو جن: گیسٹرک میوکوسا میں ٹپیک خلیوں سے پیدا شدہ اور نمک کے تیزاب کے ساتھ مل کر پیپسن میں تبدیل ہوتا ہے۔

tic *(pep-tik)* [G. *peptikos,* helping digestion] Pertaining to pepsin or to digestion generally. **eptic ulcer,** a non-malignant ulcer in those parts of the digestive tract which are exposed to the gastric secretions; hence usually in stomatch or duodenum.

Peptic ulcer

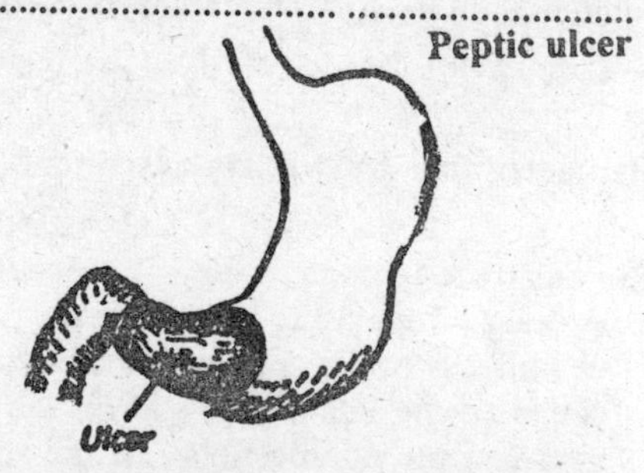

ہاضم: پیپسن یا ہاضم سے متعلق۔

Peptides *(pep-tidz)* Chemical combinations of one or more amino acids, i.e. dipeptides, tripeptides or polypeptides.

پیپٹائڈز: دو یا زیادہ امینو ایسڈز کا ایک مرکب۔

Peptone *(pep-ton)* Substance produced when the enzyme pepsin acts upon the acid metaproteins produced in the first stage of digestion of proteins.

پیپٹون: نامیاتی مادے جو معدہ میں پیپسن کے عمل کے لحمیات کی آب پاشیدگی کے ذریعہ پیدا ہوتے ہیں۔ وہ پانی میں حل پذیر ہیں اور انہیں جسم جذب کر لیتا ہے۔

Peptonuria *(pep-ton-u-ri-a)* [G.*peptos,* cooked; *ouron,* urine]. Peptones in the urine.

پیپ ٹون بولی: پیشاب میں پیپٹونز۔

Percept *(per-sept)* The mental product of a sensation; and their relationships.

مدرکہ۔ محسوس: محسوس کرنے کا ذہنی پروڈکٹ۔

Perception *(per-sep-shun)* [L. *perceptio*]. The rec- eption of a conscious impression through the senses by which distinguish objects one from another and recognize their qualities according to the different sensations they produce.

ادراک۔ احساس: ارادے کے ساتھ تاثر کی وصولی جو ان حواس سے ہوتی ہے جن سے ہم ایک دوسرے کو چیز سے ممیز کرتے ہیں۔

Percolation *(per-ko-la-shun)* [L. *percolare,* to strain through]. The process by which fluid slowly passes through a hard but porous substance.

نفوذ۔ رساؤ: وہ طریقہ جس سے سیال سخت لیکن مسامدار مادہ سے رفتہ رفتہ گزرتا ہے۔ کوئی ہوئی ادویہ سے پانی' ایتھر یا سپرٹ کو گزارا جاتا ہے اس طرح ادویہ سے جوہر حل کر کے علیحدہ کر سکتے ہیں۔

Percorten *(per-kor-ten)* De-oxycortone (q.v.)

پرکارٹن: ڈی آکسی کارٹون۔

Percussion *(per-kush-un)* [L. *percussio*, a striking]. Tapping to determine the resonance or dullness of the area examined. Normally a finger of the left had is laid on the patient's skin and the middle finger of the right hand (plexor) is used to strike the left finger.

ضرب۔ ٹھکائی: کسی جگہ کو جانچنے کے لئے آہستہ آہستہ مارنا۔ عموماً مریض کی جلد پر انگلی مارتے ہیں۔

Percutaneous *(per-ku-ta-ne-us)* [L.*per*, through; *cutis*, skin]. Through unbroken skin See CHOLANGIOGRAPHY.

جلدی: غیر شکستہ جلد میں سے۔

Perforation *(per-fora-shun)* [L. *perforare*, to pierce through]. A hole in an intact sheet of tissue. Used in reference to p. of the tympanic membrance, or the wall of the stomatch or gut, constituning a surgical emergency.

سوراخ: نسیج کی شیٹ میں سوراخ۔

Perherxiline *(per-heks-i-len)* Antianginal drug coronary vasodilator.

پرہیکسی لین: اینٹی انجینل دوا۔

Periadenitis *(per-i-ad-en-i-tis)* [G. *peri*, around; *aden*, gland; *-itis*, inflammation]. Inflammation in soft tissues surrounding glands. Responsible for the 'bull' neck in German measles.

التہاب حول الغدہ: گلینڈز کے گرد نرم بافتوں میں سوزش۔

Perianal *(per-i-an-al)* [G. *peri*, around; L. *anus*, anus,]. Surrounding an artery.

حول شریان: شریان کے گرد۔

Periarteritis *(per-i-art-e-ri-tis)* [G. *peri*, around; *arteria*, artery; *-itis* inflammation]. Inflammation of the outer sheath of an artery and the periarterial tissue. **periarteritis nodosa.** See COLLAGEN and POLYARTERITIS.

لتہاب ظہارہ شریان: پیری آرٹیریل نسیج اور شریان کی بیرونی شید کی سوزش۔

Periarthritis *(per-i-arth-ri-tis)* [G. *peri*, around *arthron*, joint; *-itis*, inflammation] Inflammation of the structures surrounding a joint. Sometimes applied to frozen shoulde (q.v.)

لتہاب حول المفاصل: جوڑ کے گرد ساختوں کی سوزش۔

Periarticular *(per-i-art-ik'-u-lar)* [G. *peri*, around; L. *articulus*, joint]. Surrounding joint.

ول المفصل: جوڑ کے گرد۔

Periacardectomy *(per-i-kard-ek-to-mi)* [G *peri*, around; *kardia*, heart; *ektome*, excision] Surgical removal of pericardium, thickene from chronic inflammation and embarrassin the heart's action.

یری کارڈیکٹومی: پیری کارڈیم کا سرجیکل خاتمہ۔

Pericardiocentesis *(per-i-kar-di-o-sen-te-sis* [G. *peris*, around; *kardia*, heart; *kentesi*. puncture]. The withdrawal of fluid from th pericardial sac by insertion of a hollow needl or cannula.

البطن تاموری: کھوکھلی سوئی داخل کر کے پیریکارڈیل تھیلی سے سیال کو کھینچنا۔

Pericarditis *(per-i-kar-di-tis)* [G. *peri*, aroun *kardia*, heart, *-itis*, inflammation Inflammation of the outer, serous covering th heart. It may or may not be accompanied b an effusion and formation of adhesion between the two layers. See BROADBENT SIGN and PERICARDECT- OMY.

م غلاف قلب: دل کے بیرونی غلاف کی سوزش۔

Pericardium *(per-i-kard-i-um)*. The doub membr- anous sac which envelops the hea The layer in contact with the heart is call 'visceral'; that reflected to from the sac called 'pariental'. Between the two is t pericardial cavity, which normally contains small amount of serous fluid--pericardial, ac

ف قلب: ڈبل جھلی دار تھیلی جو دل کو طفوف کرتی ہے۔

Perichonodrium *(per-i-knod-ri-um)* [G. *peri,* around; *chondros,* cartilage]. The membranous covering of cartilage -- perichondrial, adj.

غشاء غضروف: کارٹیلج کا جھلی دار غلاف۔

Pericolic *(per-i-kol-ik)* [G. *peri,* around; *kolikos,* suffering in the colon] Around the colon.

حول قولون: قولون کے گرد۔

Pericranium *(per-i-kran-i-um)* [G. *peri,* around; *kranion,* skull]. The perioisteal covering of the cranium--pericranial, adj.

سمحاق۔ کھوپڑی: کھوپڑی کا پیری آسٹیل غلاف۔

Pericyazine *(per-i-si-a-zen)* Phenothiazine derivative; much stronger than chlorpromazine.

پیری سیازین: فینوتھیازین سے ماخوذ۔ کلورپرومانین سے زیادہ طاقتور۔ پاگل پن کے علاج کے لئے ایک گولی صبح ایک دوپہر ایک شام۔

Perifollicular *(per-i-fol-ik-u-lar)* [G. *peri,* around; L. *folliculus,* small sac]. Around a follicle.

پیری فولیکولر: فولیکل کے گرد۔

Perilymph *(per-i-limf)* [G. *peri,* around; L. *lympha,* water]. The fluid contained in the internal ear, between the bony and membranous labyrinth.

بیرونی لمف: استخوانی اور جھلی دار لیبرنتھ کے درمیان اندرونی کان میں شامل سیال۔

Perimetrium *(per-i-met-ri-um)* [G. *peri,* around; *metra,* womb]. The peritoneal covering of the uterus--perimetrial. adj.

صفاق رحم: رحم کا پیری ٹونیل غلاف۔

Perinatal *(per-i-na-tal)* [G. *peri,* around; L. *natus,* birth] Occurring at, or pertaining to, the time of brith.

پیری نیٹل: پیدائش کے وقت سے متعلق۔

Perineorrhaphy *(per-i-ne-or-raf-i)* [G. *perineos,* space between anus and scrotum]. The operation for the repair of a torn perineum.

عجان دوزی: پھٹے پیرینیم کی مرمت کے لئے اپریشن۔

Perineotomy Episiotomy *(q.v.)*

شق عجانی: اپی سیوٹومی۔

Perinephric *(per-i-nef-rik)* [G. *peri,* around; *nephros,* kidney]. Surrrounding the kidney.

غلاف گردہ: گردے کے گرد۔

Perineum *(per-in-ne-um)* [G.perineos, space between anus and scrotum]. The portion of the body included in the outlet of the pelvis--perineal, adj.

عجان سیون: پیڑو کے بیرونی سوراخ میں شامل جسم کا حصہ۔

Perionychia *(per-i-on-ik-i-a)* [G. *peri,* around; *onyx,* nail]. Red and painful swelling around nail fold. Common in hands that are much in water or have poor circulation. Due to infection from the fungus Candida, more common now because of the use of antibiotics which subdue organisms which previously curtailed the activity of Candida Secondary infection can occur.

Periosteum *(per-i-ost-i-um)*. The membrance which covers a bone. In long bones only the shaft as far as the epiphysis is covered. It is protective and essential for regeneration -- periosteal, adj.

جھلی جو ہڈی کے گرد ہوتی ہے۔

Periostitis *(per-i-os-tis)* **perlosteitis** [G. *periosteos,* around bone; *-itis,* inflammation]. Inflammation of the periosteum. **periostitis diffuse,** that involving the periosteum of long bones. **periostitis haemorrhagic,** that accompanied by bleeding between the periosteum and the bone.

ورم ضریع: پیری آسٹیم کی سوزش۔

Periostosis *(per-i-os-to-sis)* [G. *periosteos,* around bone; *-osis,* condition]. Inflammatory hypertorphy of bone.

آماس: ہڈی کی سوزشی ہائپرٹرافی۔

Periportal *(per-i-por-tal)* [G.*peri,* around; L. *portia,* gate]. Surrounding the portal and anus.

پیری پورٹل: پورٹل ورید کے گرد۔

Periproctitis *(per-i-prok-ti-tis)* [G. *peri,* around; *proktos,* anus; *-itis,* inflammation]. Inflammation around the rectum and anus.

ورم حول دبر: ریکٹم اور مقعد کے گرد سوزش۔

Perirenal *(per-in-ren-al)* [G. *peri*, around; L.*renus*, kidneys]. Around the kidney.

حول جگری: گردے کے گرد۔

Perisplenitis *(per-i-splen-i-tis)* [G. *peri*, around; *splen*, spleen; *-itis*, inflammation]. Inflammation coat of the spleen and of the adjacent structures.

التہاب کیسہ طحال: تلی اور ملحقہ ساختوں کے پیریٹونیل کوٹ کی سوزش۔

Peristalsis *(per-i-stal-sis)* [G.*peri*, around; *stellein*, to draw in]. The characteristic movement of the intestines by which the contents are moved along the lumen. It consists of a wave of contraction preceded by a wave of relaxation peristaltic, adj.

حرکت انقباضی: آنتوں کی مخصوص حرکت جس میں خوراک آگے جاتی ہے۔

Peritomy *(per-it-o-mni)* [G.*peri*, around; *tome*, a cutting]. Excision of a protion of conjuctiva at the edge of cornea to prevent vascularization of a corneal ulcer.

غباری پردہ چشم پر عمل جراحی: قرینہ کے کنارے پر کنجنکٹیوا کے ایک حصے کو کاٹنا۔

Peritoneoscopy *(per-it-on-e-os-ko-pi)* [G. *peri*, around; *teinein*, to stretch; *skopein*, to examine]. Laparoscopy (q.v.)

پیری ٹونیوسکوپی: لپاروسکوپی۔

Peritoneum *(per-i-to-ne-um)* [G. *peri*, around; *tenein*, to stretch]. The delicate serous membrane which lines the abdominal and pelvic cavities and also covers the organs contained in them peritoneal, adj.

پیٹرو کا پردہ۔ باریطون: نازک جھلی جو بطنی اور پیڑو کے کہفوں کی دیواروں پر ہوتی ہے اور ان کے اندرونی اعضاء کو بھی ملفوف کرتی ہے۔

Peritonitis *(per-i-ton-i-tis)* [G. *peri*, around; *teinein*, to stretch; *-itis*, inflammation]. Inflammation of the peritoneum, usually secondary to disease of one of the abdominal organs.

ورم باریطون: پیریٹونیم کی سوزش۔

Peritonsillar abscess Quinsy (q.v.).

حلق کا پھوڑا: گلے کی سوزش۔

Peritrichous *(per-i-tri-kus)* [G. *peri*, around; *thrix*, hair]. Applied to bacteria which possess flagella on all sides of cell. See BACILLUS.

پیری ٹرائیکس: اس اصطلاح کا اطلاق ان جراثیم پر ہوتا ہے جن میں خلیے کے تمام اطراف پر فلیجیلا ہوں۔

Periumbillical *(per-i-um-bil-ik-al)* [G. *peri*, around; L. *umbilicus*, middle]. Surrounding the umbilicus.

حول ناف: ناف کے گرد۔

Periurethral *(per-i-u-re-thral)* [G. *peri*, around; *ourethra*, urethra]. Surrounding the urethra, as a p.u. abscess.

پیری یورتھرل: یورتھرا کے گرد۔

Perivascular *(per-i-vas-ku-lar)* [G. *peri*, around; L. *vasculum*, vessel]. Around a blood vessel.

حول عروقی: خونی رگ کے گرد۔

Perleche *(per-lesh)* Lip licking. An intertrigo at the angles of the mouth with maceration, fissuring, or crust formation. May result from use of poorly fitting dentures, bacterial infection, thrush infestation, vitamin deficiency, drooling or thumb-sucking.

بچوں کے لبوں کا مرض: لبوں کے نقطۂ اتصال یعنی منہ کے کونوں پر بعض دفعہ دانے نکل آتے ہیں۔ اکثر بخار کے ایسا ہوتا ہے۔ جراثیم یا قلت حیاتین کی وجہ سے ایسا ہوتا ہے۔

Permeability *(per-me-a-bil-it-i)* [L. *permeabilis*, that can be passed through]. In physiology, the ability of cell membrances to allow salts, glucose, urea and other solube substances to pass into and out of the cells from the body fluids.

نفوذ پذیری: کسی جسم کو ایسے مادے کے لئے نفوذ پذیر کیا جاتا ہے۔ اگر وہ اپنے آپ میں سے مادے کو گزرنے دے۔

Pernicious *(per-nish-us)* [L. *p[erniciosus*, destructive]. Deadly, noxious.

مضر۔ مہلک: خوفناک۔ تباہ کن۔

Pernicious anaemia Results from the inability of the bone marrow to produce normal red cells because of the deprivation of a protein released by gastric glands, previously called the intrinsic factor which is necessary for the absorption of vitamin B_{12}. An autoimmune mechanism may be responsible.

perniosis *(per-ni-o-sis)* [L. chilblain]. Chronic chilb- lains. The smaller arteioles go into spasm readily from exposure to cold.

پیری نیوسس: چھوٹی شریانیں سردی کی وجہ سے سپازم میں چلی جاتی ہیں۔

Peroidin *(per-o-i-din)* Potassium perchlorate (q.v.)

پرائڈن: پوٹاشیم کلوریٹ۔

Perolysen *(per-o-li-sen).* permpidine (q.v.)

Peromelia *(per-o-me-li-a)* [G. *peros,* maimed; *melos,* limb]. Teratogenic malformation of a limb.

پیرومیلیا: جوارح کی مخصوص بدصورتی۔

Peroral *(per-or-al)* [L. *per,* through; *os,* mouth]. Through the mouth, aw p. boipsy of the small bow- el.

حول دہن: منہ میں سے۔

Peroxide See HYDROGEN.

پرآکسائیڈ: ہائیڈروجن اور آکسیجن مل کر ہائیڈروجن پرآکسائیڈ بناتی ہیں۔ (۱) آکسائیڈ جو تیزاب کے ساتھ ہائیڈروجن پرآکسائیڈ بناتا ہے۔ (۲) آکسائیڈ جو ایک عنصر کے نارمل آکسائیڈ کی نسبت زیادہ آکسیجن پر مشتمل ہوتا ہے۔

Perphenzine *(per-fen-a-zen)* Antiemetic and tranquillizing agent.

Persveration *(per-sev-er-a-shun)* [L. *perseverare,* to presist]. A mental symptom consisting of an appa- rent inability for the patient's mind to detach itself from one idea to another with normal speed. Thus shown a picture of a cow, the patient repeats 'cow' when shown furthur pictures of different objects. Common in senile dementia, schizophrenia.

تکرار تصور: ایک مخصوص ذہنی علامت جس میں مریض ایک نظریہ کو چھوڑ کر دوسرا نظریہ تیزی سے نہیں اپنا سکتا۔

Personality *(per-son-al-i-ti)* [L.*personalis,* of a person]. The various mental attitudes and characteristics which distinguish a person. The sum total of the mental make-up. **psychopathic p,.** a persistent disorder or disability of mind (whether or not including subnormality of intelligence) which results in abnormally aggressive or seriously irrespon- sible conduct that requires, or is susc- eptible to, medical treatment.

شخصیت: مختلف ذہنی رویے اور خصوصیات جو ایک شخص کو ممیز کرتے ہیں۔

Perspiration *(per-spi-ra-shan)* [L. *per,* through; *spirare,* to breathe]. The excretion of the sweat glands through the skin pores. **insensible p.,** invisible, the perspiration is evaporated imme- diatley it reaches the skin surface. **sensible p.,** vis- ible drops of sweat on the skin.

عرق۔ پسینہ: جلدی سوراخوں سے پسینے کے گلینڈز کا اخراج۔

Perthes' disease (legg-Perthes-Calve's disease). Syn,. pseudocoxalgia. A vascular degeneration of the upper femoral epiphysis; revascularization occurs, but residual deformity of the femoral head may subsequently lead to arthritic changes.

مرض پرتھیز: بالائی فیمول اپی فائیسس کی واسکوتنزلی۔

Pertofran. Desipramine. See ANTIPRESANT.

پرٹوفران: ڈیسی پرامین۔

Pertussis *(per-tus-is)* Whooping cough. An infectious disease of children with attacks of coughing which reach a peak of voilence ending in an inspiratory whoop. The basis of the conditon is respiratory catarrh and the organism responsible is *Bordetella pertussis.* Prophylactic vaccination is responsible for a decrease in case incidence.

شہقہ: کالی کھانسی۔ بچوں میں چھوت کی بیماری جس میں کھانسی کا حملہ ہوتا ہے۔ اس کے لئے ویکسین استعمال کی جاتی ہے۔

Pes [L.] A foot or foot-like structure. **pescavus,** 'hollow' foot when the longitudinal arch of the foot is accentuated.Claw-foot is accentuated. Cl- aw-foot.

Pes planus. valgus-foot, flat, foot.

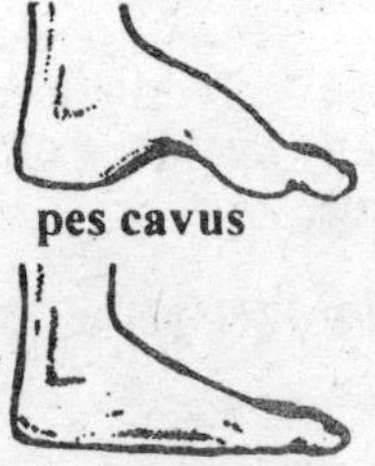

pes cavus

Pes planus

پسین پا۔ پچھلا: پیر یا پیر نما ساخت۔

Pessary *(pes-a-ri)* [L. *pessarium*]. 1. An instrument inserted into the vagina to correct uterine displa- cements. A ring or shelf p. is used to support a prolapse. A Hodge p. is used to correct a retroversion. 2. A medicated suppository used to treat vaginal infections, or as a contraceptive.

رحم بند۔شیاف مہبل: (۱) رحمی متبادلات کو صحیح کرنے کے لئے رحم میں داخل کیا جانے والا آلہ۔(۲) مانع حمل۔

Pesticides *(pes-ti-sidz)* Substances which kill pests.

Petechia *(pe-te-ki-a)* A small, haemorrhagic sp- ot--petechial, adj.

نملہ۔نمشہ۔لطخہ: چھوٹی ہیمرج والی جگہ۔ارغوانی رنگ کے باریک دانے جوتپ فرقہ ایسے بخاروں میں نظر آتے۔

Pethidine *(peth-i-din)* Synthetic analgesic and sp- asmolytic. Widely used for both pre-operative and postoperative analgesia instead of morphine. Can be given orally, intramuscularly or intravenously.

پیتھی ڈین: مصنوعی دافع درد یہ عضلاتی ٹیکہ دردزہ کے دوسرے درجے کے دوسرے دوز میں لگاتے ہیں۔کاروزی تھرامبوسز اور اس سے درد کی شدت کا احساس کم ہوتا ہے۔ہارٹ اٹیک میں شدید درد کی صورت میں اس کا ۱۰۰ ملی گرام ولایتی ٹیکہ عضلاتی ٹیکہ لگائیے۔ پتے کے درد میں بھی اس کا ٹیکہ مفید ہے۔پلمونری ایمبولزم میں درد بند کرنے کے لئے سو ملی گرام کا ٹیکہ روزانہ صبح و شام۔

Pethilorfan *(peth-il-or-fan)* Pethidine and levall- orphan tartrate, a narcotic antagonist that reduces respiratory depression without affecting analgesia.

پیتھی ڈین اور لیولورفن ٹارٹریٹ۔

Petit mal *(pet-e-mal)*. Minor epilepsy (q .v.) Momen- tary loss of consciousnes is characteristic.

خفیف مرگی: ہوش کا عارضی ضیاع۔

Petrous *(pe-trus)* [G. *petros*, stone]. Resembling st- one.

سخت۔حجر: پتھر سے مشابہ۔

Peyer's patches *(pi-ers)*. Flat patches of lymphatic tissue situated in the small intestine but mainly in the ileum; they are the seat of infection in typhoid fever; also known as 'aggregated lymph nodules.' [Johann Conrad Peyer, Swiss anatomist, 1653- 1712.].

لمفی نسیج: کے چپٹے دھبے جو چھوٹی آنت میں ہوتے ہیں۔لیکن زیادہ تر الیئم میں ہوتے ہیں۔

Peyronie's disease Deformity and painful erection of penis due to fibrous tissue formation from unkn- own cause. Often associated with Dupuytren's contracture. [Francois de la Peyronie. French surg- eon, 1678-1747.]

ریشہ دار نسیج بننے: سے آلہ تناسل درد کے ساتھ سیدھا ہونا۔

PH. The concentration of hydrogen ions expressed as a logrithm. A neutral solution has a pH 7.0. With increasing acidity the pH falls and with increasing alkalinity it rises.

پی ایچ: ہائیڈروجن آئنوں کا ارتکاز۔

Phaeochromcytoma *(fe-o-kro-mo-si-to-ma)* A cond- ition in which there is a tumour of the adrenal medulla, or of the structurally similar tissues associated with the sympathetic chain. It secretes adrenaline and allied hormones and the symptoms are due to the excess of these substances. Aetiology unknown. See TEST: ROGITINE.

ایڈرینل میڈلا کی رسولی کی حالت۔

Phagocyte *(fag-o-sit)* [G. *phagein,* to eat; *kytos,* cell]. A cell capable of engulfing other cells and debris in the tissues--phagocytic, adj.

اکالہ: سفید جیسے۔ایک خونی خلیہ خصوصاً لیکوسائیٹ جو کسی بیرونی ذرے یا جرثومے کو نگل سکتا ہے۔یہ خلیات انسان کے خون میں موجود ہوتے ہیں۔

Phagocytosis *(fag-o-si-to-sis)* [G. *phagein,* te eat; *kytos,* cell; *-osis,* condition]. The engulfment by phagocytes of foreign or other particles, or cells harmful to the body.

اکالیت۔ جراثیم خوردگی: جسم کے لئے نقصان دہ بیرونی یا دوسرے ذرات یا خلیات کو سفید جسیمے نگل جاتے ہیں۔

Phako-emulsification *(fa-ko-em-uls-i-fik-a-shun)* Ultra- sonic vibration is used to liquefy mature lens fibres. The liquid lens matter is then sucked out in an action similar to that of a vaccum cleaner.

Phalanges *(fal-an-jez)* The small bones of the finger and toes--phalanx, sing; phalangeal, adj.

پور: ہاتھوں اور پیروں کی انگلیوں کی چھوٹی ہڈیاں۔

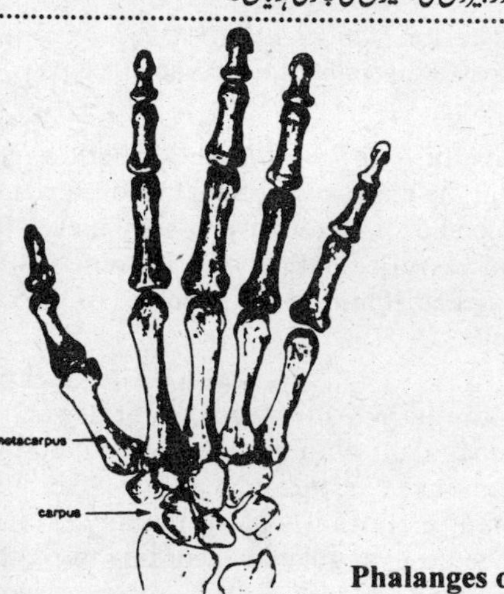

Phalanges of hand

Pharmacology *(far-ma-kol-o-ji)* [G. *pharm-akon,* drug; *logos,* discourse]. Th science dealing with drugs.

علم الادویہ: ادویات سے متعلق سائنس۔

Pharyngectomy *(far-in-jek-to-mi)* [G. *pharygx,* pharynx; *ektome,* excision]. Removal of part of the pharynx.

قطع البلعوم: فیرنکس کے حصے کا خاتمہ۔

Pharyngismus *(far-in-jis-mus)* Spasm of the phary- nx.

تشنج بلعوم: فیرنکس کا سپازم یا اینٹھن۔

Pharyngitis *(far-in-ji-tis)* [G. *pharygx,* pharynx; *-itis,* inflammation]. Inflammation of the pharynx.

ورم حلق: حلق یا فیرنکس کی سوزش یا سوج۔

Pharyngolaryngeal *(far-ing-go-lar-in-je-al)* [G. *pha- rygx,* pharynx; *larygx,* larynx] Pertaining to the pharynx and larynx.

بلعومی حنجری: فیرنکس اور لیرنکس سے متعلق۔

Pharyngolarygectomy *(far-ing-go-lar-in-jek-to-mu)* [G. *pharygx,* pharynx; *larygx,* larynx; *tome, a cutting.*]. Surgical removal of the pharynx and larynx

:فیرنکس اور لیرنکس کو اپریشن کے ذریعے کاٹ دینا۔

Pharyngoplasty *(far-ing-go-plas-ti)* [G. *pharygx;plassein,* to form]. Any plastic operation to the pharynx.

فیرنگوپلاسٹی: فیرنکس کا پلاسٹک اپریشن۔

Pharyngotomy *(far-in-got-o-mi)* [G. *pharygx,* phar- ynx; *tome,* a cutting]. The operation of opening into the pharynx.

حلق تراشی: انگلی میں تین اور انگوٹھے میں دو پوریں ہوتی ہیں۔

Phallus *(fal-us)* [G. *phallos*]. The penis--phallic, adj.

ذکر: آلہ تناسل۔

Phanquone *(fan-qwon)* Antidysentery drug.

فینکوئن: ضد پیچش دوا۔

Phantasy. See FANTASY.

سراب خیال: سوچنے والے کی خوشی یا خواہش کے مطابق عکس یا عکسوں کی زنجیر جو غیر حقیقی احساس کے ساتھ تخیل یا تصور میں آتی ہیں۔

Pharmaceutical *(far-ma-su-tik-al)* [G. *pharm-keu- tikos*] Relating to drugs.

ادویاتی: ادویات سے متعلق۔

Pharmacogenetic *(far-ma-ko-jen-et-ik)* [G.*pharmak- on,* Drug; *genesis,* descent]. Produced by drugs, usually referring to side effects.

فارمیکو جنیٹک: ادویات سے پیدا شدہ عموماً جانبی اثرات ۔ فیرنکس میں سوراخ کرنے کے لئے اپریشن۔

Pharyngotympanic tube *(far-ing-go-tim-pan-ik)* See EU-STACHIAN TUBE.

فیرنگوٹمپینگ نلی: یوسٹیشن ٹیوب۔

Pharynx *(far-ingks)* [G. *pharygx*]. The cavity at the back of the mouth. It is cone shaped, varies in len- gth (average 76 mm), and is lined with mucous membrane; at the lower end it opens into the oesophagus. The Eustachian tubes pierce its lateral walls and the posterior nares pierce its anterior wall. The larynx lies immediately below it and in front of the oesophagus--pharyngeal, adj.

حلق ۔ گلا ۔ بلعوم: منہ کی پشت پر کہفہ ۔ مخروط نما ۷۶ مم طویل، نچلے سرے پر یہ ایسوفیگس میں کھلتی ہے ۔ یہ راستہ اوپر کی طرف سے ناک سے تعلق

رکھتا ہے۔درمیان میں منہ ہے۔اس کے نیچے سانس کی نالی یا ونڈ پائپ اور غذا کی نالی یا گلٹ میں۔

Phemitone *(fem-i-ton)* Barbiturate very similar to ph- enobarbitone, but with greater antic- onyulsant act- ion. Used in epilepsy.

فیمی ٹون: مینو باربیٹون سے مشابہ باربیٹوریٹ۔

Phenacemide *(fen-as-e-mid)* Anticonvulsant useful in temporal lobe epilepsy.

فین اسے مائیڈ: مرگی میں مفید۔

Phenacetin *(fen-as-et-in)* Analgesic of great us- efulness and low toxicity. Constituent of many an -algesic preparations.

فینسیٹن: تیز ابی پائدار اور منہ کے ذریعے دی جاسکتی ہے۔پنسلین کی متبادل دوائی۔

Phenadoxone *(fen-a-doks-on)* Analgesic with considerable spasmolytic action, useful in severe pain. Can be given orally or intramu- scularly.

فیناڈوکسن،فینا کسن: ایک سفید قلمی مرکب۔نقطہ پگھلاؤ ۱۳۴ءاس درد دور کرنے کے لئے استعمال کیا جاتا ہے۔

Phenazone *(fen-a-zon)* An analgesic resembling phenacetin in effect, but is more tixic. Soluble in water.

فینازون: اثر میں فناسٹین سے مشابہ لیکن زیادہ زہریلی دوا۔پانی میں حل پذیر۔

Phenazocine *(fen-az-o-sen)* Potent analgesic for severe acute or chronic pain.

فینازوسین: شدید قدیم درد کے لئے مفید۔

Phenazopyridine hydrochloride *(fen-az-o-pir-i-den)* Urinary tract sedative, especially useful in cystitis.

فینازو پیری دین ہائیڈروکلورائیڈ: بولی راہ کو آرام پہنچانے والی مسکن دوا۔

Phenelzine *(fen-el-zen)* Antidepressant drug; a monoamine oxide inhibitor.

فینیل زین: پریشانی و مایوسی ختم کرنے والی دوا۔

Phenergan *(fen-er-gan)* Promethazine (q.v.)

فنرگان: پرومیتھازین ۔ پرومی زائے تھین کا تجارتی نام۔دردزہ کے دوسرے درجہ میں یہ دوائی دی جاتی ہے۔مقدر پچیس ملی گرام (ایک خوراک)

Phenethicillin *(fen-eth-i-sii-in)* Acid stable and can be given by mouth. Alternative t penicillin but contraindicated in penicilli sensitivity.

پنسلین کی متبادل دوا۔منہ کے ذریعے دی جاسکتی ہے۔

Pheneturide *(fen-et-ur-id)* Used in majo epilepsy, especially of temporal lobe type.

فینے ٹیورائیڈ: مرگی میں مفید۔

Phenformin *(fen-for-min)* Antidiabetic agent One of the diaguanides. Said to reduce weigh andblood cholesterol thus possibly preventin blood vessel complications. Has an insulin like action, stimu- lates the uptake of glucos by cells.

ن فارمن: ضد ذیابیطس ایجنٹ۔

Phenindione *(fen-in-di-on)* An orally activ anticoagulant with an intermediate action Widely used in thromboemblic disorders often after initial heparin therapy. Main enance doses regulated according to proth ombin time.

نڈی اون: خون جمنے نہیں دیتا۔ڈنڈی وین۔کاروزی تھرامبوسز میں اس ایک گولی صبح ایک شام ایک ماہ تک۔

Pheniodol *(fen-i-o-dol)* An iodine compoun used as a contrast agent in cholecystrography

نوڈول: ایک آیوڈینی مرکب۔

Phenmetrazine hydrochloride *(fen-met-ra-ze hi-dro-klor-id)* Appetite depressant. Dang of addiction and psychosis of a parano nature.

ن میٹرازین ہائیڈروکلورائیڈ: بھوک کم کرنے والی دوائی۔

Pheniprazine *(fen-ip-ra-zen)* A monoami oxidase inhibitor.

ی پرازین: مونوآمین آکسیڈیز۔

Phenobarbitone *(fe-no-bar-bit-on)* Long-acti barbiturate and anticonvulsant. Used general sedative, and in epilepsy.

. باربیٹون: طویل اثر والا باربیٹوریٹ۔دور دور کرنے والی دوائی اور ی میں مفید۔سفید قلمی سفوف یا مرکب۔نقطہ پگھلاؤ ۱۷۴ ڈگری سینٹی گریڈ۔ ک آور دوا عموماً حل پذیر سوڈیم نمک کی صورت میں۔گارڈی نال۔بچے اس کی ایک گولی دن میں تین دفعہ برائے مرگی یا اپی لیپسی۔

Phenol *(fe-nol)* . Carbolic acid. Powerf antiseptic, widely used as a 1 in 20 solutic

Weaker solutions occasionally used for application. Strong solutions are caustic--phenolic, adj.

فینول: کاربالک ایسڈ۔ایک سفید قلمی ٹھوس' نقطہ پگھلاؤ ۴۱ ڈگری سینٹی گریڈ' کاربالک کی مخصوص بو آتی ہے۔پانی میں حل پذیر' تباہ کن اور زہریلا' جراثیم کش کے طور پر اور پلاسٹکوں اور رنگوں کی تیاری میں استعمال کیا جاتا ہے۔

'henolphthalein *(fen-olf-tha-le-in)* Powerful non-toxic purgative, often given with liquid para- ffin.

فینالفتھلین: ایک بے رنگ قلمی ٹھوس' نقطہ پگھلاؤ ۲۶۱ ڈگری سینٹی گریڈ' رنگ کی تیاری اور بطور قبض کشا استعمال کیا جاتا ہے۔

'henoperidine Powerful analgesic that is a respi- ratory centre depressant. Useful where breating is controlled by mechanical ventilation.

فینوپیری ڈین: تنفسی مرکز کو آرام پہنچاتا ہے۔قوی دافع درد میکانکی طور پر سانس لینے کے لیے مفید۔

'henothiazines *(fen-o-thi-a-zens)* Traaquill-izing compounds. Chloropromazine and promazine belong to this group.

فینوتھیازینز: سکون بخش مرکبات۔کلورپرومازین اور پرومازین اس گروہ میں شامل ہیں۔

'henoxybenzamine *(fen-oks-i-ben-za-min)* Perip- heral vasodilator used in Raynaud's disease and as an antihypertensive agent.

فیناکسی بنزامین: جانبی باسط شرائین ریناڈ کے مرض میں مفید۔

'henoxymethlpenicillin *(fen-oks-i-meth-il pen-i-sil-in)* Oral penicillin (q.v.)

فیناکسی متھائل پنسلین: منہ کے ذریعے کھائی جانے والی پنسلین۔

'henoxypropazine A monoamine oxidase inhibitor.

فیناکسی پروپازین: ایم اے او آئی۔مونوامین آکسیڈیز۔

'hensuximide *(fen-suks'-mid)*. For petit mal

فین سکسی مائیڈ: معمولی مرگی میں مفید۔

'hensuximine *(fen-tol-a-men)* An adrenaline ant- agonist, used mainly by injection in the diagnosis and surgery of phaeochr-omocytoma, to contorl excessive variation of blood pressure. Occasionally used orally in vasospasm.

فینٹولامین: بلڈ پریشر کی زیادہ تبدیلی کو کنٹرول کرنے کے لئے مستعمل۔

Phenurone *(fen-u-ron)* Phenylacetylurea. (q.v.)

فینورون: فینائل ایسٹائیلوریا۔

Phenylacetylurea *(fen-il-as-et-il-ur-e-a)* A powerful but toxic antoconvulsant. Used in epilepsy resis- tant to other therapy.

فینائل ایسی ٹائیلوریا: ایک طاقتور لیکن زہریلا۔ضد تشنج۔

Phenylalanine *(fe-nil'-al-a-nin)* An essential amino acid associated with thyroxine and adrenaline, **phenylalanine mustard (PAM).** cytotoxic, alky- lating agent.

فینائل ایلانین: ایک قلمی حل پذیر امینوایسڈ' نقطہ پگھلاؤ ۲۸۳ ڈگری سینٹی گریڈ' انڈوں اور دودھ سے حاصل کیا جاتا ہے۔دودھ دینے والے ممالیہ جانوروں کے لئے لازمی ہے۔ایملین' سالمی وزن ۱۳ء۹۳۔جلدی انجذاب اور کھالینے سے نقصان دیتا ہے۔اس کا مائع آنکھوں کے لئے نقصان دہ ہے۔

Phenylbutazone *(fen-il-bu-ta-zon)*. Analgestic with powerful and prolonged action. Used mainly in rheumatic disorders. Toxic reactions are common and minimum mainten-ance doses are essentail. Occasionally causes salivary gland enlargement.

فینائل بیوٹازون: دافع درد دوا جس کا ایکشن طاقتور اور طویل ہوتا ہے۔جوڑوں کی خرابی میں عام مستعمل۔زہریلے تعاملات عام ہیں اس لئے اس کی کم خوراک دی جانی چاہیئے۔اس کے استعمال سے بعض اوقات سلوری گلینڈ بڑھ جاتی ہے۔بیوٹازولے ڈین۔ایکوٹ گاؤٹ' لقوہ اور پیرائی کلائی ڈائی ٹس میں اس کی ایک گولی دن میں تین مرتبہ اس کا ایک ٹیکہ روزانہ کے لئے عضلات میں پانچ دنوں تک برائے عرق النساء۔

Phenylephrine *(fen-il-ef-rin)* Vasoconstrictor and pressor drug similar to adrenaline, but more stable. Phenylephrine administrated simultaneously with isoprenaline appreciably reduces the effect on blood prssure and heart rate of isprenaline alone. Can be given intramuscularly or subcutaneously. Used as eyedrops (0.5 to 10 per cent) and as nasal spray (0.25 per cent).

فینائل ایفرین: ایڈرینالین سے مشابہ دوا لیکن زیادہ پائیدار۔آنکھوں کے ڈراپس یا ناک میں سپرے کرنے کے لئے بھی مستعمل۔

Phenylethylacetylurea *(fen-il-eth-il-as-et-il-ur-e-a)* See PHENYLACETYLUREA.

فینائل ایتھائل ایسی ٹائیلوریا: ایک طاقتور لیکن زہریلا ضد تشنج۔

Phenylketonuria *(fe-nil-ke-ton-ur-i-a)* Metabolites of phenylalanine (the best known being the phenylketones) in urine. Occurs in hyperphenylalaninaemia, owing to the lack of inactivity of the phenylalanine hydroxylase enzyme in the liver which converts dietary phenylalanine into tyrosine. Autosomal recessive disease, resu- lting in mental subnormality -- phenylke- tonuric,adj.

فینائل کیٹونیوریا: پیشاب میں فینائل ایلانین کے میٹابولائیٹس۔

Phenylpyruvic oligophrenia *(fe-nil-pi-ru-vik ol-ig-o-fre-ni-a)* See PHENYLKETONURIA.

فینائل اولیگوفرینیا: پیشاب میں فینائل ایلانین کے میٹابولائیٹس۔

Phenytoin *(fen-i-toin)* Anticonvulsant used in grand mal epilepsy, sometimes in association with phenobarbitone.

فینی ٹائن: ضد تشنج۔ اس کی سو ملی گرام کی ایک گولی دن میں تین مرتبہ برائے مرگی یا اپی لیپسی۔

Phimosis *(fi-mo'-sis)* [G.]. Tightness of the prepuce so that it can not be retracted over the glans penis.

ضیق غلفہ: آلہ تناسل کی تنی ہوئی کھچال جس کی وجہ سے وہ سر ذکر تک نہیں پہنچ سکتی۔

PHisoHex *(fi'-so-heks)* Antisepctic and antibacterial skin cleansing agent combining a detergent -- Entsufon, 3 per cent hexa- chlorophane, lanolin, cholesterols and petrolatum in an emulsion with the same pH as skin.

فائیسوہیکس: دافع تعفن اور جراثیم کش کھال کو صاف کرنے والا ایجنٹ۔

Phelebectomy *(fle-bek'-to-mi)* [G. *phelps,* vein; *ektome,* excision]. Excision of a vein **multiple cosmetic** p., (MCP) removal of varicose veins through little stab incisions which heal without scaring.

شق الورید: ورید کو کاٹنا۔

Phlebitis *(fle-bi'-tis)* [G. *phleps,* vein; *-itis,* inflammation].Inflammation of a vein-- phlebitic, adj.

ورم ورید: ورید کی سوزش۔

Phlebogram *(fle'-bo-gram)* [G. *phleps,* vein; *gramma,* letter]. See VENOGRAM.

م نبض الورید: وینوگرام۔

Phlebography *(fle-bog'-ra-fi)* See VE OGRAPHY.

Phlebolith *(fle'-bo-lith)* G. *phelps,* vein; *litho* stone]. A concretion which forms in a vein.

ید میں بننے والی پتھری۔

Phlebothrombosis *(fle-bo-throm-bo'-sis)* [*phleps,* vein; *thrombosis,* curdling Thrombosis in a vein due to sluggish flow blood rather than to inflam- mation in the ve wall, occuring chiefly in bedridden patien and affecting the deep venis of the low limbs or pelvis. The loosely attached thro bus is liable to break off and lodge in t lungs as an embolus.

ید میں تھرموبسس جس کی وجہ سے خون کا سست بہاؤ ہے۔ پیٹرو یا رزیریں رح کی گہری وریدیں زیادہ متاثر ہوتی ہیں۔

Phlegm *(flem)* [G. *phlegma*]. This secretion mucus expectorated fron the bronchi.

م: برونکائی سے میوکس کی رطوبت۔

Phlegmatic *(fleg-mat'-ik)* Emotionally stab Not easily excited.

ذباتی طور پر متوازن جسے آسانی سے جوش نہ دلایا جا سکے۔

Phlyctenule *(flik-ten'-ul)* [G. *phlyktain* blister]. A minute blister (vesicle) usual occuring on the conjunctiva or corn aphlyctenular, adj.

ک چھوٹا آبلہ جو عموماً کنجنکٹو یا قرینہ پر ہوتا ہے۔

Phobia *(fo'-bi-a)* [G. *phobos,* fear]. Morbid fea e.g. cardiac p., fear of heart disease, canc p.etc. --ph- obic, adj.

ض خوف: دہشت۔

Pholocodine *(fol'-ko-den)* Cough centre depr ssant similar to codeine.

انسی کے مرکز کو ختم کرنے والی دوا۔ کوڈین سے مشابہ۔ استھنین۔ برونکی ٹے سز میں فالکوڈین کف سیرپ کے دو چمچے صبح دو دو پہر دو شام۔

Phonocoardiogram *(fo-no-kar'-di-o-gram)* [*phone,* voice; *kardia,* heart; *gramma,* lette A graphic record of heart sounds.

کی آوازوں کا گرافک ریکارڈ۔

Phonocardiography *(fo-no-kar-di-og'-ra-fi)* [

ɔone, voice; *kardia,* heart; *gramma,* letter]. he graphic record of heart sounds.

برقی تولید سے دل کی آوازوں کی گرافک ریکارڈنگ۔

sphaturia *(fos-fa-tu'-ri-a)* [G. *phosphoros,* ght-bringer; *ouron,* urine]. Excess of ıosphates in the urine phosphaturic, adj.

فوسفاٹوریا: پیشاب میں فاسفیٹس کی زیادتی۔

spholine iodide*(fos-fo-lin-i'-o-did)* Anticho-nesterase drug; powerful miotic.

:اینٹی کولین ایسیٹر یز دوا۔

sphonates, *(fos'-fon-ats)* Chemical; when eposited in bone makes it harder for steoclasts to reabsorb that bone. Being tried r paget's deisease.

فاسفونیٹس: کیمیائی مرکب۔ جب ہڈی میں جمع ہو جائے تو آسٹیوگلاسٹ کے لئے اس ہڈی کو جذب کرنا مشکل ہو جاتا ہے۔

sphonecrosis *(fos-fo-ne-kro'-sis)* 'Fossy-jaw' ccu- ring in workers engaged in the anufacture of mathces made with white hosphorus: necrosis of the jaw with osening of the teeth.

فاسفونیکروسس: سفید فاسفورس سے تیار ہونے والی ماچس کی فیکٹریوں میں کام کرنے والوں میں جبڑوں میں دانت ڈھیلے ہو جاتے ہیں۔

sphorus *(fos'-for-us)* A non-metallic ement forming an important constituent of one and nerve tissue. Radioactive p. used in eatment of thrombocythaemia.

فاسفورس: ایک جوہری عنصر وزن ۳۰،۹۷۳۸ ' جوہری عدد ۱۵ ' یہ مختلف بہروپی اقسام میں پایا جاتا ہے سفید فاسفورس اور سرخ فاسفورس عام ہیں اول الذکر مومی سفید بہت آتش گیر زہریلا ٹھوس' نقطہ پگھلاؤ ۴۴ ڈگری گریڈ اور آخر الذکر یعنی سرخ فاسفورس غیر زہریلا' گہرا سرخ سفوف زیا آتش گیر نہیں۔ عنصر صرف مرکب حالت میں پایا جاتا ہے۔ عموماً کیل فاسفیٹ کی صورت میں پایا جاتا ہے۔ اسے برقی بھٹی میں کوک اور س (ریت) کے ساتھ گرم کرنے سے علیحدہ کیا جاتا ہے۔ فاسفورس کو اس طر ک شید کرلیا جاتا ہے۔ فاسفورس ریست کے لئے اہم ہے۔ کیلشیم فاسفی حیوانی ہڈیوں کا اہم جزو ہے۔ مرکبا فرٹیلائزر کے طور پر استعمال کیے جا ہیں۔ فاسفورس لپائڈ کا جزو ہے۔ یہ مراکز پروٹین میں ہوتا ہے۔ اس لیے تقسیم حصوں میں زیادہ پایا جاتا ہے۔ فاسفورس عمل تنفس میں اہم کردار ادا کرتا ہے۔ فاسفورس کی کمی سے پودے چھوٹے رہ جاتے ہیں۔ سرخ پگمنٹس بن جاتے ہیں اور وہ آہستہ پکتے ہیں۔ ایک غیر دھاتی عنصر جو ہڈی اور عصبی نسیج کا اہم جزو بناتا ہے۔ ریڈیو ایکٹو فاسفورس علاج میں مستعمل۔ اس کے کھانے سے منہ جل جاتا ہے۔ بدبودار اور خون آمیز الٹیاں' دل گھٹنا' پیٹ میں درد اور منہ و گلا دکھنا اس کی علامات ہیں۔ قے کرائی جاتے۔ درد کے لئے ایٹراپین کا ٹیکہ اور دل گھٹنے کے لیے کورامین کا ٹیکہ لگائیے۔ دودھ میں انڈے کی سفیدی ڈال کر دیجئے۔

Photalgia *(fo-tal'-ji-a)* [G. *phos,* light; *algos,* pain]. Pain in the eyes from exposure to intense light.

الم الضوء: زیادہ روشنی کی وجہ سے آنکھوں میں درد۔

Photochemical *(fo-to-kem'-ik-al)* Chemical changes brought about by light.

ضیاء کیمیائی: روشنی سے لائی گئی کیمیائی تبدیلیاں۔

Photocoagulation *(fo-to-ko-ag-u-la'-shun)* See LASER BEAM.

ضیائی انجماد: لیزر بیم۔

Photo-endoscope *(fo-to-end'-o-skop)* An endoscope to which a camera is attached for the purpose of making a permanent record -- photoendoscopy, n; photoendoscopic, adj; photoendoscopically, adv.

فوٹو اینڈوسکوپ: ایسی اینڈوسکوپ جس کے ساتھ کیمرہ ملحق ہوتا کہ مستقل ریکارڈ بنایا جاسکے۔

Photophia *(fo-to-fo'-bia)* [G. *phos,* light; *phobia,* fear]. Inability to expose the eyes to light -- photophobic, adj.

ضیاء ترسی۔ بغض العین: روشنی کی طرف آنکھیں کھولنے کی نااہلیت۔

Photosensitive *(fo-to-sen'-sit-iv)* Sensitive to light as the pigments in the eye.

حساس ضیاء: روشنی کے لئے حساس۔

Phototherapy *(f-to-ther'-a-pi)* [G. *phos,* light; *therapeia,* treatment]., Exposure to artificial blue light. In hyperbilirubinaemia it appears to dehydrogenate the bilirubin to biliverdin. Used for mild neonatal jaundice and to prevent jaundice in premature infants.

علاج شعاعی: مصنوعی نیلی روشنی پھینکنا۔ یرقان کے علاج میں مستعمل۔

Phren *(fren)* [G. *midriff*] The diaphragm -- phrenic, adj.

ذہن۔ دیافرغمہ: ڈایافرام۔ حجاب حاجز۔ حلق کے آخری منچلے سرے اور معدے کے درمیان پتلی سی جھلی۔

Phrenic avulsion See AVULSION.

دیافرغمی ایولسن: ایولسن۔

Phrenicotomy *(fre-ni-ko'-to-mi)* [G. *phren,* midriff; *tome,* cutting]. Division of the prenic nerve to paralyse one-half of the diaphragm.

حاجز برآری: فرینک عصب کی تقسیم تاکہ ڈایافرام کا نصف حصہ سن ہو جائے۔

Phrenoplegia *(fren-o-ple'-ji-a)* [G. *phren,* midriff; *pleg,* stroke]. Paralysis of the diaphragm.

فالج دماغ: ڈایافرام کا تشنج۔

Phrenotropic *(fren-o-tro'-pik)* Having an effect upon the mind.

فرینوٹراپک: ذہن پر اثر ہونا۔

Phthalyisulphathiazole *(tha-lil-sul-fa'-thi-a-zol)* A sulphonamide poorly absorbed from the alimentary tract, hence useful in instestinal infections, and before abdominal sugery.

تھےلل سلفاتھایازول: ایک سلفونامائیڈ۔ آنت کے امراض میں مفید۔ بطنی سرجری سے پہلے استعمال کیا جاتا ہے۔ تھےلازول۔ السریٹو کولائی ٹس میں دو گولیاں صبح، دو دوپہر، دو شام۔

Phthisis *(thi'-sis)* Old term for pulmonary tuberc- ulosis.

سل: پھیپھڑوں کی دق۔ شُشی تپ دق کے لئے قدیم اصطلاح۔

Physeptone *(fi-sep-ton)* Methadone (q.v.)

فائی سپٹون: میتھاڈون۔

Physicochemical *(fiz-i-ko-kem-ik)* Pertaining to Physics and Chemistary.

طبیعی کیمیائی: طبیعات اور کیمیا کے متعلق۔

Physiological *(fiz-i-o-loj-ik-al)* In accordance with natural processes of the body. Adjective often used to describe a normal proicess or structure, to distinguish it from an abn or pathological feature (e.g the p. lev glucose in the blood is from 3.0 to 5.0 per litre; higher and lower level pathological and indicative of dise **physiological saline** (nomal or isoton 0.9 per cent solution of sodium chlori water. **physiological solution,** a fluid iso with the body fluids isotonic with the fluids and containing similar salts.

: جسم کے قدرتی اعمال کے مطابق۔

Physiology *(fiz-i-ol-o-ji)* The sciencer w deals with the normal functions of the bo

: جسم کے عام افعال کے مطالعہ۔

Physostigmine *(fi-so-stig'-min).* An alk used in glaucoma as drops (0,25 to 1 per and to reverse the action of atro Occasionally used in paralytic ileus.

ستگمائن: ایک بے رنگ الکلائیڈ۔ نقطہ پگھلاؤ ۱۰۵ تا ۱۰۶ اس، سبز ۰،۲۵ تا ایک فیصد ڈراپس کے طور پر مستعمل اور ایٹروپین کے ایکشن کے لیے مستعمل۔

Phytomenadione. Intravenous vitamin K.

نا ڈی اون: انٹراوینس وٹامن ''کے'' ہیماپی سزیا خون تھوکنے میں روزانہ، اس کی ایک گولی صبح ایک، دوپہر ایک، شام برائے پرپرا۔

Phytomitogens *(fit-o-mit'-o-jens)* Agent appear to enhance immunity in vitro perhaps in vivo.

و جن: عوامل جو مدافعت بڑھاتے ہیں۔ جاندار اور تجربہ گاہ ں۔

Pia or pia mater *(pe-a-ma'-ter).* The inne of the meninges; the vascular meml which lies in close contact with the sub of the brain and spinal cord.

بقہ: واسکولر جھلی جو شوکی ڈور اور دماغ کے ساتھ کے بالکل قریب واقع

Pica *(pi'-ka)* [L. magpie]. Desire for e ordinary articles of food.

: خوراک میں غیر معمولی اشیاء کی خواہش۔

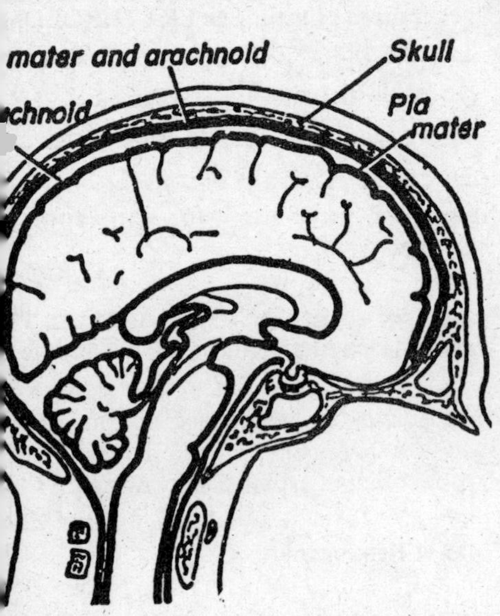

Pia mater

s diesease 1. Syndrome of ascites, hepatic lar- gement, oedema, and pleural effusion curing in constrictive pericarditis. [Friedel ck, German physician, 1867-1926]. 2. A pe of cerebral atrophy which produces ental changes similar to senescence (q.v.). rnold Pick, Czechoslovakian physician, 51-1924].

مرض پک: (۱) ایک قسم کا سنڈروم۔ (۲) سربرل اٹرافی کی ایک قسم۔

rna virus. Pico (very small) and RNA bon- ucleic acid). Small RNA viruses. The oup includes poliomyelitis virus, oxsackie, ECHO and rhinoviruses See RUS.

پکورنا وائرس: وائرس کا گروہ جن میں صرف ریبونکلیک ایسڈ ہوتا ہے۔ پولیو اور زکام کے وائرس۔

toxin *(pik-ro-toks'-in)* Central nervous stem stimulant used in barbiturate poisoning.

پکروٹاکسن: مرکزی عصبی نظام کا محرک۔ باربیٹوریٹ کے زہریلا پن مستعمل۔

Pigeon chest A narrow chest, bulging anteriorly in the breast bone region. (Pectus carintum).

کبوتر جیسی چھاتی: تنگ سینہ چھاتی کی ہڈی والے حصہ میں آگے کی طرف اوپر کو ابھرا ہوا سینہ۔

Pigment *(pig'-ment)* [L. *pigmentum*]. Any colouring matter of the body.

صبغہ۔رنگ: جسمانی رنگ۔ جسم کے رنگ والا مادہ۔

Pigmentation *(pig-men-ta'-shun)* [L. *pigmentum,* pigment]. The deposit of pigment, especially when abnormal or excessive.

قدرتی رنگت۔لونیت جلد: جسمی رنگ کا جمع ہونا خصوصاً جب غیر معمولی یا زائد ہونا۔

Piles See HAEMORRHOIDS.

بواسیر: مقعد کے گرد وریدوں کا پھیلاؤ۔ اس میں قبض رہتی ہے۔ مقعد کے مقام پر مسے بن جاتے ہیں۔ جو خون سے بھرے رہتے ہیں۔ مسے متورم ہو جائیں تو شدید درد ہوتا ہے۔ زیادہ بیٹھنے سے بواسیر ہوتی ہے۔ پیدل چلنا بہتر ہے۔ رات کو سوتے وقت لیکوئڈ پیرافین کے دو چمچے پلائیے۔ ایسٹیوفینا فتھون ایک گولی صبح ایک دوپہر ایک شام ٹیٹرا سائیکلین کپسول ہر ۶ گھنٹے بعد۔ پریڈنی سولون کمپاؤنڈ مرہم دن ۳ مرتبہ مسوں پر اندر اور باہر لگائیے۔

Pilocarpine *(pi-lo-kar'-pin).* An alkaloid used in a 0.5 to 1 percent solution as a moitic in glaucoma. Stimulates the salivary glands, and is occasionally used in high dose atropine therapy.

پلوکارپین: ایک الکلائیڈ جو سلوری گلینڈز کو تحریک دیتا ہے۔

Pilomotor nerves *(pi-lo-mo'tor)* [L. *pilus,* hair; *movere,* to move]. Tiny nerves attached to the hair follicle; innervation causes the hair to stand upright and give the appearance of 'goose flesh'.

موخر کی اعصاب: چھوٹی اعصاب جو بال کے فولیکل کے ساتھ ملحق ہوتی ہے۔

Pilonidal *(pi-lo-ni'-dal)* [L. *pilus,* hair; *nidus,* nest]. Hair containing. **pilonidal sinus,** a sinus containing hairs and which is usually found in hirsute people in the cleft between the buttocks. In this situation it is liable to infection.

کیسہ میں اجتماع شعر: بالوں پر مشتمل

Pilosebaceous *(pi-lo-se-ba'-shus)* [L. *pilus,* a hair; *sebaceus,* tallow candle]. Pertaining to the hair follicle and the sebaceous gland opening into it.

پلوسیشس : بال کے فولیکل اور اس میں کھلنے والی سیشس گلینڈ سے متعلق۔

Pilosis *(pi-lo'-sis)* [L. *pilus,* hair; G. *-osis,* condition]. An abnormal growth of hair.

پائیلوسس :بالوں غیر معمولی بڑھاؤ۔

Pimafucin, *(pim'-a-fu-sin)* Antifungal antibiotic, active against monilial infection.

پیمافیوسین :مونیلیل مرض کے خلاف عامل۔

Pimozide *(pim'-oz-id)* A long-acting neuroleptic which can be used to overcome the problem of a patient's non-compliance. Used only where there can be supervision for side effects.

Pimple *(pim'-pl)* See PAPULE.

مہاسا۔کیل :ایک چھوٹا جلدی ابھار۔

Pineal body *(pin'-e-al)* [L. *pinea,* pine cone]. A small reddish- grey conical structure on the dorsal surface of the midbrain. Its functions are not fully understood but there is some evidence that it is an endocrine gland concerned with growth.

صنوبری جسم : درمیانی دماغ کی ظہری سطح پر ایک چھوٹی مخروطی ساخت۔ اگر چہ اس کے افعال مکمل طور پر سمجھ نہیں آ سکتے تاہم چند شواہد کی رو سے یہ ایک اینڈوکرائن گلینڈ ہے جس کا تعلق نشوونما سے ہے۔لمبائی تقریباً ایک سینٹی میٹر۔

Pinguecula *(pin'-gwek-u-la)* [L. *pinqui-culus,* fattish]. A yellowish, slightly elevated thickening of the bulbar conjunctive near the lid aperture. Associated with the ageing eye.

پنکوئے کولا : پپوٹے کے سوراخ کے نزدیک کنجکٹو کی پیلی' ذرا اٹھی ہوئی دبازت۔

Pink disease Acrodynia. Disease of infants thought to be the result mercury poisoning. (The sale of mercury containing teething powders is now prohibited.) Child presents the picture of the mise- ry, with photophobia, restlessness and wasing. The extremities are swollen, and blue if child is cold, pink if he is warm. There is marked perspiration generalized pruritis. See ERYTHROEDM

گلابی: ایکروڈینیا بچوں کا مرض جس کے متعلق خیال ہے کہ پارے [ز]یلا پن سے ہوتا ہے۔ پارے پر مشتمل دانتوں کے سفوف پر پابندی [...]یئے ۔ بچہ روشنی سے ڈرتا ہے اور بے آرام رہتا ہے۔سرے متورم ہو [...]یں اگر بچہ ٹھنڈا ہو تو نیلا اور گرم ہو تو گلابی ہوتا ہے۔پسینہ بہت آتا ہے۔

Pink-eye Popular name for acute contag conjunctivitis.

[...]آنکھ: کنجکٹویٹس۔

Pinna *(pin'-a)* [L. feather]. That part of the which is external to the head; the auricle.

[...]: کان کا وہ حصہ جو سر کے باہر کی طرف ہوتا ہے۔آ ریکل۔

Pinta *(pin'-ta)* Colour changes in patches of due to *Treponema pinta,* identical with spirochaete of syphilis and yaws. (q.v.)

[...]لد کے بعض حصوں میں رنگ کی تبدیلیاں۔

Pipanol Benzhexol (q.v.)

[...]ل: بینز ہیکسول۔

Piperazine *(pi-per'-a-zen)* A highly effec anthelmintic against threadworms roundworms. Piperazine therapy car followed by incidents of unsteadiness falling; worm wobble.

[...]زین: ایک بے رنگ اساس۔نقطہ پگھلاؤ ۱۰۸° تا ۱۱۰°س کیڑوں [...]ے تباہ کن۔

Pipobromen *(pip-o-bro'-men)* Alkylating ag given orally. Used for chronic mye leukaemia.

[...]رومن: متضاد ایڈرنالین۔

Piposulfan *(pip-o-sul'-fan)* Similar structur alkyl- ating agents but its exact mod action is unkn- own. Given orally. Use chronic myeloid lenk- aemia.

[...]لفین: ساخت جو الکائیلیٹنگ ایجنٹ سے مشابہ ہو۔

Piracetam *(pir-a-set'-am)* For senile dement

Piriton *(pi'-ri-ton)* An antihistamine of [...] potency and of value in the treatmen transfusion reac- tions. Can be given orall by injection.

[...]ون: زیادہ پوٹنسی کا اینٹی ہسٹامین' کلورفزامین ایلرمین' السرینو کولائی [...]ب گولی صبح' ایک دوپہر' ایک شام۔دمہ میں یہی خوراک اسی طرح زکام

میں بھی ۔ اسی طرح مستعمل برائے سوزش گردہ' سپرنگ کٹار' الرجی چھپاکی' گرمی دانے' الیری تھیما۔

tressin *(pit-res'-in)* Vasopressin (q.v.)

پیٹریسن: واسوپریسن ۔ پیٹریسن ٹینیٹ' مرض ذیابیطس میں مستعمل۔

tting *(pit'-ting)* 1. Making an indentation in dropsical tissues. 2. Depressed scars left on the sk- in, especially after smallpox.

داغ: کھال پر رہے ہوئے نشیبی نشان مثلاً چیچک۔

tuitary extract *(pi-tu'-it-a-ri)* Vasopression. (q.v.)

نخامی عرق: ضدِ دست آور خصوصیات کا حامل۔

tuitary gland A small oval endocrine gland lying in the p. fossa of the sphenoid bone; the hypophysis cerebri. The anterior lobe secretes several homones, having an effect upon other endocrine glands. Their general overall function is to regulate growth and metabolism.

غدہ نخامیہ: سفینائیڈ ہڈی ء کے پیٹوٹری فوسا میں واقع ایک چھوٹی بیضوی' اینڈوکرائین گلینڈ' ہائپوفائیسس سربری۔

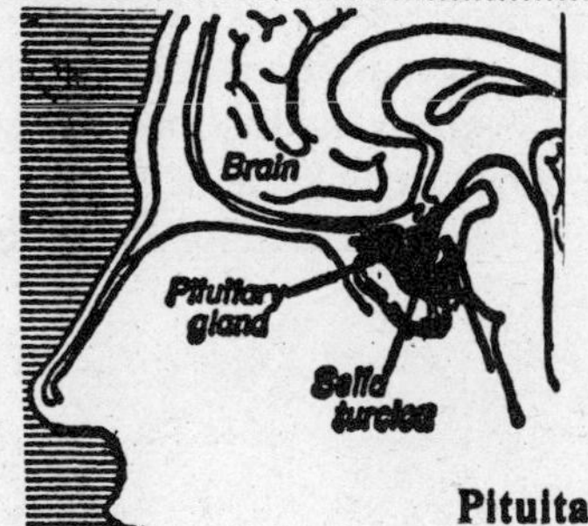

Pituitary gland

tyriasis *(pit-i-ri'-a-sis)* [G.]. Scaly (branny) eruption of the skin. **pityriasis capitis**, dandruff, **pityriasis rosea, a** slightly scaly reuption of ovoid erythemalous lesions which are widespread over the trunk and proximal parts of the limbs. There may be mild itching. It is a self-limiting condition. **pityriasis rubra**, a form of exfoliative dermatitis. **pityriasis rubra pillaris,** a chronic skin disease characterized by tiny red papules of perifollicular distribution. **pityriasis versicolor,** called also "tinea versicolor" is a fungus infection which causes the appearance of buff-coloured pathces on the chest.

بہق ابیض: جلد پھٹ کر سکیل اترنا۔ مثلاً خشکی ۔ گنج۔

Pityrosporum *(pit-i-ro-spor'-um)* A fungus associated with dandruff.

پیٹروسپورم: خشکی سے متعلق سماروغ۔

Pivhydrazine *(piv-hid'-ra-zen)* A monoamine oxidase inhibitor.

پوہائیڈرازین: مونوامین آکسیڈیز۔

PKU. Phenyldetonuria. (q.v.)

پی کے یو: فینائل کیٹونوریا۔

Placebo *(plas-e'-bo)* A harmless substance given as medicine. In experimental research an inert substance, identical in appearance with the material being tested. Neither the physician nor the patient know which is which.

پلیسیبو: ایک بے ضرر مادہ جو دوائی کے طور پر دیا جاتا ہے۔

Placenta *(pla-sen'-ta)* [L. cake]. After birth. A vascular structure developed about the third month of pregnancy and attached to the inner wall of the uterus. Through it the fetus is supplied with nourishment and oxygen and through it the fetus gets rid of its waste products. In normal labour it is expelled within an hour of the birth of the child. When this does not occur it is termed a **ratained p.** and may be an **adherent p.** The placenta is usually attached to the upper segment of the uterus; where it lies in the lower uterine segment it is called a **p. praevia,** and usually causes antepartum haemo- rrhage (now called placental abruption). See HAEMORRHAGE -- placental. adj.

Placenta praevia

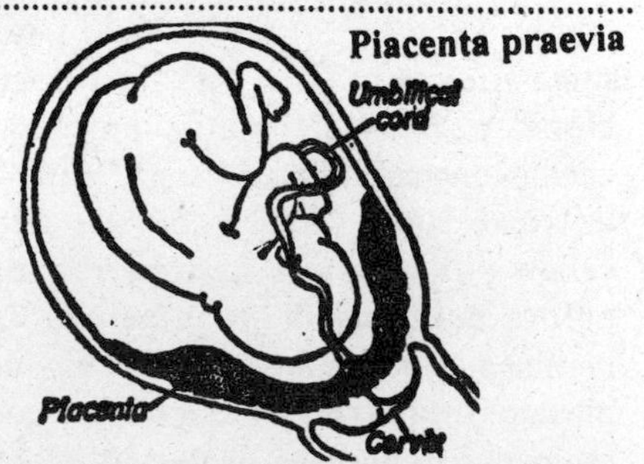

آنول: پیدائش کے بعد آنول ۔ اس کے ذریعے بچہ خوراک اور آکسیجن حاصل کرتا ہے۔

Placental insufficiency Insufficiency of the placenta. Cn occur duu to maternal disease or postmaturity of fetus giving rise to a 'small for dates' baby.

مشیمی نااہلیت: آنوں کی نااہلیت۔

Placentography *(pla-sen-tog'-ra-fi)* X-ray examination of the placenta by injection of opaque substance.

پلیسنٹوگرافی: غیر شفاف مادے کے ٹیکے سے آنول کے ایکسرے کے ذریعے ٹیسٹ۔

Plague *(plag)* [L. *plaga*]. Very contagious epidemic disease caused by *Pasteurella pestis,* and spread by infected rats. Tranfer of infection from rat to man is through the agency of fleas. The main clilnical types are buoonic, septicaemic or pneu- monic.

طاعون: چھوت کی بیماری جو چوہوں سے پھیلتی ہے پسو چوہوں سے آدمی تک پہنچتے ہیں۔

Plantar *(plan'-tar)* Pertaining to the sole of the foot, plantar arch, the union of the plantar and dorsalis pedis ateries in the sole of the foot **plantar flexion,** downward movement of the big toe.

متعلقہ ایڑی: پاؤں کی ایڑی سے متعلق۔

Plaquenil *(pla'-qwan-il)* Hydroxychloroquine. See CHLOROQUINE.

پلیکوئنل: ہائیڈروکسی کلوروکوئن۔

Plazma *(plaz-ma)* [G.]. The fluid fraction of blood. p. is used for infusion in cases of haemoconcentration of the patient's bloo, as in severe burns. Dried p. is inthe form of a yellow powder which must be 'reconstituted' before being used for infusion. Various plasma substitutes are available, e.g. dextran, plasmosan. **plasma** cell, a normal cell with arreccentric nucleus produced in the bone marrow and retiuloendothelial system, an conce- rned with the production o antibodies; abnormally produced in myelom atosis. (q.v.)

پلازما: خون مایہ۔خون کا سیالی جزو۔

Plasmapherisis *(plas-ma-fer-es-is)* Takin blood from a donor, removing some desire fraction then returning the red cells an repeating the whole pro- cess.

پلاسما فریسس: معطی سے خون لینا۔ پھر حسب منشا جزو نکال دیتے ہیں اور سرخ خلیے واپس کر کے گردش پوری کی جاتی ہے۔

Plasmin *(plaz-min)* A fibrinolysin (q.v.)

پلازمین: فائبرینولائیسن۔

Plasminogen *(plaz-min-o-jen)* Precursor o plasmin. Release of activators from damage tissue promotes the conversion o plasminogen into plasmin.

پلازمینوجن: پلازمین کا پیشرو۔

Plasmodium *(plaz-mo-di-um)* [G. *plasma,* form *eidos,* form]. A genus of protozoa. Parasites i the blood warm-blooded animals whic complete their sexual cycle in blood-suckin arthropods. Four species cause malaria in ma --- plasmodial, adj.

پلازموڈیم: یک خلوی جانور جو طفیلی ہوتا ہے ملیریا کا اصل سبب۔ پروٹوزوآ کا ایک جنس جو مچھر کے کاٹنے سے انسان کے خون میں بطور طفیلی داخل ہوتا ہے۔ وہ اپنا جنسی دور مچھر میں پورا کرتا ہے۔ اس کی چار انواع ملیریا پیدا کرتی ہیں۔

Plasmoquine See PAMAQUIN

پلازموکوئین: پاماکوئین۔

Plastazote *(plas-ta-zot)* New light weight ther- moplastic material used for splints, suppor and appliances.

پلاسٹازوٹ: نیا ہلکے وزن والا تھرمو پلاسٹک میٹریل۔ سہارا دینے کے لئے مستعمل۔

Plastic *(plas-tik)* Capable of taking a form o mould. **plastic surgery,** transfer of heatl tissue to repair damaged area and restor form.

پلاسٹک: پلاسٹکس ایسے مادے ہیں جو عام طور پر استعمال کے لئے پائیدار ہوتے ہیں۔ لیکن تیاری کی ایک مرحلہ پر پلاسٹک ہوتے ہیں اور حرارت، دباؤ یا دونوں سے ڈھل سکتے ہیں۔

latelet *(plat-let)* Syn., thrombocyte (q.v.)

دموی لوجین: یہ روانی خون کو بند کر دیتی ہے۔ یہ ایسے ذرات ہیں جن کے گرد جھلی ہوتی ہے اور خون میں گردش کرتے رہتے ہیں۔ تھرمیوسائٹس۔

latyhelminth *(plat-i-hel-minth)* [G. *platys,* broad; *helmins,* worm]. Flat worm; fluke. See SCHIS- TOSOMIASIS.

چپٹے کیڑے: جیسے چپٹے کیڑے۔ مثلاً کدو کیڑا۔ فلوک۔

leomorphism *(ple-o-mor-fizm)* [G. *pleon,* more; *porphe,* form]. Denotes a wide range in shape and size of individuals in a bacterial population -- pleomorphic, adj.

بسیار شکلیت: مختلف طریقوں پر پیدا ہونا یا پیدا ہونے والے بزرے۔ جراثیمی آبادی میں افراد کی شکل اور سائز میں کافی رینج کو ظاہر کرتا ہے۔

ethora *(pleth-o-ra)* [G.] Fullness; overloading--plethoric,adj.

کثرت الدم: بھرا ہوا۔ زیادہ ہونا۔ گنجائش سے زیادہ۔

ethysmograph *(pleth-is-mo-gral)* An instrument which meausres accurately the blood flow in a li- mb.

افراط۔ غلبہ خون: آلہ جو کسی جارح میں خون کے بہاؤ کو صحیح طور پر ناپتا ہے۔

eura *(ploo-ra)* [G.rib]. A thin serous membrance covering the surface of the lung and reflecting at the root of the lung, on the chest wall. That portion lining the chest wall is termed 'parietal p'; that closely adherent to lung tissue is 'visceral p. -- pleural. adj.

پلیورا۔ غشاء الجنب: ایک پتلی سیرس جھلی، پھیپھڑے کا پردہ۔

eurisy *(ploo-ri-si)* [G. *pleuritis*]. Inflammation of the pleura. Pleuritis. May be fibrinious (dry), be associated with an effusion (wet), or be compl- icated by empyema--pleuritic, adj.

جناب ۔ جرسام: پلیورا کی سوزش، ذات الجنب، پلیوریسی، پسلی کا درد، سٹیتھسکوپ سینے پر رکھ کر سنا جائے تو ایسی آواز آتی ہے جیسے نئے جوتے پہن کر چلتے ہوئے بعض دفعہ آتی ہے۔

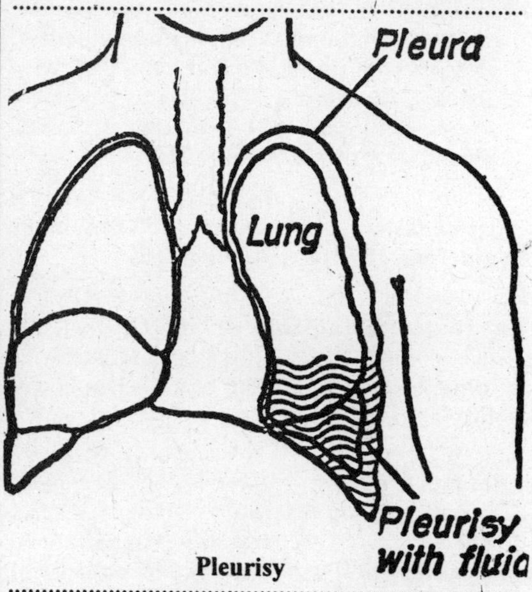

Pleurisy

Pleurodesis *(ploo-ro-de-sis)* [G. *pleura,* rib; *odyne,* pain]. Intercostal myalgia or muscular rheumatism (fibrositis). Is a feature of Bronholm disease (q.v.).

دہد پہلو۔ درد سینہ: پسلیوں کا درد۔ پھیپھڑے کے پردے کا درد۔

Pleuropulmonary *(ploo-ro-pul-mon-a-ri)* [G. *pleura,* rib; L. *pulmo,* lung]. Pertaining to the pleura and lung.

پلیورو پلمونری: پھیپھڑا اور پلیورا سے متعلق۔

Plexus *(pleks-us)* [L. a twining]. A network of vessels or nerves.

شبکہ: رگوں یا اعصاب کا جال۔

Plica *(pli-ka)* [L. *plicare,* to fold]. A fold -- plicate, adj; plication, n.

گرہ موئی: ایک تہہ۔

Plombage Extrapleural compression of the tuber-culous lung cavity.

بلبج: تپدق والے پھیپھڑے کے کہفہ کا بروں پیورال دباؤ۔

Plumbum Lead poisoning. (q.v.)

مسمومیت سربی: سیسہ کا زہریلا پن۔

Plumbism *(plum-bum)* [L.] Lead

سرب: سیسہ۔ ایک عنصر۔ ایک دھات۔

Plummer-Vinson syndrome Also Kelly Paterson syndrome. Cambination of severe glossitis with dysphagia and nutritional iron deficiency anaemia. [Henry Stanley Plummer. American Vinson. 1874-1936]. Porter Paisley Vinson. American physician. 1890-

پلمر ونسن سنڈروم: کیلی پیٹرسن سنڈروم۔

Plurigiandular *(plu-ri-gland-u-lar)* Pertaining to several glands as mucoviscidosis.

کئی غدی: مختلف غدود سے متعلق۔

Pneumaturia *(nu-mat-u-ri-a)* [G. *pneuma,* wind; *ouron,* urine]. The pasage of flatus with urine. Usually as a result of a bladder-bowel fistula.

ہوابولی: پیشاب کے ساتھ فلیٹس کا گزر۔

Pneumococcus *(nu-mo-kok-us)* [G. *pneumon,* lung; *kokkos,* berry]. *(Streptococcus pneumoniae).* A coccal bacterium arranged characteristically in pairs. A common cause of lobar pneumonia and other infections -- pneumococcal , adj.

نمونیائی نبقہ: ایک کاکسی جرثومہ جو خصوصیات کے ساتھ جوڑے کی صورت میں ہوتا ہے گرام مثبت۔

Pneumoconiosis *(nu-mo-ko-ni-o-sis)* Dust disease. Fibrosis of the lung caused by long continued inhalation of dust in industrial occupations. The most important complication is the occasional superinfection with tuberculosis. Examples are sillicosis, coal workers p., asbestosis, described else where. **rheumatoid p.,** fibrosing alveolitis occuring in patients suffering from rheumatoid arthritis -- pneumoconioses, pl.

تترب الریہ: گردوغبار والامراض۔ گردوغبار سانس کے اندر لگاتار جاتے رہنے کی وجہ سے پھیپھڑے کا فائبروسس۔

pneumoencephalogram *(nu-mo-en-kef-al-o-gram)* [F. *pneuma,* wind; *egkephalos,* brain; *gramma,* letter]. X-ray picture of cerebral ventricles after injection of air.

Pneumoencephlaography *(nu-mo-en-kef-al-og-ra-fi)* [G. *neuma,* wind; *egkephalos,* brain; *raphein,* to write]. Radiographic examination of cerebral ventricles after injection of air b means of a lumbar of cisternal puncture.

ومو انکیفالوگرافی: ہوا کے ٹیکے کے بعد سر بر ن بطینوں کی ریڈیو گرافی نچ پڑتال۔

Pneumogastric *(nu-mo-gas-trik)* Pertaining t the lungs and stomach. See VAGUS.

یوی معدی: معدہ اور پھیپھڑوں سے متعلق۔

Pneumomkoniosis See PNEUMOCONIOSIS.

ومولائی سس: دو پلیوروں پرتوں کی علیحدگی۔

Pneumolysis *(nu-mol-i-sis)* [G. *pneuma,* ai *lysis,* a loosening]. Separation of the tw pleural layers, or the outer pleural layer fro the chest wall to collapse the lung.

Pneumomediastinogram *(nu-mo-med-i-as ti-no-gr- am)* X-ray of the mediastinum aft rendering opa- que with air.

. مومیڈی اسٹینو گرام: ہوا سے غیر شفاف بنا کر میڈیا سٹائینم کا سرے۔

Pneumomycosis *(nu-mo-mi-ko-sis)* [G. *pneum* air; *mykes,* fungus; *-osis,* condition]. Fung infection of the lung such as aspergillosi actinomycosis, moniliasis -- pneumomycoti adj.

ض ریہ فطری: پھیپھڑے کا سماروغی مرض۔

Pneumonectomy *(nu-mon-ek-to-mi)* [(*pneumon,* lung; *ektome,* excision]. Excisi of a lung.

یہ براری: ایک پھیپھڑا کاٹ دینا۔

Pneumonia *(nu-mo-ni-a)* [G. *pneumon,* lung Infla- mmation of the lung with production alveolar exudate. Traditionally, two ma types were recog- nized, on an anatomical radiological basis, viz. lobar p. and broncho p. The tendency these days is to classi according to the specific bacterium or vir causing the infection (specific pneumonia on the one hand, and the aspiration of secondary pneumonias (non-specific) on t other. **hypostatic p.** is the result of stasis doccurs in the case of **debilitated patien**

'om lack of the lung. **unresolved p.** wherein ıe alveolar exudate does no liquefy but onsolidation persists -- pneumonic, adj.

نمونیہ: پھیپھڑے متورم ہو جاتے ہیں ۔ لوبر قسم کے نمونیہ میں صرف پھیپھڑے متاثر ہوتے ہیں۔ جبکہ برنکوقسم کے نمونیہ میں اعصابی تکالیف بھی ہوتی ہیں۔ کمزور افراد جلدی متاثر ہوتے ہیں۔ سینے میں درد' کھانسی' سانس تکلیف' بخار کی علامت ہیں۔ علاج کے لئے آکسی ٹیٹرا سائیکلین ہائیڈ کلورائیڈ کا ایک کیپسول ہر چھ گھنٹے بعد' پریڈنی سولون ایک گولی صبح ایک' ایک دوپہر ایک شام' سٹریٹیو مائی سین پروکین پنسلین یا آکسی ٹیٹرا سائیکلین ایک ٹیکہ روزانہ یا صبح وشام۔

umonitis *(nu-mon-it-is)* [G. *pneumon,* lung; *tis,* inflammation]. Inflammation of lung ssue.

نمونیا: پھیپھڑے کے نسیج کی سوزش۔

umoperitoneum *(nu-mo-per-it-on-e-um)* G. *pneumon,* lung; *peri,* aound; *teinein,* to retch]. Air or gas in the peritoneal cavity. an be intro- duced for diagnostic or erapeutic purposes.

خلائے تارمو میں اجتماع ریح: پرٹونیل کہفہ میں گیس یا ہوا۔

ımoradiography *(nu-mo-ra-di-og-ra-fi)* [G. ıeuma, wind; L. *radius,* ray; G. *graphein,* to irte]. Rediographic examination after injection ' air.

نیوریڈیوگرافی: ہوا کے ٹیکے کے بعد ریڈیوگرافیت جانچ۔

ımosol, An aerosol used in pneumonia.

نیوموسول: نمونیہ میں مستعمل ایروسول۔

ımothorax *(nu-mo-thor-aks)* [G. *pneumon,* ng; *thorax,* thorax]. Air or gas in the pleural vity separating the visceral from the parietal eura so that lung tissue is compressed. **tifficial p.,** induced in the treatment of lmonary tuberc- ulosis. **spontaneous p.** occurs ıen an overdilated pulmonary air scruptures rmitting commun- ication of respiratory ssages and pleural cavity. **tension p,.** occurs ıere a valve-like wound allo- ws air to enter the eural escape on expiration, thus progressively creasing intrathoracic pressure and consituting acute medical emergan- ce--pneumothoraces,

نفحہ الصدر: پلیورل کہفہ میں گیس یا ہوا جس سے ملحقہ پھیپھڑا اسکڑ جاتا ہے اور کام ختم کر دیتا ہے۔ سانس پھولنا' نیلی رنگت' گبھراہٹ' دھڑکن' صدمہ علامات ہیں۔ درد کے لئے کوڈین کمپاؤنڈ ایک گولی حسب ضرورت مریض کو بستر پر لٹا دیں۔ وجہ کا علاج کیجئے۔ ہوا دو تین ہفتوں میں جلد ہی جذب ہو جاتی ہے۔

Pneumothorax

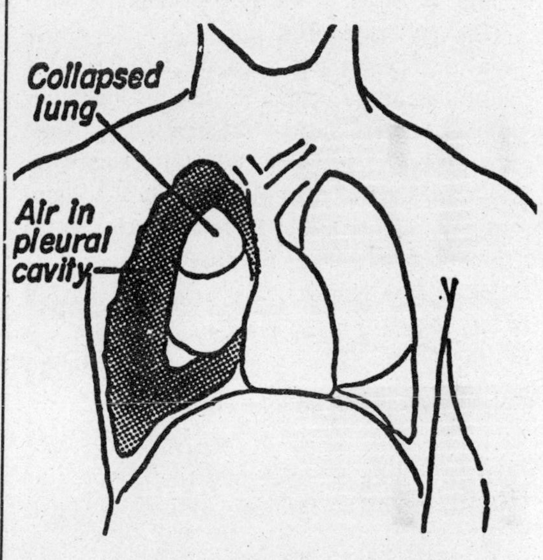

Pneumoventriculography *(nu-mo-ven-trik-u-log-ra- fi)* [G. *pneuma,* wind; L. *ventriculum,* ventricle; G. *graphein,* to write]. Examination of ecrebral ven- tricles by X-ray after injection of air directly.

نیوموونیٹر یکولوگرافی: براہ راست ہوا کے بعد ایکسرے کے ذریعے سر برں بطینوں کی جانچ۔

Poledine methylsuphate *(pol-den-meth-il-sul-fat)* Inhibits gastric secretion of acid in response to food.

پولڈین میتھائل سلفیٹ: خوراک کی وجہ سے تیزاب کے معدی اخراج کو روکتا ہے۔

Polioencephalitis *(po-li-o-en-kef-a-li-tis)*

[G.*polios*, grey; *egkephalos*, brain; *-itis*, inflammation]. Infl- ammation of the cerebal grey matter--this may or may not include the central nucleipolioencephalitic adj.

دماغ کے سفید مادہ کا ورم: سربرل گرے میٹر کی سوزش۔

Poliomyelitis *(pol-i-mi-el-i-tis)* [G. *polios*, grey; *myelos*, marrow]. Infantile paralysis. An epidemic virus infection which attacks the motor neurones of the anterior horns in brain stem (bul!bar p.) and spinal cord. An attack may or may not lead to paralysis of-the lower motor neurone type with loss of muscular power and flaccidity. Vaccination ag- ainst the disease is desirable. When it occurs with- ing two days of vaccination with any alum- cont- aining p-›phylactis, the term 'provocative paraly..c p.' is used.

فالج اطفال' پولیو: وائرس سے ہونے والی بیماری۔ اس کی حفاظتی تدابیر میں ویکسینیشن ہے۔ بچوں کا فالج معمولی بخار ہوتا ہے اور کوئی عضو (بازو یا ٹانگ) مفلوج ہو جاتا ہے۔

Polioviruses Cause poliomyelitis (q.v.)

پولیووائرس: وائرس جو پولیو کا مرض پیدا کرتا ہے۔

Politzer's bag Rubber bag for Eustachian inflation. [Adam Politzer, Austrian otologist, 1835-1920].

آلہ برائے ترویج نغنغتین: یوسٹیشن پھیلاؤ کے لئے ربڑ کا تھیلا۔ اس آلہ میں ربڑ کی تھیلی' نالی اور نوزل ہوتی ہے۔ نوزل کو نتھنے میں رکھ کر تھیلی کو دباتے ہیں۔ جس سے ہوا نغنغتین سے ہوتی ہوئی کان کے وسطی حصہ میں جا پہنچتی ہے۔

Pollenosis *(pol-en-o-sis)* Allergic condition arising formn senxitization to pollen.

زردانیت: زردانوں سے الرجی۔

Poly operation *(pol-i-a)* Partial gastrectomy. (q.v.)

پولیا اپریشن: جزوی طور پر معدے کو کاٹنا۔

Polyarteritis *(pol-i-art-er-it-is)* [G. *polys*, many; *arteria*, artery; *-itis*, inflammation]. Inflammation of many arteries. In **p. nodosa** (periateritis nodosa) aneuysmal swellings and thrombosis occur inthe affected vessels. Further damage may lead to haemorhage the clinical picture presented depends u the site affected. See COLLAGEN PERIARTERITIS.

ن کثیر شریانی: کئی شریانوں کی سوزش یا سوج۔

Polyarthralgia *(pol-i-ar-thral-ji-a)* [G.*po* many; *arthron*, joint; *-itis*, inflammati Inflammation of several joints at the time. STILL'S DISEA- SE.

مفاصل: مختلف جوڑوں میں درد۔

Polybactrin Neomycin sulphate, polymyxi and bacitracin. Antibiotic powder spr Usedn topically in sugery, burns and woun

بیکٹیرین: نیو مائی سین سلفیٹ' پولی میکسین ب اور بیسٹریسن۔ اینٹی پوڈر سپرے۔

Polycystic Protamine sulphate (q.v.)

برین: پروٹامین سلفیٹ۔

Polycystic *(pol-i-sis-tik)* [G. *polys*, ma *kystos*, bladder]. Composed of many cy Polycystic kidney disease is congenital, slowly fatal.

ردوری: کئی سسٹوں پر مشتمل۔

Polycythaemia *(pol-i-sdi-the-mi-a)* [G. *pc* many; *kytos*, cell; *haimu*, blood]. Increas the numbner of circulating red blood c This may result from dehydration or compensatory phenomenon to increas oxygen carrying capacity, as in conger heart disease. **polycythaemia v** (erythraemia) is an idiopathic conditio which the red cell count is very high. patient compl- ains of headache and lassit and there is danger of thrombosis haemorrhage. See also ERYTHROCY AEMIA.

رات خون: گردشی سرخ خونی خلیوں کی تعداد میں اضافہ۔

Polydactyly *(pol-i-dak-til-i)* [G. *polys*, ma *daktylos*, finger]. Having more than normal number of fingers or toes. polydactylism.

لاصابع: ہاتھوں اور پیروں کی انگلیوں کا نارمل تعداد سے زیادہ ہونا۔

ydipsia *(pol-i-dip'-si-a)* [G. *polys,* many; *dipsa,* thirst]. Excessive thirst.

شدت پیاس: زائد پیاس۔

lygraph *(pol'-i-graf)* [G. *polys,* many; *graphnein,* to write]. Instrument which ecords pulses simu- ltaneously.

متعدد عمل نگار: آلہ جو بیک وقت نبضوں کو ریکارڈ کرتا ہے۔

yhydramnios *(pol-i-hi-dram-ni-os)* [G. *polys,* many; *hydor,* water; *amnion,* nembrance around fetus]. An excessive mout of amniotic fluid.

پولی ہائیڈ ریمنیوس: امنیاٹک سیال کی زائد مقدار۔

y-I-C *(pol'-i-I-se)* Polysinosinic-polycytidylic cid. (q.v.)

پولی آئی سی: ایک مصنوعی نکلیک ایسڈ جو رسولیوں کو قبول نہ کرنے وا خلیوں کی قابلیت بڑھاتا ہے۔

ymyalgia rheumatical *(pol-i-mi-al-ji-a oom-mat-ik-a)* [G. *polys,* many; *mys,* muscle; *lgos,* pain, *rheumatismos,* that which flows]. syndrome occuring in elderly people omprising of a sometimes crippling ache in he shoulders, pelvic girdle muscles and pine, with pronounced morning stiffness and raised ESR. There is an association with emporal arteritis. Clinically diffe- rent from heumatoid arthritis.

ymorphonuclear *(pol-i-mor-fo-nu-kle-ar)* G. *polys,* many; *morphos,* shape; L. *nucleus,* ernel]. Having a many shaped or lobulated ucleus, usu- ally applied to the phagocytic eutrophil leuocytes (greanulocytes) which onstitute 70 per cent of the total white blood ells.

کثیر الاشکال مرکزہ: کئی شکلوں والا مرکزہ۔ اس اصطلاح کا اطلاق عم نیوٹروفل لیوکوسائیٹس (فیگو سائیٹس) پر ہوتا ہے جو کل سفید خونی خلیوں ستر فیصد پر مشتمل ہوتے ہیں۔

myxin B *(po-li-miks'-in)* An antibiotic used infections due to *Pseudomonas pyocyanea.* lso used in ear infections.

پولی میکسین ب: ایک اینٹی بایوٹک۔

Polyneuritis *(pol-i-nu-ri'-tis)* [G. *polys,* many; *neu- ron,* tedon; *-itis,* inflammation]. Multiple neuritis polyneuritic, adj.

ورم اعصاب: کئی رخی نیوٹریٹس۔

Polyoma. One of the tumour producing viruses.

پولیوما: رسولی پیدا کرنے والے وائرسوں میں سے ایک۔

Polyopia *(pol-i-op'-i-a)* [G. *polys,* many; *ops,* eye]. Seeing many images of a single object.

کثیر نظری: کسی واحد شے کے کئی عکس دیکھنا۔

Polyp-or polypus *(pol-ip(-us)* [G.*polypous,* man- y-footed] A pedunculated tumour arising from any mucous surface, e.g. cervical, uterine, nasal, etc. Usually benign but may become malignant--polypi, pl; polypous, adj.

سلعہ (غشا) مخاطی: لسی میوکس سطح سے ابھرنے والی ڈنڈی دار رسولی۔

Polypectomy *(pol-ip-ek'-to-mi)* [G. *polypous,* ma- ny-footed; *ektome,* excision]. Surgical removal of a polyp.

پولی پیکٹومی: پولپ کا سرجیکل خاتمہ۔

Polypeptides *(pol-i-pep'-tidz)* Proteins with long chai- ns of amino acids linked together.

پولی پیپٹائڈز: تین یا زیادہ امینو ایسڈز کی زنجیر جن میں سے ہر ایک اپنے پڑوسیوں سے پیپٹائڈ الحاق کے ذریعے ملا ہوتا ہے۔ پولی پیپٹائڈز زنجیریں کئی سو امینو ایسڈ اکائیوں پر مشتمل ہو سکتی ہیں۔ لحمیات پولی پیپٹائڈ زنجیروں پر مشتمل ہوتے ہیں۔ جو مختلف طریقوں سے ملی ہوتی ہیں۔

Polypoid *(pol'-i-poid)* [G. *polypous,* many-footed; *eidos,* form] Resembling a polyp(us).

چندلونیویہ: پولپ سے مشابہ۔

Polyposis *(pol-i-po-sis)* [G. *polypous,* many-footed; *-osis,* condition]. A condition in which there are numerous polypi in an organ. **polyposis coli,** a hereditary condition in which polypioccur throughout the large bowel and which leads eventually to carcinoma of the colon.

سعدانیت: ایسی حالت کہ کسی عضو میں کئی پولپ ہوں۔

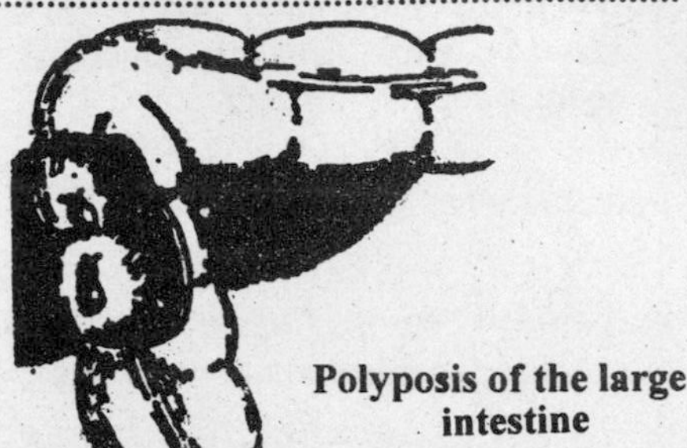

Polyposis of the large intestine

Polysaccharide *(pol--i-sak'-ar-id)* [G. *polys,* many; *sakcharon,* sugar]. ($C_6 H_{10} O_5$). Carbohydrates Co- ntainining a large number of monosaccharide groups, Starch, inulin, glyceogen, dextrin and cellulose are examples.

پولی سیکرائیڈ: قدرتی کاربوہائیڈریٹس کی ایک بڑی جماعت سادہ شکروں کی کئی سالموں کی تکثیف سے سالمات ماخوذ کیے جاتے ہیں۔ یہ جماعت سیلولوزا اورنشاستہ یاسٹارچ پرمشتمل ہے۔

Polyserositis *(pol-i-se-ro-si'-tis)* [G. *polys,* many; L. *serum,* whey; G. *-itis,* inflammation]. Inflammation of several serous membranes.

پوسیروسیٹس: کئی سیرس جھلیوں کی سوزش۔

Polysinosinic polycytidylic acid *(pol-i-sin-o-sin'- ik -pol- i-sit-i-dil'-ik)* An artificial nuclei acid that enhances the ability of cells to reject tumours in some way not yet understood.

پولی سینوسینک پولی سائیٹی ۔ ڈائیلک ایسڈ: ایک مصنوعی نکلیک ایسڈ جورسولیوں کوقبول نہ کرنے والے خلیوں کی اہلیت بڑھاتا ہے۔

Polythiazide *(pol-i-thi'-a-zid)* Diuretic, See CHLOR- OTHIAZIDE.

پولی تھیازائیڈ: پیشاب آور۔

Polyuria *(pol-i-ur'-i-a)* [G. *polys,* much; *ouron,* uri- ne]. Excretion of an excessive amount of urine. --polyuric, adj.

ذیابیطس: پیشاب کی زائد مقدار کااخراج۔

Pompholyx *(pom'-fol-iks)* [G. *bubble*]. Vesicular skin eruption on hands or feet. See CHEIROPO- MPHOLYX.

آبلہ کف: ہاتھوں اور پیروں پر کھال کا پھٹنا۔

Ponderax *(pon'-der-aks)* Fenfluramine hydrochloride (q.v.)

ریکس: فینفلوراسن ہائیڈروکلورائیڈ۔

Pons [L.]. A bridge ; a process of issue joir two sections of an organ. Pons varolii, white convex mass of nerve tissue at the b of the brain which serves to connect various lobes of the brain -- pontine, [Constantio Varolius, Italian anatom 1543-75]

یک پل۔ کسی عضو کے دوحصوں کوملانے والے نسیج کازائدہ۔ پانزویرلائی یلم کے آگے ہوتا ہے۔

Ponstan *(pon'-stan)* Mefenamic acid (q.v.)

ٹین: مفینامک ایسڈ ۔ چل ہلین میں اس کی ایک گولی دن میں تین سردرد میں۔

Pore *(por)* [G. *poros,* channel]. A mi surface ope- ning. One of the mouths of ducts (leading from the sweat glands) on skin surface; they are con- trolled by papillary muscles, contracting ans closin the cold, and dilating in the presence of he

۔منفذ: ایک چھوٹا سطحی سوراخ۔ پسینے کی نلی میں سے ایک نلی کا جلد پر ۔انہیں عضلے کنٹرول کرتے ہیں۔ سردی میں سوراخ سکڑ جاتے ہیں یا تے ہیں اور گرمی میں پھیل جاتے ہیں۔

Popliteal *(pop-lit-e'-al)* [L. *poples,* ha Pertaining to the popliteus. popliteal sp the dia- mond-shaped depression at the of the knee joint, bounded by the muscles containing the popliteal nerve and vessels.

انو: پاپلیٹس سے متعلق۔

Poradenitis *(por-ad-en-i'-tis)* [G. *poros,* p *aden,* gland, *-itis,* inflammation]. Pai mass of iliac glands, characterized by abs formation. Occurs in lymphogranul inguinale. (q.v.)

نی ٹس: الیامک۔غدودکادردوالا مادہ۔

Porphyria *(por-fi'-ri-a)* [G. *porphyra,* pu An inborn error in porphyin metabol probably hereditary, causing patholo changes in ner- vous and muscular tiss some cases of intermittent p., photosensitivity in some cases of cong p.

پورفائیریا: پوفائرن میٹابولزم میں پیدائشی غلطی جس سے عصبی اور عضلاتی نسیج میں تبدیلیاں ہوتی ہیں۔

orphyrins *(por-fi'-rins)* [G.*porphyra,* purple]. Colo- ured organic compounds; they form the basis of repiratory pigments. Naturally occuring porphyrins are uroporphyrin and coproporphyrin. They fluo- resce when exposed to Wood's light. See PORP- HYRIA.

پورفائرنز: پروں سے اخذ شدہ قدرتی طور پر پائے جانے والے جسمی رنگوں کی ایک جماعت۔ ان میں کلوروجل اور ہیموگلوبن کی ہیم شامل ہیں۔

orphyrinuria *(por-fi-rin-ur'-i-a)* [G.*porph- yros,* purple; *ouron,* urine]. Excretion of porphyrins in the urine. Such pigments are produced as a result of an inborn error of metabolism.

پورفائرینوریا: پیشاب میں پورفائرنز کا اخراج۔

orta *(por'-ta)* [L. *gate)* The depression (hilum) of an organ at which the vessels enter and leave -portal, adj. portahepatis, the transverse fissure through which the portal vein, hepatic artery and bile ducts pass on the under surface of the liver.

ناف جگر۔ باب: کسی عضو کا نشیب جہاں رگیں داخل و خارج ہوتی ہیں۔

ortacaval *(por-ta-ka'-val)* [L. *porta,* gate; *cavum,* hollow]. Pertaining to the portal vein and inferior vena cava. portacaval anastomosis, a fistula made between the portal vein and the inferior vena cava with the object of reducing the pressure within the portal vein in cases of cirrhosis of the liver. Also PORTOCAVAL.

پورٹاکیول: ادنیٰ وینا کیوا اور پورٹل ورید سے متعلق۔

ortahepatitis *(por-ta-hep-at-i'-tis)* [L. *porta,* gate; G. *hepar,* liver; *-itis,* inflammation]. Inflammation around the transverse fissure of the liver.

باب الکبد: جگر کے عرضی فشر کے گرد سوزش۔

ortal hypertension Condition when there is incre- ased pressure in portal vein (q.v.) Usually caused by cirrhosis of liver and results in splenomegaly, with hypersplenism (q.v.) and alimentary bleeding. See also BANTI'S DISEASE.

Portal vein .That conveying blood into the liver; it is about 76.2 mm long and is formed by the union of the superior mesenteric and splenic veins.

ورید جگری: جگر میں خون کے لئے جانے والی رگ۔

Portogram *(por'-to-gram)* X-ray of portal vein after splenic puncture and injection of radio-opaque liquid, or after injection of radio-opaque liquid into portal vein at operation.

پورٹوگرام: پورٹل ورید کا ایکس رے۔

Position *(po-zish'-un)* [L. *positio,* a placing]. Posture attitude. (See diagrams, pp._ . _)

وضع: طرز عمل۔ رویہ۔ کھڑے یا بیٹھے ہوئے حالت۔

Positive pressure breathing *(PPB)* Inflam of lungs to produce inspiration. Exhaled air, hand belows or more sophisticated apparatus can be used. Elastic recoil produces expiration.

پی پی بی: ہوا اندر لے جانے کے لئے پھیپھڑوں کا پھیلاؤ۔

Posseting *(pos'-et-ing)* Regurgitation of small amounts of clotted milk in infants.

پوسیٹنگ: بچوں میں کلاٹڈ دودھ کی تھوڑی مقدار کی ریگرگیٹشن۔

Possum *(pos'-sum)* Patient-Operated Selector Mech- anism. An apparatus which can be operated by a slight touch, or by suction using the mouth if no other muscle movement possible. It may transmit messages or be adapted for typing, telephoning and other activities.

Postanaesthetic *(post-an-es-thet'-ik)* [L. *post,* after; G. *anaisthesia,* loss of sensation]. After anaes- thesia.

پوسٹ اینستھیٹک: سن ہونے یا کرنے کے بعد۔

Postanal *(post-an-al)* [L. *post,* after; *anus*]. Behind the anus.

پوسٹ اینل: مقعد یا مبرز کے پیچھے۔

Postconcussional syndrome *(post-kon-kush'-on-al- sin-drom)* The association of headaches, giddiness and a feeling of suderable time after a head injury.

پوسٹ کنکشنل سنڈورم: سردرد، چکر، غنودگی اور کمزوری کا احساس جو

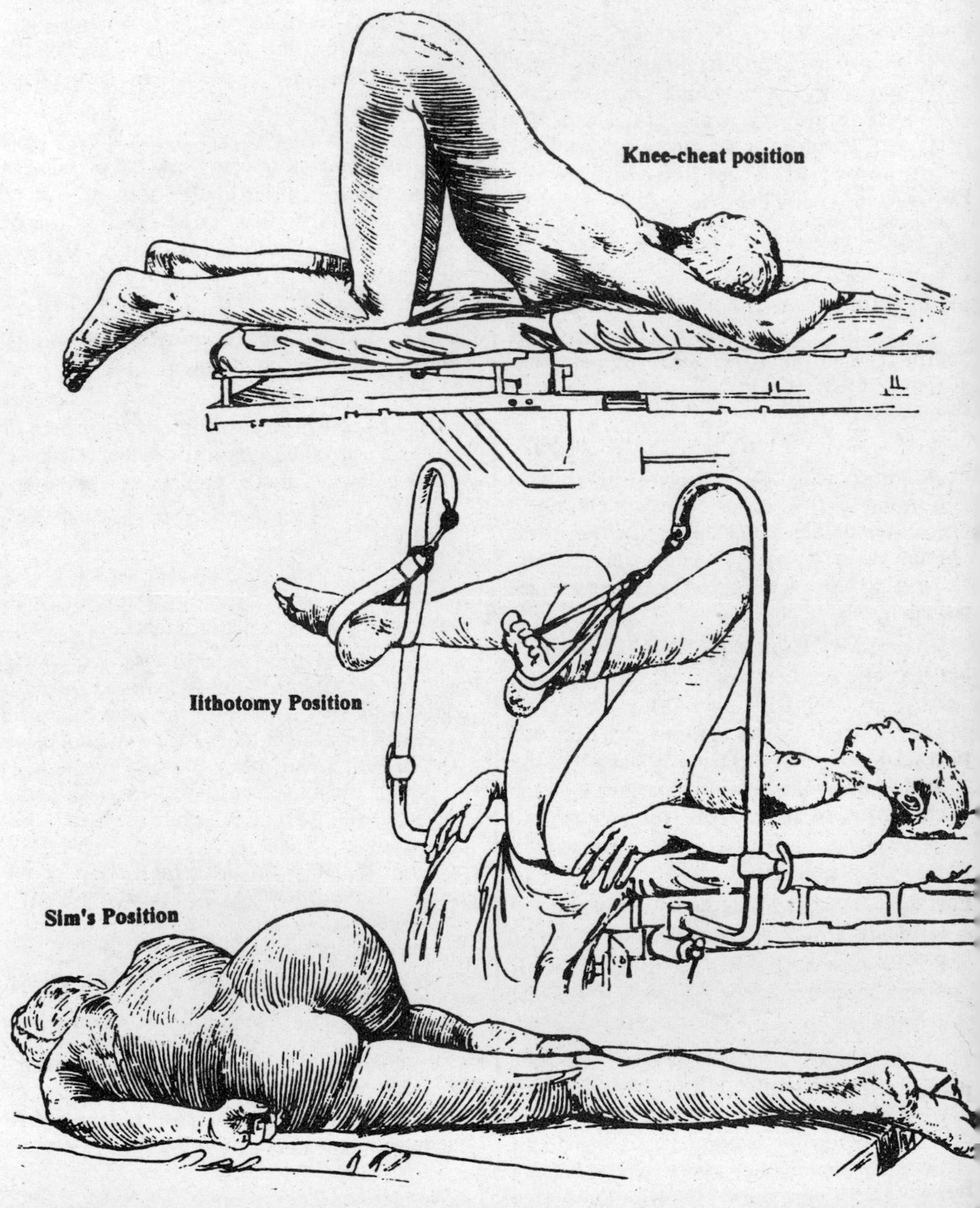
Knee-cheat position
Iithotomy Position
Sim's Position

سر کے زخم کے بعد کافی وقت رہتا ہے۔

Postdiphtheritic *(post-dif-ther-it'-ik)* [L. *post,* after; G.*dipthera,* leather]. Following an attack of diphtheria. Refers especially to the paralysis of limbs and palate.

پوسٹ ڈفتھر ٹیک: خناق کے حملہ کے بعد۔ جوارح اور پیسٹ کا خصوصا اینٹھ جانا۔

Postencephalitic *(post-en-kef-al-it-ik)* [L. *post,* G. *egkephalos,* brain; *-itis,* inflammation] Following encephalitis lethargic. The adjective is commonly used to describe the syndrome of Parkisonis, which so often results from an attack of this kind of encephalitis.

پوسٹ اینکیفالیٹک: انکفالٹس لتھارجیکا کے بعد۔

Postepileptic *(post-ep-il-ep'-tik)* [L. *post,* after; G. *ep- ileptikos*]. Following on an epileptic seizure. **postepoleptic automatism** is a fugue state, foll- owing on a fit, when patient may undertake a course of action, even involving violence, without having any memory of this (amnesia).

بعد الصرع: مرگی کے دورہ کے بعد۔

Posterior *(pos-te'-ri-or)* [L. Situated at the back]. **posterior chamber of the eye** space between the anterior surface of iris. See AQUEOUS --- post- eriorly, adv.

سرین۔ دمی۔ پچھلا۔ خلفی: پشت پر واقع۔

Postganglionic *(post-gang-gli-on'-ik)* [L. *post,* after; G. *gagglion,* tumour]. Situated after a collection of nerve cells (ganglion) as a p. nerve fibre.

پوسٹ گینگلیانک: عصبی خلیوں کے مجمع کے بعد واقع۔

Postgastrectomy syndrome Covers two sets of symptoms, those of hypoglycaemia when the patient is hungry, and those of a vasovagal attack immediately after a meal.

پوسٹ گیسٹر یکٹومی سنڈ ورم: دو اقسام کی علامت۔ جب مریض بھوکا ہو تو ہائپوگلائیسیمیا کی علامات اور کھانے کے فورا بعد واسو ویگل کا حملہ۔

Postherpetic *(post-her-pet'-ik)* [L. *post,* behind; G. *herpein,* to creep]. After shingles.

پوسٹ ہرپٹیک: شنگلز کے بعد۔

Posthitis *(pos-thi-tis)* [G. *posthe,* prepuce *-itis,* inflammation]. Inflammation of the prepuce.

ورم غلفه: پریپوس یا آلہ تناسل کے سرے کی کھال کی سوزش۔

Postmature *(post-ma-tur')* [L. *post,* behind; *maturus,* ripe]. Past the expected date of delivery. A baby is postmature when labour is delayed beyond the usual 40 weeksp- ostmaturity, n.

بچے کی پیدائش کی متوقع تاریخ کے بعد

Postmenopausal *(post-men-o-pawz'-al)* [L. *post,* after; G. *men,* month; *pausis,* a stopping]. Occurring after the menopause has been established.

مینوپاز کے بعد واقع ہونا۔

Postmortem *(post-mor'-tem)* [L. *post,* after; *mors,* death]. After death, usually inferring dissection of the body. Autopsy.

پوسٹ مارٹم بعد از موت: موت کے بعد لاش کی چیر پھاڑ۔

Postmyocardial infarction syndrome. Pyrexia and chest pain associated with inflammation of the pleura, lung or pericardium. Due to sensitivity to released products from dead muscle.

پلیورائی پھیپھڑا یا پیری کارڈیم کی سوزش کے ساتھ پائیر کسیا اور سینے کا درد۔

Postnasal *(post-na'-zal)* [L. *post,* behind; *nasus,* nose]. Situated behind the nose and in the nasopharynx--postnasally, adv.

خلف الانف: ناک کے پیچھے۔

Postnasal drip

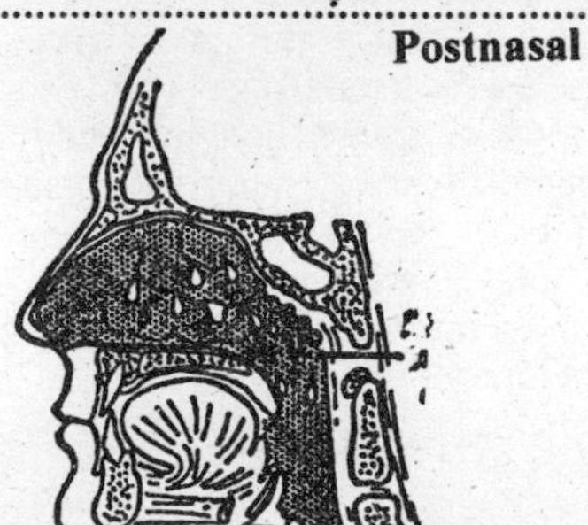

نیز دفیرنکس میں اور ناک کے عقب میں واقع۔

Postnatal *(post-na'-al)* [L. *post,* after; *natalis,* of birth]. After delivery, **postnatal examination,** routine examination 6 weeks after delivery--postnatally, adv.

بچے کی پیدائش کے بعد۔

Postoperative *(post-op'-er-at-iv)* [L. *post,* after; *operari,* to operate]. After operation-postoperatively, adv.

بعد اپریشن: اپریشن کے بعد۔

Postpartum *(post-par'-tum)* [L. *post,* after; *partus,* a birth]. After a birth (parturitionj).

بعد وضع حمل: پیدائش کے بعد۔

Postprandial *(post-pran'-di-al)* Following a meal.

بعد از طعام: کھانے کے فوراً بعد۔

Postural *(pos'-tu-ral).* Pertaining to posture. **postural drainage,** usually infers, drainage from the respiratory tract, by elevation of the foot of the bed or using a special frame.

وضعی ۔ پوسچر: یا انداز سے متعلق۔

Posture *(pos'-tur)* [L. *positura,* from *ponere,* to place]. Advice or passive arrangement of the whole body, or a part, in a definite manner.

پوسچر انداز: یقینی طریقے سے پورے جسم یا ایک حصے کی عامل یا غیر عامل تنظیم۔

Postvaccinal *(post-vak'-sin-al)* [L. *post,* after; *vaccinus,* of cows]. After vaccination.

ویکسینیشن کے بعد

Postvagotomy diarrhoea Three types: 1. Transient diarrhoea shortly after operation, lasting from a few hours to a day or two. These episodes disappear in 3 to 6 months. 2. If they recur later than this and the attacks last longer, the term, 'recurrent episodic diarrhoea' is used. 3. An increased daily bowel frequency; may be of disabling severity, but often acceptable in contrast to preoperative constipation.

اسہال کی تین اقسام۔: اپریشن کے بعد چند گھنٹے یا ایک دو روز رہتے ہیں۔ اپریشن کے کافی دیر بعد یا روزانہ زیادہ بار آنا۔

Potassium chlorate *(po-ta'-si-um klor'-at).* Mild antiseptic used in mouth-washes and gargles. Distinguish from potassium chloride.

ایک سفید قلمی حل پذیر مرکب۔ نقطۂ پگھلاؤ ۳۵۶ س' بطور تکسیدی عامل اور آتش گیر مادوں میں استعمال کیا جاتا ہے۔ ہلکے دافع تعفن کے طور پر منہ صاف کرنے اور غرغرے کرنے کے لئے مستعمل ہے۔

Potassium chloride *(po-ta'-si-um klor'-id).* Used in potassium replacement solutions, and as a supplement in chlorothiazide therapy.

پوٹاشیم میوی ایٹ۔ نقطہ پگھلاؤ ۷۷۶ س سالمی وزن ۷۴٫۵۶ ایک سفید حل پذیر قلمی مرکب۔ دوائیوں میں اور بطور فرٹیلائزر استعمال کیا جاتا ہے۔

Potassium citrate *(po-ta'-si-um sit'-rat).* Alkalinizes urine; widely used in cystitis, etc. and during sulphonamide therapy to prevent renal complications.

الکلائن پیساب آوردوا۔

Potassium deficiency Disturbed electrolyte balance; can occur after excessive vomiting, and/or diarrhoea; after prolonged use of diuretics, steroids, etc. Signs and symptoms variable, but nausea and muscle weakness ofter present Heart failure can quickly supervene.

کمی پوٹاشیم: ڈسٹرب الیکٹرولائیٹ توازن عموماً قے یا اسہال کے بعد۔

Potassium hydroxide *(po-ta'-si-um hid-roks'-id).* Caustic potash: used as liq. potassae in urine testing.

کاسٹک پوٹاش: پیشاب کو جانچنے میں مستعمل سفید ٹھوس' نقطۂ پگھلاؤ ۳۶۰٫۴ س' پانی میں حل ہو کر الکلائن محلول بناتا ہے۔ دوائیوں اور صابن کی تیاری میں استعمال کیا جاتا ہے۔

Potassium iodide *(po-ta'-si-um i'-o-did).* Used as an expectorant in bronchitis and asthma; also used in the prophylaxis of simple goitre, and pre-operatively in toxic goitre.

ایک سفید حل پذیر مرکب: نقطۂ پگھلاؤ ۶۸۶ س دوائیوں اور فوٹوگرافی میں استعمال کیا جاتا ہے۔ پرونکائیٹس اور دمہ میں مستعمل۔ مفید برائے اینکیٹومائی کوسس۔

Potassium perchlorate *(po-ta'-si-um per-klor'-at).* Suppresses trapping of iodine in thyroid gland.

: تھائیرائڈ غدہ میں آیوڈین کو کم کرنے کیلئے مستعمل۔ مفید برائے مرض ہائپر تھائیرائڈزم یعنی زہریلا گلٹھ۔

Potassium permanganate *(po-ta'-si-um per-mang'gan-at).* Purple crystals with powerful disinfectant/and deodorizing properties. Used as lotion 1 in 1000; 1 in 5000 to 10,000 for baths.

لال دوا: پرمینگنیٹ آف پوٹاش۔ایک گراجامنی قلمی حل پزیر نمک۔پانی میں حل ہوکر جامنی رنگ کا محلول بناتا ہے۔جوایک طاقتور تکسیدی عامل کے طور پر کام کرتا ہے۔یعنی واقع تعفن اور حجمی تجزیہ میں استعمال کیا جاتا ہے۔سالمی وزن۱۵۸،۰۴ جلنے میں مدد دیتا ہے۔

Potaba + 6I *(pot-o'-ba)*. Potassium paraminoben- zoate. Has an antifibrotic effect. Three g capsules orally four times daily with meals for several months.

پراٹوبا: پوٹاشیم پیراامینوبتروایٹ اینٹی فائبرونک اثر والا۔

Potter's rot *(pot'-ers rot)*. One of the many popular names for silicosis arising in workers in the pottery industry.

:برتن بنانے کی صنعت میں کام کرنے والوں میں ہونے والا مرض سلیکوسس۔

Pott's disease Spondylitis; spinal caries; spinal tuberculosis. [Percival Pott, English surgeon, 1714-88.].

مرض پوٹ۔دق نخاعی: ریڑھ کی ہڈی یا سپائن کا تپ دق۔

Pott's fracture A fracture-dislocation of the ankle joint. A fracture of the lower end of the fibula, 76 mm above the ankle joint, and a fracture of the medical malleolus of the tibia. [Percivall Pott, English Surgeon, 1714-88].

فیبولا کے نیچے سرے کا فریکچر۔

Pouch *(powch)* [F. *poche,* pocket]. A pocket or recess, **pouch of Douglas,** recto-uterine pouch.

کیسہ۔تھیلی: ایک پاکٹ۔

PPB Positive pressure breathing (q.v.).

مثبت دباؤ سے تنفس۔پوزیٹو پریشر بریڈنگ۔

PPD. Purified protein derivative. see TEST; MANTOUX.

خالص پروٹینی: ماخز۔پوریفائیڈ پروٹین۔

PPLO Pleuropneumonia-like organism similar to the virus that causes contagious pleuropneumonia in cattle. See EATON AGENT.

پی پی ایل او: مویشیوں میں چھوت کی بیماری پلیورنمونیہ کا سبب وائرس سے مشابہ پلیورنمونیہ جسمیہ۔

Prader-Willi syndrome. Described in 1956. Low birth weight, hypotonia, mental retardation, acromicria and often obesity and diabetes mellitus develop during childhood or adolescence.

پیریڈرولی سنڈروم: پیدائش کے وقت کم وزن۔ذہنی پسماندگی اور اکثر ذیابیطس۔

Praecordial See PRECODIAL

پسلی کا: دل کے بالکل اوپر سینہ کے ایریا سے متعلق۔

Praxilene *(parks'-i-len)*. Naftidrofuryl oxalate (q.v.).

Prazosin *(praz'-o-sin)*. Antihypertensive agent which is said to act peripherally by direct vasodilation.

Pre-anaesthetic *(pre-an-es-thet'ik)* [L. *prae,* before; G. *anaisthesia,* lack of sensation]. Before an anaesthetic.

پری اینستھیٹک: سن ہونے سے پہلے۔

Precancerous *(pre-kan'-ser-us)* [L. *prae,* before; *cancer,* crab]. Occurring before cancer with special reference to non-malignant pathological changes which are believed to lead on to, or to be followed by, cancer.

سرطان سے پہلے واقع ہونا۔

Precipitin *(pre-sip'-it-in)* [L. *precipitare,* to precipitate]. An antibody which forms a specific complex with precipitinogen (antigen), and under certain physiochemical conditions this results in the formation of a precipitate. This reaction forms the basis of many delicate diagnostic serological tests for the identification of minute traces of material and bacteria. See ANTIBODIES.

:اینٹی باڈی جو اینٹی جن کے ساتھ مخصوص کمپلکس بناتی ہے۔

Precordial *(pre-kor'-di-al)* [L. *prae,* before; *cor,* heart]. Pertaining to the area of the chest immediately over the heart.

پیش قلبی: دل کے عین اوپر سینہ کے ایریا سے متعلق۔

Precursor *(pre-kurs'-or)* Forerunner.

سابق۔مقدم: پیش رو۔

Prediabetes *(pre-di-abe'-tez)* [L. *prae,* before; G. *diabainerin,* to cross through]. Potential predisposition to diabetes mellitus. Preventive mass urine testing can detect the condition.

Early treatment prevents ketoacidosis and may help to prevent the more serious complications such as retinopathy and neuropathy--prediabetic, adj., n.

قبل ذیابیطس: ذیابیطس سے پہلے کی حالت۔

Predigestion *(pre-di-jest'-chun)*. Artifical digestion of protein (e.g. in peptonized foods) or amylolysis (e.g. in malt extracts or dextronized cereals) before digestion takes place in the body.

مبادی ہضم۔ ہضم سابق: پروٹین کا مصنوعی ہضم۔ یہ جسم میں ہضم سے پہلے ہوتا ہے۔

Predisposition *(pre-dis-po-zi'shunh)*. A natural susceptibility to develop or contract certain diseases.

آمادگی۔ رجحان: بعض امراض لگنے سے قدرتی مدافعت۔

Prednesol *(pred'-nes-ol)*. Prednisolone (q.v.).

پریڈنیسول: ایک تالفی ہارمون۔ پریڈنیسولون۔

Prednisolone *(pred-nis'-o-lon)*. A synthetic hormone with properties similar to those of cortisone (q.v.). but side effects, such as salt and water retention, are markedly reduced. Widely prescribed for connective tissue diseases, conditions involving immune reaction including autoimmune disorders.

پریڈنیسولون: پریڈنیسول۔ کورٹیسون سے مشابہ ایک تالیفی ہارمون۔ بواسیر میں پریڈنی سولون کمپاؤنڈ مرہم کوریا پیری کارڈائی ٹس دن میں تین مرتبہ لگائیے۔ السریٹو کولائی ٹس میں ایک گولی صبح ایک دوپہر ایک شام۔ عرق النساء کوریا پیری کارڈائی ٹس پلیوریسی، تپ دق اور نمونیا میں بھی یہی خوراک۔ اسی طرح مستعمل برائے گردہ سوزش لیوکیمیا۔ ایکوٹ ریوماٹائڈ ارتھرائی ٹس۔

Prednisone *(pred'-ni-son)*. Converted into prednisolone in the liver.

پریڈنیسون: کورٹیسون سے ماخوذ۔

Pre-eclampsia *(pre-e-klamp'-si-a)* [L. *prae,* before G. *eklampsis,* a shining forth]. A condition characterized by albuminuria, hypertension and oedema, arising usually in the latter part of pregnancy--pre-eclamptic, adj.

پری ایک لیمپیا: البومینوریا وغیرہ کی حالت۔

Prefrontal *(pre-front'-al)* [L. *prae,* before *frons,* forehead]. Situated in the anterior portion of the frontal lobe of the cerebrum. See LEUCOTOMY.

پیش جبہی: سربرم کے فرنٹل لوب کے امامی حصے میں واقع۔

Pregaday *(preg'-a-da)* Ferrous fomarate (q.v.). and folic acid (q.v.).

پرگیمل: فولک ایسڈ۔

Preganglionic *(pre-gang-gli-on'-ik)* [L. *prae,* before; G. *gagglion,* tumour]. Preceding or in front of a collection of nerve cells (ganglion) as a p. nerve fibre.

پری گینگلیانک: عصبی خلیوں کے مجمع کے سامنے۔

Pregnancy *(preg'-nan-si)* [L. *praegnans*]. Being with child, i.e. from conception to parturition normally 40 weeks or 280 days. **extrauterine p.**, see ECTOPIC P. **multiple p.**, more than one fetus in the uterus. **phantom p.**, see PSEUDOCYESIS.

حمل: بچے کا پیٹ میں ہونا۔ ۲۸۰ ایام جن میں بچہ ماں کے پیٹ میں ہوتا ہے۔

Pregnanediol Urinary excretion product from progesterone.

پریگنینڈیول: پروجیسٹرون سے بولی اخراج پروڈکٹ۔

Pregnyl *(preg'-nil)*. Chorionic gonadotrophin for undescended and ectopic testes.

پریگنل: خصیوں کے لئے کوریونک گونیڈوٹرافن۔

Prehensile *(pre-hen'-sil)* [L. *prehendere,* to seize]. Equipped for grasping.

گیرندہ: پکڑنے کے لئے مناسب۔

Preludin *(prel'-u-din)*. Phenmetrazine hydrochloride (q.v.).

پریلوڈن: فنمیٹرازین ہائیڈرکلورائیڈ۔

Premarin *(pre'-mar-in)*. Conjugated oestrogens. Can be given orally. Useful for menopausal symptoms.

پریمیرن: مینوپاز کی علامات کے لئے مفید۔

Premature *(pre'-mat-ur)* [L. *praematusrus,* too soon]. Occurring before the proper time. **premature baby,** where the birth weight is less than 2.5 kg (5½ lb) and therefore special treatment is needed. Current syns. are low weight or dysmature baby. Not all low birth weight babies are premature, but are included in a new category 'small for dates'. See PLACENTAL INSUFFICIENCY **premature beat,** see EXTRASYSTOLE. **premature labour,** expulsion of the fetus before the 280th day of gestation.

قبل از وقت: مناسب وقت سے پہلے واقع ہونا۔

Premedication *(pre-med-ik-a'-shun)* [L..*prae,* before; *medicare,* heal]. Drugs given before the administration of another drug, e.g. those given before an anaesthetic. The latter are of two types; (1) sedative, e.g. morphine; (2) drugs which inhibit the secretion of saliva and of mucus from the upper respiratory tract, e.g. atrophine.

پری میڈیکیشن: دوسری دوائی سے پہلی دی گئیں ادویات۔

Premenstrual *(pre-men'-stroo-al)* [L. *prae,* before; *menstrualis,* monthly]. Preceeding menstruation. Cyclica syndrome (q.v.). now preferred for p. symptom-complex.

قبل حیض: ماہواری سے پہلے۔

Premolars *(pre-mol'-arz)* [L. *prae,* before; *molere*, grind]. The eight bicuspid teeth, two on each side of each jaw, lying between the canine and the molars.

پیش ضرس: آٹھ بائی کسپڈ دانت۔ کینائن اور مولرز کے درمیان واقع، ہر جبڑے کی ہر ایک سائیڈ پر دو۔

Prenatal *(pre-na'-tal)* [L. *prae,* before; *natalis,* of birth]. Before birth--prenatally, adv.

قبل پیدائش: پیدائش سے پہلے۔

Pre-operative *(pre-op'-er-at-iv)* [L. *prae,* before; *operari* to operate]. Before operation--preoperat- ively, adv.

پری آپریٹو: اپریشن سے پہلے۔

Preparalytic *(pre-par-al-it'-ik)* [L. *prae,* before; G. *paralytikos*]. Before the onset of paralysis, usually referring to the early stage of polio-myelitis.

قبل تشنج: تشنج سے پہلے عموماً اولین پولیو کا مرحلہ۔

Prepatellar *(pre-pat-el'-ar)* [L. *prae,* before; *patella,* kneecap]. In front of the kneecap, as applied to a large bursa.

پری پٹیلر: گھٹنے کی چپنی کے سامنے۔

Prepubertal *(pre-pu'-bert-al)* [L. *prae,* before; *pubertas,* puberty]. Before puberty.

پیش بلوغی: سن بلوغت سے پہلے۔

Prepuce *(pre'-pus)* [L. *praeputium,* foreskin] The foreskin of the pensi.

غلفہ: سر ذکر کی کھال۔

Prerenal *(pre-re'-nal)* [L. *prae,* before; renalis, of the kidney]. Before, or in front of the kidney.

پری رینل: گردے سے پہلے یا اس کے سامنے۔

Presacral air insufflation Injection of air into retroperitoneal interstitial tissues, mainly used to demonstrate renal and adrenal outlines.

پری سیکرل ایئر انسفلیشن: مخصوص بافتوں میں ہوا کا ٹیکہ۔

Presbyopia *(prez-bi-op'-i-a)* [G. *presbys,* old man; *ops,* eye]. Long-sightedness, due to failure of accommodation in those of 45 years and onwards--presbyopic adj.; presbyope, n.

دور نظری: نزدیکی نظر کمزور ہونا۔ ۴۵ سال یا اس سے زیادہ عمر میں نزدیک کی نگاہ کمزور ہو جاتی ہے۔

Prescription *(pre-skrip'-shun)*. A written formula, signed by a physician, directing the pharmacist to prepare a remedy.

نسخہ: ڈاکٹر یا طبیب کی طرف سے تحریری نسخہ جس میں ادویات کا اندراج ہوتا ہے۔

Presenility *(pre-sen-il'-i-ti)* [L. *prae,* before; *snilis*, aged]. A condition occurring before senility is established--presenile, adj.

پری سینٹی لیٹی: بڑھاپے سے پہلے۔

Presentation *(prez-en-ta'-shun)* [L. *presentare,* to present]. The part of the fetus which first enters the pelvic brim and will be felt by the examining finger through the cervix in labour. May be vertex, face, brow, shoulder or breech.

وضع جنین۔ رخ: بچے کا وہ حصہ جو پیڑو کے کنارے میں پہلے داخل ہوتا ہے اور لیبر میں سرکس میں سے انگلی سے محسوس کیا جا سکتا ہے۔ بچے کے جسم کا وہ حصہ جو رحم کے زیریں حصے میں ہو اور پیدائش کے وقت سب سے پہلے خارج ہو اسے جنین کا رخ کہتے ہیں۔

Pressor *(pres'-sor)*. A substance which raises the blood pressure.

دوباؤافزا: بلڈ پریشر زیادہ کرنے والی شے۔

Pressure area *(presh'-er)* The bony prominences of the body, over which the flesh of bedridden patients is denuded of its blood supply as it is compressed between the bone and an external source of pressure; the latter is usually the bed, but may be a splint, plaster, upper bedclothes, chair, etc.

دباؤ کے علاقے: جسم کے استخوانی ابھار جو ہڈی اور بیرونی دباؤ کے درمیان آجاتے ہیں۔

Pressure point A place at which an artery passes over a bone, against which it can be compressed, to stop bleeding.

نقطہ ضغط: وہ جگہ جہاں سے شریان ہڈی پر گزرتی ہے اور اسے خون روکنے کیلئے دبایا جاسکتا ہے۔

Pressure sore A decubitus ulcer, arising from continual compression of the flesh over a bony prominence. The first sign is redness, then there is bruising of the skin, which finally breaks and sloughs before healing takes place by granulation. Skin grafting may be necessary.

پریشر سور: استخوانی ابھار کے اوپر گوشت کے متواتر دباؤ سے ابھرنے والا السر۔

Presystole *(pre-sis'-to-li)*. The period preceding the systole or contraction of the heart muscle--presystolic, adj.

انقباض القلب سے پہلے: دلی عضلہ کے سکڑنے سے پہلے کا عرصہ۔

Preterm delivery. When the expected date of delivery (EDD) is taken as the beginning of the 40th week rather than the end, and the mother has completed 39 weeks plus 6 days from the first day of her last menstrual period before entering the 40th week of pregnancy, then 'preterm' is delivery before the onset of the 37th week or three weeks or more before the EED.

Prevesical *(pre-ves'-ik-al)* [L. *prae,* before; *vesica,* bladder]. Anterior to the bladder.

پری ویسیکل: بلیڈر سے آگے۔

Priapism *(pri'-ap-izm)* [*Priapus,* the god of procreation]. Prolonged penile erection in the absence of sexual stimulation.

وائم خیزی: جنسی تحریک کی غیر موجودگی میں آلہ تناسل کا کافی دیر سیدھا رہنا۔

Priadel *(pri'-a-del)*. Lithium carbonate (q.v.)

پرائی ایڈل: لیتھیم کاربونیٹ۔

Prickly heat Miliaria (q.v.)

خصفہ: ملی اریا۔ گرمی دانے جو موسم برسات یا زیادہ گرمی میں نکلتے ہیں۔ ان میں خارش ہوتی ہے۔ علاج کے لئے دن میں ۳ دفعہ پری ٹون' آسٹوکیلشیم اور پت پوڈر مفید ہیں۔

Prilocaine *(pril'-o-kan)*. Local anaesthetic containing local blood vessel constrictor; synthetic; less toxic than cocaine. Basically similar to lignocaine, but less likely to cause vasodilation.

پریلوکین: مقامی طور پر سن کرنے والا۔ تالیفی' کوکین سے کم زہریلا۔

Primaquine *(prim'-a-qwin)* Antimalarial. Useful for eradication of *plasmodium vivax* from the liver.

پریما کوئین: ضد ملیریائی جگر سے پلازموڈیم ویویکس کے خاتمہ کے لئے مفید۔

Primary complex or **Ghon's focus.** The initial tuberculous infection in a person, usually in the lung, and manifest as a small focus of infection in the lung tissue and enlarged caseous, hilar glands. It usually heals spontaneously. [Anton Ghon, Austrian pathologist, 1866-1936].

پرائمری کمپلکس: کسی شخص میں تپ دق کا ابتدائی مرض' عموماً پھیپھڑے میں۔ یہ عموماً اچانک ٹھیک ہوجاتا ہے۔

Primidone *(pri'-mi-don)*. An anticonvulsant used mainly in grand mal, but is sometimes effective in petit mal.

پریمیڈون: ضد تشنج۔

Primigravida *(prim-i-grav'-i-da)* [L. *primus,* first; *gravidus,* pregnant]. A woman who is pregnant for the first time--primigravidae, pl.

پہلی حاملہ: خاتون جو پہلی دفعہ حاملہ ہو۔

Primipara *(pri-mip'-a-ra)* [L. *primus,* first; *parere,* to bear]. A woman who is giving birth to her first child--primiparous, adj.

پہلن: خاتون جو اپنے پہلے بچے کو جنم دیتی ہے۔

Primobolan *(prim-o'-bol-an)*. Methenolone enanthate (q.v.).

Primolut depot. Hydroxyprogesterone caproate (q.v.).

Primolut N. Norethisterone (q.v.).

Primordial *(pri-mor'-di-al)* [L. *primordius,* original]. Primitive, original; applied to the ovarian follicles present at birth.

اولی: اولین۔ اصل۔ اس کا اطلاق پیدائش کے وقت موجود بیضہ دانی کے فولیکلز پر ہوتا ہے۔

Primoteston depot *(pri-mo-tes'-ton)*. Intramuscular hormone preparation for male climacteric, cancer of breast and osteoporosis.

پریموٹسٹون ڈپو: آئی ایم ہارمون۔

Priscol *(pris'-kol).* Tolazoline (q.v.)

پرسکول : ٹولازولین۔

Pro-Banthine *(pro-ban'-thin)* Propantheline (q.v.).

پرو بینتھین : پروپنتھین۔ اینٹی کولی نرجک اثرات تشنج' پیٹ درد' زخم معدہ' پتے کے درد اور ورم میں مفید ایک گولی صبح ایک دوپہر ایک شام۔

Probenecid *(pro-ben'-e-sid).* A drug which inhibits the renal excretion of certain compounds, notably penicillin and paraaminosalicyclic acid, and is used to increase the blood level of such drugs. It also hinders the reabsorption of urates by the renal tubules, so increasing the excretion of uric acid, and on that account it is used in the treatment of gout.

پروبنی سڈ : دوائی۔ جو بعض مرکبات ' خصوصاً پنسلین اور پیرا امینوسیلیسائیکلک ایسڈ کے رینل اخراج کو روکتی ہے۔ جوڑوں کے درد میں مفید۔ یورک ایسڈ خارج کرنے میں مدد دیتی ہے۔ ۵۰۰ ملی گرام دن میں چار مرتبہ برائے گیوٹ گوؤٹ۔

Procainamide *(pro-kan-a'-mid).* Derivative of procaine used in cardiac arrhythmias such as paroxysmal tachycardia. Also helps to relax volountary muscle and thus overcome myotonia. Given orally or by slow intravenous injection.

پروکین امائیڈ : پروکین سے ماخوذ۔

Procaine *(pro'-kan).* Widely used local anaesthetic of high potency and low toxicity. Used mainly for infiltration anaesthesia as a 0.5 to 2 per-cent solution. Now tending to be replaced by lignocaine (q.v.). **procaine benzylpenicillin,** longer acting than benzylpenicillin.

پروکین : مقامی طور پر سن کرنے والی زیادہ استعمال ہونے والی دوائی۔ پروکین پنسلین ۴ لاکھ کا ایک ٹیکہ روزانہ دس روز تک برائے گانوکا کل ارتھرائی ٹس۔

Procarbazine *(pro-kar'-baz-en)* Drug of the nitrogen mustard group useful in Hodgkin's disease.

پروکاربازین : نائٹروجن مسٹرڈ گروہ کی ایک دوائی۔

Process *(pro'-ses)* [L. *processus*]. A prominence or outgrowth of any part.

ابھار۔ عملیہ۔ طریقہ : (۱) کسی حصے کا ابھار۔ (۲) تجربہ گاہ میں تکمیل پانے والا عمل۔

Prochlorperazine *(pro-klor-per'-a-zen)* One of the phenothiazines. Has sedative and anti-emetic properties. Useful for vertigo, migraine, Meniere's disease, severe nausea and vomiting, schizophrenia.

پروکلورپیرازین: فینوتھیازنیز میں سے ایک تے یا متلی کو روکتی ہے۔ مسکن دوا۔ سٹے مے ٹل ہچکی' درد شقیقہ' مرض مینیئر اور تے روکنے کے لئے ایک گولی صبح ایک دوپہر ایک شام۔

Procidentia *(pro-si-den'-shi-a)* [L. falling forward]. Complete prolapse of the uterus, so that it lies within the vaginal sac but outside the contour of the body.

خروج الرحم: رحم کے نیچے کی طرف مکمل جھکاؤ۔

Proctalgia *(prok-tal'-ji-a)* [G. *proktos,* anus; *algos,* pain]. The presence of pain in the rectal region.

درد مستقیم : ریکٹل حصے میں درد کی موجودگی۔

Proctitis *(prok-ti'-tis)* [G. *proktos,* anus; *-itis,* inflam- mation]. Inflammation of the rectum **granular p.,** acute p.; so called because of the granular appearance of the inflamed mucous membrane.

سوزش مستقیم: ریکٹم کی سوزش۔

Proctocaine *(prok'-to-kan)*. A solution of procaine, butyl-aminobenzoate and benzyl alcohol in almond oil. Used in pruritus ani, anal fissure, etc. Given by deep subcutaneous injection.

پروکٹوکین : بادام کے تیل میں پروکین، بٹائل امینوبنز وایٹ اور بنزائل الکحل کا محلول۔ جلد میں گہرے ٹیکے کے ذریعے دیا جاتا ہے۔

Proctoclysis *(prok-to-kli'-sis)* [G. *proktos,* anus; *klysis,* a drenching]. The administration of fluid by the rectum. See CLYSIS.

پراکٹولائی سس : ریکٹم سے سیال کا دیا جانا۔

Proctocolectomy *(prok-to-kol-ek'-to-mi)* [G. *proktos,* anus; *kolon,* colon; *ektome,* excision]. Surgical exision of the rectum and colon.

پراکٹوکولیکٹومی : ریکٹم اور قولون کی سرجیکل علیحدگی۔

Proctocolitis *(prok-to-kol-i'-tis)* [G. *proktos,* anus; *kolon,* colon; *-itis,* inflammation]. Inflammation of the rectum and colon; usually a type of ulcerative colitis.

پراکٹوکولی ٹس: ریکٹم اور قولون کی سوزش۔

Proctoscope *(prok'-to-skop)* [G. *proktos,* anus; *skopein,* to examine]. An instrument for examining the rectum, See ENDOSCOPE--proctoscopic, adj.; proctoscopy, n.

سرم بین : ریکٹم کو جانچنے کا آلہ۔

Proctosigmoiditis *(prok-to-sig-moid'-i-tis)* [G. *proktos,* anus; letter sigma; *-itis,* inflammation]. Inflammation of the rectum and sigmoid colon.

پراکٹوسگمائڈیٹس : ریکٹم اور سگمائڈ قولون کی سوزش۔

Procyclidine *(pro-sik-li-den)*. A spasmolytic drug similar in action to benzhexol, and used in the treatment of Parkinsonism. It reduces the rigidity but has little action on the tremor.

پروسائیکلی ڈین : بنزہکیسول سے مشابہ دوائی۔ پارکنسوزم کے علاج میں مستعمل۔ یہ سختی میں کمی کرتی ہے لیکن رسولی پر اس کا ایکشن کم ہوتا ہے۔
کیماڈرن اس کی ایک گولی دن میں ۳ مرتبہ برائے پارکن سوزم یا رعشہ۔

Prodexin. Antacid tablets containing aluminium glycinate and magnesium carbonate.

پروڈیکسین : ایلومینیم گلائیسیٹ اور میگنیشیم کاربونیٹ پر مشتمل گولیاں۔

Prodromal *(pro-dro'-mal)* [G. *prodromos,* running before] Preceding, as the transitory rash before the true rash of an infectious disease.,

انذاری : پہلے ہونا۔

Proflavine *(pro-fla'-ven)*. An antiseptic very similar to acriflavine (q.v.).

پروفلیون : ایکریفلیون سے مشابہ ایک دافع تعفن دوا۔

Progestasert *(pro-jes'-ta-sert)* . A flexible T-shaped unit, like an IUD; contains the natural hormone progesterone, released at a continuous rate of 65 mg daily.

Progestational *(pro-jes-ta'-shun-al)* [G. *pro-* before; L. *gestare,* to carry]. Before pregnancy. Favouring pregnancy--progestation, n.

قبل حمل : حمل سے پہلے۔

Progesterone *(pro-jes'-ter-on)*. The hormone of the corpus luteum. Used in the treatment of functional uterine haemorrhage, and in threatened abortion. Given by intramuscular injection.

پروجیسٹیرون : ایک سفید قلمی سٹرائڈ ہارمون۔ نقطہ پگھلاؤ ۱۲۸٫۵ اس؛ وضع حمل اور جنین کی حفاظت کے لئے تولید اعضا کو تیار کرنے کا ذمہ دار ہے۔
کارپس لوٹیم سے خارج ہونے والا ہارمون۔

Progestogens *(pro-jes'-to-jens)*. Substances that have an action like progesterone.

پروجیسٹوجنز : پروجیسٹیرون کی طرح کے عوامل۔

Prolottis *(pro-glot'-is)* [G. *pro,* before; *glotta* tongue]. Sexually mature segment of tapeworm--proglottides, pl.

پیش زیانہ : کدو کیڑے کا جنسی بالغ ٹکڑا۔

Prognosis *(prog-no'-sis)* [G.]. A forecast of the probable course and termination of a disease-prognostic, adj.

انذار مرض : کسی مرض کے اغلب کورس اور خاتمہ کی پیش گوئی۔

Proguanil *(pro-gwan'-il)* Synthetic anti-malaria used in prophylaxis and suppressive treatment of malaria.

پروگوانل : تالیفی ضد ملیریائی۔

Projection *(pro-jek'-shun)* [L. *projectio* throwing forward]. A mental mechanism ccurring in normal people unconsciously, nd in exaggerated form in mental illnesses, specially paranoia, whereby the person fails) recognize certain motives and feelings in imself but attributes them to others.

قلب ماہیت۔اخراج ذات: ایک ذہنی میکانیت۔

lactin *(pro-lak'-tin).* Homone secreted in the nterior pituitary gland. It acts only on the regnant woman's breasts, preparing them for ilk production. Thereafter it is secreted as a eflex response to the act of sucking, which arts the flow of milk.

پرولیکٹن : دودھ پیدا کرنے والا ہارمون۔لیکٹوجینک ہارمون بچے پیدائش کے بعد خارج ہوکر ماں کی چھاتیوں کو دودھ پیدا کرنے پر اکساتا ہے

ladone *(pro-la-don).* Analgesic. Given by ijection and suppository. Latter can be used supplement pethidine.

پرولاڈون : مسکن دوا۔

lapse *(pro-laps)* [L. *prolapsus,* a falling]. ecent; the falling of a structure. **prolapse of n intervertebral disc (PID),** protrusion of e disc nucleus (q.v.). into the spinal cord nd/or nerve roots. Most common in the mbar region where it causes low back pain nd/or sciatica. **prolapse of the iris,** the iris ulges forward through a corneal wound. **rolapse of the rectum,** the lower portion of e intestinal tract decends outside the xternal anal sphincter. **prolapse of the erus,** the uterus decends into the vagina and ay be visible at the vaginal office. See ROCIDENTA.

Pro Prolapse

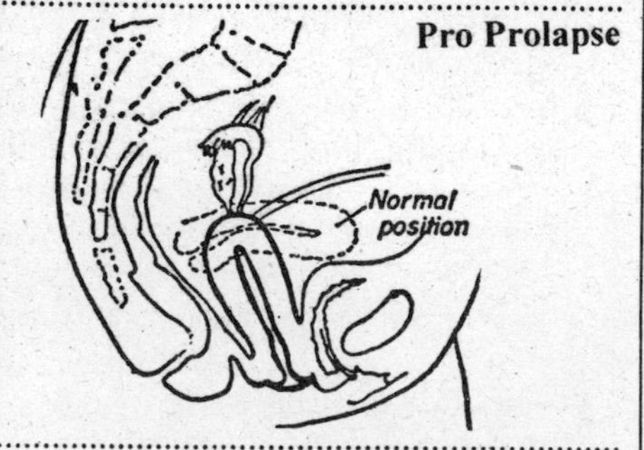

Prol **Prolapse**

حروج۔سقوط : کسی ساخت کا گرنا۔تنزلی

Degrees of prolapse oftheutrus

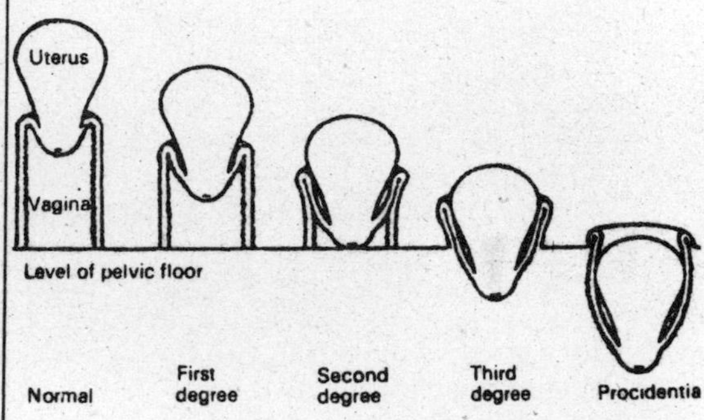

Proliferate *(pro-lif'-er-at)* [L. *proles,* off-spring; *ferre,* to bear]. Increase by cell division--proliferation, n.; proliferative, adj.

بچہ خیز، جراثیم خیز : تقسیم خلیہ کی وجہ سے بڑھنا۔

Prolific *(pro-lif'-ik).* [L. *proles,* offspring]. Fruitful, multiplying abundantly.

بچہ خیز۔بارآور : اچانک بڑھنا۔

Promazine *(pro'-ma-zen).* A tranquillizing drug similar to, but less hepatotoxic than chlorpromazine. Also useful in midwifery, treatment of alcoholism, senile agitation and for shivering attacks.

پرومازین : ایک سکون بخش دوا۔

Promethazine *(pro-meth'-az-en).* An antihistamine of the high potency and low toxicity. Very effective in urticaria. Hypnotic side effect useful in psychiatry and midwifery. Also a useful antiemetic. Given 2 hours before journey it will last for 6 to 12 h.

پرومیتھازین : اینٹی ہسٹامین۔پراثر دوا جو قے کو روکنے اور ذہنی سکون

کے لئے دی جاتی ہے۔ پرمیتھازین تھیوکلیٹ (ایومین) قے روکنے کے لئے
ایک گولی ایک شام ہچکی روکنے کے لئے بھی مذکورہ خوراکیں۔

Prominal *(pro'-min-al)*. Methylphenobarbitone (q.v.).

پرومینل : میتھائل فینوباربیٹون۔

Promontory *(prom'-on-to-ri)* [L. *promontorium*]. A projection; a prominent part.

برآمدگی : ابھار ایک نمایاں حصہ۔

Pronate *(pro'-nat)* [L. *pronare,* to bend forward] To turn the ventral surface downward, e.g. to lie on the face; to turn the palm of the hand downwards. Opp., supinate-pronation, n.

پرونیٹ : بطنی سطح نیچے کی طرف موڑنا۔

Pronator *(pro-na'-tor)* [L. *pronare,* to bend forward]. That which pronates, usually applied to a muscle. Opp. supinator.

مستدیرہ : آگے کی طرف جھکنے والا۔ اس اصطلاح کا اطلاق عموماً عضلہ پر
ہوتا ہے۔

Prondol *(pron'-dol)*. Imprindole (q.v.).

پرونڈول : اپرنڈول۔

Prone *(pron)* [L. *pronus*]. Face downwards. Opp. supine.

اوندھا : چہرہ زیریں جانب۔

Pronestyl *(pro-nes'-til)*. Procainamide (q.v.).

پرونسٹائل : پروکین امائیڈ۔

Propaderm *(prop'-a-derm)*. Beclomethasone (q.v.).

پروپیڈرم : بکلومیتھاسون۔

Propamidine *(pro-pam'-i-den)*. Antiseptic cream and jelly used for wounds and burns. Treatment for longer than 10 days in inadvisable owing to possible irritation.

پروپیمے ڈین : دافع تعفن کریم و جیلی' زخموں اور جلے ہوئے آبلوں کے
لئے مستعمل۔ دس ایام سے زیادہ علاج جاری نہیں رکھنا چاہئے۔

Propanidid *(pro-pan'-i-did)*. Non-barbiturate, short-acting i.v. anaesthetic.

Propantheline *(pro-path'-el-en)*. A synthetic compound with an atropine-like action. Used for its antispasmodic effects in pylorospasm, peptic ulcer, etc. Dryness of the mout[h] occur in some patients.

[...]لین : ایک تالیفی مرکب جس کا عمل ایٹروپین کی طرح ہوتا ہے۔
[...]تعمال سے کئی مریضوں کا منہ خشک ہو جاتا ہے۔

Properdin *(prop-er'-din).* A protein of n[...] blood serum. It can destroy certain ba[...] neutralize certain viruses and damage f[...] red blood cells.

[...]ن : نارمل خونی سیرم کی ایک پروٹین۔ یہ بعض جراثیم کو تباہ کر سکتی
[...] وائرسوں کی تعدیلی کرتی ہے اور بیرونی سرخ خونی خلیوں کو نقصان
[...]۔

Prophylaxis *(pro-fil-aks'-is)* [G. *prophyl[...]* guarding]. Prevention--prophylactic prophylactically, adv.

[...]فظ : پرہیز۔ احتیاط۔

Propicillin *(pro-pi-sil'-in)*. Oral peni[...] tablets and syrup.

[...]ن : منہ سے کھائی جانے والی پنسلین کی گولیاں اور شربت۔

Propranolol *(pro-pran'-o-lol).* Effective d[...] the prevention or correction of ca[...] arrhythmias and dysrhythmias. It re[...] frequency of anginal attacks by help[...] reduce the unnecessarily high le[...] noradrenaline activity, thus blocki[...] effects of beta-receptor activation i[...] heart and lungs. Prepared as eye dro[...] glaucoma.

[...]ول : ضد بیش طنابی' انڈرال' اختلاج القلب' نوبتی میں نصف
[...]صف گولی شام قلبی بے قاعدگی یا کارڈیک ارتھمیا میں اس کی ایک
[...]ح دو پہر شام

Proptosis *(prop-to'-sis)* [G.]. Forward [...]usion, especially of the eveball.

[...]تم : آگے کو بڑھا ہوا۔ خصوصاً آنکھ کا گولہ۔

Prophyliodone *(pro-pil-i'-o-don)*. A co[...] agent used like iodized oil (q.[...] bronchography. Has the advantage of[...] eliminated more rapidly, but is more li[...] cause coughing.

[...]ن : ایک کنٹراسٹ ایجنٹ۔

Prophylthiouracil *(pro-pil-thi-o-ur'-as-il[...]* Inhibits thyroid activity, and is u[...]

thyrotoxicosis as a less toxic alternative to methylthiouracil (q.v.).

پروپائل تھائیو یوریسل : تھائیرائڈ عاملیت کو روکتا ہے۔ مفید برائے زہریلا گلھڑ یعنی ہائپر تھائیرائڈزم۔

Proquanil *(pro'-qwan-il).* Antimalarial.

پروکوانل : ضد ملیریائی۔

Prostaglandins *(pros-ta-glan'-dins).* Share some of the properties of hormones, vitamins, enzymes and catalysts. All body tissues probably contain some p. Used to terminate early pregnancy, and prostaglandin therapy to all systems of the body is currently under investigation. Prostaglandin X (PGX) is a hormone generated in arterial walls; antithrombotic; relaxes arterial smooth muscle.

Prostate *(pros'-tat)* [L. *pro,* before; *stare,* to stand]. A small conical gland at the base of the male bladder and surrounding the first part of the urethra--prostatic, adj.

قدامیہ : یورتھرا کے اولین حصہ کے گرد اور زبلیڈر کے اساس پر ایک چھوٹی مخروطی غدہ۔ جب مردانہ عضو انتشار کی حالت میں ہوتا ہے تو پھیل کر پیشاب کی نالی کو بند کر دیتی ہے اور پیشاب خارج نہیں ہوسکتا۔ جب انتشار یا انزال ختم ہو جاتا ہے تو یہ سکڑ کر پیشاب کو خارج ہونے کا راستہ دے دیتی ہے۔ یہ گلینڈ خود بھی ایک طرح کا لعاب خارج کرتی ہے جو مادہ منویہ کے حجم کو بڑھاتا ہے۔

Prostatectomy *(pros-tat-ek'-to-mi)* [L. *pro,* before; *stare,* to stand; G. *ektome,* excision]. Surgical removal of the prostate gland. **retropubic p.,** the prostate is reached through a lower abdominal (suprapubic) incision, the bladder being retracted upwards to expose the prostate behind the pubis. **transurethral p.,** the operation whereby shreds of prostatic cautery; usually restricted to small fibrous glands or to cases of prostratic carcinoma. **transvesical p.,** the operation in which the prostate is approached through the bladder, using a lower abdominal (suprapubic) incision. See RESECTOSCOPE.

قدامیہ براری : پراسٹیٹ گلنڈ کا سرجیکل خاتمہ۔

Prostatism *(pros'-tat-ism).* General condition produced by hypertrophy or chronic disease of the prostate gland.

کبر قدامیہ : پراسٹیٹ گلینڈ کے مرض سے پیدا شدہ عام حالت۔

Prostatitis *(pros-ta-ti'-tis)* [L. *pro,* before; *stare,* to stand; G. *-itis,* inflammation]. Inflammation of the prostate gland.

ورم قدامیہ : پراسٹیٹ گلینڈ کی سوزش۔

Prostatocystitis *(pros'-ta-to-sis-ti'-tis)* [L. *pro,* before; *stare,* to stand; G. *kysits,* bladder; *-itis,* inflammation]. Inflammation of the prostate gland and male urinary bladder.

پراسٹیٹوسسٹٹس : پراسٹیٹ گلینڈ اور زبولی بلیڈر کی سوزش۔

Prosthesis *(pros'-the-sis)* [G. addition]. An artifical substitute for a missing part. **powered p.,** in electromyographic control, electrodes placed on opposing muscles transmit a signal to an electronic device which operates the prosthesis--prostheses, pl.: prosthetic, adj.

مصنوعی عضوبندی : کسی ضائع شدہ حصہ کے لئے مصنوعی متبادل۔

Prosthetics *(pros-thet'-iks)* [G. *prosthetikos,* adding]. The branch of surgery which deals with prostheses.

علم عضوبندی: سرجری کی شاخ جو متبادل اشیاء کے متعلق بحث کرتی ہے۔

Prosthokeratoplasty *(pros-tho-ke-ra-to-plas'-ti)* [G. *prosthetikos,* additing; *keras,* horn; *plassein,* to form]. Keratoplasty in which the corneal implant is of some material other than human or animal tissue.

پراستھو کراٹوپلاسٹی : کراٹوپلاسٹی جس میں قورنیہ کا پیوند انسانی یا حیوانی نسیج کے بجائے کسی دوسری شے کا ہو۔

Prostigmin *(pros-tig'-min).* Neostigmine (q.v.).

پروسٹگمین : نیوسٹگمین۔ اختلاج القلب نوبتی میں اس کی ایک گولی صبح ایک دوپہر ایک شام۔ یہی خوراک برائے انلارجڈ پراسٹیٹ یعنی پیشاب رکنا' شدید عضلاتی کمزوری یا سیاس تھنیا گریوس۔

Prostoglandins *(pros-to-glan'-dins).* Name given in 1935 to a factor in human semen which stimulated smooth muscle. Thirteen have now been isolated. Prostoglandins are secreted by a wide range of tissues and often act near the tissue producing them. They have therefore been described as 'local hormones'. They have an effect on the uterine musculature, varying with the type of prostoglandin and whether the uterus is gravid or not. Can be given by various routes-- oral, intravenous, intrauterine and intra-amniotic.

پراسٹوگلینڈنز : مقامی ہارمونز۔

Protamine sulphate *(pro'-ta-min-sul'-fat)*. A protein in simple structure used as an antidote to heparin. One ml of 1 percent solution will neutralize the effects of about 1000 units of heparin.

پروٹامین سلفیٹ : سادہ ساخت کی پروٹین۔

Protamine zinc insulin *(pro'-ta-min)*. An insoluble form of insulin, formed by combination with protamine (a simple protein) and a trace of zinc. It has an action lasting over 24 hours, and in association with initial doses of soluble insulin permits a wide degree of control.

پروٹامین زنک انسولین : انسولین کی ایک ناحل پزیر قسم جو پروٹامین اور قلیل جست کے ملاپ سے بنتی ہے۔اس کا اثر ۲۴ گھنٹے رہتا ہے۔

Protease *(pro-te'-az)*. Any enzyme which digests protein; proteolytic, adj.

پروٹین پاش: پروٹینز ز۔خامرات کا ایک گروہ جو لحمیات کو توڑ کر امینوایسڈز میں تبدیل کرنے کے اہ ہوتے ہیں۔امینوایسڈ کو لحمیات میں تبدیل کرتے ہیں اور پروٹین سالمات میں ایک امینوایسڈ کو دوسرے کی جگہ بدل سکتے ہیں۔تمام جاندار بافتوں میں پائے جاتے ہیں۔

Proteins *(pro'-te-inz)*. Highly complex, nitrogenous compounds, found in all animal and vegetable tissues. They are built up of amino acids and are essential for growth and repair of body. Those from animal sources are of high biological value since they contain the essential amino acids. Those from vegetable sources do not contain all, but some of the essential amino acids. Proteins are hydrolysed in the body to produce amino acids which are then used to build up new body proteins.

پروٹینز، لحمیے : بہت زیادہ سالمی وزن کے پیچیدہ نائٹروجنی نامیاتی مرکبات کی ایک جماعت تمام جانداروں کے لئے بہت ہی اہم، پروٹین کے سالمات سینکڑوں یا ہزاروں امینوایسڈز پر مشتمل ہوتے ہیں۔کروموسون میں بھی پروٹین پائی جاتی ہے۔خلیے کے سائیٹو پلازم میں پروٹین بنتی ہے۔خامرات بھی پروٹین میں جسم کی بالیدگی اور امراض سے ہونے والی کمی کی تلافی کے لئے لازمی ہے۔

Proteinuria *(pro-ten-u'-ri-a)* [G. *proteios*, primary]. Protein in the urine. Syn., albuminuria.

پروٹی نیوریا : پیشاب میں پروٹین۔

Proteolysis *(prc-te-ol'-i-sis)* [G. *proteios*, primary; *lysis*, a loosening]. The breaking down of proteins into simpler substancesproteolytic, adj.

پروٹین پاشی : لحمیات کی سادہ اشیاء میں تبدیلی۔

Proteose *(pro'-te-os)* [G. *proteios*, primary]. The first cleavage product in the breakdown of proteins, intermediate between protein and peptone.

پپٹون اور پروٹین کا درمیانی عنصر : لحمیات کی شکستگی میں پہلا کلیوتج پروڈکٹ۔

Proteus *(pro'-te-us)* [L. *proteus*, a Greek god who continually changed shape]. A bacterial genus. Gram-negative motile rods which swarm in culture. Found in damp surroundings. Sometimes a commensal of the intestinal tract. May be pathogenic, especially in wound and urinary tract infections as a secondary invader. Production of alkali turns infected urine alkaline.

کثیر الاشکال امیبا : لاطینی زبان کا لفظ جس کا مطلب وہ یونانی دیوتا ہے جو متواتر سکل تبدیل کرتا رہتا تھا۔ایک جراثیمی جنس، گرام منفی متحرک سلاخی جراثیم جو نمدار جگہوں پر پائے جاتے ہیں۔پروٹی اس ولگیرس مثانے میں سوزش پیدا کرتا ہے اور کئی دوسرے امراض کا سبب ہے۔پنسلین غیر موثر البتہ سٹرپٹومائی سین سیپٹران اور سگمامائی سین موثر ہیں۔

Prothionamide *(pro-thi-on'-a-mid)*. Synthetic antitubercular compound.

پرتھیوناما ئیڈ : تالیفی ضد تپ دق مرکب

Prothipendyl *(pro-thi-pen'-dil)*. Antihistaminic antiemetic and spasmolytic. Potentiates the effects of alcohol, analgesics, barbiturates and anaesthetics.

پروتھی پنڈل : ضد قے آور۔

Prothrombin *(pro-throm'-bin).* A precursor of thrombin formed in the liver. The p. time is a measure of its production and concentration in the blood. It is the time taken for plasma to clot after the addition of thrombokinase. It is inversely proportional to the amount of prothromin present, a normal person's plasma being used as a standard of comparison. Prothrombin time is lengthened in certain haemorrhagic conditions and in a patient on anticoagulant drugs.

پروتھرومبن : جگر میں بننے والی تھرومبن کا پیشرو۔

Protopathic *(pro-to-path'-ik)* [G. *protos,* first; *pathos,* disease]. The term applied to a less sensibility, as opposed to epicritic (q.v.).

مرض ذاتی۔اول تاثری : اس اصطلاح کا اطلاق کم ہوشمندی پر ہوتا ہے۔

Protoplasm *(pro'-to-plazm)* [G. *protos,* first; *plasma,* anything formed]. The complex chemical compound constituting the main part of the tissue cells; it may be clear or granulated--protoplasmic, adj.

نخرمایہ۔مادہ حیات۔پروٹوپلازم: مادہ حیات زندگی کے لئے نہایت ہی ضروری ہے۔اس کے بغیر کوئی بھی جاندار زندہ نہیں رہ سکتا۔ مادہ حیات جانوروں اور پودوں دونوں میں پایا جاتا ہے۔ایک پیچیدہ کیمیائی مرکب جو خلیوں میں موجود ہوتا ہے۔ حیرانی ونباتی خلیہ میں مرکزہ اور سائیٹو پلازم پر مشتمل ہے۔

Protozoa *(pro-to-zo'-a)* [G. *protos,* first; *zoion,* living being]. The smallest type of animal life; unicellular organisms. See AMOEBA. The commenest protozoan infestation is *Trichomonas vaginalis*--protozoon, sing.; protozoal, adj.

نخرحونیات: حیوانی زندگی کی سب سے چھوٹی قسم یک خلوی۔

Protriptyline *(pro-trip'-til-en).* Antidepressant (q.v.).

پروٹرپٹی لین : مسکن دوا۔

Protozoa

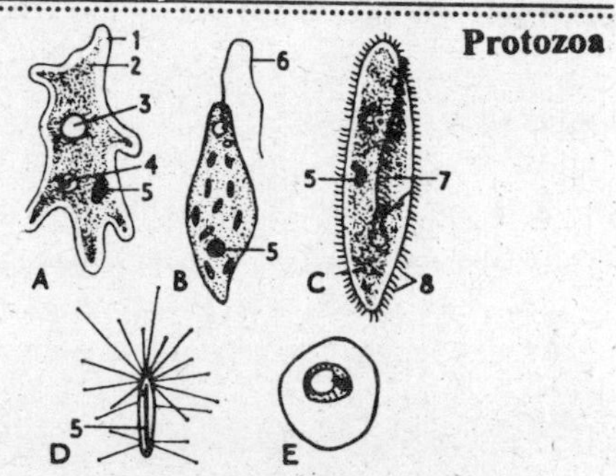

A. AMOEBA.
B. FLAGELLATE (EUGLENA).
C. CILIATA (PARAMOECIUM).
D. SUCTORIA (PODOPHRYA).
E. PLASMODIUM IN RED CORPUSCLES (ANNULAR-STAGE)

1. Ectoplasm. 2. Endoplasm. 3. Contractile vacuole. 4. Gastric vacuole. 5. Nucleus. 6. Flagellum. 7. Peristome.

Proud flesh Excissive granulation tissue.

کیرنڈ(زخم)انگور : زائدگرینولیشن نسیج۔

Provitamin *(pro-vi'-ta-min).* [L. *pro,* before; *vita,* life]. A vitamin precursor, e.g. carotene is converted into vitamin A.

بدل وٹامن : حیاتینی پیشرو۔ایک مادہ جس سے وٹامن بنتا ہے۔

Proximal *(proks'-im-al)* [L. *proximus,* nearest]. Nearest to the head or source--proximally, adv.

اتصالی۔قریبی : سریامنبع کے قریب ترین۔

Prurigo *(proo-ri'-go)* [L. itching]. A chronic, itching disease occurring most frequently in children. **prurigo aestivale,** hydroa aestivale (q.v.). **Besnier's p.,** an inherited **flexural** neurodermatitis with impaired **peripheral** circulation giving rise to dry **thickened** epidermis and outbreaks of **eczema in** childhood, Sometimes **referred to as the** atopic syndrome. See ECZEMA. **prurigo ferox,** a severe form. **prurigo mitis, a** mild form **purigo nodularis,** a rare disease of the adult female in which intersely pruritic, pea-sized nodules occur on the arms and legs.

خارشت : قدیم خارشی مرض جو عموماً بچوں میں ہوتا ہے۔

Pruritus *(proo-ri'-tus)* [L.]. Itching. Pruritus ani and p. vulvae are considered to be psychosomatic conditions (neurodermatitis) except in the few cases where a local cause can be found, e.g. worm infestation, vaginitis, Generalized p. may be a symptom of systemic disease as in diabetes, icterus, Hodgkin's disease, carcinoma, etc. It may be psychogenic, e.g. widow's itch (q.v.)--pruritic, adj.

سخت خارش : خارش کا مرض۔ پروٹیس ولوی یا شرمگاہ میں الٹرالانم دن میں دو دفعہ لگائیے یا آکسیبو پروکین مرہم (نووے سین مرہم) دن میں تین دفعہ لگائیے۔ ورگان، ویکسامیتھاسون (اورے ڈیکسان) یا کلورفنرامین۔ (پری ٹون۔ ایکرمین) ایک گولی صبح ایک دوپہر ایک شام۔

Prussic acid *(prus'-ik as'-id)* A 4 per-cent solution of hydrogen cyanide. Both the solution and its vapour are poisonous, and death may occur very rapidly from respiratory paralysis. Prompt treatment with intravenous injections of sodium nitrite and sodium thiosulphate may be life-saving.

پرسک ایسڈ : ہائیڈروسیانک ایسڈ کا انتہائی زہریلا محلول ہائیڈروجن سیانائیڈ کا ۴ فیصد محلول اور اس کے بخارات دونوں زہریلے ہیں اور موت فوری طور پر واقع ہوسکتی ہے۔ سوڈیم نائٹریٹ اور سوڈیم تھایوسلفیٹ کے انٹراوینس ٹیکے زندگی بچانے کیلئے ضروری ہیں۔

Pseudoangina *(su-do-an-ji'-na)* [G. *pseudo,* false; L. *angina,* quinsy]. False angina. sometimes referred to as 'left mammary pain', it occurs in anxious individuals. Usually there is no cardiac disease present. May be part of effort syndrome (q.v.).

کاذب دردسینہ : کاذب انجینا۔ بعض دفعہ بایاں پستانی درد جو پریشان افراد میں ہوتا ہے۔

Pseudoarthrosis *(su-do-arth-ro'-sis)* [G. *pseudo*, false; *arthron,* joint; *-osis,* condition]. A false joint, e.g. due to un-united fracture; also congenital, e.g. in tibia.

تجر مفاصل کاذب : کاذب جوڑ

Pseudoarthrosis of hip

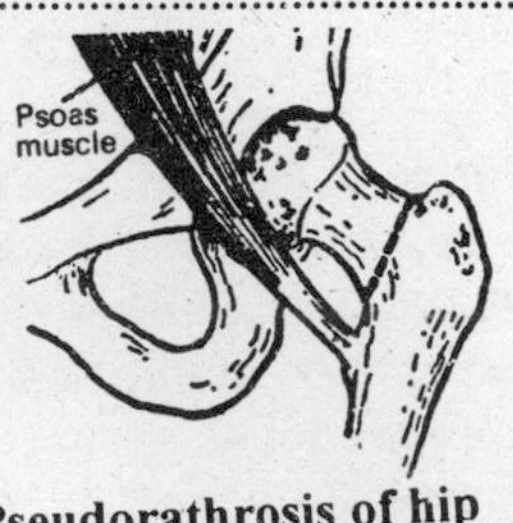

Pseudorathrosis of hip

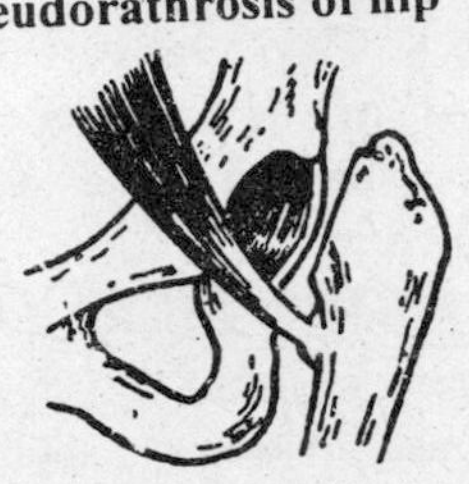

Pseudocholinesterase *(soo-do-kol-in-es'-ter-az).* A genetically inherited enzyme present in plasma and tissues (other than nerve tissue) and is synthesized in the liver. See SUXAMETHONIUM.

سیوڈوکولین ایسٹیریز: جینی طور پر توراثی خامرہ جو بافتوں (عصبی بافت کو چھوڑ کر) اور پلازما میں ہوتا ہے اگر جگر میں تالیف کیا جاتا ہے۔

Pseudocoxalgia *(su-do-koks-al'-ji-a)* [G. *pseudo,* false; L. *coxa,* hip; G. *algos,* pain]. See PERTHES' DISEASE.

مرض ورک کاذب : پرتھیز کا مرض۔

Pseudocrisis *(su-do-kri'-sis)* [G. *pseudo,* false; *krisis,* turning point]. A rapid reduction of body temperature resembling a crisis, followed by further fever.

بحران کاذب: جسم کا درجہ حرارت میں اچانک تکفیف اس کے بعد پھر بخار ہوجاتا ہے۔

Pseudocyesis *(su-do-si-e'-sis)* [G. *pseudo,* false; *kyesis,* pregnancy]. The existance of the signs and symptoms of pregnancy in the woman who believes that she is pregnant, when, in fact, this is not so.

حمل کاذب: کسی ایسی عورت میں حمل کی جملہ علامات کا ہونا جو یہ سمجھتی ہو کہ اسے حمل ہے مگر حقیقتاً ایسا نہ ہو۔

dohermaphrodite *(su-do-her-maf'-ro-dit).* person in whom the gonads of one sex are ɛsent, whilst the external genitalia comprise ɔse of the opposite sex.

کاذب دوزوجیہ : ایسا شخص جس میں صرف ایک جنس کے اعضا مو ہوں جبکہ بیرونی تولیدی اعضا جنس مخالف کے تولیدی اعضا پر مشتمل ہوں۔

dologia fantastica *(su-do-loj'-i-a* *a-tas'-ti-ka).* A constitutional tendency to l, and defend, fantastic lies plausibly, found some hysterics.

خبط دروغ گوئی: بعض ہسٹریا کے مریضوں میں جھوٹ بولنے کار جحا

domonas *(su-do-mon'-as)* [G. *pseudo,* lse; *monas,* unit]. A bacterial genus. am-negative motile rods. Found in water d decomposing vegetable matter. Some are thogenic to plants and animals and *eudomonas Pyocanea (aeruginosa)* is able produce disease in men. Found commonly a secondary invader in urinary tract ections and wound infections. Produces a e pigment (pyocyanin) which colours the date or pus.

سیوڈوموںا: ایک جراثیمی جنس۔گرام منفی متحرک سلاخی۔ جراثیم پانی اور سڑے نباتی مادہ میں پائے جاتے ہیں۔ بعض پودوں' جانوروں اور آدی بھی امراض پھیلاتے ہیں۔

domucin *(su-do-mu'-sin)* [G. *pseudo,* false; *mucus,* mucus]. A gelatinous substance t mucin) found in some ovarian cysts.

سیوڈومیوسین : بیضدانی سسٹوں میں پایا جانے والا جلاٹینی مادہ۔

doparalysis *(su-do-par-al'-i-sis)* [G. *udo,* false; *paralysis,* paralysis]. See EUDOPLEGIA.

خلج کاذب : سوڈوپلیجیا۔ ہسٹریا کے دورے۔

o-Parkinsonism *(su-do-park-in-son-izm).* signs and symptoms of paralysis (q.v.) ans when they are not postencephalitic.

کاذب پارکنسونیت : سن ہونے کی علامت۔

oplegia *(su-do-ple'-ji-a)* [G. *pseudo,* false; *ge,* stroke]. Paralysis mimicking that of anic nervous disorder but usually hyst- al in origin.

نقلی ادھرنگ : ہسٹریا کے دورے۔

Pseudopodia *(su-do-po'-di-a)* [G. *pseudo,* false; *pous,* foot]. False legs; the projectile parts of an amoeba or amoeboid cell (leucocyte) which asist it in movement--pseudopodium, sing.

کاذب پا : کاذب ٹانگیں۔ امیبا یا امیبی خلیہ کے باہر نکلے ہوئے حصے جو اسے حرکت میں مدد دیتے ہیں۔

Pseudopolyposis *(su-do-pol-i-pos'-is)* [G. *pseudo,* false; *polypous,* many-footed; *-osis,* condition]. Widely scattered polypi, usually the result of previous inflammationsome- times ulcerative colitis.

سیوڈوپولی پوسس : کافی منتشر پالپ' عموماً سابقہ سوزش کے نتیجہ میں۔

Psittacosi *(sit-a-ko'-sis)* [G. *psittakos,* parrot; *-osis,* condition]. Disease of parrots, pigeons and budgerigars which is occasionally responsible for a form of pneumonia in man. Due to an organism (Bedsonia) resembling a virus. It behaves as a bacterium though multiplying intracellularly. Sensitive to sulphonamides and antibiotics.

طوطاروگ: انسان میں نمونیہ کی ایک قسم جو طوطوں' کبوتروں وغیرہ سے لگتی ہے۔

Psoas *(so'-as)* [G.]. Muscles of the loin.

عضلہ کمر : کمرے کے عضلے۔

Psoriasis *(so-ri'-a-sis)* [G.]. A chronic skin disease in which erythematous areas are covered with adherent scales. Although the condition may occur on any part of the body, the characteristic sites are extensor surfaces, especially over the knees and elbows. When the scales are scraped they produce a shiny, silver sheen which is diagnostic. Not infectious. Cause unknown. Psoriatic arthritis--articular symptoms similar to those of rheumatoid arthritis occur in 3 to 5 per-cent of patients with psoriasis--psoriactic, adj.

چنبل : ایک قدیم جلدی مرض جس میں بعض جگہوں پر سکیل ہو جاتے ہیں۔ یہ چھوت کی بیماری نہیں وجہ نامعلوم' جسم پر نشانات جن پر چھلکوں کی تہیں ہوتی ہیں۔ خارش ہوتی ہے۔

Psoriderm *(so-ri'-derm)*. Colourless preparation of lethicin and coal tar, especially for psoriasis.

سورائی ڈرم : لیتھیسن اور کولتار سے تیار شدہ بے رنگ ۔

Psychiatry *(si-ki'-at-ri)*. The branch of medical study devoted to the diagnosis and treatment of mental illness--psychiatric, adj.

طب دماغی : طبی مطالعہ کی ایک شاخ جس میں ذہنی مرض کو تشخیص وعلاج کے متعلق بحث کی جاتی ہے۔

Paychic *(si-kik)*. Of the mind.

دماغی: ذہن کا۔

Psychoanalysis *(si-ko-an-al-i-sis)*. A specialized branch of psychiatry founded by Freud. It is a method of diagnosis and treatment of neuroses. Briefly the method is to revive past forgotten emotional experiences and effect a cure of the neurosis by helping the patient readjust his attitudes to those experiences--psychoanalytic, *adj*.

تحلیل نفسی : نفسیات کی ایک مخصوص شاخ جسے فرائڈ نے معلوم کیا۔ یہ نیوروس کی تشخیص اور علاج کا طریقہ ہے شعور اور لاشعور کے درمیان چپقلش جاننے کے لئے مریض سے بات چیت' خوابوں کی تعبیر' بحث وتمحیص اور دلائل سے مریض کو قائل کیا جاتا ہے۔

Psychochemotherapy *(si-ko-kem-o-ther-api)*. The use of drugs to improve or cure pathological changes in the emotional state--psychochemotherapeutic, adj.; psychochemotherapeutically, *adv*.

نفسیاتی کیمیائی علاج: جذباتی حالت میں مریضانہ تبدیلیوں کو بہتر کرنے یا ان کا علاج کرنے کے لئے ادویہ کا استعمال۔

Psychodrama *(si-ko-dra-ma)*. A method of psycho- therapy whereby patients act out their personal problems by taking roles in spontaneous dramatic performances. Group discussion aims at giving the patients a greater awarness of the problems presented and possible method of dealing with them.

نفسیاتی ڈرامہ : ایک نفسیاتی طریقہ جس میں ڈرامہ کیا جاتا ہے۔ اور مریض اپنے ذاتی مسائل پیش کرتا ہے ان پر بحث کی جاتی ہے اور مسائل سے آگہی ہوتی ہے۔

Psychodynamics *(si-ko-di-nam-ikz)* [G. *psych* mind; *dynamis*, power]. The science of t mental processes, especially of the causati factors in mental activity.

قوائے نفسی: ذہنی طریقوں کی سائنس۔

Psychogenesis *(si-ko-jen'-e-sis)* [G. *psych* mind; *genesis*, production]. The developme of the mind.

قائے نفس: ذہن کا ارتقاء۔

Psychogenic *(si-ko-jen'-ik)* [G. *psyche*, so *genesis*, productin]. Arising from the psyc or mind. **psychogenic symptom,** a neuro smptom.

ں زاد: دماغ یا روح سے ابھرنا۔

Psychogeriatric *(si-ko-ge-ri-at'-rik)* [G. *psych* mind; *geras*, old age; *iatrikos*, healin Psychology applied to geriatrics.

نیکو جیریاٹرک: جیریاٹرکس پر نفسیات کا اطلاق۔

Psychology *(si-kol'-o-ji)* [G. *psyche*, min *logos*, discours]. The study of the behavi of an organism in its evironment. Medica the study of human behaviour.

ات: انسانی رویہ کا مطالعہ' اس کے ماحول میں کسی جسمے کے رویے کا عہ۔

Psychometric *(si-ko-met'-rik)* [G. *psyche*, mi *metron*, a measure]. Measurement of t duration and rorce a of lmental processes.

ن پیمائی : ذہنی طریقوں کی قوت اور دورانیے کی پیمائش۔

Psychomotor *(si'-ko-mo'-ter)* [G. *psyche*, mi L. *movere*, to move]. Motor effect of psyc or cerebral activity.

ی حرکی: نفسی یا سربرل عاملیت کا موثر اثر۔

Psychoneurosis *(si-ko-nu-ro'-sis)*. Neuro (q.v.)

ی خلل اعصاب: نیوروس۔

Psychopatyh *(si-ko-path)* [G. *psyche*, mi *pathos*, disease]. One who is morally irre onsible. See PERSONALITY--psychopath adj.

نہ۔ دماغی مریض: اخلاقی طور پر غیر ذمہ دار فرد۔

Psychopathology *(si-ko-path-ol'-oj-i)* [G. *psyche,* mind; *pathos,* disease; *logos,* discourse]. The pathology of abnromal men- talproce- sses--psychopathological adj.; psyc- hopathologically, adv.

علم امراض دماغی: غیر معمولی ذہنی طریقوں کی پتھالوجی۔

Psychopathy *(si-kop'-a-thi)* [G. *psyche,* mind; *pathos,* disease]. Any disease of the mind. The term is used by some people to denote a marked immatruity in emotional development --psychopathic, adj.

دماغی عارضہ: کوئی ذہنی مرض۔

Psychopharmacology *(si-ko-far-ma-kol'-o-ji).* The use of drugs which influence the affective and emotional state.

سائیکوفارمیکولوجی: ادویات کا استعمال جو جذباتی حالت پر اثر انداز ہوتی ہیں۔

Psychophysics *(si-ko-fiz'-iks)* [G. *psyche,* mind; *physikos,* natural]. A branch of experimental psychology dealing with the study of stimuli and sensations--psychophysical, adj.

نفسی طبیعات: تجرباتی نفسیات کی ایک شاخ جس میں محرک اور حس کا مطالعہ کیا جاتا ہے۔

Psychoprophylactic *(si-ko-pro-fil-ak'-tik)* [G. *psyche,* mind; *prophylaxis,* a guarding]. That which aims at preventing mental disease.

سائیکو پروفائی لیکٹک: جو ذہنی مرض کو روکتی ہو۔

Psychosis *(si-ko'-sis)* [G. giving life to]. A mental illness arising in the mind itself, as opposed to a neurosis where the mind is affected by factors arising in the environment --psychoses, pl.; psychotic, adj.

دماغی حالت: ایک ذہنی مرض جو خود ذہن میں ابھرتا ہے۔

Psychosomatic *(si-ko-mat'-ik)* [G. *psyche,* mind; *soma,* body]. Mind-body illness, illness where emotinal factors produce physical symptoms. These arise mainly from overactivity of the autonomic nervous system which is infludenced by the emotinal state, e.g. chronic blusing may be due to feelings of guilt, the skin arterioles dilate as a result of autonomic overactivity, inflammation follows, death of some skin cells results in the development of a rash. The same 'blushing' can occur in the bowel; the p. process is t he same, resulting in ulcerative colitis. Other p. conditions include hyperthyroidism, asthma, migraine, urticaria, hayever, peptic ulcer and several skin con- ditions.

سائیکو میٹک: مرض جہاں جذباتی عوامل علامت پیدا کرتے ہیں۔

Psychosomimetic *(si-ko-so-mim'-et-ik)* [G. *psyche,* mind; *mimetikos,* imitative]. Drugs that produce psychosis-like symptoms. Hallucinogens. Also **psychotomimetic**.

سائیکوسومیٹک: سائیکوسس ایسی علامات پیدا کرنیوالی ادویات۔

Psychotherapy *(si-ko-ther'-a-pi)* [G. *psyche,* mind; *therapeia,* treatment]. Treatment of mental disorder, ranging from discussion, explanation, reassurance and psychoanalysis. group p., a priduct of World Warr II when free discussion of 'effort syndrome' produced therapeutic results. At a meeting, the anxieties of staff adnd patients are discussed and everyone is enlisted in the treatment programme--psychotherapeutic, adj.

نفسیاتی علاج: ذہنی خرابی کا علاج۔

Psychotropic *(si-ko-tro'-pik)* [G. *psyche,* mind; *trepein,* to turn]. That which exerts its specific effect upon the brain cells.

سائیکوٹراپک: جو دماغی خلیوں پر اپنا مخصوص اثر ڈالے۔

Psyllium *(si'-li-um).* The seeds of an African plant. They contain mucilage, which swells on contact with water; useful as a bulk-forming laxative.

سلیم: ایک افریقی پودے کے بیج۔ ان میں موسیلیج ہوتی ہے جو پانی میں پھول جاتی ہے۔

Pteroylglutamic acid *(ter'-o-il-gloo-tam'-ik-as-id).* Folic acid (q.v.)

ٹیروال گلوٹیمک ایسڈ: فولک ایسڈ۔

Pterygium *(te-rij'-e-um)* [G. a wing]. A degenerative conditoin of conjunctiva which encroaches on cornea--pterygial, adj.

Pterygium

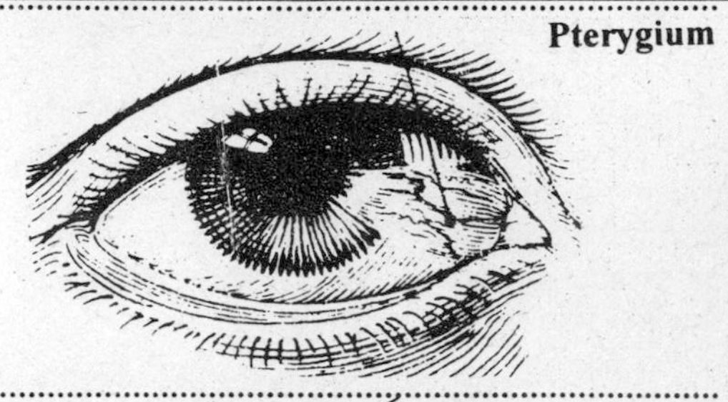

ناخنک۔ ناخونہ۔ ٹیری جیم: کجنکٹیوا کی تنزلی حالت جس سے وہ قورنیہ پر آ جاتا ہے۔ آنکھوں کے سفید حصے میں سرخ گوشت جو بڑھ کر سیاہ حصے پر چڑھنے لگتا ہے۔ آنکھوں میں خراش ہو جاتی ہے۔

Ptosis *(to'-sis)* A drooping , particularly that of the eyelid. See VISCEROPTOSIS--ptotic, adj.

سقوط جفن: نیچے جھک جانا۔ خصوصاً آنکھ کے پپوٹے کا۔

Ptyalin *(ti'-a-lin)* [G. *ptyalon,* saliva]. Salivary amylase which is a slightly acid medium (pH 6.8) converts starch into dextrin and maltose.

ٹایالن۔ لعابین: ایک خامرہ جو لعاب دہن میں پایا جاتا ہے۔ اور نشاستہ کو شکر میں تبدیل کرتا ہے۔ یعنی نشاستہ پاش ہے۔

Ptyalism *(ti'-a-lizm)* [G. *pryalon,* saliva]. Excessive salivation.

لعابیت: زائد لعاب دہن۔

Ptyalolith *(ti'-a-lo-lith)* [G. *ptyalon,* saliva; *lithos,* stone]. Salivary calculus.

ٹائیولتھ: سلوری پتھری۔

Pubertas praecox *(pu-ber'-tas-pre'-koks)* [L.] Premature (precocious) sexual development.

زودرس بلوغ: جنسی تکمیل جلدی ہو جانا۔

Puberty *(pu'-ber-ti)* [L. *pubertas*]. The age at which the reproductive organs become functionally active. It is accomaied by secondary characteristics--puberal, adj

بلوغ: تولیدی اعضاء کے فعلیاتی عامل ہو جانے کی عمر۔ اس کے ساتھ ثانوی خصوصیات بھی پیدا ہو جاتی ہیں۔

Pubes *(pu'-bez)* [L. *private* parts]. 1. Th e hairy region covering the pubic bone. 2. Os pubis.

عانہ۔ جھانٹیں۔ موئے عامہ: ۱۔ پیوبک ہڈی کو ڈھانپنے والا بالدار حصہ۔ ۲۔ اوس پیوبس۔ پیٹرو کی ہڈی، عظم عانہ۔

Pubiotomy *(pu-bi-ot'-o-mi)* [L. *pubes,* private *parts;* G. *ektome,* excision]. Cutting the pubic bone to facilitate delivery of a live child.

عانہ تراشی: زندہ بچے کی پیدائش کو آسان بنانے کے لیے پیوبک ہڈی کو کاٹنا۔

Pubis *(pu'-bis)* [N.L.] The pubic bone or os pubis, forming the centre bone of the front of the pelvis--pubic, adj.

عانہ۔ عظم عانہ پیوبس: پیٹرو کے سامنے کی سنڑ بون بنانے والی پیوبک ہڈی یا اوس پیوبس، پیٹرو کی ہڈی کو لہے کی ہڈی کا سب سے چھوٹا حصہ۔ دونوں پیوبس کے حصے پیٹرو کے سامنے آ کر ملتے ہیں اور ایک دوسرے کے ساتھ مضبوط جوڑ پیوبک سمفاسس بناتے ہیں۔

Pudendal block The rendering insensitive of the pudendum by the injection of local anaesthetic. Used mainly for epsiotomy and forceps delivery. See TRANSVAGINAL.

شرمگاہی بلاک: مقامی طور پر ٹیکے کے ذریعے سن کر کے عورت کے بیرونی اعضائے تناسل میں بے حسی پیدا کرنا۔ اس طریقے سے بچے کو شکم مادر سے چمٹی کے ذریعے باہر نکالا جاتا ہے۔

Pudendum *(pu-den'-dum)* [L. *puderre,* to be ashamed]. The external reproductive organs, especially of the female--pudenda, pl.; pudendal, adj.

شرمگاہ، ستر، خارجی عضو تناسل: بیرونی تولیدی اعضاء خصوصاً عورت کے۔

Pudenz-Hayer valve. One-way valve implanted at operation for relief of hydrocephalus.

پودنز، ہیئر ویلو: ہائیڈروکیفالس کے آرام کے لئے اپریشن کے وقت لگایا گیا یکطرفہ ویلو۔

Puerperal *(pu-er'-pe-ral)* [L. *puerperus,* childbearing]. Pertaining to childbirth, **puerperal sepsis,** infection of the genital tract occurring within 21 days of abortion or childbirth.

نفاسی: بچے کی پیدائش سے متعلق۔

Puerperium *(pu-er-pe'-ri-um)* [L. *puerperus,* childbearing]. The period immediately fol-= lowing childbirth to the time when involution is completed, usually 6 to 8 weeks --puereria, pl.

نفاس: بچے کی پیدائش کے فوراً بعد کا عرصہ جو عموماً چھ تا آٹھ ہفتے ہوتا ہے۔

moflator *(pul'-mo-fla-tor)*. Apparatus for nflation of lungs.

پلموفلیٹر: پھیپھڑوں کو پھلانے کا سامان۔

monary *(pul'-mon-ar-ri)* [L. *pulmonarius*]. ertaining to the lungs. **pulmonary distress yndrome,** see RESPIRATORY DISTRESS YNDROME.

ریوی۔ ششی: پھیپھڑوں سے متعلق۔ پلونری شریان دل کے داہنے ونٹریکل سے شروع ہوتی ہے۔ مرض پلونری ایمبولزم میں پھیپھڑے میں خون کی کو رگ بند ہو جاتی ہے۔

p [L. *pulpa*]. The soft, interior part of some rgans and structures. dentalp., found in the cavity of teeth; carries blood,nerve and ymph vessels. digital p., the tissue pad of the inger tip. Infection of this is referred to as 'p. pace infection'.

گودا۔ مغز: بعض اعضا یا ساختوں کا نرم اندرونی حصہ۔

satile *(pul'-sa-til)* [L. *pulsare,* to beat]. Beang, throbbing.

ٹپک: دھڑکنا۔ دھک دھک کرنا۔

sation *(pul-sa'-shun)* [L. *pulsare,* to beat]. eating or throbbing, as of the heart or artees.

دھڑکن۔ نبھان: دھڑکنا۔ جیسے دل کا یا شریانوں کا۔

se [L. *pulsus,* a striking]. The impulse ansmitted to arteries by contraction of the ft ventricle, and customarily palpated in the dial artery at the wrist. The p.rate is the umber of beats or impulses per minute and is bout 130 in the newborn infant, 70 to 80 in e adult and 60 to 70 in old age. the p.rhythm its regularity--can be regular or irregular; e p. voume is the amplitude of expansin of e arterial wall during the passae of the ave; the p.force or tension is its strength, timated by the force needed to obliterate it pressure of the finger. bouding p., one of rge volume and force. collapsing p. Corrigan's) , the water-hammer p.of aortic incompetence with high intial upthrust, which quickly falls away. **pulse deflcit,** the diffference in rate of the heart (counted by sttethoscope) and the pulse (counted at the wrist). It occurs when some of the ventricular contractions are too weak to open the aortic valve and hence produce a beat at th e heart but not at the wrist. **pulse pressure** is the difference between the systolic and diastolic pressures. soft p.,one of low tension. thread p., a weak, usually rapid and scarcely perceptible pulse. See BEAT.

نبض: نبض کلائی کی شریان پر دیکھی جاتی ہے بایاں بطین سکڑتا ہے تو خون شریانوں میں جھٹکے کے ساتھ داخل ہوتا ہے۔ بالغ میں نبض کی رفتار ۷۰ تا ۸۰ فی منٹ ہے۔

Pulseless' disease Progressive obliterative arteritis of the vessels arising from the aortic arch resulting in diminished r absnet pulse in the neck and arms. Thromboendarterectomy or a bypass procedure may prevent blindness by improving the carotid blood-flow at its commencement in the aortic arch.

بے نبض مرض: گردن اور بازوؤں میں نبض غائب ہوتی ہے۔

Pulsus alternans *(pul'-sus awl-ter'-nans)*. A regular pulse with alternate beats of weak and strong amplitude and of ominous inport.

پلسس آلٹرنینس: باقاعدہ نبض جس میں کمزور اور طاقت ور دھڑکن باری باری ہوتی ہے۔

Pulsus bigeminus *(pul'-sus bi-jem'-in-us)*. Double pulse wave produced by interpolation of extrasystoles. A coupled beat. A heart rhythm (usually due to excessive digitalis administration) of paired beats, each pair being followed by a prolonged pause. The second weaker beat of each pair may not be strong enough to open the aortic valve, in which case it does not produce a pulse beat and the type of rhythm can then only be detected by listening at the heart.

پلسس بائی جیمی نس: ڈبل نبض کی لہر جو زائد سسٹولز کی وجہ سے ہوتی ہے۔ دوہری دھڑکن۔

Pulsus paradoxus *(pul'-sus pa-ra-doks'-us).* Alteration of the volume of the pulse sometimes found, for example , in disease of the pericardium. The volume becomes greater with expiration, which is the reverse of the usual.

پلسس پیراڈوکسس: بعض دفعہ پیری کارڈیم کے مرض میں نبض کے حجم کی تبدیلی۔

Pulvis *(pul'-vis)* [L.]. A powder.

سفوف : سفوف یا پوڈر۔

Punctate *(pungk'-tat)* [L. *punctum,* point]. Dotted or spotted. e.g. punctate basophilia describes the immature red cell in which there are droplets of blue staining material in the cytoplasm--punctum, n.; puncta, pl.

نقطہ : نشان زدہ۔

Puncture *(pungk'-tur)* [L. *punctum,* prick]. A stab; a wound made with a sharp pointed hollow instrument for withdrawal or injection of fluid or other substace. cisternal p., insertion of a special hollow needle with stylet through the atlanto-occipital ligament between the occiput and atlas, into the cisterna magna. One method of obtaining cerebros pinal fluid. **lumbar p.,** insertion of a specia hollow needle with stylet either through th space between the third and fourth lumba vertebrae or, lower, into the subarachnoi space to obtain cerebrospinal fluid. **splenic p.** injection of radio-opaque medium prior t portogram. **sternal p.,** insertion of a specia guarded hollow needle with stylet into th body of the sternum for aspiration of a bon marrow sample. **ventricular p.,** a highl skilled method of puncturing a cerebral vent ricle for a sample of cerebrospinal fluid.

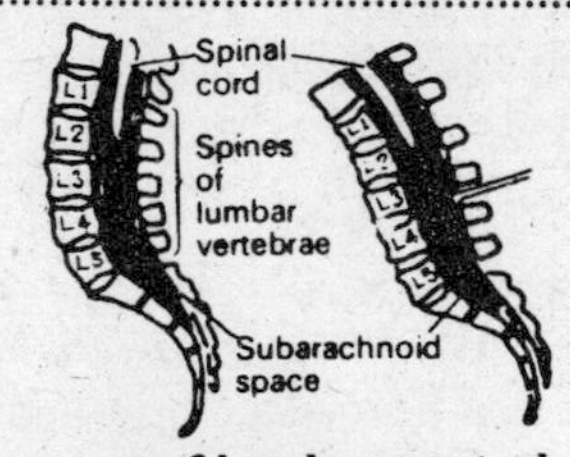

Diagram of lumbar verterbrae

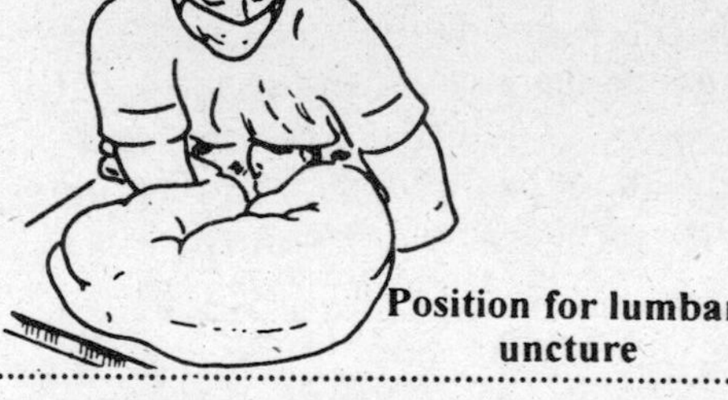

Position for lumbar uncture

سوراخ۔ جوفہ : زخم جو کسی تیز نوکیلے کھوکھلے اوزار سے کچھ نکالنے کے لئے بنایا گیا ہو یا سیال یا کسی دوسری شے کا ٹیکہ۔

Pupil *(pu-pil)* [L. *pupilla,* pupil of eye]. Th opening in the centre of the iris of the eye t allow the passage of light--pupillary, adj.

تلی : روشنی گزرنے کے لیے آنکھ کی آئیرس کے سنٹر میں سوراخ۔ تپلی پھیلنے اور سکڑنے کے قابل ہوتی ہے۔ تیز روشنی میں سکڑتی اور کم روشنی میں پھیلتی ہے۔

Pupillary *(pu-pil'-a-ri).* Pertaining to the pupil.

Purgative (pur'-jat-iv). A drug causing evac uation of fluid faeces. **drastic p.,** even mor severe in action, when the fluid faeces may b passed involuntarily.

مسہل' جلاب آور : سیالی فضلہ کو باہر نکالنے کی دوا۔ جلاب کے طور پر مستعمل۔ مثلاً کیسٹر آئل وغیرہ۔

Purin (e) s *(pu-rinz).* Constituents of nucleop roteins from which uric acid is derives. Gou is thought to be associated with the disturbe metabolism and excretion of uric acid, an foods of high purine content are excluded i its treatment.

لی مرکبات : ایک سفید قلمی نامیاتی اساس۔ نقطہ پگھلاؤ ۲۱۶° س اس کا تعلق یورک ایسڈ کے ساتھ ہے۔ سائز میں بڑے نکلیوٹائیڈ۔

Puri-Nethol. Mercaptopurine (q.v.)

ری نتھال : مرکپٹو پیورین۔ سرطان معدہ یا کینسر سٹامک کے علاج کے لئے ۵۰ ملی گرام کی ایک گولی روزانہ۔ یہی خوراک لیوکیمیا' مرض ہاجکن' سرطان کینسر۔

uromycin *(pu-ro-mi'-sin)*. Antibiotic cytotoxic agent that inhibits protein formation in cells.

پرورومائی سین: اینٹی بایوٹک سائیٹوٹاکسک ایجنٹ۔خلیوں میں پروٹین بننے کوروکتا ہے۔

urpura *(pur'-pu-ra)* [L. *purple*]. A disorder characterized by spontanecus extravasation of blood from the capillaries into the skin, or into or from the mucous membranes. Manifest either by small red spots (petechiae) or large plaques (ecchymoses) or by oozing, the latter, in the absence of trauma, being confined to the mucous membranes. It is believed that the disorder can be due to impaired function of the capillary walls, or to defectie quality or quantity of the blood platelets, and can be caused by many different conditioins, e.g. infective, toxic allergic, etc. See SCHONLEINS DISEASE. **anaphylactoid p.,** excessive reation between antigen and the protein globulin lgG (antibody). Antigen often unknown, but may be beta-haemolytic streptococci, or drugs such as sulphonamides may interact chemically with body proteins creating substances called haptens which are antigenic. **purpura haemorrhagica** (thrombocytopenic p) is characterized by a greatly diminshed latelet count. The clotting time is normal but the bleeding time is prolonges. Henochs p., a disorder mainly affecting children; characterized by purpuric bleeding into and from the wall of the gut, resulting in abdminal colic and melaena. Skin purpura and fleeting joint pains may or may not be present. Recurrences are common. [Edward Henoch, German paediatrician, 1820-1910.]

خونی دھبے۔حمیرا: خرابی کی ایک صورت جس میں خون شریانوں سے جلد یا میوکس جھلیوں میں یا ان سے نکل جاتا ہے۔جلد کے نیچے نیلے دھبے پڑ جاتے ہیں۔علاج کے لیے ملٹی وٹامن،لنکومائی سین ایسکاربک ایسڈ،فائیٹو مینا ڈی اور کیلشیم وٹامن ڈی۔

Purulent *(pu'-ru-lent)* [L. *purulentus*]. Pertaining to or resembling pus.

پیپ دار،صدیدی: پیپ سے مشابہ اس سے متعلق۔

Pus [L.] A liquid, usually yellowish in colour, formed in certain infections and composed of tissue fluid containing bacteria and leucocytes. Various types of bacteria are associated with p us having distinctive featrures, e.g. the faecal smell of p. due to *Bacterium coli;* the green colour of p. due to *Pseudomonas pyocyanea.*

پھپھولا: پیپ پر مشتمل ایک چھوٹا سوزشی ورم۔

Putrefaction (pur-ri-fak'-shun) [L. putrefacere, to rot]. The process of rotting; the destruction of organic material by bacteria--putrefactive, adj.

تعفن: گلنے سڑنے کا عمل۔جراثیم کے ذریعے نامیاتی مادے کی تباہی۔ سردیوں میں دوسرے یا تیسرے روز اور موسم گرما میں مرنے کے ۱۲ تا ۱۸ گھنٹے بعد مردہ جسم گلنا سڑنا شروع ہو جاتا ہے۔

Putrescible *(pu-tres'-ib-l)* Capable of undergoing putrefaction.

گلنے والے: گلنے سڑنے کے اہل۔

Pyaemia *(pi-e'-mi-a-)* [G. *pyon,* pus; *haima,* blood]. A grave form of septicaemia (q.v.) in which blood-borne bacteria lodge and grow in distant organs, e.g. brain, kidneys, lungs, heart, to form multiple abscesses--pyaemic, adj.

پیپ دار خون: خون کے جراثیم دور کے اعضا میں رہتے اور پرورش پاتے ہیں۔

Pyarthrosis *(pi-arth-ro'-sis)* [G. *pyon,* pus; *arthron,* joint; *-osis,* condition]. Pus in a joint cavity.

مفصل قائح: جوڑ کے کہفہ میں پیپ۔

Pycazide *(pik'-a-zid).* Isoniazid (q.v.)

پائیکازائیڈ: آئیسونیازڈ۔

Pyelitis *(pi-e-li'-tis)* [G. *pyelos,* trough; *-itis,* inflammation]. Mild form of pyelonephritis (q.v.) with pyuria but minimal involvement of renal tissue. Pyelitis on the right side is a common complication of pregnancy.

ورم حوض: پائیوریا کے ساتھ پائلونفرٹیس کی ہلکی قسم گردے کی بلغمی جھلیوں کی سوزش، کمر درد پیشاب بار بار اور لگ کے آنا، پیشاب میں پیپ۔ علاج کے لئے نائٹروفیورین ٹائن اور سوڈیم ایسڈ سٹریٹ۔

Pyelography *(pi-el-og'-raf-i)* [G. *pylos,* trough; *graphein,* to write]. Radiographic visulization of the renal pelvis and ureter by injecion of a radio--opaque liquid. The liquid may be injected into the blood stream whene it is excreted by the kidney (intravenous p.) or it may be injected directly into the renal pelvis or ureter by way of a fine catheter introduced through a cystoscope (retrograde or ascending p.)--pyelogram, n.; pyelographic, adj.; pyelographically, adv.

حوض ومثانہ نگاری: ریڈائی غیر شفاف مائع کے ٹیکے سے رینل پیٹرو اور یوریٹر ریڈیوگرافی کے طور پر دیکھنا۔

Pyeloilithotomy *(pi-el-o-lith-ot'-om-i)* [G. *pyelos,* a trough; *lithos,* stone; *tome,* a cutting]. The operation for removal of a stone from the renal-pelvis.

پائیلائیلتھوٹومی: رینل پیٹرو سے پتھری نکالنے کے لئے اپریشن۔

Pyelonephritis *(pi-e-lo-nef-ri'-tis)* [G. *pyelos,* trough; *nephros,* kidney; *-itis,* inflammation]. A form of renal infetion which spreads outwards from the pelvis to the cortex of the kidney. The origin of the infection is usually from the ureter and below, or from the blood stream--pyelonephritic, adj.

ورم حوض وگردہ: رینل مرض کی ایک قسم جو پیٹرو سے گردے کے کارٹیکس کی طرف بیرونی جانب پھیلتا ہے۔

Pyeloplasty *(pi-el-o-plas'-ti).* A plastic operation on the kidney pelvis. See HYDRONEPHROSIS.

پکنک: کرشمر کی شخصیت کی اقسام۔

Pyknolepsy *(pik'-no-lep-si)* [G. *pyknos,* thick; *lepsis,* a seizure]. A frequently recurring from of petit mal epilepsy seen in children. Attacks may number a hundred or more in a day.

پکنولیپسی: بچوں میں ہونے والے مرگی کے بار بار دورے۔ یہ حملے دن میں

یا زیادہ ہوسکتے ہیں۔

Pylephlebitis *(pi-le-fle-bi'-tis)* [G. *pyle,* g *phelps,* vien; *-itis,* inflammation]. Inflam tion of the veins of the portal system se dary to intra-abdominal sepsis.

فلے بائی ٹس: پورٹل نظام کی وریدوں کی سوزش' جگر بڑھ جاتا ہے۔ ارت باقاعدگی سے گھٹتا بڑھتا ہے۔ مہلک بیماری۔ پتے کا اپریشن فورا چاہیے۔

Pylethrombosis *(pi-le-throm-bo'-sis)* [G. p gate; *thrombos,* clot; *-osis,* condition]. ravascular blood clot in portal vein or an its branches.

ورید الباب: پورٹل ورید یا اس کی کسی شاخ میں انٹرا واسکولر خون

Pyloric stenosis *(pi-lor'-ik-sten-o'-sis)* [G. *ouros,* gatekeeper; *stenosis,* a being st ened]. 1. Narrowing of the pylorus due to tissue formed during the healing of a d enal ulcer, 2. Congenital hypertrophic p.s. to a thickened pyloric sphincter muscle, RAMSTEDTS OPERATION.

ضیق: پائیلورس کا تنگ ہونا جو ڈیئل السر کے صحت مند ہونے کے سکار سیج بننے کی وجہ سے ہوتا ہے۔ ۲۔ پائیلورک سفنکٹر کے دیز نے کی وجہ سے پائیلورس کا تنگ ہونا۔

Pyloroduodenal *(pi-lor-o-du-o-den'-al).* P ining to the pyloric sphincter and the du num.

روڈیوڈینل: پائیلورک سفنکٹر اور ڈیوڈینم سے متعلق۔

Pyloromyotomy *(pi-lor-o-mi-ot'-o-mi)* [G *louros,* gatekeeper; *mys,* muscle; *tome,* ting]. Incision of pyloric sphincter musc in pyloroplasty and Ramsted's operation.

رومایوٹومی: پائیلورک سفنکٹر عضلے کو کاٹنا۔

Pyloroplasty *(pi-lor-o-plas'-ti)* [G. *pylou* gatekeeper; *plassein,* to form]. A pl operation on the pylorus designed to w the passage.

البواب: راستہ چوڑا کرنے کے لیے پائیلورس پر پلاسٹک اپریشن۔

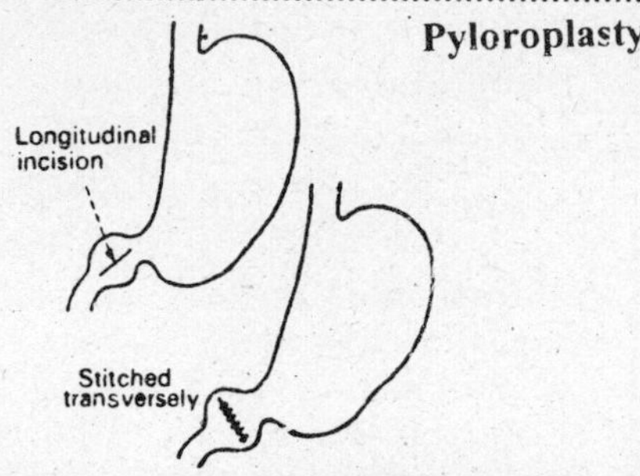

Pyloropsasm:*(pi-lor'-o-spazm)* [G. *pylouros,* gatekeeper; *spasmos,* spasm]. Spasm of the pyloric muscle; usually due to the presence of a duodenal ulcer.

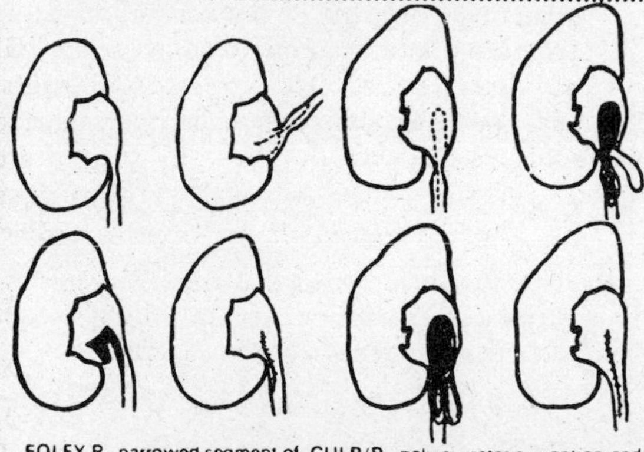

FOLEY P., narrowed segment of kidney pelvis widened by a Y-V procedure

CULP/P., pelvic-ureteric junction and upper ureter incised, narrowed segment then widened by inserting the pelvic flap into ureteric incision

Types of pyeloplasty

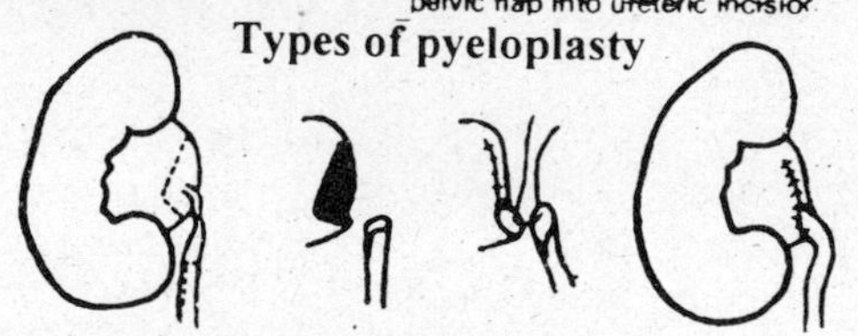

HYNES-ANDERSON P., abnormal part of ureter and adjacent pelvis excised. Enough pelvis may be removed to give appropriate reduction in size, and pelvi-ureteric junction widened with oblique anastomosis

پائیلوروسپازم: پائیلورک عضلے کا سپازم۔ عموماً ڈیوڈنیل السر کی موجودگی وجہ سے ہوتا ہے۔

Pylorus *(pi-lo'-rus)* [G. *pylouros,* gatekeeper]. The opening of the stomach into the duodenum, encircled by a sphincter muscle--pyloric, adj.

بواب۔ فم معدہ: ڈیوونیم میں معدے کا سوراخ جس کے گرد سفنکٹر عضلہ ہوتا ہے۔

Pylostrophin *(pi-los-tro'-fin).* Thin gelatin discs containing 1/750th g atropine methonitrate, and used in the treatment of pylorospasm in infants.

پائیلوسٹروفن: بچوں میں پائیلوروسپازم کے علاج میں مستعمل پتلی جلاٹینی تھالیاں۔

Pyocolpos *(pi-o-kil'-pos).* Pus in the vagina.

Pyodermia: pyoderma *(pi-o-der'-ma)* [G. *pyon,* pus; *derma,* skin]. Chronic cellulitis of the skin, manifesting itself in granulatin tissue, ulceratino, colliquative necrosis or vegetative lesions--pyodermic, adj.

پایوڈیا: جلد کا قدیم سیلولیٹس۔

Pyogenic *(pi-o-jen'-ik)* [G. *pyon,* pus; *genesis,* production]. Pertaining to the formation of pus.

پیپ زا: پیپ زا کے بننے سے متعلق۔

Pyometra *(pi-o-met'-ra)* [G. *pyon,* pus; *metra,* uterus]. Pus retained in the uterus and unable to escape through the cervix, due to malignany or atresia--pyometric, adj.

صدیدیت رحم: رحم یا یوٹرس میں رہ جانے والی پیپ جو سروکس میں سے نکلنے کے ناقابل ہو۔

Pyonephrosis *(pi-o-nef-ro'-sis)* [G. *pyon,* pus; *nephros,* kidney; *-osis,* condition]. Distension of the renal pelvis with pus --pyonephrotic, adj.

صدیدیت گردہ: پیپ کے ساتھ رینل پیڑو کا پھیلاؤ۔

Pyopen *(pi-o-pen)* carbenicillin (q.v.)

پایوپین: کاربینیسلین۔

Pyopericarditis *(pi-o-pe-ri-kard-i'-tis)* [G. *pyon,* pus; *peri,* around; *kardia,* heart; *-itis,* inflammation]. Pericarditis with purulent effusion.

التہاب التامور تقیحی: پیریکارو ڈیٹس۔

Pyopneumothorax *(pi-o-nu-mo-thor'-aks)* [G. *pyon,* pus; *pneuma,* breath; *thorax,* thorax]. Pus and gas or air within the pleural sac.

پایو نیوموتھوریکس: پلیورل سیک میں پیپ اور گیس یا ہوا۔

Pyorrhoea *(pi-o-re'-a)* [G. *pyon,* pus; *rheein,* to flow]. A flow of pus, usually referring to that from teeth sockets,p. alveolaris.

پائیوریا۔ ماخورہ: پیپ کا بہاؤ۔ عموماً دانتوں کے ساکٹ سے دانتوں کو صاف نہ کرنا اور وٹامن سی کی کمی اس کی وجوہات میں علاج کے لیے وٹامن سی کی گولیاں۔ مسوڑھوں پر لگانے کے لئے ٹینک ایسڈ گلیسرین ۵% طاقت کی دن میں ۳ دفعہ لگائیں۔ کوئی اینٹی بایوٹک دوائی بھی استعمال کرائیں۔

Pyosalpinx *(pi-o-sal'-pingks)* [G. *pyon,* pus; *salpigx,* trumpet]. A Fallopian tube containing pus.

صدیدیت بیض نالی: پیپ پر مشتمل فلوپین ٹیوب۔

Pyothorax *(pi-o-thor'-aks)* [G. *pyon,* pus; *thorax,* thorax]. Pus in the pleural cavity.

تقیح الصدر: پلیورل کہفہ میں پیپ۔

Pyramidal *(pi-ram'-id-al)* [G. *pyramis,* pyram0 id]. Applied to some conicalshaped eminences in the b ody **pyramidal cells,** nerve cells in the pre-Rolandic area of the erebral cortex, from which originate impulses to voluntary muscles. **pyramidal tracts** in the brain and spinal cord transmit the fibres arising from the p. cells.

ہرمی: جسم میں مخروط نما ابھاروں کے لیے اس اصطلاح کو استعمال کیا جاتا ہے۔

Pyrazinamide *(pir-az-in'-a-mid).* Expensive, oral, antituberculosis drug. Hepatotoxicity guarded against by SGOT tests twice weekly. Can produce gastrointestinal side effects.

پائرازیانا مائیڈ: مہنگی منہ سے کھائی جانے والی تپدق کے خلاف دوا۔ ٹیرازیڈ۔ تپ دق میں ایک گولی صبح ایک دوپہر ایک شام۔

Pyrexia *(pi-rek'-si-a)* [G. *pyressein,* to be feverish]. Fever; elevation of the body temperature above normal--pyrexial, adj.

بخار، تپ دق، تپی حالت: بخار، جسم کا درجہ حرارت نارمل سے زیادہ ہونا۔

Pyridium *(pir-id'-i-um).* Phenazopyridine hydrochloride (q.v.)

پائی ریڈیم: فینازوپائیریڈین ہائیڈروکلورائڈ۔ اس کی ایک ایک گولی صبح دوپہر شام برائے رینل کیلکولس یا گردے کی پتھری، سس ٹائی ٹس یا ورم مثانہ، پیشاب کی نالی میں درد اور جلن۔

Pyridostigmine *(pi-ri-dos-tig'-min).* Inhibitis breakdown of acetylocholine at neuromuscular junctins. Used in myasthenia gravis. Less toxic and potent, and has more prolonged action than neostigmine.

عصبی عضلاتی جنکشنوں پر ایسٹائل کولین کی شکستگی کو روکتا ہے۔ ہر ۳ گھنٹے بعد ایک یا دو گولیاں برائے شدید عضلاتی کمزوری یا میاستھنیا گریوس۔

Pyridoxin (e) *(pi-ri-doks'-in).* Vitamin B_6, may be connected with the utilization of unsaturated fatty acids or the synthesis of fat from proteins. Deficiency may lead to dermatitis and neuritic pains. Used in nausea of pregnancy and radiation sickness, muscular dystrophy, pellagra,etc.

حیاتین ب۔٦ حمل کے دوران: متلی اور تابکاری مرض وغیرہ میں مستعمل۔

Pyrimethamine *(pi-ri-meth-a-min).* A powerful antimalarial widely used in prophylaxis. suitable for administration to children.

پائیری میتھاملین: ایک طاقتور دافع ملیریا یا دوائی۔ بچوں کو دینے کے لئے مناسب۔ اس کی ایک گولی صبح ایک شام برائے ٹوکسوپلازموسز (۲ ہفتے تک)

Pyrogen *(pr'-ro-jen)* [G. *pyr,* fire]. A substance capable of producing a pyrexia- pyrogenic, adj.

پائیروجن: پائریکسیا پیدا کرنے کے قابل مادہ۔

Pyroscan *(pi'-ro-skan).* An apparatus for thermography (q.v.).Used as a screening procedure for breast cancer.

تھرموگرفی کے لیے سامان یا آلہ۔ چھاتی کے کینسر کے لئے سکریننگ کے طریق کار کے طور پر مستعمل۔

Pyrosis *(pi-ro'-sis)* [G. *firing*]. Heart brun; water- brash. Erutationof acid gastric contents into the mouth, accompanied by a burning sensation felt behind the sternum.

سوزش معدہ: دل کی جلن۔

Pyrotherapy *(pi-ro-ther'-a-pi).* Production of fever by aritfical means. See MALARIAL THERAPY.

پائیروتھیراپی: مصنوعی ذرائع سے بخار پیدا کرنا۔

Pyuria *(pi-ur'-i-a)* [G. *pyon,* pus; *ouron,* urine]. Pus in the urine (more than 3 leucocytes per high-power field)--pyuric, adj.

پیپ دار پیشاب: پیشاب میں پیپ، تین سے زیادہ لیوکوسائیٹس فی ہائی پاور فیلڈ۔

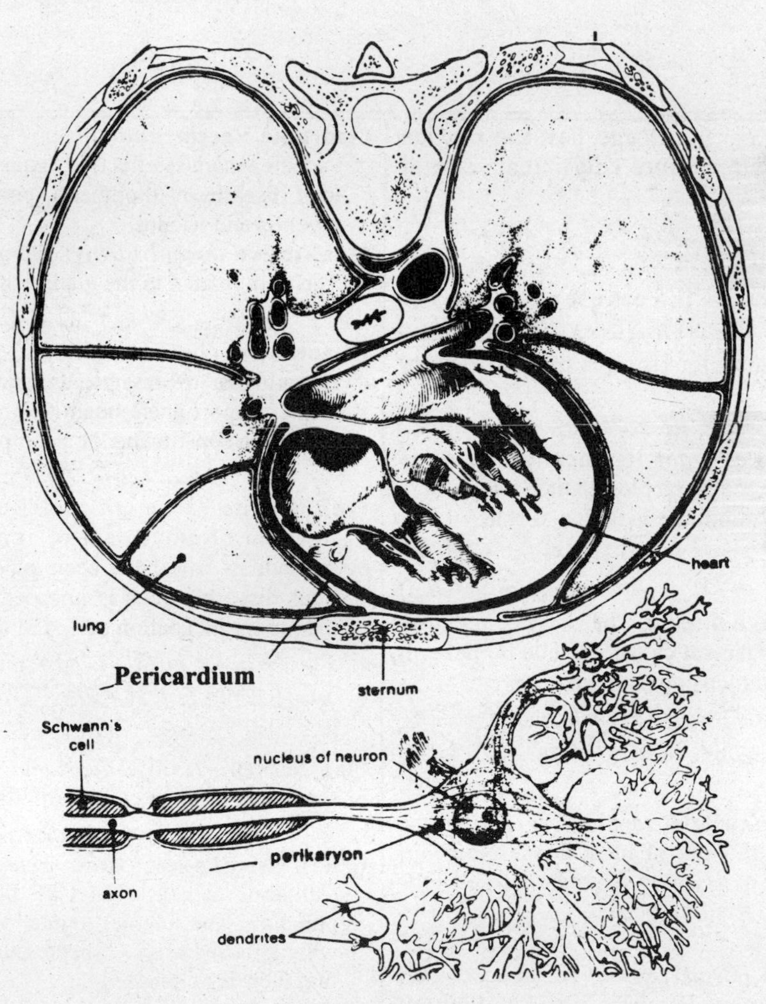

Q

Q Symbol for electric charge, heat and reaction quotient, temperature coefficient, rate of blood flow.

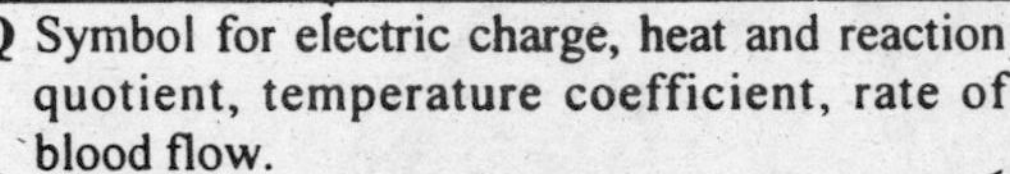

کیو: علامت ہے برقی چارج، حرارت، تعامل مستقل، درجہ حرارت اور خون کے بہاؤ کی شرح کی۔

qd. Abbreviation for [L.] qua que die (everyday).

کیوڈی: لاطینی لفظ کوا کوی ڈائی یعنی ہر روز کا مخفف۔

q.h. Abbreviation for [L.] qua que hova, every hour.

کیوایچ: لاطینی لفظ کوا کوی ہورا کا مخفف یعنی ہر گھنٹے۔

Quellede *(qwel'-ade)* Its chemical name is gammabenzene hexachloride. It is an odorless and creates minimum irritation to skin.

قوال اڈا: بنز ائل بنز وائیٹ کا متبادل۔ کم خارش والا، بے بو۔ اس کا صرف ایک دفعہ اطلاق ضروری ہے۔

Qfever This is a disease. The cause of the disease is an organism called coxielle burnelle. It is prevented by using a boiled milk.

کیو بخار: بھیڑوں اور مویشیوں سے انسان میں منتقل ہونے والی بیماری۔ اس میں جسیمہ علامات پیدا نہیں کرتا۔ دودھ ابالنا ضروری ہے تا کہ ان جسیموں کی موت واقع ہو جائے۔

Quadriceps *(kwod'ri-seps)* [L. *quadri*, four; *caput*, head]. Four headed. Possessing four heads. The q. extensor femoris muscle of the thigh which has four head.

چوسری عضلہ: ران کا عضلہ جس کے چار سر ہوتے ہیں۔

Quadriplegia *(kwod'ri-ple'ja)* [L. *quadri*, four; G. *plege*, stroke]. Paralysis of all four limbs. It is also called tetraplegia.

Qudruple Vaccine *(kwod-roop'l va'ksin)* It i vaccine which is effective against four infe ious diseases in diphtheria, pertusses, pol myelitis and tetanus.

Qualitative *(kwahli-ta-tiv)* [L. *qualitatinu* The term related to the quality of things.

ریت: کسی چیز کے معیار کے متعلق۔

Quantitative *(kwahn-ti-tativ)* [L. *quantitative* Denoting or expressible as quantity, relat to the proportionate quantities or to the an unt of the constituents of a compound.

اریت: کسی چیز کی مقدار یا اجزاء کو ظاہر کرنے والی

Quarantine *(kwor-an-ten)* Restriction freedom of movement of apparently w individuals who have been exposed to inf tious disease, which is imposed for the us maximum incubation period of the disease

گی: عام آدمی جو کسی متعدی مرض میں مبتلا ہو گیا ہو، اسے مخصوص جگہ پر رصہ کے لئے علیحدہ کر دینا۔ یہ عرصہ عموماً بیماری کے پھیلاؤ کے دن پر منحصر ہے۔

Quarten *(kworten)* [L. *quartanus*, four]. Rec ring every 72 hours i.e. fourth day.

، چوتھیا بخار: باری کا بخار جو ہر ۷۲ گھنٹے کے بعد ہوتا ہے۔

Queckenstedt's test *(kwekanshtets test)* It i technique to check the CSF flow in lum puncture. The internal jugular vein is pres which causes arise CSF pressure. This sh that their is no blockage.

Quickening The first perceptible fetal mo ments felt by the mother, usually at 16 to weeks gestation.

قوت بخش، احیا، ارتکاض: بچے کی پہلی حرکات جو ماں محسوس کرتی ہے، عموماً ۱۶ تا ۱۸ ہفتے کے حمل میں ایسا ہوتا ہے۔

uicklime Calcium oxide.

اَن بجھا چونا: کیلشیم آکسائیڈ۔ اسے تازہ چونا یا خام چونا بھی کہتے ہیں۔ انگریزی میں کوئیک لائم کہا جاتا ہے۔ ایک سفید ٹھوس، ان بجھا چونا، چونے کا پتھر بھٹی میں گرم کرنے پر تحلیل ہو جاتا ہے اور ان بجھا چونا اور کاربن ڈائی آکسائیڈ بنتے ہیں۔

کیلشیم کاربونیٹ ⟵ کیلشیم آکسائیڈ + کاربن ڈائی آکسائیڈ

uicksilver Mercury.

مرکری، پارہ، سیماب: ایک عنصر، جوہری وزن ۲۰۰٫۵۹ جوہری عدد ۸۰، ایک چاندی جیسی سفید دھات مائع، کثافت اضافی ۱۳٫۶، نقطہ پگھلاؤ ۳۹°س۔ نقطہ جوش ۳۵۷°س، تھرمامیٹر (حرارت پیما) بیرومیٹر، مینومیٹر اور دوسرے سائنسی آلات میں استعمال کیا جاتا ہے۔ اس کی بھرتیں دندان سازی میں استعمال ہوتی ہیں۔ اس کے مرکبات زہریلے ہیں اور بعض ادویات میں استعمال کئے جاتے ہیں۔

uiescent *(kwi-es'-ent)* [L. *quiescere,* to become still]. Becoming quiet. Used especially of a skin disease, which is settling under treatment.

ساکت: خاموش ہوجاتا۔ خصوصاً جلد کے متعلق مستعمل جو علاج کے ذریعے ٹھیک ہوتی جارہی ہو۔

uinalbar bitone *(kwin-al-bar'-bit-on)* A short-acting barbiturate with the general properties of the group, used in milk insomnia and anxiety conditions. Useful as 'night cap' for those with ischaemic limbs as it produces vasodilation.

کوئنل باربی ٹون: ایک مختصر العمل باربیٹوریٹ۔ نیند نہ آنے کی صورت میں اور پریشانی کی حالت میں مستعمل۔

uinthazone *(qwin-eth'-az-on)* Thiazide diuretic. See CHLOROTHIAZIDE.

کیونتھازون: تھیازائیڈ پیشاب آور۔

uinestrol *(kwin-es'-trol)* Suppresses lactation.

uinidine *(kwin'-i-din)* An alkaloid similar to quinine, but with a specific effect on the atrial muscle of the heart. Used in early artrial fibrillation, but only about 50 per cent of patients respond. Therapy should not be continued for more than 10 days adequate response has been obtained.

کیونڈین: کیونڈین ایک بے رنگ قلمی الکائیڈ ہے۔ کونین کے ساتھ ہم ترکیب۔ نقطہ پگھلاؤ ۱۷۴ تا ۱۷۵°س، ادویات میں استعمال کیا جاتا ہے۔ اختلاج القلب نوبی میں اس کی ایک ایک گولی صبح دوپہر شام۔

Quinine *(kwin-en)* The chief alkaloid of cinchona, once the standard treatment for malaria. For routine use and prophylaxis, synthetic antimalarials such as mepacrine, proguanil and pyrimethamine are now preferred. The drug also has some oxytocic action and has been employed as a uterine stimulant in labour. **quinine urethane,** sclerosing agent used for injection treatment of varicose veins. The main use is in management, of 'night cramps' where it is given as 300-600 mg of bisulphate.

کونین: ایک بے رنگ کڑوا قلمی الکلائیڈ جو سنکونا کی چھال میں پایا جاتا ہے۔ نقطہ پگھلاؤ ۵۷°س، ملیریا کے علاج کے لئے استعمال کیا جاتا ہے۔ پر میں بولی محرک کے طور پر دیا جاتا ہے۔

Quininism *(kwin-in-izm)* Headache, noises in the ears and partial deafness, disturbed vision and nausea arising from an idiosyncrasy to, or long-continued use of quinine.

تسمم کونین: سردرد، کانوں میں شور اور جزوی بہرہ پن کم بصارت اور متلی جو کونین کے زیادہ استعمال کی وجہ سے ہوتا ہے۔

Quinsy *(kwin-zi)* Acute inflammation of the tonsil and surrounding loose tissue, with abcess formation. Peritonsillar abscess.

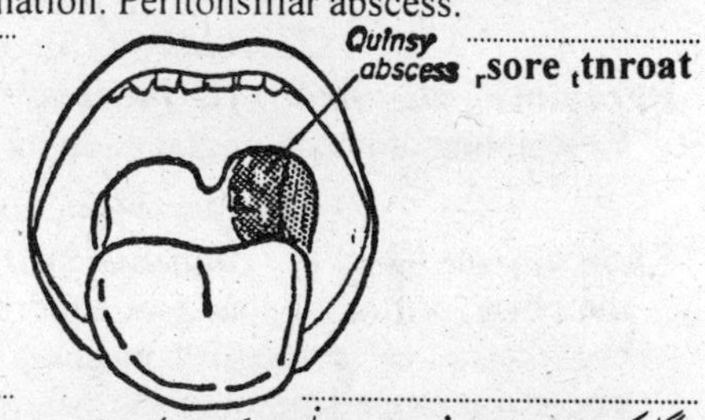

گلے کی پیپ: گلے یا ٹونسل اور ڈھیلے نسیج کے گرد انتہائی سوزش۔

Quotient *(kwo-shent)* A number obtained by division. **intelligence q., IQ,** See INTELLIGENCE. **respiratory q.,** the ratio between inspired oxygen and expired carbon dioxide during a specified time.

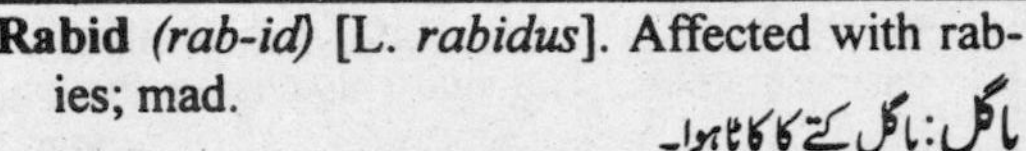

Rabid *(rab-id)* [L. *rabidus*]. Affected with rabies; mad.

پاگل: پاگل کتے کا کاٹا ہوا۔

Rabies *(ra-be'z)* [L. *rabere,* to rage]. An acute infectious disease of central nervous system affecting almost all mammals, including humans. It is caused by rhabdovirus. Usually it spreads by contamination with virus Laden saliva of bits inflicted by rabid animals like dog, cat, vampire bat etc. It is an international disease Vaccines against it are easily available.

ہلکا، پاگل پن: آب ترسیدگی یا ہائیڈروفوبیا۔ کسی پاگل جانور کے کاٹنے سے پیدا ہونے والا مرض۔ پاگل کتے کے کاٹنے سے یہ مرض ہو جاتا ہے۔ زخم کی جگہ جلن اور درد ہوتا ہے۔ مریض شور وغل سے گھبراتا ہے۔ غذا نگلنے میں دقت ہوتی ہے۔ مریض پانی دیکھ کر ڈرتا ہے۔ تشنج کے دورے پڑتے ہیں۔ منہ سے گاڑھی رال بہتی ہے۔ لوگوں کو کاٹنے لگتا ہے۔

Racemose *(ras-a-mo's)* [L. *racemus,* bunch]. Resembling of bunch of grapes on its stalk.

عنقودی: انگوروں کے گچھا سے مشابہ۔

Radical *(rad-i-kal)* [L. *radikalis*]. Directed to the cause, or root or source of a morbid process like radical surgery. It means a curative operation extending upto the root cause of disease.

بیخی: کسی چیز کی جڑ سے متعلق۔

Radioactive *(rade-o-aktiv)* Having the property of radioactivity. It is the quality of emitting of corpuscular or electromagnetic radiations consequent to nuclear disintegration. Radioactive gold, iodine and technetium are u for detection of liver, brain and visceral les respectively.

ر: تابکاری رکھنا یا تابکاری سے متعلق۔ بعض اوقات سابقہ "ریڈیو" ل کیا جاتا ہے۔ جو تابکار نکلائیڈز یا ان پر مشتمل اشیاء کو ظاہر کرتا ہے۔ مثلاً کاربن تابکاری کاربن کے لئے استعمال ہوتا ہے۔

Radiobiology *(rade-o-bi'-ol-o-je')* [L. *rad* ray; G. *bio,* life; *logos,* study]. That branc science which is concerned with the effec light and of ultraviolet and ionizing radiati upon living tissue and organisms.

ری حیاتیات: جاندار نسیج پر تابکاری کے اثرات کا مطالعہ۔

Radiocaesium *(rade-o-ke-zi-um)* It is a radic tive form of the element caesium. It is use the radiotherapy.

یوسیزیم: مرض کے تابکاری علاج میں مستعمل عنصر کیزیم کی ایک تابکار

Radiocarbon *(rade-o-kahr-bon)* A radioac isotope of carbon such as ^{14}C. Its half lif over 5000 years. It is used for metabolic search.

ری کاربن: میٹابولزم وغیرہ کی تحقیق کیلئے مستعمل عنصر کاربن کی ایک م۔

Radiograph *(rade-o-graf)* [L. *radius,* rays *graphien,* to write]. A film produced radiography.

وگراف، لاشعاعی تصویر: ایکسرے کی واضح تصویر۔

Radioiodinated human serum albumin U for detection and localization of brain lesi determination of blood and plasma volumes, circulation time and cardiac output.

ریڈیو آیوڈینیٹڈ ہیومن سیرم البومن: خون اور پلازما حجموں، گردشی وقت وغیرہ کا تعین کرنے کے لئے مستعمل۔

dioisotope *(ra-di-o-i'-so-top)* [L. *radius,* ray; G. *isos,* equal; *topos,* place]. An element which has the same atomic number as another but a different atomic weight, exhibiting the property of spontaneous decomposition. When fed or injected can be traced by a Geiger-Muller counter. **radioisotope scan,** pictorial representation of the distribution and amount of radioactive isotope present.

تابکاری ہم جا: عنصر جس کا جوہری عدد وہی ہو لیکن جوہری وزن مختلف ہو اور اچانک بوسیدگی کی خاصیت کو ظاہر کرے۔ جب اسے اس کی خوراک دی جائے یا ٹیکہ لگایا جائے تو گیگر ملر کاؤنٹر کے ذریعے معلوم کیا جا سکے۔

diokymogram *(ra-di-o-ki'-mo-gram)* [L. *radius,* ray; G. *kyma,* wave; *gramma,* letter]. A graphic record of movement of the silhouette of a part of the body.

ریڈیو کائیموگرام: جسم کے حصے کے سلہوٹ کی حرکت کا گرافی ریکارڈ۔

diologist *(ra-di-ol'-oj-ist)* Specialist in X-ray diagnosis.

تابکاری طبیب: ایکسرے تشخیص میں ماہر۔

diology *(ra-di-ol'-o-ji)* [L. *radius,* ray; G. *logos,* discourse]. The study of the diagnosis of disease by the use of X-ray—radiological, *adj.* radiologically, *adv.*

تابکاری معالجہ: ایکسریز کے استعمال سے مرض کی تشخیص کا مطالعہ۔

diomimetic *(ra-di-o-mim-et'-ik)* [L. *radius,* ray; G. *mimetikos,* imitative]. Produces effects similar to those of radiotherapy. See CYTOTOXIC.

ریڈیو ممیٹک: ریڈیو تھراپی کے اثرات سے مشابہ اثرات پیدا کرتا ہے۔

diosensitive *(ra-di-o-sen'-sit-iv)* Affected by X-rays. Applied to tumours, curable by X-rays.

ریڈیائی حساس: ایکسریز سے متاثر۔ اس کا اطلاق ایسی رسولیوں پر ہوتا ہے جن کا علاج ایکسریز کے ذریعے کیا جا سکے۔

diostoleum *(ra-di-o-sto'-le-um)* A solution of vitamins A and D (calciferol).

ریڈیوسٹولیم: حیاتین الف اور د کا محلول۔

Radiotherapist *(ra-di-o-ther'-ap-ist)* Specialist in the treatment of disease by X-rays.

ماہر معالجۂ اشعاعی: ایکسریز کے ذریعے مرض کے علاج میں ماہر۔

Radiotherapy *(ra-di-o-ther'-a-pi)* [L. *radius,* ray; G. *therapeia,* treatment]. The treatment of disease by X-rays and other forms of radiation. **endolymphatic r.,** adaptation of diagnostic lymphography, a method of introducing a radioactive substance into lymphatic channels and nodes in order to irradiate and thereby destroy maligmant cells.

تابکاری معالجہ: ایکسریز اور تابکاری کی دوسری اقسام سے مرض کا علاج۔

Radium *(ra'-di-um)* A radioactive element occurring in nature, and used in radiotherapy.

ریڈیم: قدرت میں پایا جانے والا تابکاری عنصر اور ریڈیو تھراپی میں مستعمل۔

Radon seeds *(ra'-don-seedz)* Capsules containing radon—a radioactive gas produced by the breaking up of radium atoms. Used in radiotherapy.

ریڈون سیڈز: ریڈون پر مشتمل کیپسول۔ ریڈیو تھیراپی میں مستعمل۔

Rale *(ral)* [F.] Abnormal sound heard or auscultation of lungs when fluid is present in bronchi.

رآل: برونکائی میں سیال کی موجودگی کی وجہ سے پھیپھڑوں سے غیر معمولی آواز۔

Ramstedt's operation An operation to relieve pyloric stenosis in infants by dividing the pyloric muscle, leaving the mucous lining intact. [Conrad Ramstedt, Emeritus Chief Surgeon, Rafael Clinic, Munster, 1867].

اپریشن ریمٹیڈ: بچوں میں پائیلورک سٹینوسس کے آرام کے لئے آپریشن۔

Ranula *(ran'-u-la)* [L. frog]. A cystic swelling beneath the tongue—ranular, *adj.*

ضفدع اللسان: زبان کے نیچے سسٹک ورم۔

Raphe *(raf'-e)* [G. *rhape,* seam]. A seam, suture, ridge or crease; the median furrow on the dorsal surface of the tongue.

سیون، اتصال: کریز، سلوٹ، کنارہ۔ زبان کی ڈارسل سطح پر درمیانی نشیب۔

Rapitard *(rap'-i-tard)* (Crystal II) Bovine insuline 3 parts in Actrapid (q.v.) 1 part at pH7.

راپی ٹارڈ: پی ایچ ۷ پر اکٹراپڈ حصہ میں بوون انسولین ۳ حصے۔

Rarefaction *(ra-ri-fak'-shun)* [L. *rarefacere,* to make thin]. Becoming less dense, as applied to diseased bone.

ہلکا پن: کم کثیف ہونا۔ جیسا کہ مریض ہڈی پر اطلاق ہوتا ہے۔

Rash Skin eruption. **nettle r.,** urticaria, formation of weals on the skin.

ثبوراتِ جلدی، سرخ دانے: کھال کا پھٹنا۔ پیشاب کی تیزابیت سے بچوں کی جلد پر سرخ دانے نکل آتے ہیں۔ گرمی میں یا دودھ چوسنے سے بچوں کے ہونٹوں پر یا نیچے ابتدائی ہفتوں میں آبلے پڑ جاتے ہیں۔ ان کے علاج کی ضرورت نہیں۔ گرمی دانوں پر پاؤڈر چھڑکنے سے فائدہ ہوتا ہے۔

Rashkind's septostomy When the pulmonary and systemic circulations do not communicate, an artificial atrial septal communication is produced by passing an inflatable balloon-ended catheter through the foramen ovale, filling the balloon with contrast media and pulling it back into the right atrium.

Rastinon *(ras'-tin-on)* Tolbutamide (q.v.).

رسٹی نان: ٹولبوٹامائیڈ۔

Rat-bite fever A relapsing fever caused by a *Spirillum minus* or by *Streptobacillus moniliformis.* The blood Wassermann test is positive in the spirillary infection.

چوہے کاٹے کا بخار: سپائیرلم یا سٹرپٹو بیسلس سے ہونے والا بخار۔

Rationalization *(rash-on-al-i-za'-shun)* [L. *rationalis,* reasonable] A mental process whereby a person explains his behaviour by substituting an unconscious excuse that is more acceptable than the truth, both to himself and to others. The excuse must be acceptable enough for self-deception and he feels completely justified.

تصویب۔ تاویل: اپنے آپ کو دھوکہ دینا۔ ایک ذہنی عمل جس میں ایک شخص اپنے رویہ کی وضاحت کرتا ہے اور اپنے آپ کو حق پر سمجھتا ہے۔

Rauwolfia *(rau-wol'-fi-a)* The root of an Indian plant. It is used in hypertension and as a central depressant, but the action of the drug is slow, and time is required before full response is achieved. Used mainly as the alkaloid reserpine (q.v.). Has tranquillizing property but in susceptible subjects can cause profound depression.

ؤوالفیا: ایک انڈین پودے کی جڑ۔ بیش طنابی میں مستعمل۔ سکون بخش۔

Raynaud's disease *(ra-no)* Idiopathic tropho neurosis. Paroxysmal spasm of the digital a teries producing pallor or cyanosis of finge or toes, and occasionally resulting in gang rene. Disease of young women. [Mauric Raynaud French Physician, 1834].

ض ریناڈ: نوجوان دوشیزاؤں کا مرض۔ شریانوں کا مرض۔

RDS Respiratory distress syndrome (q.v.).

ر۔ ڈی۔ ایس: سنڈروم تنفسی تکلیف۔

Reaction *(re-ak'-shun)* 1. Response to stimulus. 2. A chemical change, e.g. acid alkaline reaction to litmus paper. **allergic** (see SENSITIZATION) is a hypersensitivit disorder to certain proteins to which the pat ent is brought into contact through the me ium of his skin, his digestive or respirator tract, resulting in eczema, urticaria, hay feve etc. Inheritance and emotion contribute to th allergic tendency. The basis of the conditio is probably a local antigen-antibody reaction.

اال، ردعمل، تاثر، تیزابیت، قلویت: (۱) محرک کی طرف ردعمل (۲) ایک کیمیائی تبدیلی۔ پیشاب میں ری ایکشن کھاری۔

Reagent *(re-a'-jent)* An agent capable o producing a chemical reaction.

نعازل شے: کیمیائی تعامل پیدا کرنے کا اہل ایجنٹ۔

Reagin *(re'-ag-in)* An antibody associated wit allergic reactions. Present in the serum o naturally hypersensitive people.

یگن: الرجی کے تعاملات کے ساتھ متعلق اینٹی باڈی۔

Rebore Disobiteration (q.v.).

یبو: رکاوٹ ڈالنے والے کا خاتمہ۔

Recalcitrant *(re-kal'-si-trant)* [L. *re,* again; *ca. citrare,* to kick against the prick]. Refractory Describes medical conditions which ar resistant to treatment.

ندی: انعطافی۔ میڈیکل حالتیں بیان کرتا ہے۔

Recall *(re-kawl')* Part of the process of memory Memory consists of memorizing retention an recall.

ز کر: یادداشت کے عمل کا حصہ۔ یادداشت یاد کرنے، یاد رکھنے اور دوبارہ ں کا مظاہرہ کرنے پر مشتمل ہے۔

ecannulation *(re-kan-u-la'-shun)* Reestablishment of patency of a vessel.

ری کینولیشن: رگ کی پیٹنسی کو دوبارہ قائم کرنا۔

eceptaculum *(re-sep-tak'-u-lum)* [L. receptacle]. Receptacle, often acting as a reservoir. **receptaculum chyli,** the pear-shaped commencement of the thoracic duct in front of the first lumbar vertebra. It receives digested fat from the intestine.

کیسہ، مخزن: ریسیپٹیکل۔ اکثر ذخیرہ کرنے کیلئے مستعمل۔

eceptor *(re-sep'-tor)* [L. *recpere,* to receive]. Sensory afferent nerve endings capable of receiving and transmitting stimuli.

آخذہ: وہ حصہ جو نظامِ عصبی سے مل کر اندرونی اور بیرونی محرکات کو انجام دیتا ہے۔

ecessive *(re-ses-iv)* [L. *ecessio,* withdrawn]. Receding; having a tendency to disappear. **recessive trait,** an inherited characteristic which remains latent when paired with a dominant trait in selective mating. See MENDEL'S LAW.

رجعی: غائب ہونے کا رجحان رکھنا۔

ecipient See also BLOOD GROUPS.

گیرندہ، یابندہ: خون وصول کرنے والا۔

ecklinghausen's disease *(rek'-ling-howz-en)* Name given to two conditions. (1) osteitis fibrosa cystica - the result of overactivity of the parathyroid glands (hyperparathyroidism) resulting in decalcification of bones and formation of cysts; (2) multiple neurofibromatosis - a skin disease in which tumours of all sizes appear on the skin all over the body. [Friedrich Daniel von Recklinghausen, German pathologist, 1839-1910].

مرض ریک لنگ ہاسن: دو حالتوں کا نام: (۱) پیراتھائیرائیڈ غدود کی زائد عاملیت کا نتیجہ جس سے سست بنتے ہیں۔ (۲) ایک جلدی مرض جس میں سارے جسم پر، جلد پر رسولیاں بن جاتی ہیں۔

ecliners reflux syndrome This is due to severe disturbance of the antireflux mechanism which allows stomach contents to leak at any time whatever position the patient is in, although it is most likely to happen when the patient lies down or slumps in a low chair.

Recrudescence *(re-kroo-des'-ens)* [L. *recrudescere,* to become raw again]. The return of symptoms.

عود مرض: علامات کی واپسی۔

Rectocele *(rek'-to-sel)* [L. *rectus,* straight; G. *kele,* hernia]. Prolapse (q.v.) of the rectum, so that it lies outside the anus. Cf. procidentia. Usually reserved for herniation of anterior rectal wall into posterior vaginal wall caused by injury to the levator muscles at childbirth. Repaired by a posterior colporrhaphy.

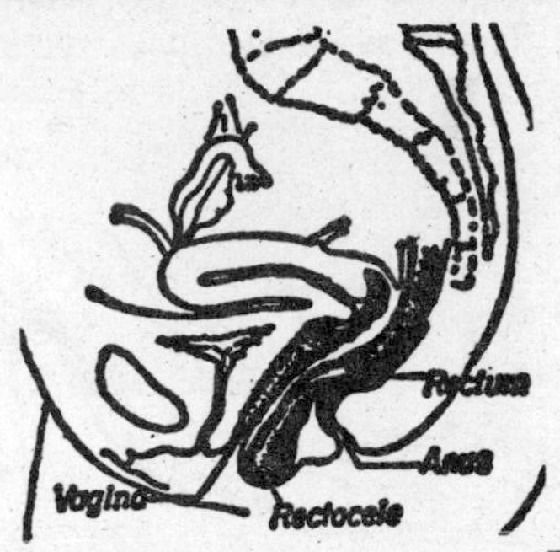

Rectocele

فتق سرم: ریکٹم کی تنزلی جس سے وہ مقعد سے باہر ہو جاتا ہے۔

Rectoscope *(rek'-to-skop)* [L. *rectus,* straight; G. *skopein,* to examine]. An instrument for examining the rectum. See ENDOSCOPE - rectoscopic, *adj.*

منظار شرجی: ریکٹم کو جانچنے کے لئے ایک آلہ۔

Rectosigmoid *(rek-to-sig'-moid)* [L. *rectus,* straight; *sigmoeides,* E shaped]. Pertaining to the rectum and sigmoid portion of colon.

ریکٹوسگمائیڈ: ریکٹم اور قولون کے سگمانما حصہ سے متعلق۔

Rectosigmoidectomy *(rek-to-sig-moid-ek'-to-mi)* [L. *rectus,* straight; G. *sigmoides,* E shaped; *ektome,* excision]. Surgical removal of the rectum and sigmoid colon.

ریکٹوسگمائیڈ یکٹومی: ریکٹم اور سگمانما قولون کو آپریشن کے ذریعے الگ کرنا۔

Rectouterine *(rek-to-u'-ter-in)* [L. *rectus,* straight; *uterus,* womb]. Pertaining to the rectum and uterus.

شرجی رحمی: ریکٹم اور یوٹرس سے متعلق۔

Rectovaginal *(rek-to-va-ji'-nal)* [L. *rectus,* striaght; *vagina,* sheath]. Pertaining to the rectum and vagina.

سرمی مہبل: ریکٹم اور ویجائنا سے متعلق۔

Rectovesical *(rek'-to-ve-sik-al)* [L. *rectus,* straight; *vesica,* bladder]. Pertaining to the rectum and bladder.

سرمی مثانی: ریکٹم اور بلیڈر سے متعلق۔

Rectum *(rek-tum)* [L. *rectus,* straight]. The lower part of the large intestine between the sigmoid flexure and anal canal - rectal, *adj.*; rectally, *adj.*

Rectum

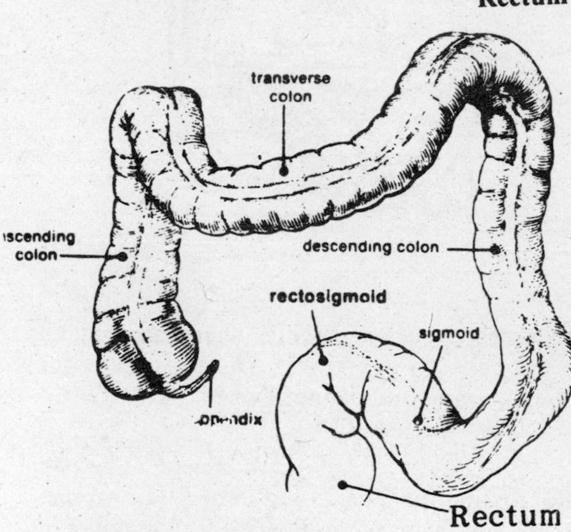

سرم، معاء مستقیم، بڑی آنت: آنت کا اختتامی حصہ جو مقعد میں کھلتا ہے۔

Recumbent *(re-kum'-bent)* [L. *recumbere,* to recline]. Lying or reclining recumbency, *n.*

افتادہ، لیٹواں: لیٹا ہوا۔

Red lotion Contains zinc sulphate which acts as an astringent and assists granulation.

لال لوشن: اس میں زنک سلفیٹ ہوتا ہے۔

Redoxon *(re-doks'-on)* Ascorbic acid (q.v.).

ی ڈاکسان: اسکاربک ایسڈ، وٹامن سی کی گولیاں۔

Redul *(red'-ul)* One of the sulphonamido pyrimidines (q.v.).

یڈل: سلفونامیڈو پائیریمیڈینز میں سے ایک۔

Referred pain Pain occurring at a distance fron its source, e.g. pain felt in the upper limb from angina pectoris; that from the gall bladder felt in the scapular region.

Reflex *(re'-fleks)* [L. *reflexus,* bent back] Reflected or thrown back. **accommodatio r.,** constriction of the pupils and covergenc of the eyes for near vision. **reflex action,** a involuntary motor or secretory response b tissue to a sensory stimulus, e.g. sneezing blinking coughing. The testing of variou reflexes provides valuable information in th localization and diagnosis of diseas involving the nervous system. **conditioned r.** a reaction acquired by repetition or practice **corneal r.,** a reaction of blinking when th cornea is touched (often absent in hysterica conditions).

ضطرار، اضطراری، عکس: منعکس یا واپس پھینکا ہوا۔ اضطراری عمل یا بفلیکس ایکشن کا مطلب ہے کہ کسی بیرونی تحریک کی وجہ سے بعض عضلات کا یر اختیاری طور پر دماغی تحریک کے بغیر حرکت میں آجانا۔ ایسا عموماً سپائنل کارڈ کے زیریں موٹر نیوران کے ذریعے ہوتا ہے۔

Reflux *(re'-fluks)* [L. *re,* back; *flux,* a flow] Backward flow.

رجعی بہاؤ: عقبی بہاؤ۔

Refraction *(re-frak'-shun)* The bending of ligh rays as they pass through media of differen densities. In normal vision, the light rays ar so bent that they meet on the retina-refractive *adj.*

نعطاف: روشنی ایک واسطے میں ہمیشہ مستقیم میں چلتی ہے۔ لیکن روشنی کی نعاع ایک شفاف واسطے سے دوسرے شفاف واسطے میں داخل ہوتی ہے تو مڑ باتی ہے۔ سمت کی اس تبدیلی کا نام انعطافِ نور ہے۔ سمت کی یہ تبدیلی صرف س وقت ہوتی ہے جب شعاع دو واسطوں کو علیحدہ کرنے والی سطح پر ترچھی گرے۔ اگر عموداً گرے تو شعاع اپنا راستہ نہیں بدلتی۔ انعطافِ نور کی وجہ سے انی سے بھرا ہوا تالاب اصل گہرائی سے کم گہرا نظر آتا ہے۔ پانی میں مچھلیاں پنی اصل جگہ سے ہٹ کر دکھائی دیتی ہیں۔ ستاروں کا ٹمٹمانا انعطافِ نور کی وجہ

سے ہے۔

کلیاتِ انعطاف: (۱) جب روشنی کی شعاع کسی لطیف واسطے سے کثیف واسطے میں داخل ہوتی ہے تو وہ عمود کی طرف مڑ جاتی ہے۔

(۲) جب روشنی کی شعاع کسی کثیف واسطے سے لطیف واسطے میں داخل ہوتی ہے تو وہ عمود سے پرے ہٹ جاتی ہے۔

(۳) شعاع وقوع، شعاع انعطاف اور نقطہ وقوع پر عمود ایک ہی مستوی میں واقع ہوتے ہیں۔

(۴) اگر روشنی کی شعاع ایک واسطے سے دوسرے واسطے میں گزر رہی ہو تو زاویہ وقوع اور زاویہ انعطاف کے سائن کی نسبت مستقل رہتی ہے۔ اس مستقل نسبت μ کو (دوسرے واسطے کا پہلے واسطے کے لحاظ سے) انعطاف نما کہتے ہیں۔ یعنی:

$$\text{انعطاف نما}\ \mu = \frac{\text{زاویہ وقوع کی سائین}}{\text{زاویہ انعطاف کی سائین}}$$

اس قانون کو سنیل کا قانون بھی کہا جاتا ہے۔ کسی واسطے کے انعطاف نما کی قیمت خلا میں روشنی کی رفتار کو اس مخصوص کثیف واسطے میں روشنی کی رفتار سے تقسیم کرنے سے بھی حاصل کی جاسکتی ہے۔ یعنی:

$$\text{انعطاف نما}\ \mu = \frac{\text{ہوا میں روشنی کی رفتار}}{\text{شے میں روشنی کی رفتار}}$$

efractory *(re-frak'-tor-i)* Resistent to treatment; stubborn, unmanageable; rebellious.

دشوار گزار: ایسا مادہ جسے بہت زیادہ گرم کرنے سے نقصان نہ پہنچے۔ ایسی اشیاء سے اینٹیں بنائی جاتی ہیں اور بھٹیوں کے اندر لگائی جاتی ہیں۔ نا قابل انتظام۔ جس پر علاج اثر نہ کرے۔

Regeneration *(re-jen-er-a-shun)* [L. *regenerare,* to beget again]. Renewal of tissue.

ولادتِ ثانیہ، نموئے ثانیہ: نسیج کی تجدید۔

Regression *(re-gre'-shun)* [L. *regressio,* turn back]. In psychiatry, reversion to an earlier stage of development, becoming more childish. Occurs in dementia, especially senile dementia.

رجوع، عمل مراجعت: تکمیل یا ارتقاء کے پہلے مرحلہ میں واپسی یعنی بچگانہ پن کی واپسی۔

Regurgitation *(re-gur-ji-ta'-shun)* [L. *re,* back; *gurgitare,* to flood] Backward flow, e.g. of stomach contents into, or through the mouth.

رجع الدم، اگل آنا: عقبی بہاؤ۔ مثلاً معدہ کے اجزاء کا منہ میں آنا۔

Rehabilitation A planned programme in which the convalescent or disabled person progresses towards, or maintains the maximum degree of physical and psychological independence of which he is capable.

بحالی: ایک مجوزہ پروگرام، جس میں ایک معذور شخص جسمانی ونفسیاتی آزادی رکھتا ہے، جس کا وہ اہل ہے۔

Reiter's syndrome A condition in which arthritis occurs together with conjunctivitis and urethritis (or cervicitis in women). It is commonly, but not always, a venereal infection and should be considered as a cause of knee effusion in young men when trauma has not occurred. [Hans Reiter, German physician, 1881-1969].

ریٹر سنڈروم: حالت جس میں یورتھریٹس، پولی ارتھریٹس اور جنکٹویٹس ہوتے ہیں۔

Relapsing fever Louse-borne or tick-borne infection caused by spirochaetes of genus Borrelia. Prevalent in many parts of the wold. Characterized by a febrile period of a week or so, with apparent recovery, followed by a further bout of fever.

رجعی بخار: برلیا جنس کے سبب مرض۔ لوٹ آنے والا بخار۔

Relaxant *(re-laks'-ant)* [L. *re,* again; *laxo,* to loosen]. That which reduces tension. See MUSCLE.

ملین: ٹینشن کو کم کرنے والی دوا۔

Relaxin *(re-laks'-in)* Polypeptides secreted by the ovaries to soften the cervix and loosen the ligaments in preparation for birth.

Remission *(re-mi'-shun)* [L. *remissio,* a sending back]. The period of abatement of a fever or other disease.

افاقہ، زمانۂ خفت: بخار یا کسی دوسرے مرض کی تخفیف کا عرصہ۔

Remittent *(re-mit'-ent)* [L. *remittere,* to send back]. Increasing and decreasing at periodic intervals.

گھٹتا بڑھتا: پیریاڈک وقفوں پر گھٹنا اور بڑھنا۔ گھٹنے بڑھنے والا بخار۔

Renal *(re'-nal)* [L. *renalis,* of the kidney]. Pertaining to the kidney. **renal asthma,** hyperventilation of lungs occurring in uraemia as a result of acidosis. **renal calculus** (q.v.), stone in the kidney. **renal glycosuria** occurs in patients with a normal blood sugar and a lowered r. threshold for sugar. **renal rickets,** see RICKETS. **renal uraemia** is uraemia (q.v.) following kidney disease itself, in contrast to uraemia from failure of the circulation of the blood (extrarenal uraemia).

گردے کا، گردوی: گردہ سے متعلق۔ رینل کیلکولس یا گردے کی پتھری عموماً کیلشیم آکسیٹ اور یورک ایسڈ وغیرہ سے بنتی ہے۔ رینل کولک یا درد گردہ شدید ہوتا ہے۔

Renin *(re'-nin)* An enzyme, released into the blood from the kidney cortex and stimulated by sodium loss. A cause of hypertension in man. See ANGIOTENSIN, ALDOSTERONE.

Sodium loss
↓
Renin
↓
Angiotensin
↓
Aldosterone from adrenal cortex
↓
Prevents sodium loss

پروٹین گردہ: ایک خامرہ جو صرف گردے کے کارٹیکس میں پایا جاتا ہے۔ آدمی میں بیش طنابی کا سبب۔

Rennin *(ren'-in)* Milk curdling enzyme of gastric juice, converting soluble caseinogen into insoluble casein.

جوہر پنیر مایہ: ایک خامرہ جو دودھ میں پروٹین کو جما دینے کی طاقت رکھتا ہے۔

Renogram *(re'-no-gram)* [L. *rena,* kidney, G. *gramma,* letter]. X-ray of renal shadow following injection of opaque medium, demonstrated in aortograph series. **isotope r.,** see TEST; RADIOISOTOPE RENOGRAM - renographical, *adj.* renographically, *adv.*

رینوگرام: غیر شفاف واسطے کے ٹیکے کے بعد رینل شیڈو کا ایکسرے۔

Reovirus *(re'-o-virus)* Respiratory enteric orphan virus (q.v.).

ریوائرس: تنفسی انٹرک یتیم وائرس۔

Replogle tube A double lumen aspiration catheter, attached to low pressure suction apparatus. It is kept patent by half hourly instillation of 1/2 ml of saline into the lumen not attached to suction.

Repression *(re-presh'-un)* [L. repressum, press back]. The refusal to recognize the existence of urges and feelings which are painful, or are in conflict with the individual's accepted moral principles. Freud called this refusal 'repression' because the painful idea was repressed into the unconscious mind.

ضبط: درد بھرے احساسات وخواہشات کے وجود کو تسلیم کرنے سے انکار۔

Resection *(re-sek'-shun)* [L. *resecare,* to cut off]. Surgical excision. **submucous r.,** incision of nasal mucosa, removal of deflected nasal septum, replacement of mucosa.

تراش: آپریشن کے ذریعے کاٹ کر الگ کرنا۔

Resectoscope *(re-sek'-to-skop)* [L. *resecare,* to cut off; G. *skopein,* to examine]. An instrument passed along the urethra; it permits resection of tissue from the base of the bladder and prostate under direct vision. See PROSTATECTOMY.

ریسیکٹوسکوپ: یورتھرا سے گزرنے والا آلہ۔

Resectotome *(re-sek'-to-tom)* [L. *resecare,* to cut off]. Instrument used for resection.

ریسیکٹوٹوم: آلہ جو آپریشن میں کاٹنے کے لئے استعمال ہوتا ہے۔

Reserpine *(re-ser'-pin)* The chief alkaloid of rauwolfia (q.v.). Used mainly hypertension, sometimes with other drugs. Severe depression has occurred after full nad prolonged therapy. Interfers with transmission in sympathetic adrenergic nerves, especially sympathetically mediated vascular reflexes and thus can lead to postural and exercise hypotension.

ریسرپین: راؤولفیا کا اہم الکلائیڈ۔ سرپاسل۔ ہائی بلڈ پریشر کے لئے ایک گولی صبح، ایک دوپہر، ایک شام۔ اگر بلڈ پریشر ہو تو یہی خوراک برائے فالج۔

Residual *(re-zid'-u-al)* [L. *residuus,* that is left behind]. Remaining. **residual air,** the air remaining in the lung after forced expiration. **residual urine**, urine remaining in the bladder after micturition.

بقیہ: بقایا۔ جو باقی بچا ہو۔

Resin *(res'-in)* A mixture of complex organic subtances which can occur naturally or be manufactured synthetically. **ion exchange r.,** administered orally, acts on the gut to effect a change in plasma ions.

رال: قدرتی رالیں نامیاتی مرکب ہیں جو بعض پودے اور حشرات خارج کرتے ہیں۔ وہ پانی میں عموماً ناحل پذیر ہوتے ہیں۔ لیکن مختلف نامیاتی محللوں میں حل پذیر ہوتے ہیں۔ لازمی تیلیوں کی تکسید سے پیدا ہوتے ہیں۔

Resistance *(re-zis'-tens)* [L. *resistere,* to withstand]. Power of resisting. In psychology the name given to the force which prevents repressed thoughts from re-entering the conscious mind from the unconscious. **resistance to infection,** the power of the body to withstand infection. See IMMUNITY. **peripheral r.,** that offered by the capillaries to the blood passing through them.

مزاحمت، مناعیت: مدافعت کی طاقت۔

Resochin *(res'-o-chin)* Chloroquine (q.v.).

ریزوچن: کلوروکوئین۔ ملیریا بخار کے لئے گولیاں۔

Resolution *(rez-o-loo'-shun)* [L. *resolvere,* to loosen]. The subsidence of inflammation; describes the earliest indications of a return to normal, as when, in lobar pneumonia, the consolidation begins to liquefy.

انحطاط: نارمل ہو جانا۔ سوزش کا خاتمہ۔

Resonance *(rez'-o-nans)* [L. *resonare,* to resound]. Themusical quality elicited on percussing a cavity which contains air. **vocal r.** is the reverberating note heard through the stethoscope when the patient is asked to say 'one, one, one, or 'ninety-nine'.

گونج، گمک: میزو، میرزم، کوانٹم کیمیائی گمک۔ کسی سالمے کی ساخت کی وضاحت اس کے جواہر کی مقررہ گرفت کی حالتوں اور جواہر کے درمیان گرفت بانڈز کے صحیح اعداد سے ہوتی ہے کیونکہ وہ سالمے کی صحیح صورتحال کی سادی تصویر پیش کرتی ہے۔ سالمے کی خصوصیات کسی بھی کلاسیکل ضابطے کے مطابق نہیں ہوتیں۔ مثلاً الیکٹرون کثافت کی تقسیم اگر اہتزاز کے اہل نظام پر ایک چھوٹی میقاتی یا دوری قوت کا اطلاق کیا جائے تو نظام عام طور پر چھوٹے حیطہ کے جبری اہتزازات میں سیٹ ہو جاتا ہے۔ گمک ایسا مظہر ہے جس میں کسی جسم کے ارتعاش کا حیطہ بڑھ جاتا ہے۔ جب اس پر ایسی دوری قوت لگائی جائے، جس کا ٹائم پیریڈ کے برابر ہو۔

Resonium *(re-so'-ni-um)* A synthetic resin that can absorb potassium. Given in hyperkalaemic states, anuria, shock and other conditions of high potassium blood level.

ریسونیم: ایک تالیفی رال جو پوٹاشیم کو جذب کر سکتی ہے۔

Resorcinol *(re-zor'-sin-ol)* A mild antiseptic derived from phenol. Used in hair lotions and antipruritic ointments. It should not be used for long periods on open surfaces.

رال پوٹاش: ایم ہائیڈروکسی بنزین، ایک ٹھوس ڈائی ہائیڈرک فینول، نقطہ پگھلاؤ ۱۱۰° س، بیروزون یا رالوں، ادویات اور دوسرے حاصلات کی تیاری میں بطور انٹرمیڈیٹ استعمال کیا جاتا ہے۔ فینول سے اخذ شدہ ایک ہلکا دافع تعفن۔ بالوں کے لوشن میں مستعمل۔ کھلی سطوح پر زیادہ عرصہ استعمال نہیں کرنا چاہئے۔

Resorption *(re-sorp'-shun)* [L. *resorbere,* to drink in]. To absorb again, e.g. absorption of (1) callus following bone fracture, (2) roots of the deciduous teeth, (3) blood from a haematoma.

انجذاب، جذب عضو: دوبارہ جذب کرنا۔

Respiration *(res-pi-ra'-shun)* [L. *respirare,* to breathe]. The act or function of breathing. **abdominal r.,** the use of the diaphragm and abdominal muscles in breathing. **anaerobic r., result,** if the availability of oxygen to the fetus is limited, with the production of lactic and pyruvic acids, and a fall in the pH value of fetal blood; this can be measured in labour once the cervix has dilated, by taking a microsample of blood from the fetal scalp. **paradoxical r.,** during inspiration air drawn into unaffected lung via normal route and from lung on affected side, during expiration air forced from lung on unaffected side, some of which enters lung on affected side, resulting in inadequate oxygenation of blood; occurs when ribs are fractured in two places. **periodic r., (Cheyne Stokes r.),** cyclical waxing and waning of respiration, characterized at the extremes by deep, fast breathing and by apnoea; it generally has an ominous prognosis. **tissue r.,** oxygen used by living cells to release the chemical energy that is stored in foodstuffs—respiratory, *adj.*

عمل تنفس: عمل تنفس سے مراد جاندار خلیوں کی تکسید ہے اور اس عمل سے توانائی حاصل ہوتی ہے۔ پودے ہوا کی آکسیجن استعمال کرتے ہیں اور بطور فاضل کاربن ڈائی آکسائیڈ چھوڑتے ہیں۔ تنفس کی دو اقسام ہیں: ہوائی تنفس اور غیر ہوائی تنفس۔ ہوائی تنفس آکسیجن کی موجودگی میں ہوتا ہے۔ ہوائی تنفس کو مندرجہ ذیل کیمیائی مساوات سے ظاہر کیا جا سکتا ہے:

گلوکوس + آکسیجن ← کاربن ڈائی آکسائیڈ + پانی + توانائی

غیر ہوائی تنفس میں آکسیجن کیمیائی طور پر کسی مرکب کے ساتھ نہیں ملتی۔ اس قسم کے تنفس میں گلائی کولی سس ہوتا ہے۔ یعنی پائیروک ایسڈ بنتا ہے۔ لیکن اس سے آگے کیمیائی عمل ہوائی تنفس سے مختلف ہو جاتا ہے۔ خمیر بہت سے سماروغ اور کچھ بڑے پودوں میں غیر ہوائی تنفس سے الکحل بنتا ہے۔ پائیروک ایسڈ سے کاربن ڈائی آکسائیڈ اور ایسٹلڈی ہائیڈ بنتے ہیں۔

پائیروک ایسڈ ← ایسیٹلڈی ہائیڈ + کاربن ڈائی آکسائیڈ

ایسٹلڈی ہائیڈ کی تخفیف ہو کر الکحل بنتا ہے۔ جیسا کہ خمیروں میں ہوتا ہے۔

$CH_3\ CHO + DN.\ H_2$

alcohol dehgodrogonose

ایسٹلڈی ہائڈ $CH_3\ CH_2OH + DN$

الکحل

غیر ہوائی تنفس میں خلیوں کو تھوڑی توانائی دستیاب ہوتی ہے۔ غیر ہوائی تنفس کو مندرجہ ذیل کیمیائی مساوات سے ظاہر کیا جا سکتا ہے۔

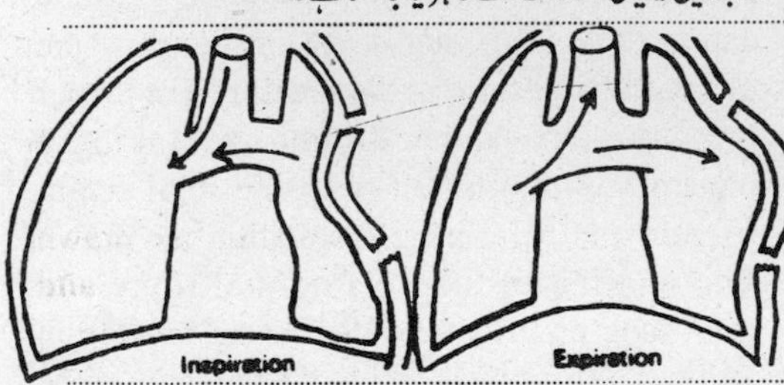

گلوکوس ← ایتھائل الکحل + کاربن ڈائی آکسائیڈ + ۱۲ کلوگرام کیلوریز

تنفس رنگ یا پگمنٹ: ایک شے جو خونی خلیوں یا خونی پلازما میں بنتی ہے جو آکسیجن کے ساتھ ملتی ہے اور دوبارہ آکسیجن سے علیحدہ ہو جاتی ہے، مثلاً ہیموگلوبین۔ سانس کی رفتار ۱۶ مرتبہ فی منٹ یعنی پھیپھڑے ۱۶ مرتبہ پھیلتے اور سکڑتے ہیں۔ ایک منٹ میں تقریباً ۵۰۰ سی سی خون پھیپھڑوں سے گزرتا ہے اور تقریباً ۴۰۰ سی سی آکسیجن گیس فی منٹ جذب ہوتی ہے اور ۳۲۰ سی سی کاربن ڈائی آکسائیڈ گیس فی منٹ خارج ہوتی ہے۔

Respirator *(res'-pi-ra-tor)* [L. *respirare,* to breathe again]. 1. An apparatus worn over the nose and mouth and designed to purify the air breathed through it. 2. An apparatus which artficially and rhythmically inflates and deflates the lungs as in normal breathing, when for any reason the natural nervous or muscular control of respiration is impaired. The apparatus may work on either positive or negative pressure or on electrical stimulation. **pump r.,** heart-lung machine by which the blood can be removed from a vein for oxygenation, after which it is returned to the vein.

آلہ تنفس: (۱) ایسا سامان جسے ناک اور منہ پر پہن لیتے ہیں اور اس میں سے ہوا صاف ہو کر سانس میں جاتی ہے۔

(۲) آلہ جو پھیپھڑوں کو مصنوعی طور پر پھیلاتا ہے جیسا کہ نارمل تنفس میں ہوتے ہے۔

Respiratory distress syndrome Dyspnoea in the newly born. Due to failure of secretion of protein-lipid complex (pulmonary surfactant) by type II pneumocytes in the tiny air spaces of the lung on first entry of air. Causes atelectasis. Formerly called hyaline membrane disease. Environmental temperature of 32-34° C (90-94 F), oxygen and infusion of sodium bicarbonate are used in treatment. Clinical features include severe retraction of chest wall with every breath, cyanosis, an increased respiratory rate and an expiratory grunt.

تنفسی تکلیف سنڈروم: نوزائیدہ بچے کا سنڈروم۔ علاج میں بیرونی درجہ حرارت ۳۲ تا ۳۴° س۔ آکسیجن اور سوڈیم بائی کاربونیٹ کا دخول شامل ہے۔

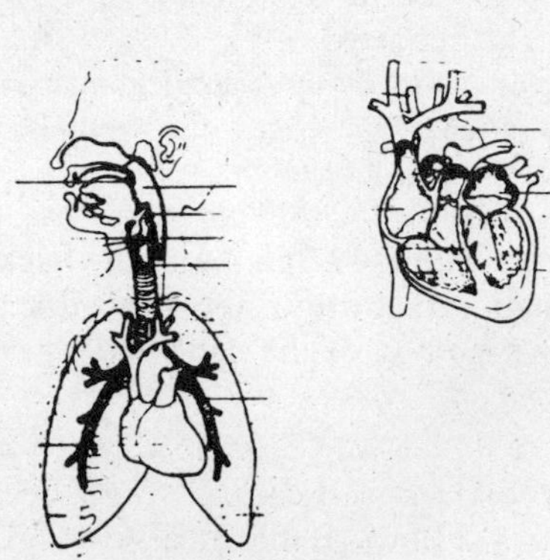

(respiratory & circulatory system)

Respiratory failure A term used to denote failure of the lungs to oxygenate the blood adequately. **acute r.f.** denotes respiratory insufficiency secondary to an acute insult to the lung; hypoxaemia develops, frequently terminating in bronchopneumonia. **acute-on-chronic r.f.,** hypoxaemia resulting from chronic obstructive airways disease such as chronic bronchitis and emphysema.

Respiratory syncytial virus Causes severe respiratory infection with occasional fatalities in very young children. Infections are less severe in old children.

ریسپی ریٹری سن سٹیل وائرس: بالائی وزیریں دونوں تنفسی امراض کا ذمہ دار۔

Responaut Person with permanent severe respiratory paralysis needing a mechanical device.

ریسپونانٹ: شخص جسے مستقل سخت تنفسی تکلیف ہو، اسے میکانکی طریق

چاہئے۔

Resuscitation *(re-sus'-i-ta-shun)* [L. *resuscitare,* to revive]. Restoration to life of one who is apparently dead (collapsed or shocked). See CARDIAC. **expired air r.,** See KISS OF LIFE — resuscitatioin, *n.*; resuscitative, *adj.*

اِحیا، ہوش میں لانا، بحالیٔ زندگی: جو بظاہر جو مر گیا ہو، اسے دوبارہ زندگی مل جانا۔

Retching Straining at vomiting.

ابکائی: قے کے وقت زور لگانا۔

Retention *(re-ten'-shun)* [L. *retinere,* to hold back]. 1. Retaining of facts in the mind. 2. Accumulation of that which is normally excreted. **retention of urine,** accumulation of urine within the bladder due to interference of nerve supply, obstruction or psychological factors.

حبس، حبس البول: (۱) ذہن میں حقائق محفوظ رکھنا۔

(۲) نارمل طور پر اخراج ہونے والے کو جمع کر کے رکھنا۔ پیشاب کا رک جانا۔

Reticular *(re-tik'-u-lar)* [L. *reticulum,* little net]. Resembling a net.

شبکی، خلوی: جال سے مشابہ۔

Reticulacyte *(ret-ik-u-lo-sit)* [L. *reticulum,* little net; G. *kytos,* cell]. A young circulating red blood cell which still contains traces of the nucleus which was present inthe cell when developing in the bone marrow.

شبکہ خلیہ: ایک نوعمر گردشی سرخ خونی خلیہ جس میں اس مرکزہ کے باقیات ہوں، جو ہڈی کے گودے میں بننے والے خلیے میں موجود تھا۔

Reticulocytoma See EWING'S TUMOUR.

رٹیکولوسائیڈو: ایونگ کی رسولی۔

Reticulocytosis *(ret-ik-u-lo-si-to'-sis)* [L. *reticulum,* little net; G. *kytos,* cell; *-osis,* condition]. An increase in the number of reticulocytes in the blood indicating active red blood cell formation inthe marrow.

شبکہ خلویت: جانبی خون میں رٹیکولوسائیٹس کی زیادتی۔

Reticuloendothelial system *(ret-ik-u-ol-end-oth-e-li-al)* A widely scattered system of cells, of common ancestry and fulfilling many vital functions, e.g. defence against infection, antibody, blood cell and bile pigment formation, etc. Main sites of r.e. cells are bone marrow, spleen, liver and lymphoid tissue.

رٹیکولوانیڈو تھیلیل نظام: خلیوں کا منتشر سلسلہ جو جاندار ٹیکہ لگانے سے رنگ پکڑنے کی خصوصیت رکھتا ہے۔ وہ گردش میں جراثیم اور دوسرے بیرونی اجسام کو بھی لیتے ہیں۔

Reticulosis *(ret-ik-u-lo'-sis)* [L. *reticulum,* little net; G. *-osis,* condition]. Term loosely used to describe conditions in which there is a reaction of reticuloendothelial cells. **malignant r.,** neoplastic disorder affecting the reticuloendothelial system; now called malignant lymphoma—reticuloses, *pl.*

رٹیکولوسیس: رٹیکولوانڈو تھیلیل نظام کا مرض۔

Retina *(ret'-i-na)* [L. *rete,* net]. The light sensitive internal coat of the eyeball, consisting of eight superimposed layers, seven of which are nervous and one pigmented. It is soft in consistency, translucent and of a pinkish colour —retinal, *adj.*

شبکیہ، پردۂ چشم، پردۂ شبکیہ: آنکھ کے گولے کا اندرونی کوٹ جو روشنی کے لئے حساس ہوتا ہے۔ یہ نیم شفاف اور گلابی رنگت کا ہوتا ہے۔

Retinitis *(ret-in-i-tis)* [L. *rete,* net; G. *-itis,* inflammation]. Inflammation of the retina. **retinitis pigmentosa,** a familial, degenerative condition which progresses to blindness.

سوزش شبکیہ: ریٹنا کی سوزش۔

Retinoblastoma *(re-in-o-blas-to'-ma)* [L. *rete,* net; G. *blastos,* shoot; *-oma,* tumour]. A malignant tumour of the neuroglial element of the retina, occurring exclusively in children.

قرصہ چشم: ریٹنا کی ایک رسولی جو زیادہ تر بچوں میں ہوتی ہے۔

Retinopathy *(ret-in-op-ath-i)* [L. *rete,* net; G. *pathos,* disease]. Any non-inflammatory disease of the retina.

ریٹنو پیتھی: ریٹنا کا غیر سوزش مرض۔

Retinoscope *(ret-in-o-skop)* [L. *rete,* net; G. *skopein,* to examine]. Instrument for detection of refractive errors by illumination of retina using a mirror.

شبکیہ بین: آئینہ کے استعمال سے ریٹنا روشن کرنے سے انعطافی غلطیوں کا تعین کرنے کے لئے آلہ۔

Retinotoxic *(ret-in-o-toks-ik)* Usually applied to drugs which may damage the retina in some instances.

Retractile *(re-trak-til)* Capable of being drawn back, i.e. retracted.

Retractor *(re-trak-tor)* A surgical instrument for holding apart the edges of a wound to reveal underlying structures.

Retrobulbar *(ret-ro-bul-bar)* [L. *retro,* behind; *bulbus,* bulb]. Pertaining to the back of the eyeball. **retrobulbar neuritis,** inflammation of that portion of the optic nerve behind the eyeball.

عقب مقلہ: آنکھ کے گولے کی پشت سے متعلق۔

Retrocaecal *(re-tro-sek-al)* [L. *retro,* behind; *coecus,* blind]. Behind the caecum, e.g. a retrocaecal appendix.

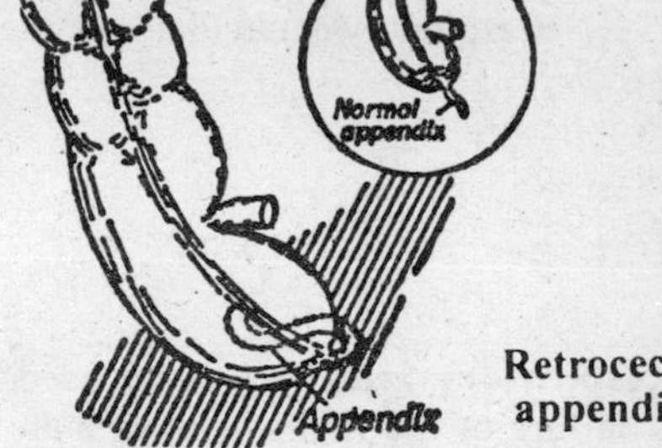

Retrocecal appendix

پس اعوری: سیکم کے پیچھے۔

Retroflexion *(ret-ro-flek-shun)* The state of being bent backwards. Opp., anteflexion.

پشت کوزی: پچھلی طرف مڑنے کی حالت۔ دوہرا ہونا۔ اندرونی معائنہ میں بچے دانی یا یوٹرس کی پوزیشن اس طرح دیکھی جا سکتی ہے۔

Retrograde *(ret-ro-grad)* [L. *retrogradi,* to go backward]. Goind backward. **retrograde pyelography** (q.v.).

پس خرام: پچھلی جانب جانا۔

Retrogression *(ret-ro-gresh-un)* See REGRESSION.

انحطاط: ریگریشن۔

Retrolental fibroplasia *(ret-ro-len-tal fi-bro plaz-i-a)* [L. *retro,* behind; *lens,* lentil, *fibra* fibre; G. *plassein,* to form]. The presence of fibrous tissue in the vitreous, from the retina to the lens, causing blindness. Noticed shortly after birth, more commonly in premature babies who have had continuous oxygen therapy.

ریٹرولینٹل فائبرو پلاسیا: ویٹریئس میں، ریٹنا سے عدسہ تک، ریشہ دار نسیج کی موجودگی جس سے اندھاپن ہوتا ہے۔

Retro-ocular *(ret-ro-ok-u-lar)* [L. *retro*, behind; *oculus*, eye]. Behind the eye.

پس چشمہ: آنکھ کے پیچھے۔

Retroperitoneal *(re-tro-pe-ri-ton-e-al)* [L. *retro*, behind; G. *peri*, around; *teinein*, to stretch]. Behind the peritoneum.

پس ثربہ: پیریٹونیم کے پیچھے۔

Retropharyngeal *(re-tro-far-in-je-al)* [L. *retro*, behind; G. *phayngx*, pharynx]. Behind the pharynx.

پس بلعومہ: فیرنکس کے پیچھے۔

Retroplacental *(re-tro-pla-se-tal)* [L. *retro*, behind; *placenta*, a cake]. Behind the placenta.

ریٹروپلیسنٹل: پلیسنٹا کے پیچھے۔

Retropleural *(re-tro-plu-ral)* [L. *retro*, behind; G. *pleuro*, rib]. Behind the pleura.

ریٹروپلیورل: پلیورل کے پیچھے۔

Retropubic *(ret-ro-pu-bik)* [L. *retro*, behind; *pubes*, the private parts]. Behind the pubis.

پس عانی: پوبس کے پیچھے۔

Retrospection *(ret-ro-spek-shun)* Morbid dwelling on the past.

Retrosternal *(ret-ro-ster'-nal)* [L. *retro*, behind; G. *sternon*, breast]. Behind the breast bone.

پس قصہ: چھاتی کی ہڈی کے پیچھے۔

Retrotracheal *(ret-ro-trak-e'-al)* [L. *retro*, behind; G. *trachus*, rough]. Behind the trachea.

وراء الجب: ٹریکیا کے پیچھے۔

Retroversion *(ret-ro-ver-shun)* [L. *retro*, behind; G. *vertere*, to turn]. Turning backward. **retroversion of the uterus,** tilting of the whole of the uterus backward with the cervix pointing forward—retroverted, *adj.*

میلانِ خلفی: پچھلی جانب مڑنا۔ اندرونی معائنہ میں بچے دانی یا یوٹرس کی پوزیشن آگے یا پیچھے جھکاؤ کو ظاہر کرتی ہے۔

Revascularization *(re-vas-kul-ar-iz-a-shun)* [L. *re*, again; *vasculum*, small vessel]. The regrowth of blood vessel into a tissue or organ after deprivation of its normal blood supply.

ری واسکولیرائزیشن: نارمل خونی سپلائی کی محرومیت کے بعد عضو یا نسیج میں خونی رگ کی دوبارہ نمو۔

Reverin *(rev'-er-in)* Broad spectrum antibiotic of the tetracyline series. Of good local and general tolerance.

ریورِن: ٹیٹرا سائیکلین سلسلے کے چوڑے طیف والی اینٹی بائیوٹک۔

Reverse barrier nursing Every attempt is made to prevent carrying infection to the patient. Used for agranulocytosis and immunosuppressive treatment.

ریورس باریر نرسنگ: کوشش کی جاتی ہے مریض کو انفیکشن نہ ہو۔ علاج کے لئے مستقل۔

Rh. Rhesus factor See BLOODGROUPS.

Rhagades *(rag'-a-dez)* [G. *rhagas*, fissure]. Sup- erficial elongated scars radiating from the nostrils or angles of the mouth and which are pathognomonic or congenital syphilis. See STIGMATA.

بوائی: نتھنوں اور منہ کے زاویوں سے باہر آتے ہوئے مصنوعی لمبے نشان۔

Rhei *(re'-i)* Genitive of Rheum, *i.e.* rhubarb (q.v.).

رئیم آفیسینیلے کی خشک جڑ

Rheomacrodex *(re-o-mak'-ro-deks)* A low molecular weight dextran (q.v.). Antithrombotic. Used to prevent clots in grafted vein.

ریومیکروڈیکس: کمسالمی وزن والا ڈیکسٹران۔

Rhesus factor See BLOODGROUPS.

بندری جز: خون کے ذرّات میں پیدا ہونے والے ذرّات جو آر، ایچ مثبت و منفی ہوتے ہیں۔

Rheumatic *(roo-mat'-ik)* [G. *rheumatikos*, subject to a flux]. Pertaining to rheumatism. See CHOREA.

گھٹیا زدہ: جوڑوں کے درد سے متعلق۔

Rheumatism *(roo'-mat-izm)* [G. *rheumatismos*, that which flows] A non-specific term embracing a diverse group of diseases and syndromes which have in common, disorder or diseases of connective tissue and hence usually present with pain, or stiffness, or swelling of muscles and joints. The main groups are rheumatic fever, rheumatoid arthritis, ankylosing spondylitis, non-articular rheumatis, osteoarthritis and gout, **acute r.** (rheumatic fever), a disorder tending to recur but initially commonest in childhood, classically presenting as fleeting polyarthritis of the larger joints, pyrexia and carditis within 3 weeks following a streptococcal throat infection. Atypically , but not infrequently, the symptoms are trivial and ignored, but carditis may be severe and result in permanent cardiac damage. **non-articular r.,** involves the soft tissues and includes fibrositis, lumbago, etc.

گٹھیا، جوڑوں کا درد: ایک غیر مخصوص اصطلاح جو کئی مختلف امراض کو ظاہر کرتی ہے۔ اس میں سنڈروم رابطی نسیج کی خرابی وغیرہ ہیں۔ عام طور پر عضلات اور جوڑوں میں درد، سختی اور ورم ہوتے ہیں۔

Rheumatoid *(roo'-mat-oid)* [G. *rheuma,* stream; *eidos,* form]. Resembling rheumatism, **rheumatoid arthritis,** a disease of unknown aetiology, characterized by a chronic polyarthritis mainly affecting the smaller peripheral joints, accompanied by general ill health and resulting eventually in varying degrees of crippling joint deformities and associated muscle wasting. It is not just a disease of joints. Every system may be involved in some way. Many rheumatologists therefore prefer the term 'rheumatoid disease'. There is some question of it being an autoimmune process. **rheumatoid factors,** macro gammaglobulins found in most people with severe r. arthritis. They affect not oonly joints but lung and nerve tissues and small arteries. It is not yet known whether they are the cause of, or the result of, arthritis. See PNEUMOCONIOSIS and STILL'S DISEASE.

گٹھیا نما: ریومانزم سے مشابہ۔

Rheumatology *(roo-mat-ol-o-ji)* [G. *rheumatikos,* subject to a flux; *logos,* discourse]. Th science or the study of rheumatic disease.

یومیٹرولوجی: ریومیٹک مرض کا مطالعہ یا سائنس۔

Rhinitis *(ri-ni-tis)* [G. *rhis,* nose; *-itis,* inflammation]. Inflammation of the nasal mucou membrane.

ک کی سوزش: نتھنوں کی میوکس جھلی کی سوزش۔

Rhynology *(rin-ol-o-ji)* [G. *rhis,* nose; *logos* discourse]. The study of disease affecting th nose—rhynologist, *n.*

م امراض ناک: ناک کو متاثر کرنے والے امراض کا مطالعہ۔

Rhinophyma *(ri-no-fi-ma)* [G. *rhis,* nose *phyma,* tumour]. Nodular enlargement of ski of nose.

ک کی رسولی: ناک کی جلد کا نوڈولر بڑھاؤ۔

Rhinoplasty *(ri-no-plas-ti)* [G. *rhis,* nose; *plassein,* to form]. Plastic surgery of the nose.

ک پیوندی: ناک کی پلاسٹک سرجری۔

Rhinorrhoea *(rin-or-e-a)* [G. *rhis,* nose; *rheein,* to flow]. Nasal discharge.

ک بہنا: ناک کا ڈسچارج یا بہاؤ۔ ناک سے رطوبت گرنا۔

Rhinoscopy *(rin-os-kop-i)* Inspection of th nose using an instrument, a nasal speculum a rhinoscope.

Rhinosporidosis *(ri-no-spor-i-do-sis)* A fung condition affectin the mucosa of the nos eyes, ears, larynx and occasionally the genitalia; characterized by persistent polypi.

ینوسپوریڈوسس: ایک سماروغی حالت۔ جو ناک، آنکھوں، کانوں، س اور بعض دفعہ تولیدی اعضاء کے میوکوسا کو متاثر کرتی ہے۔

Rhinosporidium *(ri-no-spor-id-i-um)* [G. *rhi* nose; *spora,* seed] A genus of fungi, parasit to man.

ینوسپوریڈیم: سماروغ کا ایک جنس جو آدمی پر طفیلی ہے۔

Rhinovirus *(ri-no-vi-rus)* There are about 1 different varieties which can cause the com on cold.

نو وائرس: تقریباً ۵۰ مختلف اقسام زکام پیدا کرتے ہیں۔

Rhizotomy *(ri-zot-o-mi)* [G. *rhiza,* root; *tome,* cutting]. Surgical division of a root; usual the posterior root of a spinal nerve. **chemic r.,** accomplished by injection of a chemic often phenol.

بیج اندوزی: جڑ کی سرجیکل تقسیم۔عموماً سپائنل عصب کی خلقی جڑ۔

hodopsin *(ro-dop-sin)* [G. *rhodon,* rose; *opsis,* vision]. The visual purple contained in the retinal rods. Its colour is preserved in darkness; bleached by daylight. Its formation is dependent on vitamin A.

بصری ارغوان: بصری اُودا رنگ جو ریٹنی سلاخوں میں ہوتا ہے۔اس کا رنگ اندھیرے میں محفوظ ہوتا ہے۔دن کی روشنی میں ختم ہو جاتا ہے۔اس کے بننے کا انحصار حیاتین الف پر ہے۔

homboid *(rom-boid)* [G. *rhombos,* magic wheel; *eidos,* form]. Diamond shaped.

معین نما: ہیرے کی شکل کا۔

honchus *(rong-kus)* [G. *rhogchos,* wheezing]. An adventitious sound heard on auscultation of the lung. Passage of air through bronchi obstructed by oedema or exudate produces a musical note. See SIBILUS.

خس خس: پھیپھڑے کی اتفاقیہ سنی گئی آواز۔

hubarb *(roo-barb)* The dried root Chinese Rheum officinale. It is purgative in large doses, astringent in small doses. Used in mist gent c rhei, etc.

ریوند: ریئم آفیسینیلے کی جڑ۔زیادہ خوراکوں میں دست آور۔

iboflavine *(ri-bo-fla-ven)* A constituent of the vitamin B group. Given in Meniere's disease, angular stomatitis and a variety of other conditions.

وٹامن ب، رائبوفلیون: لیکٹو فلیون۔حیاتین ب۲۔ پانی میں حل پذیر مرکب جو حیاتین بی کمپلیکس کا رکن ہے۔یہ مختلف خامرات کا حصہ ہوتا ہے جن کا تعلق خلوی تنفس کے ساتھ ہوتا ہے۔نوعمری میں نشوونما میں مدد دیتا ہے اور جلدی صحت میں اہم کردار ادا کرتا ہے۔اسے حیاتین جی بھی کہا جاتا ہے۔

ibonuclease *(ri-bo-nu'-kle-az)* Enzyme that breaks down ribonucleic acid. Has been made synthetically.

رائبو نیوکلی ایز: ایک خامرہ جو رائبو نیوکلیک ایسڈ کی آب پاشیدگی کی عمل انگیزی کرتا ہے۔

ibonucleic acid RNA. See DEOXYRIBONUCLEIC ACID.

رائبو نیوکلیک ایسڈ: نیوکلیک ایسڈ کی ایک قسم۔اسے مختصراً آر۔این۔اے لکھا جاتا ہے۔اس میں ریبوز، شکر، فاسفیٹ، ایڈنین، گوانین سائٹوسین اور یوریسل ہوتے ہیں۔ڈی این اے سے موصولہ اطلاعات یا ہدایات پیغامبر آر۔این۔اے کے ذریعے سائٹو پلازم میں جاتی ہیں اور ٹرانسفر آر۔این۔اے سائٹو پلازم سے امینو ایسڈز کو اکٹھا کرتا ہے۔

Ribosomes *(ri'-bo-somz)* Submicroscopic protein-making agents inside all cells.

Ribs The twelve pairs of bones which articulate with the twelve dorsal vertebrae posteriorly and form the walls of the thorax. The upper seven pairs are **true r.** and are attached to the sternum anteriorly by costal cartilage. The remaining five pairs are the **falser r.** The first three pairs of these do not have an attachment to the sternum but are bound to each other by costal cartilage. The lower two pairs are the **floating r.** which have no anterior articulation. **cervical r.** are formed by an extension of the transverse process of the seventh cervical vertebra in the form of bone or a fibrous tissue band; this causes an upward displacement of the subclavian artery. A congenital abnormality.

پسلیاں، اضلاع: ہڈیوں کے ۱۲ جوڑے۔ بالائی سات جوڑے اصلی پسلیاں ہیں جو اگلی طرف سے سٹرنم کے ساتھ ملحق ہوتی ہیں۔بقایا پانچ جوڑے کاذب پسلیاں ہوتی ہیں۔جن میں سے پہلے تین جوڑے سٹرنم کے ساتھ ملحق ہوتے نہیں بلکہ آپس میں جڑے ہوتے ہیں۔زیریں دو جوڑے آزاد ہوتے ہیں۔

Rice-water stool The stool of cholera. The 'rice grains' are small pieces of desquamated epithelium from the intestine.

اسہال: ہیضہ کا براز۔

Rickets *(ri'-kets)* A disorder of calcium and phosphorus metabolism associated with a deficiency of vitamin D, and beginning most often in infancy and early childhood between the ages of 6 months and 2 years. There is proliferation and deficient ossification of the growing epiphyses of bones, producing 'bossing', softening and bending of the long weight-bearing bones, muscular hypotonia, head sweating and, if the blood calcium falls sufficiently, tetany. **fetal r.,** See ACHONDROPLASIA. **renal r.,** a condition of decalcification (osteoporosis) of bones associated with chronic kidney disease and clinically simulating rickets, occurs in later age groups and is characterized by excessive urinary calcium loss. **vitamin D resistant r.**, due to disease of the lower extremities producing short legs. Genetic illness. No deficiency of vitamin D, Serum levels of phosphorus low. No associated renal disease. Thought to be due to a defect in the tubular re-absorption of phosphorus and a lowered calcium absorption from the gut causing secondary hyperthyroidism and a vitamin D abnormality.

سوکھا: وٹامن ڈی کی کمی کے ساتھ کیلشیم اور فاسفورس میٹابولزم کی خرابی۔ دو سال تک کی عمر کے بچوں میں یہ مرض ہوتا ہے۔

Rickettsia *(ri'-ket-si-aa)* Small pleomorphic parasitic micro-organisms which have their natural habitat in the cells of the gut of arthropods. Some are pathogenic to mammals and man, in whom they cause the typhus group of fevers. They are smaller in size than bacteria and larger than the viruses. Many of their physiological characters resemble the bacteria, but like the viruses they are obligate intracellular parasites. [Howard Taylor Ricketts, American pathologist. 1871-1910].

رکٹسیہ: چھوٹے پلیومورفک جیسے جو طفیلی ہوتے ہیں اور آرتھروپوڈز کی گٹ کے خلیوں میں قدرتی طور پر رہتے ہیں۔ بعض ممالیہ جانوروں اور آدمی میں امراض پیدا کرتے ہیں۔ گرام منفی، غیر متحرک سائز ۵،۰×۳،۰، ٹائیفس بخار، ٹرنچ بخار کیو بخار وغیرہ کے ذمہ دار۔ علاج کے لئے کلوریم فینی کال اور ٹیٹرا سائیکلین آزمائیے۔

Rickety rosary. Series of protuberances (bossing) at junction of ribs and costal cartilages in children suffering from rickets.

رکٹی روزری: رکیٹس کے بیمار بچوں میں پسلیوں اور کوسٹل کارٹیلجز کے جنکشن پر ابھاروں کا سلسلہ۔

Rider's bone. A bony mass in the adductor muscles of the thigh, from repeated minor trauma in horse-riding.

عظم الراکب: ران کے ایڈکٹر عضلات میں انخوانی مادہ۔

Rifadin *(ri-fa'-din)*. Rifampicin (q.v.)

ریفاڈین: ریفامپسن ادویہ سے مزاحمتی تپ دق کے علاج کے لیے ثانوی

ٹی بایوٹک دوا۔ اکثر جراثیم اور گرام مثبت کاکسی کے لیے عامل۔

Rifaldazine *(rif-al'-daz-en)*. Main indication as a secondary drug in treating drug resista tuberculosis.

یفلڈازین: تپ دق جس میں ادویہ سے مدافعت پائی جائے کے علاج ے لیے ایک ثانوی دوائی۔

Rifamycin *(ri-fa-mi'-sin)*. Antibiotic. For Streptomyces group of organisms. Useful resistant tuberculosis; also effective staphylococcal infections. Some of the drug excreted in tears and it has some antivir properties.

یفامائی سین: اینٹی بایوٹک۔ جسیموں کے سٹرپٹو مائی سیز کے گروہ سے۔ متی یا مزاحمتی تپ دق میں مفید۔ سٹیفائلوکاکسی سے پیدا شدہ امراض میں بھی ژ۔ کچھ دوا آنسوؤں میں باہر نکلتی ہے جس میں اینٹی وائرل خصوصیات ہیں۔

Rifampicin *(ri-fam'-pi-sin)*. Antibiotic. Ma indication is as a secondary drug in treati drug-resistant tuberculosis. Bacteriostati Active against a wide range of bacteria a Gram-positive cocci. *Mycobacteriu tuberculosis*, but with limited action again Gram-negative bacteria. Useful for lepros

یمپسین: اینٹی بایوٹک۔ ادویہ سے مزاحمتی تپ دق کے علاج کے لئے وی دوا۔ اکثر جراثیم گرام مثبت کاکسی کے خلاف عامل۔

Rigor *(ri'-gor)* [L. stiffness]. A sudden chi accompanied by severe shivering. The bo temperature rises rapidly and remains hi until perspiration ensues and causes a grad fall in temperature. **rigor mortis** t stiffening of the body after death.

رہ تپ: سردی سے ٹھٹھرنے کے ساتھ اچانک لرزہ جسمانی درجہ حرارت ت زیادہ ہو جاتا ہے۔ پھر پسینہ آ کر درجہ حرارت میں کمی ہوتی ہے۔

RIHSA. Radio-iodinated human serum album (q.v.)

آئی ایچ ایس اے: ریڈیو آیوڈینیٹڈ ہوین سیرم البومن

Rimactane *(ri-mak'-tan)*. Rifampicin (q.v.)

یکٹین: ریفامپسین۔ ادویہ سے مزاحمتی تپ دق کے علاج کے لیے ثانوی بایوٹک دوا اکثر جراثیموں اور گرام مثبت کاکسی کے لئے عامل۔

Rimifon *(ri'-mi-fon)*. Isoniazid (q.v.)

فون: آئیسونیازوڈ۔

Ringworm generic term used to describe contagious infection of the skin by a fungus, because the common manifestations are circular (circinate) scaly patches. See also TINEA and MYCOSIS.

داود هدر: سماروغی جلدی مرض بیان کرنے کے لیے مستعمل اصطلاح۔ موسم برسات یا زیادہ پسینے والے موسم میں ہوتا ہے کشمیر میں زیادہ ہوتا ہے۔

Risus sardonicus *(ri'-sus-don'-ik-us)*. The spastic grin of tetanus (q.v.).

تبسم تشنج: تشنج کا سپاسٹک گرن۔

Ritalin. Methyl phenidate (q.v.)

ریٹالین: میتھائل فینیڈیٹ۔

River blindness A form of onchocerciasis (q.v.)

دریائی اندھاپن: انکوسرسیاسس کی ایک قسم۔

RNA. Ribonucleic acid (q.v.)

آر این اے۔ رن (: نکلیک ایسڈ کی ایک قسم۔ اس میں ریبوز' شکر' فاسفیٹ ایڈنین' گوانین' سائٹوسین اور یوریسل ہوتے ہیں' ڈی' این' اے سے موصولہ ہدایات پیغامبر آر این اے کے ذریعہ سائٹو پلازم میں جاتی ہیں۔ اور ٹرانسفر آر این اے سے آمینو ایسڈ کو اکھٹا کرتا ہے۔

Robert Jones's' abduction frame A metal frame with a leather saddle used to treat hip disease. [Sir Robert Jones, English orthopaedic surgeon, 1858-1933]

رابرٹ جونز ایڈکشن فریم: ہپ مرض کے علاج کے لئے مستعمل چمڑے کی زین کے ساتھ ایک دھاتی فریم۔

Rondomycin *(ron-do-mi'-sin)*. Methacycline (q.v.)

رونڈومائی سین: میتھا سائیکلین۔ ٹیٹرا سائیکلین کے اثر والے کیپسول۔

Roentgen or Rontgen *(ront'-gen)* rays. X-rays. [Wilhelm Konrad von Rontgen, German physicist, 1845-1923.]

لاشعاعیں۔ اشعہ رانجن: ایکس ریز

Rogitine *(rog'-i-ten)*. Phentolamine (q.v.)

روجی ٹین: فینٹول امین

Romberg's sign. A sign of ataxia (q.v.). Inability to stand erect (without swaying) when the eyes are closed and the feet together. Also called 'Romergism. [Moritz Romberg, German neurologist, 1795-1873].

علامت رومبرگ: اٹیکسیا کا نشان۔ جب پاؤں اکھٹے اور آنکھیں بند ہوں تو سیدھا کھڑا نہیں ہوا جاتا۔

Rondomycine *(ron-do-mi-sen)* Mathacycline (q.v.).

رونڈومائی سین: میتھا سائیکلین۔ اس کے دو کیپسول صبح، دو شام برائے یرقان، زکام۔

Ronicol *(ron'-i-kol)* Nicotynyl alcohol (q.v.).

رانی کول: نکوٹینائل الکحل۔

Rosacea *(ro-za'-se-a)* A skin disease which shows on flush areas of the face, especially in women at menopause. In areas affected there is chronic dilation of superficial capillaries and hypertrophy of sebaceous follicles, often complicated by an acneiform eruption.

بادشنام، کلابیہ، ورد یہ: ایک جلدی مرض جو خصوصاً خواتین میں مینوپاز پر چہرے کے سرخ ایریا میں دکھائی دیتا ہے۔

Rose bengal *(roz-ben'-gal)* A straining agent used to detect threads of mucus in the eye afflicted with keratoconjunctivitis.

Roseola *(ro-ze-o'-la)* The earliest manifestation of secondary syphilis (q.v.). This syphilide is a faint, pink spot, widespread in distribution except for the skin over the hands and face.

سرخ بادہ: ثانوی آتشک۔ آبلہ فرنگ۔

Rotaviruses Viruses associated with gastroenteritis in children and infants. Related to, but easily disinguished from reoviruses.

Rotator *(ro-ta'-tor)* [L. *rotare,* to turn round]. A muscle having the action of turning a part.

عضلۂ دوار: کسی حصے کو موڑنے کا عمل کرنے والا عضلہ۔

Roth spots Round white spots in the retina in some cases of bacterial endocarditis; thought to be of embolic origin. [Moritz Roth, Swiss physician and pathologist, 1839-1915].

Roughage *(ruf'-aj)* Coarse food containing much indigestible vegetable. fibre, composed of cellulose. It provides bulk in the diet and by this means helps to stimulate peristalsis and eliminate waste products. Lack of r. may cause atonic constipation. Too much r. may cause spastic constipation.

موٹا جھوٹا چارہ: سیلولوز پر مشتمل ہضم نہ ہونے والے نباتاتی ریشہ کی خوراک۔

Rouleaux *(roo'-lo)* [F.]. A row of red blood cells, resembling a roll of coins.

انبار جسیماتِ خون: سکوں کے رول سے مشابہ، سرخ خونی خلیوں کی قطار۔

Roundworm *(Ascaris lumbricoides)* Look like earth worms. Worldwide distribution. Parasitic to man. Eggs passed in stools; ingested; hatch in bowel, migrate through tissues, lungs and bronchi before returning to the bowel as mature worms. During migration worms can be coughed up—which is unpleasant and frightening. Heavy infections can produce pneumonia. A tangled mass can cause intestinal obstruction or appendicitis. The best drug for treatment is piperazine. Roundworm of the cat and dog is called Toxocara.

حیہ، کلپ: اسکیرس لمبریکائیڈز۔ یہ کیچوؤں کی طرح نظر آتے ہیں۔ دنیا بھر میں پائے جاتے ہیں۔ آدمی پر طفیلی شکل میں گول اور لمبے۔ مادہ نر سے لمبی ہوتی ہے۔ عموماً لمبائی ۶ تا ۱۰ انچ۔ علاج کے لئے اینٹی سپار کا شربت سوتے وقت ایک اونس پی لیا جائے یا ایک اونس پیرازین شربت ایک دفعہ سوتے وقت۔

Rous sarcoma virus (RSV). A virus of chickens which can cause tumours (sarcomas). A typical member of the RNA tumour virus group; despite much research no viruses belonging to this group have as yet been isolated from human tumours.

آر۔ایس۔وی: اس سے پیشتر کہ یہ پروٹین بنانے اور تولید کے قابل ہو، آر۔اے۔وی کی موجودگی ضروری ہے۔

Roux-en-Y operation. Originally the distal end of divided ieiunum was anastomosed to the stomach, and the proximal jejunum containing the duodenal and pancreatic juices was anastomosed to the jejunum about 76.2 mm below the first anastomosis. The term is used to include joining of the distal jejunum to a divided bile duct, oesophagus or pancreas, in majorr surgery of these structures. [Cesar Roux, Swiss surgeon, 1857-1926].

رُواین وائی اپریشن: ڈسٹل جیجونم کو منقسم بائل ڈکٹ، ایسوفیگس یا لبلبہ کے ساتھ ملانا۔

Rovsing's sign. Pressure in the left iliac fossa causes pain in the right iliac fossa in appendicitis. [Niels Thorkild Rovsing, Danish surgeon 1862-1927].

علامت راوُ سنگ: اپنڈیسائیٹس میں بایاں الیائک فوسا میں دباؤ دائیں الیائک فوسا میں درد پیدا کرتا ہے۔

RPCF. Reiter protein complement fixation.

آر پی سی ایف: ریٹر پروٹین کمپلیمنٹ فکسیشن۔

RSV. 1. Respiratory syncytial virus (q.v.). 2. Rous sarcoma virus (q.v.).

آر ایس وی: (۱) پروٹین بنانے اور تولید کے قابل ہونے سے پہلے آر اے وی کی موجودگی لازمی ہے۔

(۲) دونوں زیریں و بالائی تنفسی امراض کا ذمہ دار۔

Rubefacients *(roo-bi-fa-shents)* [L. *ruberfacere*, to make red]. Substances which, when applied to the skin, cause redness (hyperaemia).

محمر، حمرت آور: اشیا جو جلد پر لگانے سے سرخی پیدا کرتی ہیں۔

Rubella *(roo-bel'-a)* [L. *rubellus*, red-dish]. Syn. German measles. An acute, infectious, eruptive fever (exanthema) caused by a virus and spread by droplet infection. There is pyrexia, coryza, conjunctivitis, a pink rash, enlarged occipital and posterior cervical glands. Complications are rare, except when contracted in the first three months of pregnancy it may produce fetal deformities. See HPV-77.

خسرۂ کاذب: جرمن خسرہ۔ وائرس سے پیدا شدہ بخار۔

Rubidomycin *(roo-bid-o-mi'-sin)* Daunorubicin (q.v.).

ربیڈومائی سن: ڈانوروبیسن۔

Rugae *(roo'-je)* [L.]. Wrinkles, corrugations, folds, often of an impermanent nature and allowing for distension.

Ruge of stomach

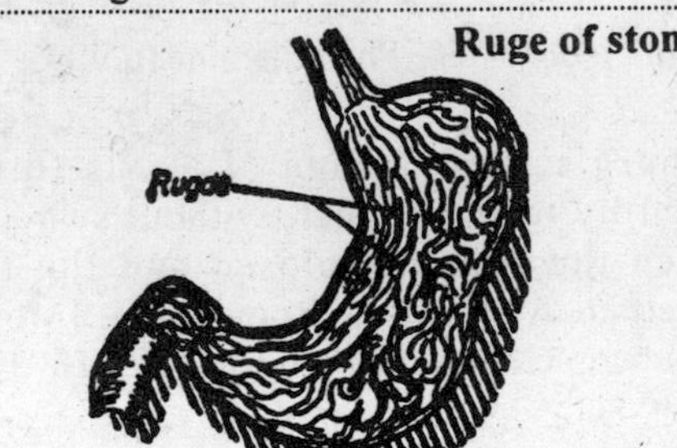

شکن غشا مخاطی: جھریاں، سلوٹیں۔

Rupia *(roo-pe-a)* [G. *rhypos,* filth]. Stuck-on crusts which look like limpets. Rupial syphilide, a late manifestation of secondary syphilis.

کھرنڈ: آتشکی دانے۔

Rapture *(rup-tur)* [L. *ruptura,* a break]. Tearing, splitting, bursting of a part. A popular name for hernia (q.v.).

فتق، شقاق: پھٹنا۔ کسی حصے کا پھٹ جانا۔ ہرنیا کا مشہور نام۔

Russell traction. Weighted skin traction using slings and pulleys. [William Russell, Edinburgh physician, 1852-1940].

Ryan virus. Identified as an amoeba of the genus Hartmannella.

ریان وائرس: جنس ہارٹ منیلا کا امیبا۔

Ryle's tube *(rilz)* A small-bore gastric tube, weighted at the tip. [John A. Ryle, British physician, 1889---].

S

Sabin's Vaccine *(sabinz vaksin)* [Albert Bruce Sabin, Russian born American virologist 1906-1993]. It is a vaccine against poliomyelitis. It is live poliovirus. It is used orally.

سابن ویکسین: امریکی ماہر حراثیم البروٹ بروس سابن کے نام پر جو ۱۹۰۶ء میں پیدا ہوا۔ پولیو کے خلاف مدافعت یا مزاحمت پیدا کرنے کیلئے ویکسین۔

Sac *(sak)* [L. *saccus*. G. *sakkos*, pouch]. Pouch, baglike organ or structure.

کیسہ، تھیلی، چھالہ: ایک چھوٹی تھیلی یا سست نما یا جوف۔

Saccharides *(saka-ri'd)* One of a series of carbohydrates, including the sugars. It contains all the three classes of saccharides.

شکری مرکبات: سادہ شکر۔ ایک مونوسیکرائیڈ۔

Saccharin *(sakarin)* A white crystalline compound several hundred times sweeter than sucrose. It is used as a sweetening agent in pharmacentical preparations.

سکرین، جوہری شکری، معدنی شکر: ایک سفید قلمی نیم حل پذیر ٹھوس، نقطہ پگھلاؤ ۲۲۷°س، جب خالص ہو تو اس میں مٹھاس، چینی یا شکر سے ۵۵۰ گنا زیادہ ہوتی ہے۔ لیکن خوراکی قدر نہیں رکھتا بلکہ زیادہ استعمال کی صورت میں نقصان دِہ ہے۔ ٹالوین سے تیار کیا جاتا ہے۔ سوڈیم نمک کی صورت میں بھی استعمال کیا جاتا ہے۔ جسے سکرین سوڈیم کہتے ہیں۔ شکر کا معروف متبادل۔

Saccharolytic *(sak-a-ro-litik)* [G. *lysis*, loosening]. Capable of breaking the glycosidic bonds in saccharides i.e. capable of fermentation.

سیکرولائیٹک: کاربوہائیڈریٹس کو تخریب کرنے کی اہلیت رکھنا۔

Sacculation *(sak-u-la'shan)* [L. *sacculus*, a small pouch]. The quality of being sacculated or pursed out with little pouches.

سیکولیشن: کئی چھوٹی تھیلیوں کا ظہور۔

Saccule *(sak-ul)* [L. *sacculus*, a small sac]. A small or little sac like sacculi alveolares.

کیسک: ایک چھوٹی تھیلی۔ یوٹریکل اور کاکلیا سے متعلق تھیلی۔

Sacral *(sak-ral)* [L. *sacralis*]. Pertaining to or situated near the sacrum.

سیکرل: سیکرم سے متعلق۔

Sacroanterior *(sa-kro-an-tere-ar)* It is a term used to show the breech presentation of the fetus. The fetal sacrum is directed to one or other acetabulum of the mother.

عجزی امامی: بچے کے سیکرم کو ماں کے ایسیٹبولم کی طرف موڑا جاتا ہے۔

Sacrococcygeal *(sa-kro-koks-ij'-e-al)* [L. *sacer*, sacred; G. *kokkyx*, cuckoo]. Pertaining to the sacrum and the coccyx.

عجزی عصعصی: سیکرم اور کاکس کے متعلق۔

Sacroiliac *(sa-kro-il'-i-ak)* [L. *sacer*, sacred;

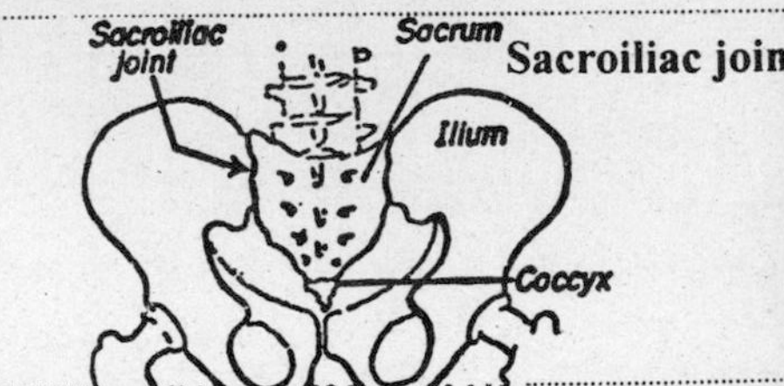

Sacroiliac joint

ilium, flank]. Pertaining to the sacrum and the ilium.

عجزی حرقفی: سیکرم اور ایلم سے متعلق۔

Sacrolumbar *(sa-kro-lum'-bar)* [L. *sacer,* sacred; *lumbus,* loin]. Pertaining to the sacrum and the loins.

عجزی قطنی: سیکرم اور کمر سے متعلق۔

Sacroposterior *(sa-kro-pos-te'-ri-er)* [L. *sacer,* sacred; *post,* behind]. Used to describe a breech presentation in midwifery. The fetal sacrum is directed to one of other sacroiliac joint of the mother—sacroposteriorly, *adv.*

عجزی حلفی: بچے کے سیکرم کو ماں کے سیکروالیائک جوڑ کی طرف گھمایا جاتا ہے۔

Sacrum *(sa-krum)* [L. *sacer,* sacred]. The triangular bone lying between the fifth lumbar vertebra and the coccyx. It consists of five vertebrae fused together, and it articulates on each side with the innominate bones of the pelvis, forming the sacroiliac joints—sacra, *adj.*

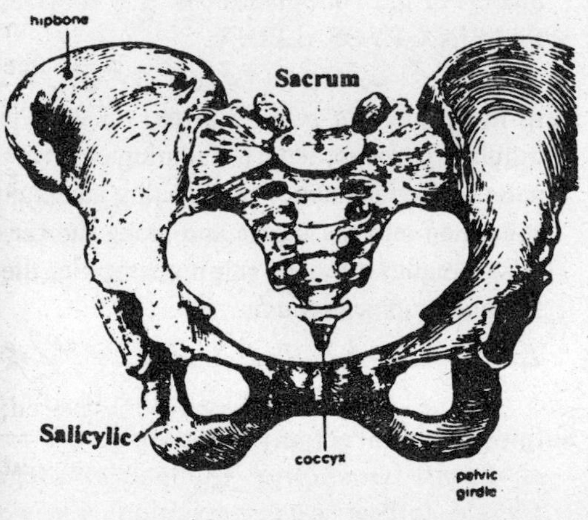

چوتڑ کی ہڈی، عظم عجز: پانچویں لمبر مہرے اور کاکس کے درمیان واقع تکونی ہڈی۔ یہ پانچ ملحقہ سروں پر مشتمل ہے۔

Saddlenose. One with a flattened bridge; often a sign of congenital syphilis.

فطس الانف، پچکی ناک: چپٹے پل کے ساتھ۔ اکثر پیدائشی آتشک کا نشان۔

Sadism *(sa-dizm)* The obtaining of pleasure from inflicting pain, violence or degradation on another person, or on the sexual partner. Opp. masochism.

لذت جلادی: دوسرے شخص یا جنسی شریک کی توہین کر کے، تشدد یا اسے دکھ پہنچا کر خوش ہونا۔

Safapryn *(sa'-fa-prin)* 'Safe' aspirin. It is claimed that it does not cause gastric bleeding.

سفا پرائن: محفوظ اسپرین۔ دعویٰ کیا جاتا ہے کہ اس کے استعمال سے معدہ سے خون جاری نہیں ہوتا۔

Sagittal *(saj'-it-al)* [L. *sagitta,* arrow]. Resembling an arrow. In the anteroposterior plane of the body. **sagittal suture,** the immovable joint formed by the union of the two parietal bones.

تیر نما: تیر سے مشابہ۔

Salazopyrin *(sal-as-o-pi'-rin)* Salicylazosulphapyridine (q.v.).

سلازو پائیرن: سیلیسائیلازوسلفاپائیریڈین۔

Salbutamol *(sal-but'-a-mol)* Bronchodilator derived from isoprenaline. Does not produce cardiovascular side effects when inhaled in the recommended dose.

سیلبیوٹامول: آئیسو پرینالین سے اخذ شدہ۔

Salicylamide *(sal-is-il'-a-mid)* Milk analgesic similar in action to the salicylates, but less likely to cause gastric dislurbance.

سیلی سیلامائیڈ: میلی ڈین۔ دافع درد دوا۔ بچے کی پیدائش کے بعد درد کے علاج کے لئے ایک گولی حسب ضرورت دیجئے۔ اس سے قبض ہوتی ہے۔ اس کی ایک یا دو گولیاں دن میں ۳ دفعہ برائے سر درد، پر ہیز ذاسٹر یا علہ منطقیہ ایک ایک گولی دن میں ۳ د . برائے جگر کا امیبی پھوڑا۔

Salicylazosulphapyridine *(sal-is- .-a-zo-sul-fa-pi-ri-den)* A sulphonamide compound which, after ingestion, is said to be distributed largely in connective tissues. It is used in the treatment of ulcerative colitis.

سیلی سائیلازوسلفاپائیریڈین: ایک سلفونامائیڈ مرکب۔

Salicylic acid *(sal-i-sil'-ik-as-id)* Has fungicidal and bacteriostatic properties, and is used in a variety of skin conditions. It is a constituent of Whitfield's ointment. The plaster is used to remove corns and warts.

صفعاف کا تیزاب: ایک سفید قلمی ٹھوس۔ نقطہ پگھلاؤ ۱۵۹° س، دافع تعفن کے طور پر اور اسپرین کے ماخذ کی صورت میں استعمال ہوتا ہے۔ جلدی حالتوں کی ورائٹی میں مستعمل۔ پلستر چھالوں کو ختم کرنے کے لئے استعمال کیا جاتا ہے۔

Saline *(sa'-lin)* [L. *sal,* salt]. A solution of salt and water. Normal or physiological s. is a 0.9 per cent solution with the same osmotic pressure as that of blood. See HYPERTONIC, HYPOTONIC, ISOTONIC.

نمکین: نمک اور پانی کا محلول۔ نمک پر مشتمل خصوصی طور پر میگنیشیم اور الکلائن دھاتوں کے نمکیات۔ ایسا محلول پانی میں نمکیات کا محلول ہوتا ہے۔ خصوصاً ایسا محلول جو جسمی سیالوں کے ساتھ آئیسوٹونک ہو۔ نارمل یا فزیالوجیکل نمکین ۰٫۹٪ محلول ہوتا ہے۔ جس کا نفوذ دباؤ خون کے برابر ہوتا ہے۔

Saliva *(sal-i'-va)* [L.]. The secretion of the salivary glands; spittle. It contains water, mucus and ptyalin (q.v.)—salivary, *adv.*

لعاب: مائع جو منہ میں لعاب کے طور پر پیدا ہوتا ہے۔ لعابی غدود کی خارج ہونے والی رطوبت اس میں پانی میوکس اور ٹایالن ہوتے ہیں۔

Salivary *(sal'-iv-a-ri)* Pertaining to saliva. **salivary calculus,** a stone formed in the salivary ducts. **salivary glands,** the glands which secrete saliva, viz., parotid, submaxillary and sublingual.

لعابی: لعاب سے متعلق۔

Salivation *(sal-iv-a'-shun)* [L. *salivare,* to spit out]. An increased secretion of saliva. Ptyalism.

کثرتِ لعاب: لعاب کا بڑھا ہوا اخراج۔

Salk vaccine *(solk-vak'-sen)* A preparation of killed poliomyelitis virus used as an antigen to produce active arrtificial immunity to poliomyelitis. By injection. [Jonas Edward Salk, American bacteriologist. 1914---].

سالک ویکسین: مردہ پولیو وائرس کو استعمال کرتے ہیں۔ پولیو کے خلاف عامل مصنوعی مزاحمت پیدا کرنے والی ویکسین۔ اس کا نام امریکی ماہر جراثیم جونس ایڈورڈ سالک کے نام پر رکھا گیا جو ۱۹۱۴ء میں پیدا ہوا۔

Salmonella *(sal-mon-el'-a)* A genus of bacteria Gram-negative rods. Parasitic in many animals and man in whom they are ofte pathogenic. Some species, such as *Salmonell typhi,* are host-specific, infecting only man, i whom they cause typhoid fever. Others, suc as *S. typhimurium,* may infect a wide range o host species, usually through contaminate foods.

سامنی عصیات: جراثیم کا ایک جنس۔ گرام منفی سلاخی جراثیم۔ کئی جانوروں ئمول آدمی میں طفیلی اور امراض پیدا کرتا ہے۔ اس کی ایک نوع سے تپ محرکہ یا ٹیفائیڈ بخار ہوتا ہے جو سالمونیکلا ٹائی فی ہے۔ سائز ۳×۶ مائیکرون، ۵۶ رجے سنٹی گریڈ پر نصف گھنٹے میں مر جاتے ہیں۔ یہ ایکٹوز کو تخمیر کرنے کی صلاحیت نہیں رکھتے۔ کلورو یم فینی کال سے ختم ہوتے ہیں۔

Salpingectomy *(sal-pin-jek'-to-mi)* [G. *salpig* trumpet; *ektome,* excision]. Excision of Fallopian tube.

نات فلوپی، براری: فلوپین نلی کو کاٹ کر الگ کرنا۔

Salpingitis *(sal-pin-ji'-tis)* [G. *salpigx,* trumpe *-itis,* inflammation]. Acute or chronic inflam mation of the Fallopian tubes. See HYDRO SALPINX, PYOSALPINX.

رم بیض نالی: فلوپین نلیوں کی قدیم یا انتہائی سوزش۔

Salpingogram *(sal-ping'-o-gram)* [G. *salpig* trumpet; *gramma,* letter]. Radiological exami nation of tubal patency by injecting an opaqu substance into the uterus and along the tube —salpingography, *n.*; salpingographic, *adj* salpingographically, *adv.*

لپنوگرام: یوٹرس میں اور نلیوں کے ساتھ ساتھ غیر شفاف مادہ داخل کر کے ں کی پیٹنی کی ریڈیالوجی کی جانچ۔

Salpingo-oophorectomy *(sal-ping-go-o-o-for ek'-to-mi)* [G. *salpigx,* trumpet; *oon,* eg *pherein,* to bear; *ektome,* excision]. Excisio of a Fallopian tube and ovary.

لپنو او فوریکٹومی: فلوپین ٹیوب اور بچہ دانی (بیضہ دانی) کو کاٹنا۔

Salpingostomy *(sal-ping-gos'-to-mi)* [G. *salpig* trumpet; *stoma,* mouth]. The operatio performed to restore tubal patency.

شق البوق: نلی کی پیلٹنی برقرار رکھنے کے لئے کیا گیا اپریشن۔

Salpinx *(sal'-pingks)* [G. *salpigx,* trumpet]. A tube, especially the Fallopian tube or the Eustachian tube.

قاذف نالی: ایک نلی یا ٹیوب، خصوصاً فلوپین ٹیوب یا یوسٹیچین ٹیوب۔

Salupres. Hypotensive. Combination of reserpine and hydrochlorothiazide.

سیلوپرس: ریزرپین اور ہائیڈروکلوروتھیازائیڈ کا ملاپ۔

Saluric *(sal-u-rik)* Chlorothiazide (q.v.).

سلورک: کلوروتھیازائیڈ

Salve *(sav)* An ointment.

مسکن مرہم: ایک مرہم

Sal volatile *(sal-vol-at'-i-li)* Aromatic solution of ammonia. A household analeptic.

نمک امونیا: امونیا کا خوشبودار محلول۔ کمرشل امونیم کاربونیٹ جو دراصل امونیم بائی کاربونیٹ امونیم کارباميٹ اور امونیم کاربونیٹ کے آمیزہ پر مشتمل ہے۔

Salyrgan *(sal-ir'-gan)* Mersalyl (q.v.).

سیلرگین: مرسیلائل۔

Sanamycin *(san-a-mi'-sin)* See ACTINOMYCIN C.

سیماما‌ئی سین: ایکٹینومائیسین سی۔

Sandfly *(phlebotomus).* Responsible for short, sharp, pyrexial fever called 'sandfly fever' of the tropics. Likewise transmits leishmaniasis (q.v.)

ریت مکھی: ایک قسم کے بخار کی ذمہ دار جسے سینڈ فلائی بخار کہتے ہیں۔

Sanguineous *(sang-gwin'-i-us)* [L. *sanguts,* blood]. Pertaining to or containing blood.

دموی، پرخون: خون پر مشتمل یا خون سے متعلق۔

Santonin *(san'-ton-in)* An anthelmintic once used for round worm, but less toxic and more reliable drugs such as piperazine (q.v.) are now preferred.

سنتونین: یہ دوا راؤنڈ ورم کے لئے مستعمل تھی لیکن اب کم زہریلی اور زیادہ بھروسہ والی ادویہ مثلاً پیپرازین کو ترجیح دی جاتی ہے۔ سنتونین ۲ گرین اور کیلومل ۲ گرین کی ایک گولی رات کو سوتے وقت اور صبح کو میگ سلفاس کا جلاب دیجئے۔ پیٹ کے کیڑے یا کیچوے نکالنے کیلئے مفید ہے۔

Saphenous *(saf-e'-nus)* Apparent; manifest. The name given to the two main veins in the leg, the internal and the external, and to the nerves accompanying them.

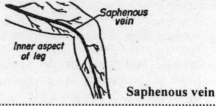

Saphenous vein

Inner aspect of leg

Saphenous vein

صافنی: ظاہری۔ ٹانگ دو بڑی وریدوں کا نام، اندرونی و بیرونی اور ان کے ساتھ ہی اعصاب۔

Saponification *(sa-pon-i-fik-a'-shun)* [L. *sapo,* soap; *facere,* to make]. Conversion into a soapy substance.

صابون سازی: ایسٹر کی آب پاشیدگی۔ یہ اصطلاح الکلی استعمال کر کے ایسڈ کی آب پاشیدگی تک محدود ہے۔ اس طرح نمک اور آزاد الکحل بنتا ہے۔

Sapraemia *(sap-re'-mi-a)* [G. *sapros,* putrid; *haima,* blood]. A general bodily reaction to circulating toxins and breakdown products of saprophytic (non-pathogenic) organisms, derived from one or more foci in the body.

فسادِ خون: گندخور جسیموں کی شکستگی کے پروڈکٹس اور گردشی زہروں یا ٹاکسنز کے لئے عام جسمانی ردِعمل۔

Saprophyte *(sap'-ro-fit)* Free-living micro-organisms obtaining food from dead and decaying animal or plant tissue—saprophytic, *adj.*

غلاظتی جرثومہ: مردہ اور گلے سڑے حیوانی و نباتی نسیج سے خوراک حاصل کرنے والے آزاد رہنے والے لخورد جسمے۔

Sarcoid *(sar'-koid)* [G. *sarkoeides,* fleshlike]. A term applied to a group of lesions in skin, lungs or other organs, which resemble tuberculous foci in structure, but the true nature of which is still uncertain.

گوشت نما: جلد، پھیپھڑوں یا دوسرے اعضاء میں زخموں کا گروہ۔

Sarcoidosis *(sar'-koid-o-sis)* [G. *sarkoeides,* flesh- like; *-osis,* condition]. A granulomatous di- sease of unknown aetiology in which histo- logical appearances resemble tuberculosis. May affect any organ of the body, but most commonly presents as a condition of the skin., lymphatic glands or the bones of the hand. See LUPUS.

سارکائیڈوسس: بظاہر تپ دق سے مشابہ مرض۔ یہ مرض جسم کے کسی بھی حصہ کو متاثر کرسکتا ہے لیکن زیادہ تر جلد، لمفی غدود یا ہاتھ کی ہڈیوں کی حالت۔

Sarcoma *(sar-ko'-ma)* [G. *sarkoma,* fleshy over-growth]. Malignant growth of mesodermal tissue (e.g. connective tissue, muscle, bone—sarcomatous, *adj.* sarcomata, *pl.*

سلعہ لحمی: واصل نسیج میں ہونے والی رسولی۔

Sarcomatosis *(sar-ko-ma-to-sis)* A condition in which sarcomata are widely spread through-out the body.

Sarcoptes *(sar-kop-tez)* Genus of Acerina. *Sar-coptes scabiel* is the itch mite which causes scabies (q.v.).

سارکاپ ٹیز۔ سکیبائی: سکیبیز پیدا کرنے والا اچائیٹ۔

Sarcopted Amitriptyline (q.v.). See ANTI-DEPRESSANT.

سیروئن: امیٹرپٹائیلین

Sartorius *(sar-tor'-i-us)* [L. *sartor,* patcher]. The tailor's muscle of the thigh, since it flexes one leg over the other.

عضلہ ران: ران کا ٹیلرز عضلہ جسم کا طویل ترین عضلہ ایلم کے سامنے کے بالائی ابھارے سے اٹھ کر ران کو ترچھا کراس کرتا ہوا ٹبیا کی اندرونی جانب کے بالائی حصے میں جڑتا ہے۔

SAT. Sodium antimony tartrate (q.v.).

ایس اے ٹی: سوڈیم اینٹی منی ٹارٹریٹ۔

Saventrine Long-acting isoprenaline. A sustained release preparation active for 8 hours. Given to raise the heart rate to more than 40 by increasing the rate of the idioventricular rhythm. Toleration may avoid artificial pacing.

سیلونٹرین: طویل العمل آئیسوپرینالین۔ دل کی دھڑکن تیز کرنے کے لئے۔

Savlon *(sav'-lon).* Chlorhexidine 1.5 per cent and centrimide 15 per cent.

سیولون: کلوہکسیڈین ۵ء۱ فیصد اور سٹریمائیڈ ۱۵ فیصد۔

Scab A dried curst forming over an open wound.

کھرنڈ: کھلے زخم پر بننے والا خشک کرسٹ۔

Scabies *(ska'-bi-ez)* [L. the itch.]. A parasiti skin disease caused by the itch mite. High contagious. See QUELLADA.

ارش تر۔ خشک خارش: ایک طفیلی جلدی مرض جو خارش جوں سے ہوتا ہے۔ چھوت کی بیماری جسم پر خارس بعض اوقات چھوٹے چھوٹے دانے۔

Scald (skawld). An injury caused by moist heat.

غ گرم آب: نمدار حرارت سے ہونے والا زخم انسان بھاپ سے جھلس تا ہے گرم پانی سے جلنا۔

Scalenus syndrome *(skal-e'-nus-sin'-drom* Pain in arm and fingers, often with wastin because of compression of the lower trunk the brachial plexus behind scalenus anteric muscle at the thoracic outlet.

نڈروم عضلہ مثلثہ: بازو اور انگلیوں میں درد۔

Scalp (skalp). The hair-bearing skin whic covers the cranium.

Scalpel (skal-pel). A surgeon's knife which ma or may not have detachable blades.

Scan See SCINTISCANNING.

قطیع کرنا: سنٹی سکیننگ۔

Scanning speech A form of dysarthria occurrin in disseminated sclerosis. The speech jumpy or staccato or slow.

نطعی تقریر: ڈس آرتھرما کی ایک قسم۔ تقریر سست یا جھٹکے دار ہوتی ہے۔

Scaphoid *(skaf'-oid)* [G. *skaphe,* boat; *eido* form]. Boat-shaped as a bone of the tarsus an carpus.

ظم زورقی: کشتی نما جیسا کہ کارپس اور ٹارس کی ہڈی۔

Scapula *(skap'-u-la)* [L.]. The shoulderblade-- large, flat, triangular bone--scapular, adj.

انے کی ہڈی: شانے کا بلیڈ۔ ایک بڑی چپٹی تکونی ہڈی۔ دھڑ کے پیچھے سری پسلی سی ساتویں پسلی تک پھیلی ہوئی ہے۔ یہ پسلیوں سے جڑی ہوئی نہیں ی۔ شانہ کی تکونی ہڈی کے بیرونی کنارے پر شانہ کا جوف ہوتا ہے۔ جس بازو کی ہڈی ہیومرس کا گول کنارہ ہوتا ہے اور شانہ کا جوڑ بناتا ہے۔ شانہ کی ی کے اسی کنارے پر ایک اور نوکیلا حصہ ہوتا ہے جس سے بازو کو حرکت ینے والے عضلات جڑے ہوتے ہیں۔ شانہ کی ہڈی کو جگہ پر قائم رکھنے کا کام

ہنسلی کی ہڈی کرتی ہے۔

Scapul

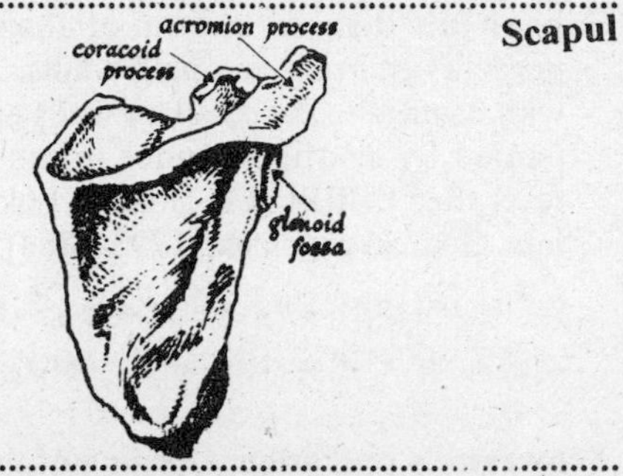

ar, The dense, avascular white fibrous tissue, formed as the end-result of healing, especially in the skin. Cicatrix,

داغ زخم: گھنا یا کثیف سفید ریشہ دار نسیج جو صحت مند ہونے کے نتیجہ میں بنتا ہے خصوصاً جلد میں۔

arification *(skar-i-fik-a'-shun)* [L. *scarificare,* to scratch open]. The making of a series of small, superficial incisions or punctures in skin.

نشتر زنی: جلد میں چھوٹے مصنوعی شگافوں یا پنکچروں کے سلسلے کا بننا۔

arlatina *(skar-la-te'-na).* Scarlet fever. Infection by haemolytic streptococcus producing a rash. Occurs mainly in children. Begins commonly with a throat infection, leading to pyrexia and the outbreak of a punctate erythematous eruption of the skin. characteristically the area around the mouth escapes (circumoral pallor)--scarlatinal, adj.

لال بخار: سکارلٹ بخار ہیمو لائیٹک سٹرپٹوکاکس سے ہونے والی انفیکشن عموماً بچوں میں ہوتا ہے۔

arlet red A dye used as a stimulating ointment (2 to 5 per cent) for clean but slow-healing ulcers, wounds and pressure sores.

گلنار: السر' زخم اور بستر کے ناسور جو صاف ہوں لیکن آہستہ آہستہ ٹھیک ہو رہے ہوں' کے لئے محرک مرہم (۲ تا ۵ فیصد) کے طور پر مستعمل ایک رنگ۔

heuermann's disease Osteochondritis of spine affecting the ring epiphyses of the vertibral bodies. Occurs in adolescents. Holger Werfel Secheuermann, radiologist and orthopaedic surgeon of Copenhagen, 1877-1960].

مرض شیورمین: یہ مرض بالغوں میں ہوتا ہے مہری اجسام کے رنگ ایپی فائیسز کو متاثر کرنے والی سپائن کی آسٹیو کونڈرائٹس۔

Schilder's disease. Genetically determined degenerative disease associated with mental subonormality. [Pul Schilder, German-American psychiatrist, 1886-1940.]

مرض شیلڈر: جینی طور پر متعین تنزلی مرض جس کا تعلق ذہنی پسماندگی کے ساتھ ہے۔

Schiotz tonometer, See TONOMETER [Hjalmar Schiotz, Norwegian physician, 1850-1927.]

شیوٹز ٹونومیٹر: ٹونومیٹر

Schistosoma *(skis-to-so'-ma)* [G. *schistos,* cleft; *soma,* body]. A genus of trematode worms or flukes which infest man. *Schistosoma* mansoni occurs in Africa, the West Indies and Brazil. *Schistosoma Japonicum* occurs in the Far East.

مشقوق البطن: ٹریماٹوڈ۔ کیڑوں یا فلوکس کا ایک جنس جو آدمی حملہ کرتا ہے۔

Schistosomiasis *(skis-to-so-mi'-a-sis)* [G. *schistos,* cleft, *soma,* body; N.L. *-iasis,* conditon]. Infestation of the human body by Schistosoma ('blod flukes') from drinking, or bathing in infected water. *Schistosoma haematobium* results in vesical schistosomiasis with haematuria as a characteristic symptom. *Schistosoma mansoni* and *Schistosoma japonicum* produce intestinal schistosomiasis characterized at first by diarrhoea and later by hepatosplenic disease.

سکسٹوسومیاسس: سکسٹوسوما کا انسانی جسم میں پہنچنا جو گندے پانی میں نہانے یا پینے سے پہنچتا ہے۔

Schistosomicides *(skis-to-so'-mi-sid)* [G. *schistes,* cleft; *soma,* body; L. *coedere,* to kill]. Lethal to Schistosoma--schistosomicidaal, *adj.*

سکسٹوسومیاسس: سکسٹوسوما کی لئے مہلک۔

Schizophrenia *(skiz'-o-fre'-ni-a)* [G. *schizein,* to cleave; *phren,* mind]. A mental disease first described by Kraepelin in 1896 as dementia pracox, Bleuler coined the names. in 1911. A group of mental illnesses characterized by disorganization of the patient's personality, often resulting in chronic life long ill-health and hospitalization. The onset, commonly in youth or early adult life, is either sudden or insidious. Bleuler described four main types, **(1) simplex, (2) catatonic s, (3) paranoid s, (4) hebephrenic s,** but the terms have disappeared from common usage. There are three elements common to all cases; a shallowness of emotional life; an inappropriateness of emotion; unrealistic thinking.

پراگندہ ذہنی: ایک دماغی عارضہ۔ شخصیت بے ربط ہو جاتی ہے اور متاثرہ شخص دائمی مریض بن کر ہسپتال میں داخل رہتا ہے۔ طویل المیعاد عارضہ۔ ایسا شخص جذبات سے عاری ہوتا ہے۔ بلیولر نے ۱۹۱۱ء میں اس مرض کو جودہ نام سے موسوم کیا۔ علامات، بلاموضوع بولنا، آدابِ مجلس کا خیال نہ رکھنا، زیادہ وہم، وقت کی پابندی نہ کرنا، معمولی واقعات کو اہمیت دینا، غیر مناسب سوال کرنا، غیر مناسب جواب، فرائض سے لاپرواہی اور خواہ مخواہ لڑائی جھگڑا ہیں۔

Schizophrenic *(skiz-o-fren'-ik)* Pertaining to schizophrenia. **schizophrenic syndrome in childhood** considered to be the best diagnostic labe, rather than autism or psychosis in childhood. A working party (1961) formulated nine diagnostic points for this condition.

پراگندہ ذہنی: سکائیزوفرینیا سے متعلق۔

Schlatter's disease. Also Osgood-Schlatter's disease. Osteochondritis of the tribial tubercle. [Carl Schlatter, Swiss surgeon, 1864- 1934]. Robert Bayley Osgood, American orthonaedic surgeon, 1873-1934].

مرض سکلیٹر: ٹیبا کے ابھار کی آسٹیوکانڈرٹیس۔

Schlemm's canal. A lymphaticovenous canal in the inner part of the sclera, close to its junction with the cornea, which it encircles. [Friedrich Schlemm, German anatomist, 1795-1858---].

قنال سکلیم: سکلیرا کے اندرونی حصہ میں لمفی وریدی قنال۔

Scholz's disease. Genetically determined degenerative disease associated with mental subnormality. [Willibald Scholz, German neurologist, 1899].

سکولز: ذہنی پسماندگی کے وابستہ جینی طور پر متعین تنزلی عارضہ۔

Schonlein's disease. A form of anaphylact purpura occurring in young adults, associa with damage to the capillary walls and acc panied by swollen, tender joints and m fever. See PURPURA. [Johann Lukas Sch lein, German physician, 1793-1864].

سکونلین: شریان سے خون نکلنا۔ یہ عارضہ نوجوان بالغوں کو لاحق ہوتا اس سے شریانی دیواروں کو نقصان پہنچتا ہے۔ جوڑ متورم ہوتے ہیں اور ار رہتا ہے۔

Schwartze's operation. Opening of the mast process of the excision of infected bone drainage of cellular suppuration. [Hermann R. Schwartzo German otologist, 1837-191

رٹز اپریشن: بیمار ہڈی کو کاٹنے کے لئے مسٹائیڈ زائدے کا کھولنا۔

Sciatica *(si-at-ik-a)* [G. *ischion,* hip joint]. F in the line of distribution of the sciatic ne (bottock, back of thigh, calf and foot).

النساء: شیاٹک عصب کی تقسیم کی لکیر میں درد۔ ساری ٹانگ میں درد۔ فینائل بوٹازو، بیوٹالجن، پریڈنی سولون اور وٹامن ب کمپاؤنڈ فورٹ وبیان) دیجئے۔

Scintillography: scintiscanning *(sin-til-og-fi-sin-ti-skan-ning)* [L. *scintilla,* spar Visual recording of radioactivity over selec areas after administration of suitable radio tope.

وگرافی: مناسب ریڈیو آئیسوٹوپ دینے کے بعد منتخب حصوں پر تابکاری ری ریکارڈنگ۔

Scirrhous *(skir'-us)* [G. *skiros,* hard]. Hard; sembling a scirrhus.

سرطانی: سخت۔

Scirrhus *(skir'-us)* [G. *skiros,* hard]. A carci ma which provokes a considerable growth hard, connective tissue; a hard carcinoma the breast.

چھاتی کا سخت سینوما۔

Scissor leg deformity. The legs are crosse walking—following double hip-joint dise or as a manifestation of Little's dise (spastic cerebral diplegia).

مقراض پا: ٹانگوں کو چلتے ہوئے کراس کرنا۔

ra *(skler'-a)* [G. *skleros,* hard]. The 'white' f the eye; the opaque bluish-white fibrous uter coat of the eyeball covering the osterior five- sixths; it merges into the ornea at the front- scleral, *adj.*; sclerae, *pl.*

سفیدہ چشم: آنکھ کی سفیدی۔ آنکھ کے گولے کا غیر شفاف نیلگوں سفید ر دار بیرونی کوٹ۔

rema *(skler'-e-ma),* **scleroderma** *(skler-o-er-ma),* **scleroedema** *(skler-e-de-ma)* [G. *kleros,* hard]. Progressive atrophy of the skin localized or diffuse patches. Localized s. is alled 'morphea'. The diffuse form leads to erve limitation of movement over joints and the face.

شمی صلابت: مقامی حصوں میں جلد کی سودی اڈانی۔

ritis *(skler-i'-tis)* [G. *skleros,* hard; *-itis,* in-amation]. Inflammation of the sclera.

ورم صلبیہ: سکلیرا کی سوزش۔

rocorneal *(skler-o-kor'-ni-al)* [G. *skleros,* ard; L. *corneus,* horny]. Pertaining to the clera and the cornea, as the circular junction f these two structures.

صلبی قرنی: قرنیہ اور سکلیرا سے متعلق۔

roderma *(skle-ro-der'-ma)* [G. *skleros,* ard; *derma,* skin]. A disease in which ocalized oedema of the skin is followed by ardening, atrophy, deformity and ulceration. ccasiona- lly it becomes generalized, roducing immob- ility of the face, ontraction of the fingers; diffuse fibrosis of e myocardium, kidneys, digestive tract and ings. See COLLAGEN and DERMATO-IYOSITIS.

تصلب جلد: ایک مرض میں جلد کے مقامی اڈیما کے بعد سختی، اٹرافی، بدشک اور السریشن ہوتے ہیں۔

roma *(skler-o-ma)* [G. *skleros,* hard; *-oma,* mour]. Hardening of a tissue.

نسیجی صلابت: نسیج کا سخت ہونا۔

rosis *(skler-o'-sis)* [G. *sklerosis,* hardening]. erm used in pathology to describe abnormal hardening or fibrosis of a tissue. **disseminated s.** (syn. **multiple s.**), a variably progressive disease of the nervous system, most commonly first affecting young adults, in which patchy, degenerative changes occur in nerve sheaths in the brain, spinal cord and optic nerves, followed by sclerosis (glial scar). The presenting symptoms can be diverse, ranging from diplopia to weakness or unsteadines of a limb; disturbance of micturition are common. See TEST; platelet stickness. **tuberose s.,** See EPILOIA—sclerotic, *adj.*

تصلب انساج: کسی نسیج کی غیر معمولی سختی یا فائبروسس۔

Sclerotherapy *(skler-o-ther'-a-pi)* [G. *skeros,* hard; *therapeia,* treatment]. Injection of sclerosing agent for treatment of varicose veins. **compression s.,** rubber pads are bandaged into position over the injection sites to increase localized compression in these areas.

Sclerotic *(skler-ot-ik)* Pertaining to sclerosis.

Sclerotomy *(skler-ot'-o-mi)* [G. *skleros,* hard; *tome,* a cutting]. Incision of sclera for relief of acute glaucoma, prior to doing a decompression operation.

صلبیہ تراشی: اپریشن سے پہلے انتہائی گلاکوما کے آرام کیلئے سکلیرا کو کاٹنا۔

Scolex *(sko'-leks)* [L.]. The head of the tapeworm by which it embeds into the intestinal wall, and from which the segments (proglottides) develop.

سر کدودانہ: کدو کیڑے کا سر جس سے وہ آنت کی دیوار میں دھنستا رہتا ہے اور ٹکڑے بنتے ہیں۔

Scoline *(sko'-len)* Suxamethonium (q.v.).

سکولین: سکسامیتھونیم۔

Scoliosis *(sko'-li-o-sis)* [G.]. Lateral curvature of the spine.

التوا: سپائن کا جانبی خم۔

Scopolamine *(sko-pol'-a-min)* Hyoscine (q.v.).

دواء صداقت، سکوپولامین: ہائیسین۔ مارفین کے ساتھ یہ دوائی ملا کردی جاتی ہے جس کے زیر اثر ہونے والے اپریشن کی یاد باقی نہیں رہتی۔ ہوش میں آنے کے بعد مریض کو یاد نہیں ہوتا کہ اس کا اپریشن ہوا ہے۔

Scorbutic *(skor-bu'-tik)* Pertaining to scorbutus,

the old name for scurvy.

اسقر بوطی: اسر بوط سے متعلق۔

Scotoma *(sko-to'-ma)* [G. *skotos,* darkness]. Blind spot in field of vision. May be normal or abnormal—scotomata, *pl.*

داغ تیرہ: بصارت کے فیلڈ میں اندھا دھبہ۔

Scotopic vision The ability to see well in poor light.

ظلمتی بصارت: مدھم روشنی میں اچھی طرح دیکھنے کی قابلیت۔

Scott's dressing Ung. hydrarg. co. An ointment containing camphor, olive oil, mercury and beeswax is spread on strips of lint and applied to swollen joints. [John Scott. English surgeon, 1799-1846].

سکاٹ کی پٹی: متورم جوڑوں پر لگانے کے لئے مرہم۔

Screening. See FLUOROSCOPY.

فلوری معائنہ: فلوروسکوپی۔

Scraple *(skra-pe)* Virus disease of sheep and goats.

سکر یپی: بھیڑوں اور بکریوں کا وائرس کا مرض۔

Scrofula *(skrof'-u-la)* Tuberculosis of bone or lymph gland—scrofulous, *adj.*

خنازیر: لمفی غدیا ہڈی کا تپ دق۔

Scrofuloderma *(skrof-u-lo-der'-ma)* An exudative and crusted skin lesion, often with sinuses, resulting from a tuberculous lesion underneath, as in bone or lymph glands.

خنازیر جلدی: جلدی زخم۔

Scrotum *(skro'-tum)* [L.]. The pouch in the male which contains the testicles—scrotal, *adj.*

صفن: نرمیں خصیوں پر مشتمل تھیلی۔

Scurf. A popular term for dandruff.

سرکی خشکی: خشکی کیلئے ایک معروف اصطلاح۔

Scurvy *(skur'-vi)* A deficiency disease caused by lack of vitamin C (ascorbic acid). Clinical features include fatigue and haemorrhage. Latter may take the form of oozing at the gums or large ecchymoses. Tiny bleeding spotson the skin around hair follicles are charac-teristic. In children painful subperiosteal haemorrhage (rather than other types of bleeding) is pathognomonic.

بوط، اسکروی: وٹامن سی (اسکاربک ایسڈ) کی کمی سے لاحق ہونے
رضہ۔اس سے تھکاوٹ اور ہیمرج ہوتے ہیں۔

Scybala *(sib'-a-la)* [G. *skybalon,* dung]. Rou ed, hard, faecal lumps. **scybalum,** *sing.*

فضلہ آنت: گول، سخت، فضلے کے تودے۔

Sea legs. Meclozine. See ANTIHISTAMINE

Sebaceous *(se-ba'-shus)* [L. *sebaceus,* a tal candle]. Pertaining to fat or suet. **sebace glands,** the cutaneous glands which secret oily substance called 'sebum'. The duct these glands are short and straight and o into the hair follicles.

دار: چکنائی سے متعلق۔ سیبے شش سسٹ سیبے شش گلینڈ کی نالی بند
سے مواد اندر جمع ہونے سے بنتی ہے۔

Seborrhoea *(seb-o-re'-a)* [L. *sebum,* tallow *rheein,* to flow]. Greasy condition of scalp, face, sternal region and elsewhere to overactivity of sebaceous glands. The orrhoeic type of skin is especially liabl conditions such as alopecia, seborrh dermatitis, acne, etc.

ن شحم، بفا: سر کی کھال کی چکنی حالت۔

Sebum *(se'-bum)* [L.]. The normal secretio the sebaceous glands; it contains fatty ac cholestrol and dead cells.

رطوبت: غدۂ شحمی کی رطوبت۔ یہ فیٹی ایسڈز کولیسٹرول اور مردہ خلیوں
ہے۔

Seclomycin *(sek-lo-mi'-sin)* Mixture of stre mycin panicillin, broad spectrum antibiotic

مائی سن: سٹرپٹو مائی سین اور پنسلین کا آمیزہ۔ پیپ ختم کرنے کیلئے
بکہ روزانہ اسی طرح برائے آسٹیو مائی لائی ٹس یعنی گھمیر۔

Seconal *(sek'-on-al)* Quinalbarbitone (q.v.).

: کوئنل باربیٹون۔ باربیچوریٹ۔ ایک خواب آور دوا۔

Secretin *(se-kre'-tin)* [L. *secernere,* to separ A hormone produced in the duodenal muc which causes a copious secretion of pan atic juice. Available as snuff.

لکیزہ: ڈیوڈینل میوکوسا میں پیدا شدہ ہارمون۔

Secretion *(se-kre'-shun)* [L. *secretio,* separation]. A fluid or substance, forme concentrated in a gland, and passed into the alimentary tract, the blood or to the exterior.

افراز: گلینڈ میں مرتکز یا بننے والا سیال یا مادّہ۔

cretory *(se-kret'-o-ri)* [L. *secernere,* to separate]. The process of secretion; describes a gland which secretes.

ریزش ساز، افرازی: اخراج رطوبت کا طریق۔ رطوبت خارج کرنے والا گلینڈ۔

dation *(se-da'-shun)* [L. sedare, to soothe]. The production of a state of lessened functinal activity.

سکون: کم فعلیاتی عاملیت کی حالت۔

dation *(sed'-at-iv)* [L. sedare, to soothe]. An agent which lessens functional activity.

مسکن۔ تسکین بخش: فعلیاتی عالمیت کو کم کرنے والا ایجنٹ نیند کی کمی، پریشانی، وہم، ذہنی اذیت وغیرہ میں مستعمل۔ مثلاً برومائیڈ وغیرہ۔

dormid *(sed'-or-mid).* A mild sedative and hypnotic. A useful alternative to barbiturates, but it may cause purpura in sensitive patients.

سیڈورمڈ: ہلکی مسکن اور خواب آور دوا باربیچوریٹس کا مفید متبادل لیکن حساس مریضوں میں شریانوں سے خون نکل آتا ہے۔

gment *(seg'-ment)* [L. *segmentum,* piece]. A small section; a part -segmental, adj.; segmentation, n.

حلقہ: ایک چھوٹا سیکشن۔ ایک حصہ۔

gregation *(seg-re-ga'-shun)* [L. *segregare,* to separate]. A setting apart, usually for a particular purpose, e.g., those suffering from the same or similar disease.

علیحدگی: الگ کرنا، عموماً کسی خاص مقصد کے لئے مثلاً وہ یکساں مرض کے شکار ہوں۔

idlitz powder *(sed'-litz)* A popular aperient. It is dispensed as two powders, one containing sodium potassium tartrate and sodium bicarbonate, the other trate and sodium bicarbonte, the other containing tartaric acid. Both powders are dissolved in water, and taken as an effervescent draught. [Named from a mineral spring in Bohemia.]

سیڈلٹز سفوف: اصل میں دو پاؤڈر ہیں ۔ ایک میں سوڈیم پوٹاشیم ٹارٹریٹ اور سوڈیم بائی کاربونیٹ اور دوسرے میں ٹارٹرک ایسڈ ہوتا ہے دونوں کو پانی میں حل کرلیا جاتا ہے۔

Seldinger Intra-arteria catheter See diagram.

Seldinger catheter

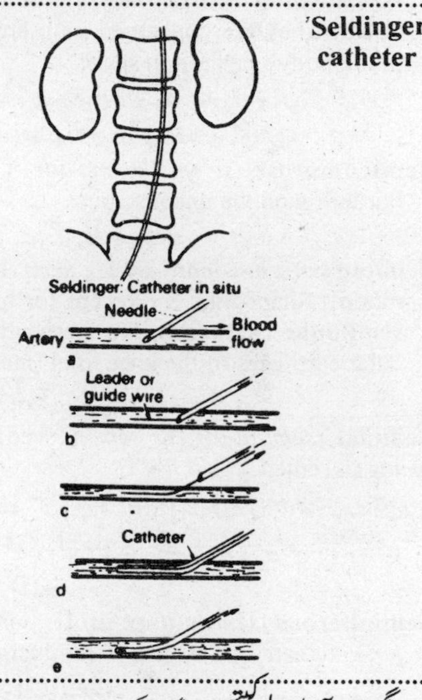

سیلڈنگر انٹرا آرٹیریل کیتھیٹر: شکل دیکھئے۔

Selenomethionine *(sel-en-o-meth-i-o-nen)* An injection in which the sulphur atom present in the amino acid methionine is replaced by radioactive selenium. Taken up selectively by the pancreas; valuable in diagnosis of pancreatic disease.

Sella turcica *(sel-a-tur-sik-a)* [L. *sella,* saddle; *turcicus,* Turkish]. Now called 'pituitany fossa'.

سیلا ٹرسیکا: اب اسے پیٹوایٹری فوسا کہا جاتا ہے۔ سیفلینا ئیڈ ہڈی میں نشیب جس میں پیٹوایٹری گلینڈ ہوتی ہے۔

Semen *(se'-men)* [L. seed]. The secretion from the testicles and accessory male organs, e.g. prostate. It contains the spermatozoa.

منی، نطفہ: خصیوں اور زائد نر اعضاء سے رطوبت کا افراز۔ مثلاً پراسٹیٹ۔ اس میں سپر میٹازوآ ہوتے ہیں۔ سفید گاڑھی سیال رطوبت، مخصوص بو، اس میں سپرم خوردبین سے نظر آتے ہیں۔ ایک سی سی میں دس کروڑ سپرم ہوتے ہیں۔

Semicircular canals *(se-mi-sir'-ku-lar ka-nalz)* Three membranous semicircular tubes contained within the bony labyrinth of the internal ear. They are concerned with appreciation of the body's positon in space.

ازابیب نیم دائری: درمیانی کان کے استخوانی لیبرنتھ میں تین جھلی دار نیم دائروی نکیال۔ وہ فضا میں جسم کی پوزیشن کو متوازن رکھتی ہیں۔

Semicomatose *(se'-mi-ko-ma-toz)* Condition bordering on the unconscious.

سیمی کوماٹوس: بے ہوشی کے قریب حالت۔

Semilunar *(sem-i-loon'-ar)* [L. *semi,* half; *luna,* moon]. Shapedlike a crescent for half moon. **semilunar cartilages,** the crescentic intrarticular cartilages of the knee joint (menisci).

عظم ہلالی، نیم قمری: ہلال یا نصف چاند کی شکل کا۔

Seminal *(sem'-in-al)* [L. *semen,* seed]. Pertaining to semen.

منوی: سیمن سے متعلق۔ منی انڈے کی سفیدی کی طرح معلوم ہوتی ہے لیکن زیادہ گاڑھی اور سفیدی مائل ہوتی ہے۔ خشک ہونے پر سفید دھبہ ہوتا ہے جسے منوی داغ کہا جاسکتا ہے۔

Seminiferous *(sem-in-if'-er-us)* [L. *semen,* seed; *ferre,* to carry]. Carrying or producing semen.

منی بر: سیمن پیدا کرنا یا لے جانا۔

Seminoma *(sem'-in-o-ma)* [L. *semen,* seed; G. *-oma,* tumour]. A malignant tumour of the testis—seminomata, *pl.*; seminomatous, *adj.*

سلعہ خصیہ: خصیہ کی رسولی۔

Semipermeable *(se-mi-per'-me-ab-l)* Used to describe a membrane which is permeable to some substances in solutions, but not to others.

نیم مسام دار: اس جھلی میں سے محلل کے مالیکیول زیادہ ارتکاز یکساں ہوجاتا ہے۔ نیم مسام دار جھلی میں سے محلول کی پرگندگی کو عمل نفوذ کہا جاتا ہے۔ عمل نفوذ میں محلل کی پراگندگی ہوتی ہے تاکہ منحل کی محلول میں پانی کی پراگندگی عمل نفوذ ہے۔

Senescene *(se-nes'-ens)* [L. *senescere,* to grow old]. Normal changes of mind and body in increasing age—senescent, *adj.*

پیرانہ سالی، انحطاط: عمر بڑھنے میں جسم و ذہن کی نارمل تبدیلیاں۔

Sengstaken tube For compression of bleeding oesophageal varices.

سنگسٹیکن نلی: روانی خون والی ایسوفیگس کی دوالی وریدوں کے دباؤ کیلئے۔

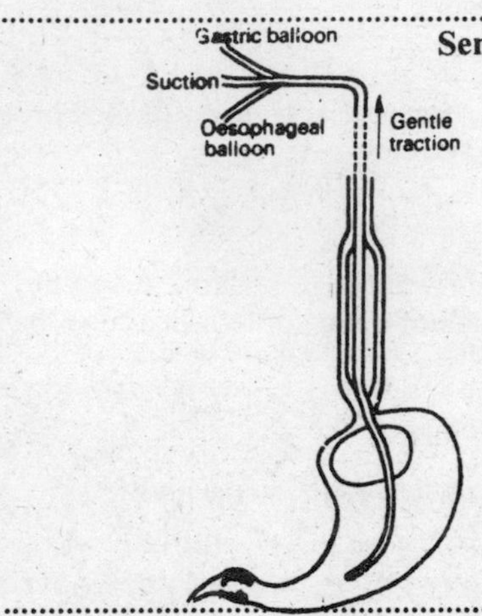

Sengstaken tub

Senile *(sen'-il)* [L. *senilis,* aged]. Senescenc complicated by morbid processes—senility,

رانہ: بڑھاپے کی طرف گامزن۔

Senna *(sen'-na)* Leaves and pods of a purgativ plant from Egypt and India. Once use extensively as Black Draught or compoun senna mixture.

ا: مصر اور انڈیا کے دست آور پتے اور پھلیاں۔

Senokot Standardized senna (q.v.).

ینوکاٹ: معیاری سنا۔

Sensible *(sen'-sib-l)* 1. Endowed with the sen of feeling. 2. Detectable by the senses.

ی حس، ذکی: (۱) محسوس کرنے کی حس ہونا۔
(۲) حواس کے ذریعے معلوم کرنے کے قابل۔

Sensitization *(sen-si-ti-za'-shun)* Rendering se sitive. Persons may become sensitive to variety of substances which may be food (e. shellfish), bacteria, plants, chemical substan es, drugs, sera, etc. Liability is much great in some persons than others. Sensitizing age acts as an antigen leading to development antibodies in the blood. See ALLERGY ANAPHYLAXIS.

اس گری: حساس بنانا۔

Sensorineural *(sen-sor-i-nur'-al)* [L. *sensu*

senses; G. *neuron,* nerve]. Pertaining to sensory neurones. **sensorineural deafness,** a discriminating term for nerve deafness.

ensory *(sen-sor-i)* [L. *senss,* sense]. Pertaining to sensationn. **sensory nerves,** those which convey impulses to the brain and spinal cord.

حساسہ، حساسوی: احساس سے متعلق۔ حساسوی اعصاب پیغامات باہر سے دماغ کو لاتے ہیں۔ ان کو افرنٹ نروبھی کہا جاتا ہے۔

entiment *(sen'-ti-ment)* [L. *sentire,* to fel]. A group of emotionally charged tendencies centred on some person or object. Sentiments increase with experience of environment.

احساس، خیال، جذبہ دل: کسی شخص یا شے پر مرکوز جذباتی رجحانات کا گروہ۔

epsis *(sep'-sis)* [G. putrefaction]. The state of being infected with pusproducing organisms--septic, adj.

تعفن: پیپ پیدا کرنے والے جسیموں سے عارضہ لاحق ہونے کی حالت۔

epticaemia *(sep'-ti-sem'-i-a)* [G. *sepsis,* putrefaction; *haima* , blood]. The persistence and multiplication of living bacteria in the blood stream--septicamic, adj.

عفونت خون، سپٹی سیمیا: خون میں زندہ جراثیم کا ہونا اور ان کی تولید اندام نہانی کی چھوت میں سوتکی بخار ہو جاتا ہے اگر علاج نہ کرایا جائے تو سارے خون میں پھیل سکتی ہے اس سے خونی سفید خلیے زیادہ ہو جاتے ہیں۔ اس میں پنسلین یا اوریینین کا ٹیکہ مفید ہے۔

ptrin *(sep'-trin).* Tablets containing 80 mg trimethoprim and 400 mg sulphamethoxazole.

سیپٹرین: گولیاں جن میں ۸۰ ملی گرام ٹرائی میتھو پرم اور ۴۰۰ ملی گرام سلفا میتھو کسازول ہوتا ہے۔

ptum *(sup'-tum).* A partition between two cavities, e.g. between the nasal cavities--septa, pl,; septal , septate , adj.

حجاب۔ حاجز: دو کھفوں کے درمیان تقسیم۔ مثلاً نتھنوں کے درمیان فاصل ناک۔

quela *(se-kwe'-la)* [L. *sequi,* to follow]. Pathological consequences of a disease, e.g. pock-marks of smallpox--sequelae , pl.

نتیجہ مرض: کسی مرض کے پیتھولوجیکل نتائج مثلاً چیچک کے نشان۔

Sequestrectomy *(se-kwes-trek'-to-mi)* [L. *sequester,* standing apart; G. *ektome,* excision]. Excision of a sequestrum (q.v.)

دمہ براری: سیقسٹرم کو کاٹنا۔

Sequestrum *(se-kwes'-trum)* [L. sequester, standing apart]. A piece of dead bone which separates from the healthy bone but remians within the tissues--sequestra, pl.

رمی۔ دمہ: مردہ ہڈی کا ٹکڑا جو صحت مند ہڈی سے الگ ہو جاتا ہے لیکن بافتوں میں رہتا ہے۔

Serenace Haloperidol (q.v.)

سیرینیس: ہیلوپیریڈول

Serenid-D (ser'-e-nid). Oxazepam (q.v.)

سیرنیڈ ڈی: اکساز پیام

Serology *(se-rol'-oj-k)* [L. *seruia,* whey ; G. *logos,* discourse]. The branch of science dealing with the study of sera--serological, adj; serologically, adv.

مصلیات: سیرا کے مطالعہ سے متعلق سائنس کی شاخ۔

Seropurulent *(se-ro-pur'-u-lent)* [L. *serum* , whey; *purulentus,* purulent]. Containing serum and pus.

خوناب و پیپ سے مرکب: آب خون یا سیرم اور پیپ پر مشتمل۔

Serosa *(se-roz'-a)* [L. *serum* , whey]. A serous membrane , e.g. the peritoneal covering of the abdominal viscera--serosal, adj.

سلی۔ غشاء مصلی: سیرم والی جھلی، مثلاً بطنی دسرا کا پیریٹونیل غلاف۔

Serositis *(se-ro-si'-tis)* [L. *serum* , whey; G. *itis,* inflammation]. inflammation of a serous membrane.

ورم بریشمہ: سیرم والی جھلی کی سوزش۔

Serotonin *(se-ro-ton-in)* A product of cell metabolism. Liberated by blood platelets after injury. Together with histamine may be concerned in allergic reaction.

سیروٹونن: خلوی میٹابولزم کا ایک پروڈکٹ۔ زخم کے بعد خونی پلیٹلیٹس خارج کرتے ہیں۔

Serous *(se'-rus)* [L. *serum,* whey]. Pertaining to serum. **serous membrane,** one lining a cavity which has no communication with the external air.

خونابی: مصلی سیرم سے متعلق۔

Serpasil *(ser'-pa-sil)* See RESERPINE.

سر پاسل: ریسرپین۔ سیبا کمپنی کی دوائی۔ ہائی بلڈ پریشر کے لئے ایک گولی صبح ایک دوپہر، ایک شام اگر بلڈ پریشر ہو تو یہی خوراک برائے فالج۔

Seriginous *(ser-pij'-in-us)* [L. *sepere,* to creep]. Snakelike, coiled, irregular and used to describe the margins of skin lesions, especially ulcers and ringworm.

سائی، تعبانیہ، دادزرہ: سانپ کی طرح، بے قاعدہ، جلدی زخموں کے کنارے بیان کرنے کے لئے مستعمل خصوصاً السر اور رنگ ورم۔

Serration *(ser-a'-shun)* [L. *serra,* saw]. A saw-like notch—serrated, *adj.*

دندانہ: آرے کی طرح کٹاؤ۔

Serum *(se'-rum)* [L. whey]. Supernatant fluid which forms when blood clots. **antitoxic s.,** prepared from the blood of an animal which has been immunized by the requisite toxin; it contains a high concentration of antitoxin. **serum sickness,** the symptoms arising as a reaction about ten days after the administration of serum; utricarial rash, pyrexia and joint pains—seta, *pl.*

سیرم، مصل: مائع جو خون جمنے کے بعد بچ رہتا ہے۔ خون سے خونی خلیوں اور فائبرن کے نکل جانے کے بعد بچنے والا مائع۔ کوئی ایسا ہی جسمانی مائع۔

Serum gonadotrophin *(se'-rum-gon-ad-o-tro'-fin)* An ovarian-stimulating hormone obtained from the blood serum of pregnant mares. It is used in amenorrhoea, often in association with oestrogens.

سیرم گونیڈوٹرافن: بیضہ دانی کو محرک کرنے والا ہارمون جسے حاملہ گھوڑیوں کے خونی سیرم سے حاصل کیا جاتا ہے۔

Sesamoid *(ses'-a-moid)* Resembling a seed. **sesamoid bones,** small bony masses formed in the tendons, e.g. the patella and the pisiform (wrist) bone.

دانہ دار، سمسم (تل) نما: بیج سے مشابہ۔

Sessile *(ses'-il)* [L. *sedere,* to sit]. Non-penduncculated; having a broad base.

بے ساقہ: بلا ڈنٹھل۔ چوڑا اساس رکھنا۔

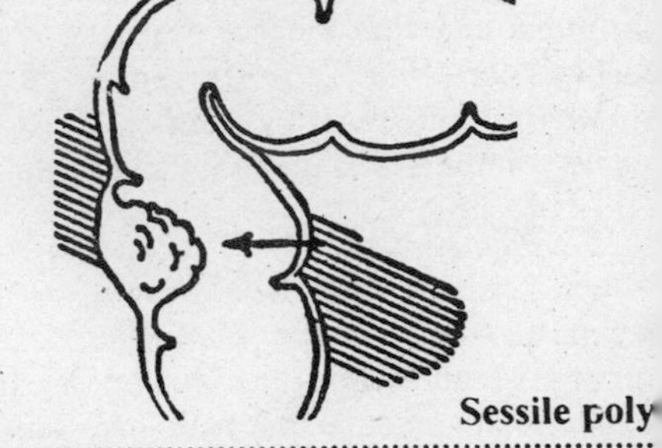

Sessile poly

Sex-linked. Refers to genes which are locate on the sexs chromosomes.

SGOT. Serum glutamic oxalacetic transaminas See TEST, ENZYME.

ایس جی او ٹی: سیرم گلوٹیمک آکسل لیسیٹک ٹرانس امینیز۔ نارمل ویلیو ۵ تا ... اکائیاں۔

SGPT. Serum glutamic pyruvic transminas See TEST, ENZYME.

ایس جی پی ٹی: سیرم گلوٹیمک پائیروک ٹرانس امینیز۔ نارمل ویلیو ۵ تا ۴۰ ... ئیاں۔

SH 420. Norethisterone (q.v.).

ایس ایچ ۴۲۰: ناراتھیسٹرون۔

Shelf operation. An open reduction of a coge ital dislocation of hip join, involving the u of a bone graft. Performed at 7 to 8 yea after failure of conservative treatment.

...ف اپریشن: چوتڑ کے جوڑ کی ڈسلوکیشن کی کھلی تخفیف۔ اس میں استخوانی ... کا تعلق ہے۔

Shigella *(she-gal'-a)* A genus of bacteria co taining some of the organisms causing dyse ry, *Shigella sonnei, S. flexneri, S. shigae.*

Shin bone. The tibia, the medial bone of t foreleg.

...ی کی ہڈی: ٹیبیا۔ پیش ٹانگ کی میانی ہڈی۔

Shingles. See HERPES.

...طقی: پرہیز

Shirodkar's operation. Placing of a pur string suture around an incompetent cerv during pregnancy. It is removed when lab starts.

...ن شروڈکر: حمل کے دوران سیو چڑ رکھنا جو دردزہ شروع ہونے پر ہٹا

دیا جاتا ہے۔

Shock. The circulatory disturbance produced by severe injury or illness and due in large part to reduction in blood volume. There is discrepancy between the circulating blood volume and the capacity of the vascular bed. Initial cause is reduction in circulating blood volume; perpetuation is due to vasoconstriction, therefore vosoconsrictor drugs are not given. Its features include a fall in blood pressure, rapid pulse, pallor, restlessness, thirst and a cold clammy skin.

صدمہ، چوٹ: سخت مرض یا زخم سے پیدا شدہ گردشی خرابی جس سے خونی حجم میں کمی واقع ہو جاتی ہے۔ اس کی علامات بلڈ پریشر میں کمی، تیز نبض، بے آرامی، پیاس اور ٹھنڈی جلد ہیں۔

Short-circuit operation. An anastomosis designed to bypass an obstruction in a conducting channel, e.g. gastrojejunostomy.

دورِ قیصر اپریشن: ایصالی راہ میں رکاوٹ کو بائی پاس کرنے کے لئے بنا ہوا جال۔

Short-sightedness. Myopia (q.v.).

قریب بصری: مائی اوپیا۔ دور کی نظر کا کمزور ہونا۔ دور کی اشیاء صاف اور واضح نظر نہیں آتیں۔ ایک ارتقائی رجحان۔ آنکھ کا ایک نقص۔

Shoulder girdle. Formed by the clavicle and scapula on either side.

نطاق شانہ: ہر سائیڈ پر سکیپولا اور ہنسلی کی ہڈی سے بنتا ہے۔

Shoulder lift. See AUSTRALIAN LIFT.

شولڈر لفٹ: آسٹریلیائی لفٹ۔

Show. A popular term for the blood-stained vaginal discharge at the commencement of labour.

نمائش: لیبر کے وقوع کے وقت خون سے رنگا ویجائنا کے ڈسچارج کے لئے معروف اصطلاح۔

Shunt. A term applied to the passage of blood through other than the usual channel.

Sialagogue *(si-al-a-gog)* [G. *sialon,* saliva; *agogos,* leading]. An agent which increases the flow of saliva.

تھوک آور: ایجنٹ جو لعاب دن کے بہاؤ کو بڑھاتا ہے۔

Sialogram *(si-al'-o-gram)* [G. *sialon,* saliva; *gramma,* letter]. Radiographic picture of the salivary glands and ducts, usually after injection of radio-opaque medium. sialography, *n.*; sialographic, *adj.*; sialographically, *adv.*

سیالوگرام: عموماً ریڈیو اوپیک واسطے کے انجکشن کے بعد سلوری غدود اور نالیوں کی ریڈیوگرافک تصویر۔

Sialolith *(si'-al-o-lith)* [G. *sialon,* salive; *lithos,* stone]. A stone in a salivary gland or duct.

حصاۃ غدہ ریقیہ: سلوری گلینڈ یا نالی میں پتھری۔

Sibling *(sib'-ling)* One of a family of children having the same parents.

بہن بھائی، ہم مادر پدر: ایک ہی والدین کے بچوں کی فیملی کا ایک بھائی اور بہن۔

Sickle-cell anaemia. Familial, hereditary haemolytic anaemia peculiar to Negroes. The red cells are crescent-shaped.

داسی خلیاتی بھس: اس میں سرخ خونی خلیے ہلالی شکل کے ہوتے ہیں۔ یہ عارضہ حبشیوں کے ساتھ مخصوص ہے۔

Side effect. any physiological change other than the desired one from drug administration, e.g. the antispasmodic drug propantheline cause the s.e. of dry mouth in some patients. The term also covers undesirabe drug reactions. Some are predictable being the result of a known metabolic action of the drug, e.g. yellowing of skin and eyes with mepacrine; thining of skin and bone and formation of striae with corticosteroid; loss of hair with cyclophosphamide. Unpredictable reactions can be: (1) Immediate; anaphylactic shock, angioneurotic oedema. (2) Erythematous; all forms of erythema, including nodosum and multiforms and purpuric rashes. (3) Cellular reactions; eczematous rashes and contact dermatitis. (4) Specific reactions; e.g. light-sensitive eruptions with Ledermycine and griseofulvin.

غیر مفید اثر: دوائی سے کوئی ایسی فزیالوجیکل تبدیلی جسکی خواہش نہ کی گئی ہو۔

Siderosis *(sid-er-o'-sis)* [G. *sideros,* iron; *-osis,* condition]. Excess of iron in the blood or tissues. Inhalation of iron oxide into the lungs can produce a s. as one form of pneumoconiosis (q.v.).

آہنیت: خون یا بافتوں میں لوہے کی زیادتی۔

Sigmamycin *(sig-ma-mi'-cin)* Capsules of tetracycline (q.v.) and oleandomycine (q.v.). The mixture is claimed to have a wider range of activity than either antibiotic alone.

سگما مائی سین: ٹیٹرا سائیکلین اور اولی بنڈو مائیسین کے کیپسول۔ ایک کیپسول ہر چھ گھنٹے بعد۔

Sigmoid *(sig'-moid)* [G. letter sigma]. Shaped like the letter **S. sigmoid flexure,** an S-shaped curve joining the descending colon above to the recturm below.

سگمائی: انگریزی حرف ایس کی شکل کا۔

Sigmoidoscope *(sig-moid'-o-skop)* [G. letter sigma; *skopein,* to examine]. An instrument for visualizing the rectum and sigmoid flexure of the colon. See ENDOSCOPE—sigmoido-

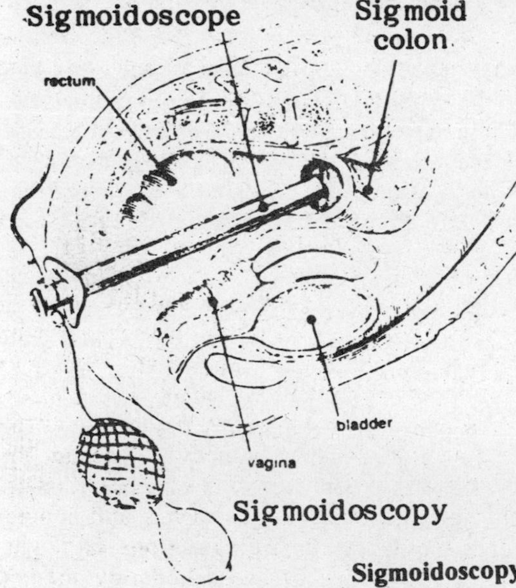

Sigmoidoscopy

دوخمہ بین: قولون کے سگمائیڈ فلیکسر اور ریکٹم کو دیکھنے کے لئے ایک آلہ۔

Sigmoidostomy *(sig-moid-os'-to-mi)* [G. letter sigma; *stoma,* mouth]. The formation of a colostomy in the sigmoid (pelvic) colon.

دوخمہ قولونی تفویہ: سگمائیڈ یا پیٹرو کے قولون میں کولوسٹومی کا بننا۔

Sign *(sin)* [L. *signum*]. any objective evidence of disease.

علامت: مرض کا کوئی معروضی ثبوت۔

Silbephylline *(sil-bef'-i-lin)* Diprophylline (q.v.).

سلبیفلین: ڈائی پروفلین۔

Silicones *(si'-li-kons)* Organic compounds which are water-repellant.

سلیکونات: پانی دھکیلنے والے نامیاتی مرکبات۔

Silicosis *(si-li-ko'-sis)* [L. *silex,* flint; G. *-osis,* condition]. Fibrosis of the lung form the inhalation of uncombined silica. A form of pneumoconiosis or 'industrial dust disease', found in metal grinders, stone-workers, etc.

سیلیکیت: خالی سیلیکا کے سانس کے ذریعے اندر جانے سے پھیپھڑے کا فائبروسس

Silver nitrate *(sil'-ver-ni'-trat)* In the form of small sticks, is used as a caustic of warts. Occasionally used as antiseptic eye drops (1 per cent), and as an application to ulcers. Now being used 1/2 per cent solution for burns to control bacterial infection in postburn period. Causes sodium and chloride loss from wound surface. Sodium chloride given orally or intravenously. Urine tested for chlorides.

سلور نائٹریٹ، سنگ جہنم: ایک سفید حل پذیر قلمی نمک، نقطہ پگھلاؤ ۲۰۹° س، مارکر کی سیاہی، ادویات اور کیمیائی تجزیہ میں استعمال جاتا ہے۔ سالمی وزن ۱۶۹٫۸۷ کھانے پر نقصان دہ ٹھوس اور محلول آنکھوں میں جلن اور جلد پر آبلے ڈالتے ہیں۔

Silver sulphadiazine *(sil'-ver-sul-fa-di'-a-zen)* Silver derivative of sulphadiazine (q.v.). Topical bacteriostatic agent.

Silverman score. A method of rating respiratory distress by assessing movement of accessory muscles and degree of expiratory grunt.

سلور مین سکور: تنفسی تکلیف کی شرح کا طریقہ۔

Simmonds' disease. Patient becomes **emaciated,** suffers from early senility; face **unduly wrinkled,** hair grey and sparse, blood pressure low, pulse slow, bones become frail. Preeviously incorrectly called hypopituitary cachexia. [Morris Simmonds, physician in Germany, 1855-1925].

مرض سمنڈز: مریض پر بڑھاپا چھایا دکھائی دیتا ہے۔ چہرے پر جھریاں، بال سفید، بلڈ پریشر کم، نبض کمزور اور ہڈیاں کمزور ہو جاتی ہیں۔ اس مرض کو جرمنی میں فزیشن موریس سمنڈز (۱۸۵۵ء تا ۱۹۲۵ء) کے نام سے موسوم کیا گیا۔ وقت سے پہلے بڑھاپا۔

Sinemet *(sin-i-met)* Levodopa (q.v.), combined with carbidopa (q.v.) in 10:1 ratio.

Sinequan *(sIn-e-qwan)* Doxepin (q.v.).

سائین کوئین: ڈوکسپین۔ ۱۰ اور ۲۵ ملی گرام کے کیپسول۔ یہ دوا دماغ اور موڈ پر اثر کرتی ہے۔ گھبراہٹ، پریشانی اور وہم دور کرنے میں کارآمد، ڈیومیکس کمپنی کی دوائی۔

Sinew *(sin-u)* A ligament or tendon.

وتر، طنب: لگمنٹ یا ٹنڈان۔

Sinoatrial node *(si'-no-at-ri-al)* See NODE.

Sinogram *(si'-no-gram)* [L. *sinus,* cavity; G. *gramma,* letter]. Radiographic picture of a sinus after injection of radio-opaque medium.

سائینو گرام: ریڈیو اوپیک واسطے کے انجکشن کے بعد سائنس کی ریڈیو گرافک تصویر۔

Sintisone *(sin'-ti-son)* Oral preparation of prenisolone that does not produce 'mooning' of face.

سنٹی سون: پریڈرنیسولوں سے تیار شدہ منہ کے ذریعے کھائی جانے والی دوا۔

Sinus *(si'-nus)* [L.]. 1. A hollow or cavity, especially the nasal sinuses. 2. A channel containing blood, especially venous blood, e.g. the sinuses of the brain. 3. A recess or cavity within a bone. 4. Any suppurating tract or channel. **coronary s., the dilated terminal part** of the great cardiac vein. It is about 25.4 mm in length and opens into the right atrium. **frontal s.,** two cavities in the frontal bone, one on each side of the medial line, which open into the upper part of the nasal cavity — See PILONIDAL CAVERNOUS.

جوف عظم، ناسور، جوف دمل: (۱) ایک کھوکھلا یا کہفہ۔ خصوصاً نتھنے۔ ان سے ہڈیوں کا بوجھ کم ہوتا ہے اور آواز میں ریزوننس پیدا ہوتی ہے۔

(۲) خون خصوصاً وریدی خون پر مشتمل چینیل مثلاً دماغ۔

(۳) ہڈی کے اندر کہف۔

(۴) کوئی سہارا دینے والا راستہ یا چینل۔

Sinusitis *(si-nu-si-tis)* [L. *sinus,* hollow; G. *-itis,* inflammation]. Inflammation of a sinus, used exclusively for the paranasal sinuses.

ورم جوف انفی: کہفہ کی سوزش۔ ناک کی ملحقہ ہڈیوں میں خلا۔ زکام لگنے کے دوران میں بلغم ریشہ اکٹھا ہو کر سوزش ہو جاتی ہے۔ سر میں درد ہوتا ہے۔ بخار بھی ہوتا ہے۔

Sinusoid *(si-nu-soid)* [L. *sinus,* hollow; G. *eidos,* form]. A dilated channel into which arterioles open in some organs and which take the place of the usual capillaries.

جوف خون: ایک کشادہ چینل جس میں چھوٹی شریانیں بعض اعضاء میں کھلتی ہیں اور جو عام شریانوں کی جگہ لیتی ہیں۔

Sitz-bath *(sits-bath)* [G. *sitzen,* to sit]. Hip bath.

نشستی غسل: ہپ باتھ۔

Sjogren-Larssonsyndrome. Genetically determined congenital ectodermosis. Associated with mental subnormality.

سجور گرین لارسن سنڈروم: جینی طور پر متعین مرض ایکٹوڈرموسس۔ ذہنی پسماندگی کے ساتھ وابستہ۔

Sjogren's syndrome *(swa'-grens)* Deficient secretion from lacrimal, salivary and other glands, mostly in postmenopausal women. There is keratoconjunctivitis, dry tongue and hoarse voice. Thought to be due to an autoimmune process. Also called **keratoconjunctivitis sicca.** [Henrick Samuel Conra Sjogren, Swodish ophthlmologist, 1899---].

سجور گرین سنڈروم: زیادہ تر پوسٹ مینوپازل خواتین میں لکریمل۔ سلوری اور دوسری غدود سے رطوبت میں کمی۔ زبان خشک اور آواز بیٹھی ہوئی۔

Skeleton *(skel-e-ton)* The bony frame-work of the body, supporting and protecting the soft tissues and organs. **appendicular s.,** the bones forming the upper and lower extremities, **axial s.,** the bones forming the head and trunk —skeletal, *adj*.

پنجر، ڈھانچہ: جسم کا ہڈی دار فریم ورک جو نرم بافتوں اور اعضاء کو سہارا دیتا

ہے اوران کی حفاظت کرتا ہے۔

Sketaton

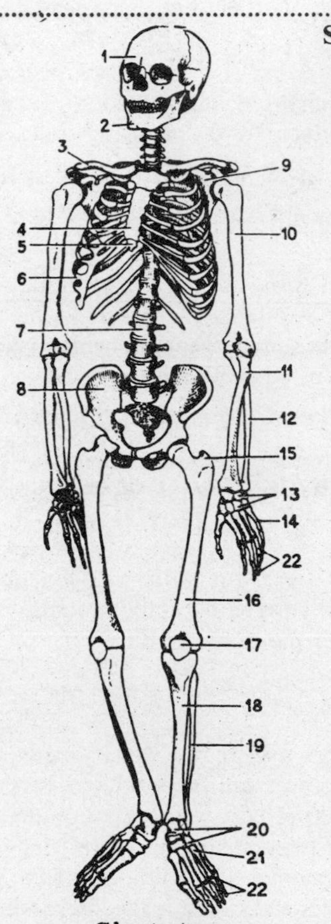

Sketaton

1. Skull, 2. Mandible, 3. Clavicle or collar-bone, 4. Sternum or breast-bone, 5. Xiphoid process, 6. Ribs, 7. spine, 8. Pelvis, 9. Scapula or shoulder-blade, 10. Humerus, 11. Radius, 12. Ulna, 13. Carpal bones, 14. Metacarpal bones, 15. Trochanter, 16. Femur, 17. Patella or knee-cap, 18. Tibia, 19. Fibula, 20. Tarsal bones, 21. Metatarsal bones, 22. Phalanges.

skene's glands. Two smallglands at the entrance to the female urethra; the paraurethral glands. [Alexander Johnston Chalmers Skene, American gynaecologist, 1838-1900].

سکینز گلینڈز: مادہ یورتھرا کے داخلے کی جگہ پر دو چھوٹی غدود۔ پیرایورتھرل غدود۔

Skin. The tissue which forms the outer covering of the body; it consists of two man layers: (1) the epidermis, or cuticle, forming the outer coat; (2) the dermis, or cuitis vera, the inner or true skin, lying beneath the epidermis.

Skin

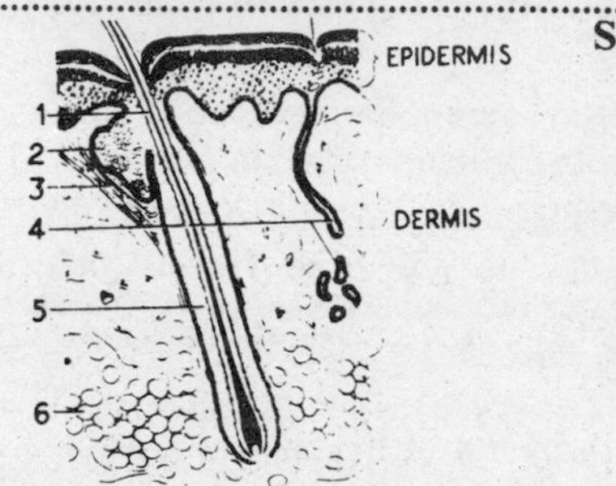

SECTION OF HUMAN SKIN

1. Hair in follicle, 2. Sebacceous gland, 3. *Erector pili* muscle 4. Sweat glands, 5. Root sheath, 6. Fat and subcutaneous tissue, 7. Pore.

جلد: نسیج جو جسم کا بیرونی غلاف بناتا ہے۔ یہ دو بڑی پرتوں پر مشتمل ہے:

(۱) اپی ڈرمس یا کیوٹیکل جو بیرونی کوٹ بناتی ہے۔

(۲) ڈرمس یا کیوٹس ویرا۔ اندرونی یا اصل جلد جو اپی ڈرمس کے نیچے ہوتی ہے۔ جلد کی چھوت یا سکن انفکشن جلد پر موجود سٹیفا ئلو کا کسی جراثیم کی وجہ سے ہوتی ہے، اس لئے غسل ضروری ہے۔

Skopyl *(skop-il)* Methylscopolamine (q.v.).

Skull. The bony framework of the head. See CRANIUM.

کھوپڑی، جمجمہ: سر کا ہڈی والا فریم ورک۔ کھوپڑی میں کاسہ سر یا کرینیئم کی ۸ چہرہ کی ۷ اور ناک کی ۷ یعنی کل ۲۲ ہڈیاں ہوتی ہیں۔ ان میں سے صرف زیریں جبڑے کی ہڈی حرکت کر سکتی ہے۔

Sleeping sickness. A disease endemic in Africa, characterizsed by increasing somnolence caused by infectionof the brain by trypanosomes. See TRYPANOSOMIASIS.

مرض النوم، نوام: ٹرائی پنوسوما سے ہونے والی دماغی بیماری نیند لانے والی بیماری۔ علاج کیلئے سورامین اور ٹرائی پارسے مائیڈ۔

Sleep-walking. See SOMNAMBULISM.

خواب خرامی: سومنیمبولزم۔

Slough *(sluf)* Septic tissue which becomes

necrosed and separates from the healthy tissue.

کھرنڈ: تعفن والانسیج جوصحت مندنسیج سے الگ ہوجاتا ہے۔

Slow K. Slow-release potassium chloride.

ست پوٹاشیم: آہستہ ریلیز پوٹاشیم کلورائیڈ۔

Smallpox. Variola. Caused by a virus eradicated from most parts of the world following WHO campaign. Headache, vomiting and high fever precede the eruption of a widespread rash which is papular, vesicular and finally pustular. The eruption follows a set pattern of dissemination, commencing on the head and face. When the final stage of desiccation is pased scars (pockmarks) are left to disfigure the skin. Prophylaxis against the disease is by vaccination. See VACCINIA.

جدری چیچک، ماتا: ایک وائرس سے ہونے والا مرض، ماتا سے مشابہہ، سر درد، متلی اور زیادہ بخار کے بعد جسم پر دانے نکل آتے ہیں۔ جب یہ مرحلہ گزر جاتا ہے تو جلد پر نشان رہ جاتے ہیں جن سے جلد بدصورت ہوجاتی ہے۔ اس کے لئے حفاظتی ٹیکہ یا ویکسین لگائی جاتی ہے۔ اب دنیا سے اس مرض کا خاتمہ کر دیا گیا ہے۔

Smear A film of meterial spread out on a glass side for microscopic examination. **cervical s.,** microscopic examination of cells scraped from the cervix to detect carcinoma-in-situ. See CARCINOMA.

سمیئر: خوردبینی جانچ کے لیے شیشے کی سلائیڈ پر پھیلائے گئے میٹریل کی فلم

Smegma *(smeg'-ma)* [G. *unguent*]. The sebaceous secretion which accumulates beneath the prepuce and clitoris.

صابونیہ: چربی دار یا سیبیش اخراج جو سر ذکر کی کھال اور کلائیٹورس کے نیچے جمع ہوجاتا ہے۔

Smelling salts A mixture of compounds usually containing some form of ammonia, which acts as a stimulant, when inhaled.

امونیم کاربونیٹ۔ لخلخہ: مرکبات کا آمیزہ جس میں کسی قسم کی امونیا بھی ہوتی ہے، جواندر سانس لینے پر محرک کے طور پر کام کرتی ہے۔

Smith-Petersen nail A frifid, cannulated metal nail used to provide internal fixation for intracapsular fractures of the femoral neck. [Marius Nygaard Smith Petersen, American surgeon, 1886-1953.]

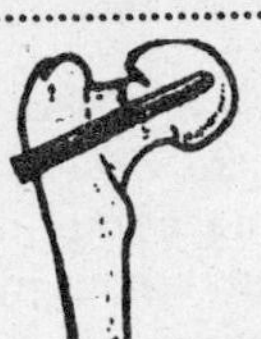

Smith-Petersen nail

سمتھ پیٹرسن کیل: ایک دھاتی کل جو فیمورل گردن کے انٹرا کیپسولر فریکچرز کے اندرونی فیکشین کے لیے استعمال کیا جاتا ہے۔ اسے ایک امریکی سرجن سمتھ پیٹرسن (۱۸۸۶ء تا ۱۹۵۳ء) کے نام سے موسوم کیا گیا۔

Snare *(snar)*. A surgical instrument with a wire loop at the end; used for removal of polypi.

رسولی کاٹ تار: ایک سرجیکل آلہ جس کے سرے پر تار کا لوپ ہوتا ہے

Snellen's test types A chart for testing visual acuity. [Hermann Snellen, Dutch ophthalmologist, 1834-1908].

سنیلنز ٹیسٹ ٹائپس: تیز نظری کو ٹیسٹ کرنے کے لئے چارٹ۔

Snow Solid carbon dioxide. Used for local freezing of the tissues in minor surgery.

یخ: ٹھوس کاربن ڈائی آکسائیڈ معمولی سرجری میں بافتوں کے مقامی انجماد کے لئے مستعمل۔

Snuffles *(snuf'-lz)*. A snorting inspiration due to congestion of nasal mucous membrane. It is a sign of early congenital (prenatal) syphilis when the nasal discharge may be purulent or bloodstained.

سوں سوں کرنا: نیزل میوکس جھلی کے اجتماع خون کی وجہ سے خراٹے کے ساتھ اندر کی طرف سانس لینا۔

Sociocultural *(so-si-o-kul'-tur-al)*. Pertaining to culture in its sociological setting.

معاشرتی، ثقافتی: سماجی سیٹنگ میں کلچر سے متعلق۔

Sociology *(so-si-ol'-o-ji)* [L. *socius*, companion; G. *logos* discourse]. The scientific study of interpersonal and intergroup social relationship--sociological adj.

عمرانیات: بین شخصی اور بین گروہی سوشل تعلقات کا سائنسی مطالعہ۔

Sociomedical *(so-si-o-med'-ik-al)* . Pertaining to the problems of medicine as affected by soc -iology (q.v.)

سماجی طبی: سوشیالوجی سے متاثر ہوکرادویہ کے مسائل سے متعلق۔

Sodium acetrizoate *(so'-di-um-a-set-tri-zo-at)*. An organic iodine compound used as a contrast agent in intravenous pyelography.

سوڈیم ایسٹری زوایٹ: ایک نامیاتی آیوڈین مرکب۔

Sodium acid phosphate *(so'-di-um-as'-id-fos'-fat)*. Saline purgative and diuretic. It increases the acidity of the urine, and is given with hexamine as a urinary antiseptic.

سوڈیم ایسڈ فاسفیٹ: نمکین جلاب آور اور پیشاب آور۔ یہ پیشاب کی تیزابیت کو بڑھاتا ہے۔

Sodium and megluminediatrizoates *(so'-di-um-meg'-lu-min-di-a-tri-zo'-atz)* Water soluble, radio--opaque form of iodine given before an X-ray using a fluorescent screen.

Sodium amytal Amylobarbitone (q.v.)

سوڈیم امائٹل: ایمائیلو باربیٹون۔

Sodium antimonylgluconate *(so'-di-um-an-tim-on-il-gloo'-kon-at)*. Used intravenously in schistosomiasis.

سوڈیم اینٹی مونائل گلوکونیٹ: سکسٹوسومیاسس میں مستعمل۔

Sodium antimony tartrate *(so'-di-um an-tim '-on- il-gloo'-kon-at)*. Used intravenously in schis- tosomiasis.

سوڈیم انٹی منی ٹارٹریٹ: ایس اے ٹی۔ سکسٹوسومیاسس میں مستعمل۔

Sodium benzoate *(so'-di-um-ben'-zo-at)*. An acidifying diuretic, given when a lowering of the urinary pH is desired.

سوڈیم بنزوایٹ: ایک سفید حل پذیر سفوف۔ دافع تعفن اور خوراک محفوظ کرنے کے لئے استعمال کیا جاتا ہے۔ تیزابیت بڑھانے والا۔ پیشاب آور۔ جب بولی پی ایچ کم کرنا ہو تو دیا جاتا ہے۔

Sodium bicarbonate *(so'-di-um-bi-kar'-bon-at)*. A domestic antacid, given for heartburn, etc. For prolonged therapy alkalis that cause less rebound acidity are preferred.

سوڈیم بائی کاربونیٹ: سوڈیم ہائیڈروجن کاربونیٹ۔ ایک سفید حل پذیر سفوف۔ بیکنگ پوڈر۔ آگ بجھانے اور ادویات میں استعمال کیا جاتا ہے

سالمی وزن ۸۴،۰۱۔ دل کی جلن وغیرہ میں گھریلو استعمال کی چیز۔

Sodium chloride *(so'-di-um-klor'-id)*. Salt present in body tissues. Used extensively in shock and dehydration as intravenous normal saline, or as dextrosesaline in patients unable to take fluids by mouth. Used orally as replacement therapy in Addison's disease, in which salt loss is high. When salt is lost from the body , there is compensating production of renin (q.v.)

سوڈیم کلورائڈ۔ نمک طعام: عام نمک یا خوردنی نمک۔ ایک سفید قلمی حل پذیر نمک' نقطۂ پگھلاؤ ۸۰۱ سم سمندری پانی میں کثرت سے پایا جاتا ہے۔ نمک کی کانیں پاکستان میں کھیوڑہ اور کالا باغ میں سالمی وزن ۵۸،۴۴۔ کانی نمک کے طور پر بکثرت ملتا ہے۔ جسمانی بافتوں میں موجود صدمہ پہنچنے اور ڈیہائیڈ ریشن میں مستعمل۔ مرض ایڈیسن میں نمک کے زیادہ ضیاع کی صورت میں منہ کے ذریعے دیا جاتا ہے۔

Sodium citrate *(so'-di-um sit'-rat)*. An alkaline diuretic very similar to potassium citrate. Used also as an anticoagulant for stored blood, and as an to milk feeds to reduce curdling.

سوڈیم سائٹریٹ: ایک الکلائن پیشاب آور۔ پوٹاشیم سٹریٹ سے مشابہ

Sodium fusidate *(so'-di-um fu'-si-dat)* Expensive drug for the treatment of staphylococcal infections.

سوڈیم فیوسی ڈیٹ: سٹیفائلوکاکسی سے ہونے والے امراض کے علاج کے لئے مہنگی دوائی۔

Sodium gentisate *(so'-di-um jen-tis'-at)*. A salicylate-like compound, used in rheumatic conditions when salicyltes are not tolerated.

سوڈیم جینٹی سیٹ: جوڑوں کے درد میں مفید دوا۔

Sodium iodide *(so'-di-um i-o-did)*. Used occasionally as an expectorant, and as a contrast agent in retrograde pyelography.

سوڈیم آیوڈائیڈ: ایک سکلیر وزنگ ایجنٹ۔

Sodium morrhuate *(so'-di-um mor'-ru-at)*. A sclerosing agent sometimes used in the obliterative treatment of varicose veins.

سوڈیم مورہوایٹ: ایک سکلیر وزنگ ایجنٹ۔

Sodium perborate *(so'-di-um per-bor'-at)*. Aqueous solutions have antiseptic properties similar to those of hydrogen peroxide, and are used as mouth-washes, etc.

سوڈیم پر بوریٹ: ایک سفید حل پذیر قلمی مرکب، نقطۂ پگھلاؤ ۶۳ سم، بطور رنگ کاٹ اور دافع تعفن استعمال کیا جاتا ہے۔ آبی محلول ہائیڈروجن پر آکسائیڈ کی طرح دافع تعفن خواص رکھتے ہیں اور ماؤتھ واش کے طور پر استعمال کئے جاتے ہیں۔

Sodium propionate *(so'-di-um pro'-pi-on-at)*. Used as an antimycotic in fungal infections as gel, ointment, lotion and pessaries.

سوڈیم پروپیونیٹ: جیل، مرہم یا لوشن کی صورت میں سماروغی امراض میں بطور اینٹی مائیکوٹک مستعمل۔

Sodium salicylate (so'-di-um sal-is'-il-at). Has the analgestic action of salicylates in general, but of particualr value in rheumatic fever. Large doses are essential. Chronic rheumatiod conditions do not respond so well.

سوڈیم سیلی سائی لیٹ: مکسن دوا۔ درد کے بخار میں مفید۔

Sodium stibogluconate *(so'-di-um stib-o-gloo'-kon-at)*. Used in treatment of leishmaniasis.

سوڈیم سٹیبوگلوکونیٹ: لشمانیاسس میں مفید۔

Sodium sulphate *(so'-di-um sul'-fat)*. A popular domestic purgative. A 25 per cent solution is used as a wound dressing. Given intravenously as a 4.3 per cent solution in anuria.

گلابری نمک ۔ گلابرز سالٹ: سالٹ کیک۔ ایک سفید حل پذیر قلمی نمک رنگوں اور صابن کی تیاری میں استعمال کیا جاتا ہے۔ سالمی وزن ۱۴۲٫۴، ایک معروف گھریلو جلاب ۲۵ فیصد محلول زخم کی ڈریسنگ کے لیے استعمال کیا جاتا ہے۔

Soframycin *(sof-ra-mi'-sin)*. Framycetin (q.v.)

سوفرامائی سین: فرامسٹن۔

Soft sore The primary ulcer of the genitalia occurring in the venereal disease chancroid (q.v.)

سافٹ سور: اعضائے تولید کی پرائمری رسولی۔

Solacen *(sol'-a-sen)*. Tybamate (q.v.)

سولیسن: ٹائیامیٹ

Solapsone *(sol-ap'-son)*. Chemically related to dapsone (q.v.)

سولیپ سون: ڈیپسون سے کیمیائی تعلق۔

Solar plexus *(so'-lar pleks'- us)*. A large network of sympathetic (autonomic) nerve ganglia and fibres, extending from one adrenal gland to the other. It uspplied the abdominal organs.

شمسی صنفیرہ: سمپتھیٹک عصبی گینگلینا اور فائیرز کا جال جو ایک ایڈرینل گلینڈ سے دوسری کی طرف پھیلا ہوا ہے۔ یہ بطنی اعضاء کو جاتا ہے۔

Solpadeine *(sol'-pa-den)*. Soluble tables of paracetamol with codeine and caffeine.

Solute *(sol-ut')* That which is dissolved in a fluid.

منحل: ایسی شے جو محلل میں حل ہو کر محلول بنائے۔

Solution *(sol-u'-shun)*. A fluid which contains a dissolved substance, saturated s., one in which as much of the solid is dissolved as will be held in solution without depositing or floating.

مُحلول: مختلف سالمی ساخت کی دو یا زیادہ اشیاء کا یکساں یا یک جان سالمی آمیزہ۔ اس لفظ کا اطلاق عموماً ٹھوس کا مائع میں حل ہونے پر ہوتا ہے۔

Solvent *(sol'-vent)*. An agent which is capable of dissolving other substances.

محلل: ایسی شے جو دوسری اشیاء کو اپنے اندر حل کرنے کی طاقت رکھتی ہو، یہ عموماً مائع ہوتا ہے۔ جس میں دوسری اشیاء حل ہو جاتی ہیں۔ محلول کا وہ جزو جس کی طبی حالت وہی ہوتی ہے، جو محلول کی ہوتی ہے۔ مثلاً پانی میں شکر کے محلول (شربت) میں پانی محلل ہے جبکہ شکر منحل ہے۔

Somatic *(so-mat'-ik)* [G. *somatikos*, of the body]. Pertaining to the body. **somatic nerves,** nerves controlling the activity of striated, skeletal muscle.

جسمانی: جسم سے متعلق۔ جسمانی خلیے وہ خلیے ہوتے ہیں جن سے کسی جسم کا جسم بنتا ہے۔ غیر تولیدی خلیے۔

Somatostain *(so-ma-to-stat'-in)* Growth hormone release-inhibiting hormone (GH-RIH). Remarkable hypothalamic tetradecapeptide.

Somatotrophin *(so-ma-to-tro'-fin)* [G. *soma*, body; *trophe*, nourishment]. The growth factor secreted by anterior pituitary gland.

سومیٹوٹرافن: امامی پیٹوٹیری گلینڈ سے خارج ہونے والا نمو کا عامل۔

Somnabulism *(som-nam'-bu-lizm)* [L. *somnus*, sleep; *ambulare*, to walk]. Sleepwalking; a state of dissociated consciousness in which sleeping and waking states are combined. Considered normal in children but as an illness having a hysterical basis in adults.

خواب خرامی: نیند میں چلنا۔ اس میں سونے اور جاگنے کی کیفیات مل جاتی ہیں۔

Sonalgin *(son-al'-jin)* Butobarbitone (q.v.), codeine (q.v.) and phenacetin (q.v.).

Soneryl *(son'-er-il)* Butobarbitone (q.v.).

سونریل: بوٹوباربیٹون۔ خواب آور۔ ایک گولی سوتے وقت۔

Sonicaid *(son'-i-kad)* Diagnostic ultrasound machine used to detect movement inside body.

Sonne dysentery *(son'-ne-dis'-en-ter-i)* Bacillary dysentery caused by infection with *Shigella sonnei* (Sonne bacillus), the commonest form of dysentery in the United Kingdom. The organism is excreted by cases and carriers in their faeces, and contaminates hands, food and water, from which new hosts are infected. [Carl Sonne, Danish bacteriologist, 1882 - 1948].

سونے پیچش: بیلری پیچش۔

Sonograph *(so'-no-graf)* Graphic record of sound waves.

سونوگراف: مادہ تولیدی اعضاء پر اطلاق شدہ صوتی لہروں کی دخل اندازی کا گرافک ریکارڈ۔

Soporific *(sop-or-if'-ik)* [L. *sopor*, sleep; *facere*, to make]. An agent which induees profound sleep.

منوم دواء: گہری نیند لانے والا ایجنٹ۔

Sorbide nitrates *(sor'-bid-nit-rat)* Improves effort tolerance in angina.

سوربائیڈ نائٹریٹ: درد دل یا انجینا میں کوشش برداشت کو بہتر بناتا ہے۔

Sorbitol *(sor'-bit-al)* Liquid for parenteral feeding.

Sordes *(sor'-dez)* [L.]. Dried, brown crusts which form in the mouth, especially on the lips and teeth, in illness.

پپڑی: خشک بھورے کرسٹ جو منہ میں بنتے ہیں، خصوصاً لبوں اور دانتوں پر، بیماری میں۔

Souffle *(soo'-fl)* [F.]. Puffing or blowing sound. **funic s.**, auscultatory murmur of pregnancy Synchronizes with the fetal heart-beat and i caused by pressure on the umbilical cord **uterine s.**, soft, blowing murmur which ca be auscultated over the uterus after the fourt month of pregnancy.

سرسراہٹ: آواز پیدا کرنا۔ مسلسل ہلکی آواز جو انگلی مارنے سے چھاتی یا رحم سے نکلے۔

Sound. An instrument to be introduced into hollow organ or duct so as to detect a stone o to dilate a stricture.

صوت، آواز: ایک فعلیاتی حس جسے کان وصول کرتا ہے۔ جب کوئی چیز ت تیزی کے ساتھ مرتعش ہوتی ہے یا لرزتی ہے تو آواز پیدا ہوتی ہے۔ یہ ب قسم کی توانائی ہے۔ آواز جانے کیلئے واسطے کی ضرورت ہوتی ہے۔ آواز ولی موجوں کی صورت میں چلتی ہے۔ جب کوئی جسم ایک ثانیہ میں کم از کم ۲۰ مرتعش ہو تو آواز پیدا ہوتا ہے۔ ۲۰ ہزار سے زیادہ تعدد کی آواز بالا صوتی ہلاتی ہے۔ کسی کھوکھلے عضو یا نلی میں داخل کرنے کے لئے استعمال کیا جاتا ہے۔

Sourdille's operation. Multiple-stage operatic for the relief of deafness. See FENESTRAT ION. [Maurice Sourdille, French otologis 1885-1961].

ورڈلیز اپریشن: بہرہ پن کے آرام کے لئے کئی مراحل والا اپریشن۔

Soya bean *(soi'-a-ben)* A highly nutritio legume used in Asiatic countries in place meat. It contains high-quality protein ar little starch. Is useful in diabetic preparation

ا دار لیگوم: ایشیائی ممالک میں گوشت کی جگہ مستعمل۔ اس میں پروٹین ده اور نشاستہ کم ہوتا ہے۔

Spansules. A chemical means of prepari drugs so that there is controlled release v oral route.

ن سیولز: ادویہ تیار کرنے کا کیمیائی ذریعہ۔

Sparine. Promazine (q.v.).

رین: پرومازین۔

Spasm. Convulsive, involuntary muscular c traction.

غ، اینٹھن: بلا ارادہ عضلے کا سکڑنا۔

Spasmolytic *(spas-mo-lit'-ik)* Current term antispasmodic drugs—spasmolysis, *n.*

دافع تشنج دواء: اینٹی سپاسموڈک ادویہ۔

actic *(spas'-tik)* [G. *spastikos,* drawing in]. In a condition of muscular rigidity or spasm, e.g. spastic diplegia (Little's disease (q.v.)).

متشنج، سخت: عضلاتی سختی یا سپازم کی حالت میں۔

actity *(spas-ti-it-i)* [G. *spastikos,* drawing in]. Condition of rigidity or spasm.

اینٹھن: سختی یا سپازم کی حالت۔

atula *(spat-u-la)* A flat flexible knife with blunt edges for making poultices and spreading ointment. **tongue s.,** a rigid, blade-shaped instrument for depressing the tongue.

کفچہ: ایک چپٹا لچک دار چاقو جس کے سرے کند ہوتے ہیں اور وہ پولٹس بنانے اور مرہم پھیلانے کے کام آتا ہے۔

ecies *(spe'-shez)* [L. kind]. A subdivision of genus. A group of individuals having common characteristics and differing only in minor details.

نوع: جماعت بندی کی سب سے چھوٹی اکائی جس کے ارکان ایک دوسرے کے ساتھ مشابہت رکھتے ہیں اور باہمی عمل تولید کرتے ہیں۔

ecific *(spe-sif'-ik)* [L. *species,* kind; *facere,* to make]. Special; characteristic; peculiar to **specific disease,** one that is always caused by a specified organism. **specific gravity,** the weight of a substance, as compared with that of an equal volume of water, the latter being represented by 1000.

نوعی، مخصوص: کسی نوع کی خصوصیت، خاص۔

ectrophotometer *(spek-tro-fo-tom'-et-er)* A spectroscope combined with a photometer for quantitatively measuring the relative intensity of different parts of a light spectrum.

طیفی ضیاء پیما: دونوری اشعاع طول موج، طول موج سے موازنہ کے لئے فوٹو میٹر۔

ectroscope *(spek-tro-skop)* An instrument for observing spectra of light.

طیف بین: طیفوں کے مشاہدہ یا طیفی تجزیہ کے لئے ایک آلہ۔

eculum *(spek-u-lum)* [L. mirror]. An instrument used to hold the walls of a cavity apart, so that the interior of the cavity can be examined—specula, *pl.*

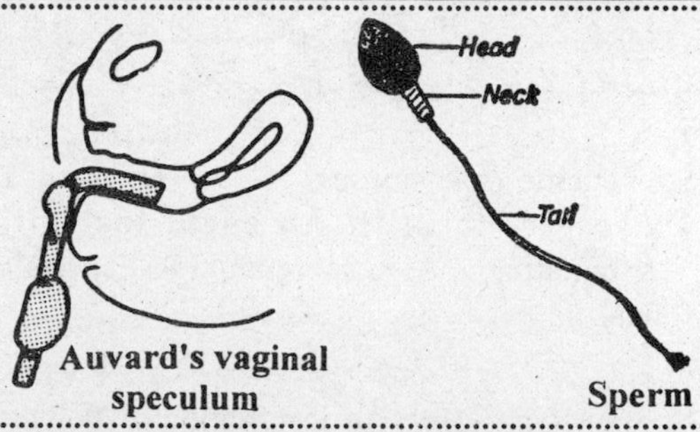

Auvard's vaginal speculum

Sperm

Sperm [G. *sperma,* seed]. Abbreviation for spermatozoon.

کرم منی، نطفہ: سپرمیٹوزون کے لیے مختصر اصطلاح۔ ہر کام کا ایک گول سر، ایک درمیانی جسم اور ایک دم ہوتی ہے ۔ یہ بہت چھوٹے ہوتے ہیں اور خوردبین سے نظر آتے ہیں۔

Spermatic *(sper-mat'-ik)* [G. *sperma,* seed]. Pertaining to or conveying semen. **spermatic cord,** supends the testicle in the scrotum and contains the s. artery and vein and the vas deferens.

منوی: منی یا سیمن سے متعلق۔

Spermaticidal *(sper-mat-i-si'-dal)* [G. *sperma,* seed; L. *coedere,* to kill]. Lethal to spermatozo.

سپرمیٹی سیڈل: سپرمیٹوزوآ کے لیے مہلک۔

Spermatogenesis *(sper-mat-o-jen'-e-sis)* [G. *sperma,* seed; *genesis,* descent]. The formation and development of sperm--spermatogenetic, adj.

تولید منی: نطفوں کی بناوٹ اور تکمیل۔

Spermatorrhoea *(sper-mat-o-re'-a)* [G. *sperma,* seed; *rheein,* to flow]. Involuntary discharge of semen without orgasm.

جریان ۔ سیلان منی: جوش کے بغیر منی کا بلا ارادہ اخراج ۔ اکثر یہ مرض کثرت مجامعت یا جلق کی عادت کی وجہ سے عضو تناسل کے ذکی الحس ہونے سے ہو جاتا ہے ۔ مریض کا دل وست' اعضاء شکنی کا شکایت' پیشاب کرتے وقت جلن اور گدگدی' پیشاب بار بار اور زیادہ کمر میں درد' چکر آنا' مزاج چڑچڑا' حافظہ کمزور' نیند نہ آنا' جماع کے خیال سے انزال تہائی پسند۔

Spermatozoon *(sper-mat-o-zo'-on)* [G. *sperma,* seed; *zoion,* living being]. A mature, male reproductive cell-spermatozoa, pl.

کرم منی: پختہ نر تولیدی خلیہ ۔ سپرم ز گیمیٹ جو ایک سپرمیٹوسائیٹ سے میاسس کے ذریعے چار بنتے ۔ مرد کے تولیدی مادے میں سپرم جو باریک

ہوتے ہیں اور خوردبین سے دکھائی دیتے ہیں۔تولیدی مادے کے ایک قطرے میں کروڑوں سپرم ہوتے ہیں۔جبکہ بچہ پیدا کرنے کے لیے صرف ایک ہی سپرم کافی ہے۔

Spermicide *(sper'-mi-sed)* [G. *sperma,* seed; L. *coedere,* to kill]. An agent that kills spermatozoa. Aiso spermatocide-- spermicidal, adj.

سپرمی سائیڈ: سپرمیٹوزوآ کو مارنے والا ایجنٹ۔

Spersin *(sper'-sin).* An insufflation of Polymyxin and Neomycin.

سپرسن: پولی مکسن اور نیومائی سین کی انفلیشن۔

Sphenoid *(sfe'-noid)* [G. *wedge; eidos,* form]. A wedge-shaped bone at the base of the skuli --sphenoidal, adj.

خانہ نما ہڈی: کھوپڑی کے اساس پر چھینی نما ہڈی۔کھوپڑی کی تلی کی ہڈی جو بے قاعدہ شکل کی ہوتی ہے کاسئہ سر کی تلی کا ایک حصہ اور سامنے آنکھوں کے حلقوں کی بیرونی دیوار بناتی ہے۔یہ ہڈی کاسئہ سر اور چہرے کی ہڈیوں کے درمیان واقع ہے۔

Spherocyte *(sfer'-o-sit)* [G. *sphaira,* shpere; *kytos,* cell]. Round red blood cell, as opposed to biconcave--spherocytic, adj.

سفیروسائیٹ: گول سرخ خونی خلیہ۔

Spherocytosis *(sfer-o-si-to'-sis)* [G. *sphaira,* sphere; *kytos,* cell; *osis,* condition]. Syn. for acholuric jaundice. A heredo of amilila genetic disorder transmitted as a dominant gene, i.e. with a one in two chance of transmission. It exists from birth but can remain in obeyance throughout life; sometimes discovered by 'accidental' examination of the blood. See JAUNDICE.

Sphincter *(sfink'-ter)* [G. *sphinggein,* to bind tight]. A circular muscle, contraction of which serves to close an orifice.

عاصرہ: ایک گول عضلہ جس کے سکڑنے سے سوراخ بند ہو جاتا ہے۔

Sphincterotomy *(sfink-ter-ot'-omi)* [G. *sphigkter,* that which binds tight; tome, a cutting]. Surgical division of a muscular sphincter.

…ی عضلئہ عاصرہ: عاصرہ عضلہ کی سرجیکل تقسیم۔

Sphygmocardiograph *(sfig-mo-kar'-di-o-gr…* [G. *sphygmos,* pulse; *kardia,* heart; *graphe…* to write]. An apparatus for simultaneo… graphic recording of the radial pulse a… heart-beats--sphygmocardiographic, a… sphygmocardiographically,adv.

…ر النبض والقلب: نبض اور دل کی دھڑکنوں کی بیک وقت گرافک …رڈنگ کے لیے سامان۔

Sphygmograph *(sfig'-mo-graf)* [G. *sphygm…* pulse; *graphein,* to write]. An apparat… attached to the wrist, over the radial arte… which records the movements of t… pulse-beat--sphygmographic, adj.

…ں نگار: آلہ جو کلائی کے ساتھ شریان پر باندھا جاتا ہے۔اس طرح نبض …فتار کو ریکارڈ کیا جاتا ہے۔

Sphygmomanometer *(sfig-mo-man-om'-et-…* [G. *sphygmos,* pulse; *manos,* rar; *metron* measure]. An instrument used for measur… the blood pressure.

…ں فشار پیما: بلڈ پریشر کی پیمائش کے لیے ایک آلہ مریض کے بازو پر …ھ کر ہوا بھرتے ہیں۔اور سٹےتھس کوپ سے نبض کی آواز سنتے ہیں۔

Spica *(spi'-ka)* [L.] A bandage applied i… tigure-of-eight pattern.

…ی پٹی: پٹی جو آٹھ کے انگریزی ہندسے کی شکل میں باندھی جاتی ہے۔

Spicule *(spi'-kul)* [L. *spica* , spike]. A sm… spike-like fragment, especially of bone.

…نی: ایک چھوٹا سپائیک نما ٹکڑا، خصوصاً ہڈی کا۔

Spigot *(spig'-ot).* Glass, wooden or plastic … used to close a tube.

Spina bifida *(spi'- na bif'-id-a).* A congeni… detect in which the vertebral neural arches … to close, so exposing the contents of … spinal canal posteriorly. The fissure usua… occurs in the lumbosacral region. T… contents of the canal may or may not protr… through the opening; this latter conditio… called'spina bifida occulta.

شوکہ ءمعشوقہ : نقص جس میں مہروی عصبی قوسیں بند ہونے میں ناکام رہتی ہیں۔اس طرح خلفی سپائینل قنال کے اجزاءنظر آتے ہیں۔

Spina bifida

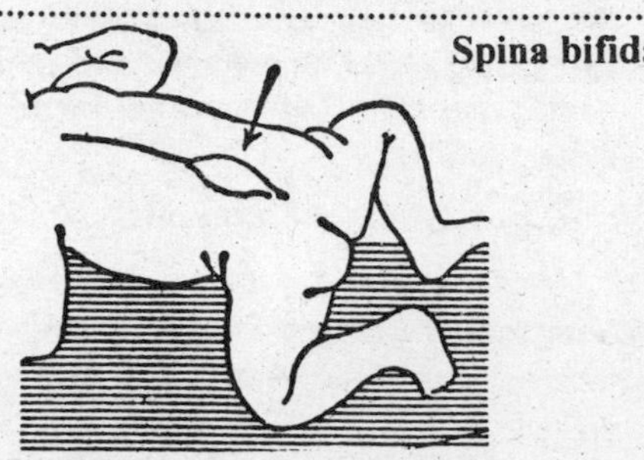

inal *(spi'-nal)* [L. *spina,* thorn]. Pertaining to the spine. **spinal anaesthetic,** a local anaesthetic solution is injected into the subarachnoid space, so that it renders the area supplied by the selected s. nerves insensitive. **spinal canal,** the central hollow throughout the s.column. **spinal caries,** disease of the vertebral bones. **spinal column,** a bony structure formed from 33 separate bones; the lower ones fuse together; the rest separated by pads of cartilage. spinal the brain down the s, canal as the level of cord, the continuation of nervous tissue of the first or second lumbar vertebra. spinal nerves, 31 pairs leave the s. cord and pass out of the s. canal to supply the periphery.

Spinal curvature

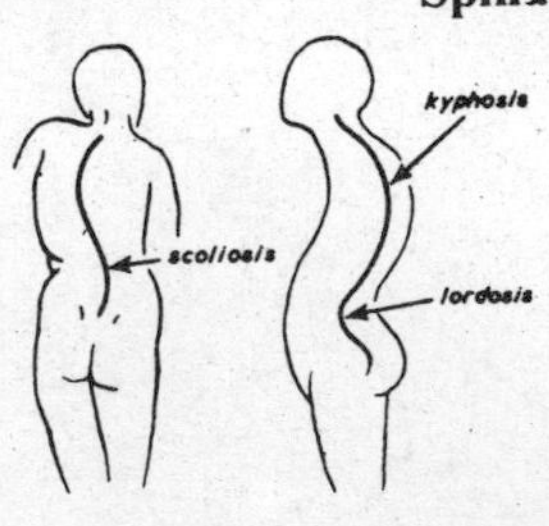

نخاعی۔شوکی: سپائن سے متعلق۔سپائنل کارڈیا حرام مغز تین پردوں میں لپٹا ہوتا ہے۔اورمیڈلا آبلانگیٹا سے شروع ہوکر ریڑھ کی ہڈی کی سپائنل کینال میں سفر کرتا ہے۔

Spine *(spin)* [L. *spina,* thorn]. A popular term for the bony spinal or vertebral column. A sharp process of bone--spinous, spinal ,adj.

شوکہ۔کانٹا: ریڑھ کی ہڈی کے لیے معروف اصطلاح۔ہڈی کا تیز زائدہ۔

Spirmaycin *(spi-ra-mi'-sin)* [L.] An orally active antibiotic with a range of activity similar to that of penicillin and erythromycin.

اسپائیرامائی سین: پنسلین اور ارتھرومائی سین سے مشابہ اینٹی بایوٹک۔

Sppirillum *(spi-ril'-um)* [L. *spira* , a spiral]. A bacterial genus. Cells are rigid screws or portions of a turn. Common in water and organic matter. *Spirillum minus* is found in rodents and may infect man , in whom it causes one form of rat-bite fever--spirilla, pl; spirillary, adj.

لولبی جرثومہ: ایک جراثیمی جنس۔پانی اور نامیاتی مادہ میں عام۔شکل میں سپرنگ کی طرح۔

Spirochaete *(spi'-ro-ket)* A bacterium having a spiral shape--spirochaetal, adj.

طویل مرغولی جرثومہ: سپائیرل شکل کا ایک جرثومہ۔سپائرو کیٹیا پیلے ڈا مرض آتشک کا سبب ہے خوردبین میں بغیر رنگ دیئے ڈارک گراؤنڈ النومینیشن کے ذریعے دیکھتے ہیں۔یعنی روشنی سلائیڈ کو ایک طرف سے دی جاتی ہے۔اور سامنے فیلڈ کو اندھیرے میں رکھتے ہیں۔اس طرح سفید چمکیلے اور متحرک سپائرو کیٹ دیکھے جاسکتے ہیں۔

Spirochaetaemia *(spi-ro-ket-e'-mi-a)* [G. *speira,* coil; *chaite,* a bristle; *haima,* blood]. Spirochaetes in the blood stream. This kind of bacteraemia occurs in the secondary stage of syphilis and in the syphilitic fetus--spirochaetaemic, adj.

سپائیروکیٹیمیا: خون کی نہر میں سپائیروکیٹس۔

Spirograph *(spi'-ro-graf)* [L. *spirare,* to breathe; G. *graphein,* to write]. An apparatus which records the movement of the lungs--spirographic, adj; spirographically, adv.; spirography, n.

تنفس نگار: پھیپھڑوں کی حرکت ریکارڈ کرنے والا آلہ۔

Spirometer *(spi-rom'-et-er)* [L. *spirare* , to breathe; G. *metron,* a measure]. An instrument for measuring the capacity of the lungs. See BRONCHOSPIROMETER--spirometric, adj. spirometry, n.

تنفس پیا: پھیپھڑوں کی گنجائش ناپنے کا آلہ

Spironolactone Aldactone-A. Antialdosterone preparation. Acts on the complex biochemical processes involved in oedematous accumulation and causes renal excretion of sodium and water.

سپائیرونول ایکٹون: اینٹی ایلڈوسیٹرون سے تیار شدہ ایلڈ یکٹون اے۔

Spittle *(spit')* Sputum; that which is expectorated.

تھوک۔ بلغم: ہائیڈروکیفالس کو نکالنے کے لیے مستعمل دماغ کے پردوں میں آنے والے پانی کے اخراج کے لیے راستے میں مستعمل جھلی یا اخراج رطوبت کا راستہ۔

Spitz-Holter valve. Used to drain hydrocephalus (q.v.).

سپٹز ہولٹر والو: ہائیڈروکیفالس کو نکالنے کے لئے مستعمل دماغ کے پردوں میں آنے والے پانی کے اخراج کے لئے راستے میں مستعمل جھلی یا اخراج رطوبت کا راستہ۔

Splanchnic. *(splangk'-nik)* [G. splagchna, inward parts]. Pertaining to or supplying the viscera.

امعائی۔ احشائی: وسرا سے متعلق۔

Splanchnicectomy *(splang-knik-ek'-to-mi)* [G. *splagchna,* inward parts; *ektome,* excision]. Surgical removal of the splanchnic nerves, whereby the viscera are deprived of sympathetic impulses; occasionally performed in the treatment of hypertension or for the relief of certain kinds of visceral pain.

سپلینک نک ایکٹومی: سپلانکنک اعصاب کا سرجیکل کٹاؤ۔ اس سے وسرا کے درد کی بعض اقسام کو آرام آتا ہے۔

Splanchnology *(splangk-nol'-o-ji)* [G. *splagchna,* inward parts; *logos,* discourse]. The study of the structure and function of the viscera.

م الاحشا: وسرا کی ساخت اور فعل کا مطالعہ۔

Spleen *(splen)* [G. *splen*]. A lymphoid, vascul organ immediately below the diaphragm, the tail of the pancress, behind the stomach. can be enlarged in reactive and neoplas conditions affecting the reticuloendothel system (q.v.)

: معدہ کے عقب میں لبلبہ کی دم پر، ڈایافرام کے عین نیچے۔ ایک لمفی' ولر عضو یہ زیادہ تکلیف میں بڑھ جاتی ہے۔ حیات کے لیے غیر ضروری۔

Splenectomy *(splen-ek'-to-mi)* [G. *splen,* sple *ektome,* excision]. Surgical removal of t spleen.

ل برآری: تلی کا سرجیکل کٹاؤ۔

Splenic anaemic See BANTT'S DISEASE.

بانتی: بنٹی کا مرض۔ اس بیماری میں تلی بڑھ جاتی ہے۔ قلت الدم کے خونی قے یا خونی دست آتے ہیں۔

Splenitis *(splen-i'-tis)* [G. *splen,* spleen; *i* inflammation]. Inflammation of the spleen.

طحال: تلی کی سوزش۔

Splenocaval *(splen-o-ka'-vel)* [G. *splen,* sple L. *Cavum,* hollow]. Partaining to the sple and inferior vena cava, usually referring anastomosis of the splenic vein to the IVC.

نوکیول: تلی اور ادنی وینا کیوا سے متعلق۔

Splenorenal sh

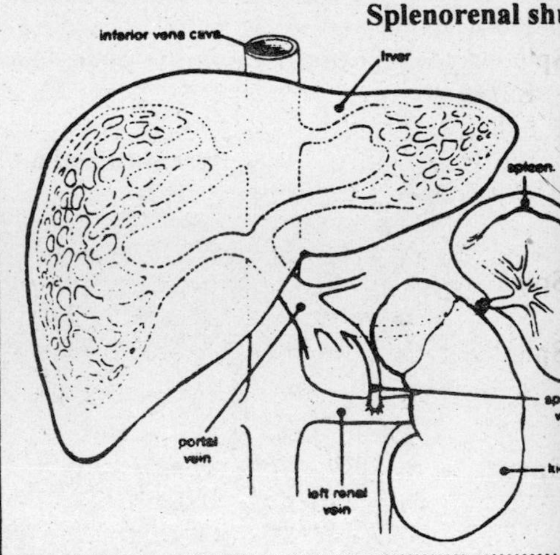

Splenogram *(splen'-o-gram)* [G. *splen,* Spleen; *gramma,* letter]. Radiographic picture of the spleen after injection of radio-opaque medium--splenograph, splenography n; splenographical, adj.; splenographically, adv.

اسپلینو گرام: ریڈیواوپیک واسطے کے انجکشن کے بعد تلی کی ریڈیوگرافک تصویر۔

Splenomegaly *(splen-o-meg'-al-i)* [G. *splen,* spleen, *magas,* large]. Enlargement of the spleen.

کبرالطحال: تلی کا بڑھنا۔مختلف امراض میں تلی بڑھ جاتی ہے۔خصوصاً ملیریا سے تلی بڑھتی ہے۔دیگر امراض یہ ہیں۔کالا آزار' لیموکیمیا' یرقان' سرہو سز لیور' مرض بنٹی' مرض ہاجکن' کینسر یا سرطان۔

Splenoportal *(splen-o-por'-tal)* [G. *splen,* spleen; L. *porta,* gate]. Pertaining to the spleen and portal vein.

سپلینو پورٹل: تلی اور پورٹل ورید سے متعلق۔

Splenoportgram *(splen-o-port'-o-gram)* [G. *splen,* spleen; L. *porta,* gate; G. *gramma,* letter]. Radiographic picture of the spleen and portal vein after injection of radio-opaque medium--splenoportograph, splenoportography, n.; splenoportographical, adj.; splenoportographically, adv.

اسپلینو پورٹوگرام: ریڈیواور پیک واسطے کے انجکشن کے بعد تلی اور پورٹل ورید کی ریڈیوگرافک تصویر۔

Splenorenal *(splen-o-re'-nal)* [G. *splen,* spleen; L. *ren,* kidney]. Pertaining to the spleen and kidney, as anastomosis of the splenic vein to the renal vein; a procedure carried out in some cases of portal hypertension.

سپلینو رینل: تلی اور گردے سے متعلق۔

Splenovenography *(splen-o-ven-og'-ra-fi).* See SPLENOGRAM.

Spondyl *(e)spon'-dil)* [G. *spondylos,* vertebra]. A vertebra.

منکا۔فقرہ: ایک مہرہ

Spondylitis *(spon-dil-i'-tis)* [G. *spondylos,* vertebra; *-itis,* inflammation].inflammation of one or more vertebrae--spondylitic, adj. **ankylosing s.,** a condition characterized by ossification of the spinal ligaments and ankylosis of sacroiliac joints. It occurs chiefly in young men.

ورم فقرہ: ایک یا زیادہ مہروں کی سوزش

Spondylolisthesis *(spon-dil-o-the'-sis)* [G. *spondylos;* vertebra; *olishesis,* a slipping and falling]. Forward displacement of lumbar vertebra (e)--spondylolisthetic, adj.

استرخار الفقرات: لمبر مہروں کا پہلے گر جانا۔

Spondylosis deformans *(spon-dil-o'-sis-de-form' -ans)* [G. *spondylos,* vertebra; *-osis,* condition ; L. misshapen]. Degeneration of the whole intervertebral disc with new bone formation at the periphery of the disc. Commonly called osteoarthrirtis of spine.

سپانڈائی لوسس ڈیفارمینس: ساری بین مہروی تھالی کی تنزلی۔تھالی کے بیرونی جانب نئی ہڈی بنتی ہے۔

Spongioblastoma multiforme *(spon-ji-o-blas-to'-ma mul'-ti-form)* A highly malignant rapidly growing brain tumour.

Sporadic *(spor-ad'-ik)* [G. *sporadikos,* scattered] Scattered ; occurring insolated cases; not epidemic--sporadically, adv.

انفرادی۔اکادکا: منتشر۔

Spore *(spor)* [G. *sporos,* seed]. A phase in the life-cycle of a limited number of bacterial genera whrere the vegetative cell becomes encapsulated and metabolism almost ceases. These spores are highly resistant to environmental conditions such as heat and desiccation. The spores of important species such as *Clostridium tetani* and *C. botulinum* are ubiquitous so that sterilization procedures must ensure their removal or death.

تخمک۔بذرہ: جراثیموں کے محدود تعداد کے دور حیات میں ایک مرحلہ۔نباتی تولیدی خلیے۔

Sporicidal *(spor-i-si'-dal)* [G. *sporos,* seed; L. *coedere,* to kill]. Lethal to spores--sporicide, n.

بزرہ کش: بذروں کے لیے مہلک۔

Sporotrichosis *(spor-o-tri-ko'-sis)* [G. *sporos,* seed; *thrixtrichos,* hair; *-osis,* condition].

Infection of a wound by a fungus (Sporotrix schenkic). There results a primary sore with lymphangitis and subcutaneous painless granulomata. Occurs amongst those working with soil.

سپروٹرائی کوسس: سماروغ سے زخم کی انفیکشن ۔ یہ سماروغ سپوروٹرائیکم ہوتا ہے۔ان افراد میں یہ مرض ہوتا جو مٹی کا کام کرتے ہیں۔

Sporulation *(spor-u-la'-shun)* [G. *spora,* seed]. The formation of spores by bacteria.

بذرک زائی: جراثیم کا بذرے بنانا۔

Spotted fever 1. Cerebrospinal fever. Organism responsible is the meningococcus transferred by droplet infection. Occurs in epidemics. 2. Rocky Mountain spotted fever is a tick-borne typhus fever.

ہذیانی میعادی بخار: ا۔سر بروسپائینل بخار ۔ یہ وبا کی شکل اختیار کر لیتا ہے۔ ۲۔راکی ماؤنٹین سپاٹڈ بخار۔

Sprain *(spran)*. Injury to the soft tissues surrounding a joint, resulting in discoloration, swelling and pain.

موچ: جوڑ کے گرد نرم بافتوں کا زخم جس سے رنگ اڑ جاتی ہے۔سوج اور درد ہوتا ہے۔کسی عضو کے اپنے جوڑ پر سے زیادہ مڑ جانے یا کھنچ جانے سے نزدیکی عضلات مجروح ہو جاتے ہیں۔اسے موچ آنا کہا جاتا ہے۔

Sprengel's shoulder deformity Congenital high scapula, a permanent elevation of th e shoulder, often associated with other congenital deformities, e.g. the presence of a cervical rib or the absence of vertebrae [Otto G.K.Sprengel, German surgeon, 1852-1915].

بدنمائی شانہ: شانے کی مستقل بلندی'سکاپولا اونچا ہو جاتا ہے۔اس سے مزید کوئی بدصورتی پیدا ہو جاتی ہے۔مثلاً مہروں کی غیر موجودگی وغیرہ۔

Sprue *(sproo)*. A chronic malabsorption disorder associated with glossitis, indigestion, weakness, anaemia and steatorrhoea.

گنج ۔ سپرو: انجذاب کی قدیم خرابی جس سے کمزوری' ہاضمہ کی خرابی اور خون کی کمی وغیرہ واقع ہوتے ہیں۔

Sputum *(spu'-tum)* [L. spittle]. Matter which is expectorated from the lungs.

بلغم ۔ تھوک: پھیپھڑوں سے نکلنے والا مادہ۔ رنگ سفیدی مائل۔ بو' خون اور پیپ نہیں ہوتے۔ بلغم کی معمولی مقدار سلائیڈ پر دوسری سلائیڈ کے کنارے سے پھیلا کر پتلی قلم بنائیے۔خشک ہونے پر زیل نیلسن سٹین دے کر خوردبین میں دیکھئے۔ایسڈ فاسٹ بے سلائی ہوں تو تپ دق ہے۔

Squamous *(skwa'-muos)* [L. *squamosus,* scaly]. Scaly, **squamous** epithelium, the non-glandular epithelial covering of the external body surfaces, **squamous carinoma,** carcinoma arising in squamous epithelium; epithelioma.

کھپرے دار: سکیلی۔

Squills *(skwillz)* . Dried bulbs of Mediterranean plant, used in Gee's linctus and other cough preparations as an expectorant.

قسم سرطان بحری: ایک پودے کے خشک بلب۔کھانسی کے شربتوں میں مستعمل۔

Squint *(skwint)*. Syn., strabismus. Incoordinated action of the muscles of the eyeball, such that the visual axes of the two eyes fail to meet at the objective point. **convergent s.,** when the eyes turn towards the medial line. **divergent s.,** when the eyes turn outwards.

بھینگا پن: آنکھ کے گولے کے عضلات کا بلا تعاون ایکشن ۔ اس طرح دونوں آنکھیں ایک ہی چیز پر مرکوز نہیں ہوتیں۔

Staccato speech *(stak-a'-to)*. With interruptions between words or syllables. The scanning speech of disseminated sclerosis and cerebellar disease.

جدا جدا التقریر: الفاظ کے درمیان تسلسل ٹوٹنا۔

Stacke's operation Plastic operation on posterior membranous wall of the aural canal. [Ludwig Stacke, German otologist, 1859-1918].

سٹیکس اپریشن: آرن قنال کی خلفی جھلی دار دیوار پر پلاسٹک اپریشن۔

Stangnant loop syndrome Stagnation of contents of any surgically created 'loop' of intestine with consequent increase in bacterial population and interference with obsorption of food.

St Anthony's fir, Erysiplas (q.v.) and sometimes used for gangrene resulting from ergotism.

Stapedectomy *(sta-ped-ek'-to-mi)* Surgical removal of stapes for otosclerosis and insertion 1. Teflon piston (Schuknecht's operation) 2. Vein graft. 3. Plug of fat. After s., staped can be replaced by a prosthesis. Normal hearing is restored in 90 per cent of patients.

رکیب براری: سٹیپر کا سرجیکل کٹاؤ۔

epedial mobilization *(sta-ped'-i-al)*. Release of a stapes, rendered immobile by otosclerosis.

رکیبی موبیلائزیشن: سٹیپز کی ریلیز۔

apediolysis *(sta-ped-i-ol'-i-sis)* See STAPEDIAL MOBILZATION.

apes *(sta'-pez)*. The stirrup-shaped medial bone of the middle ear. **mobilization of s.,** forcible pressure on s. to restore its mobility . Gain in hearing not permanent, but a stapedectomy can be done later--stapedial , adj.

رکابی ہڈی، رکیب: درمیانی کان کی میانی ہڈی۔

aphlococcus *(staf-i-lo-kok'-us)* [Gr. *staphyle,* bunch of grapes]. A genus of bacteria. Gram-positive cocci occurring in clusters. May be saprophytes or parasites. Common commensals of man, in whom they are responsible for much minor pyogenic infection, and a lesser amount of more serious infection. Produce several exotoxins. These include leucocidins which kill WBC and haemolysins which destroy RBC. A common cause of hospital cross-infection--staphylococcal, adj.

عنبی نبقہ: جراثیم کا ایک جنس۔ گرام مثبت کا کسی گچھوں کی صورت میں طفیلی یا گندخور۔

phyloma *(staf-il-o'-ma)* [G.]. A protrusion of the cornea or sclera of the eye--staphylomata, pl.

زرالعین: آنکھ کے سکلیرا یا قرنیہ کا باہر کی طرف نکل آنا۔

rch The carbohydrate present in potatoes, rice, maize, etc. Widely used as an absorbent dusting powder.

سٹارچ، نشاستہ: پالیسکرائیڈز جو ایمائیلوز اور ایمائیلو پیکٹسین میں سے ایک ہے۔ مرتب گلوکوس اکائیوں کی زنجیروں پر مشتمل ہوتے ہیں۔ پودوں میں دانوں کی صورت نشاستہ ذخیرہ ہوتا ہے اور بیجوں میں نشاستہ پایا جاتا ہے۔ یہ پانی میں ناحل پذیر ہے۔ یہ انہضام میں شکر میں تبدیل ہوتا ہے۔ یہ عمل فامرہ کے ذریعہ ہوتا ہے۔ یہ کاربوہائیڈریٹ آلو، چاول، مکئی وغیرہ میں موجود ہوتا ہے۔ اسے جاذب چھڑکنے والے سفوف کے طور پر کثرت سے استعمال کیا جاتا ہے۔

Stasis *(sta'-sis)* [G.] Stagnation; cessation of motion. **intestinal s.,** sluggish bowel contractions resulting in constipation.

سکونِ خون: حرکت کی بندش۔ ایک ہی جگہ کھڑے رہنا۔

Status (sta'-tus) [L.] State . Condition, **status asthmaticus** is a prolonged and refractory attack of asthma. **status epilepticus** describes epilptic attacks following each other almost continuously. **status lymphatlcus** is a condition found postmortem in patients who have died without apparent cause. The thymus may be found hypertrophied with increase in lymphatic tissue elsewhere.

حیثیت۔ کیفیت: حالت۔

Steapsin *(ste-ap'-sin)*. The lipase of the pancreatic juice which splits fat into fatty acids and glycerine.

ہاضم شحم: لبلبی رس کا لائپیس جو چکنائی کو فیٹی ایسڈز اور گلیسرین میں تبدیل کرتا ہے۔

Steatorrhaea *(ste-at-or-e'-a)* [G. *stear,* Fat; *rh-eein,* to flow]. A syndrome of varied aetiology associated with multiple defects of absorbtion from the gut and characterized by the pasage of pale, bulky, greasy stools.

اسہال شحمی: گٹ سے انجذاب کے کئی نقائص کا سنڈروم

Stegomyia *(steg-o-mi'-i-a)* [G. *stegos,* roof; *myia,* fly]. A genus of mosquitoes, some of which transmit the malaria parasite. Found in most tropical and subtropical countries.

زرد بخار کا مچھر: مچھروں کا ایک جنس۔ بعض ملیریائی طفیلی منتقل کرتے ہیں۔

Stein -Leventhal syndrome. Secondary amenorrhoea, sterility, bilateral polycystic ovaries and hirsutism occurring in the second or third decades of life. Treated by wedge resection of ovary.

سٹین لیونتھال سنڈروم: ایک سنڈروم۔ بانجھ پن۔

Steinmann's pin An alternative means to the use of a Kirschner wire (q.v.) of applying skeletal traction to a limb. It has its own introducer and stirrup. [Fritz Steinmann, Swiss surgeon, 1872-1932].

پن سٹائن مین: جارح میں استخوانی ٹریکشن کے تار کے استعمال کی جگہ ایک متبادل ذریعہ۔

Stelazine Trifluoperazine (q.v.).

سٹیلا زین: ٹرفلوپیرازین۔ حمل میں قے کے علاج کے لیے ایک گولی صبح ایک دوپہر ایک شام یہی خوراک پاگل پن میں بھی۔

Stellate *(stel'-at)* [L. *stella,* star]. Starshaped stellate ganglion, a large collection of nerve cells (ganglion) on the sympathetic chain in the root of the neck.

ستارہ نما: ستارے کی شکل کا۔

Stellwag's sign Occurs in exophthalmic goitre (Graves' disease). Patient does not blink so often as usual, and the eyelids close only imperfectly when he does so. [Carl Stellwag von Caroin, Austrian ophthalmologist, 1823-1904].

علامت سٹیلو یگ: مریض زیادہ آنکھیں نہیں جھپک سکتا۔ اس کی آنکھ کے پپوٹے مکمل طور پر نہیں کھلتے۔

Stemetil *(stem'-et-il).* Prochlorperazine (q.v.)

سٹیمیٹل: پروکلورپیرازین۔ قے روکنے کے لیے ایک گولی صبح ایک دوپہر ایک شام ہچکی روکنے مریض سینئر اور درد شقیقہ کے لیے بھی مذکورہ خوراکیں دیجئے۔ سر کے چکروں کے لیے ایک گولی دن میں ۳ مرتبہ۔

Stenosis *(sten-o'-sis)* [G.] A narrowing--stenoses , pl.; stenotic , adj.

ضیق: تنگ ہونا۔

Sterkobilin *(ster-ko-bi'-lin).* The brown pigment of faeces; it is derived from the bile pigments.

براز کا بھورا مادہ ملونہ: فضلے کا بھورا جسمانی رنگ

Stercobilinogen Urobilinogen (q.v.)

سٹرکوبلینوجن: یوروبلینوجن

Stercoraceous *(ster-kor-a'-shus)* [L. *stercus,* dung]. Pertaining to or resembling faeces --stercoral, adj.

برازی: فضلہ سے مشابہ یا اس سے متعلق۔

Stereotactic surgery *(ste-re-o-tak'-tik).* Electrodes and cannulae are passed to a predetermined point in the brain for physiological observation or destruction of tissue in diseases such as paralysis agitans, multiple sclerosis and epilepsy. Intractable pain can be relieved by this method. Also stereotaxic.

سٹیریوٹیکٹک سرجری: درد دور کرنے کا ایک طریقہ۔ فزیالوجیکل مشاہدہ یا بیماریوں میں نسیج کی تباہی کے لئے دماغ میں ایک متعین نقطے پر الیکٹروڈ زیادہ برقیرے گذارے جاتے ہیں۔

Sterile *(ste'-ril).* Free from micro-organism --sterility, n.

بے جراثیم: خورد جسیموں سے آزاد۔

Sterilization *(ster-il-i-za'-shun).* 1. The process of ridding material or tissue of living microbes. 2. Rendering incapable of reproduction.

تطہیر، جراثیم کشی، غیر بارود سازی: ۱۔ جاندار مائیکروبز کا نسیج نکالنے کا طریقہ اس میں ابالنا، آٹوکلیونگ اور ڈس انفیکٹنٹ شامل ہیں۔ ۲۔ تولید کے ناقابل بنانا۔

Sternoclavicular *(ster-no-klav-ik'-u-lar)* [G. *sternon,* breast; L. *calvicula,* small key]. Pertaining to the sternum and the clavicle.

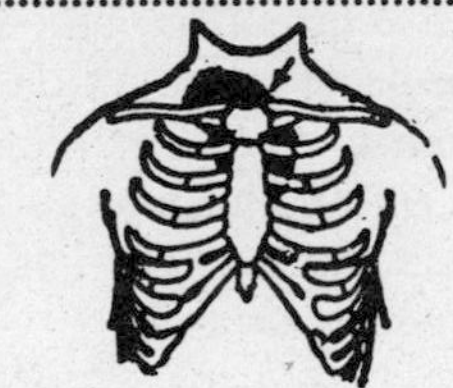

Sternoclavicular joint

قصی تر قوی: سٹرنم اور ہنسلی کی ہڈی سے متعلق۔

Sternocleidomastoid muscle *(ster-no-kli-do-mas'-toid)* [G. *sternon,* breast; *kleis,* hook; *mastos,* breast]. A strap-like neck muscle arising from the sternum and clavicle, and inserting into the mastoid process of temporal bone. See TORTICOLLIS.

سٹرنوکلیڈومیسٹائڈ عضلہ: سٹریپ نما گردن کا عضلہ جو سٹرنم اور ہنسلی کی ہڈی سے نکل کر ٹمپورل ہڈی کے مسٹائڈ زائدہ میں لگا ہوتا ہے۔

Sternocostal *(ster-no-kos'-om-i)* [G. *sternon,* breast; L. *costa,* rib]. Pertaining to the sternum and ribs.

قصی ضلعی: سٹرنم اور پسلیوں سے متعلق۔

Sternotomy *(ster-not'-om-i)* [G. *sternon,* breast; *tome,* a cutting]. Surgical division of the sternum.

سٹرنوٹومی: سٹرنم کی سرجیکل تقسیم۔

Sternum *(ster'-num)* [G. *sternon,* breast]. The breast bone --sternal, adj.

سینے کی ہڈی، قص: چھاتی کی ہڈی۔ سینے کے جوف کی سامنے کی طرف ہوتی ہے۔ یہ ہڈی بالائی چوڑا حصہ درمیانی حصہ یا جسم اور زیریں نوک پر مشتمل ہوتی ہے۔ اس ہڈی کے دونوں طرف پہلی سات پسلیاں جڑی ہوتی ہیں۔ بالائی حصہ میں ہنسلی کی ہڈی کے جوڑ کی جگہ بنی ہوتی ہے۔ زیرین نوک کے ساتھ پیٹ کی جھلی لگی ہوتی ہے۔

Sterogyl 15. Calciferol forte (NF--national Formulary).

سٹیروگائل ۱۵: کیلسیفیرول فورٹے۔

Steroids *(ster'-oidz)* [G. *stereos,* solid; *eidos,* form]. A term embracin a naturally occurring group of chemicals allied to cholestrol and including sexhormones , adrenal cortical hormones, bile acids,etc. By custom if often now implies the natural adrenal glucocorticoids, viz., hydrocortisone and cortisone, or synthetic analogues such as prednisolone and prednisone.

سٹیرائڈز: ماخوذ لائیپڈز جن میں سٹیرولز، بائیل ایسڈز بعض ہارمون اور گلوکوسائیڈز اور حیاتین ڈی شامل ہیں۔

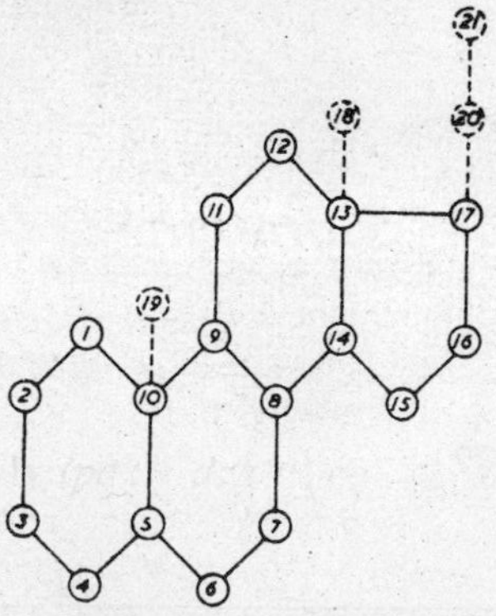

Steroids. Figure shows the basic chemical structure of steroids with the carbon atoms numbered. The distinguishing groups are attached in position 18 to 21.

Sterol *(ster'-ol)* [G. *steros,* solid; *ol,* alchol]. A solid alcohol. Cholesterol and many hormones secreted by the adrenal cortex and the gonads are examples. They all contain the same basic ring structure.

سٹیرول: سٹیرائڈ گروہ کے ماخوذ لائیپڈز۔ بہت سے جانداروں میں پائے جاتے ہیں جن میں وہ اہم کردار ادا کرتے ہیں۔

Stertor *(ster'-tor)* [L, *stertere,* to snore]. Loud snoring; sonorous breathing stertorous. adj.

شخیری: زور سے خراٹے لینا۔ خراٹے دار سا

Stethoscope *(steth'-o-skop)* [G. stethos, breast; skopein, to examine]. An instrument used for listening to the various body sounds, especially those of the heart and chest. See MEDETRON--stethoscopic, ad.; stethoscopically, adv.

صدر بلن آلہ۔ سٹیتھوسکوپ۔ جسم کی مختلف آوازیں سننے کے لئے ایک آلہ، خصوصاً دل اور چھاتی کی آواز سننے کے عمل کو آسکلٹیشن کہا جاتا ہے۔

Stevens-Johnson syndrome Sever variant of the allergic response--erythema multiforme. It is an acute hypersensitiveity state and can follow a viral or bacterial infection, drugs--such as long-acting sulphonamides, some anticonvulasants and some antibiotics. In somplications during the acute phase can be fatal. Mostly it is a benign condition, and there is complete recovery.[Albert Mason Stevens, American pacdiatrician. 1884-1945. Frank Chambliss Johnson. American paediatrician. 1894-1934].

سٹیونز جانسن سنڈروم: الرجی کی ایک قسم

Stibocaptate *(stib-o-kap'-tat).* Trivalent antimonial, effective in the treatment of intestinal schistosomiasis. Given intramuscularly. Admission to hospital essential and patient should be kept lying dion for a few hours after each injection. BAL should be available to reverse any severe toxic effects.

سٹیبو کپٹپیٹ : سرگرفتہ اینٹی مونیل، آنت کی سکسٹو سومیاسس کے علاج میں موثر ہسپتال میں داخلہ ضروری ہے۔ مریض کو ہر ٹیکے کے بعد کئی گھنٹوں تک لیٹے رہنا چاہئے۔

Stibophen *(stib'-o-fan)*. A complex antimony compound used in the treatment of schistosomiasis.

سٹیبو فین : پیچیدہ اینٹی منی کا مرکب۔ سکسٹو سومیاسس کے علاج میں مستعمل۔

Stigmata *(stig'-ma-ta)*. [G. stigma, mark or brand]. Marks of disease, or congenital abnormalities, e.g. facies of congenital syphilis--stigma, sing.

علامات مرض: مرض کے نشانات

Stilboestrol *(stil-bes'-trol)*. An orally active synthetic oestrogen, indicated in all conditions calling for oestrogen therapy. Large doses are given in prostatic carcinoma.

سٹلبو ایسٹرول: منہ کے ذریعے کھائی جانے والی تالیفی ایسٹروجن۔ نصف اور ایک ملی گرام کی گولیاں۔ ماہواری میں کمی یا بندش یا بے قاعدگی کو ٹھیک کرنے کے لئے کارآمد۔

Stilette *(stil-et')*. A wire or metal rod for maintaining patency of hollow instruments.

سٹلٹ : ایک تار یا دھاتی سلاخ جس سے کھوکھلے اوزاروں کی پیٹنسی برقرار رکھی جاتی ہے۔

Stillborn, Born dead.

پیدائشی مردہ : مردہ پیدا ہونا۔ بچہ پیدا ہوتے وقت زندہ ہوتا ہے لیکن پیدائش کے بعد سانس نہیں لیتا۔ اس لیے پھیپھڑے نہیں کھلتے۔

still's disease. A form of rheumatoid polyarthritis, involving enlargement of the spleen, lymphatic nodes and glands, occurring in infants and young children. sufferers are often retarded. Also called arthritis deformans Juvenilis [George Fredric Still, English physician, 1868-1941.]

مرض سٹل: ریوماٹائڈ پولی آرتھرٹیس کی ایک قسم۔

Stimulant *(stim'-u-land)* [L. *stimulare* , to goad]. Stimulating. An agent which excites or increases function.

محرک دوا: ایجنٹ جو فعل یا عمل کو بڑھائے۔ تحریک دینے والا۔ بلڈ پریشر کی کمی، گھبراہٹ، تنفس اور قلب کی بیشتر امراض میں مفید مثلاً سپرٹ امونیا ایرومیٹک وغیرہ۔

Stimulus *(stim'-u-lus)* [L. *stimulare,* to goad]. Anything which excites functional activity in an organ or part.

محرکہ: کوئی چیز جو کسی عضو یا حصے میں فعلیاتی عاملیت کو پر جوش کرتی ہے۔

Stitch 1. A sudden, sharp, darting pain. 2. A suture.

ٹانکا۔ ٹیس: ۱۔ اچانک، تیز، اندر تک اتر جانے والا درد ۲۔ سیوچر

Stockholmn technique A method of treating carcinoma of the cervix by radium on three succesive occasions at weekly intervals.

سٹاک ہوم تکنیک: سروکس کے کرسینوما کے علاج کا ایک طریقہ

Stokes-Adams syndrome. A fainting (syncopal) attack, commonly transient, which occurs in patients with heart block. If severe, may take the form of a convulsion, or patient may become unconscious. [William Stokes, Irish physician, 1804-78 Robert Adams, Irish physician, 1791-1875]

سنڈروم سٹوک آدم: قلبی بلاک کے ساتھ مریضوں میں ہونیوالا کمزوری کا حملہ۔ اگر حملہ شدید ہو تو مریض بے ہوش بھی ہو سکتا ہے۔

Stomach

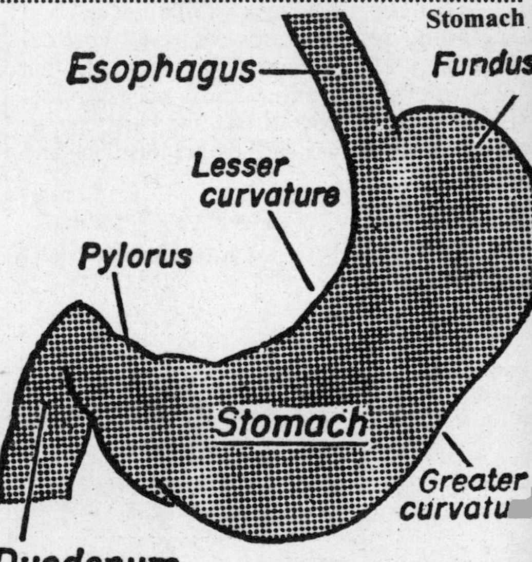

Stoma *(sto'-ma)* [G.] The mouth; any opening --stomal, adj.; stomata, pl.

دہن۔فم: منہ۔کوئی سوراخ۔

Stomach *(stum'-ak)* [G. *stomachos,* gullet]. The most dilated part of the digestive tube, situated between the oesophagus (cardiac orifice) and the beginning of the small intestine (pyloric orifice); it lies in the epigastric, umbilical and abdomen. The wall is composed of four coats; serous, muscular, submucous and mucous. **hour glass s.,** one partially divided into two halves by an equatorial constriction following scar formation.

معدہ: ابتدائی چھوٹی آنت ایسوفیگس کے درمیان واقع ہضمی نلی کا سب سے کشادہ حصہ۔ دیوار چار کوٹوں پر مشتمل ہے۔ سیرس' عضلاتی سب میوکس اور میوکس۔

Stomachics *(stom-ak'-iks)* Agents which increase the appetite, especially bitters.

محرک معدہ' ہاضوم: بھوک بڑھانے والے عوامل

Stomatitis *(sto-mat-i'-tis)* [G. *stoma,* mouth; *itis,* inflammation]. inflammation of the mouth . angular s., fissuring in the corners of the mouth consequent upon riboflavine deficiency. Sometimes misapplied to ; (1) the superficial maceration and fissuring at the labial commisures in perleche (q.v.) and (2) the chronic fissuring at the site in elderly persons with sagging lower lip or malapposition of arificial dentures. aphthous s., recurring crops of small ulcers in the mouth. Relationship to herpes simplex suspected, but not proven. See APHTHAE gangrenous s., See CANCRUM ORIS.

ورم دہن: منہ کی سوزش' منہ کا پک جانا۔ بچوں کا مرض جو منہ میں پھپھوندی لگ جانے سے ہوتی ہے منہ میں چھالے بدہضمی یا ان دھلے نپل کی وجہ سے ہوتے ہیں۔ ایک فیصد جنشن وائلٹ کا محلول لگانا مفید ہے۔

Stone *(ston).* Calculus ; a hardened mass of mineral matter.

سنگ گردہ: معدنی مادہ جو سخت ہوتا ہے۔ سٹون بلیڈر یعنی مثانے کی پتھری مردوں میں زیادہ ہوتی ہے۔ سنگ گردہ یا سٹون کڈنی کی تشخیص کے لیے سادہ ایکس رے پائیلوگرافی اور پیشاب ٹیسٹ ضروری ہیں۔

Stool The faeces. An evacuation of the bowels.

پاخانہ: فضلہ یا اس کا اخراج۔ رنگ گہرا بھورا' بوگندی' قوام سخت' خون' آنوں' پیپ یا کیڑے نہیں ہوتے۔ غیر ہضم شدہ نباتاتی مادے پائے جاتے ہیں۔ لیکن غیر ہضم شدہ چکنائیاں یا لحمی اجزاء نہیں ہوتے۔

Stovarsol *(stov-ar'-sol).* Acetarsol (q.v.).

سٹوورسول: ایسیٹارسول

Stove-in chest. There may be multiple anterior or posterior fractures of the ribs (causing paradoxical breathing) and fractures of sternum, or a mixture of such fractures.

سٹووان چیسٹ: پسلیوں کے امامی یا خلفی فریکچر اور سٹرنم کے فریکچر۔

STP. Psychedelic drug that engenders hallucinations comparabel to those experienced in schizophrenic states.

Strabismus *(strab-iz'-mus)* [G. *strabismos,* squinting]. See SQUINT.

بھینگاپن: سکوئنٹ

Stramonium *(stra-mo'-ni-um).* A plant resembling belladonna in its properties, and used as an antispasmodic in bronchitis and Parkinsonism.

دھتورہ: پودا جو اپنی خصوصیات میں بیلاڈونا سے مشابہ ہے۔

Strangulation *(strang'-gu-la-shun)* [G. *straggale,* halter]. Constricted so as to impede the circulation--strangulated, adj.

خنق: درمیان سے سکڑ جانا جس سے گردش متاثر ہوتی ہے۔ پھندا لگنا یا گلا دبا دیا جانا۔ گردن پر نشان پائے جاتے ہیں۔ مقتول جلدی بے بس ہو جاتا ہے۔ امونیا کارب سونگھائیں۔ مصنوعی سانس دیجیے۔

Strangury *(strang'-gu-ri)* [G. *stragx,* drop; *ouron,* urine]. Slow and painful micturition.

عسر البول: سست اور درد بھری مکٹوریشن۔

Strassman operation A plastic operation to make a bicornuate uterus a near normal shape. [Paul F. Strassman, German gynaecologist, 1866-1938].

سٹریس مین اپریشن: بائی کارنوایٹ یوٹرس کو قریباً نارمل شکل کا بنانے کے لیے پلاسٹک اپریشن۔

Stratified *(strat'-i-fid)* [L. *stratum,* a covering; *facere,* to make]. Arranged in layers.

طبق دار: پرتوں میں منظم

Stratum *(Stra'-tum)* [L.] A layer or lamina, e.g. the various layers of the epitelium of the skin, viz., s.granulosum, s. lucidum.

طبق خلیات: ایک تہہ یا کسمینا۔ مثلاً جلد کی اپی تھیلیم کی مختلف۔

Streptobacillus *(strep-to-bas-il'-us)*. Gram-positive , rod-shaped bacteria.

سٹریپٹو بیلس: گرام مثبت۔ سلاخ نما جراثیم۔

Streptoccus *(strep-to-kok'-us)* [G. *streptos,* curved; *coccus,* berry]. A genus of bacteria. gram-positive cocci, often occurring in chains of varying length. Require enriched media for growth and the colonies are small. Saprophytic and parasitic species. Pathogenic species produce powerful exotoxins. These include leucocidins which kill WBC and haemolysins which kill RBC. In man they are responsible for numerous infections such as scarlatina, tonsillitis, erysibpelas, endocarditis, rheumatic fever, glomerulonephritis, and wound infections in hospital--steptococal, adj.

زنجیری نبقہ: جراثیم کا ایک جنس۔ گرام مثبت کا کسی اکثر مختلف لمبائیوں کی زنجیریں بنتی ہیں۔ گند خور اور طفیلی انواع۔ اکثر اقسام انسان وحیوانات میں امراض کا سبب۔ انکے علاج میں پنسلین اور سلفا ڈرگز کامیاب ہیں۔

Streptodornase *(streplto-dor'-nas)*. An enzyme used with streptokinase (q.v.) in liquefying pus and blood clots.

سٹرپٹو دور نیز: پیپ اور خونی لوتھڑوں کو پتلا کرنے کے لیے سٹرپٹو کائینیز کے ساتھ استعمال ہونے والا ایک خامرہ۔

Streptoduocin *(strep-to-du'-o-sin)* A mixture of streptomycin and dihydrostreptomycin, said to have a lower toxicity.

سٹرپٹو ڈواسن: سٹرپٹو مائی سین اور ڈائی ہائیڈرو سٹرپٹو مائی سین کا آمیزہ۔ اس میں زہریلا پن کم ہوتا ہے۔

Streptokinase *(strep-to-ki'-naz)* . An enzyme derived from cultures of certain haemolytic streptococci. Plasminogen activator. Used with streptodornase (q.v.) .Its fibrinolytic effect has been used with thrombolytic therapy to speed removal of intravascular fibrin.

سٹرپٹو کائی نیز: بعض ہیمولائیٹک سٹرپٹو کا کسی کے کلچرز سے ماخوذ ایک خامرہ۔

Streptolysins *(strep-to-li'-sinz)* [G. *streptos,* curved; *lysis,* a loosening]. Haemolytic toxins produced by streptococci. Antibody produced in the tissues against streptolysin may be measured and taken as an indicator of recent streptococcal infection.

سٹرپٹو لائی سنز: سٹرپٹو کا کسی سے پیدا شدہ ہیمولائیٹک ٹاکسنز۔

Streptomycin *(strep-to-mi'-sin)*. An antibiotic effective against many organisms, but used mainly in tuberculosis. Treatment is usually combind with other drugs to reduce drug resistance. It is not absorbed when given orally, hence used in some intestinal infections.

سٹرپٹو مائی سین: ایک اینٹی بائیوٹک جو ایک سمارو غ سٹرپٹو مائی سیز سے بنتی ہے۔ بہت سی جراثیمی بیماریوں میں علاج کے لیے استعمال کی جاتی ہے۔ اس میں وہ بیماریاں بھی ہیں جہاں پنسلین غیر موثر ہو جاتی ہے تپ دق کے علاج میں استعمال کی جاتی ہے۔ منہ کے ذریعے دی جائے تو جذب نہیں ہوتی اس لیے بعض آنتوں کے امراض میں یہ دوا دی جاتی ہے۔ سروکس یا رحم کے منہ کی سوزش میں سٹرپٹو مائی سین پروکین پنسلین انجکشن ایک روزانہ دس دن تک تپ دق میں ایک گرام کا ٹیکہ روزانہ لگائیے پیری کارڈائی ٹس میں ایک ٹیکہ روزانہ مفید برائے ٹولاریمیا لیوپس ولگیرس۔

Streptothrix *(strep'-to-thriks)* [G. *streptos* curved; *thrix,* thread]. A filamentous bacterium which shows true branching.

سٹرپٹو تھرکس: ایک ریشہ دار جرثومہ جو صحیح شاخداری کو ظاہر کرتا ہے۔

Striatran. Emylcamate (q.v.).

سٹریاٹران: ایمائیلکیمیٹ۔

Striae *(stri'-e)* [L. furrows]. Streaks; stripes narrow bands. Striae gravidarum, lines which appear, especially on the abdomen, as a result of stretching of the skin in pregnancy; due to rupture of the lower layers of the dermis. They are red at first and then become silvery white--stria, sing.; striated, adj.

روشن دھاریاں: تنگ پٹیاں۔

Stricture *(strik'-tur)* [L. *strictura,* compression]. A narrowing, especially of a tube or canal due to scar tissue or tumour.

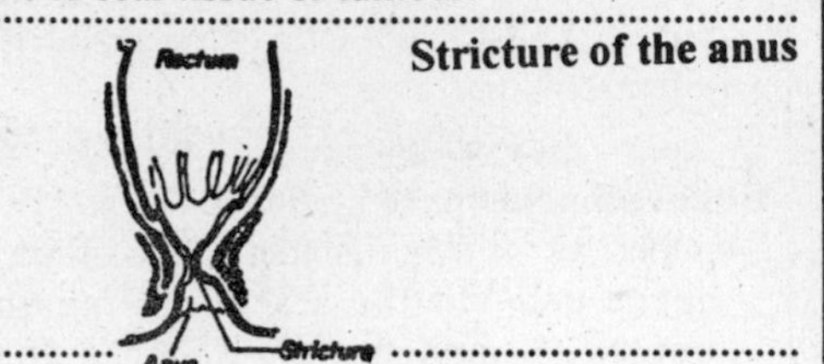

Stricture of the anus

سکڑاؤ: تنگی خصوصاً کسی نلی یا قنال کی جو کسی سکار ٹشو یا رسولی کی وجہ سے ہو سکتی ہے۔

Stridor *(stri'-dor)* [L. harsh sound]. A harsh sound in breathing, casused by air passing through constricted air passages--stridulous, adj.

خرخراہٹ: تنفس میں ایک کرخت آواز جو تنگ ہوائی راہوں میں سے ہوا کے گزرنے سے ہوتا ہے۔

Stroke *(strok)* . Popular term for apoplexy resulting from a vascular accident in the brain, usually resulting in hemiplegia. Heatstroke is hyperpyrexia due to inhibition of heat-regulating mechanism in conditions of high temperature or high humidity, or because sweating is interfered with.

فالج۔حملہ مرض: دماغ میں واسکولر حادثے کے نتیجہ میں اپوپلیکسی۔

Stroma *(stro'-ma)* [G. bed]. The interstitial or foundation sustance of a structure.

سٹروما۔اساس نسیجی: کسی ساخت کا اولین یا بنیادی مادہ۔

Strongyloides *(strong'-i-loids)*. Intestinal worms that can infest man.

سٹرونگائی لائی ڈیس: آنتوں کے کیڑے۔

Strongyloidiasis *(strong-i-loid-i'-a-sis)* Infestation with Strongyloides stercoralis, usually acquired through skin from contaminated soil, but can be through mucous membrane. At site of larval penetration there may be an itchy rash. As the larvae migrate through the lungs there may be pulmonary symptoms with larve in sputum. There may be varying abdominal symptoms. Because of autoinfective life cycle, treatment aims at complete elimination of the parasite. Thiabendazole 25 mg per kg twice daily for 2 days; given either as a suspension or tablets which should be chewed. Driving a car is inadvisable during therapy.

خیطہ زدگی: ملاوٹ شدہ مٹی سے جلد میں سٹرانگیلائیڈز سٹرکوریلس کا داخل ہوتا۔

Strontium 90 Radioactive isotope with a relatively long half-life (28 years). It is incorporated into bone tissue where turnover is slow.

سٹرونشیم ۔۹: ریڈ ایکٹو آئیسوٹوپ جس کی نصف حیات نسبتاً طویل (۲۸ سال) ہوتی ہے۔

Strophanthus *(stro-fan'-thus)*. African plant with cardiac properties similar to digitalis, but of more repid action. The active principle, strophanthin, is sometimes given by intravenous injection.

تنابی گل: افریقی پودا جس میں قلبی خصوصیات ہوتی ہیں۔

Strophulus *(strof'-ul-us)* . Prickly heat; miliaria (q.v.).

لال دانے: ملی اریا

Strychnine *(strik'-nen)*. A bitter alkaloid obtained from nux vomica. Uses as a tonic in associatoin with other bitter drugs.

سٹرکنین: الکلائڈ جو ایک پودے کے بیجوں میں پایا جاتا ہے۔ایک سفید قلمی مرکب پانی میں ذرا سا حل پذیر' نقطہ پگھلاؤ ۲۸۴° س اس کا انتہائی تلخ یا کڑوا ذائقہ ہوتا ہے۔اور اعصابی نظام پر طاقت ور اور بہت خطرناک عمل کرتا ہے۔ معمولی خوراکوں میں ادویات میں استعمال کیا جاتا ہے۔

Stupe *(stup)*. A medical fomentation (q.v.) Opium may be added to relieve pain. Turpentine may be added to produce counterirritation.

ٹکور پٹی: ایک میڈیکل فومینٹیشن درد کے آرام کے لیے افیم کا اضافہ کیا جا سکتا ہے۔

Stupor *(stu'-por)* [L]. A state of marked impairment of , but not complete loss of consciousness. The victim shows gross lack of responsiveness, usually reacting only to noxious stimuli. In psychiatry there are three main varieties of s.;depressive, schizophrenic and hysterical--stuporous, adj.

بے حسی: ہوش کے ضیاع کی حالت لیکن مکمل نہیں۔

Sturge-Weber syndrome A genetically determined congenital ectodermosis, i.e. a capillary haemangioma above eye may be accompanied by similar changes in vessles inside skull giving rise to epilepsy and other cerebral manifestations. Naevoid amentia. [William A. Sturge, English physician, 1850-1919. Frederick Parkes Weber, English physician, 1863]

سٹرج ویبر سنڈروم: ایکٹوڈرموسس کا سنڈروم۔

St Vitus, dance, See CHOREA.

سینٹ ویٹس: رقص

Stye *(sti)*. An abscess in the follicle of an eyelash. Syn., hordeolum.

شعیرہ، گوہانجنی: آنکھ کی پلک کے فولیکل تہہ، پلکوں کی جڑ میں پھوٹے کے کنارے پر ایک قسم کی پھلنی علاج کے لیے آکسی ٹیٹراسائیکلین آنکھ کا مرہم، سلفاڈایازین گولیاں۔ کرسٹامائی سین انجکشن اور سیپٹران۔

Styloid *(sti'-loid)* [G. *stylos* pillar; *eidos,* form]. Long and pointed; resembling a pen or stylus.

سہمی۔ ابریہ: لمبا اور نوکیلا۔

Styptic *(stip'-tik)*. An astringent applied to stop bleeding. Haemostatic.

حابس۔ خون بند: روانی خون روکنے کے لیے اسٹرنجنٹ۔

Stypven *(stip'-ven)* . A preparation of viper venom, used by local application as a haemostatic.

سٹیوین: سانپ کے زہر سے ماخوذ، خون روکنے کے لیے مستعمل۔

Styrion *(sti'-ri-on)*. A synthetic resin capable of absorbing acids. It is sometimes useful in peptic ulcer.

سٹائیریون: ترشوں کو جذب کرنے کے قابل ایک تالیفی رال۔

Suavitil *(su-av'-it-il)*. Benactyzine (q.v.)

سواویٹل: بینکٹائزین۔

Subacute *(sub-ak-ut')* [L. *sub,* under; *acutus,* pointed]. Moderately severe.Often the stage between the acute and chronic phases of disease. **subacute bacterial endocarditis,** septicaemia superimposed on previous valvular heart lesion. Petechiae of the skin and embolic phenomena are characteristic. **subacute combined degeneration** of the **spinal cord** is a complication of perniciou anaemia (PA) and affects the posterior an lateral columns.

ت الحاد: اکثر انتہائی وقدیم مرض کے درمیان ایک مرحلہ۔

Subarachnoid space *(sub-a-rak'-noid)* [L. *sub* under; G. *arachne* ,spider; *eidos,* form]. Th space beneath the arachnoid membrane between it and the pia mater.It contain cerebrospinal fluid.

نصہ وسط دماغ: ارکنائڈ جھلی کے نیچے جگہ۔ اس کے اوپر پایا میٹر رمیان۔ اس میں سربروسپائنل سیال ہوتا ہے۔

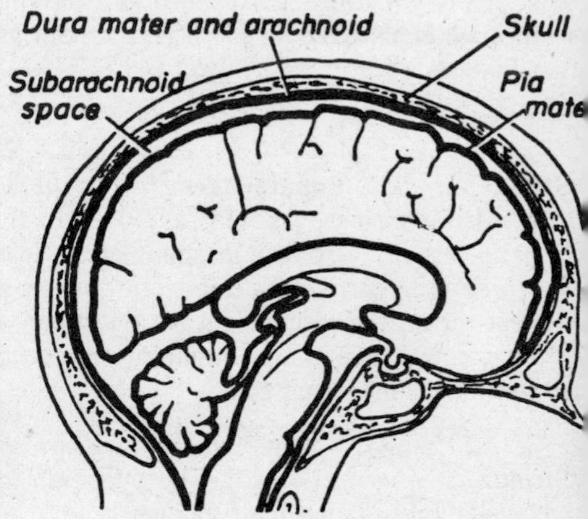

Subdural haematom

Subcarinal *(sub-kar-i'-nal)* [L. *sub,* under *carina,* keel].Below a carina, usually referrin to the carina tracheae.

ب کیرنیل: کیرائنا کے نیچے

Subclavian *(sub-kla'-vi-an)* [L. *sub,* under *clavis,* key]. Beneath the clavicle.

ریر ترقوی: ہنسلی کی ہڈی کے نیچے۔

Subclinical *(sub-klin'-ik-al)* [L. *sub,* under; G *klinikos,* of a bed]. Insufficient to cause th classical identifiable disease.

تحت سریری: کلاسیکل قابل شناخت مرض کا سبب بننے کے لیے ناکافی۔

Subconjunctival *(sub-con-junjk-ti'-val)* [L. *sub*

under; *conjunctivus,* serving to connect]. Below the conjunctiva--subconjunctivally, adv.

تحت ملتحمہ: کنجنکٹیوا کے نیچے۔

Subconscious That portion of the mind outside the range of clear consciousness, but capable of affecting conscious mental or physical reactions.

تحت الشعوری: ذہن کا وہ حصہ جو صاف اور واضح شعوریت کی رینج سے باہر ہو لیکن شعوری ذہنی یا طبعی تعاملات پر اثر کرنے کے قابل ہو۔

Subcostal *(sub-kos'-tal)* [L. *sub,* under; *costa,* rib]. Beneath the rib.

زیر ضلعی: پسلی کے نیچے

Subarachnoid space

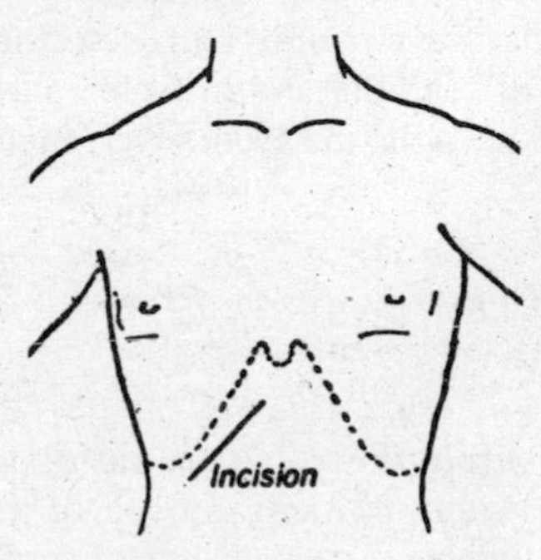

Subcutaneous *(sub-ku-ta'-ni-us)* [L. *sub,* under; *cutis,* skin]. Beneath the skin--subcutaneously, adv.

زیر جلدی: جلد کے نیچے۔ زیر جلد ٹیکہ لگانے کیلئے ابھری ہوئی جلد میں سوئی ۳۰ درجہ کے زاویہ پر چھبوئی جاتی ہے۔ یہ بالائی بازو میں لگایا جاتا ہے۔

Subcuticular *(sub-ku-tik'-u-lar)* [L. *sub,* under; *cuticula,* cuticle]. Beneath the cuticle, as a s, abscess.

تحت البشرہ: ڈیورا میٹر کے نیچے۔ ڈیورا

Subdural *(sub-du'-ral)* [L. *sub,* under; *durus,* hard]. Beneath the dura mater; between the dura and arachnoid membranes.

Subcostal incision

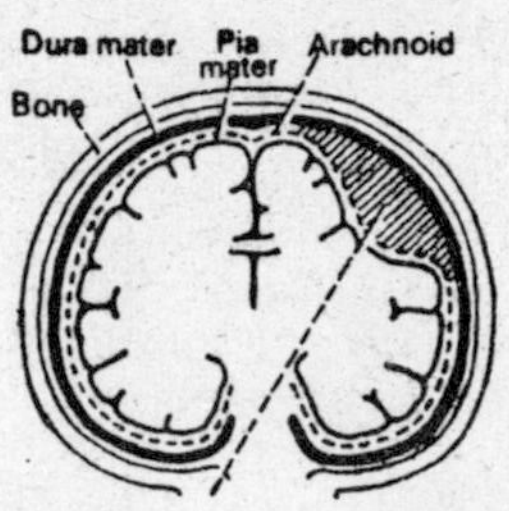

زیر جافیہ: ڈیورا میٹر کے نیچے۔ ڈیورا اور ارکنائڈ جھلیوں کے درمیان۔

Subendocardial *(sub-end-o-kar'-di-al)* [L. *sub,* below; G. *endon,* within; *kardia,* heart]. Immediately beneath the endocardium.

تحت غشاء مستبطن للقلب: اینڈوکارڈیم کے بالکل نیچے۔

Subhepatic *(sub-hep-at'-ik)* [L. *sub,* under; G. *hepar,*liver]. Beneath the liver.

زیر جگری: جگر کے نیچے۔

Subinvolution *(sub-in-vol-u'-shun)* [L. *sub,* under; *involvere,* to roll up]. Failure of the gravid uterus to return to its normal size within a normal time after childbirth. See INVOLUTION.

نامکمل کشادگی: بچے کی پیدائش کے بعد نارمل وقت میں یوٹرس کے نارمل سائز اختیار کرنے میں ناکامی۔ بچے دانی کا کم پھیلنا۔

Subjective *(sub-jek'-tiv)* [L. *subjectivus*]. Internal; personal; arising from the senses and not perceptible to others Opp., objective.

نفسی: اندرونی' ذاتی' حواس سے ابھرنے والا اور دوسروں کو نظر نہ آنے والا۔

Sublimate *(sub'-lim-at)* [L. *sublimare,* to elevate]. A solid deposit resulting from the condensation of a vapour. In psychiatry, to redirect a primitive desire into some more socially acceptable channel, e.g. strong tendency to agressiveness subliminated into sporting activity--sublimation, n.

صعید: ایسا ٹھوس جو بخاری ٹھوس کی براہ راست تکثیف سے مائع حالت میں گزرے بغیر حاصل کیا گیا ہو تصعید سے مراد کسی ٹھوس کی بخارات میں براہ

راست تبدیلی اور پگھلے بغیر تکثیف ہے۔

Subliminal *(sub-lim'-in-a)* [L. *sub,* under; *limen,* threshold]. Inadequate for perceptible response. Below the threshold of consciousness. See LIMINAL.

کششفی: شعوریت کی زیرنگرانی۔

Sublingual *(sub-ling'-gwal)* [L. *sub,* under; *lingua,* tongue]. Beneath the tongue.

زیرزبانی: زبان کے نیچے۔

Subluxation *(sub-luks-a'-shun)* [L. *sub,* under; *luxatio,* dislocation]. Incomplete dislocation of a joint. Term usually implies that joint can return to normal position without formal reduction.

جزوی خلع: جوڑ کا نامکمل ہلنا یعنی اپنی جگہ نہ رہنا۔

Submandibular *(sub-man-dib'-u-lar)* [L. *sub,* under; *mandibla,* jaw]. Belwo the mandible.

سب مینڈیبولر: مینڈیبل کے نیچے۔

Submaxillary *(sub-maks-ilL-lar-i)* [L. *sub,* under; *maxilla,* jaw]. Beneath the lower jaw.

زیرفکی: نچلے جبڑے کے نیچے۔

Submucosa *(sub-mu-ko'-sa)* [L. *sub,* under; *mucosus,* mucous]. The layer of connective tissue beneath a mucous membrane-- submucous, submucosal, adj.

زیرمخاط: میوکس جھلی کے نیچے واصل نسیج کی تہہ۔

Submucous (sub-mu'-kus). Below mucous membrane. submucous resection, straightening of a deflected nasal septum.

Subnormality A state of arrested or incomplete development of mind (not amounting to severe s.) which includes subnormality of intelligence and is of a nature or degree which requires or is susceptible to medical treatment or other special care or training of the patient. **severe s.,** a state of arrested or incomplete developm- ent of mind which includes subnormality of inteligence and is of such a nature or degree that the patient is incapable of living an independent life or of guarding himself against serious exploitation, or will be so incapable when of an age to do so.

ت طبعی: ذہن کی محدود یا مکمل ترقی جس میں ذہانت کی کمی بھی شامل ہے
ں کے لیے مریض کا علاج، خصوصی نگہداشت یا تربیت ضروری ہے۔

Suboccipital *(sub-oks-ip'-it-al)* [L. *sub,* unde *occiput,* back of head]. Beneath the occipu in the nape of the neck.

یرقذالی: آکسپٹ کے نیچے۔

Subperiosteal *(sub-per-i-os'-ti-al)* [L. *sul* under; G. *periosteos,* around the bones Beneath the periosteum of bone.

ت السمحاق: ہڈی کے پیری آسٹیم کے نیچے۔

Subphrenic *(sub-fren'-ik)* [L. *sub,* under; (*phren,* midriff]. Beneath the periosteum (bone.

یرحاجزی: ڈایافرام کے نیچے۔

Subsultus *(sub-sul'-tus)* [L. *subsultare,* to leap Muscular tremor. **Subsultus tendinum,** twi ching of tendons and muscles particular around the wrist in severe fever, such as typh oid.

شنجی حرکت: عضلاتی تشنج۔

Succinylcholine *(sucks-in-il-ko'-len).* Short-ac ing muscle relaxant.

کسی نلکولین: مختصرالعمل عضلے کو آرام پہنچانے والا۔

Succinylsulphathiazole *(suk-sin-il-sul-fa-thi a-zol)* A sulphonamide used in gastroni estinal infections and in bowel surgery. It poorly absorbed and is not effective again systemic infections.

کسی نائیل سلفاتھایازول: سلفونامائیڈ۔ معدے آنتوں کے امراض
ں مستعمل۔ سلفاسکسی ڈین ۲ گولیاں صبح ۲ دوپہر ۲ شام سپرد اور دست
کنے کے لیے کھلایئے۔ ابیائی پچس میں بھی یہی خوراک۔

Succus *(suk'-us)* [L. juice]. A juice, especiall that secreted by the intestinal glands an called's. entericus.

س: جوس یا رس خصوصاً آنتوں کی غدود سے خارج ہونے والا۔

Succussion *(suk-ush'-on)* [L. *succutere,* to flin from below]. Splashing sound produced b fluid in a hollow cavity on shaking th patient, e.g. liquid content of dilated stomac in pyloric stenosis. **hippocratic s.,** th splashing sound, on shaking, when fluid acc mpanies a pneumothorax.

زلزال : مریض کو ہلانے پر کھوکھلے کہفہ میں سیال سے پیدا ہونے والی آواز۔

Sucrose *(su'-kros).* Cane, beet or maple sugar. A disaccharide. It is normally converted into dextrose and levulose in the body.

سکروز' چینی' قند نیشکر : گنے کی شکر۔ چقندر کی شکر' سیکروز' گھروں میں مستعمل ہونے والی عام چینی ۔ایک سفید شریں قلمی ڈائی سیکرائیڈ' نقطہ پگھلاؤ ۱۶۰° تا ۱۸۶° س' یہ بہت سے پودوں میں پائی جاتی ہے۔ مثلاً گنا چقندر وغیرہ

Sucrosuria *(su-kro-su'-ri-a)* The presence of sucrose in the urine.

سکروسوریا: پیشاب میں شکروز کی موجودگی۔

Sudamina *(su-dam'-in-a)* [L. *sudare,* to sweat]. Sweat rash.

مبارکی (مرض): پسینہ آنے سے جگر پر گرمی دانے۔

Sudan blindness A form of onchocerciasis.

سوڈانی' اندھاپن: مرض کی ایک قسم۔

Sudor *(su'-dor)* [L.]. Sweat--sudoriferous, adj.

عرق : پسینہ

Sudorific *(su-dor-if'-ik)* [L. *sudor,* sweat; *facere,* to make]. An agent which induces sweating. Diaphoretic.

پسینہ آور: ایسا ایجنٹ جو پسینہ لاتا ہے۔

Suggestibility *(suj-jest'-ib-il'-it-i)* [L. *suggerere,* to suggest]. Amenable to suggestion (q.v.) is heightened in hospital patients, in the dependence on others that illness brings, in children, in the mentally subnormal and those with a tendency to hysteria.

ایماپذیری: تجویز کو ماننا۔

Sulphacetamide *(sul-fa-set'-a-mid).* A sulphonamide used mainly as eye .

Suggestion *(suj-jest'-chun)* [L. *suggestio,* suggest]. The implanting in a person's mind of an idea which he accepts fully without logical reason. Suggestion is utilized when the idea of recovery is given to ,and accepted by , a patient. In psychiatric practice. is used as a therapeutic measure sometimes under hypnosis or narcoanalysis (q.v.).

ایما' تجویز' تحریک: کسی شخص کے ذہن میں ایسا خیال ڈال دینا کہ وہ اسے بلاحیل وحجت قبول کرلے مریض کی صحت یابی پر اسے یہ خیال دیا جاتا ہے اور وہ اسے قبول کر لیتا ہے۔

Sulcus *(sul'-kus)* [L.] A furrow or groove, particularly those separating the gyri or convolutions of the cortex of the brain--sulci, pl.

ناب: نشیب' خصوصاً دماغ کی سلوٹوں کو جدا کرنے والے نشیب۔

Sulfametopyrazine *(sul-fa-met-o-pi-ra-zen)* Particularly useful for urinary infections.

Sulfamylon *(sul-fa-mi'-lon)* Mefenide acetate (q.v.)

Sulfasuxidine *(sul-fa-suks'-i-den).* Succinylsulphathiazole (q.v.).

سلفاسکسی ڈین: معدے آنتوں کے امراض میں مستعمل۔ سکسی نائیل سلفا تھیازول ۔ دست' سپرو' اور بیلری پچس روکنے کے لیے ۲ گولیاں صبح ۲ دوپہر ۲ شام

Sulphacetamide *(sul-fa-set'-a-mid).* A sulphonamide used mainly as eye drops, and systemically for urinary tract infections.

سلفاسیٹامائیڈ: سلفونامائیڈ جو زیادہ تر آئی ڈراپس میں استعمال کیا جاتا ہے۔ ایک قطرہ دن میں ۴ مرتبہ برائے ٹرے کومایا لگرے۔

Sulphadizaine *(sul-fa-di'-a-zen)* Powerful sulphonamide compound for systemic use in many infections. Often drug of choice in meningococcal infections as penetration into CSF is greater. It is less effective against staphylococcal infections.

سلفاڈایازین: کئی امراض میں مستعمل طاقتور سلفونامائیڈ مرکب' زکام نپل یا بھٹنی کے درد میں' برونکائی ٹس' ٹوکسوٹولاریمیا اور سوزاک میں ۲ گولیاں صبح ۲ دوپہر ۲ شام دیجئے اور پانی زیادہ پلائیے۔ ۲ گولیاں ہر چھ گھنٹے بعد برائے ایکٹینومائی کوسز' امپے ٹائیگو' ایری سیپلاز۔

Sulphadimidie *(sul-fa-di'-mi-den).* One of the most effective and least toxic of the sulphonamides, and reduced incidence of side effects increases its value in paediatrics. The sodium salt may be given by injection.

سلفاڈیمیڈین: موثر ترین اور کم از کم زہریلے سلفونامائیڈز سے ایک۔

Sulphaemoglobinaemia *(sulf-hem-o-glob-in-e'-mi-a)* A condition of circulating sulphmethaemoglobin in the blood.

سلفاایموگلوبی نیمیا: خون میں گردشی سلفمیتھیموگلوبن کی حالت۔

Sulphafurazole *(sul-fa-fur'-a-zol)* A sulphonamide of wide application, but used mainly in urinary infections owing to its high solubility.

سلفافیورازول: ایک سلفونامائیڈ۔ بولی امراض میں زیادہ استعمال کیا جاتا ہے۔ کیونکہ یہ بہت زیادہ حل پذیر ہے۔

Sulphaguanidine *(sul-fa-gwan'-i-den)*. Once used in gastrointestinal infections but now largely replaced by less soluble compounds such as phthalylsulphathiazole.

سلفا گوانیڈین: پہلے دوا معدے آنتوں کے امراض میں بکثرت استعمال ہوتی تھی۔ لیکن اب اس کی جگہ کم حل پذیر :و یہ استعمال کی جاتی ہیں۔

Sulphamerazine *(sulf-fa-mer'-a-zen)*. A longer acting sulphonamide, effective in 8-hourly doses, but the slow elimination may cause toxic side effects.

سلفامیرازین: ایک طویل عمل والا سلفونامائیڈ۔

Sulphamethazine *(sul-fa-meth'-a-zen)*. Sulphadimidine (q.v.)

سلفامیتھازین:

Sulphamethoxazole *(sul-fa-meth-oks'-a-zol)*. Sulphonamide that has a pattern of obsorption and excretion very similar to trimethoprim.

سلفامیتھوکسازول: سلفونامائیڈ۔ ٹرائی میتھوپرم سے مشابہ

Sulphamethoxydiazine *(suf-fa-meth-oks'-i-di-a-zen)*. A variant of the sulphonamides (q.v.)

Sulphamethoxypryridazine *(sul-fa-meth-ok'-si-pi-ri-da-zen)* A long-acting, small-dosage sulphonamide.

سلفامیتھاکسی پیری ڈازین: طویل عمل والا لیکن تھوڑی خوراک والا سلفونامائیڈ۔ لیڈرکن۔ مڈیکل۔ ایک گولی روزانہ برائے بوائل۔

Sulphapyridine *(sul-fa-pi'-ri-den)*. One of the early sulphonamides, now replaced by less toxic drugs. Occasionally used in low dose in dermatitis herpetiformis.

سلفاپائیریڈین: اولین سلفونامائیڈز میں سے ایک۔ اب اس کی جگہ کم زہریلے زیرا استعمال ہیں۔

Sulphathiazole *(sul-fa-thi'-a-zo)*. A powerful but rapidly excreted sulphonamide. Toxic effects are common with this drug, and it is now used less frequently, except in assoc iation with other sulphonamides.

لفاتھیازول: ایک طاقتور لیکن تیزی سے خارج ہونیوالا سلفونامائیڈ۔ ہریلے پن کی وجہ سے کم استعمال کی جاتی ہے یا دوسری ادویہ کے ساتھ ملا کر تعمال کی جاتی ہے۔

Sulphatriad *(sul-fa-tri'-ad)*. Contains sulph adiazine, sulphamerazine and sulphathiazol Sulphonamide mixtures reduce thr risk toxic side effects.

لفاٹرائی ایڈ: سلفاڈایازین، سلفامیرازین اور سلفاتھیازول پر مشتمل۔

Sulphinpyrazone *(sul-fin-pir'-a-zon)*. Uri osuric agent.

لفن پائیرازون: یوریکوسورک ایجنٹ۔

Sulphmethaemoglobin *(sulf- met- hem- o-glo in)*. Syn., sulphaemoglobin. A sulphid oxidation product of haemoglobin, produce in vivo by certain drugs. This compoun cannot transport oxygen or carbon dioxi and , not being reversible in the body , is indirect poison.

لف میتھیموگلوبن: یہ آکسیجن یا کاربن ڈائی آکسائیڈ کونہیں لے جا تا۔ ہیموگلوبن کا ایک سلفائیڈ تکسید پروڈکٹ۔ بعض ادویہ سے جانداروں میں راہوتا ہے۔

Sulphonamides A group of bacteriostat agents, effective orally, but must b maintained in a definite concentration in th blood. Antimetabolites. Inhibit formation folic acid, which for many organisms is essential metabolite.

لفونامائیڈز: سلفاڈرگز۔ نامیاتی مرکبات کا ایک گروہ جو سلفونامائیڈ گروہ NH SO_2 یا اس کے مشتقات (ماخوذ) پر مشتمل ہے۔ یا ایسی بیماریوں علاج کے لیے مفید ہے۔ جو جراثیم سے پیدا ہوتی ہیں۔

Sulphonamidopyrimidines *(sul-fon-a-mid'-o-p ri-mid'-enz)*. Oral blood-sugar lowerin agents.

فونا میڈو پائیری میڈینز: منہ کے ذریعے کھائی جانے والی دوا۔ یہ نس خونی شکر کو کم کرتے ہیں۔

Sulphones *(sul'-fons)*. A group of synthetic dr gs useful for leprosy.

فونز: جذام یا کوڑھ کے لیے مفید تالیفی ادویہ کا ایک گروہ۔

Sulphonylureas *(sul-fon-il-u'-re-as)* Sulphon

mide derivatives that are oral hypoglycaemic agents. They increase insulin output from the pancreas.

سلفونائل یوریاس: سلفونامائیڈ کے مشتقات جولبلبہ سے انسولین آوٹ پٹ کوزیادہ کرتے ہیں۔

ılphur *(sul'-fur)*. An insoluble yellow powder once used extensively as sulphur ointment for scabies. Still used in lotions for acne and other skin disorders, and internally as a laxative.

گندھک: ایک عنصر' جوہری وزن ۳۲ء۰۶۴ جوہری عدد ۱۶ کثافت اضافی ۳ء۰۷ نقطہ پگھلاؤ ۱۱۲ء۸° اس نقطہ جوش ۴۴۴ء۶°س' علامت S پاکستان میں آزاد گندھک کے ذخائر صوبہ بلوچستان میں پائے جاتے ہیں۔ گندھک کی متعد بہروپی شکلیں ہیں مثلاً معین نما' منشوری یا نقلمی گندھک یہ حرارت اور برق کے لیے ناقص موصل ہے۔ اسے برقی آلات میں جاجڑ کے طور پر استعمال کرتے ہیں۔ اس کی بیشتر مقدار گندھک کے تیزاب کی صنعت میں استعمال ہوتی ہے۔ یہ کاربن ڈائی سلفائڈ' بارود' رنگوں اور دیا سلائی اور ربڑ کی صنعتوں میں بھی استعمال ہوتی ہے۔ اسے طب میں بھی استعمال کیا جاتا ہے۔ ایک ناحل پذیر پیلا سفوف جو پہلے گندھک کے مرہم میں بہت زیادہ استعمال کیا جاتا ہے۔ اب لوشن میں پھنسیوں اور دوسری جلدی خرابیوں میں مستعمل ہے۔ بطور جلاب بھی استعمال کیا جاتا ہے۔ مفید برائے رنگ ورم۔

ılphuric acid *(sul-fu'-rik as'-id)*. The concentrated acid is widely employed in industry, and is very corrosive. The diulte acid (10 per cent) has been given for its astringent action, but is now rarely used.

سلفیورک ایسڈ۔ گندھک کا تیزاب : ایک بے رنگ تیلیا وزنی مائع' کثافت اضافی ۱ء۸۴' محلول میں ہائیڈروجن پیدا کرتا ہے۔ یہ دواساسی ترشہ ہے۔ مرتکز گندھک کا تیزاب گرم حالت میں طاقت ور تکسیدی عامل کے طور پر عمل کرتا ہے۔ اسے پانی کے ساتھ خاص رغبت ہے یہ اچھا خشک کندہ عامل ہے۔ نامیاتی عطری مرکبات پر مرتکز گندھک کا تیزاب عمل کرتا ہے۔ جسے سلفونیشن کہا جاتا ہے۔ اس طرح سلفونیشن بنتے ہیں۔ کیمیائی صنعتوں میں سے ہر ایک صنعت میں یہ براہ راست یا بالواسطہ استعمال ہوتا ہے۔ اس کا استعمال ان صنعتوں میں زیادہ ہے تالیفی رنگوں کی صنعت' چونے کے سپر فاسفیٹ کی صنعت' پٹرولیم کی صفائی اور دھماکو اشیاء کی صنعت' سالمی وزن ۹۸ء۰۸ زہریلا جلد کو جلا دیتا ہے۔ اب اسے ادویہ میں بہت کم استعمال کیا جاتا ہے۔

ılthiame *(sul-thi'-am)*. For temporal lobe and Jacksonian epilepsy.

سلتھی ایم: ٹمپورل لوب اور دماغ کی خراب برقی عاملیت کے نتیجہ میں شعور کے ضیاع کے لیے۔

Sunstroke Syn., heat-stroke. See STROKE.

آفتاب زدگی' دھوپ کا سرسام: ہیٹ سٹروک۔ سٹروک۔ یہ تیز دھوپ میں ناکافی لباس پہن کر چلنے پھرنے سے ہوتا ہے۔ مریض کا چہرہ لال' نبض تیز' پیاس زیادہ' کھال خشک اور درجہ حرارت زیادہ ہو جاتا ہے۔ سانس گھٹنے لگتی ہے۔ جی متلاتا ہے۔ سن سٹروک سے بچنے کے لئے سولا ہیٹ استعمال کرنا چاہیے۔

Supercilium *(su-per-sil'-i-um)* [L. eyebrow]. The eyebrow--superciliary, adj.

حاجب: ابرو۔ لاطینی لفظ بمعنی ابرو

Superior *(su-pe'-ri-or)* [L. higher]. In anatomy, the upper of two parts.

اعلی۔ بالائی: دو حصوں کا اوپر والا۔

Supernumerary *(su-per-nu'-mer-ar-i)*. IN excess of the normal number; additional.

فاضل۔ فالتو: زائد۔ عام تعداد سے زیادہ

Supernumerary digit

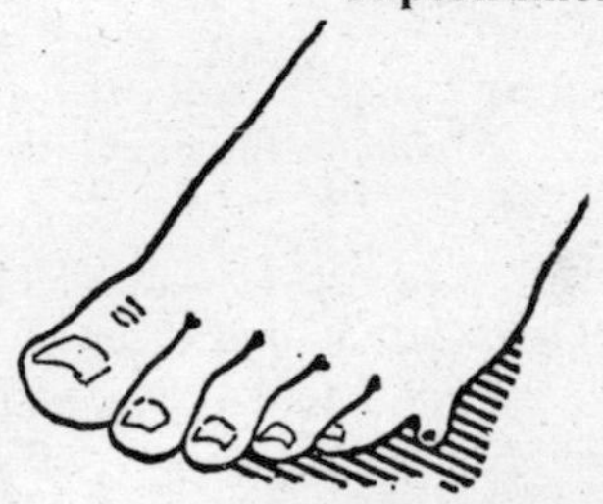

Supernumerary digit

Supinate *(su'-pin-at)* [L. *supinare,* to bend backward]. Turn face or palm upward. Opp., pronate--supination, n.

ہاتھ کو چت کرنا۔ بطح: چہرہ یا ہتھیلی اوپر کی طرف

Supinator *(su-pin-a'-tor)*. That which supinates, usually applied to a muscle. Opp., pronator.

عضلہ۔ باطح: جو چہرہ یا ہتھیلی کو اوپر کرے۔ اس کا اطلاق عموماً عضلے پر ہوتا ہے۔ یہ عضلہ زیرین بازو کی خلفی جانب ہوتا ہے۔ یہ ہیومرس اور النا سے اٹھ کر "ریڈی اس" کی بیرونی جانب پر وینٹر سے اوپر جڑتا ہے ہاتھ اور نچلے بازو کو گھماتا ہے۔

Supine *(su'-pin)* [L. *supinus,* thrown backward].

Lying on the back with face upwards, palm upwards. Opp., prone.

چت خوابی: پشت کے بل ایسے لیٹنا کہ چہرہ اوپر ہو اور ہتھیلی بھی اوپر ہو۔

Suppository *(sup-os'-i-tri)*. Medicament in a base that melts at body temperature. Inserted rectally.

شافہ: ایسے اساس میں مرہم جو جسمانی درجہ حرارت پر پگھلتا ہے۔ عموماً پاخانہ لانے کے لیے مقعد میں چڑھایا جاتا ہے۔

Suppression *(sup-resh'-un)* [L. *supprimere,* to press down]. Cessation of a secretion (e.g. urine) or a normal process (e.g. menstruation). In psychology, the voluntary forcing out of the mind of painful thoughts.This often results in the precipitation of a neurosis (q.v.).

روک۔ حبس: کسی نارمل طریقے یا رطوبت کا بند ہو جانا۔ مثلاً حیض کا بند ہونا۔ نفسیات میں تکلیف دہ خیالات کو ذہن سے زبردستی نکال دینا۔

Suppuration *(sup-ur-a'-shun)* [L. *suppurare,* to suppurate]. The formation of pus--suppurative, adj.; suppurate, v.i.

ریم: پیپ کا بننا۔

Supraclavicular *(soop-ra-klav-ik'-u-lar)* [L. *supra,* above; *clavicula,* little key]. the collar bone (clavicle).

فوق ترقوی: کاربون کے اوپر ہنسلی کی ہڈی۔

Supracondylar *(soop-ra-kond'-il-ar)* [L. *supra,* above , G. *kondylos,* knob]. Above a condyle.

فوق عقدہ عظمیہ: کنڈائل کے اوپر

Supraobital *(soop-ra-or'-bit-al)* [L. *supra,* above; *oribs,* circle]. Above the orbits. supraorbital ridge, the ridge covered by the eyebrows.

فوق محجری: دوائر کے اوپر

Suprapubic *(soop-ra-pu'-bik)* [L. *supra,* above; pubes, *private* parts]. Above the pubis.

فوق عانی: پیوبس کے اوپر

Suprarenal *(soop-ra-ren'-al)* [L. *supra,* above; *renes,* kidneys]. Above the kidney. See ADR ENAL.

برگردہ: گردے کے اوپر۔ سپرارنیل گلینڈز یا ایڈرینل گلینڈز تعداد میں ۲ ورٹبرل کالم کے دونوں طرف گردوں کے اوپر ہوتی ہیں اور پیریٹونیم کے پیچھے۔

لمبائی تقریباً چار سنٹی میٹر اور موٹائی تین سنٹی میٹر۔ رنگ زردی مائل بھورا۔

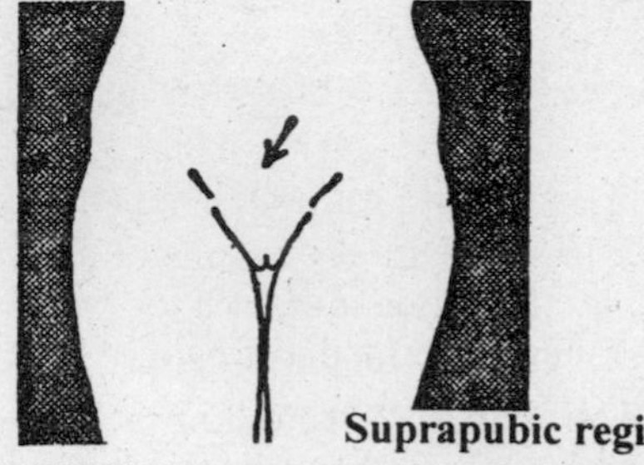

Suprapubic region

Suprapubic region

Suprasternal *(soop-ra-ster'-nal)* [L. *supra,* above; G. *sternon,* breast]. Above the breast bone (sternum).

فوق قصی: چھاتی کی ہڈی یا سٹرنم کے اوپر

Suramin *(su'-ra-min)*. Drug used i.v. in the early stages of trypanosomiasis, filariasis and onchocerciasis. Contraindications; renal disease or adrenal insufficiency.

سورامین: ایک دوا جو فلیریاسس وغیرہ میں دیجاتی ہے۔ مرض النوم میں اس کے ایک گرام کا ایک ٹیکہ ہفتے میں ایک بار رگوں میں لگایئے۔ ایسے دس ٹیکے لگایئے۔

Srugery *(sur'-je-ri)*. That branch of medicine which treats diseases, deformities and injuries, wholly or in part, by manual or operative procedures.

جراحت۔ سرجری: ادویہ کی وہ شاخ جو امراض، بدشکلیوں اور زخموں سے متعلق ہے۔ مکمل طور پر یا جزوی طور پر ہاتھ سے یا اپریشن کے طریقوں سے۔

Surmontil (sur-mon'-til). Trimipramine (q.v.)

سرمونٹل: ٹری میپرامین۔

Susceptibili *(sus-sep-tib-il'-it-i)* [L. *suscipere,* to take up]. The opposite of resistance. Usually refers to a disposition to infection.

تاثر پذیری: مزاحمت یا مدافعت کا متضاد۔

Sustac *(sus'-tak)*. Sustained action glycerly trinitrate (q.v.)

سسٹیک: گلسرائل ٹرائی نائٹریٹ۔

Suture *(su'-tur)*. The junction of cranial bones; in surgery, a stitch. See LIGATURE.

سیون ۔ ٹانکے ۔ بخیہ: کھوپڑی کی ہڈیوں کا جنکشن ۔ سرجری میں ٹانکا۔

uxamethonium *(suks-a-meth-o'-ni-um).* A muscle relaxant used in minor operative work. The action is very brief, lasting 2 to 5 min, but a longer effect can be achieved by continuous intravenous drip infusion. Usually preceded by an intravenous barbiturate to reduce initial muscular fibrillation. Normally hydrolysed by the serum enzyme pseudocholinesterase. An abnormal pseudocholinesterase affects a person's reaction to s. and can give rise to s, apnoea.

سکسا میتھونیم: عضلے کو آرام پہنچانے والا' چھوٹے اپریشن کے کام میں مستعمل ۔ ایکشن بہت مختصر ہوتا ہے۔

VC . Vaginal tablets containing acetarsol (q.v.)

ایس وی سی: ایسٹارسول پر مشتمل ویجائنا کی گولیاں۔

wab *(swob)* .1. A small piece of cotton wool or gauze. 2. A small piece of sterile cotton wool, or similar material, on the end of a shaft of wire or wood, enclosed in a protecting tube. It is used to collect material for bacteriological examination.

پھریری: ۱۔ کاٹن وول یا گار کا ایک چھوٹا ٹکڑا۔ ۲۔ کاٹن وول جو ابال لی گئی ہو' کا ایک چھوٹا ٹکڑا۔ اسے لکڑی یا تار کے سرے پر لگایا جاتا ہے اور وہ نلی میں بند ہوتا ہے۔

weat *(swet).* The secretion from the sudoriferous glands.

پسینہ: سوڈوریفرس گلینڈز کی افرازی رطوبت۔

wenson's operation. For congenital intestinal aganglionosis (Hirschsprung's disease).

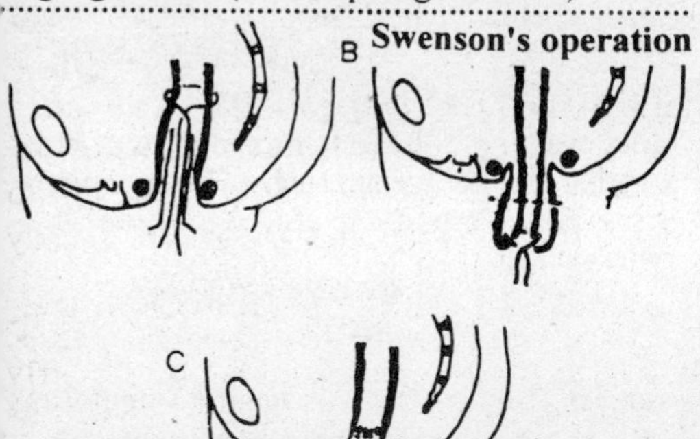

Swenson's operation

اپریشن سوینس: آنتوں کی ایگین گلیونوسس کیلئے شکل دیکھئے۔

Sycosis *(si-ko'-sis)* [G. *sykosis,* fig-likeu!cer]. Barber's itch. sycosis barbai is a pustular folliculitis of the beard area in men. sycosis nuchae is a similar folliculitis at the nape of the neck which leads to keloid thickening (acnc keloid).

انجیریہ: خارش باربر ۔ بالوں کی جڑوں میں جراثیم کیوجہ سے ورم ہو جاتا ہے اور پیپ بڑھ جاتی ہے عموماً سٹے فائیلو کا کسی کی وجہ سے مرض ہوتا ہے یہ عموماً منہ پر ہوتا ہے علاج کے لیے فیوراسین مرہم' ایک فیصد جنشن وائلٹ اور سپیٹران مفید ہیں۔

Symbiosis *(sim-bi-o'-sis)* [G. living together]. A relationship between two or more organisms in which the participants are of mutual aid and benefit to one another--symbiotic, adj.

ہم زیستی: دو جانداروں کے درمیان رشتہ جس سے وہ ایک دوسرے کے ساتھ باہمی فائدہ کے لیے اکٹھے رہتے ہیں ۔ مثلاً چرندے اور سیلولوز ہضم کرنے والے جراثیم لائیکن میں ایک ایلگا اور دوسرا فنگس ہوتا ہے ۔ ایلگا میں کلوروفل موجود ہوتا ہے اس لیے وہ اپنے اور فنگس کے لیے خوراک تیار کرتا ہے ۔ جبکہ ایلگا کے خلیے فنگس کے جسم میں رہتے ہیں۔

Symblepharon *(sim-blef'-a-ron)* [G. *syn,* with ; *blepharon,* eyelid]. Adhesion of the lid to the eyeball.

التصاق الجفن: آنکھ کے گولے کا پپوٹے کے ساتھ چپکنا۔

Syme's amputation. Amputation just above ankle joint. Provides an endbearing stump. Especially useful in primitive conditions where elaborate artificial limbs are not available. [James Syme, Scottish surgeon , 1799 -- 1870].

سائمیز ایمپوٹیشن: ٹخنے کے جوڑے ذرا اوپر قطع عضو۔

Symmetril *(sim'-et-ril)* Amantadine (q.v.).

سمیٹرل: امنٹاڈین۔

Sympathectomy *(sim-path-ek'-to-mi)* [G. *sympathein,* to feel for ; *ektome,* excision]. Surgical excision of part of the sympathetic nervous system.

مشارکی عصب شگافی: سمپی تھیٹک عصبی نظام کے ایک حصے کا سرجیکل قطع ہونا۔

Sympathetic *(sim-path-et'-ik)* [G. *sympathein,*

to feel for]. A portion of the autonomic nervous system. It is composed of a chain of ganglia on either side of the vertebral column in the thoracolumbar region, and sends fibres to all plain muscle tissue.

مشارکی: آٹونومک عصبی نظام کا ایک حصہ۔

Sympathomimetic *(sim-path-o-mim-et'-ik)* [G. *sympathein,* to feel for , *mimokos,* imitaing]. Capable of producing changes similar to those produced by stimulation of the sympathetic nerves.

سمپے تھو مائی میٹک: سمپی تھیٹک اعصاب سے پیدا ہونیوالی سے مشابہ تبدیلیاں پیدا کرنے کا اہل۔ یہ ادویات بلڈ پریشر کو زیادہ بھوک کو کم، نیند کو ختم، تنفس کو تیز، قلب کو قوی، نبض کو تیز، آنتوں کی حرکت کو کم، منہ کو خشک اور سانس کی نالیوں کا تشنج ختم کرتی ہیں۔

Symphysis *(sim'-fis-is)* [G. *symphysis,* growing together]. A fibrocartilaginous union of bones --symphyseal, adj.

ارتفاق: ہڈیوں کا فائبرو کارٹیلی جنس ملاپ۔

Symptom *(simp'-tom)* [G. *symptoma,* anything that happens]. A subjective phenomenon or manifestation of disease. symptom complex, a group of symptoms which, occurring together, typify a particular disease or syndrome--symptomatic ,adj.

علامات مرض: مرض کا ظہور۔

Symptomatology *(simp-tom-at-ol'-o-ji)* [G. *symptoma,* anything that happens; *logos,* discourse]. The branch of mdeicine concerned with symptoms. The combined symptoms typical of a particular disease.

علم علامات مرض: علامات سے متعلق طب کی شاخ۔

Synacthen *(sin-ak'-then).* Tetrocosactrin (q.v.)

سائینیکتھن: ٹیٹر کوسیکٹرن۔

Synalar *(sin'-a-lar).* Fluocinolone (q.v.)

Synapse *(si'-naps)* [G. *synapsis,* contact]. The point of communication between two adjacent neurones. Syn., synapsis.

معانقہ: نیورونز کے درمیان جنکشن جس سے حیوانات کے عصبی نظاموں میں عصبی امپاس منتقل ہوتے ہیں۔ معانقہ عموماً ایک نیوران کے ایکسون اور دوسرے کے ڈینڈرائٹ کے درمیان بنتا ہے۔

Synchysis *(sing'-ki-sis).* Degenerative condition of vitreous humor of the eye, rendering it fluid, synchysis scintillans, fine opacities in vitreous.

لینت زجاجیہ: آنکھ کے وٹریس ہیومر کی تنزلی حالت جس سے سیال بنتا ہے۔

Syncope *(sing'-ko-pi)* [G. *syngkope,* sudden loss of strength]. A faint. Caused by reduced cerebral circulation often following a fright, when vasodilation is responsible . May be symptomatic of cardiac arrhythmia, e.g. heart block--syndactylous, adj.

ضعف: کمزوری۔ طاقت کا اچانک ضیاع معمولی بے ہوشی۔ خون کی کمی یا خون ختم ہونے سے دل کا فعل رک جانا ہے۔ اور موت واقع ہو سکتی ہے۔

Syndactyly *(sin-dak'-ti-li)* [G. *syn,* with; *daktylos,* finger]. Webbed fingers or toes. Also syndactylism, syndactylia-- syndactylious, adj.

پیوستہ انگشتی: جھلی والی انگلیاں

Syndrome *(sin'-drom)* [G. *syndromos,* a running together].A group of symptoms and or signs which, occurring together, produce a pattern or symptom complex, typical of a particular disease..

اجتماع علامات: علامات کا مجموعہ

synechia *(sin-ek'-i-a)* [G. *synecheia,* continuity]. Abnormal union of parts, especially adhesion of the iris to the cornea in front, or the lens capsule behind-synechiae, pl.

التصاق: حصوں کا غیر معمولی ملاپ

Synergism *(sin'-er-jizm)* [G. *synergos,* cooperator]. The harmonious working together of two agents, such as drugs, microorganisms, muscles, etc. Alo synergy--synergic,adj.

ملی عملی: دو ایجنٹوں کا اکھٹے مل کر کام کرنا مثلاً ادویات، خوردجسیے، عضلات وغیرہ

Synergist *(sin'-er-jist).* An agent co-operating with another. One partner in a synergic action.

مل عملیہ: ایجنٹ جو دوسرے کے ساتھ تعاون کرے۔

Synkavit *(sin'-kav-it)*. A water-soluble compound possessing high vitamin K activity.

سن کیوٹ: پانی میں حل پذیر مرکب جو وٹامن "کے" عاملیت رکھتا ہے۔

Synovectomy *(si-nov-ek'-to-mi)*. [N.L. *synovia*; G. ektome, excision]. Excision of synovial membrane. Current early treatment for rheumatoid arthritis especially of the hands.

شق مفصل: سائینووئیل جھلی کا قطع کرنا۔

Synovia *(si'-no'-vi-a)*. [N.L.]. The fluid secreted by the membrane lining a joint cavity--synovial adj.

زلال: جوڑ کے کہفہ کی غلافی جھلی سے خارج ہونے والا سیال۔

Synovial membrane *(si-no'-vi-al mem'-bran)*. That lining a joint capsule; it does not cover the articular surfaces. See BURSA.

غشاء زلالی: جوڑ کے کیپسول کی غلافی پرت۔

Synovioma *(si-no-vi-o'-tis)*. [N.L.].*synovia;* G -oma, tumour]. A turnour of synovial membrane--benign or malignant.

سائینووی اوما: سائینووئیل جھلی کی رسولی۔

Synovitis *(si-nov-i'-tis)*. [N.L. *synovia;* G. *-itis,* inflammation]. Inflammation of a synovial membrane.

ورم زلالی: سائینووئیل جھلی کی سوزش۔

Synthesis *(sin'-the-sis)*. [G. a putting together]. The chemical building up of complex substances from simpler substances--synthetic, adj.

تالیف، ترکیب: اکھٹے کرنا۔ مرکب کا اس کے عناصر یا سادہ مرکبات سے بننا۔

Syntocinon. Synthetic oxytocin (q.v.).

سائنٹو سینان: تالیفی یا ترکیبی آ سیٹوسن بچے کی پیدائش کے بعد خون کو روکنے اور آنوں کو خارج کرنے کا جتن کیا جاتا ہے۔ اس میں آرگومیٹرین سائنٹو سینان کا ٹیکہ بھی دیا جاتا ہے۔ اس سے آنوں کے اخراج میں مدد ملتی ہے۔

Syntometrine *(sin-to-met'-rin)*. Ergometrine maleate 0.5 mg and synthetic oxytocin 5 units in one ampoule. Combines the rapid action of oxytocin with the more sustained action of ergometrine on the uterus.

سینٹو میٹرین: ایک ایمپول میں ارگومیٹرین ملی ایٹ ۰.۵ ملی گرام اور تالیفی آ کسیٹوسن ۵ یونٹ۔

Syphilide *(sif'-il-id)*. [N.L. syphilis]. A syphilitic skin lesion.

آتشکی جلدی مرض: آتشک کی وجہ سے جلدی دانے۔

Syphilis *(sif'-il-is)* . [Syphilus, syphilitic shepherd in poem by Fracastorius (1530), in which the term first appears]. The most severe venereal disease, caused by *Treponema pallidum.* Infection is acquired (may be accidentally) or congenital--when it is prenatal. Acquired syphilis manifests in; (1) The primary stage,appears 4 to 5 weeks (or later) after infection when a primary chance associated with swelling of local lymph glands appears. (2) The secondary stage in which the skin eruption (syphilide) appears. (3) The third stage occurs 15 to 30 years after initial infection. Gummata appear , or neurosyphilis and cardiovascular syphilis supervene. The commonest types of nervous system involvement are general paralysis of the insane and tabes dorsalis (locomotor ataxia). Cardiovascular involvement produces cerebrovascular disasters, aortic aneurysm and impairment or destruction of the aortic valve --syphilitic , adj.

آتشک: اس کا سبب ٹریپونیما پیلیڈم ہے۔ مرض لگنے کے چار پانچ ہفتوں کے اندر عضو تناسل پر پھنسی نکلتی ہے۔ پھر سارا جسم دانوں سے بھر جاتا ہے۔ ۱۵ تا ۳۰ سال میں سب اعصاب بیکار ہو جاتے ہیں۔

Syringomyelia *(si-ring-go-mi-e'-li-a)* [G. *syrigx,* pipe; *myelos,* marrow]. An uncommon, progressive disease of the nervous system of unknown cause, beginning mainly in early adult life. Cavitation and surrounding fibrous tissue reaction, in the upper spinal cord and brain stem, intefere with sensation of pain and temperature, and sometimes with the motor pathways. The characteristic symptom is painless injury, particularly of the exposed hands. Touch sensation is intact.

کہفیت نخاع: جوانی کے ابتدائی ایام میں نظام کا ایک مرض، اس کا سبب معلوم نہیں۔

Syringomyelocele *(si-ring-go-mi'-el-o-sel)* [G. *syrigx,* pipe; *myelos,* marrow]. Most severe form of meningeal hernia (spina bifida). The central canal is dilated and the thinned-out posterior part of the spinal cord is in the hernia.

نخاعی کھفی قیلہ: ہرنیاایک شدید قسم۔

Systole *(sis'-to-li)* [G. a drawing together]. The contraction phase of the cardiac cycle-- systolic, adj.

انقباض قلب: دل کی دھڑکن کا عمل جب قلبی عضلہ سکڑتا ہے۔جس سے خون شریانوں میں جاتا ہے۔

Systolic murmur. Abnormal quality of first heart sound related to the area of one of the heart valves, e.g. systolic mitral murmur.

سسٹولک مرمر: پہلی دلی صدا کی غیر معمولی خاصیت۔

Sytron *(sit'-ron)* Elixir. Sodium iron edetate. For iron deficiency anaemia.

سٹران اکسیر: سوڈیم آئرن ایڈیٹیٹ۔خون میں لوہے کا کمی کے لیے اکسیر۔

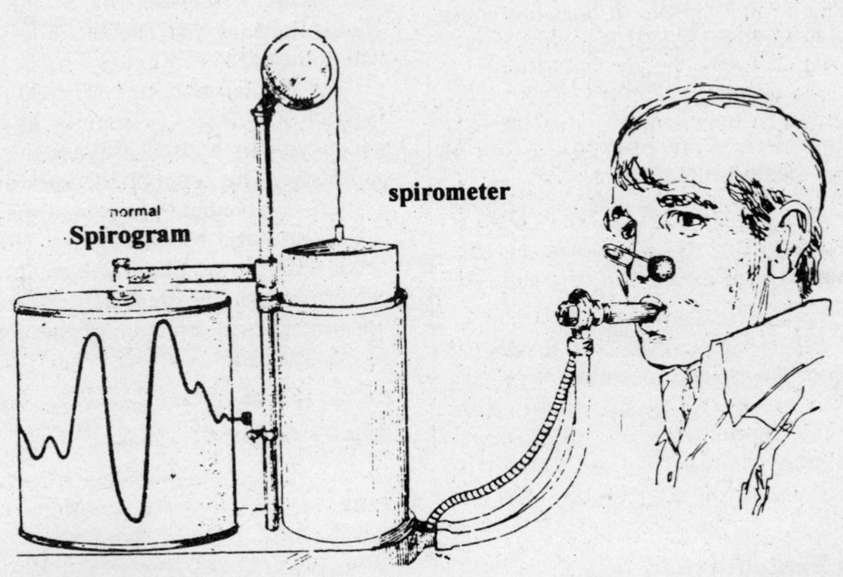

T

AB Vaccine It is a vaccine against typhoid and paratyphoid fever. This contains killed salmonelle typhi s. paratyphi A&B. Its therapeutic use is to produce pyrexia.

ٹی۔اے۔بی ویکسین: مردہ سالمونیلا ٹائفی، پیراٹائفی اے اور پیرا ٹائفی بی پر مشتمل ایک ویکسین ٹائیفائیڈ اور پیراٹائیفائیڈ بخار کے خلاف آدمی میں عامل مصنوعی قوتِ مزاحمت پیدا کرنے کے لئے مستعمل۔

abes *(ta-bez)* [L. wasting away, decaying or melting]. Any wasting of the body, progressive atrophy of the body or part of it. **t. dorcalis**, parenchymatous neurosyphillis in which there are slowly progressive degeneration of the posterior columns and posterior roots and ganglie of the spinal cord. **t. mesenterica** tuberculosis of the mesenteric glands in children.

boparesis *(tabo-pa-resis)* [L. *tabes,* wasting away; G. *paresis,* paralysis]. General paralysis occurring concomitantly with tabes dorsalis.

ٹیبو پیری سس: دیوانے کی عام اینٹھنے کی حالت۔

ce *(ta's)* Trademark for the preparation of chlorotrianisene.

ٹیس: کلوروٹرائی انیسین۔

chistoscope *(ta-kisto-skop)* [G. *tachistos,* swiftest; *scope*, to see]. A device used in physiological psychology to demonstrate iconic memory. Here the images are displayed for controlled tinies usually less than one-tenth of a second. It is used in 'word blind centres'.

توجہ نما: آریا ایل بصری فیلڈ میں پہلے سے تعین شدہ وقفوں کے لئے پیٹرن اور الفاظ بنانے کے قابل بناتا ہے۔ لفظی اندھوں کی تربیت کے مراکز میں مستعمل۔

Tachycardia *(tak-i-kahr-de-a)* [G. *tachistos,* swiftest; *cardio,* heart]. Excessive rapidity inthe action of the heart. The term is usually applied to a heart rate above 100 beats per minute in adults. **paroxysmal t.,** a condition marked by attacks of rapid action of heart having sudden onset and cessation.

اختلاجِ قلب: دل کا زائد تیز عمل۔

Tachyphasia *(taki-fa-zi-a)* [G. *phasis,* speech]. Excessive rapidity in speech. It occurs in some mental problems.

طلق اللسان، سہولت کلام: بعض ذہنی خرابیوں میں تقریر کے بہاؤ کی انتہائی تیزی۔

Tachypnoea *(takip-ne-a)* [G. *pnoia,* breath]. Excessive rapidity of respiration. A respiratory neurosis marked by quick, shallow breathing.

سرعت تنفس: تنفس کی غیر معمولی فریکوئنسی۔

Tactile *(tak-ti'l)* [L. *taktilis*]. Pertaining to touch.

لمسی: چھونے کی حس سے متعلق۔

Taenia *(te'-ni-a)* A genus of flat, parasitic worms; cestodes or tapeworms. *Taenia echinococcus,* the adult worm lives in the dog's intestine (the definitive host) and man (the intermediate) is infesed by swallowing eggs from the dog's excrement. These become, embryos in the human small intestine, pass via the blood stream to organs, particularly the liver, and develop into hydatid cysts. Taenia saginata larvae present in infested, undercooked beef. Commonest species in Britain. In man's (the definitive host) intestinal lumen they develop into the adult tapeworm, which by its four suckers attaches itself to the gut wall. Treated with two 500 mg tablets of Yomesan--chewed and swallowed with water before breakfast. This drug partially digests the worms, hence it must never be used in *T. solium* infections. *Taenia solium,* resembles *T. saginata,* but has booklets as well as suckers. Commonest species in Eastern Europe. The larvae are ingested in infested, undercoooked pork; man can also be the intermediate host for this worm by ingesting eggs which, developing into larvae in his stomach , pass via the bowel wall to reach organs, and there develop into cysts. In the brain these may give rise to epilepsy. Treatment in hospital with 1 g meparine hydrochloride via duodenal tube followed in 30 min by saline purge.

جنس کدودانہ: چپٹے طفیلی کیڑوں کا ایک جنس سسٹوڈ یا کدو کیڑے۔

Teania *(ten'-i-a)* [G. *tainia* , band]. A flat band. **teania coli,** three flat bands running the length of the large intestine and consisting of the longitudinal muscle fiibres.

فیتہ: ایک چپٹی پٹی۔

Taeniacide *(ten'-i-a-sid)* [G. *tainia,* band; L. *caedere,* to kill]. An agent that destroys tapeworms -- taeniacidal , adj.

کدودانہ کش: کدو کیڑوں کو تباہ کرنیوالا ایجنٹ۔

Taeniafuge *(ten'-i-a-fuj)* [G. *tainia,* band; L. *fugere,* to flee]. An agent that expels tapeworms.

دافع کدودانہ: کدو کیڑوں کو نکالنے والا ایجنٹ۔

Tagamet *(tag'-a-met)*. Cimetidine (q.v.).

Talampicillin *(tal-am-pi-sil'-lin)*. Hydrolysed in mucous membrane to release free ampicillin (q.v.).

Talc. A naturally occurring soft white powder, consisting of magnesium silicate. Used extensively as a dusting powder, prior to the donning of surgical gloves. K285 (q.v.) now preferred.

برق: ہائیڈریٹ میگنیشم سلیکیٹ۔ ٹالکم پوڈر میں استعمال کیا جاتا ہے۔

Talipes *(tal'-i-pez)* [L. *talus,* ankle; *pes,* foot] Congenital deformity of foot--'club-foot' Club-foot includes t. equinovarus and t calcaneovalgus.

کج پائی: پاؤں کی بدشکلی کا مرض۔ کلب فٹ۔

Talus *(tal'-us)* [L.] The astragalus; situate between the tibia proximally and th calcaneus distally, thus directly bearing th weight of the body. It is the second larges bone of the ankle.

Deformities i talipes

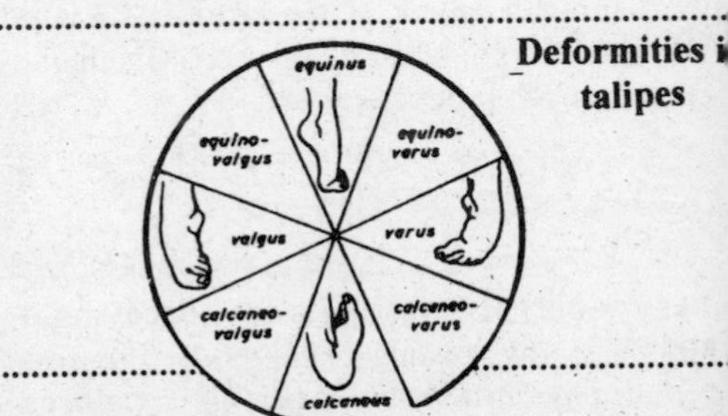

ٹخنے کی ہڈی: اسٹراگیلس۔ یہ ٹخنے کی دوسری سب سے بڑی ہڈی ہے۔

Tamponade Insertion of a tampon. See CAI DIAC.

یلہ بندی: روئی کی ڈاٹ اندر دینا (خون وغیرہ بند کرنے کے لیے)

Tanderil *(tan'-der-il)*. Oxyphenbutazone (q.v.)

نڈرل: آکسی فنبوٹازون۔ یہ گولیاں ورم اور سوزش ختم کرنے میں مفید ۔ جوڑوں کا درد، سر اور آنکھوں کی چوٹ، موچ، پاؤں کی چوٹ وغیرہ میں آمد۔

Tannafax *(tan'-a-faks)* A proprietary prepar ion containing tannic acid in jelly form. Us ful for superficial burns and scalds.

فیکس: جیلی کی صورت میں ٹینک ایسڈ کی تیاری مصنوعی آبلوں کے عمل، آگ سے جلی ہوئی جگہ پر لگایئے۔

Tanni acid *(tan'-nik as'-id)*. A brown prwd obtained from oak galls. It has astringe properties, and is used as a rectal irrigation colitis, as suppositories for haemorrhoids a as a jelly for mild burns.

دیا کسے کا تیزاب: ایک سفید ٹھوس۔ یہ گالک ایسڈ اور گلوکوس سے اخذ

شدہ کثیر ترکیبہ ایسٹر ٹائپ ہے۔ یہ رنگنے کی صنعت میں سیاہی بنانے میں استعمال کیا جاتا ہے۔ بھورا سفوف جو شاہ بلوط کے گال سے حاصل ہوتا ہے۔ ہلکے آبلوں کے لیے جیلی کی صورت میں استعمال کیا جاتا ہے۔

Tantalum *(tant'-a-lum)*. A rare metal sometimes used in the form of wire or gauze to reinforce weak areas in the body, as in the repair of a lrage hernia.

ٹنٹالم'طنطلوم: ایک عنصر' جوہری وزن ۱۸۰٫۹۲۸ جوہری عدد ۷۳ کثافت اضافی ۱۶٫۶ نقطہ پگھلاؤ ۲۹۹۶° س' ایک خاکستری سفید دھات برقی بلبوں کے فلامنٹ' بھرتوں اور دوسری اشیاء میں استعمال کیا جاتا ہے۔ بعض اوقات تا ریا گاز کی صورت میں مستعمل۔

Tapeworm. Taenia (q.v.).

کرم کدو' کدو دانہ: ٹینیا۔ کیڑے لمبے اور چپٹے، منہ کی طرف سے باریک اور دم کی طرف سے موٹے' ٹکڑے ٹوٹ کر پاخانے میں آتے ہیں۔ گوشت میں موجود ہوتے ہیں۔ علاج کے لیے اینتھی نین ایم اینڈ بی کی چھ گولیاں صبح چھ شام اور چھ اگلی صبح اور پھر جلاب دیں۔ یا نکلو سامائیڈ' (یومی سان) سوتے وقت ۴ گولیاں' صبح میگنیشیم سلفیٹ کا فروٹ سالٹ۔

Tapping Aspiration. Paracentesis (q.v.)

بزل: پیراسنٹی سس

Tar. Usually refers to wood tar, which, like coal tar, is used in a variety of skin disorders **coal t.**, a black viscid substance obtained as a by-product from coal distillation. Liq. picis carb. is an alcoholic solution of coal t., used in dermatological conditions.

تارکول: مختلف گہرے، گاڑھے نامیاتی مرکبات، مثلاً کول تار۔ جلدی خرابیوں میں مستعمل کول تار۔ ایک سیاہ گاڑھا مرکب ہے جو کوئلہ کی کشید سے حاصل کیا جاتا ہے۔

Taractan. Chloroprothixene. (q.v.).

ٹیری کٹان: کلور پروتھکسین۔

Tarsalgia *(tar-sal-ji-a)* [G. *tarsos,* flat surface; *algos,* pain]. Pain in the foot.

درد کف پا: پاؤں میں درد۔

Tarsometatarsal *(tar-so-met'-a-tar-sal)* [G. *tarsos,* flat surface; *meta,* between *tarsos*]. Pertaining to the tarsal and metatarsal region.

ٹارسو میٹا ٹارسل: ٹارسل اور میٹا ٹارسل حصوں سے متعلق۔

Tarsoplasty *(tar'-so-plas-ti)* [G. *tarsos,* flat surface; *plassein,* to form]. Any plastic operation to the eyelid.

ٹارسو پلاسٹی: آنکھ کے پپوٹے کا کوئی پلاسٹک اپریشن۔

Tarsorrhaphy *(tar'-sor-raf-i)* [G. *tarsos,* flat surface; *rhaphe,* sutrue]. Suturing of the lids together in order to protect cornea when it is anaesthetic, or to allow healing.

ٹارسرافی: صحت مند کرنے کے لئے یا جب اسے سن کیا گیا ہو تو قرنیہ کو محفوظ رکھنے کے لئے دونوں پپوٹوں کو اکٹھے سی دینا۔

Tarsus *(tar'-sus)* [G. *tarsos,* flat surface]. 1. The seven smalll bones of the foot. 2. The thin elongated plates of dense connective tissue found in each eyelid, contributing to its form and support—tarsal, *adj*.

کف پا: (۱) پاؤں کی سات چھوٹی ہڈیاں۔
(۲) آنکھ کے ہر پپوٹے میں پایا جانے والا گھنے واصل نسیج کی پتلی دراز پلیٹیں۔

Tartar *(tar-ter)* The deposit which forms on the teeth. **cream of t.**, potassium bitartrate. **tartar emetic,** antimony and potassium tartrate.

تا تار: دانتوں پر جمع ہونے والا مواد۔ چاقو کی نوک سے چھیل کر صاف کر دیا جاتا ہے۔ مسوڑھوں اور دانتوں کے اتصال پر میل۔

Tay-Sachs' disease. Primary defect appears to be a deficiency of the enzyme *β*-D-*N*-acetyl-hexosaminidase which leads to a massive acculumation on a specific lipid substance called GM_2, or Tay-Sachs ganglioside—hence the alternative name, gangliosidosis. [Warren Tay, English physician, 1843-1927. Bernard Sachs, New York neurologist, 1858-1944].

ٹے سیکس مرض: سر برل لپائڈوسس جو چربیلے میٹابولزم کی غلطی کی وجہ سے ہوتا ہے۔

Tears *(terz)* The secretion formed by the lacrimal gland. It contains the enzyme lysozome which acts as an antiseptic.

آنسو، اشک: لیکریمل گلینڈ سے بننے والی رطوبت۔ اس میں خامرہ لائیسوزائیم ہوتا ہے جو دافع تعفن کے طور پر عمل کرتا ہے۔

Tease *(tez)* To draw or pull out into fine threads, as in separating the fibres of a particle of muscle tissue.

شق نسیج: باریک دھاگوں میں کھینچنا، جیسا کہ عضلی نسیج کے ذرے کے ریشوں کو الگ الگ کرنے میں۔

Teat *(tet)* A nipple.

سر پستان: نپل، تھن۔ بھٹنی۔

Teclothiazide *(tek-lo-thi'-a-zid)* Oral diuretic. See CHLOROTHIAZIDE.

ٹیکلوتھیازائڈ: منہ کے ذریعے کھائی جانے والی دوا پیشاب آور۔

Teeth *(teth)* The structures used for mastication. The deciduous, milk or temporary set, 20 in number, is shed by the age of 7. The permanent set, 32 in number, is usually complete in the late teens. **canine** or **eye t.** have sharp fanglike edge for tearing food. **Hutchinson's t.** have a notched edge and are characteristic of congenital syphilis. **inscisor t.** have knife-like edge for biting food. **premolar** and **molar t.** have a squarish termination for chewing and grinding food. **wisdom t.** are the last molar teeth, one at either side of each jaw.

دانت: چبانے کے لئے مستعمل ساختیں۔ ۲۰ دانت دودھ کے دانت ہوتے ہیں جو سات سال کی عمر تک ٹوٹ جاتے ہیں۔ ان کی جگہ نئے دانت نکلتے ہیں۔ بیس سال کی عمر تک پورے بتیس دانت مکمل ہوتے ہیں جو مستقل ہوتے ہیں۔

Teeth

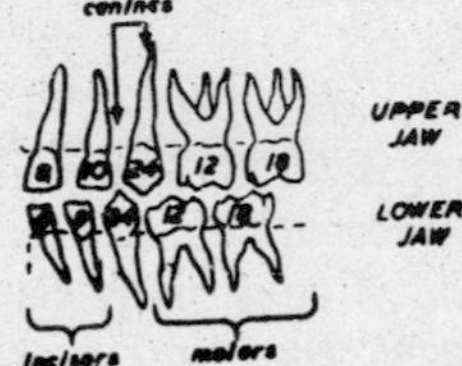

Primary dentition. The teeth are marked with the time of eruption in months.

Tegretol *(teg'-ret-ol)* Carbamazepine (q.v.).

ٹیگریٹول: کاربامیزپین۔

Tegument *(teg'-u-ment)* [L. *tegumentum,* covering]. The skin or covering of the animal body.

غلاف: حیوانی جسم کا غلاف یا کھال۔

Telangiectasis *(tel-an-ji-ek'-ta-sis)* [G. *telos,* end; *aggeion,* vessel; *ektasis,* extension]. Dilatation of the capillaries on a body surface.

تمدّدعروقِ شعریہ: جسمی سطح پر باریک نسوں کا پھیلنا۔

Telepaque *(tel-e-pak)* Iopanoic acid (q.v.).

ٹیلی پیک: آئیسوپینوئک ایسڈ۔

Teleradium *(te-le-ra'-di-um)* [G. *tele,* far off Radium whose radiation is directed into th body from an external source; radium beam.

لی ریڈیم: ریڈیم بیم۔ ریڈیم جس کی تابکاری کسی بیرونی منبع سے جسم میں ل ہوتی ہے۔

Teletherapy *(te-le-ther'-a-pi)* [G. *tele,* far of *therapeia,* treatment]. By custom refers t treatment with teleradium. Now include cobalt or caesium beams—teletherapeuti *adj.* teletherapeutically, *adv.*

لی تھیراپی: ٹیلی ریڈیم سے علاج۔ اب اس میں کوبالٹ یا سیزیم بیم شامل ں۔

TEM. Tretamine (q.v.).

۔ای۔ایم: ٹریٹامین۔

Temperament *(tem'-per-a-ment)* [L. *temperan entum,* mixing in proportion]. The habitu mental attitude of the individual. Four classi al types described originally—sanguine, ph gmatic, bilious melancholic.

اج، خصلت: فرد کا عادی ذہنی رویہ۔ اس کی چار اقسام ہیں۔ سنگوئین، میٹس، بلیئس، میلنکولک۔

Temple *(tem'-pl)* [L. *tempora*]. That part of t head lying between the outer angle of the e and the top of the ear-flap.

Temple regi

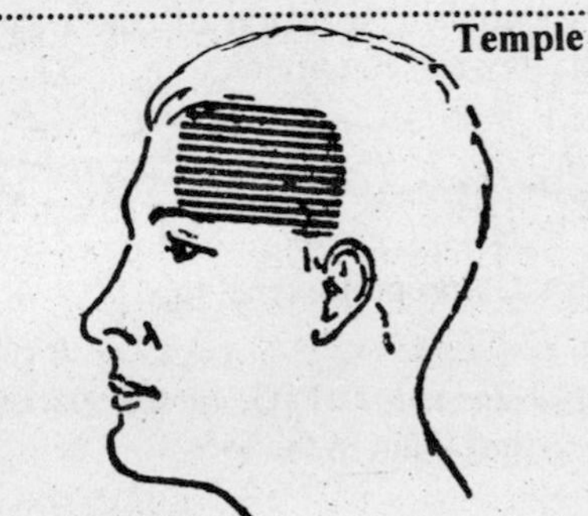

ٹی، صُدغ: سر کا وہ حصہ جو آنکھ کے بیرونی زاویہ اور کان کے فلیپ کی کے درمیان واقع ہے۔

Temporal *(tem-por-al)* Relating to the temp **temporal bones,** one on each side of the he below the parietal bone, containing the middle ear.

صدغی: کنپٹی یا ٹمپل سے متعلق۔ کنپٹی کی ہڈیاں جو سر کے دائیں و بائیں طرف کل دو ہوتی ہیں۔

Temporomandibular *(tem'-por-o-man-dib'-u-lar)* [L. *tempora,* temples; *mandibula,* jaw]. Pertaining to the temporal region or bone, and the lower jaw.

صدغی فکی اسفل: ٹمپورل ریجن یا ہڈی اور زیریں جبڑے سے متعلق۔

Temposil *(tem'-po-sil)* Analogue of disulphiram (q.v.).

TEN. Toxic epidermal necrolysis (q.v.). Tendon (ten'-don) [G. tenon]. A firm , white , fibrous inelastic cord which , attaches muscle to bone --tendinous, adj.

وتر: ایک مضبوط' سفید' ریشہ دار' غیر لچکدار ڈوری جو عضلے کو ہڈی کے ساتھ ملاتی ہے۔

Tenesmus *(ten-ez'-mus)* [G. *telnein,* to stretch]. Painful, ineffectual straining to empty the bowel or bladder.

شدید پیچش: آنتا یا بلیڈر کو خالی کرنے کے لیے تکلیف دہ غیر موثر کھچاؤ۔

Tenoplasty *(ten'-o-plas-ti)* [G. *tenon,* tendon; *plassein,* to form]. A plastic operation on a tendon--tenoplastic , adj.

ٹینو پلاسٹی: وتر یا ٹنڈان کا پلاسٹک اپریشن۔

Tenormal *(ten-orm'-al)*. Pempidine (q.v.)

ٹینورمل: پمپی ڈین

Tenorrhaphy *(ten-or'-raf-i)* [G. *tenon,* tendon; *rhaphe,* suture]. The suturing of a tendon.

وتر پیوندی: وتر یا ٹنڈان کو ٹانکا لگانا۔

Tenosynovitis *(te-no-si-no-vi'-tis)* [G. *tenon,* tendon; N.L. *synovia,* synovia; G. *itis,* inflammation]. Inflammation of the thin synovial lining a tendon sheath, as distinct from its outer fibrous sheath. It may be caused by mechanical irritation or by bacterial infection.

ورم غلاف وتر: غلاف وتر یا ٹنڈان شید کے پتلے سائینوویل غلاف کی سوزش

Tenotomy *(ten-ot'-om-i)* [G. *tenon,* tendon; *tome,* cutting]. Division of a tendon.

وتر تراشی: وتر یا ٹنڈان کی تقسیم۔

TEPP. Ethyl pyrophosphate (q.v.)

ٹی ای پی پی: ایتھائل پائیرو فاسفیٹ۔

Teratogen *(ter'-at-o-jen)* [G. *teras,* monster]. Anything capable of disrupting fetal growth and producing malformation. Classified as drugs, poisons, radiatoins physical agents such as ECT, infection--e.g. rubella, and rhesus and thyroid antibodies. See DYSMORPHOGENIC--teratogenic, teratogenetic, adj.; teratogenicity, teratogenesis, n.

ٹیریٹوجن: پیٹ میں بچے کی نشوونما میں خلل پیدا کرنے کے قابل۔ اس سے بناوٹ میں خرابی ہوجاتی ہے ان میں ادویات' شعاع' زہر وغیرہ ہیں۔

Teratoloty *(ter-at-ol'-o-ji)* [G. *teras,* monster; *logos,* discourse]. The scientific study of teratogens and their mode of action-- teratologist, n.; teratological adj.; teratologically, adv.

اعجوبیات: ٹریٹوجنز اور ان کے عمل کے طریقے کا سائنسی مطالعہ۔

Teratoma *(te-ra-to'-ma)* [G. *teras,* monster; *-oma,* tumour]. A tumour of embryonic origin and composed of various structures, including both epithelial and connective tissues; most commonly found in the ovaries and testes, the majority being malignant--teratomata , pl.; teratomatous , adj.

سلعہ ثلاثی: جنینی ماخذ کی رسولی جو مختلف ساختوں بشمول اپی تھیلیل اور رابطی بافتوں کے' پر مشتمل ہوتی ہے۔ بیضہ دانیوں اور خصیوں میں عام۔

Terra-Cortril *(ter-ra-kor'-tril)*. Terramycin, hydrocortisone and polymyxin B. Mainly used as eye, ear and nose drops and for topical application.

ٹیرا کورٹرل: ٹیرامائی سین' ہائیڈروجن کارٹی سون اور پولی مکسن ب۔ آنکھ' کان اور ناک کی قطروں کے طور پر مستعمل۔

Terramycin *(ter-ra-mi'-sin)*. Oxytertracycline (q.v.)

ٹیرامائی سین: آکسی ٹیٹراسائیکلین۔ موثر اینٹی بایوٹک دست روکنے کے لیے ہر چھ گھنٹے بعد ایک کیپسول' بچوں کو اس کا سفوف پانی میں گھول کر دن میں چار مرتبہ پلائیے۔ نفخ شکم یا فلیٹولینس جگر کا امیبی پھوڑا اور نمونیا کے علاج کے لیے ایک کیپسول دن میں ۴ مرتبہ۔ اسی طرح برائے غذائی سمیت ٹولاریمیا'

اسہال۔

Tersavid *(ter'-sa-vid)*. Pivhydrazine (q.v.)

ٹریسی وڈ: پوہائیڈرازین۔

Tertiary *(ter'-shi-a-ri)*. Third ni order.

سوم پر: ترتیب میں تیسرا

Tertroxin *(ter-troks'-in)*. A preparation of liothyronine (q.v.) that has a standerdized activity.

ٹرٹراکسن: لیوتھائیرونین کی تیاری جوایک معیاری عاملیت رکھتی ہے۔

TEST Adrenal function tests. Abnormal adrenal -cortical function can be detected by measuring the 24-hour urinary output of 17 oxosteroids and 17 hydroxycorticoids or by estimating the 11-hydroxycorticosteroids in plasma. In doubtful cases the estimations can be repeated following the administration of ACTH. See METAPYRONE TEST. Increased adrenal medullary function may be detected by measuring urinary vanyl mandelic acid (VMA) excretion.

ٹیسٹ: جانچ پڑتال۔آزمون۔ ا۔ ایڈرینل کی کارکردگی کاٹیسٹ۔غیر معمولی ایڈرینل کارٹیکل کارکردگی کاتعین گزشتہ۲۴ گھنٹوں کے پیشاب سے کیا جاتا ہے۔

Astrup test Estimates degree of acidosis by measuring gas (O_2 and CO_2) pressures in arterial blood.

۲۔ اسٹرپ ٹیسٹ: شریانی خون میں آکسیجن اور کاربن ڈائی آکسائیڈ کے دباؤ کی پیمائش کرنے سے تیزابیت کااندازہ کیاجاتا ہے۔

Augmented histamine test See HISTAMINE TEST

Basophil test. Distinguishes between immediate and delayed hypersensitivity states. There is a basophil reaction in all of the immediate allergic states.

۳۔ باسوفل کاٹیسٹ: فوری اور موخر بیش حساسیت کے درمیان فرق جاننے کے لیے کیاجاتا ہے۔

Bence-Jones' protein test See BENCEJONES' PROTEIN.

Breath-H2 (hydrogen) test For disaccharide intolerance. Indirect method for detecting lactase deficinency.

Bromosulphthalein test A test used to assess hepatic function ; 5 mg per kg body weight of bromsulpthalein (BSP) are injected intravenously. The dye is usally excreted in the bile; if more than 5 per cent of the dye is circulating in the blood 45 min after injection there is impaired hepatic function.

۴۔ بروموسلف تھالین ٹیسٹ: جگری فعل کاتعین کرنے کے لیے ٹیسٹ۔انٹراوینس ٹیکے کے ذریعے ۵ ملی گرام بروموسلف تھالین فی کلوگرام جسمی وزن کے تناسب سے جسم میں داخل کیا جاتا ہے۔ رنگ بائل سے نکل جاتا ہے۔اگر ٹیکے کے ۴۵ منٹ بعد ۵ فیصد سے زیادہ رنگ خون میں گردش کر رہا ہوتو جگری فعل میں نقص ہوتا ہے۔

Calcium test In a normal person sudden increase of calcium by i.v. infusion causes raised phosphate level in blood and urine. In hyperparathyroidism this does not occur.

۵۔ کیلشیم ٹیسٹ: ایک نارمل شخص میں کیلشیم دینے سے خون اور پیشاب میں فاسفیٹ بڑھ جاتا ہے مگر ہائیپر پیراتھائی رائڈزم میں ایسانہیں ہوتا۔

Caloric test *(ka-lor'-ik)*. The assessment of vestiblar function by means of heat. Investigation of vestibular disease.

۶۔ کیلورک ٹیسٹ: گرمی کے ذریعے ویسٹی بول کی کارکردگی کاتعین

Cosoni test Intradernal injection of 0.2 ml of fresh, sterile hydatid fluid. A white papule indicates a hydatid cyst.

۷۔ کسونی ٹیسٹ: تازہ سٹرائل ہائیڈیٹڈ سیال کا ۰٫۲ ملی لٹر کاانٹراڈرمل انجکشن۔

Colloidal gold test One of the laboratory tests of cerebrospinal fluid (CSF) with special application in the dignosis of syphilis of brain or spinal cord. Different dilutions of a colloidal gold solution show precipitation of the metal when added to an abnormal CSF. The degree of precipitation is shown by corresponding colour changes and the colours are reported as numbers from 1 to 5. Ten dilutions are commonly tested. Tabes dorsalis gives a pattern of numbers such as 001234-4321; general paralysis of the insane (GPI), demyelination diseases--e.g. multiple sclerosis, carcinomatous meningitis and subacute inclusion-body encephalitis gives a pattern of numbers such as 5554433210.

۸۔ کولائی ڈل گولڈٹیسٹ : سربروسپائینل سیال کے لیبارٹری ٹیسٹوں میں سے ایک اس کا اطلاق نخاع یا دماغ کی سفلس کی تشخیص پر کیا جاتا ہے۔

Complement fixation test. See COMPLEMENT.

Coombs' test. A highly sensitive test designed to detect immune antibodies, attached to red blood cells or present in serum; the 'direct' method detects the former; the 'indirect' method detects the latter. Especially useful in the diagnosis of the haemolytic syndromes. [R.R.A Coombs' contemporary British scientist.]

۹۔ کومز کا ٹیسٹ : یہ ٹیسٹ امیون اینٹی باڈیز کا پتہ لگانے کے لیے کیا جاتا ہے یہ حساس ٹیسٹ ہے۔ اینٹی باڈیز سرخ خونی خلیوں کے ساتھ ملحق ہوتی ہیں۔ یا سرم میں موجود ہوتی ہیں۔ ہیمولائیٹک سنڈرومز میں خصوصاً مفید۔

Cortisone suppression test. Differentiates primary from secondary hypercalcamia. Sarcodosis causes secondary hypercalcaemia. Primary hyperparathyroidism causes primary hypercalcaemia.

۱۰۔ کورٹیسون سپریشن ٹیسٹ : ثانوی ہائپر کلسیمیا سے ابتدائی کو میمز کرتا ہے۔

Creatine test. See CREATINE.

Demco test. Done on centrifuged blood for glandular fever.

۱۱۔ ڈمکو ٹیسٹ: غدودیہ بخار کے لیے مرکز گریز خون پر کیا جاتا ہے۔

Dextroxylase test See XYLOSE TEST.

Diagnex blue test A means of showing production of acid by the stomach without passing a stomach tube; tablets and granules taken orally. The findings are revealed by testing the urine.

۱۲۔ ڈیاگنیکس بلیوٹیسٹ : معدہ میں نلی گزارے بغیر معدہ میں تیزاب کی پیداوار ظاہر کرنے کا ذریعہ۔ گولیاں اور دانے منہ کے ذریعے کھائے جاتے ہیں۔

Duke's test See BLEEDING TIME. Skin pricked, blood continuously removed with absorbent paer until it ceases so flow. Normal 3 to 5 min.

۱۳۔ ٹیسٹ ڈیک : جلد کو چبھو کو جاذب کاغذ سے خون کو متواتر ہٹایا جاتا ہے۔ یہاں تک کہ اس کی روانی بند ہو جاتی ہے۔ وقت تقریباً ۳ تا ۵ منٹ۔

Echo encephalogram . A new test for detecting intracerebral space-occupying lesions causing midline shift.

۱۴۔ ایکوانکیفالوگرام: انٹراسربرل جگہ گھیرنے والے دانے معلوم کرنے کا نیا طریقہ۔

Edrophonium test For myasthenia gravis. A sinall i.m. dose of edrophonium. A chloride will immediately relieve symptoms, albeit temporarily, while quinine sulphate will increase the muscular weakness.

Enzyme tests. The presence of abnormally high concentrations of serum enzymes may indicate underlying disease. Those enzyme tests in common use and the diseases which cause high levels include.

Acid phosphatase--carcinoma of prostate.

Aldolase-muscle disease.

Alkaline phosphatase--obstructive jaundice and various forms of bone disease.

Amylase--acute pancreatitis; See DIASTASE.

Creatinephosphokinase (CPK)--raised only in acute myocardial infarction and not in other cardiopathies.

Dopamine-β-hydroxylase (DBH)--for high blood pressure.

Glutamic oxalacetic transaminase (GOT)--myocardial infarction.

Glutamic-pyruvic transaminase (GPT)--liver disease

Hydroxybutyrate dehydrogenase-- myocardial infarction.

Lactate dehydrogenase (LDH)--when tissue of high metabolic activity dies tissue necrosis is quickly reflected by increased LDH.

۱۵۔ ٹیسٹ خامرہ: سیرم کے خامرات کا زیادہ ارتکاز مختلف امراض کی نشاندہی کرتا ہے۔ ان میں سے چند حسب ذیل ہیں۔

ایسڈ فاسفیٹز۔ پراسٹیٹ کا کارسینوما۔

امائیلز۔۔ شدید پیکریائیٹس

ایلڈولیز۔۔ عضلی مرض

الکلائن فاسفیٹز۔ رکاوٹ والا یرقان اور ہڈی کے مرض کی مختلف اقسام۔

کریا ٹین فاسفو کا ئینیز ۔ سی پی کے ۔صرف مایو کارڈیل انفارکشن میں زیادہ۔
گلوٹیمک پائیروک ٹرانس امائینیز ۔ مایو کارڈیل انفارکشن ۔ جگر کا مرض ہائیڈرو
کسی بٹائریٹ ڈی ہائیڈ روجنز مایو کارڈیل انفارکشن۔
لیکٹیٹ ڈیہائیڈروجنز۔ جب زیادہ میٹابولک کارکردگی کا نسیج مرجاتا ہے تو اس
کی زیادہ مقدار نسیج نکروسس تیزی سے منعکس ہوتا ہے۔

Flocculation test Serum set up against various salts-- gold, thymol, cephalin, choleterol. Presence of abnormal serum proteins results in cloudiness. Abnormal forms of albumin and globulin made by diseased liver cells.

۱۶۔ فلا کولیشن ٹیسٹ : مختلف نمکیات کے خلاف سیٹ سیرم ۔غیر
معمولی سیرم لحمیات کی موجودگی دھندلا پن پیدا کرتی ہے ۔البومن اور گلوبولن کی
غیر معمولی اقسام بیمار جگری خلیے بناتے ہیں۔

Fluorescein string test A test used to detect the site of obscure upper gastrointestinal haemorrhage. The patient swallows a raido--opaque knotted intravenously and after a few minutes the string is withdrawn. If staining has occured the site of bleeding can be determined.

۱۷۔ فلورسین سٹرنگ ٹیسٹ : خراب بالائی معدی آنتی ہیمرج کی
جگہ کا پتہ لگانے کے لیے ٹیسٹ۔

Galactose test Forty g galactose in 500 ml water taken after fasting. Five hours later urine collected. If it contains 2 g or more g it indicates liver damage.

۱۸۔ گلیکٹوزٹیسٹ : یہ ٹیسٹ جگر کو پہنچنے والے نقصان کو ظاہر کرتا ہے۔

Glucose tolerance test Useful in the diagnosis of diabetès mellitus and other causes of glycosuria. Serial collections of blood are estimated for blood glucose following the oral or intravenous administration of 50g glucose, and urine samplès are simultaneously tested for glucose.

۱۹۔ گلوکوس کی برداشت کا ٹیسٹ : ذیابیطس اور گلائیکوسوریا کی
دوسری وجوہات کی تشخیص میں مفید۔

Gonococal complement fixation. A specific serological test for the diagnosis of gonorrhoea.

۲۰۔ گونوکاکسل کمپلیمنٹ فکسیشن ٹیسٹ : سوزاک کی تشخیص کے
لیے مخصوص سیرولوجیکل ٹیسٹ۔

Growth hormone (GH) test The effect o growth hormone that is used clinically i measurement is its reciprocal relationshi with blood glucose. Blood is therfore take for estimation of GH during a standard 50 oral glucose tolerance test. In acromegaly, nc only is the resting level of GH higher, but i does not show normal suppression wit glucose.

۲۔ گروتھ ہارمون ٹیسٹ : گروتھ ہارمون کا اثر جو پیائش میں مستعمل
ہے خونی گلوکوس سے متناسب ہوتا ہے اس لیے ٹیسٹ کے لیے خون لیا جاتا ہے

Guthrie test . Assay of phenylalanine from drop of blood dried on special filter pape Done on the sixth day of life. It is necessar to confirm the diagnosis in those infants wit a positive test.

۲۱۔ گتھری ٹیسٹ : مثبت ٹیسٹ والے بچوں میں تشخیص کی تصدیق کے
لیے ضروری ہے۔یہ چھٹے دن کیا جاتا ہے۔

Haemagglutination tests for pregnancy. Al based on the same principle , are almost a accurate as the Hogben test and can b performed more rapidly. The addition of urin from a pregnant person will preven haemagglutination occurring between re cells pretreated with human chlorioni gonadotrophin (HCG) in the presence o specific antisera.

۲۲۔ حمل کے لیے ہیمیگلوٹینیشن : یہ تمام ٹیسٹ ایک ہی اصول پر
ی ہیں۔

Haematoporphyrin test One to 3 h after inje ction haematoporphyrin localizes in rapidl multiplying cells and fluoresces unde ultraviolet light. In many instances inves tigatyors can detect the exact extent o malignant or precancerous tissue.

۲۔ ہیمٹیو پورفائیرن ٹیسٹ : انجکشن کے ایک تا ۳ گھنٹے بعد تیزی
سے تقسیم ہونے والے خلیوں میں ہیمٹیو پورفائیرن مقامی طور پر جمع ہو جاتا ہے

Heaf test. Multiple puncture of epidermis wit special gun through a layer of filter pape soaked in tuberculin strength 1 in 1000 or 1 i 100. Inflammatory reaction is positive.

۲۴۔ ہیف ٹیسٹ : مخصوص گن، کے ساتھ اپی ڈرمس کا کئی رخی پنکچر

Hess test. Sphygmomanometer cuff applied and inflated. Petechial eruption in surrounding area after 5 min denotes a positive reaction. i.e. weakness of the capillary walls. [Walter Rudolf Hess, Swiss physiologist. 1881]

۲۶۔ ہیس ٹیسٹ: نسوں کی دیواروں کی کمزوری دیکھنے کے لیے۔

Hickey-Hare test . Intravenous infusion of hypertonic saline causes increase in urinary output. Administration of 0.2 to 0.3 ml of ADH deceases output.

۲۷۔ ہکی ہیئر ٹیسٹ: اس سے پیشاب ٹیسٹ کیا جاتا ہے۔

Histamine test . Designed to determine the maximal gastric secretion of hydrochloric acid. A Levin's tube is positioned in the most dependent part of the stomach of a fasting, weighted patient. Following the collection of a control specimen and the injection of an appropriate dose of an antihistamine (100 mg mepyramine maleate) 0.04 mg per kg body weight histamine acid phosphate is injected subcutaneously and gastric secretions are collected for a further hour. By titrating the collections against a standard alkaline solution the acidity of the gastric secretions can be determined.

۲۸۔ ہسٹامین ٹیسٹ : نمک کے تیزاب کی زیادہ سے زیادہ معدی رطوبت کا تعین کرنے کے لیے۔

Hogben test. A female Xenopus toad is injected with a preparation obtained from the early morning urine of a woman suspected of pregnancy. In the case of pregnancy the toad lays eggs after 8 to 24 h. The test is over 99 per cent accurate [Lancelot Hogben, British scientist. 1895]

۲۹۔ ہاگبن ٹیسٹ: ایسی خاتون جسے حاملہ ہونے کا شبہ ہو اس کا علی الصبح پیشاب سے حاصل شدہ کا مادہ نیوپس ٹوڈ کو ٹیکہ لگایا جاتا ہے۔ حمل ہونے کی صورت میں ٹوڈ ۸ تا ۲۴ گھنٹے بعد انڈے دیتی ہے۔ یہ ٹیسٹ ۹۹ فیصد سے زیادہ صحیح ہے۔

Human chorionic gonadotrophin (HCG) test. Presence of HCG in urine detectable in early morning specimen of urine fron 6th week of pregnancy. Result can be given in 2 min and cofirmed in 2 h.

۳۰۔ انسانی کوریونک گونیڈوٹروفن ٹیسٹ : پیشاب میں انسانی کوریونگ گونیڈوٹروفن کی موجودگی۔ حمل کے چھٹے ہفتے سے پیشاب کے علی الصبح نمونہ میں معلوم کیا جا سکتا رزلٹ صرف ۲ منٹ میں دیا جا سکتا ہے۔ اور تصدیق ۲ گھنٹوں میں کی جا سکتی ہے۔

Insulin test For determining the completeness or otherwise of surgical vagotomy. Hyoglycaemia is the response to i.v. insulin when the vagus nerve is intact. Complete vagotomy gives a negative response.

۳۱۔ انسولین ٹیسٹ: سرجیکل ویگوٹومی کی تکمیل ہونے یا نہ ہونے کا پتہ لگانے کے لیے ٹیسٹ۔

Jelly test Old tuberculin in a jelly is applied to skin, usually between shoulder blades in babies. If positive, inflammation appears at site of application.

۳۲۔ جیلی ٹیسٹ : اولڈ ٹیوبرکولین جیلی میں ملا کر جلد پر بچوں کے کندھوں کے درمیان لگائی جاتی ہے۔ اگر مثبت ہو تو لگانے والی جگہ پر سوزش یا سوج ہو جاتی ہے۔

Kahn test. A serological test for the diagnosis of syphilis. The patient's serum reacts with an heterologous antigen prepared from mammalian tissue, and flocculation is produced if syphilitic antibodies are present, [Reuben Leon Kahn, American bactriologist, 1887]

۳۳۔ کہن ٹیسٹ: غلس کی تشخیص کے لیے ایک سیرولوجیکل ٹیسٹ۔

Kay's augmented histamine test. See HISTAMINE TEST.

Kidney function tests Various tests are available for measuring renal function. All require cereful collection of urine specimens. Those in common use are; paraaminohippuric acid clearance test for measuring renal blood flow; creatinine clearance test for measuring glomerular filtration rate; ammounium chloride test for measuring tubular ability to excrete hydrogen ion; urinary concentration and dilution tests for measuring tubular function; radioisotope renogram (q.v.). See INDIGOCARMINE.

۳۴۔ گردے کی کارکردگی کے ٹیسٹ: رینل کارکردگی کی پیمائش کے لیے مختلف ٹیسٹ۔ ان تمام میں پیشاب کے نمونے احتیاط سے جمع کرنے ضروری ہیں۔

Kveim test. An intradermal test for sarcoidosis using tissue prepared from person known to be suffering from the condition. [Morten Ansgar Kveim, Oslo physician, 1892-1966.]

۳۵۔ کولم ٹیسٹ: سارکائڈوسس کے لیے انٹراڈرمل ٹیسٹ۔

Levulose test See LAEVLOSE.

Leptospiralagglutination tests Serological tests used in the diagnosis of specific leptospiral infections , e.g. Weil's disease.

۳۶۔ لیپٹو سپائیرل اگلوٹینیشن ٹیسٹس: لیپٹو سپائیرل امراض کی تشخیص میں مستعمل سیرولوجیکل ٹیسٹس۔

Makari intrademal test for cancer The detection of antigen-antibody complexes in response of interaction of antigen (TPS, tumour polysaccharide substances) and serum antibodies by use of a skin test.

Mantoux test Intradermal injection of old tuberculin or PPD (purified protein derivative --a purified type of tuberculin) into anterior aspect of forearm. Inspection after 48 to 72 h. If positive there will be an area of induration and inflammation greater than 5 mm in diameter.

۳۷۔ منٹوکس ٹیسٹ: پیش بازو کی امامی طرف میں اولڈ ٹوبرکولن کا انٹراڈرمل انجکشن۔ ۴۸ تا ۷۲ گھنٹوں کے بعد اس کا معائنہ کیا جاتا ہے۔ اگر مثبت ہو تو سوزش کا ایریا قطر میں ۵ ملی میٹر سے زیادہ ہوگا۔

Match test A rough test of respiratory function. If a person is unable to blow out a lighted match held 4 inches from a fully open mouth there is significant reduction of respiratory function.

۳۸۔ میچ ٹیسٹ: تنفسی فعل کا ایک رف ٹیسٹ۔ اگر کوئی شخص کھلے ہوئے منہ سے ۴ انچ کے فاصلہ پر جلتی دیا سلائی کو پھونک مار کر نہ بجھا سکے تو اس میں تنفسی فعل کی نمایاں کمی ہے۔

Matapyrone test A test of pituitary and adrenal function. The urinary excretion of 17 hydroxycorticosteroids is estimated before and after the oral administration of metapyrone. Disease of the pituitary or adrenal cortex causes an abnormal result.

۳۹۔ میٹاپائیرون ٹیسٹ: پیٹوایٹری اور ایڈرینل فعل کا ٹیسٹ۔

Paricreatic funtion test Levin's tubes are positioned in the stomach and second part of duodenum. The response of the pancreatic gland to various hormonal stimuli can be measured by analysing the duodenal aspirate. See SELENOMETHIONINE.

۴۰۔ لبلبہ کی کارکردگی کا ٹیسٹ: لیون کی نلیاں معدہ اور ڈیوڈینم کے دوسرے حصے میں رکھی جاتی ہیں۔ اس طرح مختلف ہارمونوں کے لیے لبلبہ کی گلینڈ کے ردعمل کی پیمائش ہو سکتی ہے۔

Pandy test. For excess globulin in CSF. Only significant if total protein is normal, when it suggests a diagnosis of demyelinating disease (e.g. multiple sclerosis) or sypilis.

۴۱۔ پینڈی ٹیسٹ: سی ایس ایف میں زائد گلوبون کیلئے۔

Patch test Old tuberculin incorporated in a strapping dressing. Usually applied to skin between shoulder bladed in babies. If positive, there is inflammation at site of application.

۴۲۔ پیچ ٹیسٹ: بچوں میں کندھوں کے درمیان جلد پر اولڈ ٹوبرکولن کی ڈریسنگ کی جاتی ہے اگر مثبت ہو تو لگانے والی جگہ پر سوزش یا سوج ہوتی ہے۔

Paul-Bunnell test. A serological test used in the diagnosis of infective mononucleosis. Antibodies which occur in patients with this disease agglutinate sheep's erythrocytes. [J. R. Paul, American physician, 1893 W.W. Bunnell, American physcician, 1902]

۴۳۔ پال بنل ٹیسٹ: مانونکلیوسس کی تشخیص میں مستعمل سیرولوجیکل ٹیسٹ۔

Protein-bound iodine test Blood taken for serum protein-bound iodine which corresponds to circulating thyroid hormone levels. In preparation for test--no iodine-containing medicines and a fish-free diet.

۴۴۔ پروٹین باؤنڈ آیوڈین ٹیسٹ: سیرم پروٹین باؤنڈ آیوڈین کے لیے خون لیا جاتا ہے۔ جو گردشی تھائیرائڈ ہارمون لیولز کے مطابق ہوتا ہے۔ ٹیسٹ کی تیاری میں آیوڈین پر مشتمل ادویہ نہیں دی جاتیں اور خوراک میں مچھلی نہیں ہونا چاہیے۔

Pentagastrin test. When injected. P. causes parietal cells to secrete acid to their utmost capacity, expressed as m Eq H^+ in 1 h, for the peak 30 min after injection--PAO (peak acid output).

۴۵۔ پنیٹا گیسٹرین ٹیسٹ: پنیٹا گیسٹرین ہارمون گیسٹرین کا تالیفی متبادل ہے۔ رات بھر بھوکا رہنے کے بعد انجکشن دیا جاتا ہے۔ وقفوں وقفوں سے گیسٹرک جوس اکٹھا کیا جاتا ہے۔ اس میں الرجی نہیں ہوتی۔

Platelet stickiness test. Increased in multiple sclerosis and rapidly growing tumours. May be consequent on degradation of neural tissue, as it is rich in phospholipid, fractions of which have been shown to be potent aggregators of platelets in suspension.

۴۶۔ پلیٹلیٹ چپکنے کا ٹیسٹ: کئی رخی سکلیروسس اور تیزی سے بڑھنے والی رسولیوں میں اضافہ۔

Prognosticon test. For pregnancy.

Prothrombin test. Indirectly reveals amount of p. in the blood. To a sample of oxalated blood are added all the factors needed to bring about clotting, except prothrombin time taken for clot to form is therefore dependent on amount of p. present. Normal time, 10 to 12 seconds.

۴۷۔ پروتھیرومبین ٹیسٹ: بلاراست پروتھرومبین کی مقدار خون میں معلوم کی جاتی ہے۔ آکسیلیڈ خون میں ایسے اجزاء شامل کیے جاتے ہیں جو خون کو جما دیتے ہیں۔ خون کے جمنے کا وقت پروتھرومبین کی مقدار پر منحصر ہوتا ہے نارمل وقت ۱۰ تا ۱۲ سیکنڈ ہے۔

Radioiodine uptake test The person is given a small dose of radioactive iodine, and the radioactivity of the thyroid galnd is subsequently measured. If the gland is overactive more than 45 per cent of the iodine will be taken up by the gland within 4 h. If the gland is underactive less than 20 per cent will be taken up after 48 h.

۴۸۔ ریڈیو آیوڈین اپٹیک ٹیسٹ: شخص کو ریڈیو ایکٹو آیوڈین کی تھوڑی سی خوراک دی جاتی ہے۔ اور تھائیراڈ گلینڈ کی تابکاری کی پیمائش کر لی جاتی ہے۔

Radioisotope renogram A kidney function test in which renal blood flow, tubular function and renal excretion can be roughly estimated following the intravenous injection of a radioactive labelled substance which is rapidly accumulated and excreted by the kidneys. Simultaneous counting of the radioactivity over the kidneys allows comparison of the function of the two kidneys. Counters placed over renal tract can detect obstruction such as a stone in the ureter.

۴۹۔ ریڈیو آئیسوٹوپ رینوگرام: گردے کی کارکردگی کا ٹیسٹ۔

Rheumatoid arthritis (RA) latex test. Discerns the presence in the blood of rheumatoid factor.

۵۰۔ آر اے لیٹیکس ٹیسٹ: ریوماٹائڈ فیکٹر کی خون میں موجودگی ٹیسٹ کی جاتی ہے۔

Respiratory function tests Numerous tests are available for assessing respiratory function. These include measurements of the vital capacity (VC). forced vital capacity (FVC), forced expiratory volume (FEV) (which is the volume of air that can be expired in 1 second) and the maximal breathing capacity (MBC) which is that quantity of air that can be shifted in 1 min.

۵۱۔ تنفسی کارکردگی کا ٹیسٹ: اس کے کئی ٹیسٹ ہیں۔

Rinne's test. Testing of air condition and bone condition hearing, by tuning fork. [Friedrich Heinrich Rinne, German otologist, 1819-68.]

۵۲۔ ٹیسٹ رنے: ٹیوننگ فورک کے ذریعے ہوائی اور استخوانی کنڈکشن کا ٹیسٹ۔

Rogitine test If hypertension is permanent, an adrenalytic cobstance, Rogitine (phentolamine) 5 mg, is injected intravenously, A fall in excess of 35 mmHg in the systolic, and 25 mmHg in the diastolic pressure, occurring within 2 min of injection, is highly suggestive of phaeochromocytoma.

۵۳۔ روجٹین ٹیسٹ: فیوکروسائیٹوما کے لیے ٹیسٹ۔

Saxona test. Radioreceptor assay test for pregnancy yielding results in 1 h. Can identify those with a tendency to abort.

SCAT (Sheep cell agglutination test) Presence in the blood of rheumatoid factor detected by the sheep cell agglutination titre.

۵۴۔ ایس سی اے ٹیسٹ: ریوماٹائڈ فیکٹر کی خون میں موجودگی۔

Schick A test used to determine a person's susceptibility or immunity to diphtheria. It consists in the injection of 2 or 3 minims of freshly prepared toxin beneath the skin of the left arm. A similar test is made into the right arm, but in this the serum is heated to 75°C for 10 min, in order to destroy the toxin but not the protein. A positive reaction is recognized by the appearance of a round red area on the left arm within 24 to 48 h, reaching its maximum intensity on the fourth day, then grandully fading with slight pigmentation and desquamation. This reaction indicates susceptibility or absence of immunity. No reaction indicates that the subject is immune to diphtheria. Occasionally a pseudoreaction occurs, caused by the protein of the toxin; in this case the redness appears on both arms, hence the value of the control. [Bela Schick, Austrain paediatrician, 1877-1967.]

۵۵۔ شک ٹیسٹ: کسی شخص کی خناق کے لیے مزاحمت کا تعین کرنے کے لیے ٹیسٹ۔

Schilling test Estimation of absorption of radioactive vitamin B_{12} for confirmation of pernicious anaemia.

۵۶۔ شلنگ ٹیسٹ: حیاتین ب۱۲ کی کمی یا انجذاب کی خرابی کا پتہ لگانے کے لیے ٹیسٹ۔

Schultz-Charlton test A blanching produced in the skin of a patient showing scarlatinal rash, around an injection of serum from a convalescent case, indicating neutralization of toxin by antitoxin. [Werner Schultz, German physician, 1878-1947.]

۵۷۔ پسینہ ٹیسٹ: اگر سلور نائیٹریٹ اور پوٹاشیم کرومیٹ کی پیٹری ڈش کو ہاتھ کی ہتھیلی کے ساتھ دباتے ہیں تو پسینہ میں زائد کلورائڈز نمایاں سفید پرنٹ بناتے ہیں۔

Scriver test Remarkably efficient in detecting, by a single procedure, 22 aminocidopathies.

Secretin test A quantitative and qualitative test to estimate secretion of pancreatic juice in response to the enzyme secretin.

Sweat test. Petri dish prepared with agar, silvar nitrate and potassium chromate. With palm of hand pressed to this, excessive chorides in sweat gives distinctive white print, as mucoviscidosis.

Synacthen test Synacthen is a proprietary preparation of tetrosactrin which is synthetic ACTH. Intramuscular infusion of s. normally produces pituitary stimulation for increased secretion of steroid hormones by adrenal cortex, measured by estimation of plasma cortisol. Lack of response denotes inactivity of adrenal cortex as in Addison's diseae.

۵۸۔ سائینیکتھن ٹیسٹ: ایڈرینل کارٹیکس سے سٹرائڈ ہارمونز کا زائد اخراج کیا جاتا ہے۔ ردعمل میں کمی ایڈرینل کارٹیکس کی غیر موجودگی کو ظاہر کرتی ہے۔

Thyopac test. A resin uptake test to measure circulating thyroid hormone levels.

۵۹۔ تھائیو پیک ٹیسٹ: گردشی تھائیرائڈ ہارمون لیولز کی پیمائش کے لیے رال کا اپٹیک ٹیسٹ۔

Thyroid antibody test. Thyroid antibody levels indicate the presence and severity of autoimmune thyroid disease.

۶۰۔ تھائیرائڈ اینٹی باڈی ٹیسٹ: تھائیرا اینٹی باڈی لیولز آٹو امیون مرض کی موجودگی اور شدت کو ظاہر کرتے ہیں۔

Thyroid stimulating hormone (TSH) test. Radio- immunoassay of level of serum thyroid stimulating hormone. Useful in diagnosing mild hypothyroidism.

۶۱۔ تھائیرائڈ: تحریکی ہارمون ٹیسٹ ہلکا ہائپو تھائیراڈزم تشخیص کرنے میں مفید۔

Tolbutamide test Fasting blood sugar taken. Intravenous infusion of tolbutamide. Blood taken for glucose level 20 and 30 min later. Normal response--rapid fall of blood sugar dut to increase manufacture of insulin. Mature type diabetic response--delayed fall. Prematurity type diabetic response--none.

۶۲۔ ٹولبوٹامائیڈ ٹیسٹ: اس میں خون کو ٹیسٹ کیا جاتا ہے۔

Triple test A Dreiling tube is passed through the mouth into the duodenum and pancreatic function tests are carried out. In these, the enzymes secretin and pancreozymin are given to stimulate the pancreas and the juice is aspirated as it flows into the duodenum. It is possible to recognize a tumour in the pancreas from analysis of the volume and chemistry of this juice. Some of the juice is then examined by the pathologist using Papanicolaou's method to show cancer cells, and thirdly, the radiologist performs a hypotonic duodenogram which, unlike the conventional barium meal, frequently demonstrates tumours of the pancreas or ampulla. The test takes 2 hours to complete.

Jrea clearance test urea concentraion test. Procedures for measuring the efficiency of kidney function and both require urine collection under specified conditions.

٦٣۔ یوریا کے ارتکاز کا ٹیسٹ: گردے کی کارکردگی کی پیمائش کے لیے طریقے۔اس میں مخصوص حالتوں میں پیشاب جمع کیا جاتا ہے۔

Van den Bergh's test. Estimation of serum bilirubin. Direct positive reaction (conjugated) in obstructive and hepatic jaundice. Indirect positive reaction (unconjugated) in haemolytic jaundice. See BILIRUBIN.

٦٤۔ ٹیسٹ برغ: سیرم بلیروبن کا تخمینہ۔

Vitamin K test After injection of vitamin K, serum prothrombin rises in obstructive jaundice, remains depressed in toxic jaundice.

٦٥۔ یٹسٹ حیاتین ''کے'': حیاتین ''کے'' کے انجکشن کے بعد سیرم پروتھرومبین آلسٹر کٹو یرقان میں بڑھتا ہے اور زہریلے یرقان میں بدستور کم رہتا ہے۔

Volmer test Tuberculin jelly applied to skin and covered with adhesive. Inflammation indicates positive reaction.

٦٦۔ وولمر ٹیسٹ: ٹبرکولن جیلی جلد پر لگائی جاتی ہے۔سوج مثبت ردعمل ظاہر کرتی ہے۔

Von Pirquet's test Old tuberculin applied to cleansed skin followed by scarification. If positive, inflammation appears at site of scarification.

٦٧۔ ٹیسٹ پرکویٹ: اولڈ ٹبرکولن صاف جلد پر لگائی جاتی ہے' بعد میں نشان پڑ جاتے ہیں۔اگر مثبت ہو تو نشانوں والی جگہ پر سوج ہو جاتی ہے۔

TPI test. *Treponema pallidum* immobilization test. A modern, highly specific test for syphilis in which syphilitic serum immobilizes and kills spirochaetes grown in pure culture.

٦٨۔ ٹی پی آئی ٹیسٹ: سفلس معلوم کرنے کے لیے ٹیسٹ۔سفلس کی تشخیص میں کیا جاتا ہے۔

Wassermann test Carried out in the diagnosis of syphilis. It is a complement-fixation test and is not entirely specific. See also under **TPI test.** [August von Wassermann, German bacteriologist, 1866-1925.]

٦٩۔ واسرمن ٹیسٹ:

Weber's test. Tuning fork test for the diagnosis of conduction deafness. [Friedrich Eugen Weber, German otologist. 1832-91.]

٧٠۔ٹیسٹ ویبر: بہرہ پن کی تشخیص کے لیے۔

Weil-Felix test. An agglutination reaction used in the diagnosis of the typhus group of fevers. Patient's serum is titrated against an heterologous antigen. [Edmund Weil, German physician in Prague, 1880-1922. Arthur Felix, Prague bacteriologist, 1887-1956.]

٧١۔ ویل فیلکس ٹیسٹ: بخاروں کے ٹائفس گروہ کی تشخیص میں مستعمل۔

Wool test A test for detecting colour blindness. The person is asked to select skeins of wool of matching colours.

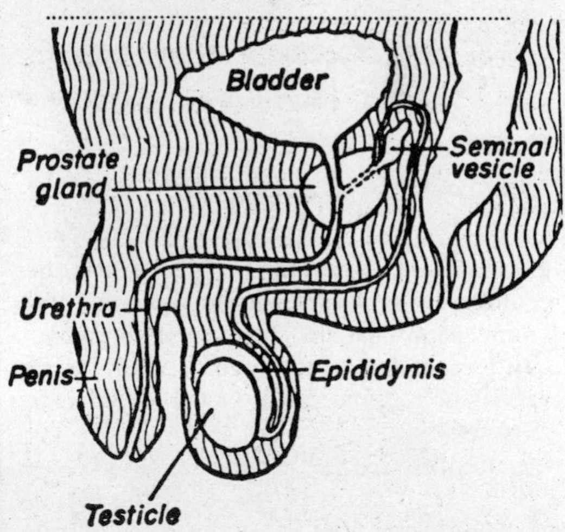

Testicle and attachments

۷۲۔ اون ٹیسٹ: اونی اندھاپن معلوم کرنے کے لیے ٹیسٹ۔

Widal test (ve'-dal). An agglutination reaction for typhoid fever. The patient's serum is put in contact with *Salmonella typhi.* The result is positive it agglutination occurs, proving the presence of antibodies in the serum. [Georges F.1. Widal, French physician, 1862-1929,]

۷۳۔ وائیڈل ٹیسٹ: تپ محرقہ کے لیے اگلوٹی نیشن ردعمل۔ مریض کے سیرم کو سالمونیلا ٹائیفی کے ساتھ رکھا جاتا ہے۔ اگر اگلوٹی نیشن ہو تو نتیجہ مثبت ہے۔ جس سے ثابت ہوتا ہے کہ سیرم میں اینٹی باڈیز موجود ہیں۔

Xylose test. More convenient than fat balance and equally as accurate. Xylose given orally and its urinary exretion measured. Normally 25 per cent of loading dose is excreted. Less than this indicates malabsorption syndrome.

۷۴۔ زائیلوز ٹیسٹ: زائیلوز دہنی طور پر دیا جاتا ہے اور اس کا بولی اخراج ناپا جاتا ہے۔ اس کی ۲۵ فیصد خوراک باہر نکل آتی ہے۔ اس سے کم انجذاب کی خرابی کو ظاہر کرتی ہے۔

Testicle *(tes'tik-l)* [L. testiculus, of testis]. Testis--testicular, adj.

فوطہ، ٹٹا: خصیہ۔ یہ دو چھوٹی اور بیضوی شکل کی منی پیدا کرنے والی سفید گلٹیاں ہیں۔ ہر ایک خصیہ پر چھ غلاف ہوتے ہیں۔ ہر ایک خصیہ جوانی میں ڈیڑھ انچ لمبا ایک انچ چوڑا سوا انچ موٹا اور قریباً نصف چھٹانک وزنی ہوتا ہے۔ بایاں حصہ نسبتاً بڑا ہوتا ہے۔ ان کی اندرونی رطوبت مرد میں ہرمونز پیدا کرتی ہے۔ اور سیدھی خون میں شامل ہوتی ہے بیرونی رطوبت میں منی ہوتی ہے جو نالیوں کے ذریعے اوپر جا کر جمع ہوتی رہتی ہے۔ مرد کے انزال کے وقت مثانہ کا منہ بند ہو جاتا ہے تاکہ منی پیشاب سے متاثر نہ ہو۔

Testis *(tes'-tis).* One of the two galndular bodies contained in the scrotum of the male; they form sperms and also the male sex-hormones. **underscended t.,** the organ remains in the pelvis or inguinal canal. Cryptorchism (q.v.) --testes, pl.

خصیہ۔ فوطہ: دو عدد غدود یہ اجسام میں ایک جوز کے سکروٹم میں ہوتا ہے وہ کرم ہائے منی اور نر جنسی ہارمون بناتے ہیں۔

Testosterone *(tes-tos'-ter-on).* The hormone derived from the testes and responsible for the development of the secondary male characteristics. Used in carcinoma of the breast, to control uterine bleeding and in male underdevelopment.

ٹیسٹوسٹیرون: خصیوں سے اخذ شدہ ہارمون اور ثانوی نر خصوصیات کی تکمیل کا ذمہ دار چھاتی کارسینوماس، یوٹرس کے روانی خون کے لیے اور نر میں کم نمو میں مستعمل۔ نامردی کے علاج کے لیے ایک ٹیکہ ہفتے میں ایک بار ٹیسٹوویرون۔

Tetanus *(tet'-an-us)* [G. tetanos]. Lockjaw. Disease caused by *Clostridium tetani,* an anaerobe which may be present in road dust and manure. Patient develops spasm and rigidity of muscles. Tetanus toxoid injection produces acitve immunity. ATS injection produces passive immunity--tetanic, adj.

چاندنی، فک بستگی۔ کزاز: یہ مرض کلاسٹریڈیم ٹیٹنی کے سبب ہوتا ہے جو ایک این ایروب ہے اور سڑک کی گرد اور کھاد میں موجود ہوتا ہے۔ مریض میں سپازم اور عضلات کی سختی پیدا ہو جاتی ہے۔

Tetany *(tet'-en-i)* [G. tetanos, convulsive spasm]. Condition of muscular hyperexcitability in which mild stimuli produce cramps and spasms (cf. carpopedal spasm). Found in parathyroid deficiency and alkalosis. Associated in infants with gastrointestinal upset and rickets.

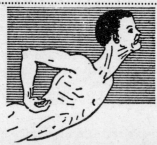

Tetany

Tetany (showing typical opisthotonos and finger and hand spasm)

نوبتی کزاز: بچوں کا مرض جو معدے کے نقائص اور رکٹس کی وجہ سے ہوتا ہے۔ اس میں ہاتھ پاؤں اکڑ جاتے ہیں۔ اینٹھن کے دورے پڑتے ہیں۔

Tetmosol *(tet'-mo-sol).* Monosulfiram (q.v.)

ٹیٹموسول: مانوسلفرم

Tetrabenazine Nitoman. Tranquillizer.

ٹیٹرابنیازین: نٹومان۔ سکون بخش دوا۔

Tetrachlor (o) ethylene *(tet-ra-klor-eth'-i-len)*. An anthelmintic given in hookworm. A single dose is used.

ٹیٹرا کلور(و) ایتھی لین: کیڑے مار دوا جو ہک ورم میں دی جاتی ہے۔ اس کی واحد خوراک استعمال کی جاتی ہے۔

Tetracoccus *(tet-ra-kok'-us)*. Coccal bacteria arranged in cubical packets of four.

چونبقہ: چار کے کیوبیکل پیکٹوں میں مرتب کاکسی جراثیم۔

Tetracycline *(tet-ra-si'-klin)*. A broad spectrum antibiotic related to both aureomycin and terramycin and used for similar purposes. As a rule it causes less gastrointestinal disturbances. There is less absorption of oral t. when the stomach is full, or contains aluminium, calcium and magnesium. Causes fluroescence in body cells. This disappears rapidly from normal cells when the drug is discontinued and is retained by cancerous cells for 24-30 h after dosage ceases. Can be used for tuberculosis.

ٹیٹرا سائیکلین: چوڑے طیف کی اینٹی بایوٹک دوا۔ آریو مائی سین اور ٹیرا مائی سین سے تعلق اور انہی مقاصد کے لیے مستعمل۔ اس سے معدے اور آنتوں میں خرابی کم ہوتی ہے۔ اسے تپدق کے لیے استعمال کیا جا سکتا ہے۔ ایکرومائی سین۔ اس کے دو ڈ کیپسول آتشک یا سفلس میں ہر چھ گھنٹے بعد بیس یوم تک نے سلری پیچش اور بواسیر کے ایک کیپسول ہر چھ گھنٹے بعد امیبائی پیچش میں ایک کیپسول ہر ۴ گھنٹے بعد ۱۰ یوم تک ڈائی ورٹی کیولائیٹس، السر یٹو کولا ئیٹس اور سپرو میں، ایک کیپسول ہر چھ گھنٹے بعد۔

Tetracyn *(tet'-ra-sin)*. Tetracycline (q.v.)

ٹیٹرا سن: ٹیٹرا سائیکلین۔

Tetradactylous *(tet-ra-dak'-a-til-us)* [G. *tetra*, four; *daktylos*, finger]. Having four digits on each limb.

چوانگشتا: ہر جارح پر چار انگلیاں ہونا۔

Tetradecapeptide *(tet-ra-dek-a-pep'-tid)* [G. *tetra*, four; *deka*, ten; *peptikos*, to cook]. A sophisticated peptide (q.v.)

Tetrahydroaminacrine *(tet-ra-hi'-dro-a-me-n'-o-kren)*. Counteracts the narcotic and respiratory depressant effect of other drugs, e.g. morphine.

ٹیٹرا ہائیڈروامینا کرین: دوسری ادویات سے خواب آور اور تنفسی کمی کو متوازن کرتا ہے۔

Tetralogy of Fallot A form of congenital heart defect which includes narrowing of the pulmonary artery, a septal defect between the ventricles, hypertrophy of the right ventricle, and displacement of the aorta to the right. [Etienne Lous Arthur Fallot, French physician, 1850-1911.]

تثلیث قلب: دل کے نقص کی ایک قسم۔ پیدائشی نقص۔ پھیپھڑے والی شریان تنگ ہو جاتی ہے۔

Tetralysal *(tet-ra-li'-sal)*. A tetracycline derivative which maintains higher blood serum lenels with fewer doses, resulting in greater efficiency in combating infections of the respiratory system.

ٹیٹرالائی سال: ٹیٹرا سائیکلن سے اخذ شدہ۔ چند خوراکوں سے زیادہ خونی سیرم لیولز برقرار رہتے ہیں۔

Tetraplegia *(tet-ra-ple'-ji-a)* [G. *tetra*, four; *plege*, stroke]. Paralysis of all four limbs. Also QUADRIPLEGIA.

ٹیٹرا پلیجیا: چاروں جوارح کی اینٹھن۔

Tetrocosactrin *(tet-ro-ko'-sak-trin)*. Synthetic ACTH. As it does not cause allergic reactions, it should replace ACTH in treatment of asthma, etc.

ٹیٹروسیکٹرن: دمہ کے علاج میں مستعمل۔

THA. Tetrahydroaminacrine (a.v.)

ٹی ایچ اے: ٹیٹرا ہائیڈروامین ایکرین۔

Thalamotomy *(thal-am-ot'-o-mi)* [G. *thalamos*, chambers; *tome*, cutting]. Usually operative (stereotaxic) destruction of a portion of thalamus. Can be done for intractable pain.

تھیلاموٹومی: تھیلامس کے ایک حصے کی اپریشن کے ذریعے تباہی۔

Thalamus *(thal'-a-mus)* [G. *thalamos*, chamber]. A collection of grey matter at the base of the cerebrum. Sensory impulses from the whole body pass through on their way to the cerebral cortex--thalami, pl.; thalamic, adj.

اندرون حرم۔عرشہ: سر برم کی اساس پر گرے میٹر کا جمع ہونا۔

Thalassaemia *(thal-as-em'-i-a)* [G. *thalassa* the sea; *haima*, blood]. Cooley's anaemia (q.v.).

Genetically transmitted haemoglobin abnromality.

تھیلسیمیا: وراثت میں منتقل ہونے والی ہیموگلوبن کی خرابی۔

Thalazole *(thal'-a-zol)*. Phthalylsulphathiazole (q.v.)

تھیلازول: فتھالائل سلفاتھیازول۔ السرٹیو کولائی ٹس میں ۲ گولیاں صبح ۲ دوپہر ۲ شام۔

THAM. Tris hydroxylmethyl aminomethane. (q.v.)

ٹی ایچ اے ایم: ٹرس ہائیڈروکسل میتھائل امینومیتھین۔ ایسیڈوسس کے علاج کے لیے مستعمل ایک الکلی۔

Thanatology *(than-at-ol'-o-ji)* [G. *thanatos,* death; *logos,* discourse]. The study of death to discover a trust worthy way of deciding that death beyond resuscitation has taken place.

علم موت: موت کا مطالعہ۔

Theca *(the'-ka)* [G. *theke,* case]. An enveloping sheath, especially of a tendon. theca vertebralis, the membranes enclosing the spinal cord--thecal adj.

غلاف: ایک غلافی شید، خصوصاً ٹنڈان کی۔

Theine *(the'-in)*. An alkaloid found in tea.

تھین۔ کیفین: چائے میں پایا جانے والا الکلائڈ۔

Thenar *(the'-nar)* [G. palm]. The palm of the hand and the sole of the foot. thenar eminence, the palmar eminence below the thumb.

Thenar

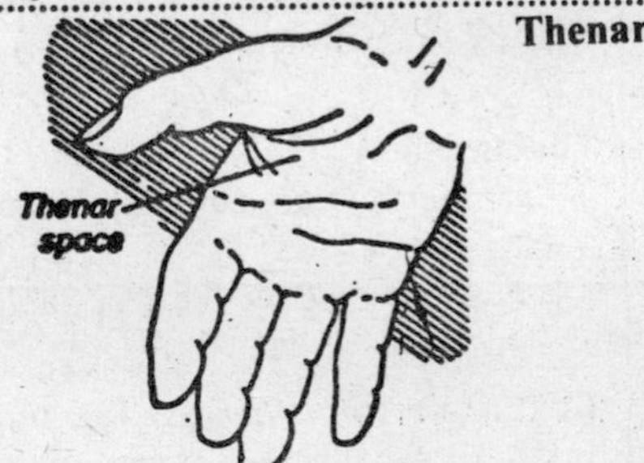

ہتھیلی۔ تلوا: ہاتھ کی ہتھیلی اور پاؤں کا تلوا۔

Theobromine *(the-o-bro'-men)*. A drug allied to caffeine, but with a less stimulating and more powerful diuretic action. Sometimes given with phenobarbitone to reduce frequency severity of anginal attacks.

برومین: ایک سفید ناحل پذیر قلمی الکلائیڈ۔ نقطہ پگھلاؤ ۳۴۳۷س' میں پایا جاتا ہے۔ اور ادویات میں استعمال کیا جاتا ہے۔ اس دوا کا تعلق سے ہے لیکن اس کم تحریک والی اور زیادہ طاقت ور پیشاب آور۔

Theo-nar *(the'-o-nar)*. Theophylline noscapine capsules that give immed release of part of dose, and delayed releas remaining dose for control of bronchospas

ر: تھیوفلین اور نوسکاپین کے کیپسول۔

Theophorin *(the-of'-or-in)*. Phenindamine (c

رن: فینِنڈامین۔

Theophyulline *(the-of'-il-lin)*. A diuretic rel to caffeine but more powerful. It is u mainly as its derivative amniophylline in treatment of congestive heart failure, dy oea and asthma. Present in mersalysl Neptal injections.

ین: نقطہ پگھلاؤ ۲۷۲°س' چائے میں پایا جاتا ہے 'اور ادویات میں کیا جاتا ہے۔ پیشاب آور۔ کیفین سے متعلق لیکن زیادہ طاقت ور اور نیپٹل انجکشنوں میں موجود۔

Therapeutics *(ther-a-pu'-tiks)* [G. *thera, tikos,* wait on, cure]. The branch of me science dealing with the treatmen disease--therapeutic adj. therapeutically, a

الجہ: مرض کے علاج سے متعلق میڈیکل سائنس کی شاخ۔

Therapy *(ther'-a-pi)* [G. *therapeia*]. Treatm

لاج: علاج۔

Thermal *(ther'-mal)* [G. *theme,* heat]. Pertai to heat.

رارتی: حرارت سے متعلق۔

Thermogenesis *(ther-mo-jen'-e-sis)* [G. *the* heat; *genesis,* production]. The producti heat--thermogenetic, adj.

زائی: حرارت کی پیداوار۔

Thermography *(ther-mog'-ra-fi)* [G. *the* heat; *graphein,* to write]. Temperature rences throughout the body are record photographic film for diagostic purpo thermographic, adj.; thermographically, thermograhp, n.

تپش نگاری: تشخیصی مقاصد کے لیے فوٹوگرافی فلم پر سارے جسم میں درجہ حرارت کے اختلافات ریکارڈ کیے جاتے ہیں۔

Thermolabile *(ther-mo-la'-bil)* [G. *therme,* heat; L. *labills,* slipping]. Capable of being altered by heat.

حرحساس: حرارت سے تبدیل ہونے کا اہل۔

Thermolysis *(ther-mol'-i-sis)* [G. *therme,* heat; *lysis,* a loosening]. Loss of heat--thermolytic, adj.

حرارت پاشی: حرارت کا ضیاع۔

Thermometer *(ther-mom'-et-er)* [G. *therme,* heat; *metron,* a measure]. An instrument containing a substance, the volume of which is altered by temperature--thermometric, adj. The low reading clinical thermometer is marked either.

Thermometers

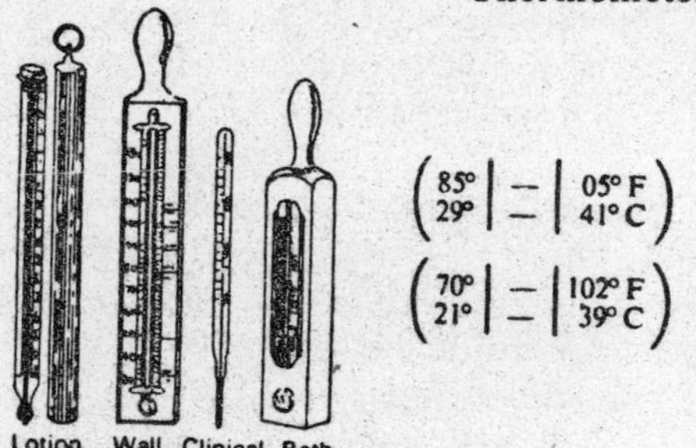

تھرمامیٹر۔تپش پیما: ایسے مادہ پر مشتمل آلہ جس کا حجم درجہ حرارت سے تبدیل ہوتا ہے۔

Thermophil *(ther'-mo-fil)* [G. *therme,* heat; *philein,* to love]. A micro-organism accustomed to growing at a high temperature-- thermophilic, adj.

حرارت پسند: زیادہ درجہ حرارت پر نمو پانے والا خوردجسمیہ۔

Thermoscan *(ther'-mo-skan).* Apparatus capable of scanning the distribution of heat over an area. Sufficiently sensitive to record temperature differentials down to 0.2° C. Among the many conditions which can be studied are blood flow disorders, viability of skin grafts, onset of malignant breast tumours and the extent of varicose veins.

تھرموسکین: کسی ایریا پر تقسیم حرارت کی سکینگ کے اہل سامان۔کئی حالتیں جو اس کی مدد سے مطالعہ کی جاسکتی ہیں۔ان میں روانی خون کی خرابی' جلدی پیون کاری' چھاتی کے ناسور وغیرہ شامل ہیں۔

Thermostable *(ther-mo-sta'-bl)* [G. *therme.* heat; L. *stabilis,* stable]. Remaining unaltered at a high temperature, which is usually specified --thermostability, n.

حرپائیدار: زیادہ درجہ حرارت پر بلا تبدیلی رہنا جو عموماً مخصوص ہوتا ہے۔

Thermotherapy *(ther-mo-ther'-a-pi)* [G. *the-rme,* heat; *therapeia,* treatment]. Heat treatment.

حرارتی علاج: حرارتی علاج۔علاج بذریعہ حرارت۔

Thesaurosis *(thes-awr-o'-sis)* [G. *thesauros,* store; *-osis,* condition]. Term currently concerned with hair sprays. Macromolecules taken up by cells of the reticuloendothelial system with a consequent inflammatory reaction. Similar to sarcoidosis.

تھیساروسس: ہیر سپرے سے متعلق اصطلاح۔

Thiabendazole *(thi-a-bend'-az-ol).* Can be used as single dose treatment for threadworms. Effective orally for larva migrans caused by some species of Ancylostoma. Best available treatment for strongyloides infestation. No starvation or purgation necessary. Stated to clear the infection in about 50 per cent of patients with trichuriasis.

تھایابینڈازول: چرنوں کے علاج کے لیے واحد خوراک کے طور پر یہ دوائی استعمال کی جاسکتی ہے۔

Thiacetazone *(thi-a-set'-a-zon).* Synthetic antitubercular compound. As effective as PAS and cheaper. Can be used in a regimen of one dose per day with isoniazid.

تھایاسیٹازون: تالیفی اینٹی ٹبرکولر مرکب۔

Thialbarbitone *(thi-al-bar'-bit-on).* A barbiturate used as an intravenous anaesthetic in a similar way to thiopentone. It is said to cause less laryngeal spasm of respiratory depression.

تھایابار بی ٹون: ایک بار بی ٹوریٹ۔ انٹراوینس سُن کرنے والے کے طور پر مستعمل۔

Thiambutosine *(thi-am-but'-o-sen)*. Antileprotic drug.

Thiamine *(thi'-a-men)*. See ANEURINE.

تھایامین: اینورین۔ حیاتین ب۔ حیاتین ب پیچیدہ کارکن۔ سفید قلمی سفوف۔ پانی میں حل پذیر الکوحل میں حل پذیر۔ بہت سے جانداروں کو اس کی ضرورت ہوتی ہے۔ یہ کلیجی، دودھ، انڈوں اور پھلوں میں پایا جاتا ہے۔ اس کی کمی سے کئی بیماریاں لاحق ہوتی ہیں۔

Thiersch skin graft *(teersh)*. Films of epidermis with a portion of dermis applied to a raw area shaved smooth from granulations. [Karl Thiersch, German surgeon, 1822-95.]

Thiethylperazine *(thi-eth-il-per'-a-zen)*. For nausea, vomiting and vertigo.

تھائی ایتھائل پیرازین: متلی یا قے کے لیے۔ ٹوری کین۔ ایک ٹیکہ صبح ایک شام حسب ضرورت۔

Thiomerin *(thi-om'-er-in)*. A mercury containing diuretic, similar in action to mersalyl, but suitable for subcutaneous injection.

تھایومیرین: پارے میں مشتمل پیشاب آور دوا۔ عمل میں مرسیلائل کی طرح لیکن جلدی ٹیکے کیلئے موزوں۔

Thiomersalate *(thi-o-mer'-sal-at)*. An organic mercurial antiseptic and fungicide. Used for skin sterilization and as a lotion.

تھایومرسلیٹ: ایک نامیاتی پارے والا دافع اور سماروغ کش۔ جلد کو پاک کرنے اور بطور لوشن مستعمل۔

Thiopentone *(thi-o-pen'-ton)*. A barbiturate given by intravenous injection as a short-acting basal anaesthetic. The effect can be extended by additional doses, and in combination with curare compounds adequate relaxation for major surgery can be achieved.

تھایاپنٹون: ایک بار بی ٹوریٹ جو انٹراوینس انجکشن کے ذریعے دیا جاتا ہے۔ مختصر العمل بنیادی سن کرنے والے کے طور پر مستعمل۔

Thiopropazate *(thi-o-pro'-paz-at)*. Sedative and antiemetic used widely for psychoneurotic states.

تھایو پروپازیٹ: سائیکو نیوروٹک حالتوں میں مستعمل۔ جذبات سرد کرنے والی اور قے روکنے والی دوائی۔

Thioquanine *(thi-o-qwan'-en)*. Antimetabolite. Interferes with synthesis of nucleoprotein, thus useful in acute luekaemia.

تھایوکوانین: اینٹی بولائٹ۔ نکلیو پروٹین کی تالیف میں خلل انداز ہوتا ہے۔ اس لیے شدید لیوکیمیا میں مفید ہے۔

Thioridazine *(thi-o-rid'-a-zen)*. Sedative, tranquillizer. Closely resembles chlorpromazine.

تھیوریڈازین: کلورپرومازین سے مشابہ۔ سکون بخش دوا۔

Thiotepa *(thi-o'-te'-pa)*. Triethylene thiophosphoramide (q.v.).

تھایوٹیپا: ٹرائی ایتھائلین تھایو فاسفورائیڈ۔

Thiothixene *(thi-o-thiks'-en)*. Antipsychotic, used in schizophrenia.

تھایوتھکسین: اینٹی سائیکوٹک۔ شائزوفرینیا میں مستعمل۔

Thoracentesis *(thor-a-sen-te'-sis)* [G. *thorax*, chest; *kentesis*, puncture]. Paracentesis (q.v.) of the pleural cavity.

صدر سوزنی: پیورل کہفہ کی پیراسینٹیسس۔

Thoracic *(thor-as'-ik)*. Pertaining to the thorax thoracic duct, a channel conveying lymph (chyle) from the receptaculum chyli in the abdomen to the left subclavian vein. **thoracic inlet syndrome**, See CERVICAL RIB.

صدری: تھیوریکس سے متعلق۔

Throacoplasty *(thro'-ak-o-plas-ti)* [G. *thorax*, *plassein*, to form]. An operation on the thorax in which the ribs are resected to allow the chest wall to collapse and the lung to rest used in the treatment of pulmonary tuberculosis.

صدر پیوندی: تھیوریکس پر اپریشن جس سے چھاتی کی دیوار ل جاتی ہے ر پھیپھڑے آرام کرسکتے ہیں۔ شریانی تپ دق میں مستعمل اپریشن۔

Thoracoscope *(thor'-ak-o-skop)* [G. *thorax*, thorax; *skopein*, to examine]. An instrument which can be inserted into the pleural cavity through a small incision in the chest wall, to permit inspection of the pleural surfaces and division of adhesions by electric diathermy.

thoracoscopic, adj.; thoracoscopy, n.

پلیورابین: چھاتی کی دیوار میں ایک چھوٹے شگاف میں سے پلیورل کہفہ میں گھسایا جانے والا آلہ تاکہ پلیورل سطوح کا معائنہ کیا جاسکے اور برقی ڈایا تھرمی سے چپٹنے کی تقسیم دیکھی جاسکے۔

Thoracotomy *(thor-a-ko'-to-mi)* [G. *thorax,* thorax; *tome,* a cutting]. Surgical exposure of the thoracic cavity.

صدر شگافی: چھاتی کے کہفہ کو اپریشن سے عریاں کرنا۔

Thorax *(tho'-raks)* [G.]. The chest cavity--thoracic, adj.

Thorax

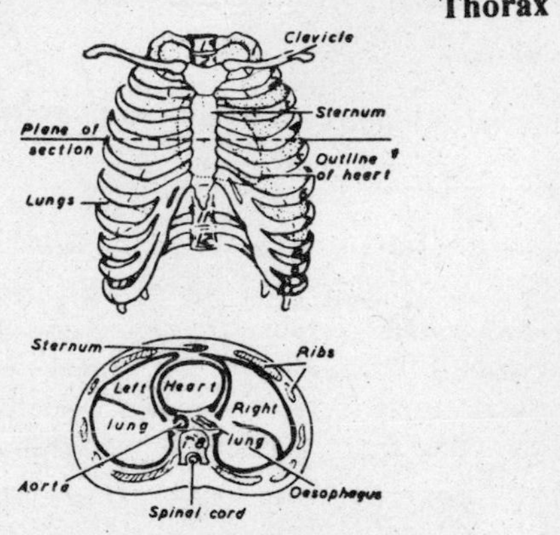

صدر۔ سینہ: یونانی لفظ۔ چھاتی کا کہفہ یا جوف۔

Thorium X *(tho'-ri-um).* A substance allied to radium, but with only a brief radioactive life. It is used as a varnish or ointment in the treatment of various skin conditions.

تھوریم ایکس: ریڈیم سے مشابہ مادہ لیکن تابکاری زندگی مختصر۔ مختلف جلدی حالتوں میں علاج کے لیے مرہم یا وارنش کے طور پر مستعمل۔

Threadworm *(thred).* Enterobius (Oxyuris) Vermicularis. Tiny thread like worms that infest man's intesine. Females migrate to anus to lay eggs, thus spread of , and reinfestation easy. The whole family should be treated simultaneously using piperazine over a week, together with hygiene measures to prevent reinfestation. A further course after 10 days interval is advisable to deal with worms that have since hatched, as the eggs are not affected by the drug.

چرنا: انٹروبیس یا آکسی یورس ورمیکولیرس چھوٹے دھاگے نما کیڑے جو آدمی کی آنت میں ہوتے ہیں۔ مادہ کیڑے مقعد کیطرف انڈے دینے کے لیے ہجرت کر جاتے ہیں۔ اس طرح ان کا انتشار آسان ہو جاتا ہے۔ پائپرازین پورے خاندان کا وایک ہفتے تک استعمال کرنا چاہیے اور صفائی کا خیال رکھنا چاہیے۔ دس ایام کے وقفہ کے بعد دوبارہ کورس کرنا چاہیے۔

Thronine *(thre'-o-nin).* An essential amino acid (q.v.)

تھریونین: ایک لازمی امینوایسڈ۔

Thrill Vibration as perceived by the sense of touch.

لرزہ: چھونے کی حس سے ارتعاش۔

Thrombectomy *(throm-bek'-to-mi)* [G. *thrombus,* clot; *ektome* excision]. Surgical removal of a thrombus from within a blood vessel.

ولمہ براری: خونی رگ میں سے تھرومبس کا اپریشن سے خاتمہ۔

Thrombin *(throm'-bin)* [G. *thrombos,* clot]. Not normally present in cirulating blood; generated from prothrombin (Factor II). See BLOOD CLOTTING. The extrinsic and intrinsic pathways lead to production of thrombin. The extrinsic pathway is tested by the prothrombin time (PT). The intrisnic pathway involves principally Factors IX and VIII among others. The partial thromboplastin time (PTT) or a modification called the partial thromboplastin time with kaolin (PTTK) detects abnormalities in this pathway. See CHRISTMAS DISEASE and HAEMOPHILIA.

خمیر خون: مادہ جو فائبرینوجن کو فائبرن میں تبدیل کرتا ہے۔

Thromboangiitis *(throm-bo-an-ji-i'-tis)* [G. *thrombos,* clot; *aggeion,* vessel; *-itis,* inflammation]. Clot formation within an inflamed vessel. **thromboangiitis obliterans** (syn., Buerger's disease), an uncommon disorder of unknown cause, occurring mainly in young adult Jewish males, characterized by patchy, inflammatory, obliterative, vascular disease, principally in the limbs (sometimes in the cardiac or cerebral vessels), and presenting usually as calf pains, or more severely as early gangrene of the toes and following a chronic progressive course.

تھرمبوانجیٹیس :رگ میں خون کالوتھڑا جمنا۔

Thromboarteritis *(throm-bo-ar-te-ri'-tis)* [G. *thrombos,* clot; *arteria,* artery; *-itis,* inflammation]. Inflammation of an artery with clot formation.

التہاب الشریان: خون کے لوتھڑے والی شریان کی سوزش یا سوج۔

Thrombocyte *(throm'-bo-sit)* [G. *thrombos,* clot; *kytos,* cell]. Syn., blood platelet. Plays a part in the clotting of blood.

خلیہ دلمی: خونی پلیٹ لیٹ۔خون کے جمنے میں حصہ لیتا ہے۔

Thrombocythaemia Syn., thrombocytosis (q.v.)

Thrombocytopenia *(throm-bo-si-to-pen'-i-a)* [G. *thrombos,* clot; *kytos,* cell; *penia,* want]. A reduction in the number of platelets in the blood--thrombocytopenc, adj.

تھرمبوسائیٹو پنیا۔: خون میں پلیٹ لیٹس کی تعداد میں تخفیف۔

Thrombocytopenic purpura *(thrombo-si-to-pe'-nik pur'-pu-ra).* A syndrome characterized by a low blood platelet count, intermittent mucosal bleeding and purpura (q.v.). It can be symptomatic, i.e. secondary to known disease or to certain drugs; or idiopathic, a rare condition of unknown cause (syn., purpura haemorrhagica) occurrring principally in children and young adults. In both forms the bleeding time is prolonges.

تھرمبوسائیٹو پینک پر پیورا: ایک سنڈروم جس میں کم خونی پلیٹ لیٹ میو کوسل روانی خون اور پر پورا ہوتے ہیں۔

Thrombocytosis *(throm-bo-sit-o'-sis)* [G. *thrombos,* clot; *kytos,* cell; *-osis,* condition]. An increase in the number of platelets in the blood.

تھرمبوسائی ٹوسس: خون میں پلیٹ لیٹس کی تعداد میں اضافہ۔

Thromboembolic *(throm-bo-em-bol'-ik)* [G. *thrombos,* clot; *embolos,* plug]. Used to describe the phenomenon whereby a thrombus or clot detaches itself and is carried to another part of the body in the blood strem to block a blood vessel there.

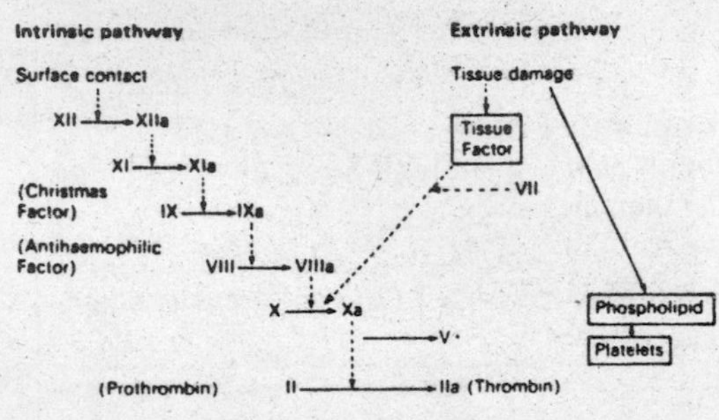

A cascade of blood coagulation reactions leading to thrombin formation.

تھرمبوایمبولک :اسے بیان کرنے کے لیے جہاں خون کا لوتھڑا الگ ہو کر جسم کے دوسرے حصے میں جا کر خونی رگ کو بند کر دیتا ہے۔

Thromboendarterectomy *(throm-bo-end-art-er-ek'-to-mi)* [G. *thrombos,* clot; *endon,* within; *arteria,* artery; *ektome,* excision]. Removal of a thrombus from an artery following reboring.

تھرمبواینڈارٹریکٹومی: شریان سے تھرومبس کو نکالنا اور سوراخ کیا جاتا ہے۔

Thromboendarteritis *(throm-bo-end-art-e-ri'-tis)* [G. *thrombos,* clot; *endon,* within; *arteria,* artery *-itis,* inflammation]. Inflammation of the inner lining of an artery with clot forma -tion.

تھرمبواینڈ آرٹریٹس: لوتھڑا بننے والی شریان کے اندرونی غلاف کی سوزش

Thrombogen *(throm'-bo-jen).* Precursor of thrombin (q.v.)

Thrombogenic *(throm-bo-jen'-ik)* [G. *thrombos,* clot; *genesis,* descent]. Capable of clotting blood--thrombogenesis, thrombogenicity, n.; thrombogenetic, adj.; thrombogenetically, adv.

تھرمبوجینک: خون جمانے کا اہل۔

Thrombokinase *(throm-bo-kin'-az)* [G. *thrombos,* clot]. Syn., thromboplastin (q.v.).

تھرمبوکائی نیز: تھرومبوپلاسٹن۔

ombolytic *(throm-bo-lit'-ik)* [G. *thrombos*, ot; *lysis*, a loosening]. Pertaining to disingration of a blood clot. thrombolytic thepy, attempted removal of preformed intrav-scular fibrin occlusions using fibrino- lytic gents--thrombolysis, n.

تھرمبولائی ٹک: خون کے لوتھڑے کے خاتمہ سے متعلق۔

ombophlebitis *(throm-bo-fle-bi'-tis)* [G. *rombos*, clot; *phleps*, vein; *-itis*, inflamation]. Inflammation of the wall of a vein ith secondary thrombosis within the invoed segment. **thrombophlebitis migrans,** current episodes of t. affecting short lengths superficial veins. Deep vein t. uncommon d pulmonary embolism rare--thrombophletic, adj.

تھرمبوفلائی ٹی ٹس: ثانوی تھرومبوسس والی ورید کی دیوار کی سوزش۔

omboplastin *(throm-bo-plas'-tin)* [G. *rombos*, clot; *plassein*, to form]. An enzyme hich converts prothrombin into thrombin. trinsic t., produced by the interaction of veral factors during the clotting of blood. uch more active than tissue thromboplastin. sue t., thromboplastic enzymes are present many tissues, and tissue extracts are used clotting experiments and in the estimation prothrombin time.

تھرمبو پلاسٹین: خامرہ جو پرو تھرومبن کو تھرومبن میں تبدیل کرتا ہے۔

mbosis *(throm-bo'-sis)* [G. *thrombos*, clot; *sis*, condition]. The intravascualr formation a blood clot--thrombotic, adj.; thromboses,

خون بستگی۔ تجمد: خون کے لوتھڑے کا انٹراواسکولر بننا۔

mbus *(throm'-bus)* [G. *thrombos*, clot]. An travascular blood clot--thrombi, pl.

دلمہ: ایک انٹراواسکولر خون کا لوتھڑا۔

sh Candidiasis (q.v.).

قلاع۔ منہ پک جانا: کینڈی ڈیاسس۔ منہ آنا بچے کے منہ میں سفید
سا نظر آتا ہے۔ تالو اور زبان پر چھالے ہوتے ہیں۔ سفید دھبوں کی در
جگہ سرخ ہوتی ہے۔ اس کی وجہ ماں کی اندام نہانی میں پھپھوندی ہوتی
جسے ایلبی کین کہا جاتا ہے۔ بچے میں علامات چوتھے روز ظاہر ہوتی ہیں۔
دھبوں کو صاف کرنے سے نیچے زخم ظاہر ہوتا ہے۔ جس پر ڈیکواڈن پینٹ

ٹسٹین محلول لگاتے ہیں۔

Thyline *(thi-lin)*. Nifenazone (q.v.).

تھائیلین: نیفینازون۔

Thymectomy *(thi-mek'-to-mi)* [G. *thymos*, soul; ektome, excision]. Surgical excision of the thymus.

تیموسیہ براری: تھائمس کا سرجیکل قطع۔

Thymol *(thi'-mol)*. The chief antiseptic constituent of oil of thyme. Widely employed in mouthwahses and dental preparations, and has been given as an anthelimintic in hookworm.

ست سعتر: تھائیم کے تیل کا بڑا دافع تعفن جزو، گلا صاف کرنے کے لیے
مستعمل اور ہک ورم کے لیے کیڑے مار دوا کے طور پر دیا جاتا ہے۔

Thymoleptic *(thi-mo-le'-tik)*. A current term for durgs primarily exerting their effect on the brain, thus influencing 'feeling' and behaviour.

تھائی لیپٹک: دماغ پر اثر کرنے والی ادویہ جن کا اثر احساس اور رویہ پر
ہوتا ہے۔

Thymoma *(thi-mo'-ma)* [G. *thymos*, soul; *-oma*, tumour]. A tumour arising in the thymus--thymomata, pl.

سلعہ تیموسیہ: تھائمس میں ابھرنے والی رسولی۔

Thymosin *(thi'-mo-sin)*. Hormone secreted by the epithelial cells of the thymus gland. Provides the stimulus for lymphocyte production within the thymus;confers on lymphocytes elsewhere in the body the capacity to respond to antigenic stimulation.

تھائموسین: تھائمس گلینڈ کے اپی تھیلیل خلیوں سے اخراج ہونے والا
ہارمون۔

Thymoxamine *(thi-moks'-a-men)*. Vasodilator drug. Blocks alpha receptors of sympathetic nervous system. Useful in Meniere's disease.

تھائی موکسامین: واسوڈائیلیٹر ڈرگ۔

Thymus *(thi'-mus)*. A gland lying behind the breast bone and extending upward as far as the thyroid gland. It is well developed in infacny and attains its greatest size towards puberty; and then the lymphatic tissue is replaced by fatty tissue. It has an immunological role. Autoimmunity is thought to result from pathological activity of this gland--thymic, adj.

تیموسیہ: چھاتی کی ہڈی کے پیچھے گلینڈ اور بالائی جانب تھائیرائڈ گلینڈ تک جاتی ہے۔ یہ گلینڈ بچپن میں ہوتی ہے اور جوانی تک سوکھ جاتی ہے۔

Thyroglossal *(thi'-ro-glos'-al)*. Pertaining to the thyroid gland and the tongue. **thyroglossal** duct, the fetal passage from the thyroid gland to the back of the tonuge where its vestigial end remains as the formen caecum. Thyroglossal cyst or fistula can occur.

ورقی لسانی: تھائیرائڈ گلینڈ اور زبان سے متعلق۔

Thyroid *(thi'-roid)*. The ductless gland found on both sides of the trachea. It secretes thyroxine, which controls the rate of metabolism. The commercial material is the t. gland to the ox, sheep or pig, dried and reduced to powder, and adjusted in strength to contain 0.1 per cent of iodine as thyroxine. Used in myxoedema and cretinism.

غدہ ورقیہ: ٹریکیا کی دونوں اطراف پر واقع بلا نلی گلینڈ یہ تھائیروکسین پیدا کرتی ہے۔ جو میٹابولزم کی شرح کو کنٹرول کرتی ہے۔

Thyroidectomy *(thi-roid-ek'-to-mi)* [G. *thureoides*, shield-shaped; *ektome*, excision]. Surgical removal of the thyroid gland.

ورقیہ براری: تھائیرائیڈ گلینڈ کا سرجیکل خاتمہ۔

Thyroiditis *(thi-roid-i'-tis)* [G. *thureoeides*, shield-shaped; *-itis*, inflmmation]. Inflammation of the thyroid gland. **lymphadenoid t.** (autoimmune t. or Hashimoto's disease), a firm goitre ultimately resulting in hypothyroidism. **Riedel's t.,** a chronic fibrosis of the thyroid gland; ligneous goitre.

ورم ورقیہ: تھائیرائیڈ گلینڈ کی سوزش۔

Thyrotoxicosis *(thi-ro-toks-i-ko'-sis)* [G. *thureoeides*, shield-shaped; *toxkikon*, poison; *-osis*, condition]. One of the autoimmune thyroid disease. A condition due to excessive production of the thyroid gland hormone (thyroxine), probably in response to stimulation by an axcessive production of pituitary thyrotrophic hormone, and resulting classically in anxiety, tachycardia, sweating increased appetite with weight loss, and a fin tremor of the outstretched hands, an prominence of the eyes. It is much commoner in women than in men. In older patients cardiac irregularities may be a prominent feature-thyrotoxic, adj.

سمومیت ورقی: آٹوامیون تھائیرائڈ امراض میں سے ایک تھائیرائڈ کے رمون' تھائیروکسین کی زائد پیداوار کی وجہ سے حالت۔ سوچ میں تیزی' رکات تیز' ہلکا رعشہ' جلد گیلی ہتھیلیوں پر پسینہ' بھوک تیز' وزن کم' جسم گرم اور بض تیز ہوتی ہے۔ یعنی ۱۰۰ تا ۱۶۰ فی منٹ رہتی ہے۔

Thyrotrophic *(thir'-o-trof-ik)*. A substanc which stimulates the thyroid gland, e.g. the hormone secreted by the anterior pituitar gland.

ھائیروٹرافک: تھائی رائیڈ گلینڈ کو تحریک دینے والا مادہ تھائیروٹرافک رمون تھا تھائیرائڈ گلینڈ کی نشوونما کرتا ہے اور اسے تھائیراکسین ہارمون پیدا رنے کے لیے تحریک کرتا ہے۔

Thyroxine *(thi-roks'-in)*. The principal hormon of the thyroid gland. It raises the basal metabolic rate.

فراز ورقیہ: آیوڈین پر مشتمل امینوایسڈ جو تھائیرائڈ گلینڈ پیدا کرتی ہے۔ لص سفید قلمی شے' نقطہ پگھلاؤ ۲۳۶س' تھائیرائڈ کمی پورا کرنے کے لیے ستعال کیا جاتا ہے۔ ایک گولی دن میں ۳ مرتبہ برائے مکسے ڈیما۔ ایکرومیگلی ر کرٹزم۔

Tibia *(tib'-i-a)* [L.] The shin-bone; the larger o the two bones in the lower part of hte leg; articulates with the femur, fibula and talus-tibial, adj.

ڈلی کی اندرونی ہڈی۔ ٹبیا: ٹانگ کے نچلے حصے میں دو ہڈیوں میں سے ایک بڑی۔ ٹبیا کا بالائی کنارہ ران کی ہڈی کے ساتھ گھٹنے کا جوڑ بناتا ہے۔ ں کنارے پر دو نشیب ہوتے ہیں جن میں ران کی ہڈی کی نوکیں آ جاتی ہیں۔ ریں کنارہ ٹخنے کی ہڈی یا اسٹرا گیلس کے ساتھ مل کر ٹخنہ بناتا ہے۔

Tibiofibular *(ti-bi-o-fib'-u-lar)* [L. *tibia*, shin-bone; *fibula*, clasp]. Pertaining to the tibi and the fibula.

یوفیبولر: ٹبیا اور فیبولا سے متعلق۔

Tic *(tik)*. Purposeless involuntary, spasmodi muscular movements and twitchings, du partly to habit, but often associated with psychological factor.

عضلہ تشنج: بے مقصد بلا ارادہ سپاسموڈک عضلی حرکات جزوی طور پر عادت کی وجہ سے لیکن اکثر نفسیاتی عامل سے متعلق۔

Tic douloureux *(doo-ler-oo')*. Trigeminal neuralgia. Spasms of excruciating pain in distribution of trigeminal nerve.

تشنج چہرہ: ٹرائی جیمینل نیورلجیا۔

Tick *(tik)*. A blood-sucking parasite, larger than a mite. Some o them are concerned in the transmission of relapsing fever, typhus, etc.

چچڑی: ایک خون چوسنے والا طفیلی۔

Timolol meleate *(time'-o-lol mal'-e-at)* Hypotensive beta-blocking agent.

Tincture *(tink-tur)*. Solution of a durg in alcohol.

ٹنکچر: الکوحل میں محلول یا الکوحل سے علیحدہ کیا گیا۔ عموماً ٹنکچروں مستعمل۔

Tinea *(tin'-e-a)* [L. gnawing worm]. See RINGWORM. **tinea barbae** (barbers' itch), ringworm of the beard. **tinea capitis,** ringworm of the head, tinea croporis (also circinata), ringworm of the body. **tinea cruris** ('Dhobie itch'), ringworm of the crutch area. tinea pedis (dermatophytosis), ringworm of the foot.

جنس بید۔ جنس کرم لباس: رنگ ورم۔

Tinnitus *(ti-ni'-tus)* [L.] A buzzing, thumping or ringing sound in the ears.

کان بجنا: کانوں میں گھنٹیاں بجنا۔

Tissue *(tis'-u)*. A collection of cells or fibers of simialr function, forming a structure.

نسیج۔ بافت: یکساں خلیوں کا ایسا گروہ جن کا فعل بھی یکساں ہو۔

Titration *(ti-tra'-shun)*. Volumetric analysis by aid of standard solutions.

معائرہ: حجمی تجزیہ کا ایک بنیادی عمل۔

Titre *(te'-ter)*. A standrad of strength per volume.

عیار: طاقت فی حجم کا معیار۔

Tobramycin *(tob-ra-mi'-sin)*. Antibiotic particularly effective against Pseudomonas aeruginosa and Staphylococcus aureus. Such infections can be lethal to those afflicted with cystic fibrosis.

توبرامائی سین: اینٹی بایوٹک۔ خصوصاً سیوڈوموناس ایروجینوزا اور سٹیفائلوکوکس آریس کے خلاف موثر۔

Tocograpby *(tok-og'-raf-i)* [G. *tokos,* birth; *graphein,* to write]. Process of recording uterine contractions using a tocograph or a parturiometer.

ٹوکوگرافی: ٹوکوگراف کے استعمال سے یوٹرس کے سکڑاؤ کو ریکارڈ کرنے کا طریقہ۔

Tocopherol *(tok-of'-er-ol)*. Synthetic vitamin E, similar to that found in wheat-germ oil. It has been used in habitual abortion, and empirically in many other conditions with varying success.

ولادت آور: تالیفی وٹامن ای۔ ایک پیلا ناحل پذیر مرکب۔ نقطہ پگھلاؤ ۲۰۰ تا ۲۱۰°س، اس کی کمی انسانی صحت کے لیے مضر ہے یہ سبزی کے پتوں میں پایا جاتا ہے۔

Tofranil. Imipramine (q.v.) See ANTIDEPRESSANT.

Tolanase *(tol'-an-az)*. Tolazamide (q.v.).

Tolazamide *(tol-az'-mid)*. Oral antidiuretic agnet. One of the sulphonylureas.

ٹولازیمائیڈ: ذہنی طور پر دیا جانے والا۔ ضد پیشاب آور ایجنٹ۔

Tolazoline *(tol-az'-o-len)*. A peripheral vasodilator, of value in circulatory disorders such as Raynaud's disease and related conditions. Has also been used in ophthalmic conditions such as keratitis.

ٹولازولین: ایک جانبی واسوڈائیلیٹر۔ گردشی خرابیوں میں اسے اہمیت حاصل ہے۔

Tolbutamide *(tol-bu'-mid)*. A sulphonamide derivative which stimulates the islets of Langerhans to pour out more insulin. Has been used with success in the oral treatment of diabetes, so that insulin injections may be reduced or withdrawn. Not suitable for juvenile or severe diabetes.

ٹولبیوٹامائیڈ: ایک سلفونامائیڈ حاصل جو آئیلیٹس آف لنگرہانز کو زیادہ انسولین پیدا کرنے کی تحریک کرتا ہے۔ ذیابیطس کے ذہنی علاج میں مفید۔ شدید ذیابیطس میں مناسب نہیں۔

Tolerance Ability to tolerate the application or

administration of a substance, usually a drug. One may have to increase the dose of the drug as t. develops, e.g. nitrites. **exercise t**, exercise accomplished without pain or marked breathlessness. American Heart Association's classification of functional capacity; Class 1--no symptoms on ordinary effort; Class 11--slight disability on ordinary effort (in Britain it is usual to subdivide this class into class 11a--able to carry on with normal housework under difficulty--and class 11b--cannot manage shopping or bedmaking except very slowly); Class111--marked disability on ordinary effort which prevents any attempt at housework; Class IV--symptoms at rest or heart failure.

تاب آوری: کسی شے عموماً دوائی دیئے جانے یا اس کے اطلاق کو برداشت کرنے کی قابلیت۔

Tolnaflate *(tol'-naf-lat)*. Antifungal agent, useful for athlete's foot.

ٹولنافلیٹ: سماروغ کش عامل۔ ایتھلیٹ کے پاؤں کے لیے مفید۔

Tolnate. Prothipendyl (q.v.).

Tomograph *(to'-mo-gra)* [G. *tomos,* cutting; *graphein,* to write]. Differential radiograph demonstrating a selected layer in a specified region of the body. A series of such films with the 'in focus' layer set at various depths allows a three dimensional impression to be built up.

Tomography

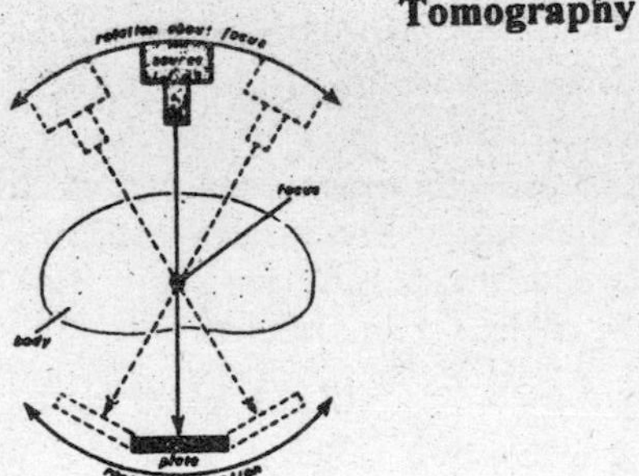

Shows extent of cysts, tubercular foci, cancer, calculi, etc.--tomography, n.; tomographic, adj., tomographically, adv.

ٹوموگراف: جسم کے مخصوص حصہ میں منتخب پرت کو ظاہر کرنے کے ممیّز ریڈیوگراف۔

Tone (ton); **tonus** *(ton'-us)*. The normal, healthy state of tension.

مزاج صحیح: تنشن کی نارمل، صحت مند حالت۔

Tongue *(tung)*. The mobile muscular organ contained in the mouth; it is concerned with speech, mastication, swallowing and state. **strawberry t.,** thickly furred with projecting red papillae. As the fur disappears the t. is vividly red, like an overripe strawberry. Characteristic of scarlet fever.

زبان: منہ کے اندر عضلی عضو۔ اس کا تعلق تقریر چبانے، نگلنے اور چکھنے سے ہے۔

Tongue

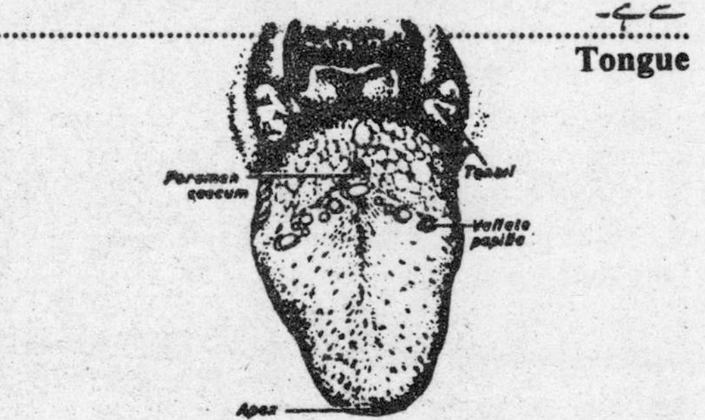

Tonic *(ton'-ik)* [G. *tonos,* tension]. Used to describe a state of continuous muscular contraction, as opposed to intermittent contraction. Cf, clonus.

مقوی (دوا)۔ لوچی: متواتر عضلی سکڑاؤ کی حالت۔ جب نوزائیدہ بچہ اپنی پشت کے بل لیٹا ہو تو ٹونک نیک رجحان کو ظاہر کرتا ہے۔ اس کا سر حرکت کرتا ہے اور جدھر وہ دیکھ رہا ہوتا ہے۔ اس کا بازو اور ٹانگ کچھ کچھ یا مکمل طور پر ادھر پھیلی ہوئی ہوتی ہے۔ یہ رجحان بچے میں اعصابی نظام کے نامکمل ہونے کی علامت ہے۔ یہ رجحان بچے میں تین یا چھ ماہ کے بعد غائب ہو جاتا ہے۔

Tonography *(ton-og'-ra-fi)* [G. *tonos,* tone; *graphein,* to write]. Continuous measurement of blood, or intraocular, pressure, carotid compression t., normally occlusion of one ommon carotid artery causes an ipsilateral all of intraocular pressure. Screening test for arotid insufficiency.

تنش نگاری: خون کے یا انٹرآ کولر دباؤ کی لگاتار پیمائش

ıometer *(ton-om'-et-er)* [G. *tonos,* tension; *ıetron,* a measure]. An instrument for ıeasuring intraocular pressure.

تنش مقلہ پیماء: انٹرآ کولر دباؤ کی پیمائش کا ایک آلہ۔

ısillectomy *(ton-sil-ek'-to-mi)* [L. *tonsillae,* ɔnsils; G. *ektome,* excision]. Removal of the ɔnsils.

لوزہ برآری: ٹانسلز کا خاتمہ

sillitis *(ton-sil-i'-tis)* [L. *tonsillae,* tonsils; G. *'tis,* inflammation]. Inflammation of the ɔnsils.

ورم ٹانسل۔ ورم لوزتان: ٹانسلز کی سوزش یا سوج۔ گلے دکھتے ہیں ا ربخار ہو جاتا ہے۔ علاج کے لیے سٹر پٹو مائی سین' پروکین پنسلین انجکش روزانہ ایک لگائیے۔ گلے میں منڈلز پینٹ لگائیے اور نمک کے غرارے ک جائیں ارتھرومائی سین کی ایک گولی ہر چھ گھنٹے بعد۔

silloliths *(ton'-sil-o-liths)* [L. *tonsillae,* ɔnsils; G. *lithos,* stone]. Concretions arising ı the body of the tonsil.

ورم لوزہ: ٹانسل کے جسم مں ابھرنے والی گلٹیاں۔

sillopharyngeal *(ton-sil-o-far-in-je'-al)* [L. *ɔnsillae,* tonsils; G. *pharynx,* pharynx]. ertining to the tonsil and pharynx.

ٹانسلوفیرنجیئل: ٹانسل اور فیرنکس سے متعلق۔

sillotome *(ton'-sil-o-tom)* [L. *tonillae,* tonls; G. *tome,* a cutting]. Instrument for xcision of tonsils.

لوزہ تراش: ٹانسلز نکالنے کے لیے آلہ۔

sils *(ton'-silz)* [L. tonsillae]. The small bo-es, one on each side, covered by mucous embrane, embedded in the fauces between e palatine arch; composed of about 10 to 18 mph follicles--tonsillar, adj.

لوزتین: پیلاٹائن آرچ کے درمیان فاسز میں دھنسے ہوئے ہیوکس جھلی ڈھکے' ہر طرف ایک' چھوٹے اجسام۔ قریباً ۱۰ تا ۱۸ لمف فولکلز پر مشتمل۔

ectomy *(top-ek'-to-mi).* Modified frontal ɔotomy. Small incisions made in thalamof-ntal tracts.

ٹوپیکٹومی: ترمیم شدہ فرنٹل لوبوٹومی۔

Tophus *(to'-fus)* [L.] A small, hard concretion forming on the ear-lobe, on the joints of the phalanges, etc. in gout--tophi, pl.

نقرس'ٹوفس: ایک چھوٹی سخت گلٹی جو کان کے لوپ یا فینجز کے جوڑوں پر یا دوسری جگہوں پر بن جاتی ہے۔

Topical *(top'-ik-al)* [G. *topos,* place]. Local--topically, adv.

محدود'مقامی: مقامی۔ وہ تکلیف جو کسی ایک عضو تک محدود ہو۔

Topography *(top-og'-ra-fi)* [G. *topos,* place; *graphein,* to write]. A description of the regions of the body--topographical, adj.; topographically, adv.

ناحیہ عضونگاری: جسم کے حصوں کی تفصیل۔

Torecan *(tor'-e-kan).* Thiethylperazine (q.v.).

ٹوری کین: تھائی ایتھائل پیرازین۔ قے روکنے کیلئے ایک ٹیکہ صبح ایک شام حسب ضرورت عضلاتی ٹیکہ۔

Torsion *(tor'-shun).* Twisting.

مروڑ: محور کے گرد ٹوسٹ جو مختلف جوڑوں کے عمل سے اس وقت پیدا ہوتا ہے جب وہ متوازی کے پلین میں عمل کر رہے ہوں۔

Torticollis *(tor-ti-kol'-is)* [L. *torquere,* to twist; *collum,* neck]. Wryneck; a painless contraction of one sternomastoid muscle. The head is slightly flaxed and drawn towards the contracted side, with the face rotated over the other shoulder.

صعر: ایک سٹرنومسٹائیڈ عضلے کا بے درد سکڑاؤ۔

Tosmilen *(tos-mil'-en).* Anticholinesterase eyedrops, useful in glaucoma. Miotic.

ٹوسملان: ضد کولین ایسٹیریز آنکھوں کے قطرے گلاکوما میں مفید۔

Toti's operation See DACRYOCYSTORHINOSTOMY. [Addeo Toti, Italian ophthalmologist and laryngologist, 1861-1946.]

ٹوٹی کا اپریشن: ڈیکرائیوسسٹورائنوسٹومی۔

Tourniquet *(toor'-ne-ka)* [F.]. An apparatus for the compression of the blood vessels of a limb. Designed for compression of a main artery to control bleeding. Is also often used to obstruct the venous return from a limb and so facilitate the withdrawal of blood from a vein. Tourniquets vary from a simple rubber band to a pneumtic cuff.

شریان بند: کسی جارح کی خونی رگوں کو دبانے کیلئے سامان ۔ اس سے شریان سے خون کی روانی کو روکا جاتا ہے۔

Two (to). Coarse flax.

ٹو: کورس فلیکس۔

Toxaemia *(toks-e'-mi-a)* [G. *toxikon,* poison; *haima,* blood]. A generalized poisoning of the body by the products of bacteria or damaged tissue--toxaemic, adj.

شریان بند: کسی جارح کی خونی رگوں کو دبانے کیلئے سامان ۔ اس سے شریان سے خون کی روانی کو روکا جاتا ہے۔

Toxic *(toks'-ik).* Poisonous.

Toxic Epidermal necrolysis *(toks'-ik-ep-i-der'-mal ne-krol'-is-si)* [G. *toxikon,* poison; *epi,* on; *derma,* skin; *nekros,* corpse; *lysis,* a loosening]. A syndrome in which the appearance is of scalded skin. It can occur in response to drug reaction, staphylococcal infection, systemic illness, and it can be idiopathic.

Tomicity *(toks-is'-it-i)* [G. *toxikon,* poison]. The quality or degree of being poisonous.

زہر آلودگی: زہریلا ہونے کا درجہ یا صفت۔

Toxicology *(toks-i-kol'-o-ji)* [G. *toxikon,* poison; *logos,* discourse]. The science dealing with poisons--toxicological, adj.; toxicologically, adv.

علم سموم ۔ سمیات: زہروں سے متعلق سائنس ۔ خودکشی یا کسی کی جان لینے کے لیے زہر کھایا یا کھلایا جاتا ہے۔

Toxicomania *(toks-ik-o-ma'-ni-a).* WHO definition; Periodic or chronic state of intoxication produced by repeated consumption of a drug harmful to the individual or society. Characteristics are;(1) Uncontrollable desire or necessity to continue consuming the drug and to try to get it by all means. (2) Tendency to increase the dose. (3) Psychic and physical dependecny as a result.

زہر مانیا: فرد یا سوسائٹی کے مضر دوا کے بار بار استعمال سے پیدا شدہ نشے کی پیریاڈک یا قدیم حالت۔

Toxin *(toks'-in).* A product of bacteria poisonous to other cells which , on injection into animal or man, stimulates the production of an antibody (i.e. antitoxin) to it . non-bacterial t., a poisonous nitrogenous compound such as that liberated from diseased or injured tissue.

عفونتی زہر: مواد ساقہ ۔ زہر ۔ یہ نام عموماً جراثیم سے پیدا ہونے والے انتہائی زہریلے مادوں کیلئے استعمال ہوتا ہے۔

Toxocara *(toks-o-car'-a).* Genus of roundworm of the cat dog. Man can be infested (toxocariasis) by eating with hands soiled from these pets. The worms cannot become adult in man (incorrect host) so the larval worms wander through the body, attacking mainly the liver and the eye. Treatment is unsatisfactory, but the condition usually clears after several months.

ٹوکسا کیرا: بلی اور کتے کا راؤنڈ ورم ۔ انہیں ہاتھ لگانے سے کھانے میں آدمی میں جاسکتا ہے ۔ جگر اور آنکھ پر حملہ کرتا ہے۔

Toxoid *(toks'-oid)* [G. *toxikon,* poison; *eidos,* form]. A toxin altered in such a way that it has lost its poisonous properties but retained its antigenic properties. Vaccines are prepared from toxins by accelerating the change to toxoid with oxidizing agents.

سم نما: ٹاکسین جو اپنے زہریلے خواص کھودے لیکن ضد جینی خواص برقرار رکھے ۔ ویکسین میں مستعمل۔

Toxoid-antitoxin *(toks-oid-an-ti-toks'-in).* A mixture of toxoid and homologous antitoxin in floccule form, used as a vaccine, e.g. in immunization against diphtheria.

ٹاکسائیڈ اینٹی ٹاکسن: ٹاکسائڈ اور یکساں اینٹی ٹاکسن کا آمیزہ ویکسین کے طور پر مستعمل۔

Toxoplasma *(toks-o-plas'-ma).* A genus of parasite which causes toxoplasmosis.

ٹاکسو پلازما: ایک طفیلی جو ٹاکسو پلازماسس کرتا ہے۔

Toxoplasmosis *(toks-o-plas-mo'-sis)* [G. *toxikon,* poison; *plasma,* anything formed; *-osis,* condition]. Infection by Toxoplasma parasite which, commonly occurring in mammals and birds, may infect man. Intrauterine fetal an infant infections are often severe, producing encephalitis, convulsions hydrocephalus and eye diseases, resulting in death or , in those who recover, mental retardation and impaired sight. Infection in older children and adults may result in pneumonia, nephritis or skin rashes. Skull X-ray reveals flecks of cerebral calcification. Skin and antibody tests confirm the diagnosis.

ٹوکسو پلازموسس: ٹاکسو پلازما طفیلی جو عموماً پستانیہ جانوروں اور پرندوں میں ہوتے ہیں۔ بعض اوقات انسان بھی مرض کا موجب بنتے ہیں۔ حاملہ عورت کو چھوت لگ جانے سے بچے کے لئے خطرناک' ہلکا بخار' سردرد' عضلات میں درد' خون میں کمی' خون کے سفید ذرات۔

Trabeculae *(tra-bek'-u-le)* [L. little beam]. The fibrous bands or septa projecting into the interior of an organ, e.g. the spleen; they are extensions from the capsule surrounding the organ--trabecula, sing; trabecular, adj.

کڑیاں: ریشہ دار پٹیاں یا پردے جو کسی عضو کے اندر تک چلے جاتے ہیں۔ مثلاً تلی

Trabeculotomy *(trab-ek-u-lot'-o-mi)*. Operation for glaucoma. It aims at creating a channel through the trabecular meshwork from the canal of Schlemm to the angle of the anterior chamber.

ٹربیکولوٹوی: گلاکوما کے لئے اپریشن۔

Trace. elements Metals and other elements that are regularly present in very small amounts in the tissues and known to be essential for normal metbolism (e.g. copper, cobalt, manganese, fluorine, etc.)

قلیل عناصر: عناصر جو تھوڑی سی مقدار میں کسی جاندار کو چاہئیں۔

Tracer *(tra'-ser)* A substance or instrument used to gain information. Radioactive tracers have extended knowledge in physiology; some are used in diagnosis.

سراغ رساں: اطلاع حاصل کرنے کے لئے مستعمل مادہ یا آلہ۔

Trachea *(trak-e'-a)* [G. *trachus*, rough]. The windpipe; the fibrocartilaginous tube lined with mucous membrane passing form the larynx to the bronchi. It is about 11.43 cm long and about 25.4 mm wide--tracheal, adj.

Trachea

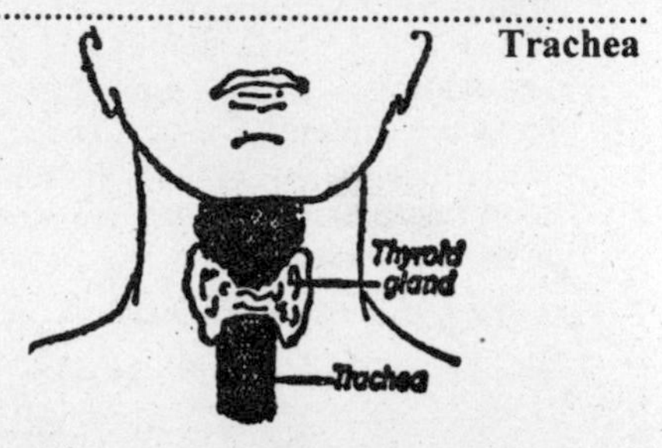

قصبۃ الریہ۔ سانس کی نالی: ہوا کی نالی۔ لیرنکس سے برونکائی تک نلی یہ قریباً ۱۱.۴۳ سم لمبی اور قریباً ۲۵.۴ مم چوڑی ہے۔ گردن میں سامنے کی طرف واقع' غذا کی نالی اس کی پشت پر ہوتی ہے۔ سینے میں داخل ہو کر اس کی دو شاخیں ہو جاتی ہیں۔ سانس کی نالی میں ۱۶ سے ۲۰ تک کرکری ہڈی کے چھلے ہوتے ہیں۔ یہ چھلے مکمل نہیں ہوتے۔

Tracheitis *(trak-e-i'-tis)* [G. *trachus*, rough; *-itis*, inflammation]. Inflammation of the trachea.

ورم قصبیہ: ٹریکیا کی سوزش یا سوج

Trachelorrhaphy *(trak-el-or'-raf-i)* [G. *trachelos*, neck; *rhaphe*, suture]. Operative repair of a uterine cervical laceration.

خم رحم پیوندی: رحم یا یوٹرس کی سرویکل لیسریشن کی اپریشن کے ذریعہ مرمت

Tracheobronchial *(trak-e-o-brong'-ki-al)* [G. *trachus*, rough; *brongchos*, bronchial tube]. Pertaining to the trachea and the bronchi.

ٹریکیو برونکیل: ٹریکیا اور برونکائی سے متعلق۔

Tracheobronchitis *(trak-e-o-brong-ki'-tis)*. Inflammation of the trachea and bronchi.

ورم قصبیہ وشعبیہ: ٹریکیا اور برونکائی کی سوزش

Tracheo-oesophageal *(trak-e-o-e-sof-aj-e-al')* [G. *trachus*, rough; *oisophagos*, gullet]. Pertaining to the trachea and the oesophagus.

قصبی مریوی: ٹریکیا اور ایسوفیگس سے متعلق۔

Tracheostomy *(tr-ke-os'-to-mi)* [G. *trachus*, rough; *stoma*, mouth]. Fenestration in the anterior wall of the trachea by removal of circular piece of cartilage from third and fourth rings, for establishment of a safe airway and reduction of 'dead space' —tracheostome, n.

ٹریکیوسٹومی: ٹریکیا کی امامی دیوار میں سوراخ۔

Tracheotomy *(tr-ke-ot'-o-mi)* [G. *trachus,* rough; *tome,* cutting]. Vertical slit in the anterior wall of the trachea at the level of the third and fourth cartilaginous rings. Usually performed in young children.

قصبیہ شگافی: تیسرے اور چوتھے نرم ہڈی والے حلقے کے لیول پر ٹریکیا کی امامی دیوار میں عمودی شگاف جب گلے کے راستے سانس بند ہونے لگے تو اپریشن ضروری ہو جاتا ہے۔

Trachoma *(tra-ko'-ma)* [G.] Contagious inflammation affecting conjunctiva, cornea and eyelids. Due to Bedsonia, which resembles a virus. It behaves like a bacterium, though it multiplies intracellularly. Sensitive to sulphonamides and antibiotics. If untreated it leads to blindness. Medical Research Council's Trachoma Research Unit is trying out a vaccine--trachomatous, adj.

ککرے: کنجکٹوا، قرینہ اور آنکھ کے پپوٹوں کو متاثر کرنے والی سوزش۔

Traction *(trak'-shun).* A drawing or pulling on the patient's body to overcome muscle spasm, and to reduce or prevent deformity. A steady pulling exerted on some part (limb or head) by means of weights and pulleys. See BALKAM BEAM. BRAUN'S FRAME, BRYANTS TRACTION. RUSSELL TRAC- TION.

انقباض: عضلی سپازم کو روکنے اور بدشکلی کو ختم کرنے یا روکنے کے لئے مریض کے جسم کو کھینچنا۔ اوزان اور چرخیوں کے ذریعے کسی جسمانی حصے پر مستقل کھچاؤ۔

Halo-pelvic traction

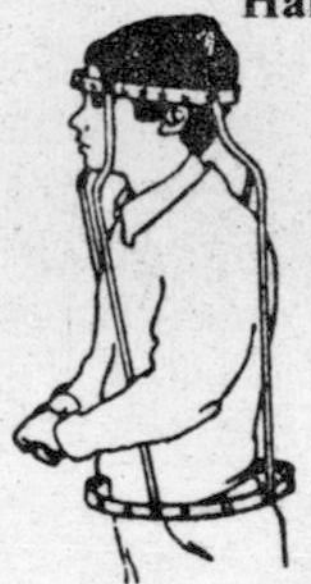

Tractotomy *(trak-tot'-o-mi).* Incision of a ne tract. Surgical relief of intrac- table pa Using stereotactic measures this operatio now being done for some forms of mer illness.

ٹوٹومی: عصبی ٹریکٹ کا شگاف۔

Tragus *(tra'-gus)* [G. *tragos,* a goat]. The p ection in front of the external auditory m tus--tregi, pl.

۔: بیرونی سمعی می ایٹس کے سامنے پروجیکشن۔

Trait *(tra).* An individual characteristic form part of the whole personality.

ہ: ایک انفرادی خاصیت جو پوری شخصیت کا حصہ ہوتی ہے۔

Trance *(trans)* [L. *transire,* to pass over]. A rm used for hypnotic sleep and for cert self-induced hysterical stuporous states.

سبات۔سکتہ: (تنویمی) بے خوف نیند کے لئے مستعمل اصطلاح۔

Tranquillizers *(tran'-kwi-li-zers)* [L. *tranquil* calm]. These drugs do not affect a ba disease, but reduce symptoms so that pati feels more comfortable and is more accessi to help from psychotherapy. Greatly exagg ate the effects of alcohol. Chlordiazepox (Librium), meprobamate (Equanil, Miltow hydroxyzine (Atarax) and methylepenty (Oblivon). Syn., ataractic, neuroleptic, an olytic, thymoleptic.

ن بخش: پریشانی میں تخفیف کے لئے استعمال کی جانے والی دوائی۔ ے سستی نہیں ہوتی اور نہ ہی چستی پر اثر انداز ہوتی ہے۔

Transabdominal *(trans-ab-dom'-in-al)* [L. *tra* through; *abdomen,* belly]. Through abdomen as the t. approach for nephrectom transabdominally, adv.

س ایبڈمینل: بطن میں سے۔

Transamniotic *(trans-am-ni-ot'-ik)* [L. *tra* through; G. *amnion,* membrane round fetu Through the amniotic membrane and fluid at. transfusion of the fetus for haemoly disease.

س امنیاٹک: امنیاٹک جھلی اور سیال میں سے۔

Transection *(tran-sek'-shun)* [L. *trans,* throu *sectio,* a cutting]. The cutting across or m hanical severance of a structure.

عرضی تراش: کسی ساخت کے میکانکی طور پر کاٹنا۔

Transfrontal *(trans-front'-al)* [L. *trans,* through; *frons,* forehead]. Through the frontal bone; an approach used for hypoph- ysectomy.

ٹرانس فرنٹل: فرنٹل ہڈی میں سے۔

Transfusion *(trans-fu'-zhun)* [L. *transfundere,* to transfuse]. The introduction of fluid into the tissue or into a blood vessel. **blood t.,** the transfer of blood into a vein. **intrauterine t.** of the fetus endangered by rhesus incompatibility. Red cells are transfused directly into the abdominal cavity of the fetus, on one or more occasions. This enables the induction of labour to be postponed until a time more favourable to fetal welfare. Also called **intraabdominal prenatal t.**

انتقال خون: نسیج یا خونی رگ میں سیال کا دخول۔

Transillumination *(trans-il-u-min-a'-shun).* The transmission of light through the sinuses for diagnostic purposes.

تنویر عبوری: تشخیصی مقاصد کی لئے خالی جگہوں میں سے روشنی کا گذر۔

Transirrigation *(trans-ir-ri-ga'-shun)* [L. *trans,* through ; *irrigare,* to irrigate]. Diagnostic puncture and lavage, as performed in maxillary sinusitis.

ٹرانس اریگشن: تشخیصی پنکچر

Transithal *(trans'-i-shal).* Buthalitone (q.v.)

ٹرینسی تھل: بوتھلیٹون۔

Translocation *(trans-lo-ka'-shun).* Transfer of a segment of a chromosone to a different site on the same chromosome or to a different one. Can be the cause of congenital abnormality.

Translucent *(trans-lu'-sent)* [L. *trans,* through; *lucere,* to shine]. Intermediate between opaque and transparent.

نیم شفاف: غیر شفاف اور شفاف کے درمیان انٹرمیڈیٹ۔

Translumbar *(trans-lum'-bar)* [L. *trans,* through; *lumbus,* loin]. Through the lumbar region. Route used for injecting aorta prior to aortography,

ٹرانس لمبر: لمبر ریجن میں سے۔

Transmigration *(trans-mi-gra'-shun)* [L. *trans,* through; *migrare,* to migrate]. The transit of a cell through a membrane.

ہجرت: جھلی میں سے خلیے کی ٹرانزٹ۔

Transmural *(trans-mu'-ral)* [L. *trans,* through; *murus,* wall]. Through the wall, e.g. of a cyst, organ or vessel--transmurally, adv.

ٹرانس میورل: دیوار میں سے مثلاً رگ، عضو کا سسٹ کا۔

Transonic *(tran-son'-ik).* Allowing the passage of ultrasound. See ULTRASONIC.

انتقال صوتی: الٹراساؤنڈ کے گزر کی اجازت۔

Transperitoneal *(trans-per-it-on-e'-al)* [L. *trans,* through; G. *peri,* around; *teinein,* to stretch]. Across or through the peritoneal cavity. See DIALYSIS.

ٹرانس پیری ٹونیل: پیری ٹونی سے کہفہ میں سے یا پار۔

Transnasal *(trans-na'-zal)* [L. *trans,* through; *nasus,* nose]. Through the nose--transnasally, adv.

ٹرانس نیزل: ناک میں سے۔

Transplacental *(trans-pla-sen'-tal)* [L. *trans,* through; *placenta,* cake]. Through the placenta--transplacentally, adv.

ٹرانس پلیسنٹل: پلیسنٹا میں سے۔

Transplantation *(trans-plan-ta'-shun)* [L. transplantare, to transplant]. Grafting on to one part, tissue or an organ taken from another part or another body.

انتقال عضو: کسی دوسرے حصے یا دوسرے جسم میں سے لے کر عضو، نسیج یا حصے کی پیوندکاری۔

Transrectal *(trans-rek'-tal)* [L. *trans,* through; *rectus,* straight]. Through the rectum as a t. injection into a tumour--transrectally, adv.

ٹرانس ریکٹل: ریکٹم میں سے۔

Transsphenoidal *(trans-sfen-oid'-al)* [L. *trans,* through; *sphenoeides,* wedgeshaped]. Through the sphenoid bone; an approach used for hypophysectomy.

ٹرانس فینائڈل: سفینائڈ ہڈی میں سے۔

Transthoracic *(trans-thor-as'-ik)* [L. *trans,* through; G. *thorax,* thorax]. Across or through the chest.

ٹرانس تھیوریسک: چھاتی میں سے ایک کے پار۔

Transudate *(trans'-u-dat)* [L. *trans,* through; *sudare,* to sweat]. A fluid that has passed out of the cells either into a body cavity (e.g. ascitic fluid in the peritoneal cavity) or to the exterior (e. g. serum from the surface of a burn)--transudation, n.

رساؤ: سیال جوخلیوں سے باہر چلا جائے۔ کسی جسمی کہفہ میں یا باہر۔

Transurethral *(trans-u-reth'-ral)* [L. *trans,* through; G. *ourethra,* urethra]. By way of the urethra.

ورائے احلیل: احلیل یا یورتھرا کی راستے سے۔

Transvaginal *(trans-va-jin'-al)* [L. *trans,* through; *vagina,* sheath]. Through the vagina as an incision to drain the uteromanily in cardiac surgery--transventricularly, adv.

ٹرانس ویجائنل: ویجائنا میں سے۔

Transventricular *(trans-ven-trik'-u-lar)* [L. *trans,* through; *ventriculum,* ventricle]. Through a ventricle. Term used mainly in cardiac surgery--transventricularly, adv.

ٹرانس وینٹریکولر: بطین میں سے۔

Transvesical *(trans-ves-ik-al)* [L. *trans,* through; *vesica,* bladder]. Through the bladder, by custom referring to the urinary bladder--transvesically, adv.

ٹرانس ویزیکل: بلیڈر میں سے۔

Tranylcypromine *(tran-il-si-pro'-min).* Monamine oxidase inhibitor (q.v.)

ٹرینائل سائپرومین: ایم۔اے۔او۔آئی آکسیدامین آکسیڈ

Trasylol *(tra'-sil-ol).* Aprotinin (q.v.)

ٹریسیلول: اپروٹینن۔

Trauma *(traw'-ma)* [G.] Bodily injury; emotional shock--traumatic, *adj.*

زخم: جسم کا زخم۔ جذباتی صدمہ۔

Traumatoloty *(traw-mat-ol'-o-ji).* The branch of surgery dealing with injury from accident.

علم زخم: حادثہ سے زخم کے متعلق سرجری کی ایک شاخ۔

Trematoda *(trem-a-to'-da).* A class of parasitic worms which include many pathogens of man such as the Schistosoma of bilharziasis.

وشیعات: طفیلی کیڑوں کی ایک جماعت جن میں کئی کیڑے انسان میں امراض پیدا کرتے ہیں۔

Tremor *(trem'-or)* [L. *tremere,* to tremble]. Involuntary trembling. **coarse t.,** violent trembing. fine t., slight trembling as seen in the outstretched hands or tongue of a patient suffering from thyrotoxicosis, **intention t.,** only occurs on voluntary movement; characteristic of disseminated sclerosis.

رعشہ۔کپکپی: بلاارادہ کپکپاہٹ۔

Trendelenburg's operation Ligation of the long saphenous vein in the groin at its junction with the femoral vein. Used in cases of varicose veins. [Friedrich Trendelenburg, German surgeon, 1844-1924.]

اپریشن،ٹرینڈیلن برگ: فیمورل ورید کے ساتھ اس کے جنکشن پر۔

Trendelenburg's sign A test of the stability of the hip, and particularly of the ability of the hip abductors (gluteus medius and minimus) to steady the pelvis upon the femur. Principle; normally when one leg is raised from the ground the pelvis tilts upwards on that side, through the hip abductors of the stan- ding limb. If the abductors are inefficient (e.g. in poliomyelitis, severe coxa vara, and congenital dislocation of the hip), they are unable to sustain the pelvis against the body weight, and it tilis downwards instead of rising. [Friedrich Trendelenburg, German surgeon, 1844-1924.]

علامت ٹرینڈیلین برگ: چتون کے توازن کا سیٹ۔

Trephine *(tre-fin')* [G. *trypaein,* to bore]. An instrument with sawlike edges for removing a circular piece of tissue, such as the cornea or skull.

ترفین: کسی نسیج کا گول ٹکڑا اتارنے کے لئے آری کے کناروں والا آلہ۔ جیسا کہ قرنیہ یا کھوپڑی کے لئے استعمال کیا جاتا ہے۔

Treponema (G. *trepein,* to turn; *nama,* thread]. A slender spiral-shaped bacterium which is actively motile. Best visualized with dark-ground illumination. Cultivated in the laboratory with great difficulty. *Treponama pallidum* is the causative organism of syphilis; *T. perienue* the spirochaete that causes yaws (q.v.); *T. carateum* the spirochaete that causes pinta (q.v.)xdse

ٹریپو نیما پلیڈم: آتشک پیدا کرنے والا جسیمہ۔ایک متحرک جرثومہ۔تجربہ گاہ میں مشکل سے کاشت ہوتا ہے۔

Treponematosis See YAWS.

Treponemicide *(trep-on-em'-i-sid)* [G. *trepein,* to turn; L. *coedere,* to kill]. Lethal to Treponema --treponemicidal, adj.

ٹریپونیمی سائیڈ: ٹریپونیما کے لئے مہلک۔

Trescatyl *(tres'-kat-il).* Ethionamide (q.v.).

ٹریسکاٹائل: ایتھیونامائیڈ۔

Tretamine *(tret'-a-men).* A cytostatic drug with an action similar to that of mustine, but active orally. Used in leukaemia and Hodgkin's disease.

ٹریٹامین: سائیٹوسٹیٹک ڈرگ۔ایکشن میں مسٹین سے مشابہ۔ذہنی طور پر عامل۔

Trevintex *(trev'-in-teks).* Prothionamide (q.v.)

ٹریونٹیکس: پرتھیونامائیڈ۔

Triamcinolone Steroid with good anti-inflammatory effect and very little electrolyte retaining activity. Due to stimulation of protein breakdown it can cause muscle wasting.

ٹرائی ایم سینولون: سٹیرائڈ۔اس سے لحمی تخریب کے وجہ سے عضلے کا ضیاع ہوسکتا ہے۔اس کی ایک ایک گولی صبح دوپہر شام برائے ٹرائی جیمینل نیورلجیا یا ابرد کا عصبی درد۔

Triamterene *(tri-am'-ter-en).* Diuretic that increases excretion of sodium chloride but lessens potassium loss at distal kidney tubule.

ٹرائی ایمٹرین: پیشاب آور دوا جو سوڈیم کلورائیڈ کے اخراج کو بڑھاتی اور گردے کے ٹیوبول پر پوٹاشیم کے ضیاع کو کم کرتی ہے۔

TRIC agent. Trachoma inclusion conjunctivitis. Responsible for infections of eye, genital tract and urethritis. See CONJUNCTIVITIS.

ٹی۔آر۔آئی۔سی عامل: آنکھ کے امراض کے لئے ذمہ دار۔

Triceps *(tri'-seps)* [L. *having* three heads]. The three-headed muscle on the back of the upper arm.

سہ راسی: بالائی بازو کی پشت پر تین سروں والا عضلہ کہنی کو سیدھا کرنے میں کام آتا ہے۔

Trichiasis *(trik-i'-a-sis)*[G.]. Abnormal eyelashes causing irritation from friction on the eyeball.

پڑبال: غیر معمولی پلکیں جو آنکھ کے گولے پر رگڑ سے خارش پیدا کرتی ہیں۔

Trichinosis *(trik-in-o'-sis)* [G. *trichinos,* hair-like; *-osis,* condition]. A disease caused by eating undercooked pig meat infected with *Trichinella spiralis* (the trichina worm). The female worms living in the small bowel produce larvae which invade the body and, in particular, form cysts in skeletal muscles; the usual symptoms are diarrhoea, nausea, colic, fever, facial oedema, muscular pains and stiffness.

ترخینا (مرض): ٹرائیکنیلا سپائیریلس والے کم پکے ہوئے سور کے گوشت کے کھانے سے ہونے والا مرض۔

Trichloracetic acid *(tri-klor-as-et'-ik).* Powerful caustic and astringent. Used as a crystal for application to warts and ulcers.

ٹرائی کلورایسی ٹک ایسڈ: طاقتور کاسٹک۔آبلوں اور السرز پر لگانے کے لئے قلم کے طور پر مستعمل۔

Trichlorethylene *(tri-klor-eth'-i-len).* Liquid similar to chloroform, and also used as an inhalation anaesthetic. Inhand in small doses, it is useful in relieving the pain of trigeminal neuralgia.

ٹرائی کلورتھائیلن: کلوروفارم سے مشابہ مائع۔

Trichomonacide *(tri-ko-mo'-na-sid).* Lethal to the protozoa belonging the genus Trichomonas.

ٹرائیکوموناسائیڈ: پروٹوزوآ کے جنس ٹرائیکوموناس کیلئے مہلک۔

Trichomonas *(tri-ko-mo'-nas).* A protozoan parasite of man. *Trichomonas vaginalis* produces infection of the urethra and vagina often associated with profuse discharge (leucorrhoea). The organism is best recognized by microsopic examination of the discharge. See PROTOZOA, AMOEBA.

ٹرائیکوموناس ویجائینیلس: آدمی کا پروٹوزون طفیلی، یورتھرا اور ویجائنا کو متاثر کرتا ہے۔

Trichomoniasis *(tri-ko-mon-i-a'-sis)* Inflammation of the vagina (urethra in males) caused by *Trichomonas vaginalis.*

ٹرائیکومونیاسس : ٹرائیکوموناس ویجائینلیس سے ہونے والی ویجائنا (مردوں میں یوتھرا) کی سوزش۔

Trichomycin. An antibiotic trichomonacide. Vaginal and oral tablets. Ointment relieves pruritis.

ٹرائیکومائی سین: اینٹی بایوٹک ٹرائیکوموناسائیڈ' ویجائنل اور دہنی گولیاں۔

Trichophytosis *(tri-ko-fi-to'-sis).* Infection with a species of the fungus Trichophyton, e.g. ringworm of the hair or skin.

داد: سماروغ کی ٹرائیکوفائیٹن نوع کا مرض۔ مثلاً بالوں یا جلد کا رنگ ورم۔

Trichuris *(tri-ku'-ris)* [G. *thrixtrichos,* hair; *oura,* tail]. A genus of nematodes. *Trichuris trichiura,* the whipworm (q.v.)

ٹرائی کیورس ٹریکی یورا: وہپ ورم۔

Trichuriasis *(trik-u-ri'-a-sis)* [G. *thrixtrichos,* hair, *oura,* tail]. Infestation with whipworm *(Trichuris trichiura).*

سوطی مرض: وہپ ورم کی انفیسٹیشن۔

Triclofos *(tri'-klo-fos).* Derivative of chloral hydrate causing less gastric irritation.

ٹرکلوفوس: کلورل ہائیڈریٹ کا حاصل جو کم معدی جلن پیدا کرتا ہے۔

Tricloryl *(tri-klor'-il).* Triclofos (q.v.)

ٹرائی کلورل: ٹرکلوفاس۔

Tricuspid *(tri-kus'-pid)* [L. *tri-,* three; *cuspis,* point]. Having three cusps. **tricuspid valve,** that between the right atrium and ventricle of the heart.

سہ کنگری: تین کپسول والا۔

Tridione *(tri'-di-on).* Troxidone (q.v.)

ٹرائی ڈی اون: ٹروکسیڈون۔

Triethylene thiophosphoramide Alkalylating cytotoxic agent.

ٹرائی ایتھائیلین تھایو فاسفورامائیڈ: الکلائی اینٹنگ سائیٹو ٹاکسک ایجنٹ۔

Trifluoperazine *(tri-floo-o-per'-zen).* Tranquillizer and antiemetic. More potent and less sedative than chlorpromazine.

ٹرائی فلو پیرازین: سکون بخش اور صدقے آور۔ سٹیلازین' حمل میں قے کے علاج کے لئے ایک گولی' صبح ایک دوپہر ایک ایک شام' یہی خوراک پاگل پن میں بھی۔

Trigeminal *(tri-jem'-in-al)* [L. *trigeminus,* triplet]. Triple; separating into three sections. e.g. the t, nerve , the fifth cranial nerve, which has three branches, supplying the skin of the face, the tongue and teeth. trigeminal neuralgia, see TIC DOULOUREUX.

تربغی: تکنا تین حصوں میں تقسیم۔ تربغی زوِیا عصب ملا جلا ہے۔

Trigger finger A condition in which the finger can be actively bent but cannot be straighteaned without help; usually due to a thickening on the tendon which prevents free gliding.

بلی انگل: حالت جس میں انگلی موڑی جا سکتی ہے۔ لیکن بغیر مدد کے سیدھی نہیں ہو سکتی۔

Trigone *(tri'-gon)* [G. *trigonos,* three-cornered]. A triangular area, especially applied to the bladder base bounded by the ureteral openings at the back, and the urethral opening at the front--trigonal, adj.

مثلث مثانہ۔ مثلثہ: تکونی ایریا۔

Tri-iodothyronine *(tri-i-o-do-thi'-ro-nen).* A thyroid hormone that plays a part in maintaining the body's metabolic process.

ٹرائی آیوڈوتھائیرونین: تھائیرائڈ ہارمون جو جسم کے میٹابولزم میں اہم کردار ادا کرتا ہے۔

Trilene *(tri'-len).* Trichlorethylene (q.v.)

ٹرائی لین: ٹرائی کلورا یتھائیلین۔

Trimeprazine *(tri-mep'-ra-zen).* Antihistamine with sedative action. Phenotriazine derivative. Used in treatment of pruritis, urticaria and pre-operatively for children.

ٹرائی میرازین: اینٹی ہسٹامین۔ فینوٹرایازین سے ماخوذ۔

Trimester *(tri-mes'-ter)* [L. *trimestris,* of 3 months]. A period of 3 months.

سہ ماہی: تین ماہ کا عرصہ۔

Trimettaphan *(tri-met'-a-fan)* Brief-acting blocking agent used by i.v. injection to produce a fall in blood pressure during bloodless field surgery.

ٹرائی میٹافین: گینگلیاں بلاکنگ ہائیپوٹنسو ایجنٹ ارفونڈ۔

Trimethadione *(tri-meth-a-di-on).* An anticonvulsant with a specific action in petit mal. M produce toxic effects such as agranulocytosis and drug rash, and some patients experience visual disturbances.

ٹرائی میتھڈون: دورے یا بے حوشی کوختم کرنے والی دوا۔

Trimethoprim *(tri-meth'-o-prim)*. Antibacterial agent. Has selective inhibiting action on the enzyme that converts folic acid into folinic acid, needed by many bacteria. When used with sulphonamides the ensuing action is bactericidal. The sulphonamide must have a similar pattern of obsorption and excretion.

ٹرائی میتھو پرم: جراثیم کش عامل۔اس خامرہ پرمنتخب روکنے والا ایکشن جوفو لک ایسڈ کوفولینک ایسڈ میں تبدیل کرتا ہے۔موخرالذکر کی ضرورت جراثیم کو ہوتی ہے۔ جب سلفونا مائیڈز کے ساتھ استعمال کیا جاتا ہے۔تو جراثیم کش ہوتا ہے۔

Trimipramine *(trim-ip'-ra-men)*. Antidepressant similar to imipramine (.v.).

ٹرائی مائیپر امین: ضدبیزاری۔امپر امین سے مشابہ۔

Trinitrine caffeine *(tri-nit'-ren kaf'-en)*. Glyceryl trinitrate (q.v.).

Triostam *(tri-os-tam)*. Sodium antimony gluconate (q.v.)

ٹرائیوسٹیم: سوڈیم اینٹی منی گلوکونیٹ۔

Tripelennamine *(tri-pel-en'-a-men)*. Antihistamine, useful in treatment of allergy.

ٹرائی پیلین امین: اینٹی ہسٹامین الرجی کے علاج میں مفید۔

Triple antigen. Contains diphtheria, whooping-cough and tetanus antigens.

سہ گونا اینٹی جن: خناق۔کالی کھانسی اور تشنج کے اینٹی جنز پر مشتمل۔

Triplopen *(trip'-lo-pen)*. Benethamine penicillin G, procaine penicillin G and sodium penicillin G. Used for acute localized infectins.

ٹرپلوپین: بنیھامین پنسلین جی۔ پروکین پنسلین جی اور سوڈیم پنسلین جی۔شدید مقامی امراض

Triptafen *(trip'-ta-fen)*. Amitriptyline (q.v.)

ٹریٹافین: امیٹرپٹیلائن۔

Tris-hydroxylmethylaminomethane *(tris-h-i-droks'- il-meth'-il am-in-o-me'-than)*. An alkali used to treat acidosis.

Trismus *(triz'-mus)* [G. a grinding]. Spasm in the muscles of mastication.

کزاز: چاب عضلات میں اینٹھن۔

Trisomy *(tri'-so-mi)*. Division into three giving an extra chromosome, i.e. 47 in man.

ٹرائی سومی: تین میں تقسیم سے ایک زائد کروموسوم یعنی آدمی میں ۴۷

Trocar *(tro'-kar)*. A pointed rod which fits inside a cannula.

مبزل: ایک نوکیلی سلاخ جو کنولا میں فٹ ہوتی ہے۔

Trochanters *(tro-kan'-terz)*. Two processes, the larger one (t. major) on the outer, the other (t. minor) on the inner side of the femur between the shaft and neck; they serve for the attachment of muscles--trochanteric, adj.

طروخا: دوزائدے۔فیمر کے بیرونی جانب بڑا اور اندرونی جانب دوسرا۔ یہ عضلات کوملانے کا کام کرتے ہیں۔

Trochlea *(trok'-le-a)* [G. *trochilia*, pulley]. Any part which is like a pulley in stucture or function--trochlear, adj.

غضرف: کوئی حصہ جو ساخت یا فعل میں چرخی کی طرح ہوتا ہے۔

Tromexan *(tro-meks'-an)*. Ethyl biscoumacetate (q.v.).

ٹرومیکسان: ایتھائیل بسکم ایسٹیٹ۔

Trophic *(tro'-fik)* [G. *trophe*, nourishment]. Pertaining to nutrition.

غذائی: تغذیہ سے متعلق۔

Trophoblastic tissue *(tro-fo-blas'-tik-tis'-u)* [G. *trophe*, nourishment; *blastos*, germ]. Cells covering the embedding ovum and concerning with the nutrition of the ovum.

ٹروفو بلاسٹک نسیج: خلیے جو دھنے ہوئے بیضے کے اوپر ہوتے ہیں اور بیضے کے تغذیہ سے متعلق۔

Trophoneurosis *(tro-fo-nu-ro'-sis)* See RAYNAUDS DISEASE.

غذائی خلل اعصاب: مرض ریناڈ۔

Trouseau's sign. See CARPOPEDAL SPASM [Armand Trousseau, French physician, 1801-67].

علامت ٹروسیو: کارپوپیڈل اینٹھن۔

Troxidone *(troks'-i-don)*. Trimethadione (q.v.).

ٹروکسیڈون: ٹرائی میتھاڈی اون۔

Trypanosoma *(tri-pan-o-so'-ma)*. A genus of parasitic protozoa. Their life cycle alternates between blood-sucking arthropods and vertebrate hosts, and in the latter they appear frequently in the blood stream as fusiform, actively motile structures some 12 to 40 m in length. A limited number of species are pathogenic to man.

جسم ترفانی: طفیلی پروٹوزوآ کا ایک جنس۔اس کے میزبان آرتھوپوڈ اور مہرے ہیں۔اسکی محدود انواع انسانی امراض پیدا کرتی ہیں۔سائز ۸ تا ۳۰ مائیکرون۔دم کی موجودگی کی وجہ سے حرکت کرتا ہے افریقہ میں اس کی وجہ سے مرض النوم ہوتا ہے۔انسانی جسم میں مکھی کا کاٹنے سے داخل ہوتا ہے۔

Trypanosomiasis *(tri-pan-o-som-i'-a-sis).* Disease produced by infestation with Trypanosoma. In man this may be with *Trypanosoma rhodesiense* in East Africa ro *T. gambiense* in West Africa, both transmitted by the tesets fly, and with *T. cruzii,* transmitted by bugs in South America. In West Africa infection of the brain commonly produces the symptomatology of 'sleeping sickness'.

مرض النوم: ٹرائی پینوسوما کی وجہ سے مرض۔مغربی افریقہ میں دماغ متاثر ہوتا ہے۔اور عام طور پر نومی مرض ہوتا ہے۔

Tryparsamide *(tri-par'-sa-mid).* An organic arsenic compound of value in the treatment of trypanosomiasis. It is usually given by intravenous injection, as it is more irritant and less effective orally.

ٹرائی پارساما ئیڈ: ایک نامیاتی آرسینک مرکب۔ٹرائی پینوسومیاسس کے علاج کے لئے۔یہ دوا عموماً انٹراوینس انجکشن کے ذریعے دی جاتی ہے۔

Trypsin *(trip'-sin).* A proteolytic enzyme present in pancreatic juice. Given in digestive disorders. Specially purified forms are used to liquefy clotted blood and other secretions, and in ophthalmology to facilitate removal of cataracts.

عصیر ہاضم: لبلبی رس میں موجود خامرہ۔انہضام میں پروٹین کو امینو ایسڈ میں تبدیل کرتا ہے۔ہضمی خرابیوں میں دیا جاتا ہے۔خصوصاً خالص اقسام جمے ہوئے خون اور دوسری رطوبتوں کو مائع بنانے کے لئے استعمال کیا جاتا ہے۔

Tryptizol. Armitriptyline (q.v.) See ANTIDEPRESSANT. In small doses can be used to prevent bed-wetting in adults. Not suitable for the elderly. Makes one aware of full bladder even though one is sleeping soundly.

ٹرپٹی زول: امیٹرپٹائیلین۔ضد بیزاری۔تھوڑی خوراکوں میں بالغوں میں تربستری روکنے کے لئے مستعمل ہے۔معمر کے لئے موزوں نہیں۔

Tryptophane *(trip'-to-fan).* One of the essential amino acids necessary for growth.

ٹرپٹوفین: لازمی امینو ایسڈز میں سے ایک جو نشوونما کے لئے ضروری ہے۔

Tsetse fly *(tset'-se)* A fly of the genus Glossina. A common vector of Trypanosoma in Africa. The Trypanosoma live part of their life cycle in the flies and are transferred to new hosts, including man, in the salivary juices when the fly bites for a blood meal.

سی سی مکھی: گلوسینا پلپلیس۔افریقہ میں ٹرائی پینوسوما اس میں پایا جاتا ہے۔جب یہ مکھی کی نئے میزبان بشمول انسان کو کاٹتی ہے۔تو اس میں منتقل ہو جاتا ہے۔

Tubal *(tu'-bal).* Pertaining to a tube **tubal pregnancy see** ECTOPIC PREGNANCY

Tubarine *(tu'-bar-en).* Tubocurarine (q.v.).

ٹیوبارین: ٹیوبوکیورارین۔

Tubegauz *(tub'-gawz).* A special type of woven circular bandage, applied with a special applicator.

ٹیوب گاز: گول پٹی کی مخصوص قسم۔

Tubercle *(tub'-er-kl)* [L. *tuberculum,* small lump]. 1. A small rounded prominence usually on bone.2. The specific lesion produced by *Mycobacterium tuberculosis.*

دانہ سل۔درنہ: ا۔ عموماً ہڈی پر پایا جانے والا ایک چھوٹا گول ابھار ۲۔ مائیکوبیکٹریم ٹیوبوکولوسس سے پیدا شدہ مخصوص زخم۔

Tuberculide *(tu-ber'-kul-id)* [L. *tuberculum,* small lump]. Also tuberculid. Mstastatic manifestation of tuberculosis producing a skin lesion, e.g. papulonecrotic t., rosacelike t. (Cf. syphilide.)

ٹیولبرکولائیڈ: تپ دق کی وجہ سے جلدی زخم۔

Tuberculin A sterile extract of either the crude (old t.) or refined (PPD) complex protein constituents of the tubercle bacillus. Its commonest use is in determining whether a person has or has not previously been infected with the tubercle bacillus, by injecting a small amount into the skin and reading the reaction if have **escaped previous infection.** See MA

NTOUX.

سلیں: ٹیوبرکل بیلس کے پیچیدہ لحمی اجزاء کا بے اثر عرق۔

Tuberculoid *(tu-ber'-ku-loid)*. Resembling tuberculosis. Describes one of the two types of leprosy.

درنہ نما: تپ دق سے مشابہ۔

Tuberculoma *(tu-ber-ku-lo'-ma)*. A caseous tubercle, usually large, its size suggesting a tumour.

سلعہ دق: عموماً بڑا ٹیوبرکل۔

Tuberculosis *(tu-ber-ku-lo'-sis)* [L. *tuberculum,* small swelling; G. *-osis,* condition]. A specific, infective disease caused by *Mycobacterium tuberculosis* (Koch's tubercle bacillus). **avian t.,** endemic in cattle and transmitted to man via infected cow's milk, causing disease of the glands and rarely of the lungs and joints. **human t.,** endemic in man and the usual cuase of plumonary and other forms of tuberculosis. **miliary t.,** a generalized acute form in which, as a result of bloodstream dissemination, minute, multiple tuberculous foci are scattered throughout many organs of the body--tubercular, tuberculous, adj.

تپ دق۔ سل: ایک مخصوص چھوت کی بیماری جو مائیکو بیکٹریم ٹیوبرکولوسس سے ہوتی ہے۔

Tuberculostatic *(tu-ber-ku-lo-stat'-ik)*. Inhibiting the growth of the tubercle bacillus *(Mycobacterium tuberculosis)*.

ٹیوبرکولوسٹیٹک: مائیکوبیکٹریم۔ ٹیوبرکولوسس کی نمو روکنا۔

Tuberose *(tuberous)* sclerosis See EPILOIA.

آماسی تصلب: اپی لویا۔

Tuberosity *(tu-ber-os'-it-i)* [L. *tuber,* swelling]. A bony prominence.

بصلہ دار: ایک استخوانی ابھار۔

Tubigrip *(tu'-bi-grip)*. Supporting hose. Can be worn during a operation and early postoperative period to prevent deep vein thrombosis.

ٹیوبی گرپ: سہارا دینے والا۔ اپریشن کے دوران۔ اور فوراً بعد گہری وریدی تھرومبوسس روکنے کے لئے پہنا جاسکتا ہے۔

Tubocurarine *(tu-bo-ku-rar'-en)*. The muscle-relaxing drug obtained from the South American arrow poison curare. Action reversed by neostigmine given intravenously together with atropine which depresses vagus nerve and so quicknes the heart beat.

ٹیوبوکیورارین: عضلے کو آرام پہنچانے والی دوا۔

Tubo-ovarian *(tu-bo-ov-ar'-i-an)* [L. *tubus,* tube; *ovum,* egg]. Pertaining to or involving both tube and ovary , e.g. tubo-ovarian abscess.

بوقی مبیضی: دونوں نلی و بیضدانی سے متعلق۔

Tubular necrosis *(tu'-bul-ar ne-kro'-sis)*. Degenerative change resulting from renal ischaemia. May terminate fataly with uraemia. Syndrome occurs in shock such as the cruch syndrome (q.v.), severe burns, hypotension, intrauterine haemorrhage and dehydration. Represents a type of acute renal failure.

نلی نما یا انبوبی نیکروسس: بولی اسکیمیا سے ہونے والی تخریبی یا تنزلی تبدیلی۔

Tubule *(tu'-bul)* [L. *tubulus,* small tube]. A small tube. **collecting t.,** straight tube in the kidney medulla conveying urine to the kidney pelivs. **convoluted t.,** coiled tube in the kidney cortex. **seminiferous t.,** coiled tube in the testis. **uriniferous t.,** syn. nephron (q.v.).

قنات صغیر: ایک چھوٹی نلی۔

Tuinal *(tu'-in-al)*. Hypnotic. A mixture of quinalbarbitone (q.v.) and amylobarbitone (q.v.).

ٹوئنل: خواب آور۔ کوئنل باربیٹون اور امائیلو باربیٹون کا آمیزہ۔

Tularaemia *(tu-lar-e'-mi-a)*. Syn., deer-fly fever; tick fever; rabbit fever, etc. An endemic disease of rodents, caused by Pasteurella tularensis; transmitted by biting insects and acquired by man either in handing infected animal carcases or by the bite of an infected insect. Suppuration at the inoculation site is followed by inflammation of the draining lymph glands and by severe constitutional upset--tularaemic, adj.

ہرن مکھی بخار: خرگوش بخار۔ کترنے والے حیوانات کا مرض۔ چوہوں گلہریوں اور دوسرے جانوروں کی بیماری۔ جانوروں کی مکھیوں میں پی بیٹو کار

نیس ہے۔ جوکھیوں کے کاٹنے سے انسان تک انفیکشن پہنچتی ہے۔ بخار سردی' غدود متورم' کاٹنے والی جگہ پر زخم اس کی علامات ہیں۔

Tulle gras *(tul'-gra)*. Non-adhesive dressing for wounds. Gauze impregnated with soft paraffin, and sterilized.

ٹیول گرا: زخموں کے لئے نہ چپکنے والی ڈریسنگ۔

Tumescence *(tu-mes'-ens)* [L. *tumescere,* to swell]. A state of swelling; turgidity.

خفف سوجن: سوج ہونے کی حالت۔ متورم۔

Tumour *(tu'-mor)* [L.] A swelling. A mass of abnormal tissue which resembles the normal tissues in structure, but which fulfils no useful function and which grows at the expense of the body. Benign, simple or innocent tumours are encapsulated, do not infiltrate adjacent tissue or cause metastases and are unlikely to recur if removed. **malignant t.,** not encapsulated, infiltrate adjacent tissue and cause metastases. See CANCER--tumorous, *adj.*

رسولی۔ سلعہ: سوج یا ورم۔ غیر معمولی نسیج کا مادہ۔ ساخت میں عام نسیج سے مشابہ۔ لیکن فعل میں غیر مقدار اور جسم سے خوراک لے کر بڑھتا ہے۔

Benign tumor of the prostate

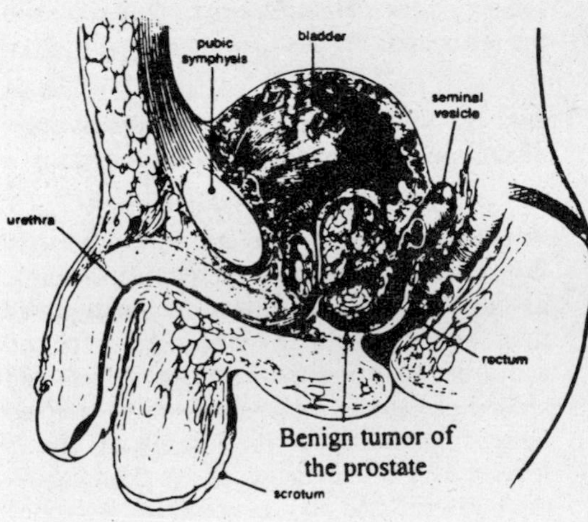

Benign tumor of the prostate

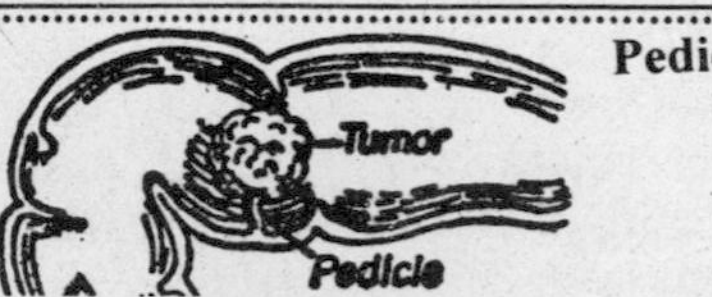

Pedicle

Pedicle

Tunica *(tun'-ik-a)* [L. a tunic]. A lining membrane; a coat. **tunica adventitia,** the outer coat of an artery. **tunica intima,** the lining of an artery, **tunica media,** the middle muscular coat of an artery.

غلاف: غلافی جھلی۔ کوٹ۔

Tunnel reimplatation operation. See LEADBETTER-POLITANO OPERATION.

ٹنل ری ایپلانٹیشن اپریشن: لیڈبیسٹر پولیٹانو اپریشن۔

Tubrinate *(tur'-bin-at)* [L. *turbinatus*]. Shaped like a top or inverted cone. **tubinate bone,** one on either side forming the lateral nasal walls.

معکوس مخروطی: لٹو کی شکل کا یا الٹی مخروط۔

Turbinated *(tur'-bin-a-ted)* [L. *turbinatus,* cone- shaped]. Scroll-shaped, as the three ethmoidal t. processes which project from the lateral nasal walls.

لٹونما: سکرول کی شکل کا۔

Tubinectomy *(tur-bin-ek'-to-mi)* [L. *turbo,* whirled; *ektome,* excision]. Removal of turbinate bones.

مفتول براری: ٹربینیٹ ہڈیوں کا ڈھانچہ۔

Turgid *(tur'-jid)* [L. *turgescere,* to swell]. Swollen; firmly distended, as with blood by congestion--turgescence, n.; turgidity, n.

پھولا: متورم۔ سوجا ہوا۔ مکمل کھچا ہوا۔

Turner's syndrome Gonadal dysgenesis. Can be identified at birth; 45 chromosomes instead of 46; one sex chromosome missing. Brought up as girl though genetic male. Such an individual has small female gentialia, scanty pubic hair. atrophic ovaries, webbed neck and valgus of the elbows. [Henry H. Turner, American, endocrinologist, 1892]

ٹرنرز سنڈروم: ۴۶ کروموسوموں کے بجائے ۴۵۔ ایک جنسی کروموسوم کم۔

اگر چہ جینی طور پر نر ہوتا ہے۔ لیکن اسے لڑکی کے طور پر پالا جاتا ہے۔

Tussis *(tus'-sis)* [L.]. A cough.

سعال: کھانسی

Tybamate *(ti'-bam-at)*. Analogue of meprobamate (q.v.)

ٹائیبامیٹ: میروبامیٹ کا اناکوگ۔

Tympanic *(tim-pan'-ik)*. [G. *tymponon,* durm]. Pertaining to the tympanum. **tympanic membrane** (membrane tympani), the eardrum.

طبلی: طبل یا ٹمپینم سے متعلق۔

Tympanites *(tim-pan-it'-ez)* [G. *tympanon,* drum]. Abdominal distension due to accumulation of gas in the intestine. Also called 'tympanism'.

نفخ شکم: آنت میں گیس جمع ہونے سے بطنی کھچاؤ۔

Tympanitis *(tim-pan-i'-tis)* [G. *tympanon,* drum; *-itis,* inflammation]. Inflammation of the tympanum.

ورم طبل: طبل یا ٹمپینم کی سوزش۔

Tympanoplasty *(tim'-pan-o-plas'-ti)*. Any reconstructive operation on the middle ear designed to improve hearing. Normally carried out in ears damaged by chronic suppurative otitis media with associated conductive deafness--tymponoplastic, adj.

Talipes

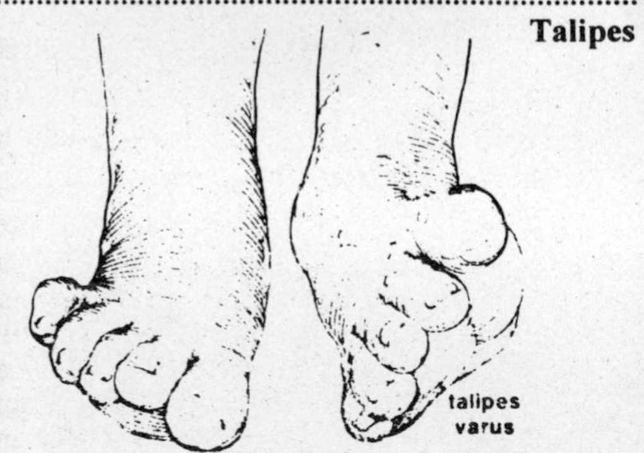

Talipes

ٹمپینو پلاسٹی: قوت سماعت بہتر کرنے کے لئے درمیانی کان کا اپریشن۔

Tympanum *(tim'-pan-um)* [G. *tympanon,* drum]. The cavity of the middle ear.

طبل۔ درمیانہ کان: درمیانی کان کا کہفہ۔

Typhoid fever *(ti-foid)*. An infectious fever usually spread by contamination of food, milk or water supplies with *Salmonella typhi,* either directly by sewage, indirectly by flies, or by faulty personal hygiene. Symptomless carriers harbouring the germ in the gall-bladder and excreting it in their stools are the main source of outbreaks of disease in this country. The average incubation period is 10 to 14 days. A progressive febrile illness marks the onset of the disease, which develops as the germ invades lymphoid tissue, including that of the small intestine (Peyer's patches) to profuse diarrhoeal (pea soup) stools which may become frankly haemorrhagic; ultimately recovery usually begins at the end of the third week. A rose-coloured rash may appear on the upper abdomen and back at the end of the first week. See TAB.

تپ محرقہ: سالمونیلا ٹائیفی کی وجہ سے بخار۔ یہ خوراک دودھ اور پانی میں ہوتا ہے۔ چھوت کی بیماری۔

Typhus *(ti'-fus)* [G. *typhos,* delusion]. An acute infections disease characterized by high fever, a skin eruption, and severe headache. It is disease of war, famine or catastrophe, being spread by lice, ticks or fleas. It is only sporadic in Britian. Infecting organism is *Rickeitsia prowazekii,* sensitive to sulphona- mides and antibiotics.

تیفوس: چھوت کی بیماری جس میں بخار سر درد اور جلد کا پھٹنا شامل ہیں۔

Tyramine *(ti'-ra-men)*. An enzyme present in several foodstuffs. See MONOAMINE OXIDASE.

Tyrosine (e) *(ti'-ro-sin)*. An amino acid associated with growth. Combines with iodine to form thyroxine.

ٹائیروسین : ایک سفید قلمی امینو ایسڈ۔ زیادہ تر لحمیات سے حاصل کیا جاتا ہے۔نقطہ پگھلاؤ ۳۱۰تا ۳۲۰°س۔

Tyrosinosis *(ti-ro-sin-o'-sis)*. Due to abnormal metabolism of tyrosin, phydroxyphenylp-yruvic acid is excreted in the urine.

ٹائیروسائی نوسس: ٹائروسن کے غیر معمولی میٹابولزم کی وجہ سے پیشاب میں پی ہائیڈروکسی فینائل۔

Tyrothricin *(ti-ro-thri'-sin)*. A mixture of gramicidin and other antibiotics. Itr is too toxic for systemic therapy, but is valuable in number of infected skin conditions.

ٹائیروتھریسین : گریمیڈن اور دوسرے اینٹی بایوٹکس کا آمیزہ۔ متعدد جلدی حالتوں سے مستعمل پائیریوک ایسڈ کا اخراج۔

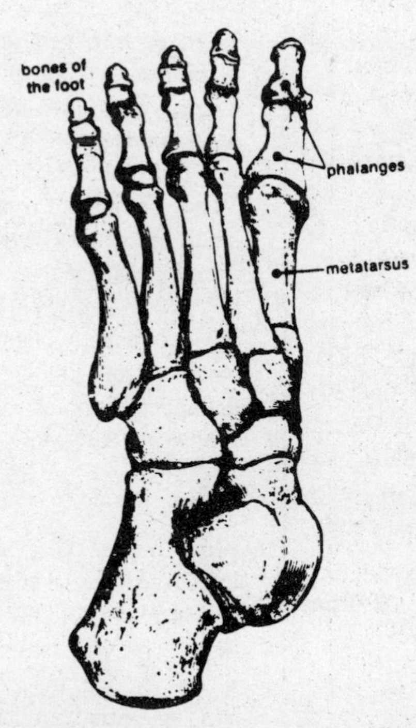

U

UCB 1549 It is a drug name used for the disease Parkinsonism.

یوسی جی ۱۵۴۹: پارکنسونزم کے لئے دوا۔

Ulbreval *(ul-bre-val)* Buthalitone a drug.

البریویل: بتھالیٹون۔

Ulcer *(ul'sar)* [L. *ulcus*; G. *helkosis*]. A local defect or excavation of the surface of an organ or tissue which is produced by sloughing of inflammatory necrotic tissue. **cushing's u.,** a peptic ulcer associated with manifest or occult lessons of the central nervous system. **decubital u.,** an ulceration caused by prolonged pressure in a patient allowed to lie two still in bed for a long peiod of time, called also decubitus bed sore, and pressure sore. **dendritic u.,** ulcer caused by herpes simplex infection. It is branching in nature and of cornea. **peptic ul,** ulceration of the mucous membrane of the esophagus, stomach or duodenum, caused by the action of of acid gastric juice. **perforating ulcer,** an ulcer which involves the entire thickness of an organ as the foot, or the wall of the stomach or intestine, creating an opening on both surfaces. **vodent u,** ulcerating basal cell cancinoma of the skin. **varicose u,** one that is due to varicose veins, as a stasis ulcer.

زخم۔ السر۔ ناسور۔ قرحہ: جسمی سطح میں ایک کھلا زخم۔

lcerative *(ul-ser-a-tiv)* Pertaining to or characterized by ulceration.

قرحی: السر کی نیچر کا۔ السر سے متعلق۔ السریٹو کولائیٹس مرض جس میں بڑی آنت میں ورم ہو جاتا ہے۔

Ulcer

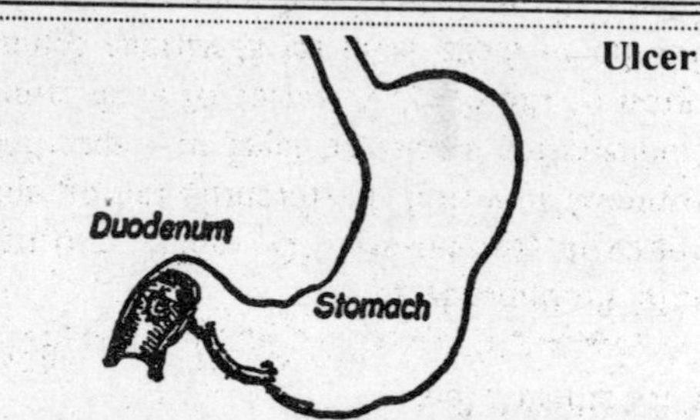

Ulcerogenic *(ul-ser-o-jen-ik)* [L. *ulcus*; G. *genesis,* to produce]. Causing ulceration; leading to the production of ulcers.

السیروجینک: السر پیدا کرنے کا اہل۔

Ultramicroscopic *(ul-tra-mi'kro-skopik)* Too small to be seen with an ordinary microscope.

الٹرامائیکروسکوپک: وراء خورد بینی۔ اتنا چھوٹا کہ خورد بین سے بھی نہ دیکھا جاسکے۔ ٹنڈل اثر کے استعمال سے دکھانے والی وراء خورد بین سے نظر آنے والا۔

Ultrasonic *(ul'tra-son'ik)* [L. *somes,* sound]. Pertaining to mechanical radiant energy having a frequency beyond the upper limit of perception by the human ear, that is, beyond about 20,000 Hz (Hertz - cycles per second).

بالاصوتی، الٹراسونک: ۳۰,۰۰۰ سائیکلز فی سیکنڈ سے زائد تعدد کے میکانکی اور ارتعاشات سے متعلق۔

Ultrasonography *(ul-tra-son-og'-ra-fi).* [L. *ultra,* beyond; *sonus,* sound; G. *grapheink* to wirte]. Production of visual image from application of ultrasound, sound waves with a frequency of over 20,000 Hz (cycles per second) and inaudible to the human ear--ultrasonographically, adv.; ultrasonograph, n.

الٹراسونوگرافی: بالاصوت کے اطلاق سے مرئی عکس کی پیداوار۔

Ultrasound *(ul-tra-sownd).* Can be used for cleansing and nebulizing.

بالاصوت: اسے صفائی کے لیے استعمال کیا جاسکتا ہے۔

Ulbilicated *(um-bil'-i-ka-ted)* [L. *umbilicus,* middle]. Having a central depression, e.g. smallpox vesicle.

ناف نما: مرکزی نشیب رکھنا۔

Umbilicus *(um-bil-i'-kus)* [L. middle]. The abdominal scar left by the separation of the umbilical cord (q.v.) after birth; the naval—umbilical, *adj.*

ناف: پیدائش کے بعد امبلیکل کارڈ کی علیحدگی سے بننے والا بطنی نشان۔

Uncinate *(un'-sin-at)* [L. *uncinus,* hook]. Hook-shaped. Unciform.

ہک نما: ہک کی شکل کا۔

Unconsciousness *(un-kon'-shus-nes)* [A.S. *un,* not; *conscire,* to know, be aware]. State of being unconscious; insensible.

بے ہوشی: بے ہوش۔ بے ہوشی کی حالت۔ بے ہوشی کا تعلق دماغ سے ہے۔ اگر دماغ کا فعل کمزور ہوجائے تو بے ہوشی طاری ہوجاتی ہے۔

Undine *(un'-den)* [L. *unda,* a wave]. A small, thin glass flask used for irrigating the eyes.

چشم شویہ: آنکھ دھونے کے لئے چھوٹی پتلی شیشے کی صراحی۔

Undulant fever *(un'-du-lant)* [L. *unda,* a wave]. The condition is also called 'abortus f.', 'Malta f.' and 'Mediterranean f.' See BRUCELLA, BRUCELLOSIS.

لہریا بخار: اسے مالٹا بخار بھی کہتے ہیں۔

Unguentum *(ung-gwen'-tum)* [L.]. Ointment.

مرہم: مرہم۔

Unicellular *(u-ni-sel'-u-lar)* [L. *unus,* one; *cellula,* cell]. Consisiting of only one cell.

واحد خلویہ، یک خلوی: صرف ایک خلیہ پر مشتمل۔

Unilateral *(u-ni-lat'-e-ral)* [L. *unus,* one; *latus,* side]. Relating to or on one side only —unilaterlally. *adv.*

یک طرفہ: صرف ایک طرف ہونا یا ایک طرف ہونے کے متعلق۔

Uniocular *(u-ni-ok'-u-lar)* [L. *unus,* one; *oculus,* eye]. Pertaining to, or affecting, one eye.

وحید العین، یک چشمہ: ایک آنکھ سے متعلق یا ایک آنکھ کا متاثر ہونا۔

Uniovular *(u-ni-ov'-u-lar)* [L. *unus,* one; *ovum,* egg]. Pertaining to one ovum, as u. twins (identical). (Cf. binovular.)

وحید البیض: ایک بیضہ سے متعلق۔

Unipara *(u-nip'-a-ra)* [L. *unus,* one; *parere,* to bring forth]. A woman who has born only one child—uniparous, *adj.*

ایک بچہ جننے والی: خاتون جس نے صرف ایک بچے کو جنم دیا ہو۔

Unna's paste *(un'-nas)* A glycogelatin and zinc oxide preparation, used in the treatment of varicose veins in association with supportive bandaging. [Paul Gerson Unna, German dermatologist, 1850-1929].

ضماد اُناس: گلائیکو جیلاٹن اور زنک کی تیاری۔ مرض دوالی میں مستعمل۔

Urachus *(u'-rak-us)* [G. *ouron,* urine; *echein,* to hold]. The stemlike structure connecting the bladder with the umbilicus in the fetus; in postnatal life it is represented by a fibrous cord situated between the apex of the bladder and the umbilicus, known as the median umbilical ligament—urachal, *adj.*

رباط نال، یوریکس: تنے کی طرح ساخت جو پیٹ کے اندر بچے میں بلیڈر کو امبلیکس کے ساتھ ملاتی ہے۔

Uracil mustard *(u'-ra-sil mus-tard)* Uramustine (q.v.).

یوریسل مسٹرڈ: یوراسٹین۔

Uraemia *(u-re'-mi-a)* A clinical syndrome due to renal failure resulting from either disease of the kidneys themselves, or from disorder or disease elsewhere in the body which induces kidney dysfunction, and which results in gross biochemical disturbance in the body including retention of urea and other nitrogenous substances in the blood. Depending on the cause it may or may not be reversible. The fully developed syndrome is characterized by nausea, vomiting, headache, hiccough, weakness, dimness of vision, convulstions and coma—uraemic, *adj.*

یورے میا، یوراتیت خون: گردوں کے کسی مرض یا خرابی کی بنا پر بولی یا رینل ناکامی کی وجہ سے کلینکل سنڈروم۔ اس کی علامات سر درد، متلی، قے، کھانسی، کمزوری، نگاہ میں دھندلاہٹ، دورے اور بے ہوشی ہیں۔ مریض کو ٹھنڈ سے بچایئے۔ علاج کے لئے گلوکوس ۵ فیصد ۴۰ قطرے فی منٹ وریدی ڈرپ، بیٹامیتھاسون، ڈیکسامیتھاسون، وٹامن ب کمپلیکس اور فیرس فیوم یٹ، کیلیم وٹامن ڈی اور ہائیڈروکلورتھایانائیڈ۔

Uramustine *(u-ra-mus'-ten)* Antimitotic agent occasionally used in cancer.

یورامسٹین: ضد مائیٹوسس ایجنٹ۔ سرطان میں مفید۔

Uraemic snow. See URIDROSIS.

یوریمک سنو: یوریڈروسس۔

Urate *(u'-rat)* A salt of uric acid; such compounds are present in the blood and urine.

یوریٹ: یورک ایسڈ کا نمک۔ ایسے مرکبات خون اور پیشاب میں موجود ہوتے ہیں۔

Uraturia *(u-rat-ur'-e-a)* [G. *ouron,* urine]. Excess of urates in the urine—uraturic, *adj.*

بول یورائی: پیشاب میں یوریٹس کی زیادتی یا کثرت۔

Urea *(u-re'-a)* The end waste product of protein metabolism; it is excreted in the urine of which it is the main chemical constituent. Can be given orally as a diuretic.

یوریا، مادۂ بول: ایک سفید قلمی نامیاتی مرکب۔ پیشاب میں پایا جاتا ہے۔ نقطہ پگھلاؤ ۱۳۲ °س۔ پہلا نامیاتی مرکب جو مصنوعی طور پر تیار کیا گیا، فرٹیلائزر اور دوائیوں میں استعمال ہوتا ہے۔ پیشاب آور کے طور پر ذہنی طور پر دی جاسکتی ہے۔

Ureaphil *(u-re'-a-fil)* Urea compound used to produce dehydration in cerebral oedema, raised intraocular pressure, and as a diuretic in resistant cases. Has a low potential for sodium retention, thus increases urinary output.

یوریافل: یوریا کا مرکب۔ پیشاب آور کے طور پر مستعمل۔

Ureter *(u'-re-ter)* [G. *oureter*]. The tube passing from each kidney to the bladder for the conveyance of urine; its average length is from 25.00 to 30.48 cm—ureteric, ureteral, *adj.*

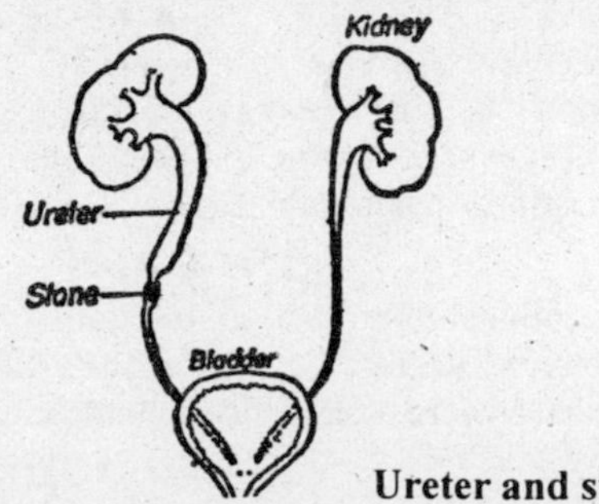

Ureter and stone

حالب، قناتِ گردہ: بزخ پیشاب کے لئے ہر گردے سے بلیڈر کی طرف آنے والی نلی۔ اس کی اوسط لمبائی ۲۵ تا ۳۰٫۴۸ سم ہے۔ تعداد میں ۲۔ گردے کے پاس نلی چوڑی ہوتی ہے اور پیلوس آف کڈنی کہلاتی ہے۔ یہ نالیاں پیٹ کی خلفی دیوار کے ساتھ ساتھ سوآئیں عضلے کے سامنے اور پیری ٹونیم جھلی کے عقب سے ہوتی ہوئیں یورنری بلیڈر یا مثانے کی عقبی جانب جاکر کھلتی ہیں۔ ان کی بیرونی دیوار میں فائبرس گوشت، اس کے اندر غیر اختیاری عضلات کی تہہ اور بالکل اندر میوکس جھلی ہوتی ہے۔ یہ نالی اپنے عضلات کی وجہ سے سکڑ کر پیشاب کو آگے دھکیلنے کی طاقت رکھتی ہے اور اس کا کام پیشاب کو گردوں سے مثانے تک پہنچانا ہے۔

Ureterectomy *(ur-et-er-ek'-to-mi)* [G. *oureter,* ureter; *-itis,* inflammation]. Inflammation of a ureter.

حالب۔ برداری: یوریٹر کا قطع۔

Ureteritis *(u-ret-er-i'-tis)* [G. *oureter,* ureter, *-itis,* inflammation]. Inflammation of a ureter.

ورم حالب: یوریٹر کی سوزش۔

Ureterocolic *(ur-et-er-o-kol-ik)* [G. *oureter,* ureter; *kolon,* colon]. Pertaining to the ureter and colon.

یوریٹروکولک: یوریٹر اور قولون سے متعلق۔

Ureterocolostomy *(ur-et-er-o-kol-os'-to-mi)* [G. *oureter,* ureter; *kolon,* colon; *stoma,* mouth]. Surgical transplantation of the ureters from the bladder to the colon so that urine is passed by the bowel; sometimes carried out to relieve strangury in tuberculosis of the bladder, or prior to cystectomy for bladder tumours.

یوریٹروکولوسٹومی: بلیڈر سے قولون تک یوریٹر کی سرجیکل پیوند کاری تا کہ

پیشاب مقعد سے خارج ہو سکے۔

Ureteroleal *(ur-et-er-o-il-e-al)* [G. *oureter,* ureter; L. *ilia,* flanks]. Pertaining to the ureters and ileum as the anastomosis necessary in ureteroileostomy.

یوریٹروالیل: الیم اور یوریٹرز سے متعلق۔

Ureteroileostomy *(ur-et-er-o-il-e-os-to-mi)* [G. *oureter,* ureter; L. *ilia,* flanks ;G. *stom,* mouth]. More usually 'ileoureterostomy' (q.v.)

یوریٹروالیوسٹومی: الیو یوریٹروسٹومی۔

Ureterolith *(u-ret-er-o-lith)* [G. *oureter,* ureter; *lithos,* stone]. A calculus in the ureter.

حصات حالبیہ: یوریٹر میں پتھری۔

Ureterolilthotomy *(ur-et-er-o-lith-ot'-o-mi)* [G. *oureter,* ureter; *lithos,* stone; *tome,* a cutting]. Surgical removal of a stone from a ureter.

اخراج حصات حالب: یوریٹر سے پتھری کا سرجیکل خاتمہ۔

Ureterosigmoidostomy *(ur-et'-er-o-sig-mo-id-os-to-mi).* See URETEROCOLOSTOMY.

Ureterostomy *(u-ret-er-os'-to-mi)* [G. *oureter,* uerter; *stoma,* mouth]. The formation of a permanent fistula, through which the ureter discharges urine. **cutaneous u.,** transplantation of the ureter to the skin. See BLADDER.

حالب شگافی: مستقل فثولا کا بننا جس میں سے یوریٹر پیشاب خارج کرتا ہے۔

Ureterovaginal *(u-ret-er-o-vaj-i'-nal)* [G. *oureter,* ureter; L. *vagina,* sheath]. Pertaining to the ureter and vagina.

حالبی مہبلی: یوریٹر اور ویجائنا سے متعلق۔

Ureterovesical *(u-ret-er-o-ves'-ik-al)* [G. *oureter,* ureter; L. *vesica,* bladder]. Pertaining to the ureter and bladder.

یوریٹروویزیکل: یوریٹر اور بلیڈر سے متعلق۔

Urethane *(ur'-eth-an).* This compound has diuretic, hypnotic and cytostatic properties.

یورتھین: یہ مرکب پیشاب آور خواب آور اور سائیٹوسٹیٹک خصوصیات کا حامل ہے۔ بعض اوقات لمفی اور مائلا ئڈ لیو کیمیا میں مستعمل۔ پالیم زکی ایک جماعت کیمیائی طور پر یورتھین رالیس کہا جاتا ہے۔ یورتھینز کاربالک ایڈ کے ایسٹرز ہیں۔ اس نام کا اطلاق عموماً ایتھائل کاربامیٹ پر کیا جاتا ہے۔

Urethra *(u-re'-thra)* [G. *ourethra*]. The passage from the bladder through which urine is excreted; in the female it measures 25.4 to 38.1 mm; in the male 25.00 cm--urethral, *adj*.

مبال۔ پیشاب کی نالی۔ احلیل: شانہ یا [بلیڈر سے باہر راستہ جس میں سے پیشاب خارج ہوتا ہے۔ مادہ میں اس کی پیمائش ۲۵٫۴ تا ۳۸ مم اور نر میں ۲۵ سم ہے۔ نالی پراسٹیٹ گلینڈ کے درمیان سے گزر کر آتی ہے۔ مردوں میں آلہ تناسل کے اندر سفر کی وجہ سے زیادہ طویل ہوتی ہے۔ عورتوں میں یہ نالی ویجائنا یا اندام نہانی کے منہ کے آگے کھلتی ہے۔

Urethral syndrome Symptoms of urinary infection although the urine is sterile when withdrawn by catheter. Suggests that infection is confined to the urethra and adjoining glands.

مبالی سنڈروم: بولی مرض کی حالت۔

Urethritis *(u-re-thri'-tis)* [G. *ourethron,* urethra; *-itis* inflammation]. Inflammation of the urethra. **non-specific u.** (NGU), now listed by the DHSS as a venereal disease.

ورم مبال: پیشاب کی نالی یا یورتھر کی سوزش۔

Urethrocele *(ur-eth'-ro-sel)* [G. *ourethron,* urethra; *kele,* hernia]. Prolapse of the urethra, usually into the anterior vaginal wall.

فتق مبال: پیشاب کی نالی یا یورتھرا کا خروج عموماً امامی ویجائنل دیوار میں۔

Urethrogram *(ur-eth'-ro-gram).* X-ray of urethra. Can be part of cystography (q.v.) or the dye may be inserted into bladder by catheter. X-ray taken on voiding bladder.

Urethroscope *(ur-eth-rog'-ra-fi)* X-ray examination of the urethra. See UROGRAPHY.

یورتھروگرافی: پیشاب کی نالی یا یورتھر کا ریکس رے ٹیسٹ۔

Urethrography *(ur-eth-rom-et-ri)* [G. *ourethron,* uretron, a measure]. Measurement of the urethral lumen using urethrometer--urethrometric, adj,; urethrometrically, *adv.*

یورتھرا پیمائی: یورتھرومیٹر کے استعمال سے یورتھرا کے لیومن کی پیمائش۔

Urethrometry *(ur-eth-ro-plas'-ti)* [G. *ourethra,* urethra; *plassein,* to form]. Any plastic operation on the urethraurethroplastic, *adj*.

یورتھروپلاسٹی: پیشاب کی نالی یا یورتھرا کا کوئی پلاسٹک اپریشن۔

Urethroplasty *(ur-eth'-ro-skop)* [G. *ourethra,* urethra; *skopein,* to examine]. An instrument designed to allow visualization of the interior of the urethra--urethroscopic, adj.; urethroscopically, adv.; urethroscopy, n.

مبال بین: پیشاب کی نالی یایورتھرا کے اندر جھانکنے کے لئے ایک آلہ۔

Urethrostenosis *(ur-eth-ro-sten-o'-sis)* [G. *ourethra,* urethra; a narrowing]. Urethral stricture.

تشنج یورتھرا: پیشاب کی گزرگاہ کی تنگی۔

Urethrotomy *(ur-eth-rot'-o-mi)* [G. *ourethra,* urethra; *tome,* a cutting]. Incision into the urethra; usually part of an operation for stricutre.

مبال شگافی: یورتھرا میں شگاف عموماً تنگی کے لئے اپریشن کا ایک حصہ۔

Urethrotrigonitis *(ur-eth-ro-tri-gon-i'-tis)* [G. *ourethra,* urethra; *trigonos,* three-cornered; *-itis,* inflammation]. Inflammation of the bladder. See TRIGONE.

یورتھروٹرائیگو نائیٹس: بلیڈر کی سوزش۔

Uric acid *(ur'-ik-as'-id).* An acid formed in the breadown of nucleoproteins in the tissues, and excreted in the urine. It is relatively insoluble and liable to give rise to stones. Present in excess in the blood in gout and a gout-like syndrome occurring in male infants, manifesting as early as 4 months with self-destructive behaviour, cerebral palsy and mental retardation.

تیزاب بولی: ایک نامیاتی ترشہ' اس کا تعلق پیورین گردہ سے ہے۔ ایک بے رنگ قلمی ٹھوس جو پانی میں ہلکا ساحل پذیر ہے۔ بعض جانوروں کے پیشاب میں معمولی سی مقدار پائی جاتی ہے۔ جوڑوں کے درد کی بیماری میں جوڑوں تیزاب کے سوڈیم اور پوٹاشیم نمکیات جمع ہو جاتے ہیں۔ اس سے پتھری بن سکتی ہے۔ جوڑوں کے درد میں خون میں زائد مقدار میں موجود۔

Uricosuric *(u-ril-o-su-rik).* Enhances renal excretion of uric acid due to impairment of tubular reabsorption. Such substances used in chronic gout.

یوریکوسیورک: یورک ایڈ کے رنل اخراج کو بڑھاتا ہے۔

Uridrosis *(u-ri-dro'-sis)* [G. *ouron,* urine; *hidrosis,* sweating]. Excess of urea in the sweat; it may be deposited on the skin as fine white crystals. 'Uraemicsnow'.

یورائی پسینہ: پسینہ میں یوریا کی زیادتی۔ یہ جلد پر باریک سفید قلموں کی صورت میں جمع ہوتا ہے۔

Urinalysis *(u-rin-al'-i-sis)* [L. *urina,* urine; G. *lysis,* a losening]. Examination of the urine.

تحلیل البول: پیشاب کا ٹیسٹ یا معائنہ۔

Urinary *(ur-in'-ar-i).* Pertaining to urine. **urinary diversion,** see BLADDER.

Urination *(u-rin-a'-shun)* [L. *urina,* urine]. Mict- urition (q.v.)

تبویل: پیشاب کرنا۔ پیشاب کرنے کا عمل۔

Urine *(u'-rin)* [L. urina]. The ambercoloured fluid which is excreted from the kidneys at the rate of about 1500 ml every 24 hours in the adult; it is slightly acid and has a specific gravity of 1005 to 1030.

بول پیشاب: گردوں سے خارج ہونے والا سیال جو بالغ میں ۲۴ گھنٹوں میں ۱۵۰۰ ملی لیٹر ہوتا ہے۔ اس کا نارمل رنگ ذرا سی زردی اور پیلاہٹ رکھتا ہے۔ مخصوص بدبو، تیزابی خواص۔ اس میں پانی ۹۶ فیصد' یوریا ۲ فیصد اور باقی ۲ فیصد یورک ایسڈ' کریاٹی' نین' فاسفیٹ' سلفیٹ' آکسلیٹ اور کلورائیڈز ہوتے ہیں۔ وزن مخصوص ۱۰۱۵ مقدار ۴۰/۴ اونس ہوتی ہے۔

Uriniferous *(u-rin-if'-er-us)* [L. *urina,* urine; *ferre,* to carry]. Conveying urine.

بول بردار: پیشاب لے جانا۔

Urinogenital *(u-rin-o-jen'-it-al)* See URENOGENITL.

بولی تناسلی: بولی اور تولیدی اعضاء سے متعلق۔

Urinometer *(u-rin-om'-e-ter)* [L. *urina,* urine; G. *metron,* a measure]. An insrument for estimating the specific gravity of urine.

بول پیما: پیشاب کے وزن مخصوص کے تخمینہ کے لئے آلہ۔

Urispas *(ur'-is-pas)* Flavoxate (q.v.).

Urobilin *(u-ro-bil'-in)* [G. *ouron,* urine; L. *bilus,* bile]. A pigment formed by the oxidation of urobilinogen and excreted in the urine and faeces.

یوروبلین: یوروبینوجن کی تکسید سے بننے والا پگمنٹ۔ پیشاب اور فضلے میں خارج ہوتا ہے۔

Urobilinogen *(u-ro-bil-in'-o-jen)* A pigment formed from bilirubin in the intestine by the actio⁻ of bacteria. It may be reabsorbed into the circulation and converted back to bilirubin in the liver or excreted in the urine.

یوروبلینو جن: جراثیم کے عمل سے آنت میں بلیروبن سے بننے والا پگمنٹ ۔ یہ گردس میں دوبارہ جذب ہوسکتا ہے اور جگر میں دوبارہ بلیروبن میں تبدیل ہوجاتا ہے یا پیشاب میں خارج ہوجاتا ہے۔

Urobilinuria *(u-ro-bil-in-ur'-i-a)* The presence of increased amounts of urobilin in the urine. Evidence of increased production of bilirubin in the liver, e.g. after haemolysis.

یوروبلین بولی: پیشاب میں یوروبلن کی بڑھی ہوئی مقداروں کی موجودگی۔

Urochrome *(u'-ro-chrom)* The pigment which gives urine its normal colour. Its chemical composition and origin are unknown.

Urogenital *(u-ro-jen'-it-al)* [G. *ouron,* urine; L. *genitalis,* genital]. Pertaining to the urinary and the genital organs.

بولی تناسلی: بولی اور تولیدی اعضاء سے متعلق۔

Urogram *(u'-ro-gram)* [G. *ouron,* urine; *gramma,* letter]. Radiograph of urinary tract after injection of contrast media.

یوروگرام: کنٹراسٹ میڈیا کے انجکشن کے بعد بولی راہ کا ریڈیوگراف۔

Urografin *(ur-o-graf'-in)* Sodium and meglumine diatrizoates (q.v.).

Urography *(ur-og'-ra-fi)* [G. *ouron,* urine; *graphein,* to write]. X-ray examination of urinary tract by means of contrast media, e.g. pyelography, cystography, cystourethrography, urethrography.

یوروگرافی: کنٹراسٹ میڈیا کے ذریعے بولی راہ کا ایکسرے ٹیسٹ۔

Urokinase *(u-ro-kin'-as)* An enzyme which dissolves fibrin clot. Used for traumatic and postoperative hyphaema. It has been tried in hyaline membrane disease.

یوروکائی نیز: خامرہ جو فائبرن کے لوتھڑے کو حل کرلیتا ہے۔

Urologist *(u-rol'-o-jist)* [G. *ouron,* urine; *logos,* discourse]. A person who specializes in disorders of the female urinary tract, and the male genitourinary tract.

ماہر بولیات: ایسا شخص جو مادہ بولی راہ اور نر تولیدی بولی راہ کی خرابیوں میں مہارت رکھتا ہے۔

Urology *(u-rol'-o-ji)* [G. *ouron,* urine; *logos,* dis- course]. That branch of science which deals with disorders of the female urinary tract and the male genitourinary tract—urological, *adj.*, urologically, *adv.*

بولیات: مادہ بولی راہ اور نر تولیدی بولی راہ کی خرابیوں سے متعلق سائنس کی شاخ۔

Urolucosil *(ur-o-luk'-o-sil)* A sulphonamide highly effective in urinary infections. the low dose (0.1g) markedly reduces the risk of renal complications.

یورولیوکوسل: ایک سلفونامائیڈ جو بولی امراض میں از حد مؤثر ہے۔

Uropac *(ur'-ro-pak)* Iodoxyl (q.v.).

یوروپیک: آیوڈوکسل۔ اس کا وریدی ٹیکہ خاص ایکسرے کے لئے لگایا جاتا ہے۔ اس ٹیکے سے حوض گردہ گردے کی نالیاں اور مثانہ نظر آتے ہیں۔

Uroselectan *(ur-ro-se-lek'-tan)* Iodoxyl (q.v.).

یوروسلیکٹین: آیوڈوکسل۔

Urticaria *(ur-ti-ka'-ri-a)* Syn., nettle-rash or hives. An allergic skin eruption characterized by multiple, circumscribed, smooth, raised, pinkish, itchy weals, developing very suddenly, usually lasting a few days, and leaving no visible trace. Common provocative agents in such as shellfish, injected sera, and contact with, or injection of, antibiotics such as penicillin and streptomycin. See ANGIO-HEUROTIC OEDEMA.

پتی کا اچھلنا، چھپاکی: الرجی سے جلد کا پھٹنا۔ کثرت جس سے ہوتا ہے۔ جسم پر دھپڑ پڑجاتے ہیں اور خارش ہوتی ہے۔

Uteroplacental *(u-ter-o-plas-en-'tal)* Pertaining to the uterus and placenta.

رحمی مشیمی: رحم یا یوٹرس اور پلسنٹا سے متعلق۔

Uterorectal *(u-ter-o-rek'-tal)* [G. *uterus,* womb; L. *rectus,* straight]. Pertaining to the uterus and the rectum.

یوٹیروریکٹل: رحم یا یوٹرس اور ریکٹم سے متعلق۔

Uterosacral *(u-ter-o-sa'-kral)* [L. *uterus,* womb; *sacer,* sacred]. Pertaining to the uterus and sacrum.

رحمی عجزی: رحم یا یوٹرس اور سیکرم سے متعلق۔

Uterosalpingography *(u-ter-o-sal-ping-go'-raf-i)* [L. *uterus,* womb; G. *salpigx,* trumpet; *graphein,* to write]. X-ray by means of injection of contrast media (for patency of Fallopian tubes).

یوٹیروسیلپنگوگرافی: کنٹراسٹ میڈیا کے انجکشن کے ذریعے ایکسرے۔

Uterovaginal *(u-ter-o-vaj-in'-al)* [L. *uterus,* womb; *vagina,* sheath[. Pertaining to the uterus and the vagina.

رحمی مہبلی: رحم یوٹرس اور ویجائنا سے متعلق۔

Uterovesical *(u-ter-o-ves'-ik-al)* [L. *uterus,* womb; *vesica,* bladder]. Pertaining to the uterus and the bladder.

رحمی گیسوی: رحم یا یوٹرس اور بلیڈر سے متعلق۔

Uterus *(u'-ter-us)* [L.]. The womb; a hollow muscular organ into which the ovum is received through the uterine tubes, and where it is retained during development, and from which the fetus is expelled through the vagina. **bicornuate u.,** a uterus with two horns. **gravid u.,** a pregnant uterus —uterine, *adj.*; uteri, *pl.*

Uterus

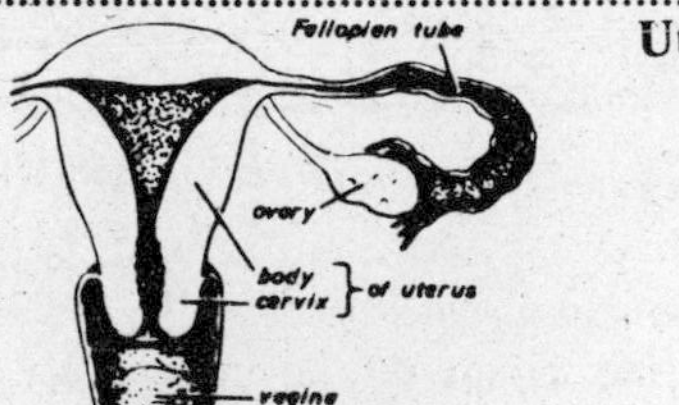

رحم، بچہ دان، مہبل: رحم یا بچہ دانی۔ کھوکھلا عضلے دار عضو جس میں نلکیوں میں سے آتا ہوا بیضہ وصول کیا جاتا ہے اور تکمیل کے دوران یہیں رکھا جاتا ہے اور جہاں سے بچے کو ویجائنا میں سے باہر کی طرف دھکیلا جاتا ہے۔ رحم پیڑو کے جوف کے اندر مثانہ اور رووہ مستقیم کے درمیان واقع ہے اور باطات کے ذریعہ اپنی جگہ پر قائم ہے۔ زماو بکارت میں یہ عضو تین انچ لمبا، دوانچ چوڑا، ایک انچ موٹا اور قریبا نصف سے پون چھٹانک وزنی ہوتا ہے۔ رحم کے درمیانی حصے راستہ کشادہ ہو جاتا ہے۔ اس کے آخری سرے پر رحم کا منہ ہوتا ہے۔ رحم یا یوٹرس سے نکلنے والا حیض کا خون اسی راستے سے باہر جاتا ہے۔ ویجائنا یا اندام نہانی ایسی ٹیوب ہے جو ویسٹی بیول سے ۴۵ درجے کے زاویہ پر پیچھے اور اوپر کو جاتی ہے۔ جماع کے وقت مردانہ عضو تناسل ویجائنا میں داخل ہوتا ہے۔

Utrical *(u'-trik-al)* [L. *utriculus,* small bag]. A little sac or pocket.

ابنالچہ: ایک چھوٹی تھیلی یا جیب۔ ایمپیولی کا تعلق اس تھیلی کے ساتھ ہوتا ہے۔

Uvea *(u'-vi-a)* [L. *uva,* grape]. The pigmented part of the eye, including the iris, ciliary body and choroid—uveal, *adj.*

عنبیہ: آنکھ کا پگمنٹ والا حصہ جس میں آئرس، ہدبی جسم اور کورائڈ شامل ہیں۔

Uveitis *(u-ve-i'-tis)* [L. *uva,* grape; G. *-itis,* inflammation]. Inflammation of the uvea.

ورمِ عنبیہ یا یودیا کی سوزش۔

Uvulva *(u'-vu-la)* [L. *uva,* grape]. The central, tag-like structure hanging down from the free edge of the soft palate.

Uvula

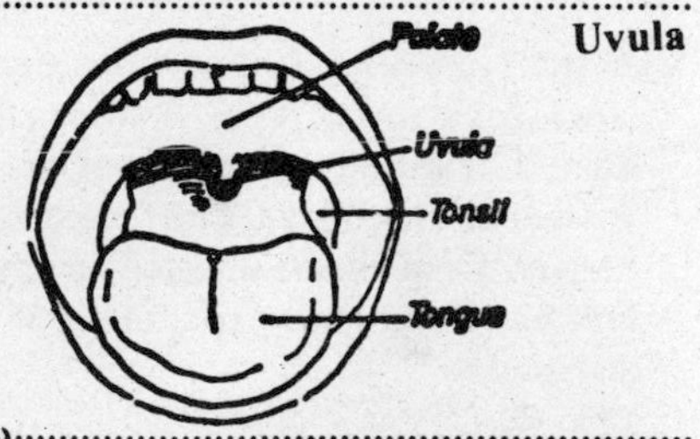

تالو، کوا، لہاۃ: یوولا ایک مرکزی ٹیگ نما ساخت ہے جو نرم پیلیٹ کے آزاد کنارے سے نیچے لٹکتی ہے۔

Uvulectomy *(u-vul-ek'-to-mi)* [L. *uva,* grape; G. *ektome,* excision]. Excision of the uvula.

لہاۃ شکافی: یوولا کا قطع۔

Uvulitis *(u'-vul-i-tis)* [L. *uva,* grape; G. *-itis,* inflammation]. Inflammation of the uvula.

ورمِ لہات: کوے یا یوولا کی سوزش۔

V

Vaccination *(vak'si-na'shan)* [L. *vacca,* low]. The introduction of vaccine into the body for the purpose of inducing immunity. Coined originally to apply to the injection of small pox vaccine. The term has come to mean any immunizing procedure in which vaccine is injected.

عامل: مصنوعی مزاحمت پیدا کرنے کے مقصد کے لئے کسی اینٹی جینک مادہ کا جسم میں داخل کرنا۔

Vaccine *(vak-sen)* [L. *vaccinus,* pertaining to cows, from *vacca,* cow]. A suspension of attenuated or killed micro-organisms (bacteria, viruses or vickettsiae) or of antigenic proteins derived from them, injected for the prevention, ameliovation or treatment of infectious diseases.

ویکسین: وائرس یا دوسرے خوردبینی جسیموں سے تیار کر کے انسانی جسم میں داخل کی جاتی ہے تاکہ اینٹی باڈیز بن جائیں اور جسم میں بیماری کے خلاف قوت مدافعت پیدا ہو جائے۔ اسے ایڈورڈ جینر نے سب سے پہلے معلوم کیا تھا۔

Vaccinia *(vak-sin-e-a)* [L. *vacca,* cow]. The cutaneous and sometimes systemic reactions associated with vaccination with small pox vaccine.

جدریُ البقر: ماتا۔ مویشیوں میں چھوت کی بیماری۔ یہ انسان میں بھی منتقل ہو جاتی ہے لیکن چیچک کے خلاف قوت مدافعت پیدا کرتی ہے۔

Vaccinotherapy *(vak-sino-therape')* Therapeutic use of vaccines. It is a non-specific, as TAB vaccine is used to produce artificial pyrexio.

ویکسینو تھراپی: مرض کے علاج کے لئے ویکسین کا استعمال۔

Vagal *(va-gal)* Pertaining to the vagus nerve.

ویگل: ویگس سے متعلق۔

Vagine *(va-ji'n)* [L.]. A sheath or sheath-like structure. The canal in the female extending from the value to the cervix uteri. In copulation, it receives the penis. Posterior mesasurement is 88.9 mm while the anterior wall measurement is 76.2 mm.

شرمگاہ، اندام نہانی، مہبل، فرج: ایک شید۔ عضلی جھلی دار راستہ جو سروِکس یوٹرائی سے ڈلوا تک ہوتا ہے۔ امامی دیوار کے ساتھ ۷۶٫۲ مم اور خلفی کے ساتھ ۸۸٫۹ مم۔ اس کے دہانے پر شریانیں ختم ہوتی ہیں، جو اسے حساس بناتی ہیں۔ اسی لئے مردانہ عضو کے دخول کے وقت عورت اس جگہ لذت محسوس کرتی ہے۔ اس کی نالی لچکدار ہوتی ہے۔ اس کی اندرونی جلد کے نیچے پٹھے ہوتے ہیں جو بچے کی پیدائش کے وقت پھیل جاتے ہیں۔

Vaginismas *(vaj-i-niz-mas)* [L.]. Painful spasm of the vagina due to involuntary contraction of vaginal musculature severe enough to prevent intercourse, the cause may be organic or psychogenic.

Vaginitis *(vaj-i-nitis)* Inflammation of the vagina. It is marked by pain and by a purulent discharge inflammation of the sheath. **Senile v.,** It is marked by the formation of superficial erosions which often adhere to opposed surfaces, sometimes causing obliteration of the vaginal canal. **Trichomonas v.,** Vaginitis produced by the protogoan trichromonas. This organism has cilia.

Vagolytic *(va-go-lit'-ik)* [L. *vagus,* wandering;

G. *lysis,* a loosening]. That which neutralizes the effect of a stimulated vagus nerve.

ویگولائی ٹک: تحریک شدہ ویگس عصب کے اثر کی تعدیل کرنے والا۔

Vagotomy *(va-got'-o-mi)* [L. *vagus,* wandering; G. *tome,* a cutting]. Surgical division of the vagus nerves; done in conjunction with gastroenterostomy in the treatment of peptic ulcer or pyloroplasty.

تقطیع عصب راجع: ویگس اعصاب کی سرجیکل تقسیم۔

Vagus *(va'-gus)* [L. wandering]. The parasympathetic pneumogastric nerve; the tenth cranial nerve, composed of both motor and sensory fibres, with a wide distribution in the neck, thorax and abdomen, sending important branches to the heart, lungs stomcah, etc.—vagal, *adj.*; vagi, *pl.*

عشریہ، عصب تائیہ: پیراسمیتھٹک نیوموگیسٹرک عصب۔ دسویں کرینیل عصب جو موٹر اور سنسری ریشوں پر مشتمل ہے۔ سینے اور پیٹ میں کئی اعضاء کو سپلائی ہوتی ہے۔ یہ میڈلا آبلانگیٹا سے شروع ہو کر کھوپڑی کے نیچے ایک مخصوص سوراخ سے نکل کر گردن کے راستے خونی رگوں کے ساتھ ساتھ سینے میں داخل ہوتی ہے اور بعد میں پیٹ میں داخل ہوتی ہے۔

Valgus *(val'-gus)* [L.]. Displacement or angulation away from the midline of the body, e.g. hallux valgus.

روح القدم: لاطینی لفظ۔ جسم کی میانی لکیر سے دور ہٹاؤ۔

Valine *(va'-len)* One of the essential amino acids (q.v.).

ویلین: لازمی امینو ایسڈز میں سے ایک۔

Valium *(val'-i-um)* Diazepam (q.v.).

ویلیم: ڈایازیپام۔ خواب آور دوا۔ دل کے دورے میں ۲ تا ۵ ملی گرام۔ مالی خولیا اور پریشانی میں مفید۔

aloid *(val-oid)* Cyclizine (q.v.).

allergan. Trimeprazine (q.v.).

ویلرگان: ٹرائی میپرازین۔ خارش بند کرنے کے لئے کارآمد۔ ایک گولی صبح، ایک دوپہر، ایک شام۔

alve *(valv)* [L. *valva,* fold]. A fold of membrane in a passage or tube permitting the flow of contents in one direction only. **valvular repiacement,** operation for insertion of prosthetic mitral or aortic valve—valvular, *adj.*

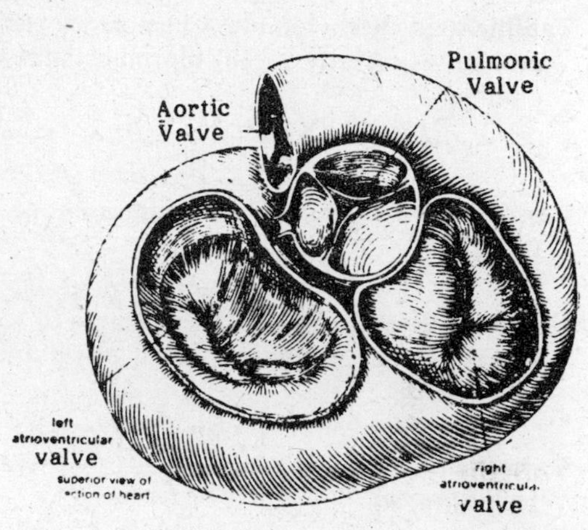

Valve

والو: راستے یا نکی میں جھلی کی تہہ جو اس میں موجود اشیا کا بہاؤ ایک ہی سمت میں رکھتی ہے۔

Valvoplasty *(val-vo-plas'-ti)* [L. *valva,* fold; *plassein,* to form]. A plastic operation on a valve, usually reserved for the hearth; includes valve replacement and valvulotomy—valvoplastic, *adj.*

والوو پلاسٹی: ویلو کا پلاسٹک اپریشن۔ عموماً دل کے لئے مخصوص۔

Valvotomy *(val-vot'-om-i)* See VALVULOTOMY.

ویلووٹومی، قطع ویلو: ویلووٹومی۔ ویلو میں شگاف۔

Valvulitis *(val-vu-li'-tis)* [L. *valva,* fold; G. *-itis,* inflammation]. Inflammation of a valve, particularly in the heart.

ورم باب دل: ویلو کا سوزش، خصوصاً دل میں۔

Vamin. Scientifically prepared sulution for parenteral feeding.

Vancomycin *(van-ko-mi'-sin)* Antibiotic for overwhelming staphylococcal infections. Natural resistance to v. rare. Has to be given intravenously Ototoxic.

وینکومائی سین: سٹیفائلوکاکسی امراض کے لئے اینٹی بایوٹک۔

Vandid *(van-did)* Vanillic acid diethylamide

(q.v.).

وینڈ ڈ: وینلک ایڈ ڈائی ایتھائل امائیڈ۔

Vanillic acid diethylamide. Chemorepetor stimulant, especially useful inpromoting respiration.

وینلک ایسڈ ڈائی ایتھائل امائیڈ: کیموریسپٹر تحریک کرنے والا۔ خصوصاً تنفس بڑھانے میں مفید۔

Vanquin *(van'-qwin)* Viprynium embonate (q.v.).

وین قوئین: وپرائنیم آمبونیٹ۔

Vaquez's disease. Polycythaemia vera (q.v.). [Louis Henri Vaquez, French physician, 1860-1936].

مرض ویکوویز: پولیسا ئتھیمیا ویرا۔

Varicella *(va-ri-sel'-ia)* Chickenpox (q.v.)—varicelliform, *adj.*

کاکڑا: ماتا۔ چکن پوکس۔

Varices *(var'-i-sez)* [L.]. Dilated, tortuous (or varicose) veins—varix, *sing.*

دوالی وریدین: پھیلی ہوئی وریدیں۔

Varicocele *(va'-ri-ko-sel)* [L. *varicosus,* full of dilated veins; G. *kele,* tumour]. Varicosity of the veins of the spermatic cord.

ویری کوسیل: سپری ڈوری کی وریدوں کا پھیلاؤ۔ فوطوں کی رگوں کے پھولنے سے بنی ہوئی گانٹھ۔

Varicose *(va'-ri-kos)* [L. *varicosus,* full of dilated veins]. Dilated varicosity, *n.* **varicose veins,** dilated veins, the valves of which become incompetent so that blood flow may be reversed. Most commonly found in the lower limbs, rectum (haemorrhoids) or lower oesophagus (oesophageal varices).

دوالی، پھولی ورید: پھیلی ہوئی کشادہ۔

Varicotomy *(va-ri-kot'-o-mi)* [L. *varicosus,* full of dilated veins; G. *tome,* cutting]. Excision of a varicose vein.

قطع الدوالی: کشادہ ورید کا قطع۔

Varidase. Streptokinase (q.v.) and streptodornase (q.v.).

ویری ڈیز: سٹرپٹو کائینیز اور سٹرپٹو ڈورنیز۔

Variola *(va-ri-o-la)* [L.]. Smallpox (q.v.).

چیچک: سمال پوکس

Varioloid *(va'-ri-o-loid)* [L. *variola,* small pox]. Attack of smallpox modified by previous vaccination.

لی چیچک: چیچک کا حملہ۔

Varistab *(va-ri-stab')* Ethyloleamine (q.v.).

یری سٹیب: ایتھائیلولیامین۔

Varix *(va'-iks)* [L.]. A dilated and tortuous vein—varices, *pl.*

والی، متمدد ورید: کشادہ ورید۔

Varus *(var'-us)* [L.]. Displacement or angulation towards the midline of the body, e.g. coxa vara.

ع القدام: جسم کی میانی لکیر کی طرف ہٹاؤ۔

Vas [L.]. A vessel—vasa, *pl.*

قنات، عرق: چھوٹی رگ۔ جسم میں چھوٹی رگ نالی جس کے ذریعے بت بہتی ہے۔

Vas deferens *(vas-def'-er-enz)* The excretory duct of the testis.

ل المنی، ناقل دعاء، ناقل قنات: خصیے کی اخراجی نالی۔ ان کی تعداد ہوتی ہے۔ ہر نالی قریباً دوفٹ طویل ہوتی ہے۔ خصیوں میں منی پیدا ہو کر ان وں کے ذریعہ کیسۃ المنی میں جا کر جمع ہو جاتی ہے۔

Vasa vasorum *(va'-za-vaz-or'-um)* The minute nutrient vessels of the artery and vein walls.

روق درعروق: شریان اور ورید دیواروں کی باریک تغذیہ دار رگیں۔

Vascular *(vas'-ku-lar)* [L. *vasculum,* small vessel]. Supplied with vessels, especially referring to blood vessels.

روقی قنات دار: جس میں رگیں ہوں۔ خصوصاً خونی رگیں۔

Vascularization *(vas-ku-lar-i-za'-shun)* [L. *vasculum,* small vessel]. The acquisition of blood supply. The process of becoming vascular.

وقی سازی: واسکولر ہونے کا عمل۔

Vasculitis *(vas-kul-i'-tis)* [L. *vasculum,* small vessel; G. *-itis,* inflammation]. Inflammation of a blood vessel. Also angiitis.

وقی سوزش: خونی رگ کی سوزش۔

Vasectomy *(vas-ek'-to-mi)* [L. *vas,* vessel; G. *ektome,* excision]. Surgical excision of part of the vas deferens.

وے سیکٹومی: واس ڈیفرنز کے حصے کا سرجیکل قطع۔

scoconstrictor *(va-so-kon-strik'-tor)* [L. *vas,* vessel; *contringere,* to draw tight]. Any agent which causes a narrowing of the lumen of blood vessels.

قابض شرائین: عامل جو خونی رگوں کے لیومن کی تنگی کا سبب بنتا ہے۔

sodilator *(va-so-di'-la-tor)* [L. *vas,* vessel; *dilatare,* to dilate]. Any agent which causes a widening of the lumen of blood vessels.

باسط شرائین: عامل جو خونی رگوں کے لیومن کی چوڑائی کا سبب بنتا ہے۔

soepididymostomy *(va'-so-ep-i-did-i-mos-'o- mi)* [L. *vas,* vessel; G. *epi,* on; *didumoi,* wins; *stoma,* mouth]. Anastomosis of the vas leferens to the epididymis.

دموی اپیڈ یموسٹومی: اپیڈیڈایمس کی طرف واس ڈیفرنز کا جال۔

somotor nerves *(va-so-mo'-ter)* [L. *vas,* vessel; *movere,* to move]. Nerves which cause changes in the calibre of the blood vessels.

اعصابِ عروق حرکی: اعصاب جو خونی رگوں کی اہلیت میں تبدیلی کا باعث بنتے ہیں۔

sopressin *(vaz-o-pres'-in)* Formed in the ypothalamus. Passes down the nerves in the ituitary stalk to be stored in the posterior obe of the pituitary gland. It is the antidiure-ic hormone (ADH). Can be given by inject-on or as snuff in diabetes insipidus. Synthetic reparation available—Pitressin.

ویسوپریسن: ہائپوتھیلامس میں بننے والا۔

ospasm *(va'-so-spazm)* [L. *vas,* vessel; G. *pasmos,* spasm]. Constricting spasm of essel walls—vasospastic, *adj.*

دموی تشنج: رگ کی دیواروں کی رگ دار اینٹھن۔

ovagal attack. Faintness, pallor, sweating, eeling of fullness in epigastrium. When part f the post-gastrectomy syndrome it occurs a w minutes after a meal.

واسواویگل حملہ: کمزوری، پسینہ آنا، اپی گیسٹریم بھرا ہونے کا احساس۔

oxine *(vaz-oks'-en)* Methoxamine (q.v.).

ویسوکسین: میتھوکسامین۔

nsol *(vat'-en-sol)* Guanoclor (q.v.).

وٹین سول: گوانوکلور۔

VBI. Vertebrobasilar insufficiency (q.v.).

وی۔بی۔آئی: خلفی دماغ میں خون کی کمی کی وجہ سے سنڈروم۔

Vector *(vek'-tor)* [L. *vehere,* to carry]. Carrier of disease.

حامل مرض: مرض لے کر جانے والا۔

Veganin *(vej'-a-nin)* A preparation similar to tab. codeine co. (BNF), containing aspirin, phenacetin and codeine.

ویگانین: ایک دوا اے پی سی کے علاوہ کوڈین شامل ہے۔سر درد کے لئے کارآمد۔ایک گولی دن میں تین مرتبہ۔

Vegetations *(vej-e-ta'-shuns)* [L. *vegetare,* enliven]. Growths or accretions composed of fibrin and platelets occuring on the edge of the cardiac valves in endocarditis.

پھنسیاں: کارڈیاٹک ویلوز کے کنارے پر واقع فائبرن اور پلیٹلیٹس پر مشتمل بڑھاؤ۔

Vegetative *(vej-e-ta'-tiv)* [L. *vegetare,* enliven]. Pertaining to the non-sporing stage of a bac-terium.

نموی: جرثومہ کے بذرے نہ بنانے والے مرحلہ سے متعلق۔

Vegolysen *(vej-o-li'-sen)* Hexamethonium (q.v.).

ویگولائیسن: ہیکسامیتھونیم۔

Vehicle *(ve-i-kl')* [L. *vehiculum,* conveyance]. An inert substance in which a drug is administered, e.g. water in mitures.

واسطہ: ایک غیر عامل مادّہ جس میں دوا ڈالی جاتی ہے۔مثلاً آمیزوں میں پانی۔

Vein *(van)* [L. *vena,* vein]. A vessel conveying blood from the capillaries back to the heart. It has the same three coats as an artery, the inner one being fitted with valves—venous, *adj.*

ورید: رگ جو خون کونسوں سے واپس دل میں لے جاتی ہے۔

Velactin *(vel-ak'-tin)* A substitution for milk in milk-free diets.

Velbe *(vel'-be)* Vinblastine (q.v.).

Venepuncture *(ve-ni-pungk-tur)* [L. *vena,* vein; *punctura,* a puncture]. Insertion of a needle into a vein.

وینی پنکچر: ورید میں سوئی گھسانا۔

Venereal *(ven'-e-re-al)* [L. *venereus,* from

Venus, goddess of love]. Pertaining to or caused by sexual intercourse. **venereal disease,** gonorrhoea, non-specific urethritis, syphilis and soft sore.

جماعی: جنسی ہم بستری سے متعلق۔ وینرئل امراض جنسی امراض ہیں جو مردوں میں پائے جاتے ہیں۔

Venereology *(ven-e-re-ol'-o-ji)* The study and treatment of venereal disease.

زہراویات: جنسی ہم بستری کے مرض کا علاج اوراس کا مطالعہ۔

Venesection *(ve-ni-sek'-shun)* [L. *vena,* vein; *sectio,* cutting]. A clinical procedure, formerly by opening cubital vein with scalpel (now usually by venepuncture), whereby blood volume is reduced in congestive heart failure.

ورید شگافی: ایک کلینیکل طریقہ۔ڈرپ لگانے کے لئے ضروری۔

Venoclysis *(ve-no-kli'-sis)* [L. *vena,* vein; G. *klysis,* a drenching]. The introduction of nutrient or medicinal fluids into a vein. See CLYSIS.

تطعیم وریدی، احتقان وریدی: ورید میں دوائیوں یا غذا کے سیال کا دخول۔

Venogram *(ve'-no-gram)* [L. *vena,* vein; G. *gramma,* letter]. A radiograph of venous system after opaque media injection.

وینوگرام: غیر شفاف واسطے کے ٹیکے کے بعد وریدی نظام کا ریڈیوگراف۔

Venography *(ven-og'-ra-fi)* [L. *vena,* vein; G. *graphein,* to write]. X-ray examination of venous system by injection of opaque media —venographically, *adv.*

وینوگرافی: غیر شفاف واسطے کے ٹیکے سے وریدی نظام کا ایکسرے ٹیسٹ۔

Venous *(ve'-nus)* [L. *vena,* vein]. Pertaining to the veins.

وریدی: وریدوں سے متعلق۔

Ventolin *(ven'-tol-in)* Salbutamol (q.v.).

وینٹولن: سلبوٹامول۔

Ventous extraction. Use of the vacuum extractor in obstetrics.

وینٹوس ایکسٹریکشن: آبسٹیٹرکس میں ویکوم ایکسٹریکٹر کا استعمال۔

Ventral *(ven'-tral)* [L. *venter,* belly]. Pertaining to the abdomen or the anterior surface of the body—Ventrally, *adv.*

یمی: جسم کی امامی سطح یا بطن سے متعلق۔

Ventricle *(ven'-trik-'l)* [L. *ventriculum*]. A sı belly-like cavity. **ventricle of the brain,** cavities filled with cerebrospinal fluid wi the brain. **ventricle of the heart,** the two l er muscular chambers of the heart—ver cular, *adj.*

Ventr

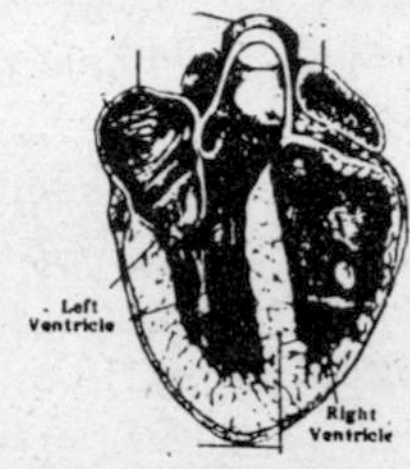

ن، بطین: ایک چھوٹا بطن نما کہفہ۔ دل کا ایک خانہ۔

Ventriculocysternostomy *(ven-trik'-u-lo-tern-os'-to-mi)* [L. *ventriculum,* ventri *cisterna,* cistern; G. *stoma,* mouth]. Artif commmunication between cerebral ventri and subarachnoid space. One of the drai operations for hydrocephalus.

یکولوسسٹرنوسٹومی: سربرل وینٹریکلز اور سب ارکنائڈ جگہ کے مصنوعی ذرائع آمد ورفت۔

Ventriculography *(ven-trik-u-log'-ra-fi)* *ventriculum,* ventricle; G. *graphein,* to wı X-ray examination of ventricles after injec of an opaque medium—ventriculograp *adj.*

نگاری: غیر شفاف واسطے کے ٹیکے کے بعد وینٹریکلز وینٹریکلز کا ے امتحان۔

Ventriculoscope *(ven-trik'-ul-o-skop)* An in ment via which the cerebral ventricles ca examined.

Ventriculostomy *(ven-trik-ul-os'-to-mi)* [L. *triculum,* ventricle; G. *stoma,* mouth] artificial opening into a ventricle. Usu refers to a drainage operation for hy cephalus.

کولوسٹومی: وینٹریکل میں ایک مصنوعی سوراخ۔

Ventrosuspension *(ven-tro-sus-pen'-shun)*

ion of displaced uterus to anterior abdominal wall.

ویٹرو سسپینشن: ہٹے ہوئے یوٹرس کی امامی بطنی دیوار میں فکسیشن۔

ule *(ven'-ul)* [L. *venula*]. A small vein. A yringe-like apparatus for collecting blood om a vein.

وریدک: چھوٹی ورید۔ورید سے خون جمع کرنے کے لئے آلہ۔

amon *(ve'-ra-mon)* See AMIDOPYRINE.

apamil *(ver-a-pam'-il)* Synthetic drug which ppears to have a quindine-like action on the yocardium. Useful for angina of effort.

colate *(ver-e-ko'-lat)* Cholagogue (q.v.).

ویریکولیٹ: ایک دوا جو آنت میں بائل کے بہاؤ میں اضافے کا سبب ہے۔

iloid *(ve'-ri-loid)* Preparations of green elle- bore. Useful in hypertension, articularly in association with similar drugs.

ویریلائیڈ: ہائپر ٹنشن میں مفید۔

nicide *(ver'-mi-sid)* [L. *vermis*, worm; *co-lere*, to kill]. An agent which kills intestinal orms—vermicidal, *adj*.

کرم کش: آنت کے کیڑوں کو مارنے والا عامل۔

miform *(ver'-mi-form)* [L. *vermis*, worm; *rma*, form]. Wormlike. **vermiform appen-x**, the vestigial, hollow, wormlike structure tached to the caecum.

دردی: کیڑے کی طرح کا۔ درمیفارم اپنڈکس ایک فضول، کھوکھلی، کیڑے ساخت جو سیکم کے ساتھ ملحق ہوتی ہے۔

mifuge *(ver'-mi-fuj)* [L. *vermis*, worm; *greer*, to flee]. An agent that expels intestin- worms.

دافع دیدانِ معا: ایسا ایجنٹ جو آنت کے کیڑوں کو باہر نکال دے۔

ix caseosa *(ver'-niks ka-zi-o-za)* The fatty bstance which covers the skin of the fetus birth and keeps it from becoming sodden the liquor amnii.

پردۂ جنین: چربیلا مادہ جو پیدائش کے وقت بچے کی جلد کو ڈھانپتا ہے۔

nal *(ve'-ron-al)* Barbitone (q.v.), one of the st compounds of this type to be used ther-eutically.

ویرونل، منوم دوا: ایک سفید قلمی مرکب۔ نقطہ پگھلاؤ ۱۹۱° س، بار بیٹوریٹ

خواب آور دوا کے طور پر مستعمل۔

Verruca *(ve-roo'-ka)* [L.]. Wart. Non-venereal warts of the genitals are called 'condylomata acuminata' (q.v.). **verruca necrogenica,** post-mortem wart, develops as result of accidental inoculation with tuberculosis. **verruca plana juvenilis,** the common multiple, flat, tiny warts often seen on children's hands and knees. **verruca plantaris,** a flat wart on the sole of the foot. Highly contagious. **verruca seborrhoeica,** the brown, greasy wart seen in seborrhoeic subjects commonly on chest or back. **verruca vulgaris,** the common wart of the hands, of brown colour and rough pitted surface—verrucous, verrucose, *adj.*; verrucae, *pl.*

مسا: آبلہ۔دانہ۔

Versapen *(ver'-sa-pen)* Hetacillin (q.v.).

ورساپین: ہیٹاسلین۔

Versene EDTA. A chelating agent, the calcium and sodium salts of which have been used to remove harmful substances from the body, e.g. lead, radioactive heavy metals. The newly formed stable chelate compounds are excreted in the urine.

ورسین: جس کے کیلشیم اور سوڈیم نمکیات جسم سے ضرررساں مادے ختم کرنے کے لئے استعمال کئے جاتے ہیں۔ مثلاً سیسہ، ریڈیو ایکٹو بھاری دھاتیں نئے بننے والے مرکبات پیشاب میں خارج ہوتے ہیں۔

Version *(ver'-shun)* [L. *vertere*, to turn]. Turning —applied to the manoeuvre to alter the posit- ion of the fetus *in utero*. **cephalic v.,** turning the child so that the head presents. **external v.** is turning the child by manipulation through the abdominal wall. **internal v.** is turning the child by one hand in the uterus, and the other on the patient's abdomen, **podalic v.,** turning the child to a breech presentation. This v. may be external or internal.

سرک رحم: موڑنا۔ پیٹ میں بچے کا رخ پھیرنا۔

Vertebrobasilar insufficiency. Syndrome caused by lack of blood to the hindbrain. May be progressive, episodic, or both. Clinical manifestation include giddiness and vertigo, nausea, ataxia, drop attacks and signs of cerebellar disorder such as nystagmus.

ورٹبرو بیسیلر انسفی شینسی :خلفی دماغ کوخون کی کمی کے سبب سنڈروم۔

Vertex *(ver'-teks)* [L. top]. The top of the head.

چوٹی، راس: سر کا اوپر والا حصہ۔

Vertigo *(ver-ti'-go)* [L.]. Giddiness, dizziness—vertiginous, *adj*.

دورانِ سر: لاطینی لفظ۔ سر چکرانا۔

Vesical *(ves'-i-kal)* [L. *vesica,* bladder]. Pertaining to the bladder.

مثانی: بلیڈر سے متعلق۔

Vesicant *(ves'-i-kant)* [L. *vesica,* bladder]. A blistering substance.

آبلہ انگیز: چھالوں والا مادّہ۔ ادویات جن کے لگانے سے آبلے پڑ جائیں۔

Vesicle *(ves'-ik-l)* [L. *vesicula*]. A small bladder, cell or hollow structure. A skin blister—vesicular, *adj.*; vesiculation, *n*.

آبلہ، چھالا: ایک چھوٹا بلیڈر، خلیہ یا کھوکھلی ساخت۔ ایک جلدی چھالا۔

Vesicostomy *(ve-si-kos-to-mi)* [L. *vesica,* bladder; G. *stoma,* mouth]. Syn., cystostomy. **cutaneous v.,** the bladder is drained on to the anterior abdominal wall to which an ileostomy bag is attached. A tube of bladder muscle conducts urine from bladder to surface.

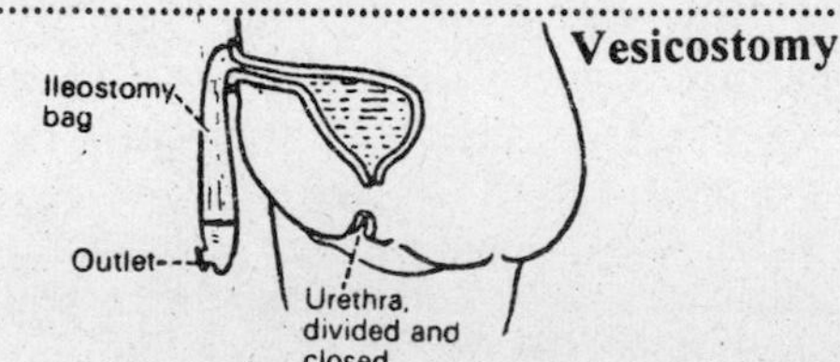

مثانہ شگافی: سسٹو سٹومی۔

Vesicoureteric *(ve-si-ko-u-ret-er'-ik)* [L. *vesica,* bladder; G. *oureter,* ureter]. Pertaining to the urinary bladder and ureter. Vesicouretic reflux can cause pyelonephritis.

ویز یکو یورٹیرک: بولی بلیڈر اور یوریٹر سے متعلق۔

Vesicovaginal *(ve-si-ko-vaj-in'-al)* [L. *vesica,* bladder; *vagina,* sheath]. Pertaining to t urinary bladder and the vagina.

نی مہبلی: بولی بلیڈر اور ویجائنا سے متعلق۔

Vesiculitis *(ves-ik-u-li'-tis)* [L. *vesicula,* vesic G. *-itis,* inflammation]. Inflammation o vesicle, particularly the seminal vesicles.

کیہ ءِ منی: ویزیکل، خصوصاً سیمینل ویزیکل کی سوزش۔

Vesiculopapular *(ves-ik-u-lo-pa-pu-lar)* *vesicula,* vesicle; *papula,* pimple]. Pertaini to or exhibiting both vesicles and papules.

یکیولو پیپولز: ویزیکلز اور پیپولز سے متعلق۔

Vessel *(ves'-el)* [L. *vascellum*]. A tube, duct canal, holding or conveying fluid, especia blood and lymph.

، دعا: نکی، نالی یا قنات جس میں سیال ہو، خصوصاً خون اور لمف۔

Vestibule *(ves'-ti-bul)* [L. *vestibulum,* passag 1. The middle part of the internal ear, ly between the semicircular canals and cochlea. 2. The triangular area between labia minora-vestibular, *adj*.

ٹ، دہلیز: (ا) درمیانی حصہ جو نصف دائروی قنالوں اور کاکلیا کے ان واقع ہوتا ہے۔

لیبیا مائینورا کے درمیان تکونی ایریا۔ یہ عضو بادام کی شکل کا ہے اور یا کلائی ٹورس سے اوپر واقع ہے۔

Vestigial *(ves-tij'-i-al)* [L. *vestigium,* trac Rudimentary; indicating a remnant of sor thing formerly present.

ئی: تخفیف شدہ۔ پہلے سے موجود کو ظاہر کرنے والی ذرا سی ساخت۔

Viable *(vi-a-bl')* Capable of living a separ existence—viability, *n*.

ی، ذیستنی: الگ وجود کے طور پر زندہ رہنے کے قابل۔

Viacutan *(vi-a-kut'-an)* Available as tulle dre ing and emulsion. Promotes healing under aseptic cover. Active against Gram-posit and Gram-negative bacteria, including Ps domonas and Proteus. Activity enhanc rather than diminished inpresence of seu pus and tissue debris. Bacterial resistance not occur and local sensitivity reactions uncommon.

کیوٹین: بطور ڈریسنگ اور ایملشن مہیا ہے۔ گرام منفی جراثیم کے خلاف

عامل۔

'ibramycin *(vib-ra-mi-sin)* Doxycycline (q.v.).

وبرامائی سین: اس اینٹی بایوٹک کی روزانہ دہی خوراک خون کے موزوں ارتکاز کو برقرار رکھتی ہے۔

'ibration syndrome. Impotency and paralysis of the arm and hands in workers using vibrating machines. Syn., Raynaud's phenomenon.

ارتعاشی سنڈروم: مرتعش مشینیں استعمال کرنے والے کارکنوں میں بازوؤں اور ہاتھوں کا سن ہو جانا۔

'ibrio *(vib-ri-o)* [L. *vibrare,* to vibrate]. A genus of curved, motile, micro-organisms. *Vibrio cholerae* or *comma* causes cholera.

ارتعاشیہ: خمدار متحرک خورد جسمیوں کا ایک جنس۔ وبریو کالری ہیضہ کا سبب ہے۔ یہ انگریزی علامت 'کوما' یا اردو کے حرف ''و'' کی شکل کے ہوتے ہیں۔

'icarious *(vi-kar-i-us)* [L. *vicarius,* substituted]. Substituting the function of one organ for another. **vicarious menstruation,** bleeding from the nose or other part of the body when menstruation is abnormally suppressed.

عوضی: ایک عضو کے فعل کی جگہ دوسرے کا تبادلہ۔

'illus *(vil-us)* [L. shaggy hair]. A microscopic fingerlike projection, such as found in the mucous membrane of the small intestine, or on the outside of the chorion of the embryonic sac—villi, *pl.*; villous, *adj.*

خملہ: ایک خوردبینی انگشت نما ابھار۔ چھوٹی آنت میں میوکس جھلی میں پایا جانے والا امبریانک یعنی جنینی تھیلی کے کوریون کے باہر کی طرف۔

'inblastine *(vin-blas'-ten)* Alkaloid from periwinkle. Antimitotic used mainly in Hodgkin's disease and choriocarcinoma resistant to other therapy. Given intravenously.

ونبلاسٹین: ایک الکلائیڈ۔ ضد مائیٹوسس۔

'incristine *(vin-kris-ten)* Antileukaemic drug. Derived from an extract of the periwinkle plant. Given intravenously.

ونکرسٹین: ضد لیوکیمیا دوائی۔

'ineberg operation. For angina pectoris. Internal mammary artery dissected from chest wall and implanted with bleeding side holes into the wall of the left ventricle. Established vascular connections with the coronary circulation. First performed by Vineberg in 1950.

وائن برگ اپریشن: انجینا پکٹورس کے لئے۔

Vinesthene *(vin-es-then)* Vinyl ether (q.v.).

وینستھین: ونائیل ایتھر۔

Vinyl ether *(vi-nil-eth-er)* An inhalation anaesthetic similar to ether, but more rapid and less sustained in effect.

وینائل ایتھر: سانس کے ذریعے اندر لے جانے والا، سن کرنے والا۔ ایتھر سے مشابہ۔ ڈائی وینائل ایتھر، ایک بے رنگ آتش گیر مائع۔ نقطہ جوش ۳۹° س۔

Viocin *(vi-o-sin)* Viomycin (q.v.).

وائیوسین: وائیومائیسن۔

Viomycin *(vi-o-mi-sin)* An antibiotic used in the treatment of tuberculosis when the disease is resistant to other drugs.

وائیو مائی سین: اینٹی بایوٹک جو تپ دق کے علاج میں اس وقت استعمال کیا جاتا ہے جب دوسری ادویہ کے لئے مزاحمت ہو۔

Vioactone *(vi-on-ak-ton)* Viomycin (q.v.).

وائیونیکٹون: وائیومائیسین۔

Viprynium *(vip-rin-i-um)* Anthelmintic effective against threadworms. Stools become red.

وپرائی نیم: چرنوں کے خلاف مؤثر دوا۔ فضلہ ضائع ہو جاتا ہے۔

Viraemia *(vir-em-i-a)* [L. *virus,* poison; G. *haima,* bleed]. The presence of virus in the blood. **maternal v.,** can cause fetal damage —viraemic, *adj.*

ویریمیا: خون میں وائرس کی موجودگی۔

Viricidal *(vi-ri-si'-dal)* [L. *virus,* poison; *caedere,* to kill]. Lethal to a virus—viricide, *n.*

وریسیڈل: وائرس کے لئے مہلک۔

Virilism *(vir'-il-izm)* [L. *virilis,* manly]. The appearance of secondary male characteristics in the female.

نریت: مادہ میں ثانوی نرخصوصیات کا ظہور۔

Virology *(vi-rol'-o-ji)* [L. *virus,* poison; G. *logos,* discourse]. The study of viruses and the diseases caused by them—virological, *adj.*

وائرولوجی: وائرس اوران سے پیدا ہونے والی بیماریوں کا مطالعہ۔

Virugon *(vir-u'-gon)* Antiviral drug effective in

influenzal type illness.

ویروگون: ضد وائرس دوا۔ انفلوئنزا قسم کی بیماریوں میں موثر۔

Virulence *(vir'-u-lens)* [L. *virulentus*, poisonous] Infectiousness; the disease producing power of micro-organism; the power of a micro-org- anism to overcome host resistance—virulent, *adj*.

سمیت: خورد جسیمے کی بیماری پیدا کرنے کی میزبان کی قوتِ مزاحمت پر غالب آنے کی طاقت۔

Virus *(vi'-rus)* [L.]. Very small micro-organisms parasitic within living cells. Differ from bacteria in having only one kind of nucleic acid, either DNA or RNA, in lacking the apparatus necessary for energy production and protein synthesis, and by not reproducing by binary fission but by independent synthesis of their component parts which are then assembled. Cause many kinds of acute and chronic diseases in man, can cause tumours in animals. Some of the more important groups are: (1) **poxviruses,** e.g. smallpox, molluscum contagiosum. (2) **herpesviruses,** e.g. herpes simplex v., cytomegalovirus, varicella zoster v., EB virus. (3) **adenoviruses**. (4) **papovaviruses,** e.g. polyomavirus, which can cause tumours in laboratory animals. (5) **reoviruses,** e.g. rotaviruses. (6) **togaviruses,** yellow fever v. (7) **picornaviruses**. (8) **myxoviruses**. (9) **paramyxoviruses**. (10) **rhabdoviruses,** e.g. rabies v. (11) **coronaviruses,** e.g. some common cold viruses. (12) **arenaviruses,** e.g. Lassa fever v. Groups 1-4 are DNA viruses, groups 5-12 are RNA viruses. Viruses spread by arthropods—insects and ticks—are known as arboviruses, these include reoviruses, togaviruses and rhabdoviruses.

وائرس، سمی مادد. یہ طاقتور خوردبین سے دیکھے جاتے ہیں، زندہ خلیوں میں پرورش پاتے ہیں اور طفیلی ہیں۔ ان کی مختلف اقسام پودوں، جانوروں اور انسان میں بیماریاں پھیلاتی ہیں۔ وائرس میزبان خلیے کے خامرہ کو استعمال کرتا ہے۔ ان کی تولید خلیہ میں ہی ہوتی ہے۔ جب خلیہ پھٹتا ہے اور وائرس خارج ہوتے ہیں تو کئی بیماریاں لاحق ہوتی ہیں۔ وائرس کو سب سے پہلے تمباکو کے پودے میں دیکھا گیا۔ یہ تمباکو کے پتوں میں بیماری پیدا کرتا ہے۔ وائرس جراثیم پر بھی حملہ آور ہوتے ہیں، ایسا وائرس جرثومہ کے خلیے میں داخل ہو کر تولید کرتا ہے، جس سے وائرس کی تعداد بڑھ جاتی ہے اور بعض دفعہ جراثیمی خلیہ پھٹ جاتا ہے اور وائرس باہر آ کر نئے جراثیمی خلیوں پر حملہ آور ہوتے ہیں۔ یہ کئی امراض کا سبب ہیں۔ مثلاً چیچک، خسرہ، کاکڑا، کن پیڑ، متعدی ورم دماغ، پولیو مائی لائی ٹس، وبائی انفلوئنزا، یرقان، نکرے وغیرہ۔ سمائیے یا وائرس گرمی سے مرجاتے ہیں۔

Viscera *(vis'-er-a)* [L. inner organs]. The internal organs—viscus, *sing.*; visceral, *adj*.

اعضاء شکم، امعا: اندرونی اعضاء۔

Visceroptosis *(vis-e-rop-to-sis)* [L. *viscero*, inner organs; G. *ptosis*, a falling]. Downward displacement or falling of the abdominal organs.

استرخانے احشا: بطنی اعضاء کا گرنا یا نیچے کی طرف آ جانا۔

Viscid *(vis-kid)* Sticky, glutinous.

Viscopaste *(vis-ko-past)* A medicated bandage impregnated with Unna's paste (q.v.).

وسکو پیسٹ: پٹی جس میں پیسٹ اُنا ہوتا ہے۔

Visual *(viz'-u-al)* [L. *visus*, sight]. Pertaining to vision. **visual field,** the area within which objects can be seen. **visual purple,** the purple pigment in the retina of the eye. Rhodopsin.

بصری: دیکھنے سے متعلق۔

Vital capacity. The amount of air expelled from the lungs after a deep inspiration.

اہلیت حیات: اندر کی طرف گہرا سانس لینے کے بعد پھیپھڑوں سے خارج شدہ ہوا کی مقدار۔

Vitallium *(vi-tal'-li-um)* An alloy which can be left in the tissues in the form of nails, plates, tubes, etc.

وٹیلیم: ایک بھرت جو پلیٹوں، نلکیوں وغیرہ کی صوت میں بافتوں میں رہ سکتی ہے۔

Vitamins *(vi'-ta-mins)* [L. *vita*, life; and 'amine']. Essential food factors, chemical in nature, present in certain foodstuffs. Some can now be synthesized commercially. Their absence causes deficiency diseases.

وٹامن، حیاتین: زائد غذائی عوامل، نامیاتی مرکبات کا گروہ جو مختلف قسم کی

خوراکوں میں پائے جاتے ہیں اور عام غذا میں ان کا موجود ہونا ضروری ہے۔ چند حیاتین مصنوعی طور پر تیار کیئے جاتے ہیں۔ حیاتین کی بدن میں کمی یا قلت متعدد امراض کا موجب بن جاتی ہے۔ وٹامن الف آدمی اور جانوروں کے لئے لازمی ہوتا ہے۔ وٹامن ب کمپلیکس پانی میں حل پذیر ہے۔ وٹامن ڈی حل ہونے والی چکنائی میں پائے جاتے ہیں۔ انسان کو ان کی اشد ضرورت ہوتی ہے۔ بچپن میں ان کی کمی سے رکٹ کی بیماری ہو جاتی ہے یہ جگر میں ذخیرہ ہوتے ہیں۔ مصنوعی طور پر بھی تیار کئے جاتے ہیں، وٹامن ای کی مہریوں کو ضرورت ہوتی ہے، وٹامن کے پرندوں اور پستانیوں بشمول آدمی کے لئے ضروری ہے، اس کی کمی جریان خون کا سبب بنتی ہے۔ پروتھرومبن پیدا کرنے کے لئے ضروری۔ صرف بائیل کی موجودگی میں جذب ہوتا ہے۔ وٹامن پی (سٹیرین) ان مادوں کا گروہ ہے جو سٹرس پھلوں میں پائے جاتے ہیں۔ نسوں کی دیواروں کے توازن کے لئے ضروری خیال کئے جاتے ہیں۔ سکروی روکنے میں وٹامن سی کے ساتھ مل کر عمل کرتا ہے۔ ہیماپٹی سز یا خون تھوکنے میں وٹامن 'کے' کا ایک انجکشن روزانہ یا ایک گولی دن میں تین مرتبہ۔ زکام میں وٹامن اے ڈی کا ایک کیپسول ہر ۴ گھنٹے بعد۔

Vitamin E deficiency syndrome. Occurs in small infants, less than 2 kg and under 35 weeks gestation. At diagnosis between 6 and 11 weeks, low haemoglobin; there is good response to vitamin E including a rise in haemoglobin and loss of oedema.

Vitiligo *(vit-il-i-go)* [L.]. Leucoderma (q.v.).

Vitiligo

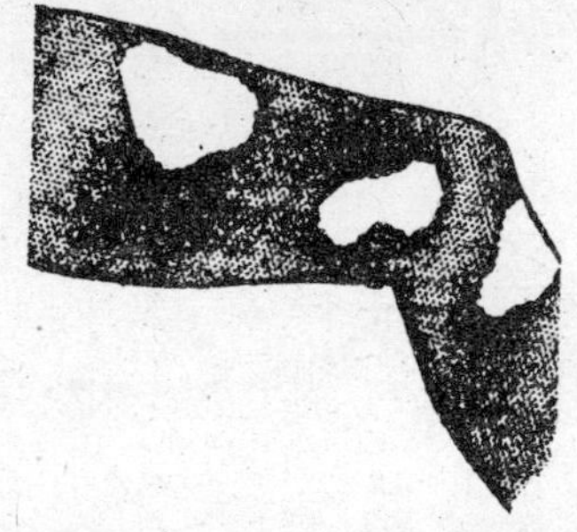

لبھاق: لیوکوڈرما۔

Vitreous *(vit'-ri-us)* [L. *vitreus,* of glass]. Resembling jelly. **vitreous chamber,** the cavity inside the eyeball. **vitreous humor,** the jelly-like substance contained in the vitreous chamber.

Vitreous humor

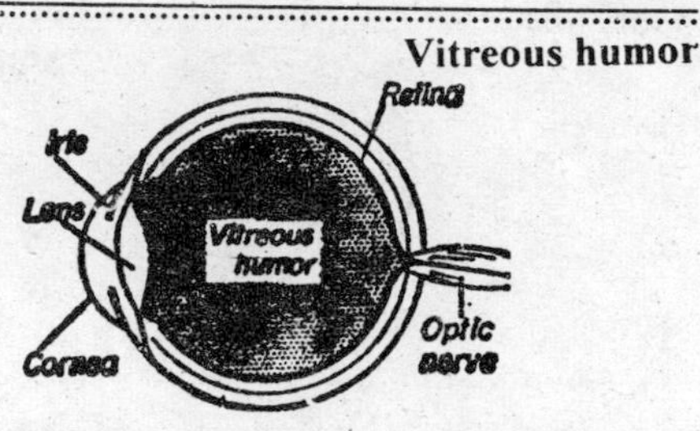

زجاجی: جیلی سے مشابہ۔

Vocal cords. Membranous folds stretched anteroposteriorly across the larynx. Sound is produced by their vibration as air from the lungs passes between them.

اوتارصوت: لیرنکس کے پاس جھلی کی تہیں۔ ان کے ارتعاش سے آواز پیدا ہوتی ہے کیونکہ پھیپھڑوں سے ہوا ان کے درمیان سے گزرتی ہے۔

Volatile *(vol'-a-til)* [L. *volatilis,* flying]. Evaporating rapidly.

طیران پذیر: تیزی سے بخارات بننا۔

Volition *(vo-lish-un)* [L. *vo-lish-un)* [L. *velle,* wish]. The will to act—volitional, *adj*.

اِرادہ: عمل کرنے کا ارادہ۔

Volkmann's ischaemic contracture *(is-ke-mik)* A flexion deformity of wrist and fingers from fixed contracturee of the flexor muscles in the forearm. The cause is ischaemia of the muscles by injury or obstruction to the brachial artery, near the elbow. [Richard von Volkmann, German surgeon, 1830-89].

وو کمینز اسکیمک کنٹریکچر: ہتھیلی اور انگلیوں کی فلیکسن بدشکلی۔

Voluntary *(vol-un-ta-ri)* [L. *voluntarious*]. Under the control of the will; free and unrestricted; as opposed to reflex or involuntary.

عمدہ، قصدی، ارادی، اختیاری: مرضی یا ارادے کے کنٹرول میں۔ آزاد اور غیر محدود۔

Volvulus *(vol-vu-lus)* [L. *volvere,* to roll]. A twisting of a section of bowel, so as to occlude the lumen.

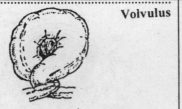

Volvulus

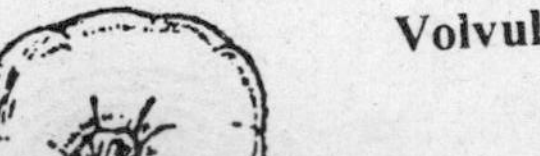

آنت کی مروڑ: آنت کے ایک حصے میں مروڑی۔

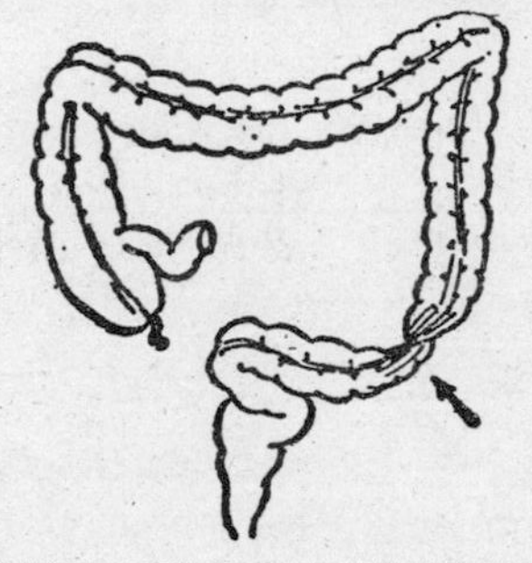

Vomit *(vom'-it)* [L. *vomere,* to vomit]. Ejection of the stomach contents through the mouth; sickness.

قے: منہ میں سے معدے کی اشیاء کا باہر آنا۔ پرکلورپیرازین (سٹے ٹل) یا کلورپرومازین (لارجیکٹل) ایک گولی صبح، ایک دوپہر، ایک شام۔

Vomiting of pregnancy. See HYPEREMESIS.

حمل کی قے: ہائپرایمیسس۔ حمل میں قے آنا۔ علاج کے لئے پرومیتھازین تھیوکلیٹ (ایومین) ایک گولی صبح، ایک شام یا پروکلوپیرازین یا ٹرائی فلوپیرازین (سٹیلازین) ایک گولی صبح، ایک دوپہر، ایک شام۔

Vomitus *(vom'-i-tus)* [L.]. Vomited matter.

مواد ے: لاطینی لفظ۔ قے۔ الٹی کا مادہ۔

Von Recklinghausen's disease. Multiple neurofibromatosis of the skin. The picture is one of multiple soft tumours in the skin, their origin being the connective tissue of cutaneous nerves. Molluscum fibrosum. [Friedrich Daniel von Recklinghausen, German pathologist; 1833-1910].

مرض وان ریک لنگ ہاسن: جلد کی کئی رخی نیوروفائبرومیٹوسس۔

Von Willebrand's disease. Bleeding disease with capillary defect, with or without AHG deficiency. [E.A von Willebrand, Finnish physician, 19th century].

مرض وان ولی برانڈ: نسوں کے نقص کے ساتھ روانی خون کا مرض۔

Voss operation. Described in 1956 for relief of pain in early degenerative disease of the hip joint. Divisonof surrounding main muscles allows healing of articulating surfaces and increases the joint space.

Vulva *(vul-va)* [L.]. The external genitalia of the female—vulval, *adj.*

Vulva

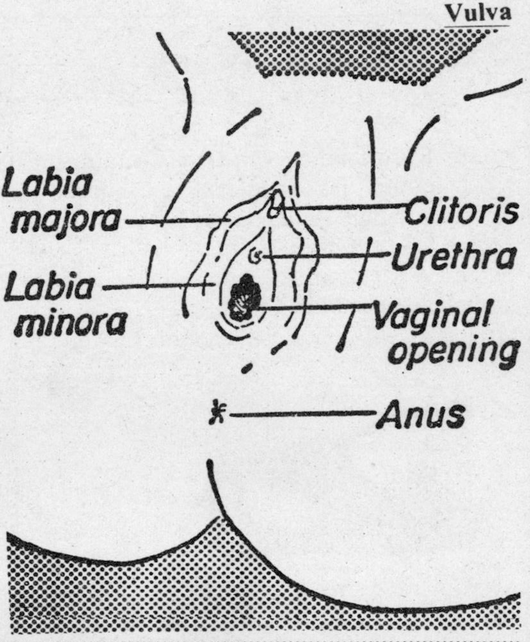

فرج، کس، شرمگاہ: مادہ کے بیرونی تولیدی اعضاء۔ اس میں سے بیامنورا، کلائی ٹورس یا بظر، ویسٹی بیول اور دہانہ فرج یا اندام نہانی کا سوراخ شامل ہیں۔

Vulvectomy *(vul-vek'-to-mi)* [L. *vulva,* covering; G. *ektome,* excision]. Excision of the vulva.

ولویکٹومی، فرج تراشی: فرج یا ولوا کی چیر پھاڑ۔

Vulvitis *(vul-vi-tis)* [L. *vulva,* covering; G. *-itis,* inflammation]. Inflammation of the vulva.

ورم فرج: فرج یا ولوا کی سوزش یا سوج۔

Vulvovaginal *(vul-vo-vaj-in'-nal)* [L. *vulva,* covering; *vagina,* sheath]. Pertaining to the vulva and the vagina.

فرجی، مہبلی: فرج یا ولوا اور ویجائنا سے متعلق۔

Vulvovaginitis *(vul-vo-vaj-in-i-tis)* [L. *vulva,* covering; *vagina,* sheath; G. *-itis,* inflammation]. Inflammaiton of the vulva and vagina.

ورم فرج و مہبل: فرج یا ولوا اور ویجائنا کی سوزش یا سوج۔

Vulvovaginoplasty *(vul-vo-vag-in-o-plas-ti)* [L. *vulva,* covering; *vagina,* sheath; G. *plassein,* to form]. Recently devised operation for congenital absence ofthe vagina, or acquired disabling stenosis—vulvovaginoplastic, *adj.*

شفری مہبلی پلاسٹی: مہبل یا ویجائنا کی خلقی غیر موجودگی کے لئے اپریشن۔

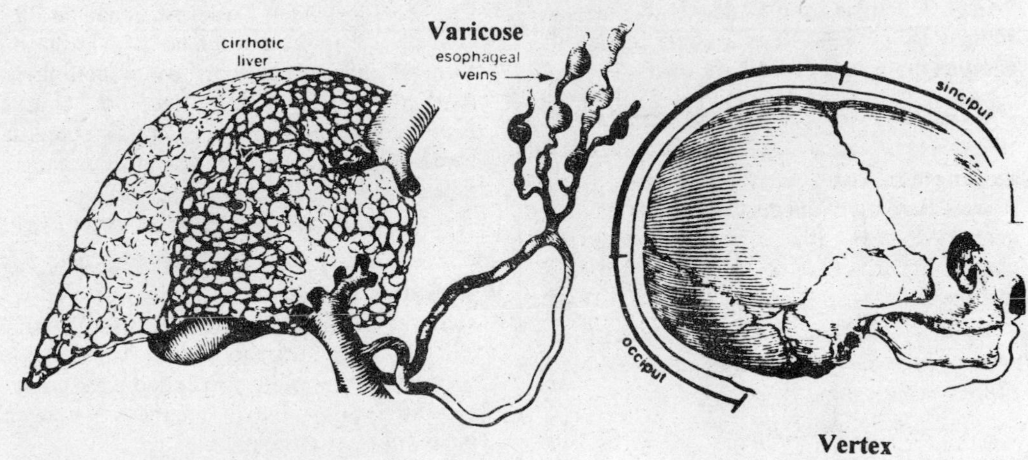

Varicose

Vertex

W

Waldeyer's ring *(vahl-di-erz ring)* [Heinrich Wilhelus Gottfried von Waldeyer, German anatomist 1836-1921]. It is a circle around the pharynx made up of lymphatic ducts.

حلقۂ والڈرے ار: گلے یا فیرنکس کے گرد ایک لمفی دائرہ یا حلقہ ولہلم فان والڈرے ارہارنز ایک جرمن ماہر تشریح کے نام پر ہے۔

Wangensteen tube *(wang'gan-ste'n tu'be)* [Owen Harding Wangensteen, American surgeon 1898-1981]. It is an apparatus with radio opaque tip. It is used to aspirate gastrointestinal fluid.

وینگیسٹین ٹیوب: بالائی سرا ریڈیو اوپیک ہوتا ہے۔

Warfarin *(war-far-in)* It is onee of the synthetic coumarin anticoagulants.

وارفیرین: دہنی طور پر مستعمل۔ جمنے کے خلاف۔

Wart *(wart)* [L. *vervuca*]. A labulated hyper plastic epidermal lesions with rough surface and viral origin.

مسہ، مہاسہ: دڑ دکا، گومڑی، وائرس کا مرض۔ جلد کھردری ہو کر ابھرنے لگتی ہے اور مہاسہ بن جاتا ہے۔

Washing soda *(wa-shing soda)* It is a common name of sodium carbonate.

سوڈا، سجی: سوڈیم کاربونیٹ۔

Water brash *(waw'ter-brash)* Heart burn with regurgitation of sour fluid or almost tasteless saliva into the mouth.

آبی قے، کھٹی ڈکار: پائیروسس۔ آروغ ترش۔ سوزش معدہ۔

Water-house Friderichsen syndrome *(waw-tar hows fridar-ik-sen sind-rom)* [Rupert Waterhouse, British physician 1873-1958, Carl Friederichsen Danis pediatrician 20th century]. It is the malignant or fulminating form of epidemic cerebrospinal meningitis, marked by sudden onsel and short course, fever, coma and collaps cyanosis, petechial hemorrhages of the skin and mucous membranes and bilateral adrenal hemorrhage.

واٹر ہاؤس فرائی ڈیرکسن سنڈروم: جلدی ہیمرج سے صدمہ۔ ایڈرینل گلینڈ میں روانی خون ہو جاتی ہے۔

Waterston's operation *(waw-tar-sten awp-ra'-shan)* [David J. Waterston, British Thoracic and pediatric surgeon 1910]. Anastomosis between the ascending aorta and right pulmonary artery as palliative treatment of congenital pulmonary stenosis.

Weal *(we'l)* It is blister appearing superficially, marked by urticaria and nettle stings.

لاس: سطحی یا مصنوعی چھالا۔

Weil's disease *(vilz dize'z)* [Adolf Weil, German physician 1848-1916]. A severe form of leptospirosis marked by jaundice usually alongwith azotemia, hemorrhages, anemia, disturbances of consciousness and continued fever. It is the disease of miners, sewer workers.

مرض ویل، یرقان وبائی: یرقان کی ایک قسم جس میں بخار ہوتا ہے۔ گندے پانی میں کام کرنے والوں کا مرض۔ جرمن معالج ایڈولف ویل کے نام پر ہے۔

Wharton's jelly. A jelly-like substance contained in the umbilical cord. [Thomas Wharton,

English physician, 1616-73].

وارٹنی جیلی: امبلیکل کارڈ میں موجود ایک جیلی نما مادہ۔ نال کے باہر آتے ہی اس کے خلیے ہوا کے دباؤ سے پھولتے پھیلتے ہیں۔ اس پر وارٹن جیلی پھیل جاتی ہے جس سے بچے کا ماں کے دورانِ خون کے ساتھ تعلق قطع ہو جاتا ہے اور بچے کے اپنے دورانِ خون کے نظام میں تبدیلیاں شروع ہو جاتی ہیں۔ دل دھڑکتے ہوئے خون پھیپھڑوں میں بھیجنے لگتا ہے۔

Wheelhouse's operation. External urethrotomy for impassable stricture. [Claudius Galen Wheelhouse, English surgeon, 1826-1909].

خارجی مبال شگافی: بیرونی یورتھروٹومی۔ ایک انگریز معالج کلاڈیس گیلن وہیل ہاؤس کے نام پر ہے۔

Whipworm *(Trichuris trichiura)* A roundworm which infests the intestine of man in humid tropics. Eggs are excreted in the stools. The worms do not normally produce symptoms, but heavy infestations of over 1000 worms cause bloody diarrhoea, anaemia and prolapse of the rectum. Treatment unsatisfactory but recently thiabendazole has cleared the infestation in about 50 per cent of patients treated.

چابک کرم، چرنے، دود الخل: ٹرائی کورس ٹرائیکیورا۔ ایک گول کیڑا جو آدمی کی آنت میں ہوتا ہے۔ انڈے فضلے میں خارج ہوتے ہیں۔

Whitehead's varnish. A solution of iodoform, benzoin, storax and tolu in ether, used as an antiseptic and protective application to wounds. [Walter Whitehead, English surgeon, 1840-1913].

محلول وہائٹ ہیڈ: آیوڈوفارم، بنزوئن، سٹوریکس اور ٹولو کا ایتھر میں محلول۔ دافع تعفن کے طور پر مستعمل۔ اس کا نام ایک انگریز سرجن والٹر وہائٹ ہیڈ کے نام پر ہے۔

White fluids. Emulsions of taracids and phenols in water, widely used for general disinfectant purpose.

سفید سیال: پانی میں ٹارایڈز اور فینولز کے ایملشن۔ دافع تعفن مقاصد کے لئے مستعمل۔

White leg. See THROMBOPHLEBITIS.

ورم نفاسی: تھرمبوفلیبیٹس۔ بچے کی پیدائش (زچگی) کے بعد دسویں دن بائیں ٹانگ متورم ہو جاتی ہے۔ ٹانگ میں درد ہلکا بخار، حرکت میں تکلیف، عضلات کی سختی اس کی علامات ہیں۔ علاج کے لئے ہیپارین ۱۰ ہزار یونٹ عضلاتی ٹیکہ ایک صبح، ایک شام پیراسیٹامول ایک گولی صبح، ایک دوپہر، ایک شام۔ ۲ ہفتے تک۔ کائموٹرپسن (کائمورل) ایک گولی صبح ایک دوپہر، ایک شام۔ کوٹرائی ماکسازول (سیپٹران) ۲ گولی صبح ۲ ہفتے تک۔

Whites. A popular term for leucorrhoea (q.v.).

سیلان الرحم: لیکوریا کے لئے معروف اصطلاح۔ پرسوت۔

White's tar paste. Zinc paste with the addition of about 6 per cent coal tar. Valuable in infantile eczema. [James C. White, American dermatologist, 1833-1916].

وہائیٹ کی ٹار پیسٹ: زنک پیسٹ قریباً ۶ فیصد کول تار کے اضافہ کے ساتھ۔ اکزیما میں مفید۔

Whitfield's ointment. An antifungal preparation containing salicylic and benzoic acids. [Arthur Whitfield, English dermatologist, 1867-1947].

مرہم وہٹ فیلڈ: سیلیسائیلک اور بنزوک ایسڈز پر مشتمل ایک ضد سماروغ۔ داد، خارش، چنبل اور اکزیما کے لئے کارآمد۔

Whitlow *(wit'-low)* Paronychia (q.v.).

اماس انگشت، چندرا: پیروناتیکیا۔ انگلی کی آخری پور میں درد ہوتا ہے۔ بعض اوقات پیپ ناخن کی جڑ میں جمع ہو جاتی ہے۔

Whooping-cough. Pertussis (q.v.).

کالی کھانسی: پرٹسس۔

Widow's itch. Pruritus (q.v.) and secondary skin eruptions occuring shortly after bereavement.

وڈوزاچ: پرورٹس اور ثانوی جلدی گرمی دانے۔

Wilms' tumour. A congenital, highly malignant, kidney tumour. [Max Wilms, German surgeon, 1867-1918].

گردوی خبیث خلقی رسولی: گردے کا ناسور۔ اس کا نام ایک جرمن سرجن میکس ولیمز کے نام پر رکھا گیا ہے۔

Wilson's disease. Hepaticolenticular degeneration with choreic movements. Due to disturbance of copper metabolism. No urinary catecholamine excretion. Associated with mental subnormality. Can be treated with BAL and penicillamine. A symptomatic relatives can be given prophylactic penicilliamine. [Sir William J.E. wilson, English dermatologist, 1809-84].

مرض ولسن: کورک حرکات کے ساتھ ہیپٹیکولنٹکولر تنزلی۔ تانبے کے میٹابولزم

میں خلل اندازی کی وجہ سے۔

Windpipe. The trachea (q.v.).

ہوا کی نالی: ٹریکیا۔

Wintergreen, oil of. Methyl saliclate (q.v.).

بتول کا تیل: میتھائل سیلیسائیلیٹ۔

Winter vomiting disease. Caused by a ubiquitous, yet still unidentified virus. Symdrome simulates food poisoning.

مرض سرمائی قے: وائرس سے ہونے والا مرض۔

Witch-haze'. See HAMAMELIDIS.

وچ بندوق: ہاملیڈس۔

Womb *(woom)* The uterus (q.v.).

رحم، بچہ دانی: یوٹرس۔

Wood's glass (or light). Special glass (or light) used for the detection of ringworm.Hailed as 'God's gift to dermatologists'. [Robert W. Wood, American physicist, 1868-1955].

شیشہ وڈ: رنگ ورم معلوم کرنے کے لئے مخصوص شیشہ یا روشنی۔

Woolsorter's disease. Anthrax (q.v.).

جمرۂ بلخیہ: انتھریکس۔

Worms, See ASCARIDES, TAENIA and TRICHURIS.

کیڑے: اسکیر یڈز، ٹیبیا اور ٹرائی کورس ٹرائیکیو را فضلے میں کیڑے نہیں ہوتے۔

Woulfe's bottle. A special bottle for washing gases. [Peter Woulfe, British chemist, 1727-1803].

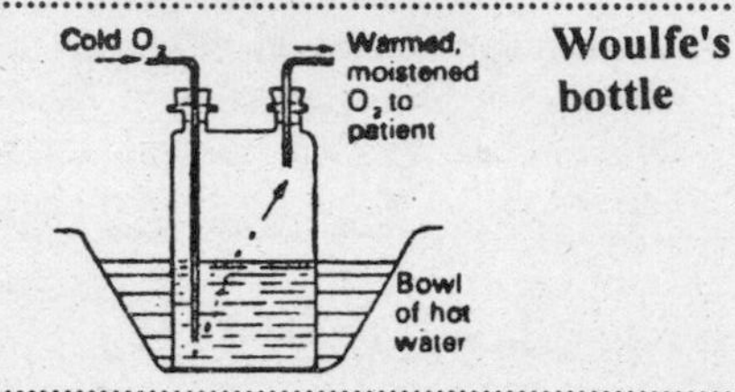

Woulfe's bottle

وولفی بوتل: گیسیں دھونے کے لئے مخصوص بوتل۔

Wrist *(rist)* [A.S. *writham,* to twist]. The carpus (q.v.).

کلائی: کارپس۔

Wryneck *(ri-nek)* See TORTICOLLIS.

گردن سیخی: ٹوریٹیکولس۔

Wyovin *(wi-o-vin)* Diclyclomine (q.v.).

وایوون: ڈائی سائیکلومین۔

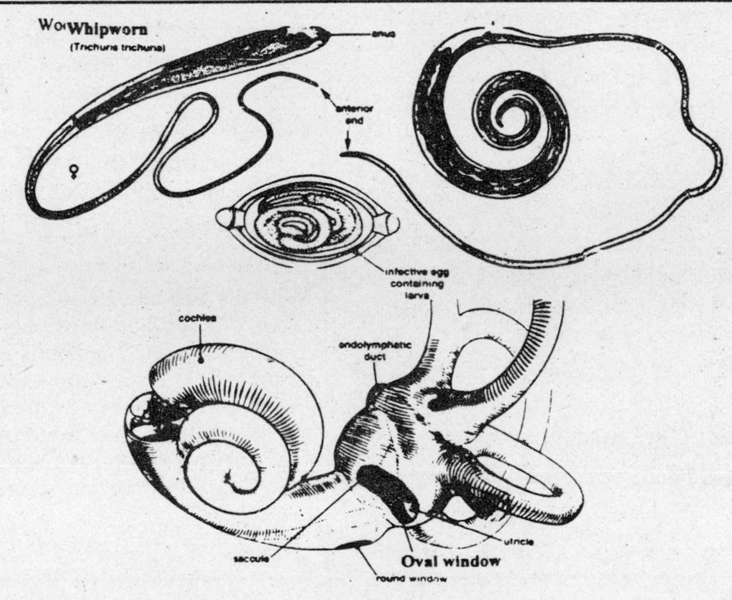

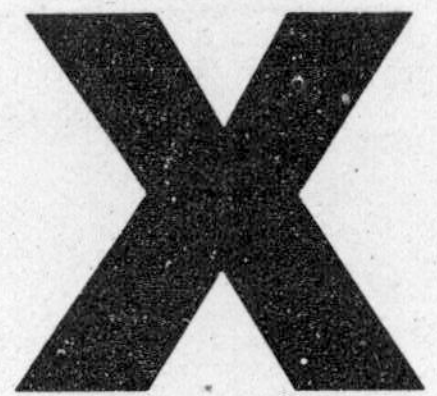

Xanthelasma *(zan-thel-az-ma)* [G. *xanth,* elasmaplate]. Planer xanthome involving the eyelids called also x. papebrarum and xanthome palpebrarum.

زردانہ، جفن: زینتھوما کی ایک ورائٹی۔

Xanthine *(zan-then)* [G. *xanthos,* yellow-named fromthe yellow color of its intrate]. A purine base found in most body tissues and fluids and urinary calculi. The meethylated xanthine compounds and their derivatives are used in medicine for their bronchodilator effects.

صفور افراز: ایک پیلا احل پذیر ہیٹر وسائیکلک مرکب ڈائی آکسیپورین جو جگہ، عضلہ، لبلبہ اور پیشاب میں پایا جاتا ہے۔ اس کے بعض حاصلات پیشاب آور ہیں۔

Xanthoma *(zan-thoma)* A tumor composed of lipid laden foam cells, which are histrocytes containing cytoplasmic lipid material.

زرد رسولی: جلد کے نیچے کولیسٹرول کا مجموعہ۔

Xenon *(ze-non)* [G. *xenos,* stranger]. A chemically inreactive gaseous element found in atmosphere. Its atomic number is 54, atomic weight is 131.30 and symbol is Xe. It is an anaesthetic agent.

زینان: ایک عنصر۔ جوہری وزن ۱۳۱٫۳، جوہری عدد ۵۴، ایک غیر عامل گیس۔ ہوا میں بالکل معمولی مقدار میں ہوتی ہے۔ بعض تھرمیانک والو، روشنی دینے والی ٹیوبیں اور روشنی والے بلب اس سے بھرے جاتے ہیں۔ سن کرنے کے لئے مستعمل۔

Xenopsylla *(zenop-sila)* [G. *psylle,* flea]. A genus of fleas including more than 30 species, many of which transmit disease producing micro-organisms. **X-cheopis**, a rat flea of worldwide distribution. It transmits plague and murine typhus.

Xantheiasma of eyelids

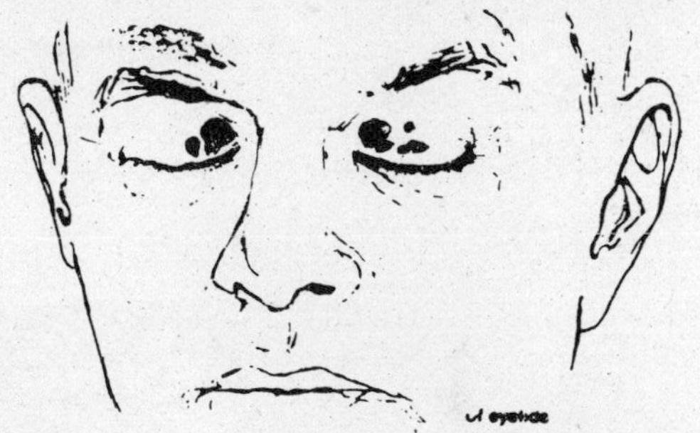

چوہے کا پسو: چوہے کا پسو جو طاعون پھیلاتا ہے۔

Xeroderma *(zero-der-ma)* [G. *derma,* skin]. A mild form of ichthyosis, markeed by a dry, rough, discolored state of the skin, with the formation of a scaly desquamation. **X-pigmentosum,** a rare pigmentary and atrophic autosomal recessive disease, due to extremocutaneous photosentivity to ultraviolet light. It begins in childhood with excessive freckling, telangiectases keratoses, papillomas and malignancies.

خشکی جلد: جلد کی خشکی اور کھردراپن۔

Xerosis *(zer-o-sis)* [G. *xeros,* dry; *osis,* condition]. Abnormal dryness as of the eye, mouth and skin.

جفاف، رمد خشک: خشکی۔

Xerostomia *(ze-ros-to-mi-a)* [G. *xeros,* dry; *stoma,* mouth]. Dry mouth.

خشکی دہن: خشک منہ۔

X-rays. Short rays of electromagnetic spectrum.

لاشعاعیں، ایکس ریز: برقی مقناطیسی طیف کی چھوٹی شعاعیں۔ وہ اس وقت پیدا ہوتی ہیں، جب کسی مادی شے کے ساتھ الیکٹرون ٹکراتے ہیں۔ ایکسریز فولڈ جسم کے تقریباً ہر حصے کا لیا جا سکتا ہے اور مرض کی تشخیص ہو سکتی ہے۔

Xylene *(zi-len)* A clear inflammable liquid resembling benzene. Has been used as an ointment in pediculosis.

زائیلین: زائیلول۔ ڈائی میتھائل بینزین ٹالوین سے مشابہ مائع جو کولتار، میں ہوتا ہے۔

Xylocaine *(zi'-lo-kan)* Lignocaine (q.v.).

زائیلوکین: لگنوکین۔

Xylol *(zi-lol)* Xylene (q.v.).

زائیلول: زائیلین۔ ڈائی میتھائل بنزین۔ ٹالوین سے مشابہ مائع جو کولتار میں ہوتا ہے۔

Xylotox *(zi-lo-toks)* Lignocaine (q.v.).

زائیلوٹاکس: لگنوکین۔ گوشت سن کرنے کے لئے مستعمل۔ دانت نکالنے اور چھوٹے اپریشنوں میں اس کا ٹیکہ لگایا جاتا ہے۔

XYY syndrome. Syn., Klinefelter's syndrome (q.v.).

ایکس وائی وائی سنڈروم: سنڈروم کلائین فیلٹر۔

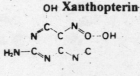

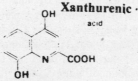

Xanthopterin

Xanthurenic acid

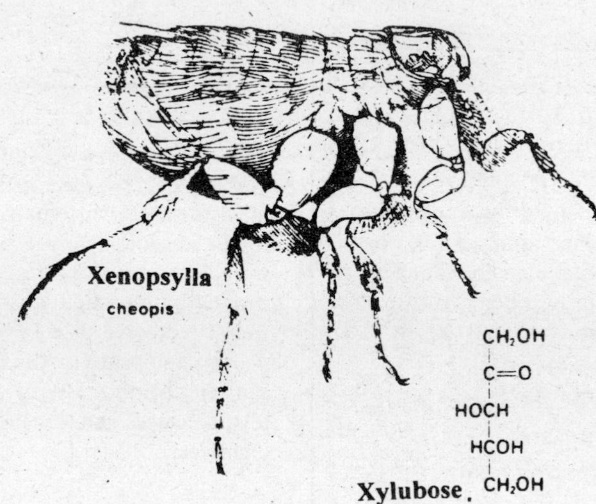

Xenopsylla cheopis

Xylubose

Y

Yaws *(yawz)* An endemic, infectious, tropical disease caused by treponema pertenue, usually affecting persons under the age of 15. It is characterized by the appearance at the site of inoculation of the spirochete which enters the body through abraded skin of a painless papule that grows into a papillome. This heals, leaving a scar. This produce of positive wassermann test in blood.

خط استوائی مرض: ایک ٹراپیکل مرض جو آتشک سے مشابہ ہے۔

Yeast *(ye'st)* It is a single celled rounded fungi that produce by budding. Fermentation is caused by the yeast.

خمیر، ییسٹ: یک خلوی فنگس، اس کی جماعت ایسکو مائی سیٹس ہے۔ تولید بڈنگ کے ذریعہ ہوتی ہے۔ اسے تجربات کے لئے فضا میں لے جایا جاتا ہے۔ سیکرومائیسیز تخمیر کرتا ہے۔

Yellow fever It is a disease of tropical areas. Arbo-virus B is the cause and spread by mosquitoes. It is markedy by jaundice, black vomit and anuria. A variant killed virus is used for vaccine preparation.

زرد بخار: ٹراپیکل علاقوں کا ایک مرض جو مچھر کے ذریعے پھیلتا ہے۔ یہ مرض ایک مخصوص وائرس کی وجہ سے ہوتا ہے۔ ۵ روز تک تیز بخار، پیشاب میں البومن، نبض ست، کمزوری، کالا پاخانہ، کالی الٹیاں، اس کی علامات ہیں۔

Yersinia *(yar-sin-e-a)* [A. E. Yersin, Swiss bacteriologist in Paris 1863-1943]. (It is an alternative name for Pasteurella).

یرسینیا: سوئیڈن کے ماہر بیکٹریالوجی اے ای یرسن کے نام پر۔ یہ دراصل پاسٹوریلا کے متبادل نام ہے۔

Yomesan *(yo me·san)* Trademark for the preparation of niclosamide.

یومیسین: نکلوساما ئیڈ۔

Yttrium 90 ***(90y)*** *(i'tre-am 90)* A very rare metal, allied to cerium symbol Y, atomic number 39, atomic weight 88.205. 90y is a radioactive isotope of yttrium that has an atomic mass of 90 and a half life of 64 hours and emits beta radiation. It is used for cancer therapy.

اٹریم ۹۰: مادّہ جو ۶۴ گھنٹوں کی نصف حیات کے ساتھ بیٹا ذرّات خارج کرتا ہے۔

Z

Zactane *(zak-tan)* Zactirin; Trade mark for the preparation of ethoheptazine citrate.

زیکٹرین: ایتھوہیپٹازین۔

Zarontin *(zaron-tin)* Trademark for the preparation of ethosuximide.

زیرونٹن: ایتھوسکسمائیڈ۔

Zinamide *(zena-mt'do)* Trademark for the prepa- ration of pyrazinemide.

زینامائیڈ: پائیرازنامائیڈ۔

Zinc Oxide *(zingk oksi'd)* A powder used topically as an astringent and protectant in various cutaneos conditions. It is added in all skin relievers, like Calamine, Lassar's paste and Unna's paste.

زِنک آکسائیڈ: سفید قلمی سفوف۔ نقطہ پگھلاؤ ۱۹۷۵ °س۔ کاسمیٹکس، ادویات اور شیشے کی صنعت میں کثرت سے استعمال ہوتا ہے۔

Zinc peroxide *(zingk par-oksi'd)* A white to yellowish white odorrless powder used in pharmaceuticals. It is a good antiseptic of long duration.

زِنک پرآکسائیڈ: دافع تعفن عمل والا سفید سفوف، ہائیڈروجن پرآکسائیڈ سے مشابہ لیکن ایکشن میں طویل اور آہستہ۔ مرہم، لوشن اور ماؤتھ واش کے طور پر مستعمل۔

Zinc stearate *(zingk ste-ar-at)* A compound of zinc with variable proportions of stearic acid and palmitic acid, containing 12.5 to 14.0 percent of zincoxide. It is used as a dusting powder.

زِنک سٹیئریٹ: ایکزیما میں ڈسٹنگ پوڈر کے طور پر مستعمل۔

Zinc sulfate *(zingk sal-fa't)* The heptehydrat zinc salt of sulfuric acid, used as an astringen for the mucous membranes, especially fo those of the eye, being considered specific fo conjunctivitis due to Hemophilus duplex. I has been used in various dermatological prep arations and internally as an antiemetic.

فید توتیا: سفید حل پذیر قلمی سفوف۔ پلیٹنگ، ادویات اور کاغذ کی صنعت ں استعمال کیا جاتا ہے۔

Zingibar *(zin-ji-bar)* It is the chemical name c ginger.

رک: ادرک۔ سونٹھ۔

Zollinger Ellison Syndrome *(zol-in-jar-eli-so sindrom)* [Robert Millon Zollingar, America surgeon 1903-1992, Edwin H. Ellison, Amer can surgeon 1918-1970]. It is a triad compris ing (i) intractable, sometimes fulminating an in many ways atypical peptic ulcers (2) extre me gastric hyperacidity and (3) gastrin-secre ing, non-beta islet cell tumors of the pancrea which may be single or multiple, small c large, benign or malignant. The gastrinom sometimes occurs in site (duodenum) othe than the pancreas. Diarrhoea may be one c symptoms. Peroral biopsy may help in dia nosing.

ولنکر ایلی سن سنڈروم: لبلبی آئیلیٹس آف لینگر ہانز کا السری ناسور۔

Zona *(zo-na)* [G. *zone,* belt]. A zone; a girdl herpes zoster. **zone pellucida,** the vitellin membrane surrounding the ovum.

حلقہ، منطقہ: ایک زون، گرڈل۔ ہر چیز زا سٹر۔ گول ساخت۔

Zonula ciliaris *(zon'-u-la-si-li-ar-is)* Suspensory ligament attaching periphery of lens of eye to ciliary body (q.v.).

حلقیزہ مژگاں: متعلق لیگامنٹ جو آنکھ کے عدسے کی جانب کو ہدبی جسم کیساتھ ملحق کرتا ہے۔

Zonule *(zon'-ul)* Small zone, belt or girdle. Zonula.

حلقہ، گھیرا، منطقہ صغیرہ: چھوٹا زون، بیلٹ یا گرڈل۔ گول ساخت۔

Zonulolysis *(zon-ul'-ol-is-is)* [L. *zone,* belt; G. *lysis,* a loosening]. Breaking down the zonula ciliaris—sometimes necessary before intracapsular extraction of the lens—zonulolytic, *adj.*

زونولولائی سس: زونولا سلی اریس کی شکستگی۔

Zoonosis *(zo-on-o'-sis)* [G. *zoon,* animal; *-osis,* condition]. Disease in man transmitted from animal. Abbattoir and farm workers at risk—zoonoses, *pl.*

مرض حیوانی: حیوان سے انسان میں منتقل ہونے والا مرض۔

Zygoma *(zi-go'-ma)* The cheekbone—zygomatic, *adj.*

زائیگوما: رخسار کی ہڈی۔

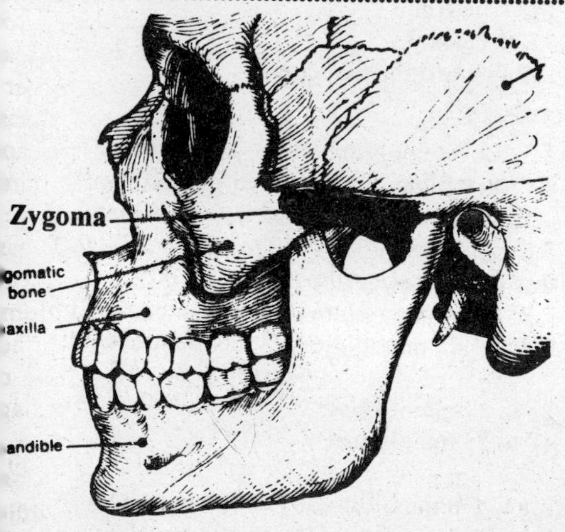

Zygote *(zi'-got)* [G. *zygon,* yoke]. The fertilized ovum.

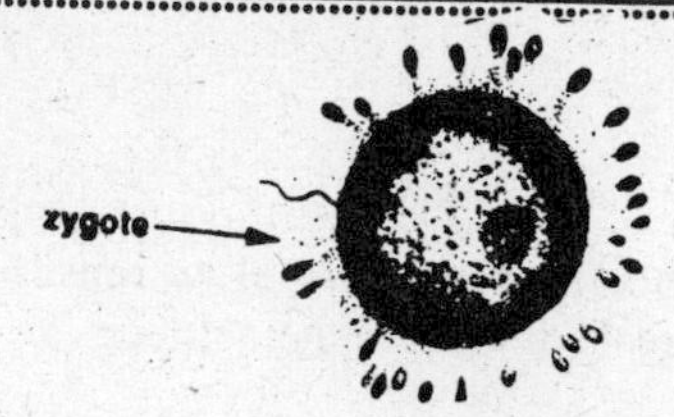

زائیگوٹ: بارور بیضہ۔ گیمیٹوں کے ملاپ سے زائیگوٹ وجود میں آتا ہے جو بلاواسطہ نیا فرد بناتا ہے۔ زنانہ عضو تناسل کے اندر داخل ہو کر سپرم کا نوک دار سر رحم کے بیضہ میں داخل ہوتا ہے۔ جب سپرم بیضہ میں داخل ہوتا ہے تو زائیگوٹ بنتا ہے جو فلوپین ٹیوب سے رحم کی طرف سفر کرتا ہے اور مختلف حصوں میں تقسیم ہوتا چلا جاتا ہے۔ ایک سے دو پھر دو سے چار اور چار سے آٹھ خلیے بنتے ہوئے خلیوں کا ایک گچھا سا بن جاتا ہے جسے مورولا کہتے ہیں۔ وہ ٹیوب میں سے گزر کر رحم میں آجاتا ہے۔ یہ سفر تقریباً تین چار روز میں مکمل ہوتا ہے۔

Zyloric *(zi-lor'-ik)* Allopurinal (q.v.).

Zymogen *(zi'-mo-jen)* The granular precursor, within the secretory cell, of enzymes.

خمیر زا مادہ، زائموجن: اخراجی خلیے میں ہی خامرات کا دانہ دار پیشرو۔

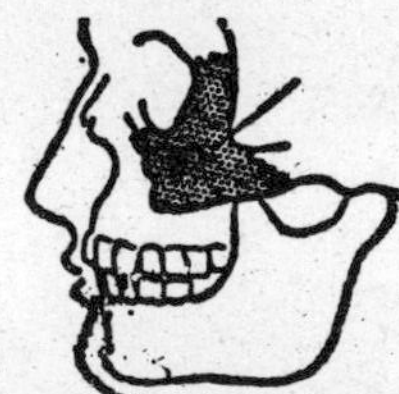

Zygomatic Bone

Appendices

Appendix 1

Blood

The figure given below represent the approximate ranges of normal values for the constituents of the peripheral blood.

RED CELLS

Haemoglobin	12 to 16 g per 100 ml
Red Cells	4.5 to 6.0 millon per mm^3
Reticulocytes (new formed red cells)	less than 1 percent of total red cells
Mean cell volume (MCV)	75 to 90 um^3 is the average volume of a single red cell
Packed cell volume (PCV or Haematocrit)	35 to 55 percent
Mean cell dianeter (MCD)	6.7 to 7.7 um
Mean cell haemolglobin concentration (MCHC)	30 to 38 percent

WHITE CELLS

Total white cells	4,000 to 11,000 per mm^3
Neutrophils	60 to 70 percent
Lymphocytes	25 to 35 percent
Basophils	1 percent
Eosinophils	1 to 4 percent
Monocytes	4 to 8 percent
Platelets (thrombocytes)	150,000 to 350,000 per mm^3

Blood Chemistry

Urea	2.5 to 7.5 mmol/litre (15 to 45 mg/100 ml)
Uric acid (men)	0.15 to 0.4 mmol/litre (2.5 to 7 mg/100 ml)
Uric acid (Women)	0.1 to 0.35 mmol/litre (1.5 to 6 mg/100 ml)
Cholesterol (at 20 years of age)	3.6 to 5.7 mmol/litre (140 to 220 mg/100 ml)
Bilirubin1	less than 17 umol/litre (1 mg/100 ml)
Calcium	2.25 to 2.6 mmol/litre (9.0 to 10.4 mg/100 ml).
Phosphate	0.8 to 1.45 mmol/litre (2.5 to 4.5 mg/100 ml)
Bicarbonate (CO_2)	
(Adults)	23 to 31 mmol/litre)
(Children)	18 to 23 mmol/litre)
Fasting blood sugar (glucose)	
(Adults)	3.6 to 5.6 mmol/litre (65 to 100 mg/100 ml)
(Children)	2.2 to 5.6 mmol/litre (40 to 100 mg/100 ml)
Potassium	3.5 to 5.5 mmol/litre
Sodium	133 to 144 mmol/litre
Chloride	96 to 106 mmol/litre

Total Plasma Proteins	6 to 8 g/100 ml
Albumin	3.3 to 5.5 g/100 ml
Globulin	1.5 to 3.3 g/100 ml
Fibrinogen	0.2 to 0.4 g/100 ml

Appendix 2

A Guide to the use of Drugs

Control over the use of drugs

Modern drugs are often powerful chemical products which can be highly effective in the treatment or control of human diseases, but may also be dangerous if used inexpertly. Trials of a new drug can take place on animals but only on humans after the drugs are shown to be safe. Even then untoward side - effects may become apparent after some years of use or possibly effects on the fetus if the mother takes the drug during pregnancy. Other side-effects can only be linked with the causative drug if a careful record is kept of all unexpected signs and symptoms occurring during the treatment of an illness with any drug.

The use of a number of drugs at the same time may be complicated not only by the identification of side-effects but also by the interaction of one drug wiht another,

The possibility of addiction to a drug or depondence on it must be considered. It has been known for a long time that such dependence could develop to powerful narcotics such as morphine and heroin when used nedically. It is now also known to occur with barbiturates, amphetamines and to an increasing extent with tranquillizers and non-barbiturate sedatives.

Drugs provided in good faith by a doctor may be abused in various ways by a patient. The doses may be taken in the wrong amount or at the wrong times. The medicine may be stopped too soon. Tra nquillizers, anti-depressants and sedatives are increasingly taken in overdoses as part of a suicidal intent.

Descriptions of drugs

The availability of drugs changes from one month to the next and the proprietary names of the drugs differ from one country to another. In all countries up-to-date indexes are available of drugs and their dosags. No attempt will be made here to give a comprehensive list drugs but some indication is given of the types of drugs in general use.

Dosage of drugs

The recommended dosage of any particular drug will normally be provided by the manufacturer; this may be given in a state d number of mg or ml per kg body-weight of the patient in 24 hours. This dose may be expected to produce a certain level of the drug in the blood strem.

There are idiosyncrasies in the absorption of drugs and the same dose may produce different blood levels in two patients of the same weight. It must also be remembered that diseases of the liver and kidneys may slow the breakdown and excretion of the drug from the body and result in a dangerously high level in the blood stream.

DRUGS ACTING AGAINST INFECTION

There are now drugs which are active against all bacteria; but some bacteria become resistant become resistant to many drugs and also the drugs often have side-effects as well as showing interaction with other drugs.

The main groups of antibiotics are the penicillins, the cephalospins the aminoglycosides and the tetracyclines.

The *pencillins* act by interfering with the formation of the bacterial cell wall. Pencillins are commonly used in infections with Gram positive organisms. The dose depends on the type and site of infection and on the partivular penicillin being used. Penicillin is often effective when given orallyh but may be used intramuscularly of intravenously. The penicillines used include benzylpencillin, methicillinm amoxycillin and ampicillin.

The most serious side-effect of penicillin is hypersensitivity which can cause rashes, an anaphylactive reaction or death. Once a person has developed a hypersensitivity to pencillin it will remain not only to the particular penicillin used but to all other drugs in the group of penicillins. any patient who develops such a sensitivity should be informed and his case records should be clearly mark.

The cephalosporins act in a similar way to penicillin but are active against Gram negative as well as Gram positive organisms. Those used include cephaloridine, cephalothin and cephalexin. They are often the first alternative drug used if the infection is resistant to penicillin.

Hypersensitivity is the main side-effect and a few patients who are sensitive to the penicillin are also sensitive to the cephalosporins.

The *aminoglyccsides* are active against Gram positive and Gram negative infections. They include streptomycin, kanamycin, neomycin and gentamicin. These drugs can cause deafness and kidney damage. They should be avoided if there is impaired function of the kidneys, in the elderly and in pregnant women.

The tetracyclines include tetracycline, oxtetracycline and chloretracycline and are active against Gram positive a nd Gram negative organisms. This group is used less than formerly because of increasing knowledge about side-effects.

Tetracyclines are laid down in bones and teeth and can cause discoloura tion of the teeth. They should not be given to children or to pregnant women. Diarrhoea due to changes in the bacterial content of the bowel can be a troublesome side effect.

Other groups of antibiotics

The macrolydes, of which erythromycin is the most important member. It is active mainly against Gram positive organisms and is useful in respiratory and middle ear infections. If can often be used as an alternative to penicillin if a patient is sensitive to penicillin.

The lincomycins include lincomycin and clindamycin. They are active against Gram positive organisms and being well concentrated in bone are useful for the treatment of bone and joint infections.

Diarrhoea is common with lincomycin and can be very severe and difficult to treat.

Chloramphenicol is a dangerous antibiotic because it can cause fatal aplastic anaemia. It should only be used in the treatment of typhoid fever or severe infections with *H. influenzae*.

The sulphonamides are bacteriostatic rather than bacteriocidal. The most commonly used sulphonamide is sulphadimidine. It is useful for treating urinary infections. Co-trimoxazole, which contains a sulphonamide, may be used on a long-term basis for the control of recurrent urinary infections.

Toxic side-effect include reashes and allergy to sunlight.

ANTIFUNGAL AGENTS

Griseofulvin is effective when taken by mouth in the treatment of fungal infections of the hair and nails.

Nystatin is used in the local treatment of candida infections of the skin and nucous membranes. *Clotrimazole* can also be used locally for the trea tment of candida infections.

ANTI-TUBERCULOSIS PREPARATIONS

Streptomycin, sodium aminosalicylate, isoniazid, ethambutol and rifampicin are the usual lrugs available for the treatment of tuberculosis. It is customary to use a combination of three of hese drugs until reports on the drug sensitivity of the causative organism are available. The course of drugs is usually completed with a combination of two effective drugs. The cost of these drugs in he correct dosage for a period of up to 18 months may preclude their use.

ANTI-AMOEBIC PREPARATIONS

Metronidazole is most commonly used for the trea tment of amoebic dysentery. If nausea is roublesome emetine may be used as an alternative. Emetine must be given by subcutaneous njection.

ANTIMALA RIALS

TREATMENT

Chloroquine is frequently used for the initial treatment of most forms of malaria, but quinine nay still be used.

After the initial treatment, primaquine may be used for 14 days in the benign forms of malaria.

PROHYLAXIS

Various drugs including chloroquine and proguanil are used. The recommended drugs, dosage and period to take them varies according to current reports and advice from the World Health Organiza tion. In most instances it is advised that the drug should be taken from the day before entering a mala nal zone until at least 30 days after leaving it.

TAPEWORMS

Niclosamide or dichlorophen kill the worm which is then partially digested adn excreted.

ROUNDWORMS

Piperazine is the most commonly used drug for the treatment of roundworm infesta tion in both adults and children. Bephenium granules or thiabendazole are aqlternative drugs.

HOOKWORMS

Bephenium granules or tetrachloroethylen may be used. The anaemia which is associated with hookworm infections must also be treated.

THREADWORMS

These are a common occurence in children and cause itching round the anus particularly at night. The whole family should be treated with viprynium or piperazine.

DRUGS ACTING ON THE ALIMENTARY SYSTEM

Antacids

These are the most effective drugs in relieving the pain due to gastric or duodenal inflammation or ulcera tion. The drugs most commonly used include sodium bicarbonate, aluminium hydroxide and magnesium trisilicate or magnesium carbonate.

Ulcer healing drugs

Various derivatives of the liquorice plant are used to speed up the healing of an ulcer. The use of these drugs must be limited and carefully supervised because they have serious side-effects.

Antispasodics cause a reduction of secretions and movements in the alimentary canal. Those used include belladonna and dicyclomine. Their use is limited by side-effects which include blurrec vision and an increased heart ratte.

Pancreattin

Strong pancreation preparations are used to make up for reduced or absent secretions from the pancreas which can occur following surgical removal of the pancreas or in cystic fibrosis in infants.

Drugs used to relieve diarrhoea

Antibiotics are now used less frequently for the treatment of diarrhoea even when the cause is known to be bacterial. The most important part of treatment, particularly in the infant, is the replacement of lost fluid.

Drugs used to control the symptoms of diarrhoea include kaolin, codeine phosphate and methy cellulose.

Laxatives

Laxatives are frequently misused and many patients with constipation would be more suitably treated by changing their diet and increasing its bulk.

Liquid paraffin softens hard stools and eases their passage. methyl cellulose increases the bulk of stools and also softens them. Cascara, rhubarb and senna active as irritant of the bowel muscle and none of these drugs should be sued for a prolonged period of time.

Drugs acting on the rectum and anus

Prednhisolone enema is useful in the treatment of ulcerative colitis.

Ittching of the anus should be diagnosed before treatment is given. the symptom can be controlled by the use of a steroid-contaning ointment or suppository. Preparations containing a loca anaesthettic can be used for a very short time to relieve the pain caused by a crack but should not be continued because they are likely to cause sensitization.

DRUGS ACTING ON THE CARDIOVASCULAR SYSTEM

Heart failure

Digoxin is used in nearly all cases of heart failure because it increases the force of the contraction of the heart muscle and reduces the heart ra te. In excessive doses it can cause nausea loss of appetitte and slowing of the heart rate to an undesirable extent.

DIURETICS

Retention of fluid in the tissues is often caused by heart failure but can also be caused by othe diseases including liver or kidney failure.

The tthiazides, which include chlorothiazide and hydrochlorothiazide, are effective for abou 12 hours. Potassium should be given when using these diuretics because they cause an excessive loss.

Frusemide has a more rapid action than the thiazides and also a stronger action, it may be useful for initial but not for maintenance treatment.

DRUGS WHICH DECREASE MYOCARDIAL EXCITABILITY

These drugs can be used when there is irregularity of the heart beat but should only be used after a precise diagnosis has been made. The drugs include lignocaine, procainamide, propranolo and exprenolol.

Drugs reducing blood pressure or antihypertensives

There are many views about how frequently and to what extent a raised blood pressure shoul be reduced by drugs. In the elderly the disadvantages may outweigh the advantages. A reduction in body-weight and giving up cigarette smoking may be more beneficial than the use of drugs.

Methyldopa, clonidine, propranolol, bethanidine or guanethidine may be used, sometimes in addition to diuretics, to cause a reduction in blood pressure.

The amount of drug necessary must be checked regularly by taking the blood pressure while the patient is standing, sitting and lying, and also before and after exercise.

DRUGS FOR ANGINA PECTORIS

Glyceryl trinitrate is usually the most effective drug in relieving the pain of angina pectoris. The drugs causes relaxation of all smooth muscle and is best taken prophylactically before the patient carries out any activity likely to provoke the pain.

Propranolol, oxprenolol and clofibrate may also be used.

Anticoagulants

These drugs are more useful in controlling venous rather than arterial thrombosis. The drugs may be used prophylactically to prevent clotting or for treatment after a clot has been diagnosed.

Heparin can be used initially but must be given intravenously and carefully controlled.

The oral anticoagulant drug most commonly used is warfarin.

DRUGS ACTING ON THE RESPIRATORY SYSTEM

Cough expectorants and suppressants combination.

Expectorants, which aid the coughing up of sputum, include potassium iodide and ipecacanha. Suppressants, which are used to stop a persistent cough, include codeine and pholcodine.

Bronchodilators

These are drugs which imitate sympathetic or adrenergic action. They may be used in asthma to dilate the bronchi and aid the passage of air.

The drugs used include adrenaline, which may be given subcutaneously or in an aerosol, ephedrine, which can be given by mouth but which can cause urinary retention and sleep disturbance and isoprenaline which can be given sublingually or in an aerosol. The dosage of isorprenaline in an aerosol must be carefully controlled because too large a dose to toxic to the heart muscle and can be fatal.

Salbutamol is used commonly either in tablets or as an aerosol. It is less dangerous than isoprenaline but aerosol dosage should be controlled.

Aminophylline can be given by intravenous injection or rectal suppository.

Corticosteroid drugs

These drugs are sometimes life-saving in the treatment of a severe attack of asthma or in status asthamitcus. They may sometime be used in the long-term management of asthma.

Hydrocortisone can be given intravenously in emergencies in the treatment of asthma.

Prednisolone may be given orally in a short course in the treatment of asthma or used for a more prolonged period in the management of severe asthma, if prednisolone is used for a long time the side-effects can include growth retardation in children.

The aerosol, beclomethasone dipropionate, is now being used successfully for many asthmatics. It provides the advantages of steroids in its direct action on the branchial mucosa without the problems of the side-effects when taken by mouth.

Sodium cron.oglycate is a prophylactic drugs which must be taken regularly and not kept until an attack of asthma starts, it must be inhaled but a child a of 5 years can usually be taught how to manage.

DRUGS ACTING ON THE NERVOUS SYSTEM

Analgesics

These may be of the following kinds:

1. Acting peripherally and used for mild or moderate pain.
2. Acting centrally and used for severe pain.
3. Acting at a specific site, such as ergotamine tartrate for migraine.

1. PERIPHERALLY ACTING ANALGESICS

Aspirin is one of this type of analgesic, it is also an anti-pyretic and has anti-inflammatory properties. Its side-effects include indigestion, anaemia from acute or chronic blood loss from the wall of the intestine and pasthma.

Paracetamol does not cause indigestion or intestinal bleeding but is toxic to the liver when taken in excessive doses.

The drugs are better taken alone rather than in combination with other analgesic drugs.

2. CENTRALLY ACTING ANALGESICS

Morphine is a very effective analgesic when given subcutaneously but it also causes respiratory depression and is potentially a drug of addiction.

Diamorphine is shorter acting, there is more danger of addiction and it is usually only used for pain relief in terminal illnesses. Pethidine can be given orally or subcutaneously. It is not as potent an analgesic as morphine and there is also the possibility of addiction.

3. SITE-SPECIFIC PAIN RELIEF

Ergotamine tartare, clonidine or methysergide can be used for the relief of pain in migraine.

Trigeminal neuralgia may be relieved by carbamazepine.

Hyponttics, sedatives and minor tranquillizers

Sleep difficulties are better resolved by finding the cause and treating that than by giving drugs.

Barbiturates are effective hypnotics but their use is now discouraged because they can cause addiction and may be taken in overlarge doses. Their action is increased by alcolol.

Benzodiazepines may be used either during the day as sedatives or at night as a hypontic. They are replacing the barbiturates.

Other sedactives include chloral preparations and some antihistamines.

Major tranquilizers

The most important group of these drugs are the phenothiazines which include chlorpromazine, prochlorperazine and trifluoperazine. Their main use is in the treatment and control of psychotic mental illness.

Chlorpromazine may be used with analgesics to control severe pain during terminal illness.

Antidepressants

TRICYCLIC ANTIDEPRESSANTS

These drugs are useful in the treatment of severe depression and may be used instead of, or with, electroconvulsive therapy. The drugs used include imiprmine and amitriptyline. The total daily dose of the drugs can be given at night when their main side-effect of causing drowsiness can be an advantage. These drugs need to be taken for about a fortnight before there is obvious clinical improvement.

Monoamine oxidase inhibitors (MAOI) which include phenelzine are used in depressive states infrequently because they have potentially fatal side effects when taken with some foods and other lrugs.

.ITHIUM CARBONATE

This compound is sometimes used for the control and prevention of recurrent attacks of lepression or for swings from depression to mania.

Anticonvulsants

If possible an accurate diagnosis of the type of epilepsy should be made before drugs are started having selected a suitable drug the patient must be supervised regularly to make sure that the fits are controlled without causing unpleasant side-effects.

Phenobarbitone may still be used to control grand mal attacks of epilepsy but phenytoin and sodium valproate are now more commonly used.

Ethosuximide can be used in petit mal and sulthiame in temporal lobe epilepsy.

The benzodiazepines may be useful in the control of fits.

Drugs used in Parkinsonism

Drugs are used which restore a correct balance between dopamine effects and cholinergic effects in the brain. The drugs which increase the dopamine effect include levodopa and amantadine. The drugs which reduce the cholinergic effect include benzhexol, benztrolpine and orphenadrine.

ORAL CONTRACEPTIVES

These are tablets containing an oestrogen or a progestogen which, when taken orally the required number of days each month, prevent conception. A combination of the drugs is more effective than either alone. The amount of oestrogen in each tablet should not exceed 50 micrograms and many preparations contain 30 micrograms.

Oral contraceptive increase the risk of vascular thrombosis particularly in women over the age of 35 years, those who are overweight and those who are cigarette smokers.

DRUGS AFFECTING ALLERGIC REACTIONS

Adrenaline may be given subcutaneously in acute allergic reactions including anaphylactic shock and severe asthma.

Antihistamines are useful when taken by mouth in the control of hay fever and cause sensitization. The main side-effect is drowsiness and a warning should be given to thos taking them about driving a car of operating machinery.

Corticosteroids can be given by mouth or in an emergency by intravenous injection. They can also be used locally in the eye, nose or on the bronchial mucosa. They are the most effective drugs in suppressing allergic reactions.

ENDOCRINOLOGICAL PREPARATIONS

Thyroid

Thyroid hormones are used in the congenital or acquired, including surgical, loss of the secretion from the thyroid gland.

Thyroxine sodium or liothyronine sodium are most commonly used.

Antithyroid substances are used to counteract the effects of an overactive thyroid glands. The drugs used include carbimazole, propylthiouracil and propranolol.

Adrenal cortex

When secretion from this area fails due to Addison's disease or surgical removal, the deficiency may be controlled by hydrocortison tables, prednisone or prednisolone. In acute failure of the adrenal cortex cortex coritsone injections may be used for a limited time.

If the secretion from the adrenal cortex is excessive, it may be controlled by dexamethasone or metyrapone.

Good control of either a deficiency or excess needs very careful control.

Insulin

A deficiency of insulin secretion from the pancreas cause diabetes mellitus with impaired digestion of food stuffs, particularly or carbohydrates. The deficiency can sometimes be counteracted by reducing the amount of carbohydrate in the diet but diabetes which occurs in children, young adults and sometimes older adults will need insulin replacement for control of the disease.

Insulin is produced mainly from the pancreas of an animal and in usually of mixed cow and pig origin.

Insulin must be injected subcutaneously, it may be of shortacting duration, soluble insulin, or of longer-acting duration, insulin zinc suspension or protamine zinc insulin.

In a diabetic coma soluble insulin can be injected intravenously or given in a drip.

ORAL HYPOGLYCAEMIC PREPARATIONS

These may be used if diet alone does not control diabetes mellitus in older and usually overweight patients. The drugs used include tolbutamide, chloropropamide and glibenclaimied. Other drug including phenformin and metformin increase the action of remaining insulin.

Female sex hormones

Oestrogen may be given as stilboestrol to stop lactation, it may also be used to control unpleasant menopausal symptoms such as hot flushes.

Progestogen may be given as norethisterone in the treatment of endometriosis.

Male sex hormones

Androgens may be given after castration of the male or in testicular deficiency from other causes. Methyltestosterone can be given by a depot injection.

Posterior pituitary preparations

If the antidiuretic hormone or vasopression is not produced by the posterior pituitary the result will be diabetes insipidus. Vasopressin can be given in various ways including nasally as desmorpressin.

APPETITE SUPPRESSANTS

These drugs should not be used for the control overweight; it is better to instruct the patient about different eating habits. Fenfluramine may be given for a limited time but is best avoided. Amphetamines must never be used because they can cause addition.

DRUGS FOR THE MANAGEMENT OF MALIGNANT DISEASE

The three groups of drugs which can be used are the cytotoxic drugs, the sex hormones and the corticosteroids.

Cytotoxic drugs

These drugs interfere with the reproduction of both cancer cells and norma l body cells. A careful watch must be kept on the cells in the blood while such drugs are being used. The drugs in this group include cyclophosphamide, mercaptopurine, methotrexate, vincristine, chlorambucil and cytarabine. It is usual to give short controlled courses of different combinations of these drugs.

Sex Hormones

Cancer of the prostate can usually by controlled by stilboestrol.

Some cancers of the breast may be helped by mandrolone which is a type of androgen.

Corticostteriods

Prednisone may be used in the acute leukaemias or in breast cancer which has metastasised.

DRUGS USED IN THE TREA TMENT OF ANAEMIA

The type of anaemia and if possible, its cause must be diagnosed before treatment is sta rted with drugs. Ferrous sulphate or ferrous gluconate may be given in iron deficiency anaemias.

For megaloblastic anaemia, vitamin B12 is necessary and can be given as hydroxocobalamin or cyanocobalamin by injection. Folic acid may be necessary to correct some types of anaemia.

APPENDIX 3

Diet

The human does not eat nutrients but food and the type of food eaten varies a great deal from culture to culture. However, certain basic nutrients are necessary for the production of energy, for adequate growth, the replacement of tissues and the maintenance of health.

The basic nutrients include:

1. Carbohydrates. 2. Proteins 3. Fats 4. Vitamins 5. Minerals

1. Carbohydrates

These contain carbone, hydrogen and oxygen, carbohydrates may be eaten as starch or as sugars. Sugars may be disaccharides or monosaccharides. The disaccharides are sucrose, containing one moleclue of glucose and one of fructose; maltose which contains two molecules of glucose, and lactose, which contains gluose and galactose. During digestion carbohydrates are broken down to the monoaccharides, glucose, fructose and galactose. These are used in the body for the production of energy or stored as glycogen.

Carbohydrate is the only nutrient in sugar but is also present in such foods as bread, potatoes, rice and pasta. In these foods'they are other nutrients including protein and vitamins.

The carbohydrates in the food supply from 50 percent to 80 percent of the total daily intake of calories. In weather fat and protein account for a relatively greater number of calories but in poorer countries a larger proportion of calories is obtained from carbohydrates.

Fat-Sluble **Vitamins Table**

Vitamin	Functions	Properties	Deficiency	Sources	Daily Requirements
A	Antiinfective. Essential for healthy skin and mucous membranes. Aids night vision.	Within the body vit. A can be synthesized from carotene, a yellow pigment (provitamin) present in food. Can be stored in the liver.	Poor growth. Rough dry skin and mucous memberane. Liability to infection of skin and mucous membranes. Lessened ability to see in the dark. In severe defieiency xeropthalmia which can lead to bindr ess	All animal fats Carrots Apricots Tomatoes Spinnach Water cress	3000, 5000 iu

D D_2 Calciferol $D_3$7-dehyd-rotachysterol	Antirachite. Assists absorption and metabolism calcium and phosphorus	Prtoduced in the bo-dy by action of sun-light on the ergoste-rol in the skin.	Rickets in children Osteomalacia and osteoporosis in adu-lts.	Oily fish Prepared from the livers of cod and halibut Da-iry Produce	400 800 iu This livel essential for children and nur-sing mothers
E Alpha toc-opherol	Necessary for the re-production of rats; not proven that this is so in human beings		Thought to inter-fere with reprodu-ction; also thought to cause certain egenerative disea-ses of the nerv-ous system and damage to the liver	Wheat germ Milk Cereals Egg Yolk Liver.	
K Menadione K, Phytome-nadione	Antihaemorrhagic Essential for the prod-uction of prothrombin.	Only absorbed in the presence of bile	Delayed clotting time, Liver dam-age	Vegetables with green leaves Peas	
WATER-SOLUBLE					
B Complex B_1 Aneurine or Thiamine B_2 Riboflavin Nicotinic acid	Antineuritic. Antiber-iberi, Health of nervous syst-em. Steady and continuous release of energy from carbohydrates. Antipellagra	Destroyed by exc-essive heat and ba-king soda Can withstand no-rmal cooking	Poor growth. Neuritis. Beri-beri Fissures at corners of mouth and o ı ton-gue. Corneal opacities. Skin manifest-ations (dermatitis). Diarrhoea. Mental symptoms. possibly dementia. Pellagra	Brewer's yeast Cereals Vegetables Eggs Fruit Liver Meat	1 15 mg 1.5 2.5 mg 10.17 mg
B_6 Pyridoxine	Protein metabolism	Relieves postradi-otyherapy	Nervousness and in-somnia		
Folic acid	Assists production of red blood cells		Some forms of macrocytic anae-mia	Green vegetables Liver	
B_{12} Cyanocobalamin	Essential for red blood	Can only be abso-rbed in the prese-nce of the intrinsic factor secreted by gastric cells. Stor-ed in the liver.	Pernicious anae-mia	Liver and all other foods containing B complex	
Cytamen		Maintenance ther-apy for patients with pernicious anaemia.		Prepared from gro-wth of Streptomy-ees	

C Ascorbic acid	Formation of bones. teeth and collagen	Destroyed by cooking in the presence of air and by plant enzymes released when cutting and granting raw lood Lost by long storage	Sore mouth and gums. Capillary bleeding. Scurvy. Delayed healing of wounds	Fresh fruit Fresh vegetables Rosehip and blackcurrant syrups	30 50 mg

2. Proteins

These contain oxygen, hydrogen, nitrogen and sometimes sulphur. They are necessary to the body for growth and repair. Opinions about the amount of protein necessary daily for a human differ widely and the amount suggested has varied from 40 grams to 100 grams. At present in the United Kingdom it is recommended that a fully adult should eat between 60 and 70 grams of protein a day which will supply about 10 percent of his total daily intake of calories. It is possible that humans would be healthier with a smaller amount of protein in the diet. Pregnant and lactating mothers need more protein than other adults.

Protein is made up of twenty-three amino acids and of these eight are called 'essential' amino acids and a further two are 'essential' in children. The term 'essential' is used because the body is unable to synthesize these amino acids and must have them in the food. Proteins were formerly known as first class, or animal, proteins which contained all the essential amino acids, and second class or vegetable proteins which contained some of the essential amino acids. This categorization has now stopped because it is realized that a varied intake of vegetable proteins including cereals and pulses can contain all the essential amino acids. The quantity and this can be a disadvantage.

Protein is used in the body for growth and repair and any excess is used up for energy or stored as fat.

3. Fats

All fats are made up of a mixture of glycerol and fatty acids but the characteristics of the fatty acids differ. A fatty acids but the characteristics of the fatty acids differ. A fatty acids is formed from a chain of carbon atoms with hydrogen and oxygen. A saturated fatty acid is one in which all the bonds is double; a poly-unsaturated fatty acid is one in which there are two or more double bonds.

Fat is found in dairy products such as milk, cream, cheese and butter; but it is also present in and around meat, in nutts, pulses and in some fish including herring and salmon.

There are three poly-unsaturated fatty acids esential for health and these are linoleic acid, linolenic acid and arachidonic acid.

The amount of fat tha t is necessary in the diet for health is not known. Cultural factors and the family income cause a wide variation in intake.

Fats are emulsified by the bile salts in the digestive tract and then broken down by lipase into glycerides, glyceerol and fatty acids.

Fats form the main supply of stored energy in the body. When it is metabolized one gram of fat produces twice as many calories as a gram of protein or a gram of carbohydrate. Fat is also a source of vitamins A.D.E and K.

4. Vitamins

These are a small but necessary part of the diet. The results of vitamin deficiencies were recognized in most cases before the chemical structure of the vitamin had been established. They were called A, B, C etc., but this, in the light of later knowledge, has led to some confusion in the nomenclature.

FAT SOLUBLE VITAMINS

Vitamin A is uspplied to the body in food as retinol and carotene. It is present in animal fats such as halibut and cod liver oil, milk, butter and cheese. It is also present in carrots and green vegetables with dark green leaves such as spinach.

2500 International Units (IU) are necessary each day. Deficiency causes night blindness, hardening of the skin and the covering of eye which can cause blindness. A deficiency is rare in the developed countries.

An excess of vitamin A, which can occur if children are given too large an amount, can cause irritability, loss, of appetite, an itching skin and swellings over the bones.

Vitamin D is supplied to the body in animal fats including milk, butter and cheese, it can also be made by the body when the skin is exposedc to ultraviolet light.

The recommended daily intake of vitamin D for infants is 400 International Units and for adults 100 International Units.

A deficiency of vitamin D in children causes rickets; and in malnourished women who have a number of pregnancies it can cause osteomalacia.

An excess of vitamin D occurs through overdosage of small children and can cause irritability, loss of appetite, loss of weight and occasionally death.

Vitamin E is associated with fertility in rats but in humans its use is still uncertain.

Vitamin K. A deficiency of vitamin K in the human is associated with impaired clotting of the blood. The deficiency is unlikely to be caused by a low intake and is probably due to a defect in its use by the body.

THE WATER SOLUBLE VITAMINS

Vitamin B is now known to be a collection of different vitamins.

Vitamin B^{1} or thiamine is necessary for the metabolism of glucose in the body and is probabgly of particular importance in the nourishment of nerve cells. A regular supply of this vitamin is needed because very little is stored in the body. It is present in a wide variety of foods including unrefined cereals, potatoes, green vegetables and milk.

A deficiency of this vitamin is very rare in the United Kingdom unless a patient is not taking food. A deficiency is common in poorer countries particularly if rice or other cereals are refined. Beriberi is the result of deficiency.

There used to be a vitamin known as B^{2} but it is now know to be a group of vitamins of which the most important is riboflavine. It source and used are similar to those of thiamine. Deficiency, which is rare in the United Kingdom, causes cracks at the corners of the mouth, a sore, red tongue and a dry, scaly skin.

Nicotinic acid is present in unrefined cereals and dairy products.

Deficiency is most common in rice-eating countries and causes pellagra. Exposed areas of the skin become pigmented and scaly, there is diarrhoea and there may be severe mental symptoms including depression.

Vitamin B^{6} is rather like vitamin E. its use is established in animals but in humans it is not yet understood. It is widely available in vegetables.

Vitamin B^{12} is present in meat and is necessary for the formation of blood cells.

A deficiency occurs because it is not absorbed through the stomach wall and its lack causes pernicious anaemia. Replacement must be by repeated injections.

Folic acid is also necessary for the formation of blood cells.and it, is widely acaible in vegetables.

A deficiency may occur in pregnant women and iron and floic acid may be given routinely during pregnancy to prevent anaemia.

Vitamin C or ascorbic acid is necessary for the healthy development of collagen in the body; this invludes bones, teeth and the lining of blood vessels.

It is present in all fruits and vegetables particularly citrus fruits.

The human adult needs about 30 mg a day and in the United Kingdom a quarter of this amount is normally supplied by potatoes.

A deficiency of vitamin C causes survey and the disease is most commonly seen in elderly people who have an insufficient dientary intake.

5. Minerals

There, like vitamins, are essential in the human diet for normal development and health; less, however, is known about many of them than about some vitamins.

Sodium or salt is to be found in all body fluids and the greater amount of it is in the extra-cellular fluid. The amount remains constant in the healthy adult. Sodium acts with potassium to stablize food may eat up to 10g.

The daily intake necessary is about 1g but some people who like salty food may eat up to 10g.

Potassium acts with sodium to keep a constant acid base balance in the bldy. Potassium is found mostly in intra-cellular fluid. Potassium is present in most foods that humans ea th including fruit, vegetables a nd cereals.

A deficiency is unlikely to be due to a low intake but to an excessive loss from the body as may occur in severe diarrhoea or while taking diuretics.

Calcium is present in the greatest quantity of all minerals in the body. Most of it is in the teeth and bones.

The daily intake necessary is probably about 500mg but it has been suggested tha t 1000mg could be necessary. It is present in large amounts in dairy foods, particularly cheese, and in hard water and in many vegetables.

A deficiency of calcium is sedom due to a lack in the dietary intake but to a defective use in the body as may occur in diseases of the parathyroid.

Phosphorus forms compounds with calcium in the bones and teeth. It also takes part in cell metabolism and reproduction. It is widely available in the diet and the body can deal with an excess by excretion in the stools or urine.

Iron is necessary in the body for the forma tion of haemoglobin. The daily intake needs to be about 10mg and probably up to 20mg in pregnant women. It is present in meat, liver, bread and vegetables.

A decficiency intake causes one type of anaemia but in the United Kingdom this type of anaemia is more often due to an acute or chronic loss of blood than to a low intake of iron.

Iodine is vital to the body for the production of thyroxin by the thyroid gland. In most parts of the world it is present in the earth and water and vegetables in in the diet have absorbed it. In areas where there is a shortage of iodine in the soil, humans may develop enlargement of the thyroid gland.

Fluorine occurs naturally in some soils and therefore in some water supplies. If it is present in a quantity of about one part per million of water it lessens the incidence of dental caries. If present in amounts of 4 or 5 p.p.m it can cause mottling of the teeth.

DIET FOR OBSETY

The problem of being overwight is largly one of more affluent countries. It is usually caused by eating more than is necessary coupled with a sedentary way life. Crash diets are of iittle use and a change in eating habits is necessary for the maintenance of permanent weight reduction.

During weight reduction the total intake of calories should be limited to 1000 calories a day and a steady weight loss of 1 to 2lb a week is sufficient.

A normal pattern of eating should be observed and the total calories divided between three or four meals. The following foods should be omitted entirely:

Sugar, cakes, biscuits, sweet puddings
Alcohol
Fried foods
Chocolate, sweets, etc.
Jam, honey, marmalade, syrup, etc.
Dried fruits
Potato crisps
Sweet canned or bottled drinks

When the target weight has been reached the daily diet may be increased but the above foods are better omitted. A weekly check should be kept and a stricter diet started if the weight is increasing.

DIABETIC DIETS

A detailed description of a diabetic diet will not be given because physicians managing diabetes usually have their own methods of controlling diet.

The principles of any diabetic diet are the restiction of starches and sugars. The quantity allowed in the diet each day must be eaten and at regular intervals; this is important if insulin is being used. In children it is more difficult to keep an exact control of these food but it is best to encourage the diabetic child to take an early, responsible sha re in the management of his diet.

In all diabetic diets it is usual to aim at a daily fixed total calorie intake which may be about 1800 kcal. This amount will vary with the sex, size and occupation of the patient. The diet is usually made up of about 210g of carbohydrate, 80g of protein and 70g of fat.

Carbohydrate is the nutrient which must be most carefully controlled and it is common to work out system of diet 'exchanges' based on the quantity of a food which contains 10g of carbohydra te.

The daily intake of milk will be controlled at about 3/4 pint and of butter at 1/2 oz.

It is usual to give the patient guidance about the following groups of foods which may also be controlled by the 'exchange' system.

1. Food which may be eaten in an unlimited quantity, including tea and coffee without sugar and with milk from the daily allowance, clear soups, cheese, fish, meat, eggs and most vegetables.
2. Foods which may be eaten in moderation including all carbohydrate foods, fresh and dried fruit, pasta, thick soups, 'diabetic' foods and dry wines and sherry.
3. Foods to be avoided include sugger, sweets, jum, syrup, sweet puddings, ice-cream, sweet wines and sherry, spirits and liquenrs.

This diet is increasingly used in constipation and in diverticulitis. It should include a large proportion of foods which are rich in fibres and relatively low in calories. These foods include:

Porrindge and muesli
Bran which can be used in baking
Wholemeal flour and bread
Fresh and dried fruit
Vegetables and pulses
Unrefined rice

GLUTEN FREE DIET

This diet is used in the management of coeliac disease and in other condition in which the bowel is unable to deal with glutein. Gluten; a plant protein, is found in wheat, rye and garley. It is made of two parts, glutemin and gliadin, and it si the latter which is harmful. Flour can be produced which is free of gluten and this flour must be used in all baking for a patient who is unable to tolerate gluten. Very small amounts of gluten can be harmful, tinned foods, sauces, etc, which contain normal flour must be excluded from the diet.

LOW SATURATED FAT DIET

This diet may be used in the management of diseases of the blood vessels and in multiple sclerosis. Fats to be avoided are those of animal origin and those which are solid at room temperature. Structurally the fats to be avoided are those that are saturated and the fats to be included in the diet are the mono-unsaturated or preferably the poly-unsaturated fats. The fats to be avoided a re fa t on meat, butter, lard, cream, cheese and bacon. Milk should be skimmed and not more than two eggs should be eaten a week.

Sunflower see oil is the best oil to use in the preparation of food and one of the varieties of poly-unsaturated margarine must be used instead of butter on bread and in baking.

Fatty fishes to be avoided include mackerel, herring and salmon; also all fish canned in oil such as sardines and tuna fish.

LOW RESIDUE AND HIGH PROTEIN DIET

This diet may be used in the management of ulcerative colitis. All food that are high in fibre content should be avoided. These include urefined cereals, wholemeal bread, vegetables, fruit and dried fruit and units. Fried food should also be avoided.

There should be an increased intake of lean meat, milk, fish, cheese (apart from cream cheese), eggs and refined cereals.

INTRAVENOUS FLUIDS

Fluid may be given intravenously to replace losses of body fluid, to replace lost blood and to keep a balance of fluid and electrolytes in those patients who are unable to take solid or liquid food by mouth.

Great care must be taken in children and in those patients with heart or kidney disease when giving intravenous fluids.

For infants and children the exact requirements of fluid must be calculated from the child's weight and the composition of the fluid must be adjusted in association with the acid base balance of the blood which should be menitored every 4 hours, together with the electrolyte measurements.

The following intravenious solution may be used in adults according to need:

1. Sodium chloride solution when there is fluid and salt loss. Sodium lactate may be added.

2. Dextrose 5% solution can be used to replce wa ter loss and provide some nourishment. Sodium chloride and dextrose may be used together.
3. Potassium chloride may be added to sodium chloride or dextrose solution to replace potassium lost in the urine or in diarrhoea.
4. Sodium bicarbonate solution and sodium lactate are used to correct acidosis after estimation of the acid base balance in the blood.
5. Dextran solution can be used for the emergency increase of the blood volume after haemorrhage and when blood is not immediately available.

If intravenous feeding needs to be continued for a period of time the caloric needs of the patient can be supplied by the addition of a solution of synthetic amino acids and emulsdied fats to the intravenous fluids.

Some drugs can be added to intravenous fluid; others have undesirable side-effects or lose their potency when added to intravenous fluids. These action should be checked before any drug is added in this way.

APPENDIX 4

Poisoning; some common causes, symptoms and treatment

In all cases of poisoning, certain general principles should be followed. It is a common misconception that for each poision there is a specific antidote. In practice, a true pharmacological antagonist is available in only 2.0 percent on poisonings. In the great majority of instances, therefore, the treatment consists primarily in the application of basic principlies of supportive treatment. If the poison is a gas, or the vapour of a volatile liquid, the patient must be removed at once to fresh air and given oxygen and artificial respiration if needed. Subsequent treatment is supportive to maintain vital functions. If the poison has been ingested in most cases it is necessary to remove as much as possible of the unabsorbed substance from the stomach. Outside hospital this is best achieved by aspiration and lavage should be given provided the patient retains an adequate cough and gagreflex, or is sufficiently unconscious to allow the introduction of a cuffed endotracheal tube to protect the airway. These procedures should only be performed with the patient lying on his side with the head dependent. An adequate size of tube must be used, e.g. if an adult 30 English gauge, and 300 ml quantities of lukewarm water should be used for lavage until the recovered fluid runs clear. As a general rule nothing should be left in the stomach after lavage for fea r of subsequent vomiting and pulmonary aspira tion. Emetic drugs have been enthusiastically recommended to avoid the use of gastric aspiration and lavage. A pomorphine may cause prolonged vomiting which may result in shook and should not be used. Copper salts have been advised as an emetic in children but are uncertain in their effects, slow in action, and as significant absorption may result in toxicity are best avoided. Syrup of ipecacuanha is quite widely used in a dose of 15 ml followed by 200 ml of water, and provided its limitations are recognized is the treatment of choice in children. The onset of its emetic effect is usually delayed for about 18 min and occasionally it may produce undesirable toxic effects after absorption.

Common errors in treatment

1. Analeptic therapy. Bemegride is not a specific barbiturate antagonist and its use in poisonings due to hypnotic drugs is associated with frequent serious side effects including cardiac arrhythmias, convulsions and even irreversible brain damage. The use of analeptics cannot be jsutified.

2. *Bladder Catheterization.* This highly dangerous procedure is seldom necessary even in deeply unconscious patients. With adequate nursing care, there should be no undue risk of skin breakdown due to incontinence of urine. Bladder catheterization is justified in prolonged bladder distension and occasionally when forced diuresis therapy is being given.
3. *Prophylactic Antibiotics.* With good nursing care, including frequent turning of the patient and careful attention to mouth hygiene prophylactic administration of antibiotics is unnecessary. These drugs should be given only when there is clear clinical or X-ray evidence of infection.

Sinstamce	Clinical Features	Treatment
Acids Strong hydrochloric acid. Spirits of salts. Strong sulphuric acid (oil of vitriol). Strong nitric acid. (See separate heading for oxalic acid) **Alkalis** Caustic soda (sodium hydroxide). Caustic potash (potassium hydroxide). Strong ammonia.	Severe burning of mouth and throat, causing dyspnoea due to oedema of glottis. Severe abdominal pains, thirst, shock, dark and bloodstained vomit, gastroenteritis	Plenty of water to dilute the poison. *Acids:* Neutralize with cream of magnesia or calcium hydroxide (56g to 1/2 litre of warm water). Carbonates, as chalk, sodium bicarbonate and washing soda also effective, but cause liberation of carbon dioxide. Soap can be used if no other alkalia available. *Alkalis:* Neutralize with acetic acid (56 g to 1/2 litre), or vinegar (112 g to 1/2 litre); lemon juice also effective, if available in sufficient quantity. General measures include morphine for pain, and arachis or olive oil as demulcent.
Amphetamine and related substances	Alertness, tremor, confusion, delirium, hallocinations, panic attacks, lethargy, exhaustion, headache, sweating, cardiac arrhythmias, hypertension or hypotension, dryness of mouth, diarrhoea and abdominal colic, ulcers of the lips in addicts, convulsions and deep unconsciousness.	Gastric aspiration and lavage. If markedly excited chlorpromazine i.m. is the most effective treatment. Intensive supportive therapy. Forced acid diuresis.

Anticoagulants Pheninione Warfarin Rodenticides	Haematuria, haemoptysis, bruising and haematemesis; occasionally bleeding elsewhere. Orange yellow urine. Prolonged prothrombin time.	Gastric aspiration and lavage. Vit. K_1 25 mg i.v. Blood transfusion if necessary.
Antidepressants Amitriptyline Impiramine Nortriptyline Desipramine Nortriptyline Desipramine Trimipramine Doxepin Protriptyline	Dryness of the mouth, dilated pupils tachycardia leading to bizarre cardiac arrhythmias, hypotension, caridac failure or arrest, urinary retention, varying degrees of unconsciousness, pressure of speech, increased limb reflexes, convulsions, torticollis and ataxia. Respiratory failure. Cardiac complications are common and particularly dangerous in children.	Gastric aspiration and lavage. Intensive supportive therapy. In the majority of patients these measures are all that are necessary. The central nervous system effects and some of the cardiac abnormalities can be abolished by the slow i.v. injection of physostigmine salicylate 1-3 mg, which may be repeated once after 10 mm. If ineffective, convulsions may be controlled by diazepam 10 mg i.v. or sodium phenobarbitone 300 mg i.m. *B*-Adrenergic blocking drugs may correct difficult caridac arrhythmias.
Antihistamines	In adults, toxic doses cause deep central depression. In children and infants, the effect is often stimulatory, and confusion and convulsions may result. Hypotension, tachycardia and occasionally cardiac arrhythmias. Respiratory depression. Dryness of the mouth, nausea and constipation. Hyperpyrexia. Agranulocytosis and aplastic anaemia may develop.	Intensive supportive therapy. Gastric aspira tion and lavage. Sedation may be required in the form of diazepam. Antibiotics, steroid drugs and blood transfusion may be necessary in severe blood dyscrasia.
Atropine Belladonna Scopolamine Homatropine Propantheline Deadly Nightshade Barbiturates	Blurring of vision, ataxia, mental confusion, hallucinations. Tachycardia, hypertension, cardiac arrhythmias. Dyness and burning of the mouth with marked thirst, nausea and	Intensive supportive therapy Gastric aspiration and lavage. Peripheral effects may be relieved by subcutaneous injection of neostigmine 0.25 mg When central nervous stimulation is marked', sedation

Long-acting: Barbitone Phenobarbitone *Medium-acting:* Allobarbitone Butobarbitone Amylobarbitone *Short-acting:* Pentobarbitone Cyclobarbitone Quinalbarbitone *Ultra-short-acting:* Hexobarbitone Thiopentone	vomiting. Urinary urgency and possible acute retention. Hyperpyrexia. Death usually results from respiratory failure. Impaired level of consciousness. Limb reflexes very variable. Withdrawl fits and delirium during the phase of recovery occur in patients habituated the drug. Cardiovascular depression with hypotension and 'shock'. Respiratory depression. Hypothermia. Renal failure. Bullous lesions occur in 6 percent of patients with this condition.	with a short-acting barbiturate or diazepam may bc necessary. Physostigmine salicylate (1-4 mg) i.m. or i.v. will rapidly antagonize the central nervous complications, but repeat doses may be required every 1 to 2 hours. Intensive supportive therapy. Gastric aspiration and lavage. Forced osmotic alkaline diuresis and/or haemodialysis are of value in patients sreverely poisoned with longacting barbiturates but are less effective with the other types.
Benzodiazepins	Physical dependence may occur when the drug has been taken for sometime. Also an additive effect occurs when taken in combination with alcohol, barbiturate, phenothiazine, monoamine oxidase inhibitors and imipramine. Loss of consciousness, bradycardia and hypotension. Respiratory depression.	Intensive supportive therapy. Gastric aspiration and lavage.
Bleaches (a) Containing sodium hypochlorite	If inhaled: Cough and pulmonary oedema. If ingested: Irritation of the mouth and pharynx; oedema of pharynx a nd larynx. Nausea and vomiting.	Gastric aspiration and lavage using 2.5 percent sodium thisulphate (if not available milk or milk of magnesia). If severely ill sodium thiosulphate (1 percent) 250 ml i.v.
b) Containing oxalic acid	Irritation of the mouth and throat. Nausea and vomiting. Muscular twitchings and convulsions. Shock and cardiac arrets. Acute renal failure the onset of which may be delayed.	Intensive supportive therapy. Gastric aspiration and lavage adding 10 g calcium lactate to the lavage fluid. Calcium gluconate 10 percent 10 ml i.v. and repeat as necessary. Provided the renal output is adequate at least 5 litres of fluid should be given for three days.

Carbamates Meprobamate Ethinamate Methylpentynol	Impairment of consciousness, muscle weakness and incorr- dination, nystagmus. Respira tory depression. Hypotension. Hypothermia. With drawal fits may occur.	Intensive supportive therapy. Gastric aspiration and lavage. Forced osmotic alkaline diuresis in severely poisoned patients and, if ineffective, haemodi- alysis.
Carbon monoxide and coal gas	Vertigo and ataxia; acute agitation and confusion; deep coma may develop. Papiloe- dema, increased limb reflexes and possible extensor plantar responses. Acute myocardial infarction, tachycardia, arrhy- thmias and hypotension. Resp- iratory stimulation, which may progress to respiratory failure. Nausea, vomiting, haematemesis and faecal incontinence are common. Bullous lesions may occur. Sequelae include Parkin- sonism, hemiparesis and imp- airment of higher intellectual function.	Urgent. Remove from exposure. Intensive supportive therapy. Give a mixture of 95 percent O_2 and 5 percent CO_2. In the presence of cerebral oedema 500 ml of 20 percent manifol i.v. over 15 min followed by 500 ml 5 percent dextrose over the next 4 hours.
Chlorate salts	Nausea, vomiting, colic and diarrhoea. Jaundice and hepatic failure. Methaemoglobinaemia. Oliguria or anuria. Initial confusion followed by convul- sions and coma.	Intensive supportive therapy. Gastric aspiration and lavage. If .cyanosis severe, methylene blue 2 5 ml of 1 percent solution, slowly intravenously. Forced diuresis and/or haemodialysis in severe poisoning. Conventional treat- ment for hepatic or renal failure
Contraceptive-pills	Mild nausea or vomiting. Withdrawal bleeding in girls may occur.	Intensive supportive therapy. Gastric aspiration and lavage.

Cresol Phenol Lysol	Strong smell of carbolic acid in patient's breath or vomit. Corrosion of lips and buccal mucosa but little pain. Marked abdominal pain, nausea and vomiting. Haematemesis or gastric perforation. After absor- ption, initial excitement then impaired consciousness. Hypotension. Dark urine, oliguria and renal failure. Liver failure may common cause of death.	Intensive supportive therapy. Gastric aspiration and lavage with care. Wash ulcers with copious water or 50 percent alcohoi. Medical measures for hepatic and renal failure. Haemodialysis may be required.
Cyanide	Very toxic. *Mild Poisoning:* Headache, dyspnoea, vomiting, ataxia and loss of consciousness occur gradually. *Severe poisoning:* The above fea tures develop very rapidly and the patient becomes deeply unconscious. The smell of bitter almonds is not necessarily present. The skin remains pink unless breathing has ceased. Rapid, thready pulse. Hypotension. Limb reflexes are often absent and the pupils are dilated.e	Speed is essential. As long as the heart sounds are audible, recovery may be anticipated with appropriate treatment. Four forms of treatment are available: (1) if the poisoning is due to inhalation, remove from contaminated atmosphere. (2) Break an ampoule of amyl nitrite under the patient's nose whilst applying artifical respiration where this is necessary. Also inject 10 ml 3 percent sodium nitrite intravenously. (3) Very slow infusion of 25 ml 50 percent sodium thiosulphate. (4) If the poison has been ingested, gastric aspiration and lavage should also be done and 300 ml 25 percent sodium thiosulphate should be left in the stomach. An emergency kit containing the above solution is commercially available and should

		be part of the equipment of al causualty Departments. An alternative to nitrit treatment is the use of Keloc yanor (cobalt edetrate). Many consider this to be the treatmen of choice. Initially 40 ml (60 mg) is given i.v. over 1 min Hypotension and nausea may be produced but recovery usually i very rapid. If this does not occu within 1 to 2 min a further 20 m (300 mg) is given i.v. immediately followed by 50 ml 5 percent doxtrose i.v.
Detergents	Nausea, vomiting and diarrhoea. Most are not very toxic	Supportive therapy.
Digitalis	Nausea and vomiting, diarrhoea. Bradycardia. Cardiac arrhythmias. Mental confusion.	Intensive supportive therapy. Gastric aspiration and lavage. Potassium chloride 1.0 orally every 20 min; if vomiting occurs 1 g in 200 ml 5 percent dextrose infused over 30 min. Lignocaine 500 mg in 500 ml saline dextrose i.v. administered at a rate depending on the clinica response is the best treatment fo ventricular ectopics. Atropine sulphate 0.6 mg i.m repeated as necessary for bradycardia. Cardiac pacing may occasionally be required.
Glutethimide	Similar to barbiturate poisoning, but depth of coma may vary considerably. Suddent apnoea may occur, probably due to sudden raised intracranial pressure. Pupils dilated and unresponsive to light. Hypotension may be severe. Myocardial infarction may occur.	Intensive supportive therapy Gastric aspiration and lavage. I there is any suspicion of raise intracranial pressure give 500 m 20 percent mannitol i.v. over 2 min followed by 500 ml 5 percent dextrose over next hourse.

Iron salts	*Stage 1.* Epigastric pain, nausea and vomiting. Haematemesis. Tachypnoea and tachycardia. *Stage 2.* An interval of hours or even several days may elapse during which there are no further signs and symptoms. Then severe headache, confusion, delirium, convulsions and loss of consciousness. Respiratory and circulatory failure. *Stage 3.* If patient survives, liver failure and renal failure may occur.	water. Afterwards 10 g desferrioxamine should be left in the stomach. Immediately inject desferrioxamine 15 mg/kg per hour to a maximum dose of 80 mg/kg per 24 hours. Medical measures for hepatic and renal failure may be necessary.
Laburnum	Burning in mouth, nausea, intractable vomiting, diarrhoea, exhaustion and collapse. Delirium, convulsions and coma.	Intensive supportive therapy. Gastric aspiration and lavage.
Lead	Severe abdominal pain, vomiting, diarrhoea, oliguria, collapse, coma. 'Shock' and hepatic failure may occur. Acute haemolytic anaemia	Intensive supportive therapy. Gastric aspira tion and lavage. When colic is severe calcium gluconate (10 percent) 10 ml i.v. Calcium disodium versenate (Versene) 75 mg per kg body weight i.v. in 24 hours plus BAL 24 mg per kg in 24 hours. This regimen should be continued for 3 to 5 days. Peritoneal or haemodialysis in severe poisoning.
Methyl aicohol Methanól Wood alcohol	Headache, blurring of vision which may lead to blindness, dilatation of pupils and papilloedema, loss of consciousness. Nausea and vomiting Hyperventilation.	Intensive supportive therapy. Gastric aspiration and lavage. Ethylalcohol 50 percent 1 ml per kg stat. then 0.5 ml per kg every 2 hours. If impaired vision, peritoneal dialysis or haemodialysis is essential.

xMethaqualone	Hypertonia, myoclonia, extensor plantar responses, papilloedema and impairment of level of consciousness. Tachycardia, acute myocardial infarction. Respiratory depression. Bleeding tendencies may occur.	Intensive supportive therapy. Gastric aspiration and lavage. Haemodialysis in severe poisoning.
Opium alkaloids Diamorphine Morphine Pethidine Codeine Dipipanone Pentazocine Propoxyphene	Impaired level of consciousness; pinpoint pupils. Convulsions may occur particularly in young children. Respiratory and circulatory depression. Methaemoglobinaemia may occur	A true antidote is available. Intensive supportive therapy. Gastric aspiration and lavage. Naloxone 0.4 mg i.v. and 0.8 mg repeated i.v. 3 min later is usually sufficient to re-establishment normal respiration and conscious level.
Organophosphorous compounds	These insecticides are very toxic. Headache, restlessness, ataxia, muscle weakness, convulsions. Salivation, nausea, vomiting, colic and diarrhoea. Bradycardia, hypotension, peripheral circulatory failure. Bronchospasm, cyanosis, acute pulmonary oedema. Respiratory failure is the usual cause of death.	Intensive supportive thereapy. Gastric aspiration and lavage if ingested. As soon as cyanosis is corrected, atropine sulphate 2 mg i.v. and repeated at 15-min intervals until fully atropinized. Pralidoxime 30 mg per kg i.v. slowly and repeat half-hourly as necessary. If sedation or control of convulsions is required, short-acting barbiturates may be used but with the greates caution.
Paracetamol	Pallor, nausea and sweating. Hypotension tachycardia and other cardiac arrhythmias. Excitement and delirium progressing to CNS depression and stupor. Hypothermia, hypoglycaemia and metabolic acidosis. Tachypnoea. Haemolysis. Renal failure. Jaundice and hepatic failure,	Intensive supportive therapy. If the plasma paracetamol half-life is greater than 4 hours cyteamine hydrochloride 2.0 g i.v. over 10 min followed by three 400 mg doeses in 500 ml of 5 percent dextrose i.v. over 4, 6 and 8 hours has been shown to reduce and even prevent liver damage. Intravenous infusion of

	which is the commonest mode of death. Seventy of poisoning best assessed on blood levels. If the plasma paracetamol level is above 2000 mol per litre and especially if the plasma half- life is great than 4 hours hepatic damage is likely.	sodium bicarbonate to correct acidaemia, i.v. glucose for hypoglycaemia, and if haemolysis is severe corticosteroids and blood transfusion may be necessary. Haemodialysis may be required for renal failure.
Paraquat	Burning sensation in mouth at time of ingestion. After a few hours painful buccal ulceration develops. Several days after ingestion a progressive alveolitis and bronchiolitis is probable and is the usual cause of death. Severe renal and hepatic impairment may occur.	Careful gastric aspiration and lavage. If paraquat ingested within 2 hours leave 500 ml of 7 percent bentonite suspension in stomach. Intensive supportive therapy. Immediate forced diuresis is safe before renal damage occurs.
Petroleum distillates	Nausea, vomiting and diarrhoea. If inhaled or aspirated, intense pulmonary congestion and chemical pneumonitis. Depression of consciousness and respiration with occasionally convulsions.	No gastric aspiration or lavage. 250 ml liquid paraffin orally. If pneumonitis, hydrocortisone 100 mg i.m. 6-hourly for 48 hours with antibiotics as indicated. Mechanical ventilation may be necessary.
Phenothiazines	Impaired level of consciousness, Parkinsonism, torticollis, oculogyric crises, restlessness and convulsions. Hypotension, tachycardia, cardiac arrhythmias. Hypothermia. Respiratory depression in severe poisoning.	Intensive supportive therapy. Gastric aspiration and lavage. Convulsions should be treated with diazepam and if this fails, with barbiturates. Cogentin (benztropine mesylate) 2 mg. i.v. is effective for Parkinsonism
Phenytoin	Stimulation and possibly euphoria, vertigo, headache, cerebellar ataxia, nystagmus, tremor, loss of consciousness. Nausea, and vomiting. Respiratory depression	Intensive supportive therapy. Gastric aspiration and lavage.

Primidone	Similar to phenytoin but loss of consciousness tends to be more marked.	Intensive supportive therapy. Gastric aspira tion and lavage. Forced alkaline osmotic diuresis or haemodialysis may be necessary in severe poisoning.
Quinine and quinidine	Tinnitus; blurred vision; headache and dizziness. Impaired consciousness; rapid, shallow breathing, cardiac arrhythmias and arrest may occur. Acute haemolysis and renal failure	Intensive supportive therapy. Gastric aspiration and lavage. ECG monitoring is required and cardiac arrhythmias treated with appropriate drugs. In marked visual impairment stellate ganglion block may produce drama tic improvement. Forced acide diuresis may be of value in severe poisoning.
Sallicylate Acetyl sallicylate Methyl salicylate Sodium salicylate	Alertness and restlessness, tinnitus, deafness. Hyperventilation. Hyperpyrexia and sweating. Nausea and vomiting. Dehydration and oliguria. Unconsciousness may occur in severe poisoning; hypoprothrom binaemia occurs in some patients. Hypokalaemia may be severe. Metabolic acidaemia and hypoglycaemia are often marked in children.	Gastric aspiration and lavage in all patients. Forced alkaline diuresis if the plasma salicylate is above 3.6 mmol per litre. In very severe poisoning haemodialysis. Intensive supportive therapy.
Snake bite Adder bite (Viper berus)	Local features; Swelling, pain and redness. General features: Agitation, restlessness, abdominal colic, vomiting and diarrhoea. Collapse an drespiratory failure may result	Specific antivenom should not be used as serious anaphylactic shock may result unless in the severly ill patient when only the Zagreb antivenom should be given by i.v. infusion. Cleanse the site and immobilize the bitten part. Hydrocortisone 100 mg i.m. Antibiotics and tetanus antitoxin should be given. Intgensive supportive therapy.

Thiazides	Polyuria, dehydration, hypokalaemia hyponatraemia, hypochloraemia and alkalaemia. Acute renal failure may occur. Also acute hepatic failure is occasionally found and in susceptible patients an acute attack of gout may result.	Intensive supportive therapy. Gastric aspiration and lavage. Potassium chloride 2 g 3-hourly depending on the degree of hypokalaemia Intravenous fluids may be necessary to correct dehydration.

APPENDIX 5

Side-room Testing

Tests that are carried out in ward side-rooms, surgeries and other places without full labora tory facilities are mainly concerned with urine, but some quick tests are available for use on blood, serum, plasma and faeces. This section, therefore, starts with urine analysis, and has two shorter sections a t the end dealing respectively with tests for glucose, ketones and urea in blood, serum or plasma, and for blood and sugars in faeces.

A. Urine testing

COLLECTION OF URINE SPECIMEN

Fresh specimens of urine should be used for all tests, because changes in the composition occur when the urine is allowed to stand, especially if it is infected. The complete specimen should be well mixed, but not centrifuged or filtered, before taking out a portion for testing.

The specimen container should be absolutely clean and free from contaminants, e.g. antiseptics or detergents, and nothing should be added to the specimen before analysis.

PHYSICAL EXAMINATION

Physical examination of the urine should include noting its quentity, colour, odour, sediment after a portion has been left to settle, and specific gravity.

Quantity The output of urine of a normal adult over 24 hours averages between 1200 and 1500 ml, and depends on fluid intake and the amount of fluid lost from the body by routes other than the kidney, such as perspiration. The amount excreted can very also in nervous and hysterical states, in various diseases and according to climatic conditions. Some drugs can increase or decrease the volume of urine.

Colour The colour of normal urine is usually amber but can vary from pale straw to brown. It is caused by various pigments, primarily urochrome which is always present in normal urine. The colour may be affected by various factors in the following ways.

Greenish-orange, caused by bile

smoky or pale reddish, caused by blood

whitish opalescent, caused probably by pus

Very pale amber, caused by dilution as a result of polyuria

Various shades resulting from igestion of drugs.

Odour In certain diseases the characteristic smell of normal urine may be altered. For examples, in diabetic ketoacidosis the urine smells of acetone and in cystitis it has a fishy odour.

Sediment A pinkish curdy deposit is caused by an excess of urates, and a white sediment usually indicates phophates.

Specific gravity The specific gravity (sp.gr.) of normal urine varies between 1.015 and 1.025. As a general rule, the greater the volume of urine passed the lower is its sp. gr., and where there is diminished volume of urine, as a febrile states, the sp. gr. will be higher. Occasionally, as in diabetes milhtus, there is increased volume of urine with a high sp. gr.

The sp. gr. is taken with a urinometer (hydrometer) as shown in the diagram. This is floated in the urine, care being taken to prevent it touching the side of the test glass used. The urine must be allowed to reach room temperature before its sp. gr. is read. The reading taken is the level of the bottom of the meniscus of the urine on the scale up the stem of the urinometer; it is important that this is done with at eye level with the liquid surface.

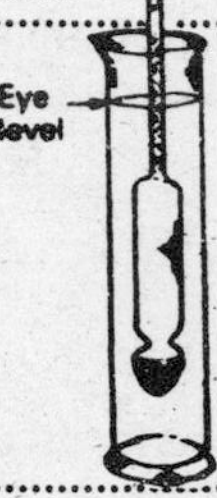

If there is insufficient urine to float the urinometer, either use a narrower urinometer or, after the chemical testing has been done, dilute the urine with an equal amount of water, measure the sp. gr. of this and correct it by doubling the last two figures of the reading.

The osmolaity of urine may sometimes be more informative than its sp. gr., but is less easily measured.

CHEMICAL ANALYSIS

Routine chemical analysis of urine generally includes testing for pH (acidity), protein, reducing sugars, glucose, ketones, blood, bilirubin, urobilinogen and nitrite (as an indication of infection). In some instances other tests may be required as well, and these are mentioned at the end of the section, e.g., tests for phenylketones, chlorides.

Usually it is sufficient to obtain semiquantitative or even qualitative estimates of urinary components. The older 'side-room' tests are described, and the Ames strip or tablet tests. Ames strip tests for pH, proteins, glucose, ketones, blood, bilirubin, urobilinogen and nitrite are available, singly (in most cases) or in varous combination on multiple-test strips up to N-Multistix strips, which carry all the above eight; for simplicity, the single tests will be described under the heading for each substance to be investigated. When using any Ames test it is important to follow exactly, the instructions for use and for preservation of the product in good condition, and to check that the product is within its expiration date shown on the label. Instructions for the Ames tablet tests are given individually in the sections which follow; those for the strip tests are similar for all of them and can be summarized thus;

(a) Completely immerse all reagent areas of the strip in fresh, well-mixed, uncentriduged urine and remove immediately.

(b) Tape edge of strip against the side or urine container to remove excess urine. Hold the strip in a horizontal position to prevent possible soliling of hands with urine or mixing of chemicals from adjacent reagent areas, making sure that the test areas face upwards.

(c) Compare test areas closely with corresponding colour charts on the bottle label at the times specified. Hold strip close to colour blocks and match carefully.

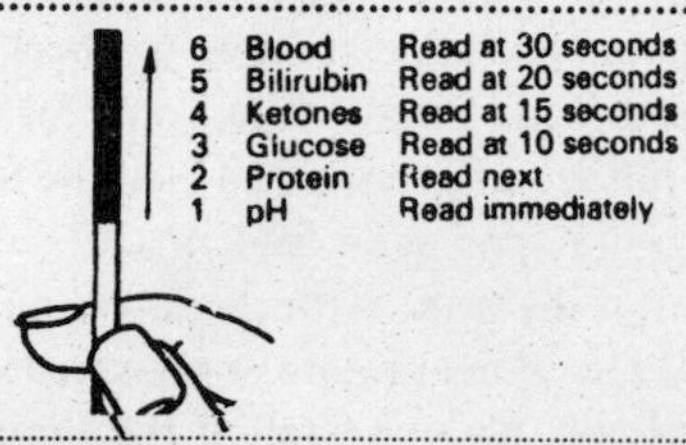

Regula quality control checks are now standard practice in the analysis of clinical specimens. For Ames tests this is easily done with Tek-Chek controls for routine urinalysis (also from Ames). These synthetic solutions provide positive and negative checks, and their use is recommended when a new bottle of reagents is opened and also each day, hidden among the batch of urines to be tested. The negative control gives confidence that not false positives are obtained and provides an appropriate negative reaction to make sure that comparison to the 'negative'. colour blocks is being made properly. The appropriate positive control gives confidence that the reagents are reacting properly with positive specimens.

pH

Ames pH test (on Hema-Combistix, Labstix, Bili-Labstix, N-Labstix, Multistix and N-Multistix strips, but not available singly).

The ames pH test covers the range 5-9 units and can be read to one unit. It should be read immediately after dipping the strip.

It is not affected by variations in the urinary buffer concentra tion, but care should be taken, by tapping the strip to remove excess urine and by holding it level while reading it, to avoid contamination from reagents from the adjacent protein, which would tend to cause an underestimate of an alkaline or neutral pH.

Protein

The excess protein excreted as a result of most of the common causes of proteinuria is mainly albumin, but globulins also may be present.

1. **Albustix strips (and all Ames multiple - test strips except Keto-Diastix)**

This test is based on the 'protein error of indicators' principle using buffered tetrabromophenol blue, and may be read immediately. It has colour blocks marked negative, trace, 30 mg/dl (+), 100 mg/dl (+ +), 300.mg/dl (+ + +), 1000 or more mg/dl (+ + + +), the figures referring to albumin. Its sensitivity is 5-20 mg/dl a lbumin. It is more sensitive to albumin than to globulin, haemoglobin,

Bence-Jones protein and mucoprotein. Clinical judgement must determine the significance of 'trace' results; particularly in urines of high specific gravity, the test area may most closely. match 'trace' despite only physiological concentrations of protein. Falsely positive results can be obtained from alkaline and/or highly buffered urines, or from contamination with quaternary ammonium salts.

2. Boiling test (heat plus asetic acid test)

(a) Check that the urine. pH is midly acidic (5 or 6 units) or just acidic to litmus paper; if it is not so, add 10 percent acetic acid solution until it is. Failure to check the initial pH and adjust it if necessary can invalidate this test. If the urine is cloudy, filter some for this procedure.

(b) Fill a boiling tube about 3/4 full with the urine and heat the top inch of liquid gently over a spirit lamp, turning the tube while heating to prevent it from cracking. Let it boil for a few moments.

(c) Compare the top, boiled, part of the urine with the lower part to see if any cloudiness has appeared. If so, it may have been caused by either protein or phosphates.

(d) Add 3 drops of 10 percent acetic acid and reboil the top portion. If cloudiness persits, proteins are indicated. If cloudiness disappears, phosphates are indicated.

3. Salicysulphonic acid test

(a) If the urine is cloudy, filter some for this test.

(b) Add 5 drops of 25 percent salicysluphonic acid to about 5 ml urine in a test tube.

(c) Shake the tube and look for cloudiness in the urine. Cloudiness indicates protein and the degree o cloudiness gives some idea of the relative protein concentration.

4 Eshach test

(a) All the urine passed by the subject over a period, say 6 hours, is collected in a cloeanstoppered bottle and mixed. Measure its sp. gr.; if this exceeds 10.010, dilute a portion with an equal volume of water. If the urine is alkaline, acidify it with a few drops of 10 percent acetic acid.

(b) Add urine to an Esbach tube (see diagram) to the level marked U. Add Esbach's reagent up to the level marked R. Cork the tube and invert it gently several times to mix the contents.

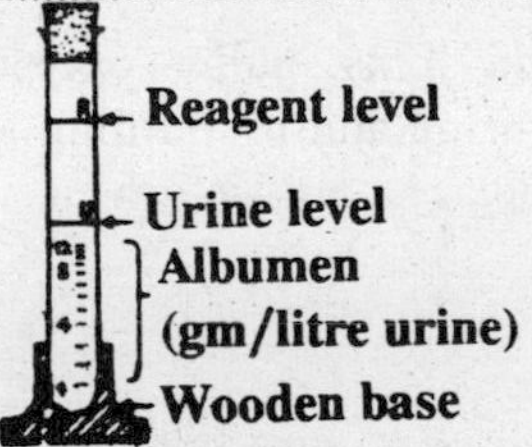

(c) Stand the tube upright and leave it in a constant temperature for 24 hours. The read the level of the precipitate of protein on the tube's scale, with the eye on a level with the top of the sediment. This gives the protein concentration of the urine in parts per 1000 (g/l).

Reducing Sugars

Although glucose is the commonest reducing sugar found in urine, more rarely galactose, lactose, fructose, pentose and maltose may be found. Because of these possibilities routine urine screening, especially for infants, should not rely on the enzymic tests specific for glucose but should include a test for reducing sugars.

Such tests are based on the reduction of hot alkaline copper sulphate to give cuprous oxide. They can react with other moderately strong reducing substances besides the abovementioned sugars, e.g. metabolities of aspirin, nalidixic acid, metaxalone, cephalothin and with ascorbic acid, etc. The precise composition of the reagent will determine the degree of nonspecificity of various tests based on copper reduction. The result will represent the sum of the effects of whatever substances that can affect the test are present in the urine. If the urine gives a positive result for reducing sugars but a nega tive result to a test specific for glucose, further investigation may be needed to find what the non-glucose reducing substance is, or possibly whether the specific enzyme test for glucose has been inhibited.

1. Clinitest reagent tablets. (Caution: these tables are caustic)

Always use the Ames test tubes and droppers provided for the test; other equipment may give incorrect results.

(a) Holding dropper upright, put 5 drops of urine into the clean dry test tube, Rinse dropper.

(b) Using the same dropper, add 10 drops of wa ter.

(c) Drop one clinitest tablet. Watch the test carefully until boiling stops and for 15 seconds longer. Do not shake the tube during this period.

(d) Now shake the tube gently and compare the colour of the colour of the contents with the colour chart. If durikng the test a bright orange colour appears (even for a moment) and then changes to a brownish colour, more than 2 percent sugar is present.

To estimate sugar concentration above 2 percent, dilute the urine being tested with normal urine (negative to clinitest) and repeat the test. Multiply the result obtained by the dilution to give the percentage to sugar.

The sensitivity of clinitest to glucose is about 150 ml/dt. It will react with reducing sugars, ascorbic acid, nalidixic acid, metaxalone, cephalothin, probenecid and salicylate metabolites if present in sufficient quantity, but not with uric acid, creatinine, penicillin, streptomycin, isoniazid, or chloral hydrate in the quantities in which these are likely to be found in urine; (these lists are not exhaustive).

2. Bendict's qualitative test

(a) To 5 ml of Benedict's qualitative reagent in a boiling tube add 8 drops of urine.

(b) Boil the mixture virorously for 2 minutes over a flame, or place the tube in a boiling waterbath for 5 minutes.

(c) In the presence of reducing substances the mixture will turn bluis-green, green, yellow, orange or brick red, depending on the nature and quantity of reducing substances present.

3. Benedict's quantitative test

This is a more elaborate version of the foregoing test using benedict's quantitative reagent designed to give semiquantitative results by titration.

Glucose

Tests for glucose based on glucose oxidase involve two reactions, firstly the oxidation of glucose by atmospheric oxygen, catalysed by glucose oxidase, to gluconic acid and hydrogen peroxide, and secondly the oxidation by hydrogen peroxide, catalysed by peroxidase, of a chromogen system such as o-tolidine or potassium oidide. The first reaction is specific for glucose and is not given by other sugars. The second is not; positive results can be given by strong oxidizing agents such as sodium hypochlorite or bleachers contasining hydrogen peroxide. The second can be inhibited by strong reducing substances which compete with the chromogen for oxygen from the hydrogen peroxide. This inhibition, e.g. from ascorbic acid, will vary with different chromogens according to the reducing power of the chromogen relative to tha t of the inhibitor.

It should be noted tha t strong reducing agents like ascorbic acid *inhibit* enzymic tests for glucose but *enhance* the results of copper reduction tests. Thus they a re a common cause of discrepant results between the two types of test for glucose, the reduction test being positive and the enzymic negative.

The enzymic tests are generally more sensitive than copper reduction tests. Thus it is possible in certain urines whose glucose concentration lies between the sensitivities of the two tests to get a positive result with the enzymic, more sensitive one and a negative with the coppern reduction, less sensitive one.

1. Clonistix strips

This test uses glucose oxidase and peroxidase, with o-tolidine puls a red dye as its chromogen system. It is qualitative only. When the colour developed at 10 seconds resembles any of the positive colour blocks, presence of glucose is indicated 'Light' generally indicates 1/4 percent or less. 'Dark' generally indicates 1/2 percent or more. 'Medium' indicates that glucose is present but does not denote amount. On average, the strips will detect about 0.1 percent glucose in urine (100 mg/dl, 5.5 mmol/l).

2. Diastix strips (and glucose portions of Ames 'improved' multiple test strips)

This test uses glucose oxidase and peroxidase, with potassium iodide plus a blue dye as its chromogen system. It is less affected by strong reducing substances like ascorbic acid and by sp. gr. of the urine than is Clinistix, and so can give semiquantitative results over the ranger 0.1 to 2 percent if rea d at 30 seconds.

Large concentra tions of ketones (80 mg/dl or greater) ma y decrease the colour development of this glucose test. It is unlikely tha t the presence of ketones simultaneously with glucose in the urine is sufficient to produce false-negative glucose results. However, when the Ames ketones test shows a 'medium' or 'large' result, the amount of glucose present may be greater than the amount shown by this test, and Clinitest tablets should be used to estimate the glucose. Diatix strips should not be used when ketonuria is likely to be present; in that circumstance Keto-Diastix strips would be preferred.

The strips will detect approximately 0.1 percent glucose in urine (100 mg/dl, 5.5 mmol/l).

Ketones

The abnormal metabolities present in the urine a s. a result of ketoacidosis are B-hydroxybutyric acid, acetoacetic acid a nd acetone. They are related chemically by oxidation, the first being the reduced from which can e oxidized to the second and on to the third. Of these three.

B-hydroxybutyric acid is not a ketone and no test for ketones detects it or includes it in its estimate of ketones.

Ketones in urine are mustable; chilling the specimen is the best way to preserve ketones if there must be a delay before testing for them.

Tests for ketones are based either on their reaction with sodium nitroprusside to give a purple colour (Ames tests and Rother's test) or with ferric chloride to give a deep red colour given with sodium nitroprusside by acetoacetic acid is stronger than that by acetone; the reaction is specific for ketones. Ferric chloride does not react with acetone, but can give reddish colours with several chemicals other than acetoacetic acid, and other colours with various other substances.

1. Ketostix strips (and ketones portions of Keto-Diastix, Labstix, Bili-Labstix, N-Labstix, Multistix and N-Multistix strips)

The reagent portion of Ketostix is impregnated with sodium nitroprusside, glycine and buffers.

This test react with acetoacetic acid and acetone but not B-hydroxybutyric acid. It should be read at 15 second. It detects 5 to 10 mg acetoacetate per dl of urine (0.5 to 1 mmol/l), and is less sensitive to acetone. The results may be interpreted as small, moderate or large. Colours which are sufficiently similar to that produced by kitones can be confusing and may be obtained from urine specimens containing bromosulphthalein or large amount of phenylketones or metabolities of L-dopa.

2. Acetest reagent tablets

Acetest tablet contain sodium nitroprusside, glycine and buffers.

(a) Place an Acetest tablet on clean, dry, white paper.

(b) Put l drop of urine on the tablet.

(c) Compare colour of the tablet with the colour chart exactly 30 seconds later.

This test resembles Ketostix strips in chemistry, sensitivity and specificity.

3. Rothera's test

(a) Saturate a portion of urine with ammonium sulphate by shaking about 5 ml of urine in a test tube with about the same volume of crystals of this salt.

(b) Add 10 drops of a freshly prepared 2 percent solution of sodium nitroprusside.

(c) Add 10 drops of strong ammonia solution (sp.gr. 0.880).

(d) Allow to stand for 15 minutes. The development of a purple colour indicates ketones.

This test is generally considered to be too sensitive, as it often gives a positive on a well subject who has not eaten for several hours.

4. Gerhardt's test

(a) Put 2 ml urine in a test tube.

(b) Add 10 percent ferric chloride solution drop by drop. A precipitate may fc m if phosphates are present but will redissolve on addition of more ferri chloride.

(c) A reddish-brown colour indicates acetoacetic.

This test is generally considered too incensitive, as clinically significant ketonuria can be present when the test is negative.

Gerhardt's test will not react with acetone or B-hydroxybutyric acid, but will give similar colour to that produced by acetoacetic acid with the urinary metabolites of number of drugs including salicylates.

Blood

Chemical tests for blood in urine are based on the peroxidase-like activity of haemoglobin, myoglobin and some of their degradation products, which can catalyse the oxidation of a chromogen system by hydrogen peroxide to give a colour. They, will react with free haemoglobin and witherythrocytes, which are lysed by the reagents used in the test, but are usually a little less sensitive to the latter.

The alternative test for blood in urine is microscopy, looking for and counting the erythrocytes in a known volume, in which the sediment has been concentrated by centrifugation. This test does not detect free haemoglobin, whether excreted as such (haemoglobinuria resulting form in vivo haemolysis) or lysed from excreted erythrocytes in urine left to stand (haematuria followed by in vitro haemolysis). As it may be more sensitive to intact erythrocytes that a chemical test, the two complement each other.

Thus the presence of free haemoglobin in the absence of intact erythrocytes in the urine is a cause of a positive result from a chemical test and negative result by microscopy. Urine for testing for blood should be stirred immediately before testing (or withdrawing a portion for testing) and microscopy should be carried out on fresh urine).

It should be noted that a negative result to a test for protein does not preclude a positive result for blood in the same urine, although haemoglobin is a protein. This is because urine normally contains up to about 5 mg per dl of protein (mainly as albumin), and a test for proteinuria must have its sensitivity adjusted to give a negative a t this physiological level. Concentrations of haemoglobin that are pathological are much lower than this, about 150 *u*g per dl, and therefore tests for haemoglobin must give positives with concentrations of this order which would be negative to a protein test. Urine should be tested for both protein and blood, regardless of the result of either.

1. Hemastix strips (and the blood portion of Hema-Combistix, Labstix. Bili-Labstix, N-Labstix, Multistix and N-Multistix strips)

   The reagent portion of Hemastix contains a peroxide, buffers and o-tolidine.

This test gives results which can be graded as 'small', 'moderate' or 'large'. Any blue spots or blue colour developing on the reagent area within 30 seconds is significant. Its sensitivity is 0.015 mg per dl for free haemoglobin, or 5-10 intact erythrocytes per *u*l at the time of manufacture for urines with low specific gravity and ascorbic acid concentrations of less than 5 mg per dl (0.28 mmol/l). The sensitivity may be expected to be less in urines of high specific gravity and ascorbic acid content. The test is slightly more sensitive to free haemoglobin and myoglobin that to intact erythrocytes.

Certain oxidizing contaminants such as hypochlorite may produce falsely positive results, as also may microbial peroxidase, associated with urinary tract infection.

2. **Guaiac test**

   (a) Ensure tha t no flame is near when this test is carried out.

(b) Put about 5 ml or urine in a test tube and add 1 or 2 drops of freshly prepared tincture of guaiacum.

(c) Carefully overlay this with about half the volume of oxonic either (*which is highly inflammable).*

(d) Hold the tube in the hand for a few minutes to warm it a little. The appearance of a blue line at the junction of the fluids indicates blood.

3. Microscopy

Techniques for this test vary in detail from laboratory. Essentially, one takes a known volume of fresh well-stirred urine (usually 10 ml,) centrifuges it, pours off most of the supernatant liquid and resuspends the sediment in a known volume of the liquid. A known quantity of this suspension is then put on a microscope slide, covered with a cover slip and examined under the high power of a microscope.

The number of erythrocytes visible are counted, the slide moved slightly and the erythrocytes in the new field counted. This is repeated for, say, 10 fields and the numbers avedraged.

The result is commonly expressed as the number of erythrocytes 'per high-power field'. With constant use of the same technique, this gives comparative results which are meaningful within that laboratory can be interpreted in the light of what is 'normal' for it. But results obtained from even a slightly different techniques will be numerically different for the same urine and probably 'normal' range will be different. It is only possible to compare results between different techniques and laboratories if each arbitrary unit 'per high-power field' is related to a scientific unit e.g., 'per mm^3'.

Bilirubin

Many tests for bilirubin in urine have been devised; the two main groups depend on coupling with a diazotized compound and on oxidation respectively. Diazotization methods can be specific for bilirubin, whereas oxidation methods are not and can give positive results on urine in which bilirubin was present initially but has oxidized to biliverdin on standing. Tests for bilirubin should be made on fresh urine.

1. Ictostix strips (and the bilirubin portion of Bili-Labstix, Multistix and N-Multistix strips)

This test depends on the reaction of bilirubin with diazotized dichloroaniline. It should be be read at 20 seconds, and give readings which can be graded as 'negative', 'small', 'moderate' or 'large'. Its sensitivity is 0.2 - 0.4 mg per dl (3.4 - 6.8 mmol/l) of bilirubin as assayed by the procedure of Golden and Snavely (J. Clin. Lab. Med. 1948, 33, 890). This is 2 to 4 times le s sensitive than lctotest tablets (see below), which may be preferred when very small concentration of bilirubin are sought.

The test is considered specific for bilirubin if the colour developed at 20 seconds matches one of those shown on the chart. Different colours may indicate that other bile reaction to bilirubin, are present in the sample, and they may mask the reaction to bilirubin. Large doses of chlorpromazine may give rise to reactions which could be confused with those for bilirubin. Metabolites of drugs which give a colour at low pH, such as pyridium and serenuim, may give a red or other colour on this test portion. If atypical colours are seen on the bilirubin test portion, the urine should be tested further (e.g. with Ictotest tablets).

2. **Ictotest reagent tablets**

(a) Place 5 drops of urine on one square of the absorbent test mat provided.

(b) Place an Ictotest tablet in the middle of the moist are.

(c) Flow 2 drops of water onto the tablet so that the water runs off onto the mat.

(d) Observe the colour of the mat around the tablet after 30 seconds. A bluish-purple colour indicates bilirubin.

Ictotest tablets employ a similar reaction to that of Ictostix strips but a different diazonium salt. The use of an absorbent mat has a chromatographic effect of concentrating the bilirubin, and so Icotest tablets are 2 to 4 times more sensitive than Ictostix strips. Because even trace amounts of bilirubin in urine are abnormal, the tablets should be preferred to the strips when seeking very low concentrations, e.g. in the earliest phase of viral hepatitis.

Urobilinogen

Urobilinogen is even less stable than bilirubin in urine which has been left to stand; it oxidizes to urobilin, which does not react with some tests for urobilinogen, i.e. those based on p-dimethylaminobenzaldehyde, such as Ames Urobilistix and most of the laboratory methods. Another test (Schlesinger's), however, first oxidizes urobilinogen to urobilin and then estimates the latter by its ability to produce a fluorescent compound with a zinc salt. This would give a positive even after urobilinogen initially present had disappeared on standing.

1. **Urobilistix strips (and the urobilinogen portion of Multistix and N0Multistix strips)**

This test is based on the development of an orange colour from the reaction of urobilinogen with p-dimethylaminobenzal-dehyde. It must be performed on fresh urine.

The colour scale permits assessment of the urobilingoen content as 0.1, 1, 4, 8 or 12 Ehrlich unit per dl, and the absence of urobilinogen from the specimen being tested cannot be detected with the strip.

The test is not completely specific for urobilinogen, and will react with some other substances known to interfere with its reagent, e.g. porphobilinogen and p-aminosalicylic acid, but the test is not a reliable method for the detection of porphobilinogen. Drugs containing an azo dye (e.g. azo gantrisin) may give a masking golden colour.

Nitrite

The production of nitritie from nitrate ion in urine is brought about by the activity of many of the common species of bacteria, but not all. Those species that do produce nitritie do so at different rates for different rates for different species. The production of nitrite depends also on the amount of nitirate available (from dietary sources) in the urine and on the time that the bacteria have had to work in that specimen of urine since the bladder was last emptied.

Thus, while the presence of nitrite in a urine specimen implies bacterial infection, it does not indicate the degree of infection, and the absence of nitrite from the specimen does not imply that there is no bacterial infection.

1. Ames nitrite test (on N-Labstix and N-Multistix strips but not available singly).

This test converts the nitrite in to nitrous acid, diazotizes that and then converts the product to an azo dye. It is sensitive to 0.075 mg per dl (0.007 mmol/l) of sodium nitrite at the time of manufacture, in urines having low specific gravity and less than 5 mg per dl (0.28 mmol.l) ascorbic acid; the sensitivity will be reduced in urines or high specific gratvity and ascorbic acid content. It assesses the concentration of nitrite as 'negative' cr 'positive'. Any shade of pink is positive and suggestive of the presence of 10^5 or more organisms per ml, but the degree of the reaction cannot be correlated with the degree of bacteriuria. A 'negative' result indicates that the nitrite concentration is below the test's sensitivity, but does not indicate that bacteriuria is absent, as expla ined above. Where there is bacterial infection the test is more likely to give a positive result if the urine has been in the bladder of about 4 hours at least. Comparison of the reagent area with a white background may help to detect very pale pink reactions. The test is specific for nitrite and will not react with any other substance normally excreted in urine.

This test has the advantages that its result is available in one minute and that it does not require the specimen to have been obtained using 'clean-catch' techniques.

Phenylketones (and metabolities of salicylates and phenothiazines)

Testing of infants' urine for phenylketones is carried out less commonly now tha t many Health Authorities test infant's blood for phenylalaninaemia (and other abnormalities) instead, as this sign is more reliable than phenylketonuria as an indication of the disorder. However, Phenistix reagent strips, which were developed to screen for plenylketonuria, still have a use for this, and additional ones for checking on the ingestion of prescribed does of paraminosalicylic acid (PAS) or for detecting overdoses of salicylates or phenothiazines.

1. Phenistix strips

The reagent area of Phenistix is impregnated with ferric ammonium sulphate, magnesium sulphate and cyclohexylsulphamic acid. Ferric ions give various volours with a number of substances in acidic conditions.

(a) As a test for phenylketonuria

The strip is dipped in urine, or pressed against a freshly wet napkin (not merely damp), and removed immediately. If the test end turns a greenishgrey similar to the shades on the colour chart within 30 seconds, the test is positive for phenylketonuria. If it turns off-white or cream within 30 seconds, the test is negative. The sensitivity of the strip to phenylpyruvic acid is 8 mg per dl.

(b) As a test for the ingestion of prescribed PAS

The strip is dipped in urine and removed immediately. A brownish-red colour appearing at once indicates that the subject has taken PAS within 12-18 hours (or possible some other salicylate). The sensitivity of Phenistix strips to PAS is 5-10 mg per dl.

(c) As a test for overdoses of salicylates or phenothiazines

The test is dipped in urine and removed immediately. If the test end turns brownish red or a shade within dull pink-red-purple colour range, the ingestion of salicylates or phenothiazines is indicated.

To ascertain which of these classes of drug was responsible, add a small volume (about 1 ml) of concentrated sulphuric acid slowly and with stirring to an equal volume of wa ter and cool it. Pur one drop of the mixture on the reagent pad of the used strip. If the colour is bleached, it was caused by a salicylate; if it is enhanced, it was caused by a phenothiazine.

The test gives a light brownish-red colour with 50 mg per dl of 'free' salicylate. The colours given by metabolites of phenothiazines are not usually sufficiently intense to be used as a check on whether a patient has taken the prescribed dose of one of this group of drugs, but the colour in the case of an overdose would be more difinite.

Chlorides

1. Fantus test

(a) Rinse a test tube and pipette with distilled water and put 10 drops of urine in the tube.

(b) Rinse the pipette with distilled water and add 1 drop of 20 percent potassium chromate solution.

(c) Rinse the pipette with distilled water and add 2.9 percent silver nitrate solution drop by drop, counting the drops and shaking the tube after each addition, until the misture changes colour sharply from yellow to reddish-brown.

The number of drops denotes the chloride in the urine, in g per l of sodium chloride; a normal result in 3 to 5 drops.

B. BLOOD, SERUM AND PLASMA TESTING

Quick test are available in the form of Ames strips or tablets for glucose, ketones and ureea in blood (Dextrostix strips, Acetest tablets and Azostix strips respectively) and for ketones in serum or plasma (Ketostix strips and Acetest tablets). They are intended for immediate use on one drop of fresh specimen, e.g. blood from a fingertip or ear prick,or from the tip of a syringe used to withdraw a large specimen for laboratory testing. Thus there is no occasion to add preservatives to the blood use for these ont he spot' test, even if the rest of the specimen may require it. In particular, Dextrostix strips should not be used on blood to which a fluorcide has been added because this will inhibit the test to some degree, depending on its concentration, and Azostix strips should not be used on blood containing a fluoride or an ammonium salt.

These quick test give semiquantitative results. They are not intended to replace quantitative laboratory analyses but to give a guide to the patient's condition in circumstances where spread is of more importance than exctitude.

Glucose

1. Dextrostix strips

The chemistry of Destrostix is similar to that of clinistix (see under Glucose in urine testing) but the chromogen system is slightly different, and the reagent area is covered with a semipermeable membrane to hold back erythrocytes, etc.

(a) Compare Dextrostix reagent area against 'O' block on colour chart. Do not use if colour of unreacted strip does not closely match that of 'O' colour block.

(b) Freely apply a large drop of capillary or venous blood sufficient to cover *entire* reagent area on *printed side* of strip.

(c) *Wait exactly 60 second* (Use sweep seconds hand or stopwatch for timing).

(d) quickly wash off blood (in 1 or 2 seconds) with a sharp stream of water, *using a wash bottle,* derected just above reagent area.

(e) Read immediately after washing (within 1 or 2 second). Hold the strip close to the colour chart.

(f) Interpolate if necessary.

The colour blocks are labelled 0, 25, 45, 90, 130, 175 and 250 mg per dl or more respectively. the test cannot give numerical values for concentrations above 250 mg per dl (unless read instrumentally, see the following items). It is specific for glucose in blood and does not react with other reducing substances as do methods depending on, for example, potassium ferriyanida. Glucose concentrations are lower in whole blood than in the serum or flasma from that blood. In blood of unusually high haematocrit (e.g. from some neonates) the strip may give a slight underestimate.

Dextrostix strips should not be used on blood to which a fluoride has been added; however, no anticoagulant is needed for the application of this test to one drop of fresh blood from a prick. A Tek-Chek synthetic control set is available for Dextrostix, similar to those described previously for the Ames urine tests.

This test will not give numerically correct results on serum or plasma

2. Dextrostix Eyetone System

It has been found that a major factor in the overall error of estimating blood glucos with Dextrostix is the visual comparison of the strip's reagent area with the colour chart. To improve this factor, instrument reading was introduced, first with the Ames reflectance meter and then with the Eyetone instrument.

Eyetone is a small mains-operated instrument which provides a more objective and precise interpretation of the colour developed on Dextrostix strips. It has a range of reading fronm 10 to 400 mg per dl (0.55 to 22.2 mmol/l glucose in whole blood). It gives a better degree of quantitation than the visual test, but makes even more important the correct technique for using the strip. A calibra tion and control set is available to standardize the Dextrostix Eyetone or Dextrostix reflectance meter systems.

Full details and instructions accompany the instruments and their calibra tion and control set or are available from Ames Company.

Ketones

1. Acetest tablets

This test has been described under Ketones in Urine Testing.

(a) Place an Acetest tablet on clean dry white paper.

(b) Put 1 drop of whole blood on top of the tablet.

(c) About 10 minutes later, remove the blood clot a nd compare the colour of the tablet below it to the colour chart.

in instruction (b) above and substituting (c) above:

(d) Two minutes later compare colour of the tablet with the colour chart.

2. Ketostix strips

This test has been described under Ketones in Urine Testing. It is not suitable for use on whole blood, but may be used on serum on plasma thus:

(a) Dip test area in fresh serum or plasma and remove it immediately.

(b) Gently tap edge of strip against the side of the specimen container, to remove excess specimen.

(c) Compare test area with colour chart, exactly 15 seconds later.

This test is sensitive to 5-10 mg/dl of acetoacetic acid; it is less sensitive to acetone, and does not react with *B*-hydroxybutric acid.

Urea

1. Azostix strips

The reagent area of Azostix is impregnated with a mixture of urease, buffers and bromothymol blue, under a semi-permeable membrane to hold back erythrocytes etc. Urea is hydrolysed by urease and produces ammonium ions which cause a colour change in the indicator.

(a) Freely apply a large drop of capillary or venous blood sufficient to cover entire reagent area on printed side of strip.

(b) Wait exactly 60 seconds. (Use sweep seconds hand or stopwatch for timing).

(c) Quickly wash off blood (in 1 or 2 seconds) with a sharp stream of water using a wash bottle and directing the stream just above the reagent area.

(d) Read the result within 1 or 2 seconds after washing. Hold the strip close to the colour chart. Interpolate if colour produces falls between colour blocks. Any delay in reading will give erroneously low results due to rapid fading of the colour reaction.

The colour blocks are marked 20, 45, 85, and 130 mg per dl of urea. To convert from blood urea to blood urea nitrogen, divide by 2.14.

Fluoride preservatives may cause erroneously low results, and ammonium salts from anticoagulants will give false elavation of the result. As with Dextrostix strips, anticoagulants will give false elevation of the result. As with Dextrostix strips, norpreservative is needed for this 'on the spot' test. In a minor proportion of patients in severe alkalosis, the pH and buffers of the blood may be sufficiently extreme to cause a slight overestimate of blood urea concentration by Azostix. In a minor proporation of patients in severe acidosis, an underestimate may be caused.

C FAECES TESTING

Faeces a re more difficult to analyse than blood or urine because they are very non-homogeneous and one cannot mix them adequately by merely stirring, as one can a liquid. Thus when a small portion is taken for testing it is unlikely to be representative of the whole, i.e. there is a large sampling error. This can be decreased either by blending the whole specimen (usually with water to make an emulsion) in a homogenizer or by replicate testing of several portions withdrawn from different parts of the specimen. The latter is probably somewhat less effective, but quicker and simpler. If there test are made on differne tportions and the results agree, one can have more confidence in the finding than if it is based on one test only and if the results disagree one can either consider the specimen to be 'borderline' or make, say, two more tests and accept the majority finding. (see Ross and Gray, Br. med J. 1964, i. 1351).

On account both of the sampling error and of the wide variation in composition of faeces, and hence in factors which may interfere with various analyses, tests on faeces are inherentlyless reliable than tests on urine or blood.

Blood

By far the most commonly requested test on faeces is that for occult blood. This is an extremely difficult analysis, because faecal samples are not very suitable for microscopy for intact red cells (which in any case would probably be disrupted unless they had come from low down in the gastrointestinal tract), and chemical tests for haemoglobin, such a s are used on urine, are liable to much interference. They can be inhibited to a variable degree by the specimen (faecal material generally has mildly reducing properties) and enhanced by several factors, e.g.

Haemoglobin from dietary sources such as rare steaks, liver, black puddings Peroxidases of bacterial origin

Peroxidases of vegetable origin, e.g. from lettuce, turnips, bananas.

Blood from the Patient not originating from gastrointestinal bleeding but from, for example, vigorous brusing of the teeth and gums.

Thus it is not surprising that a large number of tests for blood in faeces has been proposed and that there is no consensus of opinion as to the desirable sensitivity for the test. A test of low sensitivity will miss some specimens containing a little blood, whereas a test of higher sensitivity will give many positive results from the causes listed above in patients who may or may not have gastrointestinal bleeding.

To decrease the number of such 'false' positives, it is helpful to put the patient on a diet free from, or very low in, items which might contribute to a positive result, and possibly to probibit tothbrushing, for a few days before the test. For more informa tion see illingworth, D.G., 'influence of diet on occult blood test, Gut 1965, 6, 595.

Interference by peroxidases of vegetables and bacterial origin can be removed, wholly or partially, by emulsifying a portion (or preferably several portions from different parts of the specimen) with water and boiling it. However, this obviously lowers the concentration of blood to be detected.

1. Hematest reagent tablets

The chemistry of Hematest tablets is similar to that of Hemastix strips (see under Blood in Urine Testing).

(a) Make thin smear of faeces on filter paper square provided. Do not use emulsion.

(b) Place Hematest tablet across edge of smear.

(c) Flow one drop of water on top of tablet, wait 5 to 10 seconds, and flow second drop on tablet sot that it runs down sides onto filter paper.

(d) Observe colour of filter paper around tablet exactly 2 minutes later.

A positive is indicated by the appearance within 2 minutes of a blue colour. The concentration of blood is roughly proportional to the intensity of blue colour and the spreed with which it develops. Ignore any colour appearing on tablet or smear, and colour appearing in filter paper after 2 minutes.

This test is relatively insensitiveand is intended for use on undieted patients.

2. Occultest reagent tablets

The chemistry of Occultest tablets is similar to that of hemastix strips (see under Blood in Urine Testing).

These tablets, although developed originally for testing urine for blood, may be used on faeces in the same way as Hematest reagent tablets. They are about 5 times more sensitive than Hematest and are suitable for use on patients who have been dieted suitable for the previous 3-5 days. If used on the faeces of undieted pateints they must be expected to give positive results from other causes besides gastrointestinal bleeding, as indicated above.

3. Hemastix strips

This test has been described under Blood in Urine Testing. It is intended for the detection of blood in urine, and the manufacturers do not recomend its use on faeces, in which it is less reliable than in urine. However, various workers have tried it in this application using various techniques and have found it at least as reliable as some routine quick tests for occult blood (e.g. Lehmann and Kitchin, Lancet 1971, ii, 258).

Techniques vary in detail, but substantially consist of either putting a dry strip into an emulsion, if used, or applying a piece of the dry specimen to the reagent area of the strip, previously wetted briefly with distilled water. In both cases the reagent pad should be only half-covered with the specimen, so that the test can be read by observing the colour developing on the unsoiled remainder of the reagent area. A blue colour is positive; no change from cream colour is negative.

The sensitivity of the test can be varied by altering the time at which the reading is made, e.g. 15, 20 or 30 seconds, or by altering the dilution of the emulsion if used. Hemastix strips are more liable to inhibition from reducing substances in the faeces than are Hematest or Occultest, because more of the reagents can be put in a tablet than in a reagent pad.

4. Tests using solutions, nor commercial products

There are too many of these to give in detail. They are all based on the peroxidase like activity of haemoglobin to catalyse the oxidation of a chromogen by hydrogen peroxide. The preferred chromogen was benzidine until its carcinogenicity became known, since when a number of other chromogens has been tried. Some methods employ the faecal sample as it is, others use an emulsion, others an emulsion which has been boiled and cooled.

The following papers describe tests for occult blood in faeces, the chromogen being given in brackets after the reference.

Kohn and kelly (1955), *J. clin. Path.* 8,249 (o-tolidine)

Ross and Gray (1964), *Br. med J. i.* 1351 (o-tolidine)

Benson (1968), *Proc, Ass. clin. Biochem,* 5,31 (Phenolphthalein)

Wilkinson and Penfold (1969), *Lancet ii,* 847 (*guaiac)*

Deadman and Timms (1969, *clin, chim. acta* 20, 396 (2,-dichlorophenol indophenol)

Woodman (1970), *Clin, chim, acta* 29, 249 (*diphenylamine)*

Crossely (1970), *J. med, lab. Techn,* 27, 340 (aminopyridine)

Clarke (1971), *Med. lab. Tech.* 28, 187 (reduced thymolphthalein)

SUGARS

Disorders of sugar metabolism any result in the presence of reducing sugars such a lactose in the patient's faeces, for which a simple quick test would be useful routinely.

1. Clinitest tablets (Caution: These tablets are caustic).

This test has been described under reducing Sugars in Urine Testing. Kerry and Anderson (Lancet 1964, i, 981) proposed the use of Clinitest tablets as a qualitative test for sugars in faeces. Their technique was to mix thoroughly 1 volume of the faecal specimen with 2 volumes of water (these can be measured easily using a measuring cylinder), and then to perform the CLINITEST test on 15 drops of the resulting suspension, using the AMES dropper and tube without additional water. The result was read by matching the colour blocks of the chart provided for urine interpreted as follows:

Upto and including ¼%	negative
Over ¼% to ½%	suspect
Over ½%	positive

(These percentages should not be taken an numerically correct for sugars in faeces).

Clinitest tablets will react with glucose, fructose, lactose, galactose, pentose and maltose, but not with sucrose (unless this is previously hydrolysed to glucose and fructose). Their results will include a contribution from other reducing substances present in faeces, which accounts for the interpretation, in this context, being negative up to a match to the colour block that indicates ¼ percent glucose in urine. Other reference to this application of the tablets :

Anderson et al. (1966), *Lancet* i, 1322

Townley (1966), *Pediatrics* 38,127

Davidson and Mulinger (1970), *Pediatrics* 46,632

Soeparto et al. (1972). *Archs. Dis. Chidh.* 47.56

APPENDIX 6

Desirable Weights of Aduylts according to Height and Frame

Height (metres)		Small frame	Weight in kg Medium Frame	Large frame
Men	1.550	51-54	54-59	57-64
	1.575	52-56	55-60	59-65

1.600	53-57	56-62	60-67
1.625	55-58	58-63	61-69
1.650	56-60	59-65	63-71
1.675	58-62	61-67	64-73
1.700	60-64	63-69	67-75
1.725	62-66	64-71	68-77
1.750	64-68	66-73	70-79
1.775	65-70	68-75	72-81
1.800	67-72	70-77	74-84
1.825	69-74	72-79	76-86
1.850	71-76	74-82	78-88
1.875	73-78	76-84	81-90
1.900	74-79	78-86	83-93
Women 1.425	42-44	44-49	47-54
1.450	43-46	45-50	48-55
1.475	44-48	46-51	49-57
1.500	45-49	47-53	51-58
1.525	46-50	46-54	52-59
1.5850	48-51	50-55	53-61
1.575	49-53	51-57	55-63
1.600	50-54	53-59	57-64
1.625	52-56	54-61	59-66
1.650	54-58	56-63	60-68
1.675	55-59	58-65	62-70
1.700	57-61	60-67	64-72
1.725	59-63	62-69	66-74
1.250	61-65	63-70	68-76
1.757	63-67	65-72	69-79

APPENDIX 7

Weights and heights

Weights for Age, birth to 5 years, sexes combined (Jelliffe, 1966)

		Standard				Weight (kg)	
Age (Months)	**Standard ***	**80% Standard**	**60% Standard**	**Age (Months)**	**Standard***	**80% Standard**	**60%**
0	3.4	2.7	2.0	31	13.7	11.0	8.2
·1	4.3	3.4	2.5	32	13.8	11.1	8.3

2	5.0	4.0	2.9	33	14.0	11.2	8.4
3	5.7	4.5	3.4	34	14.2	11.3	8.5
4	6.3	5.0	3.8	35	14.4	11.5	8.6
5	6.9	5.5	4.2	36	14.5	11.6	8.7
6	7.4	5.9	4.5	37	14.7	11.8	8.8
7	8.0	6.3	4.9	38	14.85	11.9	8.9
8	8.4	6.7	5.1	39	15.0	12.05	9.0
9	8.9	7.1	5.3	40	15.2	12.2	9.1
10	9.3	7.4	5.5	41	15.35	12.3	9.2
11	9.6	7.7	5.8	42	15.5	12.4	9.3
12	9.9	7.9	6.0	43	15.7	12.6	9.4
13	10.2	8.1	6.2	44	15.58	12.7	9.5
14	10.4	8.3	6.3	45	16.0	12.9	9.6
15	10.6	8.5	6.4	46	16.2	12.95	9.7
16	10.8	8.7	6.6	47	16.35	13.1	9.8
17	11.0	8.9	6.7	48	16.5	13.2	9.9
18	11.3	9.0	6.8	49	16.65	13.35	10.0
19	11.5	9.2	7.0	5	16.8	13.5	10.1
20	11.7	9.4	7.1	51	16.95	13.65	10.2
21	11.9	9.6	7.2	52	17.1	13.8	10.3
22	12.05	9.7	7.3	53	17.25	13.9	10.4
23	12.2	9.8	7.4	54	17.4	14.0	10.5
24	12.4	9.9	7.5	55	17.6	14.2	10.6
25	12.6	10.1	7.6	56	17.7	14.3	10.7
26	12.7	10.3	7.7	57	17.9	14.4	1075
27	12.9	10.5	7.8	58	18.05	14.5	10.8
28	13.1	10.6	7.9	59	18.25	14.6	10.9
29	13.3	10.7	8.0	60	18.4	14.7	11.0
30	13.5	10.8	8.1				

* **Means of the Boston standards for boys and girls (Stuart and Stevenson, 1959). Means for boys are 0.05 to 0.15 kg heavier and for girls 0.05 to 0.15 kg lighter.**

Standard heights and weights of boys and girls 5 -18 years old

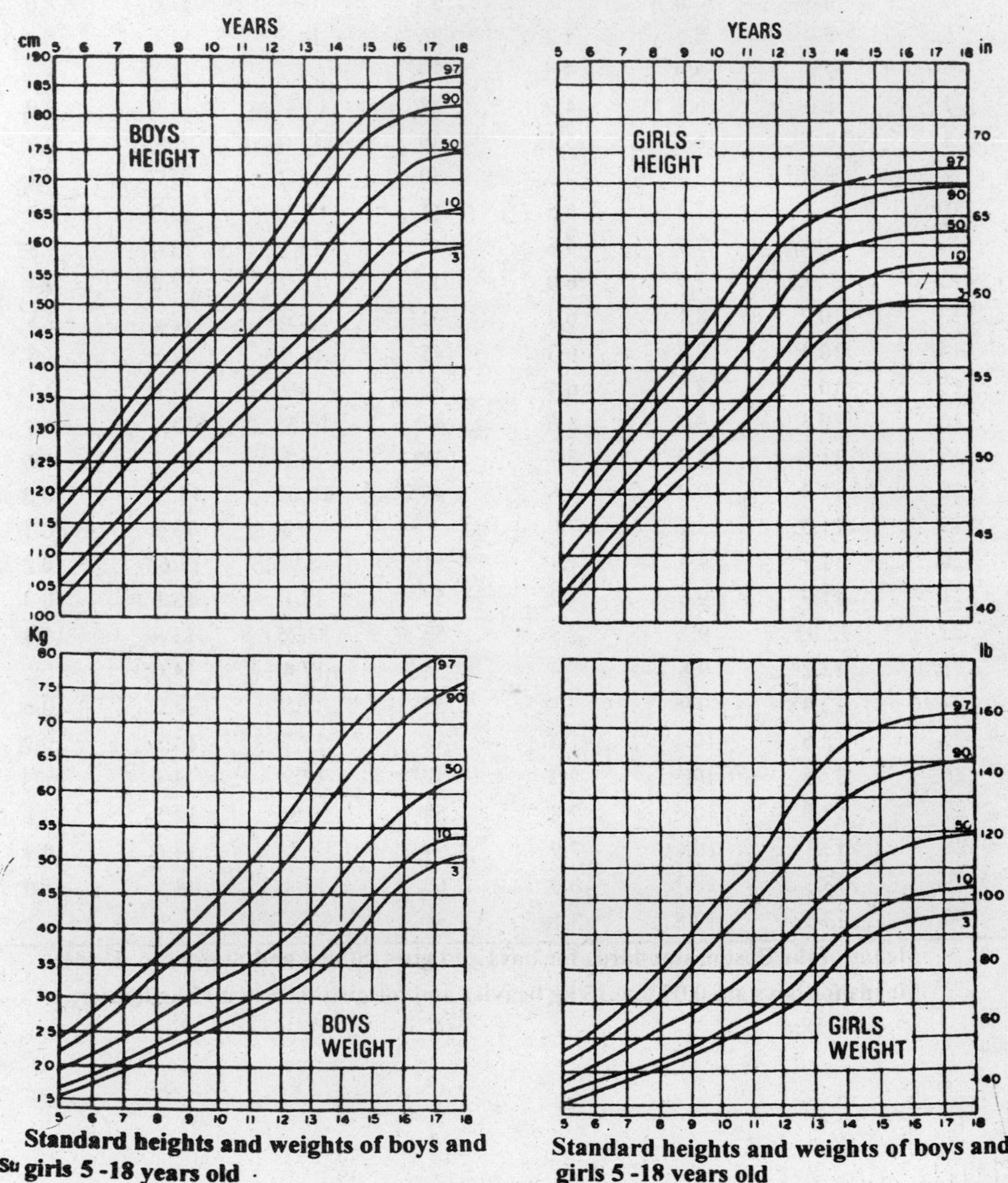

Standard heights and weights of boys and girls 5 -18 years old

Standard heights and weights of boys and girls 5 -18 years old

Coversion scales for certain chemical pathology testes and units of measurement (From D. Goodsell, (1975) Coming to terms with Si metric. Nursing Mirror. 141, 55-59. Reproduced by kind permission of the author and the Nursing Mirror.)

APPENDIX 8

Chemical pathology Blood plasma

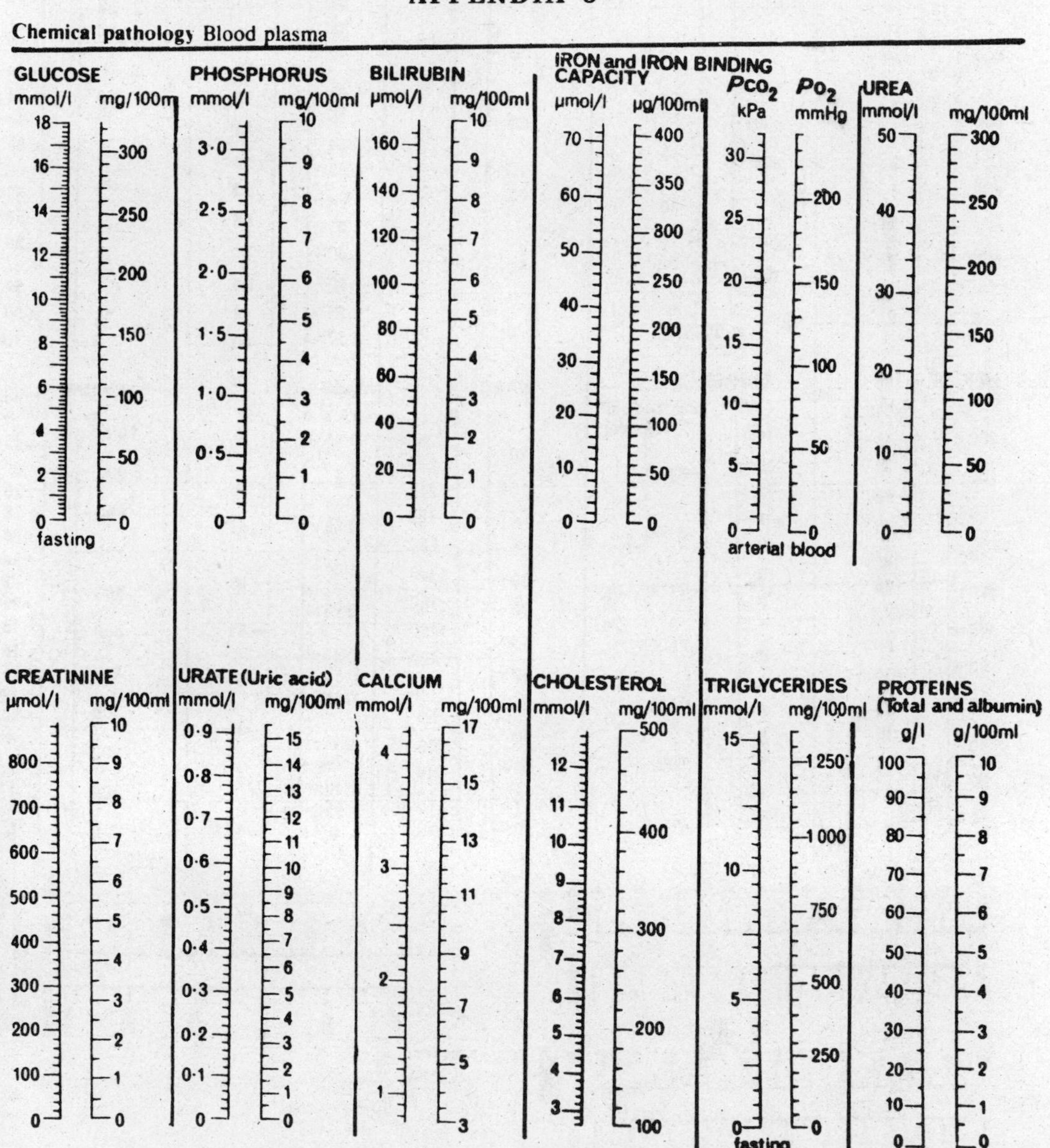

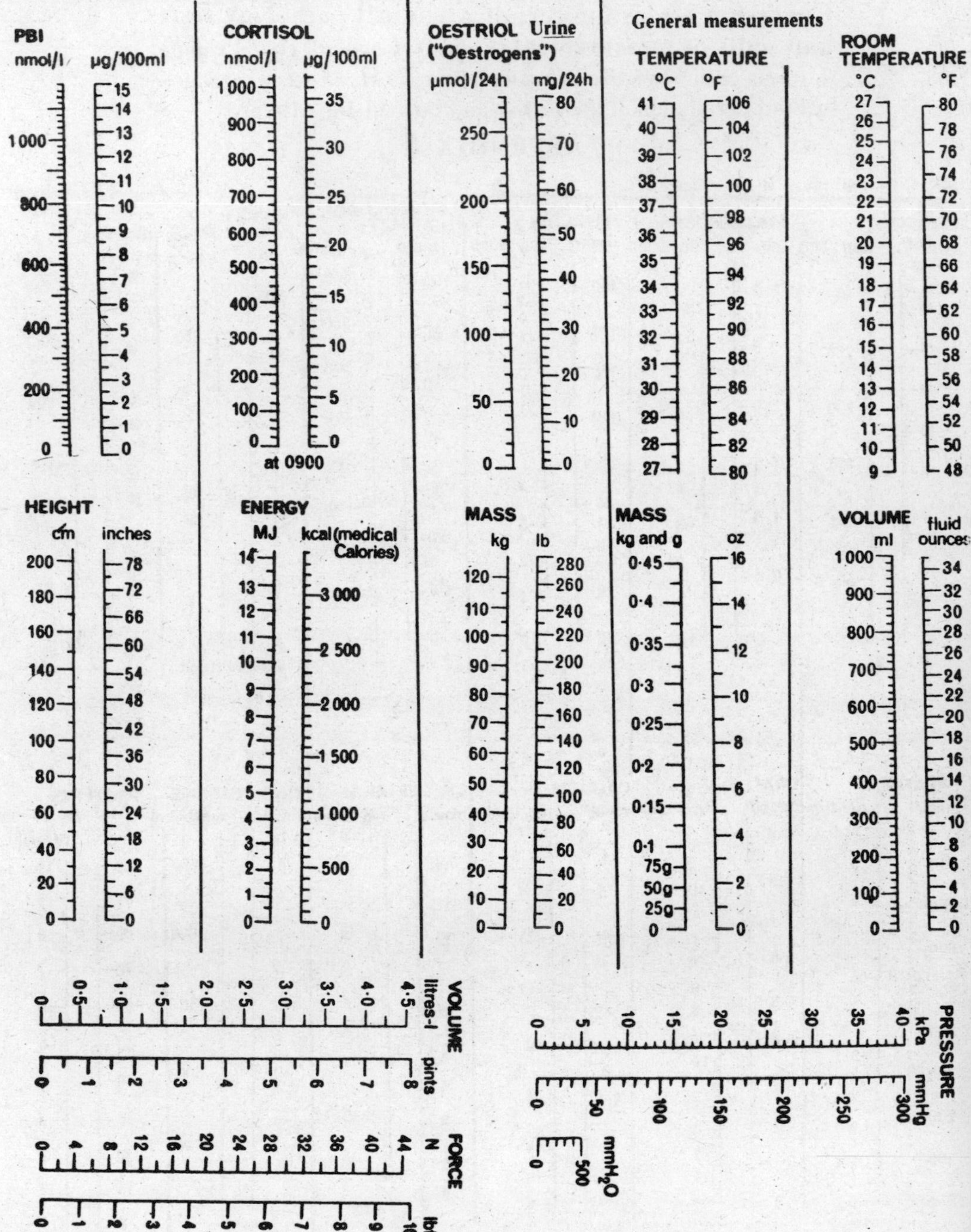
PBI
nmol/l
µg/100ml
CORTISOL
nmol/l
µg/100ml
at 0900
OESTRIOL Urine
("Oestrogens")
µmol/24h
mg/24h
General measurements
TEMPERATURE
°C
°F
ROOM TEMPERATURE
°C
°F
HEIGHT
cm
inches
ENERGY
MJ
kcal (medical Calories)
MASS
kg
lb
MASS
kg and g
oz
VOLUME
ml
fluid ounces
VOLUME
litres-l
pints
FORCE
N
lbf
PRESSURE
kPa
mmHg
mmH2O

APPENDIX 9
First Aid

The AIMS of first aid are:

1. To save life.
2. To prevent the injury and the effects of the injury getting worse.
3. To get a live patient to hospital or into other medical care.
4. To reduce the anxiety of the patient.

First aid may be done by a doctor but can be done effectively by anybody trained in the art of giving first aid and practised in applying it.

ALCOHOL should never be given

NO DRINKS should be given any patient apart from the conscious severely burned adult.

Priorities

The first aider must identify and treat urgently all life- threatening conditions. To this end the following questions should be asked about each causlty and answered as rapidly and accurately as possible in order that the appropriate steps may be instigated.

1. Should the patient be removed from a position of danger such as a live source of electricity?
2. Is the Patient breathing or not breathing? The brain can live for only about 4 minutes without a supply of oxygen reachin it in the blood. Do not waste time splinting or bandaging a patient who is not breathing. A hospital can treat a live causlty but not a dead one.
3. Is the patient bleeding severely? Both internal and external bleeding need to be recognized and immediate attention paid to stopping any visible bleeding; a causlty with internal bleeding needs urgent transfer to hospital.
4. Is the patient conscious or unconscious? Diagnosing the cause of unconsciousness is not of immediate concern to the first aider but the correct positioning of the patient will save life and must be practised by all those who study first aid.

REMOVING THE PATIENT FROM A POSITION OF DANGER

This may involve turning off an electric supply with a well-insulated device or dragging the patient out of water. A causlty trapped in a car should be left until a doctor and, if possible, the fire brigade arrive. The first aider should only attempt to carry out this manoeuver if the car is on fire. If you are dragging a casualty out of water, artificial respiration can and should be started before you have the patient in an ideal place and position.

IS THE PATIENT BREATHING?

If the casualty is not brea thing artifical respiration should be started with the minimum delay. The following measures should be carried out as rapidly as possible because there is no time to waste.

a. Put the casualty flat on his back, arch his neck and lift his lower jaw upwards and forwards.

This will lift his tongue away from the back of his throat and provide an airway (Figs. 57 and 58).

b. Clean the mouth of any debris including pieces of food and false teeth.

c. Keeping the jaw in the correct position with one hand under the patient's chin, take a deep breath in. Place your open mouth firmly over the patient's nose while keeping his mouth shut with upward pressure under his chin. Breath out steadily and firmly

The tongue blocking the throat of an unconscious patient.

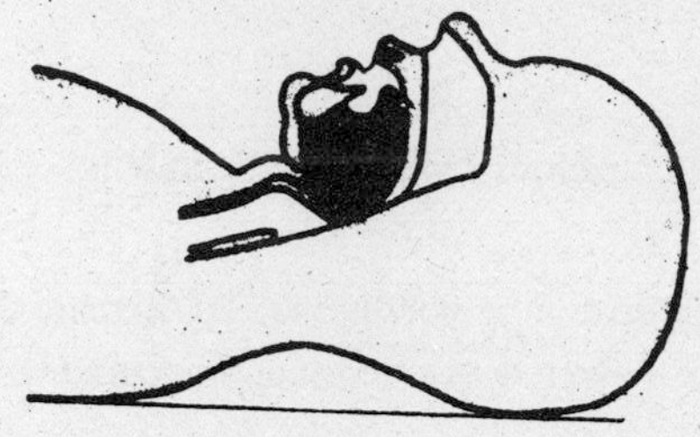

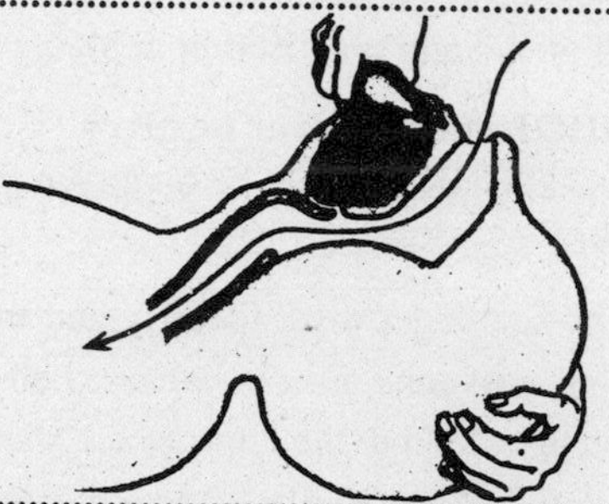

The low jaw lifted upwards and forwards thus lifting the tongue from the back of the throat.

until you see the patient's chest rise. Lift your head, turn it to one side, take a deep breath in and repeat the manoeuver (Figs. 59 and 60). If mouth - to nose respiration is impossible mouth-to-mouth respiration should be carried out.

d. Artifical respiration should be continuted until either the patient breathes spontaneously, or a doctor says that he is dead, or if a doctor is not available it should be continued for at least an hour.

The most common cause of difficulty in getting air into the lings is an obstructions in the air passage; the most common obstruction

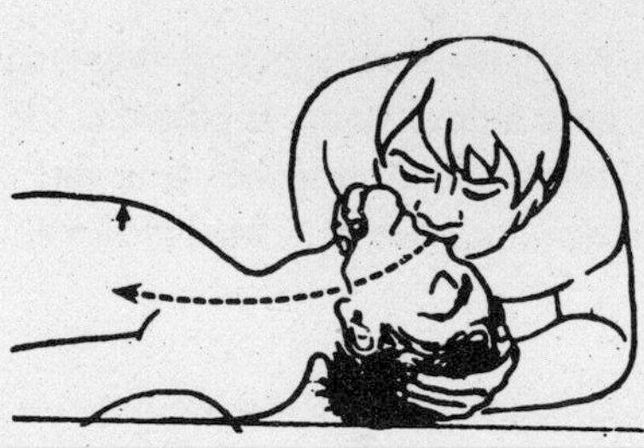

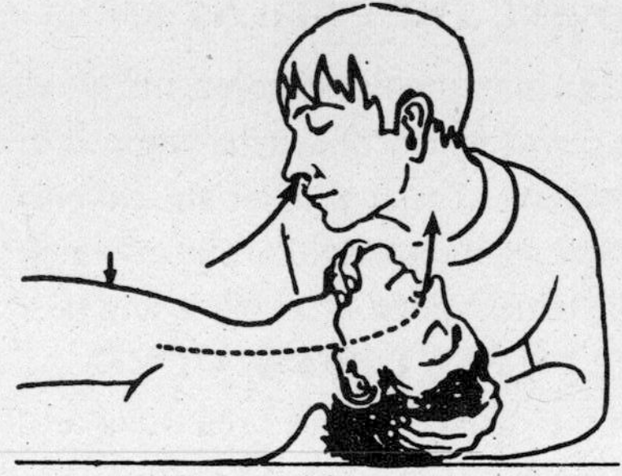

Mouth-to-nose respiration. The chest of breathes in

Operator takes away his mouth and

the causually rises as it fills with air expiration *himself. The chest of the causlly falls on*

is the tongue which due to the malpositioning of the head falls backwards and effectively blocks the passage at the back of the nose and mouth. Have a quick look in the mouth to make sure that bone further debris has appeared and then lift the lower jaw and pull it forward. Correct the extension of the neck by putting one hand under the nape of the neck and pulling the head backwards with the other hand. Continue mouth-to-nose or mouth-to-mouth respiration.

If you are using this method of artifical respiration on a child, care must be taken in the amount of air blown into the lungs. The chest must be watched constantly because damage can be done to the lungs by over-vigorous inflation. If the patient is a small child it is usually casier for the first aider to put his mouth over the child's nose and mouth.

Vomiting may occur while artifical respiration is being carried out. The patient's artifical respira tion available to the fiorst aider. It is impossible to practise on a live person but should be practised on on e of the models available for this purpose.

IS THE PATIENT BLEEDING SEVERELY?

Bleeding may be external or internal.

External bleeding can be seen on the outside of the body.

Internal bleeding may be hidden within the body or show its presence when passed in urine, ccoughed up, etc. Internal bleeding may be severe around a fracture, particularly that of the femur or thigh bone.

The diagnosis of severe bleeding must be made quickly because the loss of a litre of blood is serious.

External bleeding will be seen if looked for. Press on the area from which the blood is coming. As sterike pad is best but a bare hand is better that nothing. Put a pad over the area and bandage firmly. Raise the limb which is injured in order to decrease the blood supply to it. If blood apears through the bandage, do not remove the dressing but put another on top and bandage again more firmly.

If there are pieces of glass or other foreign bodies in a wound remove the loose ones but do not touch those that are firmly embedded. If you think that there may be a fracture under the wound build up a pad around the wound before bandaging firmly.

Internal bleeding. The patient will be pale, cold and sweating. There may be seeling from an injury such as a fractured femur. No time should be lost trying to make an accurate diagnosis. The casualty should be sent to hospital because he will need replacement of the blood lost as well as treatment of his injuries.

IS THE PATIENT CONSCIOUS OR UNCONSCIOUS?

A conscious patient makes some effort to answer a question or obey a command.

If the casualty is breathing but unconscious he should be put in the unconscious position (Fig. 61). Clear the debris from the patient's mouth. Turn the patient on to his front and his face towards you. Bend his leg, nearest to you, at the knee and bring it towards you over the other leg. Bend the arm nearest to you, at the elbow and bring the forearm towards you and let it rest on the ground parallel to the casualty's face. Finally lift his chin upwards. If possible arrange the casualty so that he has a slight head down tip.

An unconscious patient must not be left alone. A constant watch must be kept to make sure that the continues to brea the, does not choke and is gently controlled if he becomes restless.

If the patient is unconscious and not breathing artifical expira tion must be commenced immediately. If he starts breathing but remains unconscious he must then be put in the unconscious position.

ALL CAUSALTIES who have needed treatment for FAILURE TO BREATHE or for UNCONSCIOUSNESS must be seen by a doctor at a hospital.

The unconscious position

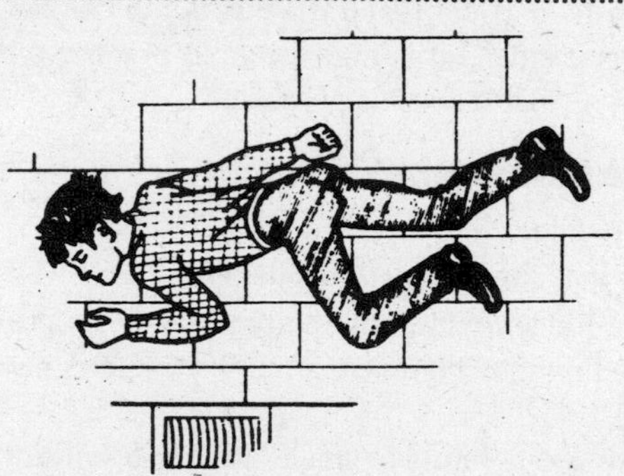

The unconscious position

Organization

At some point while dealing with a number of causalties who have life-threatening conditions you must also get an estimate of the total number of causalties and send somebody to arrange for ambulances and a doctor if possible. You will need to decide which patients need hospital treatment most urgently. Use all the available help in carrying out this organization. Calm organization is an important function of a trained first aider.

Burns

After life-saving measures have been applied, burns must be given first aid treatment. The seriousness of a burn depends to a large extent on the amount of the surface area of the body affected.

TREATMENT

1. *Extinguish the fire.* If necessary lay the casualty down and roll him in a blanket or rug to put out flames.
2. *Cool* the burnt area with cold water, if available, for at least ten minutes. This procedure lessens the damage done to the body tissues by the burn area and also relieves to pain.
3. *Cover the burnt area.* Use a sterile dressing if possible; if such dressing are not available use

any clean pieces of cloth.

DO NOT USE ANY OINTMENT OR LOTION.
DO NOT BURST ANY BLISTERS.

Keep the casualty lying down until he reaches hospital. A large amount of fluid is lost from burnt arewas and to remedy this loss conscious adult causalties should be given frequent small drinks of liquid.

DO NOT GIVE ALCOHOL.

Burns of the eye should be washed under running water for at least ten minutes and then covered with a clean dry dressing until medical help can be obtained.

A SEVERELY BURNT PATIENT NEEDS QUIET, CALM HANDING AND A GREAT DEAL OF REASSURANCE.

Fractures and dislocations

A frecture is any break or crack in a bone. A fracture may be either closed or open.

1. *A closed fracture.* The skin is intact over the area of the fracture.
2. *An open fracture.* The skin is broken over the area of the fracture. This is important because germs can enter and cause infection.

A dislocation is the disruption of a joint and occurs most commonly at the shoulder joint and the jaw. Again this may be closed or open.

Diagnosis of a fracture or dislocation can only be make conclusevely by an x-ray. This is beyond the scope of the first aider but the following sings are suggestive;

1. History of a fall other violent injury.
2. Pain
3. Tenderness on examination
4. Swelling
5. Loss or power
6. Deformity

TREATMENT

Always remember that the fracture of large bone such as the femur can be a major cause of blood loss and a blood transufison may be the most urgent treatment. Never waste time on elaborate splinting; concentrate on getting a live patient to hospital but remember the following principles:

1. A closed fracture must never become an open fracture through careless handling.
2. An open fracture must be covered to prevent infection.
3. The fracture must be prevented from getting worse during the journey to hospital.
4. *Never* cause the casualty greater pain during the diagnosis or treatment. The fractured area will be very tender and must be handled with great care.
5. No attempt must be made to restore a dislocated joint to its normal position.

The two basic principles to be observed in the treatment of all frractures dislocations are:

1. Immobilization to increase the comfort of the patient and prevent the injury getting worse.
2. Speedy removal to hospital for expert diagnosis and treatment.

If you are in doubt about the diagnosis of a fracture treat the injury as a fracture.

If one arm or one leg is fractured the uninjured limb can be used as a standard of normality and the injured limb compared with it for size and shape. Elaborate splinting is unnecessary and may do more harm than good by causing undue movement of the casualty and delaying his removal to hospital.

BASIC PRINCIPLES OF SPLINTING

1. tThe site of the fracture must be immobilised together with the joints above and below it.
2. The natural contours of the body should be levelled out by soft padding or a rolled up woolen scarf, rags, etc.
3. No badages should be put on so tightly that the blood circulation is hindered.

Fractures for the shoulder blade and upper arm: Loose padding should be put be between the arm and the body. The chest can be used as a splint and the arm places is the most confortable position against it-usually with the elbow bent and the forearm in a sling. This position immobilizes both the shoulder and elbow joints.

Fractures of the elbow and lower arm: Padding should be placed between the arm and the body but the elbow should not be bent. The casualty will usually be more confortable lying on a stretchet with the injured arm gently tied to the side of his body.

Fractures of the thigh bone or fimur: These are serious injuries because of the large amount of blood that can be lost around the site of the fracture. It is important that the casualty should be sent to hospital as soon as possible. Lay the casualty flat on a stretcher. Put padding between the knees, ankles and contours of the legs. Genttleness is important. Tie the feet together with the figure - of-eight bandage (Fig. 62). Tie the knees together and place bandages around both legs above and below the fracture. Always remember that the casualty will be severly ill with this fracture and be gentle, calm and reasuring.

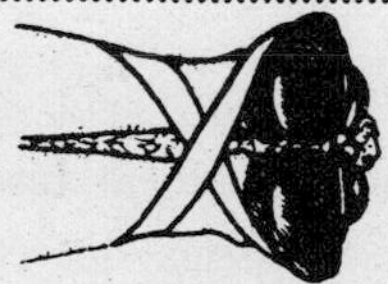

A figure of eight bandage around the feet and ankles

Fractures below the knee: Remember that in all fractures of the shin bone or tibia the injury is likely to be or to become an open fracture. If one leg is fractured the sound leg may be used as a splint for the injured one. Lay the casualty flat Place padding between the thighs, knee and ankles. Tie the feet together with a fingure-of-eight bandage. Tie the knee together and both legs together with bandages above and below the fracture.

. If both legs are fractured the injury is a very severe one. It possible two long splints should be used, one on each side of the body, long splints should be sued, one on each side of the body, long enough to reach from the armpits to beyond the feet. If such splints are not available one splint should be used from the level of the groin to beyond the feet and put between the two legs and the splints are being used additional bandages should be put around the lips and chest.

Fractures for the jaw: Bandaging is unnecessary. If both sides of the jaw are fractured passage of air into the lungs may be affected. An unconscious casualty should be put in the unconscious position. A conscious casualty should be in sitting position with the head titled slightly forward. The casualty must be taken to hospital.

Fracture of the hip bone or pelvis: This can be a serious injury depending on the amount of damage that is done inside the body. The casualty msut be put on his back on a stretcher. Put Padding between his knee and ankles. Tie his feet together with a fingure-of-eight bandage. Warn the casualty not to pass water on his way to hospital.

Fractures of the spine: This can be a very serious injury and be both life-threatening and the caused of paralysis below the site of the fracture. Send for help, a stretcher and an ambulance.

No attempt should be made to move the casualty until at least four and preferably five people are present. The movement of the casualty on to a stretcher is a job for an expert because the position of the spine must not be changed at any time during the maneover. Minor flexion or beding forward of the spine is the most dangerous change of pisition because it can compress the spinal cord and cause irreversible damage to the nerves below the level of the fracture.

Dislocations: Any dislocation is a very painful and frightening injury and the casualty needs reassurance and calm treatment.

No attempt must be made to restore the joint to its normal position. The injured area must be spoorted in the position which is most comfortable for the casualty. The casualty must taken to hospital.

Poisoning

Poisoning is a hazard that should be prevented rather than treated. There are so many poisonous substances now in general use that it is impracticable to give the treatment of each one. A general outline will be given. In the United Kingdom there are poison reference centres to which as urgent telephone call can be made for information. The number are as follows:

TELEPHONE UMBERS OF POISON REFERENCE CENTRES

Belfast	0232 40503	London	01 407 7600
Cardiff	0222 33101	Manchester	061 740 2254
Edinburgh	031 229 2477	Newcastle	0632 25131
Leeds	0532 32799		

ALWAYS KEEP A CONTAINER FROM WHICH THE POISON IS BELIEVED TO HAVE BEEN TAKEN AND SEND IT TO HOSPITAL WITH THE PATIENT

If the patient is not breathin artifical respiration must be given. When the patient starts breathing put him in the unconscious position. Send him to hospital.

If the casualty is conscious but shows signs of burning in or around the mouth send him urgently to hospital and do not make him vomit.

If casualty is conscious and shows no signs of burning in or around his mouth make him vomit. This can usually be achieved by giving him two tables spoons of salt in a cup of warm water or putting your finger down the back throat. If you are trying to make a child vomit put a spoon handle down the back of his throat and not your finger. After he has vomited give him at least a litre of water, milk, weak tea or coffee while for him to be taken to hospital, or on the way.

APPENDIX 10

Prefixes which can be used as combining forms in compounded words

Prefix	Meaning	Prefix	Meaning	Prefix	Meaning
a-	without,not	chemo-	chemical	extra-	outside
ab-	away from	chol-	bile	ferri-	
abdo-	abdominal	cholecysto-	gall bladder	ferro-	iron
abdomino-		choledocho-	common bile duct	fibro-	fibre, fibrous tissue
acro-	extermity	chondro-	cartilage	flav-	yellow
ad-	towards	chrom-	colour	feto-	fetus
adeno-	glandular	cine-	film	fore-	before, in front of
amb-		circum-	around	gala-	milk
ambi	both,no both side	co-		gastro-	stomach
amido-	NH_2 group united to a aicd radical	con-	together	genito-	genitals, reproductive
amino-	NH_2 group united to a radical other than acid radical	coli-	bowel	glosso-	tongue
amphi-	on both sides, around	colpo-	vagina	glyco-	sugar
amyl-	starch	contra-	against	gnatho-	jaw
an-	not, without	costo-	rib	haema-	
andro-	male	crani-		haemo-	blood
angi-	vessel (blood)	cranio-	skull	hemi-	half
aniso-	unequal	crypt-	hidden	hepa-	
ant-	against, counteracting	cysto-	bladder	hepatico	liver

anti-		cyto-	cell	hepato	
antè-		dacryo-	tear	hetero-	unlikeness, fis-similarity
antero-	before	dactyl-	finger	hexa-	six
antro-	antrum	de-	away, from, reversing	histo-	tissue
aorto-	aorta	deca-	ten	homeo-	like
arthro-	joint	deca-	tenth	homo-	same
auto-	self	deci-	half	hydro	water
bi-	twice, two	dent-	tooth	hygro	moisture
bili-	bile	derma-		hyper-	above
bio-	life	dermat-	skin	hystero-	uterus
blenno-	mucus	dextro-	to the right	iatro-	physician
bleph-	eyelid	dip-	double	idio-	peculiar to the individual
brachio-	arm	dis-	separation, against	ileo-	ileμm
brady-	slow	dorso-	dorsal	ilio-	ilium
broncho-	bronchi	dys-	difficult, pain-ful, abnormal	immuno-	immunity
cardio-	heart	electro-	electricity in	in-	not, in, into, within
carpo-	wrist	em-		infra-	below
cata-	down	en-	in	inter-	between
centi-	a hunderdth	end-		intra-	within
cephal-	head	endo-	in, into, within	intro-	inward
cerebro-	brain	ent-	within	ischio-	ischium
cervico-	cervix	entero-	intestive	iso-	equal
cheil-	lip	epi-	on, above, upon	karyo-	nucleus
cervico-	cervix	ery-	red	kerato-	horn, skin, cornea
cheil-	lip	eu-	well, normal	kypho-	rounded, hum-ped
cheir-	hand	ex-		lact-	milk
laparo-	flank	exo-	away from, out, out of	salpingo-	fallopian tube
laryngo-	larynx	osteo-	bone	sapro-	dead, decaying
lepto-	thin,soft	oto-	ear	sarco-	flesh
leuco-		ovari	ovary	sclero-	hard
leuko-	white	pachy-	thick	scota	darkness
lympho-	lymphatic	pan-	all	semi-	half
macro-	large	para-	beside	sero-	serum

mal-	abnormal, poor
medi-	middle
mega-	large
melano-	pigment, dark
meso-	middele
meta-	between
metro-	uterus
micro-	small
milli-	a thousandth
mio-	smaller
mono-	one, single
muco-	mucucs
multi-	many
myc-	fungus
myelo-	spinal cord, bone marrow
myo-	muscle
narco-	stupor
neo-	new
nephro-	kidney
neuro-	nerve
noct-	night
normo-	normal
nucleo-	nucleustooth
nyc-	night
oculo-	eye
odonto-	tooth
oligo-	deficiency, diminution
onycho-	nail
oo-	egg, ovum
oophor-	ovary
ophthalmo-	eye
opisth-	backward
orchido-	testis

patho-	disease
ped-	child, foot
penta-	
pento	five
per-	by, through
peri-	around
perineo-	perineum
pharyngo-	pharynx
phlebo-	vein
phono-	voic
photo-	light
phren-	diaphragm, mind
pleuro-	pleura
pluri-	many
peneumo-	lung.
podo-	foot
polio-	grey
poly-	many, much
post-	after
pre-	
pro-	before
proct-	anus
proto	first
pseudo-	false
psycho-	mind
pyelo-	pelvis of the kidney
pyo-	pus
pyr-	fever
quadri-	four
radio	radiation
re-	again, back
ren-	kidney
retro-	backward

socio-	sociology
spleno-	spleen
steato-	fat
sterno-	sternum
sub-	below
supra-	above
syn-	together, union, with
tabo-	tabes
tachy-	fast
tarso-	foot, edge of eyelied.
teno-	tendon
tetra-	four
thermo	heat
thoraco-	thorax
thrombo-	blood clot
thryo-	thyroid gland
tibio-	tibia
tox-	poison
tracheo-	trachea
trans-	across, through
tri-	three
trich-	hair
tropho-	nourishment
ultra-	beyond
uni-	one
uretero-	ureter
urethro-	urethra
uro-	unrin, urinary orgams
utero-	uterus
vaso-	vessel
veno-	vein
vesico-	bladder
xanth-	yellow

oro-	mouth	rhin	nose	xero-	dry
ortho-	straight	sacchar-	sugar	xiphi-	ensiform cartilage of
os-	bone, mouth	sacro-	sacrum	xipho-	sternum

Suffixes which can be used as combining forms in compounded words

Suffix	Meaning	Suffix	Meaning	Suffix	Meaning
-able	able to, capable of	-gram	a tracing	-phagia	swallpwomg
-aemia	blood	-graph	description, treastise, writing	-phasia	speech
-aesthesia	sensibility, sensepercept	-iasis	condition of, state	-philia	affinity for, loving
-agra	attack, severe pain	-iatric	practice of healing	-phobia	fear
-al	characterizaed by, pertaining to	-itis	inflammation of	-phylaxis	protection
-algia	pain	-kinesis	motion	-plasty	reconstructive surgery
-an	belonging to, pertaining to	-lith	calculus, stone	-plegia	paralysis
-ase	catalyst, enzyme, ferment	-lithiasis	presence of stones	-pnoea	breathing
-blast	cell	-logy	science of, study of	-poiesis	making
-caval	pertaining to venae cavase	-lysis (lytic)	breaking down, disintegration	-ptosis	falling
-cele	tumour, swelling	-malacia	softening	-rhage	to burst forth
-centesis	to puncture	-megaly	enlargement	-rhaphy	suturing
-cide	destructive, killing	-meter	measure	-rhoea	excessive discharge
-clysis	infusion, injuction	-ogen	precursor	-rhythmia	rhythm
-coccus	spherical cell	-oid	likeness, resemblance	-saccharide	basic carbohydrate molecule

-cule	little	-ol	alcohol	-scope	instrument for visual examination
-cyte	cell	-ology	the study of	-scopy	to examine visually
-derm	skin	-oma	tumour	-somatic	pertaining to the body
-desis	to bind together	-opia	eye	-somy	pertaining to chromosomes
-dynia	pain	-ose	sugar	-sonic	sound
-ectasis	dilation, extension	-osis	condition, disease, excess	-stasis	stagnation, cessation of movement
-ectomy	removal of	-ostomy	to form an opening or outlet	-sthenia	strength
-form	having the form of	-otomy	incision of	-stomy	to form an opening or outlet
-fuge	expelling	-ous	like, having the nature of	-taxia	arrangment,
-genesis		-pathy	disease	-taxis	co-ordination, order
-genetic	forma tion, origin	-penia	lack of	-taxy	
-genic	capable of causing	-pexy	fixation	-tome	cutting instruement
-gogue	increasing flow	-phage	ingesting	-tomy	incision of
				-trophy	nourishment
				-uria	urine

APPENDIX 11

Abbrevisations of some Degrees, Diplomes, other Tities and Organizations

AHA	Area Health Authority
AIMSW	Associate of the Institute of Medical Social Workers
AMO	Area Medical Officer
ANO	Area Nursing Officer
ARRC	Associate of the Royal Red Cross
ARSH	Associate of the Royal Society of Health
BA	Bachelor of Arts
BCH, BS, BCB	Bachelor of Surgery
BCHD, BDS	Bachelor of Dental Surgery
BM	Bachelor of Medicine
BSc	Bachelor of Science
CHC	Comminity Health Council
CM, ChM	Master in Surgery
CMB	Central Midwives Board
CNAA	Council for National Academic Awards
CQSW	Certificate of Qualifica tion in Social Work
DA	Diploma in Anaesthetics
DCH	Diploma in Child Health
DCP	District Community Physician
DDS	Doctor of Dental Surgery
DHSS	Department of Health and Social Security
DM	Doctor of Medicine
DMR(D)	Diploma in Medical Radiology; Diagnostic
DMR(T)	Diploma in Medical Radiology: Therapy
DMT	District Management Team
DN, DipN	Diploma in Nursing
DNE	Director of Nurse Education
DNO	District Nursing Officer
DO	Diploma in Opthalmology

DON	Diploma in Orthopaedic Nursing
DPH	Diploma in Public Health
DPM	Diploma in Psychological Medicine
Dip PysMed	Diploma of Physical Medicine
DSc	Doctor of Science
DTM&h	Diploma in Tropical Medicine and Hygiene
DivNo	Divisional Nursing Officer
FCSP	Fellow of the chartered Society of Physiotherapy
FCHs	Fellow of the Society of Chiropodists
FFARCH	Fellow of the Faculty of Anaesthetists of the Royal College of Surgeons
FPS	Fellow of the Pharmaceutical Society
FRCGP	Fellow of the royal College of General Practitioners
FRCN	Fellow of Royal College of Nursing
FRCOG	Fellow of the Royal College of Obstetricians and Gynaecologists
FRCP	Fellow of the royal College of Pathologists
FRCPath	Fellow of the Royal College of Pathologists
FRCHE,FRCP(Ed)	Fellow of the Royal College of Physicians m Edinburgh
FRCPI	Fellow of the Royal College of Physicians of Ireland
FRCPsych	Fellow of the Royal College of Psychiatrists
FRCR	Fellow of the Royal College of Radiologists
FRCS	Fellow of the Royal College of Surgeons
FRCSE, FRCS(Ed)	Fellow of the Royal College of Surgeons, Edinburgh
FRCSI	Fellow of the Royal College of Surgeons of Ireland
FRFPSG	Fellow of the Royal Faculty of Physicians and Surgeons, Glasgow
FRS	Fellow of the Royal Society
FRSE	Fellow of the Royal Society Edinburgh
GNC	General Nursing Council
HV	Health Visitor
LDS	Licentiate in Dental Surgery

LMSSA	Licentiate in Medicine and Surgery. Society of Apothecaries, London
MA	Master of Arts
MAO	Master of the Art of Obstetrics
MB	Bachelor of Medicine
MBAOT	Member of the British Association of Occupational Therapy
MC, MS, MCH, MChir	Master of Surgery
MChD, MDS	Master of Dental Surgery
MCHS	Member of the Pharmaceutical Society
MRCGP	Member of the Royal College of Obstetricians and Gynaccologists
MCSP	Member of the Chartered Society of Physiotherapy
MRCPath	Member of the Royal College of Pathologists
MRCS	Member of the Royal College of Surgeons
MS	Master of Surgery
MSA	Member of the Society of Apothecaries
MSR(T)	Member of the Society of Radiographers (Therapy)
MTD	Midwife Teacher's Diploma
NO	Nursing Officer
ONC	Orthopaedic Nursing Certificate
OND	Ophthalmic Nursing Diploma
QHNS	Honorary Nursing Sister to the Queen
QHP	Honorary Physician to the Queen
QHS	Honorary Surgeon to the Queen
RAMC	Royal Army Medical Corps
RCM	Royal College of Midwise
RCNT	Registered Clinical Nurse Tutor
RFN	Registered Fever Nurse
RGN	Registered General Nurse
RHA	Regional Health Authority
RMN	Register Mental Nurse
RMO	Resident Medical Officer

RN	Registered Nurse (Americal)
RNMS	Registered Nurse for the Mentally Subnormal
RNO	Regional Nursing Officer
RNT	Registered Nurse Tutor
RRC	Royal Red Cross
ScD	Doctor of Science
SCM	State Certified Midwife
SMO	Senior Medical Officer
SNO	Senior Nursing Officer
SRN	State Registered Nurse